COMMON VERTEBRAL
JOINT PROBLEMS

COMMON VERTEBRAL JOINT PROBLEMS

Gregory P. Grieve FCSP Dip TP

Honorary Fellow of the Chartered Society of Physiotherapy
Post-Registration Tutor, Department of Rheumatology and
Rehabilitation, Norfolk and Norwich Hospital
Former Supervisor and Clinical Tutor, Spinal Treatment Unit,
Royal National Orthopaedic Hospital, London

Foreword by

PHILIP H. NEWMAN CBE DSO MC FRCS

Lately Consultant Orthopaedic Surgeon to the Middlesex
Hospital, and Consultant Surgeon to the Royal National
Orthopaedic Hospital and Institute of Orthopaedics,
London
Past President of the British Orthopaedic Association and
formerly Chairman of the British Council of Management of
the Journal of Bone and Joint Surgery

CHURCHILL LIVINGSTONE
EDINBURGH LONDON MELBOURNE AND NEW YORK 1981

CHURCHILL LIVINGSTONE
Medical Division of Longman Group Limited

Distributed in the United States of America by Churchill Livingstone
Inc., 19 West 44th Street, New York, N.Y. 10036, and by associated
companies, branches and representatives throughout the world.

First published 1981

ISBN 0 443 02106 6

British Library Cataloguing in Publication Data
Grieve, Gregory P.
    Common vertebral joint problems.
    1. Spine—Diseases
    1. Title
    617'375   RC400

Library of Congress Catalog Card Number 81–67465

Printed in Great Britain by Butler & Tanner Ltd, Frome and London

Foreword

Modern advance in prevention and treatment has eliminated or brought under control many of the severe illnesses which, a generation or so ago, afflicted man. The medical profession now has greater opportunity to pay attention to the challenge of chronic arthritis and the effects of trauma, stress and strain and wear and tear of the musculoskeletal system.

The population of the Western world of today, its average age and demand for physical comfort gradually increasing, presents an expanding and exacting problem. In hospital practice, to which the more difficult cases are referred, it is the consultant who examines, investigates, attempts to diagnose and prescribes treatment and having excluded a serious cause or the need for inpatient treatment may refer the patient to the department of physical medicine for supervision and care. The therapist who carries out these instructions spends much time with the patient and learning from experience develops an unparalleled understanding of the nature of skeletal pain.

Greg Grieve has dedicated his professional life to an extensive study of these physical problems and has devoted his attention in particular to the multiple syndromes arising from the intervertebral and sacroiliac joints.

So impressed was he by the work of Mennell, Marlin, Cyriax, Stoddard and others that he energetically became involved, with other Chartered physiotherapists, in founding a school of instruction in the basic sciences as applied to the spine and of the problems of derangement and to train physiotherapists in the art of treatment by manipulation. Following the initial courses, with other teachers, between 1965 and 1967 he was the pioneer who carried the torch of planning the curriculum and progressive development of the annual courses during the eight especially formative years, 1968 to 1975.

During this time Grieve delved deeply into the vast literature that has accumulated on this subject. The variety and extent of this field is aptly expressed in this book: 'The mountain of literature on spinal pathology is massive enough to have become all things to all men.' This book lists no less than 1400 references and its text is astoundingly reverent to the galaxy of opinions and conclusions and the conflicting hypotheses that they contain.

Derangement of the vertebral column is covered in all its aspects and it soon becomes obvious that the value of this monograph is unique. It unfolds the nature of the problem as seen by a person who has spent much time communicating with and actively treating patients. There is much to learn both from a diagnostic and therapeutic angle which is not found in the many textbooks written by the medical profession.

This is a comprehensive aggregation of the whole subject but there is nothing pedestrian in its teaching. It is provocative and doubtless the more conservative reader would now and again catch his breath.

Above all it provides stimulation for thought on a subject which is apt to be bogged down by tradition and hampered by interdisciplinary contention.

It is a brave and brilliant endeavour to translate the jargon of the various schools into a language with a scientific basis. It cannot fail to appeal to all those interested in the vertebral column whatever their clinical status.

Aldeburgh, Suffolk 1981

P.H.N.

Preface

Is there anything whereof it may be said, 'See, this is new? It hath been already of old times, which was before us.' (Ecclesiastes i, 10)

There is little new in this book, only a different voice saying the old things, yet gathered together in a form which I hope will be useful to my colleagues.

A commonly expressed regret of therapists who strive to improve their handling of common joint problems is that some of those whose prerogative it is to diagnose and prescribe at times appear to have only a limited conception of the capabilities of modern therapists. Such is the speed with which the technology and capabilities of *all* disciplines has risen, this circumstance probably now applies to all interdisciplinary relationships.

Since it is incumbent upon us to keep our own house in order, therapists must do something about their own situation. We must provide opportunities for our peers and colleagues to know about our work, aspirations and capabilities.

In any case, it is really no more than enlightened self-interest to comprehend as much as we can about the *context* of our work because if we do not, its value and our worth will fall away. Wright and Hopkins (1978)[1353] have emphasised that some 30 per cent of physiotherapists' time is devoted to rheumatic and orthopaedic conditions.

I have attempted to formulate a guide, a vocabulary of basic information for those spending much of the day handling vertebral joint conditions. As a foundation for improving our knowledge we must know something of this if we aspire to become competent in the conservative treatment of common vertebral joint problems, and to know in which direction our knowledge must be expanded.

The easily portable knapsack-and-bedroll information and rule-of-thumb clinical methods of times past are no longer enough. Today's workers must gather knowledge from many fields, and train themselves to apply it quickly and accurately when assessing the multitude of facts obtained by a good clinical examination.

As the more successful treatment of respiratory, nervous and metabolic disease, for example, has naturally evolved from a deeper understanding of the nature of the functional abnormality concerned, it is surely axiomatic that abnormalities of the musculoskeletal system are more effectively treated when the nature of the abnormal movement is understood, since bodily movement is the function concerned. There is nothing incongruous or unacceptable in applying this basic law of progression in therapeutics equally to the treatment of diseases of the blood, for instance, and degenerative joint disease of the vertebral column.

To treat musculoskeletal pain, whether by manipulation, acupuncture, hydrocortisone injection, transcutaneous nerve stimulation, the 'back school', relaxation techniques, exercises, ultrasound or whatever, without first making a comprehensive attempt to understand the clinical nature of the musculoskeletal abnormality as it affects each patient, is the road to Erewhon.

The basic physical examination of common vertebral and peripheral joint conditions has now been developed to the stage of a modern technology, and given this as increasingly standard practice, the steady accumulation of further knowledge is certain. Without this basis, low back pain, fibrositis, muscular pains, sciatica and tension headache, etc., will remain classically associated with patent medicine advertisements, rubifacient unctions, generalised exercises, other 'shot-gun' regimes like generalised relaxation or whatever piece of gleaming chromium-plated machinery happens currently to be in vogue. There is nothing sadder than yesterday's machine.

While we make no real effort to understand the myriad clinical presentations of joint abnormality, troublesome joint pains will thunder on unabated.

Since the level of useful knowledge in the world increases horrendously, individuals have great difficulty in keeping up with advances in their own small sphere; there are the problems of assimilation and especially organisation of the available information. I have had in mind the need for a new structural framework, perhaps serving as a skeleton around which increasingly better-informed successors will build yet more meat, the whole remaining organised in the sense that the skeletal framework is never lost from sight.

The volume of information requires that many contributors are needed, and this implies my hope that others will share in formulating succeeding and better forms of this text. Unless they be monsters of omniscience, individuals who singlehandedly attempt to write on the many and diverse aspects of vertebral joint conditions must deal with some aspects about which they have little or no first-hand knowledge.

Without divine dispensation one's own view of what is important cannot be acceptable to more than a handful, and for this reason alone, I would be very grateful for information about omissions, contradictions and ambiguities; suggestions from like-minded colleages would help to make a more suitable bony framework for the new meat and help to eradicate the inevitable defects of a first attempt.

One could have written entirely on 'Manipulation', yet this presupposes that manipulation is the primary interest. This is not so—the more we understand about the genesis of these conditions, the temperament and life-habits of the patients in whom they are occurring and more especially the infinite variety of presentation from patient to patient, the better we help them; 'manipulation' is but one of our treatments, albeit a subject in itself.

The text is addressed to the members of no particular discipline other than like-minded professional colleagues, by whatever academic route they may have developed an interest in the conservative treatment of the ubiquitous, frustrating and depressing spinal joint problems suffered by such multitudes of people.

I have not attempted to categorise, or elaborate on, the pathology and syndromes of common musculoskeletal abnormalities other than in a general way, for these excellent reasons:

1. I already know of at least three different solutions to the problem of syndrome classification, which is a highly artificial business, anyway.
2. There is not space for such a full dissertation, should I be competent to provide it, if there is also to be some general attention to treatment techniques.
3. Knowledge of the subject is expanding and changing with such speed that a text purporting to be up-to-date and written by even the best authorities has little chance of meeting such a claim.

Hence, principles only are important, and do not change with the years. In *The History of Impressionism*[1029] Renoir is quoted as observing, '... though one should take care not to remain imprisoned in the forms we have inherited, one should neither, through love of progress, imagine that one can detach oneself completely from past centuries.'

Further, if we look to our experience we find that it is by thoroughly familiarising ourselves with the inventions of others that we learn to make inventions of our own, particularly in regard to clinical examination procedures and treatment techniques.

While physiotherapists should not attempt to write comprehensively on problems of diagnosis, or the disciplines of pathology, medicine, surgery, neurology, radiology and epidemiology, etc., perhaps in the devotion of a professional lifetime to this field of minor orthopaedics one may have acquired the competence to touch upon these disciplines as they concern the group of conditions under discussion here.

When students approach their training in 'clinical conditions' as diseases of the various systems, the conditions tend to assume a sort of social pecking order in their minds. Regrettably, the largely benign and humble rheumatic disorders have a habit of being relegated to the lower orders and boring peasants of this hierarchy. I believe this to be a profound mistake, since by meticulous examination and enlightened assessment each one of the 'old (and young) necks and backs' becomes an exciting detective story of absorbing interest and amply repays informed and accurate treatment, which need not be vigorous or aggressive. The ample repayment lies in the pure pleasure of relieving chronic and often disabling pain and other symptoms and in one's slowly increasing awareness of the infinite variety of ways in which movement-abnormalities of the vertebral column can present.

Degenerative joint disease of the spine is perhaps best regarded as a family of physiological ageing processes, with pathological changes intervening sooner or later *as a consequence*, the process being influenced by direct and indirect trauma or stress, and coexistent disease. Patients rarely attend because their spines are undergoing gradual and silent degeneration with gradual diminution of movement, but because they have pain and other troublesome symptoms in a specified area, and sometimes two or three.

'There is in medicine a natural law that any single manifestation, subjective or objective, may have behind it a multiplicity of organic causes, just as any single pathological event is bound to project itself into a number of different clinical manifestations' (Steindler, 1962).[1171] It is convenient to use generalised treatment procedures for 'the arthrosis' or 'the spondylosis' as the basic reason for the patient's attendance, yet always more rewarding to broaden an understanding of the infinite variety of ways in which patients can be troubled and try to perceive the nature of the causes and to adapt treatment for the unique form in which the disease affects each one.

With regard to affections of the cranial nerves, for example, Brodal (1965) has pointed out that it is somewhat unreliable to attempt fitting a given series of symptoms to one of the many syndromes described, since these syndromes rarely occur in typical form. The same applies to migraine, of course (p. 218), and especially so to all clinical presentation of musculoskeletal joint problems.

Attempts to eradicate this annoying untidiness, by seeking to impose artificial order and regularity, where none can yet exist, are foolish. Plato observed that man never legislates, but destinies and accidents happening in all sorts of ways, legislate in all sorts of ways (see p. 205). There are too many factors involved; very many of the so-called typical syndromes are surprisingly uncommon. This becomes more apparent in direct relationship to the comprehensiveness of history-taking, initial examination and careful palpation.

Because there appears to be a gross imbalance among the weight of literature on degenerative change, in that the lumbar disc has cornered a fashionable and ridiculously large share of attention, I have devoted more space than may be customary to arthrosis, and to seemingly less-visited districts of the vertebral column. The subjects of vertebral traction and the sacroiliac joint have also been given rather more space, since they currently attract considerable interest.

The opposite end of the spine, in the form of therapy for headache, already suffers from an embarrasssment of riches—academic debates over migraine become more erudite and the drugs more exotic with an increasing ball-and-chain paraphernalia of side-effects.

A very great deal more is being learned about what appears to a clinical therapist to be, in many cases, of little shopfloor clinical value, and we wistfully hope that more time will be devoted to comprehensively examining and palpating the bit that holds the headache up—the cervical spine and the craniovertebral junction.

With regard to pathological changes, it has been necessary to restrict discussion to those aspects which are of first importance in the field of musculoskeletal joint problems; where convenient to do so, reference as is necessary is made in the 'Clinical presentation' section rather than in the more detailed section on 'Pathological changes' (cf. ankylosing spondylitis).

Where it has seemed to me appropriate I have not hesitated to cross the somewhat 'watertight' descriptive boundaries of aetiology, pathology and clinical features, for the more effective presentation of important aspects in particular spinal regions, e.g. in the section on 'whiplash' injuries, the discussion of surgical problems in the section on biomechanics of the cervical cord and meninges, and the discussion of soft tissue changes.

Bourdillon (1973)[105] expressed a salient feature of spinal musculoskeletal problems:

> The paucity of clinical signs and the diversity of symptoms produced by spinal joint disorders confused the medical profession to such an extent that they were not always recognised as having their origin in spinal joints.

Occasionally, because the clinical therapist may only partially appreciate what the patient is complaining about, or fully appreciates it but does not know what to do about it, or the facilities for help are not as adequate as desired, the patient is given a few generalised exercises and told to 'live with it'. There is the paradox that while musculoskeletal abnormalities are the most frequent cause of depressing aches and pains, they tend to be regarded as the least rewarding to treat and thus may be the worst provided-for. The run-of-the-mill standard of clinical examination of these 'uninteresting' conditions is perhaps not always as painstaking as it might be, and the patience of patients is at times unbelievable. The amount of real need is calamitous, and the clinical wherewithal to cope with it ethically, knowledgeably, effectively and with a minimum of vigour, has been sadly thin on the ground.

For this reason, the energetic attack with limited means on the important lumbar spine problems by the Society for Back Pain Research will do much good; the cervical region of the vertebral column, and the ubiquitous problems of cervical spondylosis, have also received an increasing volume of expert attention[117] and, together with the advances in the understanding of pain behaviour, today's clinical workers are immeasurably better equipped than those of two decades ago. It may be that the word 'manipulation' will conjure in the minds of many the 'rogue-elephant' manipulator, banging away in a vigorous manner at whatever joint condition may present itself; it may also be that (happily a small) minority of authors with a manipulative bent, who have acquired authoritative voice and responsibility over the years, have tended to alienate the moderately minded by an habitual style of unbuttoned rhetoric and noisy self-aggrandisement.

I quote F. Dudley Hart[514]:

> In medicine the authority in the past for some theory of aetiology or drug action or pathological or physiological process was often some (often professorial) God-like figure and was sometimes based on precious little evidence, but it was accepted as true because (1) it seemed to explain things nicely and often relatively simply and (2) the gentleman who said or wrote it was a great authority. ... The God-like physician, proven repeatedly right in the past and venerated and respected accordingly, can hold back for years afterwards medical progress by an ... utterance based on inadequate evidence. ... It is so much easier for us all to believe in somebody reputable than to work it out for ourselves and see if he was right. ... Most of us perform our medical duties acting on working hypotheses rather than on fixed beliefs, but it is very easy for the one gradually and very insidiously to become the other, particularly if one is teaching and lecturing. What I say three times is true, is true, is very true.

Having travelled the long road from cocksure ignorance to thoughtful uncertainty, I am mindful of the prime need for the younger clinical workers to develop their vocabulary of anatomical information and their capacities for assessment, because superficial conclusions derived from casually observed phenomena are not always justified. The fact that most strip-clubs audiences are said to comprise baldheaded old men should not lead to a 'logical' conclusion that looking at ladies without any clothes on makes the hair fall out.

The patient who presents as 'just another old disc lesion' may have a pain behaviour and more subtle clinical signs which only reveal themselves on careful examination.

Those who have the wit and the stamina to adopt the attitude of intellectual explorers, rather than opting for an easier and safer pathway as passive recipients of orthodox knowledge, will get more interest and fun out of the proceedings and will find the work more absorbing; the overall profit exceeds the pain by a handsome margin. For myself, one of the hardest things I had to learn was concentration on treating the signs and symptoms and not unwittingly trying to treat the X-ray appearance, the textbook, the dogma or mechanical concepts of what was believed to have occurred, important though three of these may be.

I plead that the medical and physiotherapy schools might devote much more attention to the teaching of vertebral anatomy and the comprehensive management of benign articular pathology of the spinal column because, like the common cold, there's a lot of it about and its depredations interfere with our economic and social affairs to a sad extent. This is a pity, because a truly remarkable amount of the population's money syphons itself into research of one kind and another and it is plain that a minor proportion of it might acquire considerable cost-effectiveness by being channelled into teaching very many more clinicians and therapists how to recognise and treat by relatively simple means the early painful manifestations of vertebral degenerative joint disease.

A summary (Wood, 1980)[1340a] of the proceedings of a Workshop on undergraduate education in rheumatology, suggests that while the musculoskeletal system is one of the major systems of the body, its status is only infrequently recorded in patients' casenotes.

Although considerable progress has been evident since the 1971 survey, nevertheless there were still grounds for concern about the adequacy of rheumatological teaching in many undergraduate medical schools; the situation in regard to rehabilitation is less satisfactory.

Under the heading of 'Educational objectives' is suggested the fostering of an attitude of 'cooperation in regard to the contributions that can be made by various health professionals and other members of the team'.

The summary also observes that:

... the persisting neglect of the musculoskeletal system is cause for serious concern, and tends to be encouraged by the fact that patients are usually aware of their problem, in contrast to the occult nature of many visceral lesions; much effort is required to encourage all medical colleagues to examine joints properly ...

It has been suggested that because the conundrum of rheumatoid arthritis will probably be solved within the decade, rheumatology must look to new fields and should turn its main energies to backache. Together with these logical and reasonable observations is included:

Sufferers who are sufficiently alarmed by their symptoms and whose pains are severe will seek help, some from family doctors and some from heterodox healers, the osteopaths, chiropractors, manipulating physiotherapists, unqualified bonesetters or others of the host described as 'fringe medicine'.

The writer of such phrases about ethical and competent paramedical workers in the health care team could not have more plainly bared his deep anxieties. Those who profess to handle the vertebral column must be awake to all aspects at all times. Problems, a few of them highly disconcerting, have a habit of looming suddenly and the more so as one slides into an easy familiarity of handling after a 'routine' history-taking. The possibility of serious pathology, and sometimes malignancy, hangs over *all* clinical presentations of vertebral pain. That which presents as a simple joint problem can be the seemingly innocent augury of something more sinister. Not often, but often enough. For this reason alone, the therapist must be soundly and comprehensively informed, always awake and always economical in the use of vigour. There is no other way to avoid serious or catastrophic manipulation accidents.

Should there be a message in this book, it lies in the sections on assessment. In its coordinated activity and use of stored patterns the mind is like a group of prime movers and synergic muscles and its ability to grasp, sort and organise information can reach an artistry as perfect as an outfielder's leap for a back-hand catch. In his essay on Sir Isaac Newton, J. M. Keynes describes the mind-muscle as much like a lens; the ability to gather unrelated bits of knowledge in a new pattern varies from person to person. This ability is an essential quality for the accurate and detailed assessment of joint problems. Anatomical information, painstaking clinical method and basically simple things done carefully and well are more important than the facile acquisition of exotic manipulation techniques. Since we tend, at times, to take ourselves much too seriously I hope the mild irreverence here and there in the text does not make my more sober colleagues too unhappy.

The late Sir Winston Churchill once said that short words were better than long ones and the old words were best of all. I hope there are not too many long words.

G.P.G.

Acknowledgments

We climb on the shoulders of those who have gone before, and those who follow will climb on our own; we also lean on the shoulders of colleagues and I express with pleasure a debt of gratitude to John Conway (from whom I learnt much about the value of treating patients in the side-lying position) and Joe Jeans (whose friendly but incessant demands that I produce a book have now been met), also Freddie Preastner, Brian Edwards, Peter Edgelow, Marjorie Bloor, Sue Adams, Freddy Kaltenborn, Beryl Graveling, Sue Barker, Shelia Philbrook, Chris Coxhead, and Jill Guymer.

I wish to acknowledge the fruitful working relationship between Geoffrey Maitland and myself, extending over eighteen years and dating from his visit to St Thomas' Hospital in London during 1961. We have both had the privilege of developing the use of mobilisation and manipulation techniques by physiotherapists in our respective countries, and the free exchange of information and ideas between us has afforded me pleasure as well as profit.

Figures 2.18, 2.19 and 2.20 are reproduced from *Vertebral Manipulation* (4E) by kind permission of Geoffrey Maitland, AUA FCSP MAPA, and Messrs Butterworth, London.

There is an especial place in my regard for Mr P. H. Newman, in whose Tuesday clinics at the Royal National Orthopaedic Hospital I learnt so much about orthopaedic patients. He graciously lent his immense teaching authority to the 1973, 1974 and 1975 CSP Manipulation Courses, and has very kindly honoured me by writing the foreword to this book.

All therapists will join me in recording our considerable debt to Professor R. E. M. Bowden, Dr D. A. Brewerton, Mr R. Campbell Connolly, Dr J. Ebbetts, Mr A. W. F. Lettin, Dr R. O. Murray, Dr A. Stoddard, Dr J. D. G. Troup, Professor P. D. Wall and Dr B. D. Wyke. To our debt I add my warm personal thanks, also to Dr Basil Christie, Dr Ian Curwen, Dr Desmond Newton and Mr Hugh Phillips; they have more than once guided my wandering notions.

I am grateful to Professor D. L. Hamblen, Mr P. H. Newman, Mr H. Phillips, Dr W. G. Wenley and Dr B. D. Wyke for kindly looking at sections of the text and advising me; faults which remain are my own, of course.

Dr A. Burnell's enthusiasm has been a constant encouragement to physiotherapists and we owe much to Dr J. Cyriax, who brought some order to the examination of musculoskeletal problems and upon whose work further developments have been based. Also to Mr W. J. Guest, Principal of the West Middlesex Hospital School of Physiotherapy; his capacity for doing good unobtrusively has benefited physiotherapy more than it knows and I take pleasure in publicly recording my appreciation of his encouragement and support of the CSP Manipulation Courses in the early days, and of myself over 30 years of professional association.

Members of the Manipulation Association of Chartered Physiotherapists have been most fortunate to enjoy access to the great and important volume of continental medical literature in this specialist field, and for this are in major debt to the multilingual erudition of my classmate of years now sadly past, Mr H. J. C. Cooper, and to his unfailing willingness to burn the midnight oil on our behalf with French, German and if need be Russian translations.

It is a pleasure to record my debt to the technical skills of Dr John Graves of the Graves Audiovisual Medical Library, Miss Uta Boundy, Medical Photographer to the Institute of Orthopaedics, London, Mr John Tydeman of the Department of Medical Illustration, Norfolk and Norwich Hospital, and to Anglia Photographics, Halesworth; they have devoted much care and technical skill to the illustrations.

To those who patiently modelled during the long and tedious photographic sessions, viz. the late Moira Pakenham-Walsh, Sarah Key, Jenifer Horsfall, Kathleen Winter, Denise Poultney and Fiona Percival, I am very grateful.

To Mrs M. Moore, Librarian of the Norfolk and Norwich Institute of Medical Education, and to Mr C. Davenport and Mr P. Smith, respectively the previous and present Librarians of the Institute of Orthopaedics, London, I gratefully acknowledge the efficient help I have been given.

I thank Mr G. T. F. Braddock for generously providing photographic evidence of a unique experiment, which raised my interest when described, and for allowing me to publish it.

Professor Peter R. Davies has been especially generous with advice on expression of magnitudes in S-I units.

Mrs J. Whitehouse, The CSP Journal Editor, has kindly allowed me to reproduce very many figures and passages from my writings in *Physiotherapy*. I thank Mr B. Holden of Carters Ltd, Mr N. Peters of The Tru-Eze Co. Inc. and Mr J. Maley of the Chattanooga Pharmacal Co. for promptly sending me the illustrations I had requested.

Every care has been taken to make the customary acknowledgment to holders of copyright, but if any copyright material has inadvertently been used without due permission or acknowledgment, apologies are offered to those concerned.

Contents

For

Barbara Grieve—the other half of the team

*and to our mentor, Ted Goldblatt, with affection
and regard*

1. Applied anatomy—regional

A short general summary of vertebral structures and their function may usefully precede descriptions of degenerative change and its consequences. Where individual features require more extended discussion, this has been included in the appropriate sections throughout the text.

Because structural variations have considerable importance in this clinical field, and their likelihood always worth bearing in mind, some anomalies have been included with regional descriptions; reference should sooner or later be made to fuller and more detailed accounts.[315, 881, 1274, 1093]

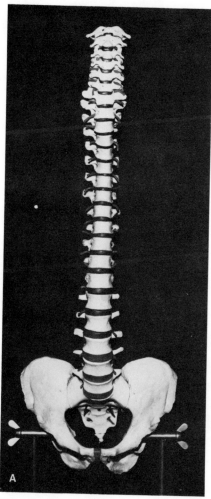
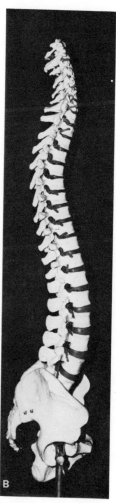

Fig. 1.1 (A) Anterior aspect of the vertebral column. Note the variations in length of transverse processes. (B) Lateral aspect. Note the varying configurations and size of spinous processes.

Patients with congenital spinal malformation have a very high incidence of associated visceral abnormalities; frequently, cardiac and renal abnormalities occur, and there may be congenital malformations of the gastro-intestinal and respiratory system.[1090]

The joints of the vertebral column (Figs 1.1, 1.2 and 1.3) *are of three kinds:*

1. *Symphyses*, i.e. secondary cartilaginous joints, between the vertebral bodies, with their interposed discs. The upper two synovial joint segments have no disc and are therefore not symphyses, besides showing other atypical features.

2. *Synovial* joints, also called zygapophyseal or facet joints, between the articular processes of the vertebral arches. The anterior symphysis together with the 2 posterior facet joints typically form one of the 'mobile segments' of the spine, totalling 25 including the upper 2 atypical segments.

3. In the cervical spine only, a further group of small articulations requires consideration (Fig. 1.4): these are the paired *joints of Luschka*,[1093] the uncovertebral or neuro-central articulations, situated in the uncovertebral region on each side between the outer posterior margins of the vertebral bodies, at the five segments between the second and seventh vertebrae.[548]

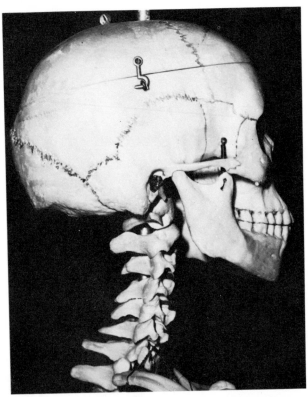

Fig. 1.2   Lateral aspect of cervical spine. Note the large and prominent spinous process of C2, the distance between the posterior tubercle of the arch of atlas and the C2 spinous process, and the somewhat depressed spinous processes of C3, C4 and C5. Tip of lateral mass of atlas is palpable between mastoid process and mandibular angle.

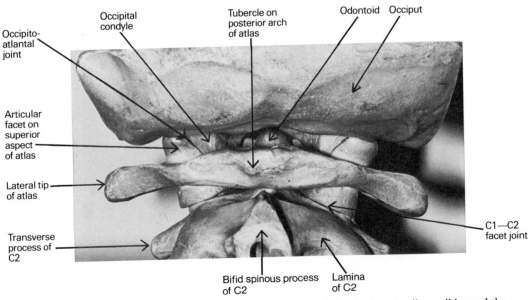

Fig. 1.3   Posterior aspect of the craniovertebral region. Note the lateral tip of atlas extending well beyond the transverse process of C2. The mastoid process of the temporal bone would lie laterally to the margins of the illustration.

CERVICAL SPINE

Because the consequences of arthrotic and spondylotic changes in the neck are usually more marked and widespread than degeneration of other spinal regions, the salient facts of anatomy and articular function in this area need careful consideration.[94, 475, 1354, 1355, 1357, 1364, 967, 1242]

A. UPPER CERVICAL SPINE (Fig. 1.5)

The craniovertebral region is of importance, as some of the most essential afferent impulses for the static and dynamic regulation of body posture arise from receptor systems in the connective tissue structures and muscles around the upper vertebral synovial joints. The importance of their functional role is clearly demonstrated, for example, in consideration of the tonic neck reflexes. Head posture governs body posture and limb control; abnormalities of afferent impulse traffic from joint receptors, because of degenerative changes, can be expected to reduce the efficiency of postural control and produce the alarming symptoms of defective equilibration.

Experimental cervical lesions in monkeys, involving unilateral section of upper cervical dorsal nerve roots, produce body dysequilibrium; and positional nystagmus, in rabbits, is caused by blocking the articular receptors in the intervertebral joints and ligaments.[586, 587, 188, 238, 1363]

Occipitoatlantal joint

The convex occipital condyles, and reciprocally concave articular surfaces of the atlas, have their long axes con-

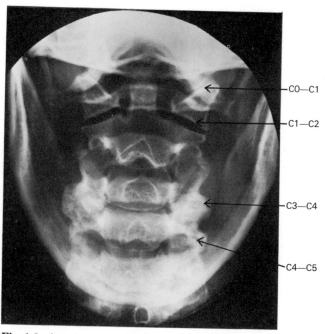

Fig. 1.5 Anterior aspect of upper cervical region. There is chondro-osteophytosis at C3-4 facet-joints on either side, and also at C4-5 on patient's left side.

verging anteriorly, with the lateral edges of the facets on the atlas banked up like a saucer, which somewhat restricts other than sagittal movements (Figs 1.3, 1.5).

Atlantoaxial joint[488, 558]

The roughly circular facets of both atlas and axis are not quite reciprocally curved; the convex upper axial surface receives the irregularly concave inferior facets of the atlas 'like the epaulettes on a pair of sloping shoulders'; the facet-planes being about 110° to the vertical. The posterior face of the anterior arch of atlas abuts against the front of the odontoid, a small synovial cavity intervening; a similar small bursa or synovial joint intervenes between the posterior face of the odontoid and its strong retaining

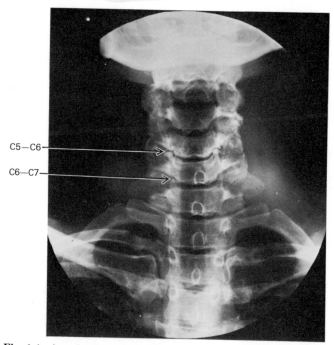

Fig. 1.4 Anterior aspect of cervicothoracic region. The uncovertebral region at C5-6 level shows the sclerosis of bony margins and flattening of the C6 uncus on the patient's right side. Compare with uncovertebral region of C6-7 space.

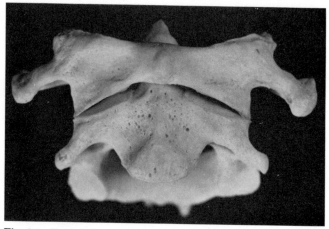

Fig. 1.6 Frontal view of the atlas and the axis.

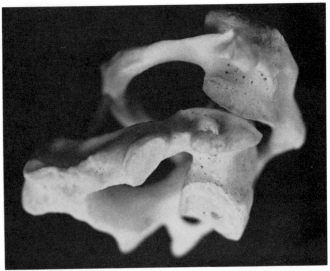

Fig. 1.7 The lateral atlantoaxial joint appears biconvex.

(Figures 1.6 and 1.7 are reproduced from Hohl M, Baker HR 1964 The atlanto-axial joint—roentgenographic and anatomical study of normal and abnormal motion. Journal of Bone and Joint Surgery 56A: 1739, by kind permission of the authors and the Editor.)

fibrous band, the transverse ligament (see below) (Figs 1.5, 1.6, 1.7).

The craniovertebral ligaments

These shared by both articulations are of much functional importance, as osteoarthrotic changes are common in this region following stress and trauma, and the dangers of possible ligamentous insufficiency must be borne in mind during treatment (Fig. 1.8).[598] From before backwards, they are:

1. The *anterior occipitoatlantal membrane*, continuous below with the anterior longitudinal ligament and blending laterally with the capsules of the facet-joints.

2. The thin *apical ligament*, attaching the tip of the odontoid to the anterior margin of the foramen magnum (Fig. 1.9).

3. The more laterally placed and tougher *alar ligaments*, attaching the posterior part of the odontoid tip to the lateral margin of the foramen magnum on each side.

4. The *transverse ligament of the atlas*, a strong fibrous band connecting each lateral mass across the front of the neural canal and passing behind the odontoid; it is a vital retaining structure stabilising the odontoid in the bony ring of atlas, and is mainly responsible for the integrity of the atlantoaxial joint. The ligament has a cruciate form, with small vertical bands of less functional importance extending upward and downward.

5. The *accessory atlantoaxial ligaments*, which pass upward and laterally from the base of the inferior vertical band of the cruciate ligament and connect the base of the odontoid process with the inferomedial part of the lateral masses of atlas. The median atlantoaxial (or atlantodental)

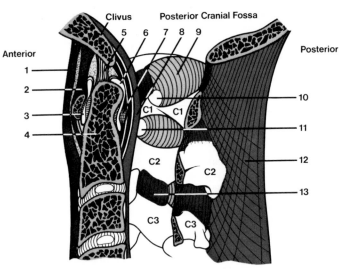

Fig. 1.8 Median and paramedian section of cervical structures.

1. Anterior longitudinal ligament
2. Anterior atlanto-occipital membrane
3. Synovial joint between anterior arch of atlas and odontoid
4. Odontoid process
5. Apical ligament of odontoid
6. Synovial joint between transverse ligament and odontoid. *NB.* 3 and 6 comprise the median atlantoaxial joint (q.v.)
7. Transverse ligament of atlas
8. Membrane tectoria—the upward continuation of the posterior longitudinal ligament
9. Posterior longitudinal ligament
10. Foramen for first cervical nerve and vertebral artery
11. Foramen for second cervical nerve
12. Ligamentum nuchae
13. Capsule of facet joint between the right side articular processes of C2 and C3.

(Reproduced from Kapandji IA 1974 The Physiology of the joints III (the trunk and vertebral column) p 187, by kind permission of the author and Librairie Maloine S.A. Paris.)

joint is very frequently the seat of arthrotic change, more so than in the two lateral articulations.[1274]

6. The *membrana tectoria*, being the upward prolongation of the posterior longitudinal ligament, covers the preceding structures posteriorly; it is attached below to the base of the odontoid, and above to the clivus of the basiocciput.

7. The *posterior occipitoatlantal membrane* completes

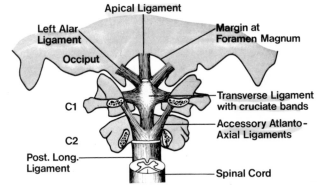

Fig. 1.9 Posterior view with vertebral arches removed.

the circle of connective tissue between occiput and atlas, blending laterally with the capsules of the facet-joints, and representing the ligamentum flavum at this segment of the spine.

8. The articular capsules between cranium and atlas are reinforced by the *lateral occipitoatlantal ligaments*, which extend from the jugular processes of the occiput to the lateral mass of the atlas on each side. In the two sets of paired joints considered above, the capsules permit relatively free movement, that of the atlantoaxial joint being the looser of the two.

N.B. The strong transverse ligament, alar ligaments, and accessory atlantoaxial ligaments mainly provide the stability between the first and second cervical vertebrae. Degenerative attenuation, or tearing, of the transverse ligament is a serious injury, allowing the possibility of the odontoid impinging on the spinal cord. When the transverse ligament is cut, the atlas is seen to displace forward up to 7 mm, and if the alar ligaments are then cut, the atlas moves forward a further 3 mm.[352]

The alar and accessory atlantoaxial ligaments are important structures in checking rotation of the head with atlas on axis, becoming taut at 30°–40° of rotation. They also restrict lateral flexion.

B. CERVICAL SPINE (C2–C7) (see Vertebral movement, p. 38)

The *intervertebral discs* contribute more than one-quarter of the length of the cervical column and this proportion is a factor in the comparatively free movement in the region.[117] By their function of withstanding the distortion imposed during movement, by their flexibility, elasticity and resilience, the discs form the anterior, weight-bearing link of each vertebral 'mobile segment'. Despite this important function, they have virtually no blood supply, as befits non-osseous, weight-bearing structures. The nucleus is avascular and only the peripheral part of the annulus enjoys a somewhat meagre blood supply during the first decade of life; even this diminishes to virtual avascularity in the young adult.[981]

The cervical interbody joints are a form of saddle articulation, convex above in the anteroposterior direction and concave from side to side (Fig. 1.4), thus forming the upward projecting uncus or lateral margins of the vertebral bodies.

C. UNCOVERTEBRAL REGION

The uncovertebral joints (or the so-called joints of Luschka) are formed between the uncinate processes, the elevated lateral edge of the upper surfaces of vertebral bodies three to seven, and the bevelled lower border of the vertebral body above (Fig. 1.4). These small horizontal cleft-like cavities or fissures[548] which appear macroscopically after the first or second decade of life but which can be recognised microscopically much earlier, are bounded anteromedially by the intervertebral disc and posterolaterally by a small capsular ligament, part of the annulus fibrosus; opposed surfaces are covered by hyaline cartilage and the space is lined by a synovium which sends small projections into the cavity as 'meniscoid' structures.[981] Shearing occurs here, especially during flexion and extension movements, and the importance of the cleft-like spaces lies in their special tendency to degenerative change, with the consequent formation of thickened soft-tissue and bony outgrowths in the neighbourhood of both the nerve root and the vertebral artery.

Jung and Kehr (1972)[623] have emphasised the especially damaging effects of uncoarthrosis in the aetiology of cervicoencephalic syndromes. The strong fibroelastic septum of the *ligamentum nuchae* (Fig. 1.8) is much more than the homologue of the supraspinous and interspinous ligaments in other parts of the column; by its attachment to all bony segments from occiput to the seventh cervical spinous process, it is an important non-contractile structure contributing to postural stability of the head and neck and also to the graduation of flexion movements.

In flexion-acceleration injuries of the neck, the amount of damage to the more intrinsic joint structures depends upon whether the degree of applied force was sufficient first to tear this thick septum, one of the first lines of defence when these injuries are sustained. Its degeneration in advanced age is one of the reasons for the lowering forward of the head in the elderly, when standing.

The facet-joints

As the paired posterior components of each movement-segment, the facet-joints are enveloped in a baggy capsule which covers them like a hood and has a degree of elasticity. This allows free movement, the *nature* of which the facet-planes largely govern. Imaginary lines joining the planes of these joints would roughly converge on the region of the eye, so that a 55° angle with the vertical of the upper cervical spine facet-planes becomes a 25° angle at the upper thoracic facet-planes.

The total surface area of these joints is about two-thirds of the articular area of the vertebral bodies, and the joint planes are approximately 45° to the vertical, thus especially at the more horizontally placed upper joints but also in the rest of the cervical column the articular cartilage bears a degree of weight, sharing the load of the head with the vertebral bodies and discs. All the posterior joints contain small 'meniscoid' structures, which project into the joint space similarly to the alar folds of the knee, and are formed of tongue-like or semilunar fringes of synovium; the subsynovial tissue is richly innervated according to Kos (1972).[677] With all other weight-bearing joints, the facet-joints inherit a marked tendency to degenerative change and suffer as much of this as any other joints in the body.[362, 643]

VESSELS

The vertebral arteries

Arising from the subclavian vessels, these run the gauntlet of many hazards in their passage through the foramina transversaria of the upper six cervical vertebrae, before

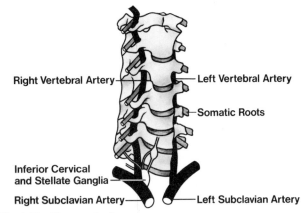

Fig. 1.10 The vertebral arteries.

they pierce the posterior atlanto-occipital membrane, enter the foramen magnum and unite on the front of the brain stem to form first the basilar artery, and then by dividing again, the two posterior cerebral arteries[437] (Figs 1.10, 1.11).

The vertebrobasilar arterial system supplies the spinal cord, the meninges, nerve roots, plexuses, muscles and joints of the neck and, intracranially, the medulla with its vital centres, the cerebellum, the vestibular nuclei and

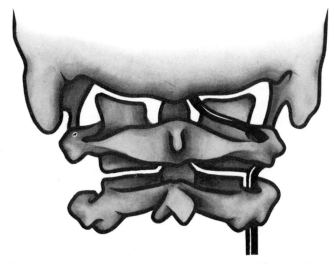

Fig. 1.11 Posterior aspect of craniovertebral region. After emerging through the foramen transversarium of the atlas, the vertebral artery winds around the articular pillar and, together with the first cervical nerve and veins, pierces the posterior atlanto-occipital membrane, to unite with its fellow on the front of the brain stem to form the basilar artery.

their connections with the equilibratory organs and the visual cortex; in the lower cervical spine other arteries contribute to the supply of extracranial structures such as muscles and nerve roots. Transient compression of the vertebral artery by bony outgrowths and soft tissue thickening during upper cervical movements, especially rotation and extension, or permanent narrowing due to exostoses from uncovertebral and facet-joint margins in the rest of the region, can produce the alarming symptoms of vertebrobasilar insufficiency. A degree of atheroma of the vessel wall increases this possibility.

A branch of the vertebral artery passes directly backwards at each segment to supply the facet-joint structures, and it is especially likely to be affected if the vertebral artery itself is distorted by degenerative processes.

The blood supply of the cervical spinal cord is derived in part from the radicular arteries, whose segmentally arranged branches from the vertebral artery lie on the front of the spinal nerve roots, enter each intervertebral foramen, give off branches to nerve roots, ganglia, facet joints and other structures, and then proceed inwards to form free anastomoses with the anterior and posterior spinal arteries. The former of these is derived from the vertebral arteries as they unite above to form the basilar artery near the foramen magnum, and the latter from the posterior inferior cerebellar arteries in the same region.

These two apparently continuous longitudinal vessels are really no more than inefficient anastomoses. Flow is downwards in the anterior spinal artery in the upper cervical region, but succeeding arteries supply a length of spinal cord both below and above their level of entry. The arteries on the cord surface are largely immune to atheromatous changes, but this complex and *highly variable* system (Fig. 1.12) of spinal cord supply is especially subject to remote effects by pressure, e.g. the radicular arteries are at hazard as they traverse the intervertebral foramina with the cervical nerve roots, and despite a certain degree of collateral supply, the vertebral artery itself is subject to compression as described, producing a pattern of cord and nerve root ischaemia with signs and symptoms *which will depend upon the pattern of supply in particular cases.*[167, 184, 384, 704, 656]

When the ischaemia is due to vessel constriction a few segments removed, the cord areas most likely to suffer are those lying more centrally, the 'watershed' areas at the boundary of adjacent territories of supply of two end-artery systems, i.e.

The terminal distribution of arterial supply accounts for many apparent anomalies in level of the lesion relative to the cause, e.g. compression at the foramen magnum can cause wasting of the hands by interruption of the downward flow in the anterior spinal artery.[704]

It should be apparent that degenerative change in the cervical region can be a matter of some importance, because in

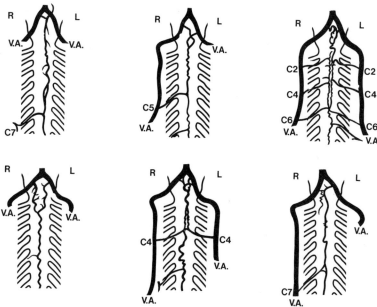

Fig. 1.12 Anterior aspect of cervical spinal cord and brain stem. Examples of the highly variable arrangement of spinal cord and nerve root arterial supply. The numbers and arrangement of radicular arteries are very inconsistent (see text). (After Dommisse GF 1974 The blood supply of the spinal cord. Journal of Bone and Joint Surgery 56B: 225.)

addition to local pain and joint stiffness, the ischaemic changes frequently involving the spinal cord due to spondylosis may lead to clinical features which can be puzzling, and to cervical myelopathy, one of the most common, if not the commonest, neurological diseases of the middle-aged and elderly (see p. 228).

Venous drainage

This is extensive, as befits the haemopoietic function of the vertebral bodies; lying in the extradural space, the internal venous plexus receives the large basivertebral veins, which drain the spongiosa of vertebral bodies, and then forms a rich anastomosis with the external venous plexus. The two plexuses form the intervertebral veins, accompanying the spinal nerves through the intervertebral foramina and draining into the vertebral vein of the neck.[532, 535]

Following its formation in the suboccipital triangle, the vertebral vein, which is connected to the intracranial venous system (see p. 62), enters the foramen transversarium of the first cervical vertebra and descends to C6 as it gathers the tributaries described; it empties into the brachiocephalic vein of the same side.

The rhythmic, pulsatile activity of veins in the cervical canal observed during myelography (after contrast medium is injected into the subarachnoid space) is vigorous, and a sudden single rise in pressure (and thus venous distension) also occurs during a cough[315] (see p. 62).

NERVE SUPPLY

An understanding of the function of receptor endings in vertebral joints and blood vessels helps a better understanding of the clinical features of degenerative disease.

Details of the complex innervation of the vertebral column are of practical importance in terms of the likely level of origin of the pain resulting from tissue changes, the areas to which pain is commonly referred, the abnormalities of posture and changes in the quality of movement, and the confusing *concomitant* symptoms and signs

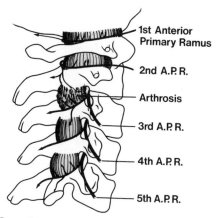

Fig. 1.13 Lateral aspect of upper five cervical vertebrae. The first two cervical roots emerge behind the facet-joints; all others emerge in front of the facet-joint. Arthrosis of the joint between C2 and C3 frequently involves the nerve root and rami by trespass upon it of degeneratively thickened tissues. (After Lazorthes G 1972 Ann. de Méd. Physique 15: 192.)

other than pain (see p. 299), some of which are certainly due to involvement of the autonomic system and which often accompany vertebral pain syndromes.

At the upper *two segments* the spinal nerve roots emerge posterolaterally behind the articular pillar and above the posterior arch of the numerically corresponding vertebra; the first cervical nerve root shares a foramen in the posterior atlanto-occipital membrane with the vertebral artery and vein (Fig. 1.13). All the other spinal nerve roots down to the level of the 5th lumbar emerge in front of the facet-joints.

Shore (1935)[1125] mentions that while the skin does not receive a direct supply from the first cervical nerve, because of a communication with the second cervical nerve

C1 has a share in supply of the cutaneous area to which the greater occipital nerve is distributed.

C2–C8

During their passage *towards* the foramina, the fibres of the roots leave the spinal cord at the level of the numerically corresponding vertebral body, and do not pass laterally in such close relationship to the disc as do the lumbar nerve roots (see p. 24). Consequently, although spinal cord and nerve root compression can occur by pathological changes in the discs, its mode of production differs somewhat to that in the lumbar region. During their passage *through* the intervertebral foramen, the roots are bounded in front and behind by structures very likely to

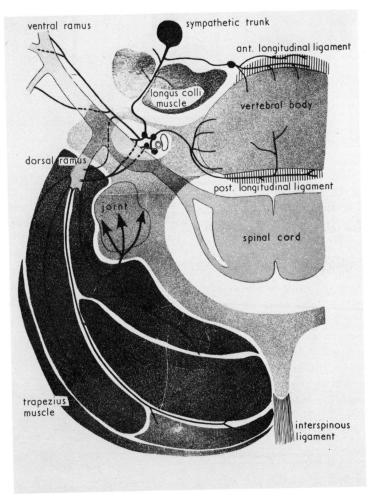

Fig. 1.14 Innervation of related cervical vertebral structures in transverse section. Muscular branches of the dorsal ramus supply the articular capsule. Parts of the vertebral plexus are seen within the foramen transversarium, together with vertebral vein and artery, and showing smaller but macroscopic ganglia in this situation. Communications of the plexus are seen with the spinal ganglion, dorsal and ventral rami, and the sympathetic trunk (and via this branch to the periosteum and marrow of the vertebral body and the anterior longitudinal ligament). Other branches are directed medially to the periosteum and spongy bone of the body and via the meningeal ramus to the dura mater and posterior longitudinal ligament. (After: Stillwell DL 1956 The nerve supply of the vertebral column and its associated structures in the monkey. Anatomical Record 125: 139. Reproduced by courtesy of the Director, Wistar Press.)

produce pressure or irritation by exostosis, these being the facet-joint structures posterolaterally and the 'neuro-central joints' anteromedially.

Cervical spine nerve roots have a rough segmental identity, i.e. after union of the ventral and dorsal rootlets, the roots emerging from the intervertebral foramina correspond numerically with the vertebra below (excepting that of the 8th cervical) and the appropriate segment of the spinal cord. Nevertheless, a few rootlets of the cord may ascend or descend to join and emerge with the spinal root numbered one above or one below the cord segment giving rise to them, and the lowest spinal cord rootlets contributing to a spinal root may be lower than the foramen for that nerve, and therefore have to ascend slightly to reach their exit from the neural canal.[537]

Paradoxically, the nerve supply to the vertebral column structures themselves is much less segmentally arranged, being derived from *the paravertebral plexus*,[1177] a rich network of fibres occupying the region of the somatic nerve roots and the sympathetic ganglia (Fig. 1.14).

Wyke (1979)[1363] observed that,

Each cervical apophyseal joint is innervated not only through articular branches of its own segmentally related spinal nerve but also by articular nerves that descend to it from the nerve root rostral to it and ascend to it from the caudally located nerve root.

There are plentiful interconnections with the sympathetic grey rami communicantes, the inferior, middle and superior cervical ganglia, the spinal posterior root ganglion and the anterior and posterior primary rami. Mixed efferent autonomic fibres and afferent somatic fibres, derived from this plexus, form 'the sinuvertebral nerve' (ramus meningeus), usually comprising two or more branches which re-enter the foramen to supply structures within the vertebral canal (Fig. 1.15). Mixed branches from the paravertebral plexus also pass externally to the sides, front and back of the vertebral bodies, supplying periosteum and ligaments; many join with the medial branch of the posterior primary rami of each spinal root, thereby reaching and serving the rich and varied receptor population of the facet-joint structures (see p. 10).

Each 'mobility segment' receives fibres derived from three adjacent spinal nerves, together with sympathetic postganglionic fibres innervating the blood vessels therein, and these approach from a variety of directions; in addition to this segmental overlap, from outside, the branches of the sinuvertebral nerve within the neural canal may wander up and down for two or three or more segments before they terminate in receptor endings (Fig. 1.15). The extension of nerves supplying the vertebral column beyond their segment of origin is comparable to the overlap of the dermatomal innervation on the body surface.

Ascending branches of mixed nerves within the neural canal, derived from the upper three cervical segments, supply the dura mater of the posterior cranial fossa, and may be concerned at times in the production of occipital headaches.[657]

The autonomic nerve supply

The supply to the head and neck is derived (a) from the three cervical sympathetic ganglia in this region, with (b)

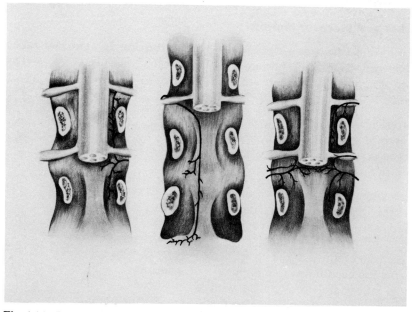

Fig. 1.15 Posterior aspect of spinal canal. The sinuvertebral nerve (ramus meningeus) may wander up and down for two, three or more segments before terminating in receptor endings. (After: Wiberg G 1949 Back pain in relation to the nerve supply of the intervertebral disc. Acta orthopaedica scandinavica 19: 211.)

parasympathetic connections contributed by cranial nerves (particularly the glossopharyngeal and vagus) (Fig. 1.14).

Although it is customary to regard the first thoracic segment as the uppermost level for emergence from the neuraxis of preganglionic sympathetic neurones, the work of Laruelle,[699] Guerrier,[461] Delmas and Laux[247] indicates that the ventral roots of C5, C6, C7 and C8 segments also contain preganglionic sympathetic efferent neurones, and that there is a deep chain of macroscopically visible ganglia along the course of the vertebral vessels in the foramen transversarium (Fig. 1.14). Similarly, clusters of intermediate sympathetic ganglia have been[550] demonstrated along the cervical nerve roots. There is experimental evidence in man that pain afferents from the face pass back to upper thoracic segments and thus the spinal cord via the cervical sympathetic chain, i.e. in addition to the multitude of afferent neurones which descend in the spinal tract of the fifth cranial nerve before synapsing in the dorsal region of C1, C2, C3 and C4 segments.[656]

The plexus which surrounds the vertebral artery enters the posterior cranial fossa with the vessels and supplies, among other structures, sympathetic fibres to the blood vessels in the vestibular portion of the inner ear; that surrounding the carotid artery contributes to the autonomic supply of the eye, assisted by the oculomotor nerve (III) which contributes parasympathetic fibres.[598]

Pathological trespass by neighbouring tissues can irritate or damage the autonomic nerve filaments with the likelihood of contributing to disturbance of function of the intracranial structures they supply, in addition to the ischaemia resulting from vertebral artery narrowing.

Details of nerve supply and receptor endings

Articular receptor distribution and function are essentially the same in all mammalian synovial joints. While omitting the detailed morphology of nerve endings, there are four types of articular systems:

Type I, II, III are corpuscular mechanoreceptors
Type IV (nociceptive) receptors subserve pain, and are distributed as capsular and perivascular plexuses, and (in ligaments) as free nerve endings.[1354, 1357, 1361b, 1363]

Unmyelinated postganglionic sympathetic vasomotor fibres are distributed to the arterial systems of joints. No nerve endings are located in articular cartilage or synovial membrane.

The importance of mechanoreceptors in the upper two or three cervical segments has been noted (see p. 3).

Intervertebral discs in adults are not supplied with nerves; nociceptive endings only are found close to the posterior part of the annulus (in the connective tissue that binds it to the posterior longitudinal ligament) as unmyelinated free and plexiform endings.

Although perivascular nerve fibres accompany the blood vessels that penetrate into new, young connective tissue formed with 'healing' of a damaged annulus, these are efferent sympathetic neurones accompanying the associated angioblast activity and supplying the blood vessels as vasomotor fibres.

In *vertebral bodies* and *arches*, perivascular nociceptive plexuses accompany the blood vessels of cancellous bone, the rich network being formed by small diameter fibres which are either poorly myelinated or unmyelinated. Similarly, the walls of periarticular arteries and arterioles, and of epidural and paravertebral veins and venules, all contain plexuses of unmyelinated nociceptive nerve filaments.

The periosteum of vertebral bodies and neural arches, and the tendons, fasciae and aponeuroses attached to them, are supplied with unmyelinated plexiform endings which are part of the nociceptive system.

The longitudinal ligaments, flaval ligaments, ligamentum nuchae and the rudimentary intertransverse ligaments are supplied with a nociceptive system of unmyelinated free nerve endings only. This is most dense in the posterior longitudinal ligament.

The dura mater has a rich supply of unmyelinated plexiform endings anteriorly and in the dural sleeves surrounding the nerve roots, but its posterior aspect is not innervated.

The cervical epidural adipose tissue is also served by a population of unmyelinated plexiform nociceptive endings which is more dense in the cervical than in other vertebral regions.

Distribution to synovial facet joints

Superficial capsule	Type I Mechanoreceptors
	Type IV Plexiform nociceptive receptors
Deep capsule	Type II Mechanoreceptors
	Type IV Plexiform nociceptive receptors
Fat pads (and in foramina)	Type II Mechanoreceptors
	Type IV Plexiform nociceptive receptors (very rich supply)
Ligaments	Type IV Free nerve endings only
Synovial membrane	No nerve endings of any kind
Cartilage	No nerve endings of any kind

Functions: Type I are especially numerous in the facet-joint capsules of the cervical spine, and are very sensitive to *changing* mechanical stress. Some of them display a constant resting low-frequency discharge due to the pressure-difference of 5–10 mmHg (0.67–1.33 kPa) between the inside and outside of the joint capsules, and to the capsular stress produced by the static tension in related muscles and elastic connective tissues. Thus they contribute to awareness of static joint position, even in immobile joints. Other receptive groups are active within certain ranges of the angle of movement of the joint. These change-of-stress sensors report dynamic joint status, and thus the direction, degree and speed of joint movement (kinaesthesis)—whether actively or passively produced. They also monitor atmospheric pressure change. They have a low threshold, are slowly adapting and also exert powerful reflexogenic effects on the muscles.[1354, 1363]

Type II end-organs lie in the deeper capsule layers, and on the surface of all fat-pads in and around synovial joints. These low-threshold, rapidly adapting sensors have no resting discharge, and only fire off at the beginning and end of joint movement, however produced. Thus, they are acceleration and deceleration sensors. They are reflexogenic only, and do not contribute to awareness of joint position or movement. Type III mechanoreceptors, which occur solely in intra- and extra-articular ligaments of other joints, are absent from all longitudinal vertebral joint ligaments. Type IV end-organ function (nociception) has been noted above, and is further discussed on p. 161.

It is important to note that: (a) the maintenance of posture, and the performance of voluntary movement, are highly integrated and co-ordinated functions of groups of skeletal muscles; appropriate changes of tone are controlled by patterns of efferent impulses which are themselves based in part on rich and complex patterns of afferent sensory impulse traffic from Type I mechanoreceptors in joint tissues and from cutaneous receptors in the skin overlying joints. This is the consciously perceived (or perceptual) system subserving postural and kinaesthetic sensation.

Degenerative disease and trauma severely affect joint capsular tissue, and careful examination will often reveal the extent to which postural sensation and kinaesthesis have been impaired by damage to or irritation of the receptor population; (b) an equally rich volume of reflexogenic, afferent (but *non-sensory*) impulses from Type I and Type II receptors plays a major part, at brain-stem and segmental levels, in producing and integrating patterns of facilitatory and inhibitory bias in the motoneurone pools of the cervical, limb, eye and jaw muscles; and it is these which underlie the functional groupings of muscle during postural control and voluntary movements. Voluntary movement is only as good as reflexogenic efficiency. These arthrokinetic reflexes are defective in diseased and trau-

matised joints, and are also disturbed when joints are immobilised, as in splints and supports, e.g. cervical collars; (c) the involvement of Type IV nociceptors by the same tissue changes is more plainly manifest during examination of patients by awareness of pain and abnormal patterns of muscle reflexes.

Dee (1978)[245] in a well-referenced summary, has reviewed the structure and function of joint innervation, and makes the suggestion that articular reflexes may have an important role in maintaining articular congruity—

possibly distributing the load in a suitable way and not merely acting to resist the gross forces that may cause subluxation or dislocation, although this is doubtless an important function.

The implications are obvious: if degenerative change has grossly disturbed afferent impulse traffic from capsular mechanoreceptors, the partial loss of 'the governor' for joint congruity has increased the susceptibility of such joints to minor articular strains from normally trivial stress.

Spinal nucleus of the fifth cranial nerve

A neuroanatomical fact of significance, when considering mechanisms of pain production from diseased or damaged joints in the upper neck, is the extent to which this brain-stem nucleus descends in the spinal cord (Figs 1.16, 1.17). Reaching from the pons to the 3rd or 4th cervical spinal segment, it receives all the nociceptive (and thermal) afferent inputs from:

5th cranial nerve
7th cranial (facial) nervus intermedius fibres
IX cranial nerve (glossopharyngeal)
X cranial nerve (vagus)
C1 ⎫
C2 ⎬ dorsal nerve roots
C3 ⎭

The extreme lower pole of the nucleus (C2 to C3 segments of the cord) receives pain afferents from the region of the mandibular angle and from the retroauricular, occipital and submandibular region, which descend to the level of the C2 and C3 dorsal nerve roots, before they synapse to give rise to the second neurones ascending to the thalamus in the bulbothalamic tract. Where the spinal cord becomes continuous with the medulla, the substantia gelatinosa is continuous with the spinal tract of the 5th cranial nerve.[109, 1355, 1180b, 130, 1281, 1277, 553, 496] The convergence of these cervical and upper spinal afferents is of clinical importance. There are good reasons for holding the view that an increase in afferent impulse traffic, originating in Type IV nociceptors in the upper cervical joints, may produce facilitatory excitation of neurones in the associated cord segments, upon which the synaptic terminals are subtended from afferents innervating relatively distant tissues of the face and cranium, and initiating symptoms of pain and

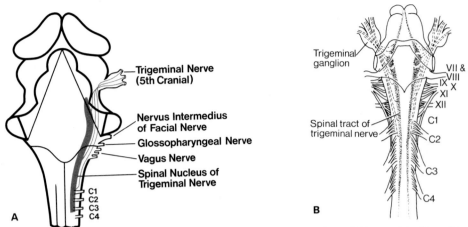

Fig. 1.16 (A) Posterior aspect of brain stem and schematic view of floor of 4th ventricle. Note the extent to which the spinal tract of the 5th cranial nerve descends in the upper cervical spinal cord (see text). (B) Posterior aspect of brain stem with cerebellum removed. The semilunar ganglia of trigeminal nerves are depicted above cut edge of middle cerebellar penduncle. Upper four cervical cord segments lie at levels indicated. (Reproduced from Wyke BD 1979 Manipulation therapy for neck pain. Physiotherapy 65: 5, by kind permission of B. D. Wyke and the Editor.)

paraesthesiae, projected or referred, to those areas which are uninvolved in the articular changes. Further, the spinal tract of the 5th cranial nerve occupies a 'watershed' area (Fig. 1.17), i.e. it lies more centrally and at the boundary of adjacent territories of supply of two end-artery systems (see p. 6) and may frequently be subject to the effects of ischaemia produced by lesions that trespass upon vessels at segments remote from that suffering the main effects of it.[656]

ANOMALIES OF BONE AND SOFT TISSUES, PERIPHERAL INNERVATION, AND VASCULAR SUPPLY

Asymmetry of the craniovertebral bony and ligamentous structures is almost the rule rather than the exception.[220]

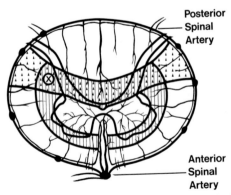

Fig. 1.17 Scheme of upper cervical spinal cord. 'Watershed' areas between territory supplied by:
▲ —anterior and posterior spinal arteries
||| —peripheral and central arterial supply
⊗ —area occupied by the spinal tract of the 5th cranial nerve.
(After: Keuter EJW 1970 Vascular origin of cranial sensory disturbance caused by pathology of the lower cervical spine. Acta neurochirurgica 23: 229.)

Infrequently, there may be congenital absence of the odontoid—the lateral mass of C1 and the body of C2 retaining their normal relationships.

A degree of platybasia or basilar impression may be present, sometimes slight and occasionally marked.[1274] Absolute values do not exist, and the condition may be unilateral or bilateral. The last occipital sclerotome sometimes forms a separate entity.[315]

Basilar impression may occur with remnants of the occipital vertebra,[315] and is often combined with other occipitocervical malformations, particularly with varying degrees of assimilation of atlas. Defective fusion of the arch of atlas (spina bifido atlanto),[738] and os odontoideum (in which the odontoid is divided transversely) may occur. The latter may rarely be an acquired lesion.[519, 1035] Fused or separate accessory bony elements may be in apposition to or united with the edge of the foramen magnum, and scattered islets of bone may be embedded in connective tissue around the foramen magnum. A third occipital condyle may be present.[220]

The various irregularities may occur together or in isolated form.[932] Sometimes a bony arch or a complete bony tunnel (ponticulus ponticus) is formed around the vertebral artery on the superior surface of atlas. While the frequency of such frank craniovertebral malformations is small, minor asymmetry is very common indeed.[220] For example, one occipital condyle is frequently smaller than its fellow, and may project further from the basiocciput, or the two condyles may not lie in the same coronal plane.

Wood (1972)[1336] has briefly surveyed the embryology of vertebral bodies and intervertebral discs, and describes an atlas vertebra in which there was an absent anterior arch, a failure of the posterior arch to unite (spina bifida atlanto) and a bilateral costal element defect in that the foramen transversarium was just a deep notch, open anteriorly. The superior facets of atlas commonly show the same asymmetrical disposition, as well as difference in size; the inferior facets articulating with the axis often show similar differences.

Below C2, there may be accessory articulations of spinous processes, and marked asymmetry of the normally bifid spines very commonly occurs. Cleavage of the cervical spinous processes has been frequently described. Congenital block vertebra is sometimes seen at C2 and C3.[1093]

Lawrence (1976)[701] studied the prevalence of cervical rheumatoid arthritis in twelve population samples, and noted that 'congenital' block vertebra had a prevalence of 0.9 per cent in those born before 1935. None was observed in those born since. Thus it appears that environmental factors predisposing to the combination of cervical arthritis and 'block vertebra' have changed since the last 40 years. Lower in the cervical column, the foramen transversarium may be incomplete, subdivided or imperforate,[117] and cervical ribs may be present unilaterally, or bilaterally in various forms.[1336] A separate centre of ossification may appear as the costal element of C7 vertebra, and produce variations from an enlarged and beaked transverse process to a fully developed and sometimes quite long rib. The incidence of cervical rib appears much greater than the incidence of vascular and neurological symptoms arising from its presence. The presence of supernumary fascial bands, variations in a normally situate first rib (see p. 131) and anomalies of the scalene muscles (scalenus minimus) have also been described.[117]

A cervical vertebral pedicle may be absent[824] and congenital elongation of the pedicles of C6 in identical twins has been reported.[162, 874]

NB. The high incidence of minor asymmetry at the craniovertebral junction and in other parts of the spine has important implications for theories of manipulative treatment which may hold that 'symmetry is all' and that asymmetry detected by palpation must always be 'normalised'.

Spinal stenosis

Since the spinal cord, its meninges and the narrow extradural space lie immediately behind the posterior longitudinal ligament, they are very easily compressed by gross bony and fibrocartilaginous projections at the level of each disc. The normal cervical vertebral canal has a sagittal diameter of about 17 mm, while that of the normal spinal cord is about 10 mm.[117] Smaller projections are frequently present in mature people without causing serious symptoms, but a factor accentuating the likelihood of spinal cord interference is a narrow neural canal, i.e. congenital spinal stenosis, when normally insignificant backward projections at disc level may cause signs and symptoms of cord pressure reasonably associated with more marked degenerative change. These are aggravated on cervical flexion, when the length of the neural canal is increased

and the neural canal contents are drawn more tightly against the prominences of degenerative, thickened tissue.[130, 120] The available space may be the decisive element in the complex of trespass by arthrotic facet joints, spondylotic spurring with osseocartilaginous bosses or bars, congenital stenosis of the spinal cord and neurological disturbances.[315]

Anomalies of innervation

The textbook patterns of root and plexus formation, and innervation of peripheral tissues, are subject to variation in a significant proportion of cases.[117] The range of the segmental contributions to the brachial plexus is not uniform, it varies from person to person and between the two sides of one individual. About 11 per cent of brachial plexuses are prefixed, that is, receive a major contribution from the C4 root at the expense of the lower roots of the plexus, and a similar percentage are postfixed, receiving a major contribution from the T1 root with the T2 contribution always present and a very small or entirely absent contribution from C4.[1101, 896, 598]

Frykholm (1971)[392] has drawn attention to the wide variations of cervical root formation; in some instances the ventral root piercing the dura at a lower level than the dorsal root. He observes that nature seldom provides a completely perfect anatomy from all functional points of view, except to a small privileged group of individuals. Even in young people there are many cases of malformed root pouches, occasionally together with radicular nerves sharply angulated upwards, or nerves eccentrically located in the intervertebral foramen.

Variations in spinal rootlet formation, roots of the plexus, distribution of the roots within trunks and cords and innervation of peripheral structures should be borne in mind, e.g. anomalous innervation of the hand occurs in at least 20 per cent of the population. The cutaneous supply of the little finger may be derived from the sixth sensory root, for example.

Anomalies of vessels

In less than 25 per cent of the population are the vertebral arteries of equal size. Irritation, compression or distortion of the larger of the two vessels will be likely to have more serious effects than interference with the vessel of smaller lumen. Variations in arterial supply of the spinal cord have already been noted (see p. 6).

THORACIC SPINE AND RIBS

The thoracic spine is the least mobile part of the spinal column, the attachment of the rib cage, together with the thin discs comprising only one-seventh of the height of this region, combining to reduce its movement considerably.

The vertebral bodies, in effect short waisted tubes,

diminish in size from T1 to T3 and then progressively increase to T12, the body of which shares the general kidney-shaped mass of the lumbar vertebrae. The bodies are slightly deeper behind; the two demifacets for articulation with the heads of the ribs are situated at the posterior aspects of the bodies in the upper region, but in the lower half of the thorax they have migrated backwards to be borne almost entirely by the bases of the pedicles.

The thin bony plates bearing the superior and inferior facets orientate the plane of the facet-joints at about 15°–20° to the vertical, often less in the lower segments; the superior facets face backwards, and a little outward and upward. The strong transverse processes have clubbed extremities and in the uppermost segments may extend laterally for 4–5 cm; they steadily diminish in size from above downwards. The concave costal facet, for reception of the tubercle of the corresponding rib, is placed anteriorly on transverse processes 1 to 6, and then steadily migrates to the superior surfaces of the transverse processes 7 to 10, becoming much flatter as it does so. Thus during respiratory movement, the upper ribs rotate on the transverse processes, while the lower ones glide.

JOINTS OF VERTEBRAL BODIES AND ARCHES

The vertebral bodies and their apophyses are connected by the intrinsic ligamentous structures common to the whole column, with the difference that they are not so thick and dense as in the lumbar region, but are more developed than in the cervical spine.

The costovertebral joints

Reception of the head of the typical ribs into the concavity formed by adjacent vertebral body margins and the disc between, is secured by a closely applied fibrous capsule, by the fan-shaped radiate ligament which covers the anterolateral aspect of the joint and by a short horizontal band of fibres, the intra-articular ligament, which connects the crest on the head of the rib to the disc and thus divides the small synovial joint into two cavities.

The costotransverse joints

These are formed by articulations of the typical ribs, halfway between head and angle of rib, with the front aspect of transverse processes of the numerically corresponding vertebrae, by the capsular and the three costotransverse ligaments; these are an important factor in restricting thoracic movements as compared to other regions.

Although the first and second ribs take little part in quiet respiratory movement, and somewhat more in forced inspiration, they have more mobility than is sometimes appreciated.

The facet-joints

These take only a very small part in weight-bearing, gravity now exerting its effect almost entirely upon the discs and vertebral bodies in this spinal region. The practically vertical set of the facet-planes also contributes to the marked limitation of thoracic movement in the sagittal plane. They contain meniscoid structures as in the cervical spine.

The thoracolumbar mortise joint

Macalister (1889)[771] stated that the thoracolumbar junction was the point most exposed to injury. The transition from thoracic to lumbar characteristics may occur at segments T10–T11 or T11–T12 or T12–L1. The transition is most marked by a singular configuration of articular processes of one vertebra which has the effect of forming with the subjacent vertebra a mortise and tenon joint when under compression or extension; this is one of the very few examples of complete bone-to-bone 'lock' in the body. The transitional vertebra is thoracic in type in its upper half, i.e. the superior facets face backwards, upwards and a little outwards, and begins to show lumbar characteristics in its lower half, i.e. the inferior articular processes begin to turn laterally, with facets slightly convex from side to side and facing laterally and forwards. On extension, the lower facets of the transitional vertebra lock into the upper facets of the uppermost 'lumbar-type' vertebra, and no movement other than flexion is then possible.

In a series of 67 adult columns,[228] the site of the mortise joint was variously at:

T10–T11	5 columns
T11–T12	46 columns
T12–L1	16 columns
Total	67 columns

The importance of this characteristic is that if manual techniques of any vigour are applied with the intention of mobilising this junction when in extension, they will certainly be fruitless, probably painful, and may even do the patient a mischief.

VESSELS

The spinal cord, with its meninges, is supplied by dorsal branches of the posterior intercostal arteries, having a variable arrangement and contributing to the likewise variable longitudinal anastomotic channels lying on the cord surface. The dorsal branches also supply the vertebral column and its articulations, and provide radicular branches to the ventral and dorsal nerve roots.

The thoracic spinal canal is consistently narrowest in that part of the vertebral column extending from T4 to T9. This narrow zone of the bony tube corresponds almost exactly with that part of the spinal cord with the poorest blood supply.[266, 82]

A more or less constant and relatively large artery—the arteria radicularis magna, or the artery of Adamkiewicz—

is always found among the lower thoracic or upper lumbar roots; it is the largest of the lower thoracic/upper lumbar branches supplying the spinal cord, and is the main nutrient vessel of the lumbar cord. It is usually near the diaphragm.

1. When the arteria magna is in the thoracic region there are fewer radicular vessels, but the longitudinal anastomosis is richer.

2. When the arteria magna is in the lumbar region, the local segmental blood supply is relatively well preserved but the anastomosis along the cord surface is poor.[533]

The significance of these observations lies in remembering the hazards of handling any patient who reports lower limb symptoms in association with thoracic spinal joint problems. In clinical treatment sessions, there is no way of knowing how narrow the margin of safety may be.

As in the cervical column, the internal and external venous plexuses unite to form the intervertebral vein, which in this region drains into the posterior intercostal veins, the tributaries of the azygos system.

NERVE SUPPLY

An important characteristic of the thoracic column is that the costovertebral and costotransverse joints share intimately in the distribution of the 'mixed' nerves from the paravertebral plexus (cf cervical spine) as well as being supplied from the related intercostal nerves (Figs 1.18, 1.19).[1361a]

Vrettos and Wyke (1974)[1276] have demonstrated by microdissection that the costovertebral joints are innervated both from the posterior primary rami and the intercostal nerves. Type I and Type II corpuscular mechanoreceptors (see p. 10) are embedded in a plexus of Type IV nociceptors, whose unmyelinated afferent neurones enter the related articular nerves.

The reflex response to electrical stimulation of these articular nerves was powerful and co-ordinated hypertonus of thoracic musculature; a simultaneous stimulus of the nociceptors altered normal respiration (see p. 385).

The sympathetic supply to the blood vessels in the region is derived from the ganglia resting against the heads of the ribs, and in this part of the spine they are components of the rich paravertebral plexus developed along the length of the column.

Branches of the sinuvertebral nerve (ramus meningeus) may wander up and down the neural canal for four or five segments before terminating as end-organs.

The sympathetic neurones accompanying the somatic nerves to upper limb may be gathered from as far caudally as the T8 segment.[635]

Branches from T2, T3 and very occasionally T4 supply the inside and back of upper arm and axillary area, joining with the medial cutaneous of the arm. T3 can frequently

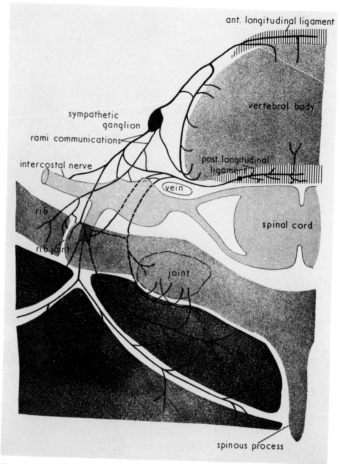

Fig. 1.18 Horizontal section at a thoracic level showing the main branches of the spinal ganglion and of the dorsal ramus. A paravertebral nerve plexus is shown, made up of communications between the spinal and sympathetic ganglia, with branches to the longitudinal ligaments, dorsal and ventral (intercostal) rami, periosteum, spongy bone of the rib, the vertebral body and arch, and to costotransverse and intervertebral joints. The sources of the meningeal ramus ('recurrent' nerve) are shown. Muscular branches of the dorsal ramus give off nerves to the intervertebral joints. (After: Stillwell DL 1956 The nerve supply of the vertebral column and its associated structures in the monkey. Anatomical Record 125: 139. Reproduced by courtesy of the Director, Wistar Press.)

be traced out to the shoulder region. The subcostal nerve (T12) often anastomoses with the lumbar plexus and gains connection thereby with the ilioinguinal and genito-femoral nerves.[164]

With regard to the lateral branches of the posterior primary rami:

1. That of the second thoracic nerve has an extensive distribution, descending paravertebrally until it emerges at the level of T6, and then climbing up to the level of the acromion area before it terminates (Fig. 1.20).[788]

2. The lateral branch of the posterior primary ramus of the 12th thoracic nerve descends as far as the postero-lateral iliac crest, and then crosses it to supply the skin over the lateral buttock (Fig. 1.20).[788,437]

The discrepancy between spinal cord segments and

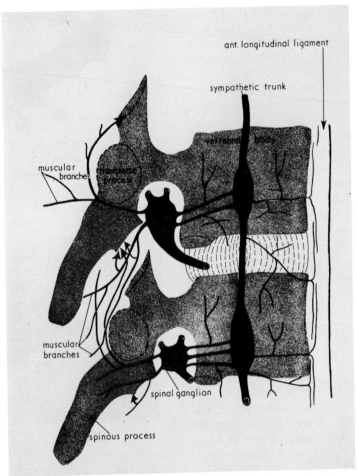

Fig. 1.19 Dorsal and ventral ramus branches in the thoracic region. A cranially directed branch of the dorsal ramus supplies deep oblique muscles and an articular capsule cranial to its level of origin. Another dorsal ramus branch supplies a joint one segment caudal, continuing into dorsal muscles. Ventral rami (not labelled) have been severed. Autonomic rami, two or more in number, give off branches to periosteum and areolar connective tissue on the surface of the intervertebral disc. The anterior longitudinal ligament and nearby periosteum receive nerves which arise from the sympathetic ganglia. (After: Stillwell DL 1956 The nerve supply of the vertebral column and its associated structures in the monkey. Anatomical Record 125: 139. Reproduced by courtesy of the Director, Wistar Press.)

vertebral body segments begins to be apparent at the lower cervical levels, and the disproportion between cord length and column length means that upper thoracic roots now have to travel downwards about 3 cm to reach their foraminal exit. At the thoracolumbar junction, the distance is about 7 cm[537] (Fig. 2.13).

ANOMALIES

Thoracic spinous processes are frequently asymmetrical, and the tips of one or more may be congenitally deviated from the mid-line by as much as 0.5 cm. Manipulative attempts at 'correction' of these 'positional defects' are less likely to be made if movement-testing during examination is careful and normal mobility confirmed thereby.

Thoracic laminae are much more uniform in configuration; in the absence of frank malformations, asymmetry detected by careful palpation may have significance, especially so when the localised area is unduly tender, also feels thickened and is reasonably associated with the symptoms reported.

Para-articular processes, as bony spicules or spurs, occur almost exclusively in the thoracic spine, and are located on the inner surfaces of the laminae very close to the articular processes.[898] They may have some clinical significance as a factor in spinal nerve root compression.

Developmental stenosis of a thoracic vertebra is not unknown[430] and in one patient severe thickening of T9 laminae was responsible for spastic paralysis of lower limbs.

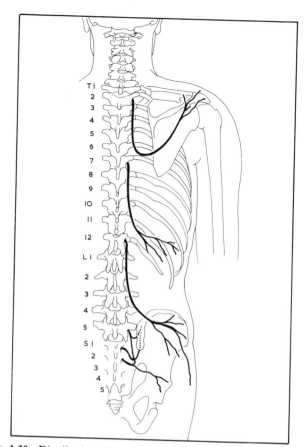

Fig. 1.20 Distribution of lateral branches of posterior primary rami of lower thoracic nerves. Extent traversed by T12 is of clinical interest.

Block vertebra, or congenital synostosis, is occasionally seen in the thoracic spine, as a partial or complete fusion of two segments.[315]

Sagittally cleft vertebra ('butterfly vertebra'), and congenital wedge vertebra with failure of development of the anterior nucleus, may also be encountered. The latter produces a prominent postural kyphus or gibbus.

A unilateral anomalous joint in a normally situate first rib has been reported[1060, 1310] and the sternal end of the 3rd or 4th rib and its cartilage is sometimes bifid. As well as a cervical rib (p. 13), an extra rib may attach to the 1st lumbar vertebra. The lowest cartilage to reach the sternum may be the 6th, 7th or 8th, therefore ribs should be counted from above downwards by their prominent angles.[434]

LUMBAR SPINE

The massive vertebral bodies are developed to sustain greater weight and other stresses than the regions above.

They are a bit deeper in front, and the fifth markedly so, accounting in part together with the similar shape of the fifth lumbar disc, for the lumbosacral angle; this is highly variable within normal limits (see p. 273).

The vertebral arches are thicker and stronger than in other regions and are buttressed with extra bone, as for example in the mamillary processes which strengthen the bony face of the posterior facets.

Unlike the bifid cervical and rather pointed thoracic spines, the lumbar spinous processes are quadrangular and project horizontally backwards (Fig. 1.21). They may exhibit a shallow depression at the middle of their subcutaneous bony ridges, a factor to be borne in mind during palpation. The fifth lumbar spinous process is frequently the smallest of the five, and its transverse process the most massive.

THE FACET-JOINTS

The plane of the vertebral arch joints is now vertical, usually but by no means always anteroposterior and gently concave medially.[726] The inward-facing concave facets of the superior articular processes therefore clasp from below the inferior, convex and outward-facing facets of the vertebrae above (Fig. 1.21).[441] A somewhat loose, fibroelastic capsule allows the opposed surfaces to separate during flexion, this movement widening the intervertebral foramen considerably. The joints contain 'meniscoid' structures as in the cervical and thoracic regions.

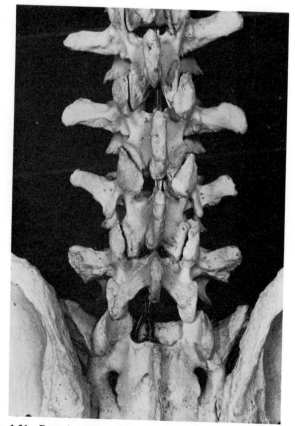

Fig. 1.21 Posterior aspect of lower lumbar spine. The facet-planes at the L3–L4 segment are anomalous, the left more than the right. The fifth lumbar spinous process is small.

The lumbar vertebral canal may be demonstrated on radiographic measurement to be narrower than usual, i.e. congenital stenosis, or the dimensions of a normal canal may be reduced by acquired stenosis, sometimes due to ligamentum flavum thickening and buckling forward into the extradural space, for example.[1088]

The typical lumbar vertebral foramen is generally triangular, but is subject to marked variations of configuration which may have important consequences (see Anomalies) (Figs 1.32, 1.33).

THE INTERVERTEBRAL DISCS

The intervertebral discs are thick enough to account for about one-third of the total height of the lumbar spine. As in all vertebral joints they are separated from the adjacent spongiosa or cancellous bone of the vertebral bodies above and below by a plate of hyaline cartilage, the circumference of which is bounded by the margins of cortical bone of the vertebral body.

1. The annulus fibrosus
This forms a fibrocartilaginous ring, more fibrous and elastic peripherally, more cartilaginous in the inner part; it encloses and retains the gel of the nucleus pulposus. The many elastic fibres of the young, healthy annulus gradu-

ally disappear during the ageing process.[223] The annular fibres are gathered in concentric lamellae, successive layers overlapping in alternately oblique directions; each lamella is also convex in the vertebral plane and its fibres form about one-half of the disc circumference (Fig. 1.22). The amount of connection or binding between each lamella is small, implying a degree of movement relative to each other.

The most laterally placed fibres of the lamellae become more slender and bifurcated as they sweep posteriorly. At the upper and lower margin of vertebral bodies the fibres may be separated into three groups by reason of their mode of attachment (Fig. 1.23).

According to McNab (1977),[780] (a) the outermost fibres are much more numerous anteriorly, and attach to the periosteum and vertebral body just beyond the epiphyseal ring of cortical bone. These are the fibres adjacent to the anterior and posterior longitudinal ligaments. (b) The epiphyseal group of fibres are the next deepest layer, attaching to the opposed superior and inferior epiphyseal bony rings of adjacent vertebral bodies. Like the foregoing, there are many of them anteriorly. (c) The innermost fibres attach above and below to the hyaline cartilaginous plate, and the majority by far of posterior annular fibres are of this type.

Ghadially (1978)[405] observed that under electron micro-

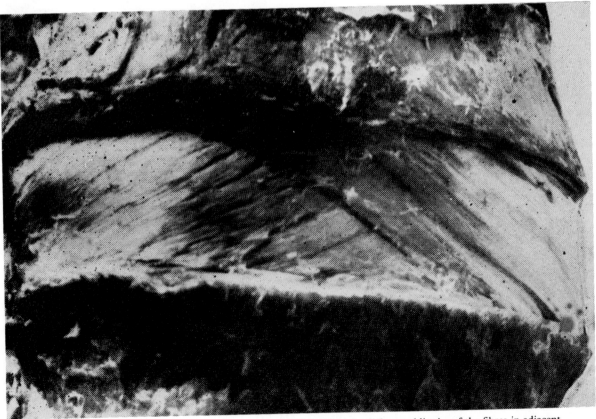

Fig. 1.22 Photograph of a dissection of the annulus fibrosus which shows the different obliquity of the fibres in adjacent laminae. (Reproduced by courtesy of the Editor, *Scottish Medical Journal.*)

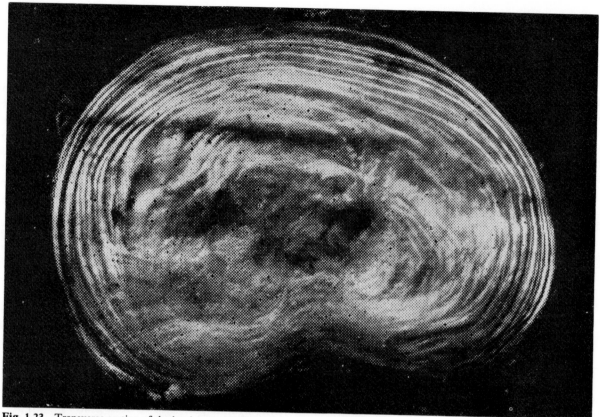

Fig. 1.23 Transverse section of the lumbosacral intervertebral disc of a young adult. The intricate pattern of the laminae of the annulus is apparent and is in contrast to the appearance of the nucleus which is nearer the back than the front. (Reproduced by courtesy of the Editor, *Scottish Medical Journal.*)

scopy the elongated fibroblast-like cells of the annulus resemble chondrocytes more than any other cell type.

Despite assumptions to the contrary, knowledge of the fine structure of intervertebral discs, particularly the annulus fibrosus, is still far from complete. For example, it is unlike any other connective tissue in the body, in that its content of proteoglycans is high. Also, the collagen content of the disc also helps to maintain its high fluid content, and plays an important part in this aspect of its biochemistry.

Functions of the annulus: (a) Forms the chief structural unit between vertebral bodies, and provides a mobile segment. (b) Encloses and retains the nucleus pulposus. (c) Restricts and regulates movement, e.g. sagittal lumbar movement is restricted almost entirely by the tough annulus. *In full flexion,* when the articular processes are more separated, some half of the diagonal lamellae *restrict rotation* to a degree and are thus under stress during this movement. (d) By virtue of an inherent elasticity, the annulus fibrosus helps to absorb the shock of compression forces, which are sustained as a circumferential tensile stress in the annulus. The diagonal strapping effect of the fibrous lamellae is important here.

The posterior part, and especially the posterolateral part, of the annulus is a site of potential weakness because: (a) of the thinning and bifurcation of annular fibres posteriorly; (b) fibrous tissue is adapted to withstand tension rather than pressure, and in the lordotic lumbar spine gravitational compression falls most heavily on the posterior aspects of the vertebral body joints; (c) the posterior longitudinal ligament is attenuated, thin and expanded at the level of the disc; (d) the eccentric position of the nucleus pulposus, which lies closer to the posterior aspect of the disc; (e) the susceptibility of this locality to succumb under the stress of rotation strains.[326]

2. The nucleus pulposus

The nucleus pulposus comprises about 40 per cent of the disc and is a semifluid gel, readily deformable but incompressible. Collagen fibres form a three-dimensional honeycomb network, enmeshing the mucoprotein gel with its rich content of mucopolysaccharide, or proteoglycans; these large molecules are strongly hydrophilic—the protein-polysaccharide gel exerts an imbibition pressure which will bind about 8.8 times its volume of water—and are mainly responsible for the high water content of the pulp, which decreases steadily with age because the disc literally dries up as the years advance. In effect, the inflated proteoglycans keep the disc blown up with water.

Although the molecular weight of proteoglycans is very

high, the hydrophilic properties depend upon its capacity as an 'ion exchanger', and thus its charge density, rather than its molecular weight. In degenerative disc disease, the proteoglycans' molecular weight becomes smaller, but this does not of itself affect the hydrophilic properties to any degree, since the essential factor is the 'ion exchanger' function and not the molecular weight.

Proteoglycans swelling is in balance with the pressure upon the disc.

The hydrophilic attraction is not biochemical bonding because appreciable amounts of water can be expressed from the nucleus by continued mechanical pressure, which may explain the diurnal variation of body height according to posture.

When there is a lower fixed-charge-density, the amount of water which can be squeezed out of the disc, under a given pressure, is much greater.

Functions of the pulp: (a) Its fluidity permits the formation of a mobile segment, and allows an even distribution of compression forces over the opposed surfaces of vertebral discs. (b) The viscid gel acts like a dynamic hydraulic suspension system.

Differences in composition between discs

The normal distribution of the population of macromolecular proteoglycans in lumbar discs is of interest.

From a detailed study[4] of the intervertebral discs, undertaken to assess the quality, and the hydrodynamic size of proteoglycan extracted from human annulus and nucleus in 8-, 16- and 44-year-old spines, it was evident that:

1. The nature of proteoglycans differs between annulus and nucleus.

2. The molecular size of the proteoglycans from both regions decreases with age, and their content of keratin sulphate increases.

3. The interaction of proteoglycans with collagen—the fibrous content of the disc—changes markedly with advancing age.

4. The composition, and thus the nature and characteristics of individual discs *differ from each other in mature lumbar spines.*

Unlike the older discs, there was uniformity between discs of the 8-year-old in the extraction of proteoglycans, and only small differences between discs of the 16-year-old spine; there was between them a general resemblance. The 44-year-old disc showed some major differences, in that:

1. A much higher proportion of the total proteoglycans was extractable from the annuli as well as the nuclei, and

2. There was a distinct difference in this respect between discs.

3. The collagen content of the discs increased from upper to lower segments.

4. The proteoglycans of the lowest disc (L5–S1) were less extractable compared with the higher segments, and

5. The proteoglycans initially extracted were on average of much smaller molecular size than those extracted subsequently.

Results suggested that ageing and/or mild degeneration is accompanied by changes in the quality of the proteoglycans family leading to closer association with collagen of some, and a diminished capacity of the remainder to form aggregates; the observed changes are likely to considerably modify the mechanical performance of the disc. In general, very much more is known about the biochemistry of intervertebral discs than the *effect* of biochemical changes on disc function as a whole.

A few elastic fibres are also found in the matrix of the nucleus pulposus.[139]

The hyaline cartilage plate

In life, the upper and lower surfaces of a vertebral body between the marginal bony rings comprise a cribriform, hyaline cartilaginous plate; there is no closure by compact bone between the cartilage and the vascular, cancellous spongiosa of the vertebral body.[508]

In effect a vertebral body is a short vertical tube of cortical bone, nipped slightly at the waist, sealed at each end by the hyaline plate and enclosing the spongiosa with its rich blood supply.

The plates have three functions:

1. They are the growth zone of the immature vertebral bodies.

2. They help to anchor the disc.

3. They provide a barrier, not impermeable, between the nucleus pulposus and the spongiosa of the bodies.

During the first decade of life, the plate is perforated by blood vessels which communicate between the pulp and the spongiosa; after their obliteration during childhood the sites of these perforations are evident as small, scarred areas on the surface of the plate, and these remain as sites of potential weakness, sometimes allowing tiny herniations of the nuclear pulp into the spongiosa. These should not be confused with macroscopic and comparatively massive vertical herniations of pulp into the vertebral bodies which are radiologically evident (as Schmorl's nodes) and observed in spines which have withstood much compression in daily living; neither do they necessarily give rise to symptoms.[1093]

There is evidence that the rhythmic compression occurring during body movements, besides exerting a centrifugal force sustained and absorbed by the elasticity of the pulp-retaining annulus, exerts vertical forces which slightly bulge the hyaline plate into the spongiosa of the vertebral bodies, thereby distorting the trabeculae to a degree, i.e. the plate acts like a diaphragm (see Vertebral movement, p. 49).[138a]

With these facts in mind, the occurrence of microscopic

and macroscopic herniations is presumably evidence of a degree of failure of the hyaline plate, or of excessive applied force, or both. Large herniations would be expected to interfere with the normal mechanics of the disc.

Detailed ultrastructural studies of the hyaline cartilaginous endplates are still needed.[405]

Nutrition of the disc

The adult disc is virtually avascular, also the interfibrillar pores of the gel will admit particles no larger than 15 Å (1.5 nM). Hence, blood cannot enter healthy pulp, after the first decade.[1202]

Nutrition appears to depend upon imbibition of fluid into it from the vertebral bodies, and from the sparse vessels of the peripheral annulus during the first years of life. This process must obviously be assisted by the rhythmic movements and compression of daily activities and it is of interest that there is a diurnal variation in body height, probably due to variable turgidity of discs, amounting to a decrease in the evening of one-quarter to three-quarters of an inch and a corresponding increase in the morning.[240]

Astronauts in space are not subject to gravitational stress, and their discs imbibe water to such a degree that they return to earth measuring 10 cm taller than when they left.[633]

There is reason to suppose that active movement assists normal fluid imbibition processes between spongiosa and pulp, and this may be a factor in delaying the slow inevitable desiccation of discs with ageing.

Nachemson (1976) provides a summary of the pathways of disc nutrition as presently understood, expressed in the accompanying schemes (Fig. 1.24).

By reason of the lack of directly penetrating vessels from the age of 15 years or so, the intervertebral disc becomes the largest avascular structure in the body. There remain vascular buds between the spongiosa of the vertebral body and the end-plates; these vascular contacts are significantly fewer in discs showing advanced degenerative changes. Diffusion of solutes can take place through the central portion of the hyaline cartilaginous end-plates as well as through the annulus fibrosus. Posteriorly, the area available for diffusion is smaller, thus the posterior part of the nucleus–annulus junctional zone receives fewer negatively charged ions. The central part of the disc, and particularly the boundary zone between nucleus pulposus and annulus fibrosus, is exposed to possible deficiency of nutrition.

It has been demonstrated that glucosaminoglycan turnover in a dog's disc is very slow, about 500 days; the turnover of collagen is even slower, hence healing of disc rupture is very slow indeed, when it occurs.

The disc appears to live and thrive on movement and change, and die slowly through lack of it.[497] There is now a shift of emphasis from the idea that disc disorders result from purely mechanical derangement, to the view that nutrition and metabolism of the disc, and the biochemistry of degenerative change, are of equal importance.[212, 811, 908]

A high concentration of hydrogen ions in the tissues is a cause of pain. The mucoprotein gel contains a variety of glucosaminoglycogens, some of which are acid and lately believed capable of causing the pain associated with degenerative disc disease.

In a proportion of those patients who exhibited much scarring and adhesion around the nerve root, postsurgical studies[886] revealed a very high pH, which was due to an increased amount of lactate. Large amounts of lactate are produced when fibroblasts and other cells are metabolising in anaerobic conditions. Yet among many of those concerned every day with the conservative treatment of

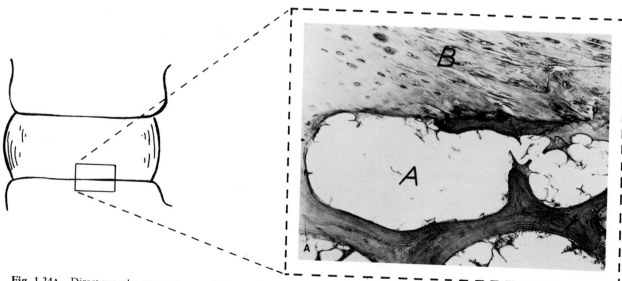

Fig. 1.24A   Direct vascular contracts, so-called vascular buds (A) between the marrow spaces of the vertebral body and the hyaline cartilage (B) of the end-plates are of importance for the nutrition of the disc.

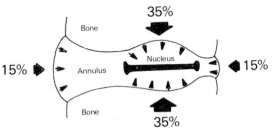

Fig. 1.24B Diffusion of small uncharged solutes such as glucose and oxygen occurs mainly through the end-plates. The area exposed to possible nutrient deficiency is shaded.

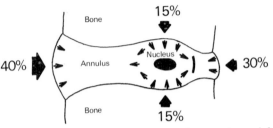

Fig. 1.24c Diffusion of negatively charged solutes, such as sulphate, occurs mainly through the annulus fibrosus. The area that receives less of such solutes is shaded.

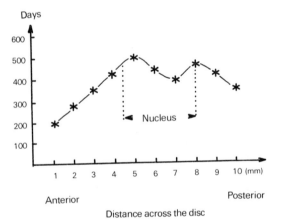

Fig. 1.24D The turnover time of glucosaminoglycans, as measured by the turnover of radioactively labelled sulphate ions in the dog's discs, is rather slow, especially in the nucleus pulposus.

(Figs. 1.24A–D with legends, are reproduced from *The Lumbar Spine: an Orthopaedic Challenge* (1976), Spine 1: 59, by kind permission of A. Nachemson and the Editor.)

musculoskeletal problems, there remains a tendency to regard the disc as a sort of badly packed suitcase, in that any untidy bits sticking out should ideally be stuffed back in again, or failing that lopped off, like a Laurel and Hardy haircut. The conception that man's erect posture is the direct cause of disc abnormality is attractive, but is certainly not substantiated by the frequency with which very similar disc abnormalities occur in four-legged animals. The first known disc lesion (1893) occurred in a dog, and was described by a veterinary surgeon.[256]

Variations of posture will alter the amount of pressure, and thus the degree of annular tension, being sustained by the disc. Direct *in vivo* measurement[883] of nucleus pulposus pressures in a 35-year-old female revealed, for example, that the total forces exerted on the L3 disc were as follows:

Sitting	15.3 kg/cm² (1500 kPa)
Standing	9.6 kg/cm² (941 kPa)
Standing with *tight corset*	7.0 kg/cm² (686.5 kPa)
Reclining	3.5 kg/cm² (343.2 kPa)

During lifting the compression acting on vertebral bodies and discs rises to very high levels, such is the degree of tension developed in deep muscles when controlling the forces accumulated during various movements and by using the spine, as it were, like a derrick.

While a tight lumbosacral support or cummerbund reduces the intradiscal pressure by approximately 30 per cent, it also reduces or modifies the gravitational and functional stress on all *other* lumbar structures, of course, and in the case of the vertebral venous plexuses the pressure may possibly be raised to a degree.

Expressed as percentages, with the figure for standing erect taken as 100 per cent. the relative pressure or load sustained by L3 disc[890] are as follows:

Lying supine with complete muscle relaxation	25
Reclining	75
Standing erect	*100*
Sitting	140
Standing, stooped forward	150
Sitting, stooped forward	185
Standing, stooped and holding weight	220
Sitting, stooped and holding weight	275

The pressures recorded, on the same basis, for classical physiotherapy exercises and postures, are interesting:

Fowler's position (lying supine with calves resting on stool)	35
Standing erect	*100*
Lying prone with feet fixed and raising head and shoulders	130
Resisted bilateral hip flexion in Fowler's position	140
Bilateral straight-leg raise in supine lying	150
Prone lying, trunk and leg extension combined	180
Supine lying with knees bent—trunk and hip flexion with thighs and legs stationary	210

These ergonomic considerations are important in the management of low back pain, and postural advice to patients.[888]

THE LIGAMENTS

The ligaments of the lumbar region are for the most part stronger and denser than elsewhere, the intertransverse ligaments and ligamentum flavum being especially well developed. Tension tests on the interlaminar ligamentum flavum[885] at the 3rd lumbar segment in 10 postmortem subjects between 13 and 80 years, showed the ligament to be almost perfectly elastic, the proportion of elastic fibres to collagen being 2:1. When the disc is normal or moderately degenerated, the ligamentum flavum has been found to prestress the disc by forces ranging from 1500 g in the young to 400 g in the elderly. Exerting these effects at a distance from the motion centre of the disc, the ligament therefore creates an intradiscal pressure of about 0.7 kg/cm² (71 kPa) in standing, at least in the young.

At lumbar segments which are not degenerated, the ligament appears to contribute to intrinsic stability of the spine, preventing the nerve roots from mechanical impingement and also prestressing the discs.

The supraspinous ligament and lumbosacral attachments of the erector spinae musculature

Previous descriptions of ligamentous arrangements at the low lumbar region appear to require modification. In careful dissections of the posterior lumbar structures of 28 specimens from subjects aged 1 month to 98 years (Heylings, 1978),[538] the *supraspinous ligament* was observed to terminate between L4 and L5; it never reached the sacrum. Below L5 spinous process, the fibres of the right and left lumbodorsal fascia decussated across the midline; after removal of the lumbodorsal fascia, the median attachments of the erector spinae musculature were seen to be variable according to the presence or absence of the supraspinous ligament. Where the ligament was present, from segments L5 upwards, the tendons attached to the lateral edge of the posterior part of the spinous process, but below this the most medial tendons decussated to cross the mid-line and attach to the opposite side of the posterior edge of spinous processes L5 and S1.

The *interspinous ligament* was seen to cross the interspinous spaces in a posterocranial direction, and consisted of ventral, middle and dorsal parts. The ventral part was clearly a posterior extension of the ligamentum flavum; the interspinous ligament was bilateral anteriorly, the slit-like median cavity being filled with fat. The middle part was plainly the major component of the ligament.

In the neutral posture the fibres had a curved disposition, becoming straight when the spine was flexed.

The band of tissue posterior to the spinous processes was thickest between the segments L5 and S1; there was no supraspinous ligament at this level and the thickness reflects the presence of the decussating erector spinae tendons and the other structures mentioned (see Vertebral movement, p. 51).

The posterior longitudinal ligament generally narrows between the levels of L1 and the sacrum, when it is merely a narrow strip of fibrous tissue, widened and further attenuated at its blending with the posterior annulus. The fifth lumbar vertebra is additionally stabilised by the iliolumbar ligament, which attaches the tip and lower anterior surface of the transverse process to (a) the adjacent iliac crest, and (b) to the roughened lateral area of the adjacent upper surface of sacrum.[437]

VESSELS

The lumbar vertebral structures are supplied by a spinal branch of the lumbar arteries, which arise from the back of the aorta. A fifth pair may branch from the median sacral or iliolumbar arteries.

After entering the foramen and supplying the nerve roots in this situation, anastomoses are formed with the longitudinal arterial network in the subarachnoid space and with the vessel of the opposite side. (See also the arteria radicularis magna', p. 14.)

The intrinsic venous drainage is arranged similarly to other parts of the column, a multitude of large veins forming tributaries of the lumbar veins in this region; the lower three usually enter the inferior vena cava and the first often joins the lumbar azygos system, but the arrangement is variable.

NERVE SUPPLY

The lumbar vertebral structures are supplied by mixed nerves from the paravertebral plexus as in other regions (see p. 9, Cervical spine), with the exception that (a) the ganglionated sympathetic trunk now lies against the medial margin of the psoas major, and below the L2 level there are no preganglionic fibres emerging from the spinal cord with the anterior roots, the sympathetic supply to spinal nerves below this level being derived as grey rami communicantes from the neighbouring ganglia, and (b) the population of nociceptor free nerve endings in ligaments is greatest in the posterior longitudinal ligament, less in other longitudinal and sacroiliac ligaments, and least in the ligamentum flavum and interspinous ligament.

A good example of the intracanal wandering of nerve fibres from the ramus meningeus is provided by a recurrent branch from the L2 segment, which after re-entering the intervertebral foramen, descends within the dorsal aspect of the posterior longitudinal ligament to the L5 level. Irritation of this branch may explain the common occurrence of low back pain in spondylotic changes anywhere between L2 and L5.[130]

This system of very fine nerves is much too fine for medical students to see in the dissecting room and accordingly is not well known among members of the profession. It belongs to that enormous field of anatomy which is really never learned in the medical course and in fact is not at all well known yet and in which a great deal more research work is needed.[1100]

Obliquity of the spinal roots

Because the spinal cord terminates at the level of L1 or L2, the lumbosacral nerve roots have to travel some distance (upper lumbar roots 9 cm, lower lumbar roots 16 cm) within the canal before they reach and emerge from their respective intervertebral foramina, and consequently their course is progressively more oblique from above downwards when compared, for example, with the more horizontal cervical nerve roots[537] (Fig. 2.13).

Immediately before the lumbar nerve roots emerge from their respective foramina, they are intimately related to the posterior and posterolateral aspects of the numerically corresponding intervertebral discs; a consequence of this intimate proximity is irritation or compression of nerve roots by movement of disc material, either backwards, or to one side, or both. These herniations and prolapses of disc substance often compress two adjacent spinal nerve roots, so closely are the lumbosacral-coccygeal roots gathered together to form the cauda equina in this part of the spine.

ANOMALIES

The transitional or junctional regions of the spine are 'ontogenetically restless'[1093] and more subject to variations and malformation than any other part of the column. Keith[638] refers to the 'physiological unstableness' of the lumbosacral area. Asymmetry of the posterior lumbar and lumbosacral joints is common, and occurs to a varying degree in approximately one-quarter of human spines. In a series of 3000 pre-employment X-ray examinations of the lumbosacral region over a two-year period, a large number of asymptomatic conditions, including degenerative processes and developmental anomalies, were encountered.

Epstein's review (1969[315]) of a long series of spinal studies in patients admitted for conditions other than back pain showed that many normal individuals have minor congenital variations at the lumbosacral junction. Likewise, radiologically evident narrowing of the lumbosacral interspace is not necessarily significant.

One facet-plane may be sagittally orientated, and its opposite fellow of the same segment be disposed with a slightly coronal angulation (Figs 1.21, 1.25, 1.31). In the segments above and below, similar asymmetry may be present, but with the sides reversed. Where evident, this alternating tropism occurs almost always as a variant in the lower half of the lumbar region.[92, 113]

A single facet on one side may be angulated downwards and inwards, while remaining sagittal in general disposition (Fig. 1.25).

Arthrosis at the anomalous synovial joint is plain, and it may be significant that this patient developed arthrosis of the hip on that side.

Congenital absence of a pedicle,[936] accessory laminae,[350]

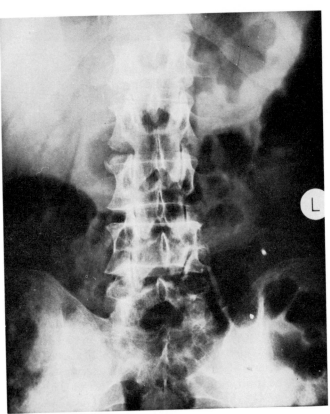

Fig. 1.25 depicts, on the a-p view, an anomalous L4–L5 facet-joint on the left side, with radiographic evidence of frank arthrosis of that joint. (The white spots are shrapnel.) His buttock and anterior thigh pains were emanating from an arthrotic left hip with marked clinical signs, and less so from his back. In some 17 per cent of cases, this type of spondylolisthesis is complicated by arthrosis of the hip. See Fig. 6.9.

osseous bridging of transverse processes, dysplasia or absence of spinous processes and clefts in pedicles of L3 and L4 have been reported.[1093]

Sagittal clefts in the vertebral arches—bifid spines—are common.[605]

Spina magna, a much enlarged spinous process of L5 coexisting with spina bifida of S1, may also occur.[1253] This part of the axial skeleton tends also to present anomalies like the lumbarised first sacral segment or the sacralised fifth lumbar vertebra, which may be either partially or completely fused to the sacrum (Figs 1.26–1.28). The large 'transverse process' of a transitional and partially sacralised L5 may form an anomalous adventitious joint with the ala of the sacrum on that side, the joint being subject to degenerative change like any other and perhaps more so because of the malformation. In at least two of the author's patients, mobilising techniques for intractable backache were unavailing until movement was specifically localised to affect the adventitious joint.[450]

The sacrum may sometimes develop with its upper surface higher on one side than the other, and a trapezoidal-shaped fifth lumbar vertebral body may be present (Figs 1.28–1.30).

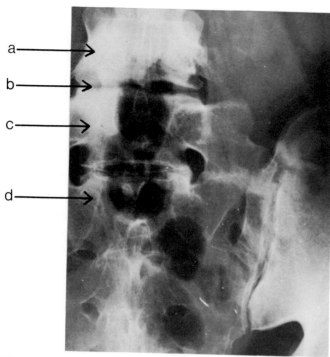

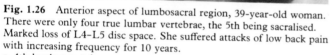

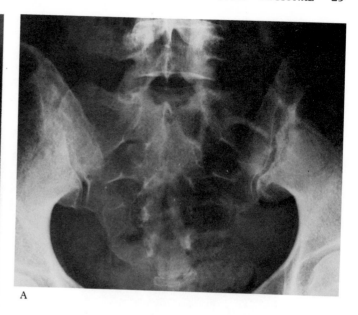

A

B

Fig. 1.26   Anterior aspect of lumbosacral region, 39-year-old woman. There were only four true lumbar vertebrae, the 5th being sacralised. Marked loss of L4–L5 disc space. She suffered attacks of low back pain with increasing frequency for 10 years.
a 4th lumbar vertebra
b Marked loss of L4–L5 disc space
c Sacralised 5th lumbar vertebra
d 1st sacral segment.

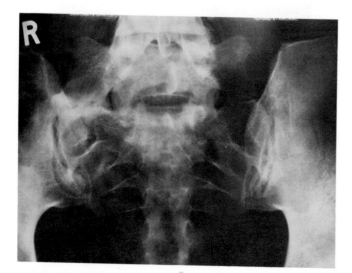

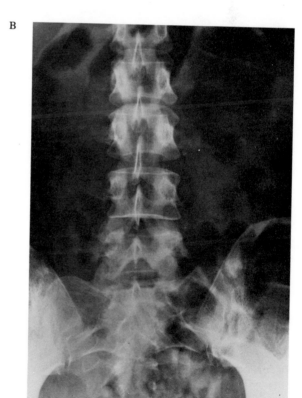

Fig. 1.27   Transitional and partly sacralised L5 with 'adventitious' joints between enlarged transverse processes and ala of the sacrum. Degenerative changes on the patient's right side.

Fig. 1.28   (A) This 35-year-old woman's sacrum is congenitally tilted upwards on her left side, and the lumbosacral junction there is partly transitional.
(B) The a-p view of her lumbar spine shows it to be virtually straight, despite a lop-sided base. Clinical assessment revealed that her right-sided haunch and groin pain on movement were emanating from the L1–L2 segment, and her low lumbar ache, on sitting, from the lumbosacral segment. Her haunch and groin symptoms were relieved by several sessions of manipulation of that segment, and her residual symptom of lumbar ache on sitting was relieved by rhythmic lumbar traction. The radiographic appearance, of course, remains unchanged.

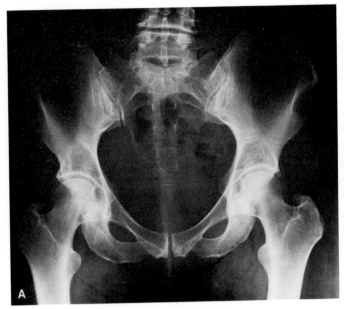

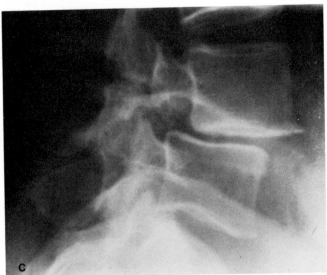

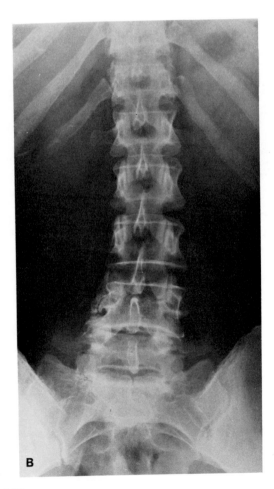

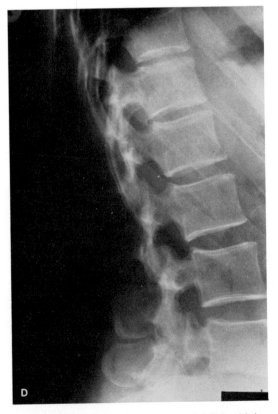

Fig. 1.29
(A) This lady's right upper sacral surface is higher than the left and she is consequently listing to the left, despite having a slight lateral pelvic tilt *upwards* on the left.
(B) The uneven sacral surface is more apparent; also apparent are the anomalous L3–L4 facet-joints. The twelfth ribs are asymmetrical.

(C) Group IIa spondylolisthesis (1st degree) at L4–L5, with bony contact of L3–L4 spinous processes.
(D) Bone-to-bone contact of L3–L4 spinous processes is shown more clearly. It was not possible, by manual or mechanical passive movement techniques, or exercises, or support, to modify this patient's right buttock pain when standing.

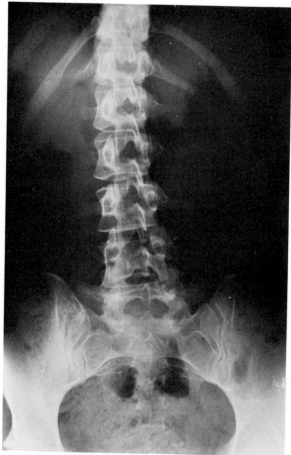

Fig. 1.30 Because of a trapezoidal and partially sacralised L5, this 22-year-old girl's spine listed to the right on a level pelvis. All movements hurt her in the low back, and flexion was limited to touching her knees. All signs were relieved by repetitive grade III pressures on the left PSIS—no other technique was effective. While now asymptomatic, she of course remains deviated.

Frequent dysplasia of the pars interarticularis of L5 has been reported.[1093]

These structural anomalies are often well tolerated until the additional insult of degenerative spondylosis is added to further narrow the lumbar canal. Surgical decompression may then be required.

Spondylolisthesis (Figs 1.29, 6.8, 6.9) has many causes[923, 927] and the general factor of mechanical weakness predisposes to the forward slip. This tendency is resisted by the bony hook comprising the pedicle, the interarticular portion of the neural arch (pars interarticularis) and the inferior facet; this hooks over the superior facet of the vertebra below.

The constant tendency cannot prevail so long as the integrity of the bony hook and the subjacent superior facet remain. The intersegmental soft tissue structures, i.e. annulus fibrosus, longitudinal and other ligaments, and muscles, make it more secure.

The resisting bony mechanism can be upset, among

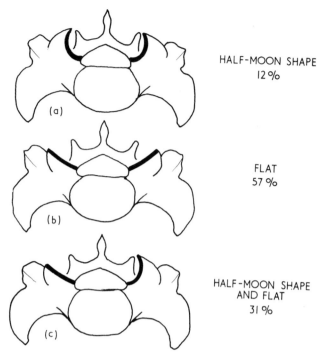

Fig. 1.31 Superior aspect of sacrum, showing main varieties of lumbosacral facet-plane orientation. (After Goldthwait, 1952.)

other causes (see p. 145) by congenital aplasia of the superior facets of the sacrum.

Lumbosacral facet-planes disposed in the coronal plane probably comprise a more efficient bony hook to resist the influence of body weight acting on the lumbosacral angle. If the facet-plane is sagittal, the integrity of the joint may be more at risk.

The differences are important because of the potential of some configurations for giving rise to signs and symptoms. The facet-planes of the lumbosacral joint frequently vary between sides, and there is also a wide variation between individuals (Fig. 1.31). Where asymmetry exists with one joint disposed in the coronal plane and the other more sagitally, naturally symmetrical regional movements of the back and pelvis may tend to exert asymmetrical forces at this segment, but excessive wear and tear with an increased likelihood of low back pain does not necessarily follow as a consequence.[1327]

Farfan[326, 324] draws attention to the potency of rotation strains in initiating the degenerative process, particularly on the side of the more oblique facet in asymmetrical joints (Fig. 1.25), yet the shape and orientation of lumbosacral facet-planes seem to have no effect on the symmetry of lumbar rotation.[769, 1093, 421]

A further factor is variation of sacral disposition; the more horizontally disposed the sacrum, the greater is the need for the strong bony hook, resisting the constant forward-slipping tendency of L5 on the sacrum under the influence of gravity. The plane of the upper surface of S1 vertebral body forms an angle with the horizontal of about 30°. The more the sacrum is horizontally disposed, the greater the angle, and vice versa. Variations of sacral disposition in the lateral view, when the angle may vary from 20° to almost 90°, and of the sacral profile itself, have frequently been considered together with abnormalities of sagittal spinal curvature, and a diathesis to one or more joint conditions of the lumbar spine, pelvic girdle and hip joints has been postulated on the basis of these observations.

Schmorl and Junghanns assert,[1093]

The differing degrees of angulation play an important role and influence the statistics and dynamics of the spine as well as the birth canal. ... Critical evaluation of all available investigative results makes it difficult to diagnose an 'abnormal' lumbosacral angle and it is even more difficult to consider it as a cause of pain.

Spinal stenosis

During the last two decades, increasing attention has centred on developmental reduction of the dimensions, together with altered configuration, of the lumbar vertebral canal (Figs 1.32, 1.33),[1088, 1267, 52, 315, 618, 1292, 1127, 660, 911] although the first account of clinical affects appeared in 1900.[1072]

All forms of stenosis show consistent abnormalities on a plan view of the vertebra: smaller interfacetal distance; shorter pedicles; reduced dorsoventral diameter; shallowness of the lateral recess.

The lateral recess, bounded by the medial portion of the superior articular facet and the lamina above, by the pedicle laterally and by the vertebral body, its superior lip and the adjacent disc below, contains the nerve root and it is in this limited space that the root is most vulnerable to compression.[1088]

In stenotic lumbar spines the cauda equina is very frequently compressed by a degree of degenerative trespass

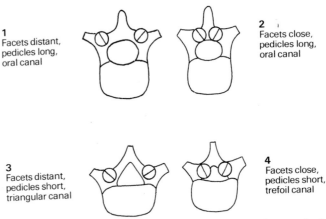

The disposition of the facets determines the shape of the vertebral foramen and spinal canal

1 Facets distant, pedicles long, oral canal

2 Facets close, pedicles long, oral canal

3 Facets distant, pedicles short, triangular canal

4 Facets close, pedicles short, trefoil canal

Fig. 1.33 The factors determining the shape of the lumbar vertebral foramina. (Reproduced from *The Lumbar Spine and Back Pain*, 1976, by kind permission of H. Baddeley and the Pitman Medical Publishing Co. Ltd.)

which could easily be accommodated without symptoms by a more roomy vertebral canal.

The incidence shows a male preponderance; it can be evident on plain films, part of this being a relative flattening of the intervertebral foramina and shortened pedicles, evident on lateral radiographs.[911]

Kirkaldy-Willis *et al.*[660] state that the condition is much more common than has been appreciated over the past 70 years.

Porter *et al.* (1980)[1001a] have highlighted the clinical importance of a trefoil-shaped lumbar canal. By studying three skeletal populations altogether comprising 240 adult, and 27 children's, spines and comparing the results with *in vivo* ultrasound measurements of the spinal canals of nearly 1500 subjects and patients from two pathological groups, they suggest that patients with disc symptoms and those with neurogenic claudication may have not only narrow but also trefoil canals. They noted that the degree of 'trefoilness' increased from L1 to L5.

In general terms, congenital malformations of weight-bearing bones might be expected to produce wear and tear, and thus symptoms, earlier than would normally symmetrical structures subjected to the same stress; this follows at times, yet as has been mentioned, many patients without symptoms exhibit a variety of skeletal abnormalities.[1327]

Soft tissues

Abnormal variations of lumbosacral root and plexus formation have been reported[651, 11] and nerve fibres forming intersegmental anastomoses in the dorsal lumbosacral rootlets have also been described;[965] these appear similar to those in the cervical region.[598]

Agnoli[11] reported on 20 personal observations and ana-

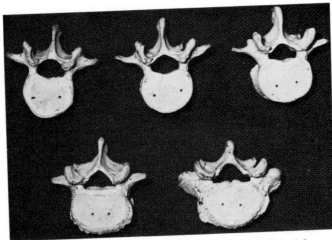

Fig. 1.32 Plan view of the lumbar vertebrae (L1 to L5, from left above to right below). The shape of the neural canal at L1 progressively changes to a trefoil shape at L5. There is relative constriction of the lateral recess of L4 vertebra on the subject's left. The apparent unilateral constriction at L3 is due to slight tilting of the vertebra.

lysed 18 cases from the literature. The most frequent anomalies were the common dural origin of two nerve roots and the common exit of two roots via one foramen. Interradicular connections, and Y-shaped or horizontally disposed nerve roots, were seen in 9 of the 20, and 6 of the 18; operation revealed only the anomalies, although the history and clinical findings suggested prolapsed intervertebral disc. Decompression produced positive results. Transforaminal ligaments[422] may be present; the frequency of anomalous fibrous bands might be higher than estimated, since many soft-tissue anomalies would escape radiological detection.

THE SACROILIAC JOINT

Because this articulation, together with the craniovertebral region and other transitional areas, is of prime importance in the understanding and conservative treatment of vertebral joint problems, a fuller account of salient features is given (Fig. 1.35).

STRUCTURE

The joint and the mechanism of the pelvis are fully described in many texts, and this description concentrates on special aspects of our concern.

The nature of the cartilage covering the opposed articular surfaces seems a matter of debate rather than agreed fact, and descriptions differ between hyaline cartilage, fibrocartilage and a reddish-grey cartilage with villous prolongations as covering one or both surfaces; the cartilage on the sacral surface is thicker than on the ilium. It is probably not of immediate clinical importance, except for a tendency for the condensation or sclerosis which appears as a result of stress (osteitis condensans ilii) to be almost invariably on the iliac side of the joint and not the sacral side; the nature and thickness of cartilage may be a factor here.[437, 790, 1082, 1095]

The sacral articular surface, a letter L lying on its side, has the shorter and vertically disposed cephalic limb borne by the first sacral segment, while the longer and horizontally disposed caudal limb is borne by the second and third sacral segments. Dorsally, the median, intermediate and lateral sacral crests represent fused spinous, articular and transverse processes respectively, and it is noteworthy that, in about 30 per cent of cases, accessory sacroiliac articulations exist between the lateral sacral crest and adjacent ilium.[1244, 1093]

In childhood both sacral and iliac articular surfaces are plane, but from puberty every conceivable combination of small ridges and furrows is seen on the two surfaces. The size, shape and roughness of the articular surfaces vary greatly between individuals, as do the small ranges of movement. In more gross terms, irregularities of the sacral surface are cephalic and caudal elevations bounding a central depression; in elderly people a third elevation lies dorsally to the central depression.[437] The configurations of the iliac articular surface are not necessarily a faithful mirror-image of the sacral surface, and great irregularity prevails in the surface formations. Similarly, the articular slits are not orientated in space as fairly uniform paramedian planes converging posteriorly; each joint exhibits at least two planes slightly angulated to one another, and often three—their disposition and area are not always similar when sides are compared in the same individual.[1157] Thus the assertion that movement, albeit small, between the two bones is primarily rotation, in an inclined parasagittal plane, requires some qualification; likewise the notion that manipulations with a rotatory component are the most important.

RELATIONS

Anteriorly, the joint is crossed above by the obturator and femoral nerves, the lumbosacral cord and the medial edge of the psoas major. The internal iliac artery and the iliac veins lie in front of it. The first sacral nerve and the piriformis muscle cross its lower part. Laterally and below the joint, the greater sciatic foramen is partially filled by the emerging piriformis muscle, above which the superior gluteal vessels and nerve emerge from the pelvis. Below the piriformis, the inferior gluteal vessels and nerve, the internal pudendal vessels and the pudendal, sciatic and posterior femoral cutaneous nerves emerge.

LIGAMENTOUS ATTACHMENTS AND EFFECTS OF GRAVITY

In an AP view, the sacrum seems inserted like a wedge between the two ilia, as the keystone of an arch. But in the lateral view, the true dependence of the joint's integrity upon the strength and efficiency of its principal ligaments is immediately apparent (Fig. 1.34).

While the anterior concavity of the sacrum serves to increase the capacity of the true pelvis, the sacral promontory projects into the pelvic cavity to form the apex of the sacrovertebral angle; gravitational stress tends to project the sacral promontory ever forward, thus tending to reduce the sagittal dimensions of the pelvic inlet and also to increase the lumbar lordosis by anterior pelvic tilt. The latter tendency is, of course, resisted extrinsically by abdominal and gluteal musculature.

Forward movement of the sacral base and backwards movement of its apex, relative to the ilia, are resisted intrinsically by the strongest ligaments in the body (Figs 1.34, 1.35). Dorsally to the sacral articular surface lies a rough deeply pitted craggy area which, together with the laterally adjacent craggy surface of the iliac tuberosity, gives attachment to the massive interosseous sacroiliac

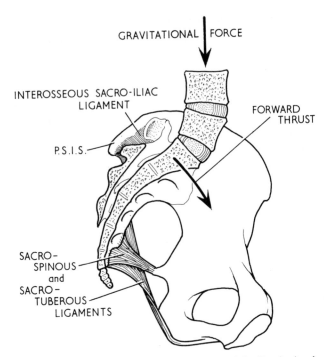

Fig. 1.34 Medial aspect of sagittal section of pelvis. Gravitational stress tends to increase sacrovertebral angle and reduce sagittal dimensions of pelvic inlet.

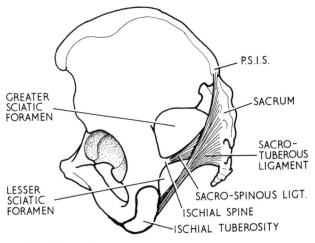

Fig. 1.36 (See text.)

ligament (Fig. 1.35) forming the chief bond of union between the two bones; it also converts the sacroiliac articulation into a part synovial joint and part syndesmosis. Interosseous ligament fibres do not tear in the cadaver when the bones are forcibly separated; the fibres detach themselves from one bone and remain fixed to the other.[838, 1082]

Below and laterally, the strong sacrotuberous and sacrospinous ligaments (Fig. 1.36) firmly attach the non-articular lower part of the sacrum and its apex to the ischial tuberosity and spine respectively. Thus a mechanical 'couple' is provided to resist the effect of gravity in the erect position. The more superficial posterior sacroiliac ligament is also very strong, but its anterior fellow is a thin weak structure which stretches and tears easily upon slight pubic separation.[1082]

The iliolumbar ligaments, attaching the fifth lumbar

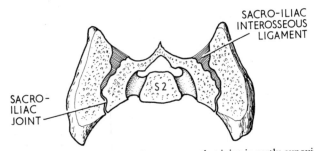

Fig. 1.35 Horizontal section demonstrates that joint is partly synovial and partly a syndesmosis. Short but very thick interosseous ligament is a principal factor in resisting excessive forward movement of sacral base.

transverse processes to the adjacent iliac crest, may give origin to some fibres of sacrospinalis and multifidus muscles.

MUSCLES

While the strongest muscles of the body surround the sacroiliac joint, none are intrinsic to it or act upon it directly as the quadriceps extends the knee, for example. It will be apparent, even to the first-year student, that this does not mean that by its attachments the surrounding muscle mass may not markedly influence the mechanical behaviour of the joint, or the stresses sustained by it. On studying the gross anatomy of the joint surfaces, it will also be apparent that since these comprise two and often three planes angulated to each other, whatever movement may be powerfully but indirectly imposed by the muscle mass, it cannot be rotation (see p. 280). The joint may be likened to the superior tibiofibular joint, disorders of which are frequently a covert cause of anterolateral leg and ankle pain. In some important respects, this little articulation is a microcosm of the sacroiliac joint and, weight-bearing strains apart, the comparative anatomy, function during walking and susceptibility to local and referred pains after what appear to be 'shuffling' lesions, are worth our consideration. The suggestion is not as incongruous as it may seem. European authors sometimes speak of piriformis spasm, and of the muscle being stretched and painful on pressure during rectal examination.[961, 736, 940]

NERVE SUPPLY

The intra-articular innervation is more abundant than macroscopic examination indicates. Segmental derivation of its nerve supply is not always the same on each side. Behind, the lateral branches of L5, S1 and S2 posterior primary rami form a plexus between the posterior and interosseous ligaments; from these loops branches ramify to the ligaments, and skin of the medial and lower buttock. Anteriorly, the joint is supplied by nerves variably derived from roots L3 to S1, and by the superior gluteal nerve (L5 to S2).[437, 110, 399, 955, 1157]

BLOOD SUPPLY

The median sacral artery branches from the aorta above its bifurcation, descending on L4 and L5 vertebral bodies to anastomose on the front of the sacrum with the lateral sacral branches from the internal iliac artery. Branches enter the anterior sacral foramina, supplying the sacral vertebrae and cauda equina in the sacral canal, and then emerge via the posterior foraminae to anastomose posteriorly with branches of the gluteal arteries. Venous drainage is by vessels accompanying the arteries, as tributaries of the lateral sacral and median sacral veins; these are tributaries of the common iliac veins.[437]

ANOMALIES

Of 30 sacra, Solonen (1957)[1157] found variations in width of the lateral part in 25 cases; the left lateral was wider in 19, the right in 6, and in only 5 cases were the two sides similar.

Variations in the height of sacral alae and the body of Sl (Figs 1.31, 1.37), [1093] transitional vertebrae, a laterally tilted upper surface of the sacrum, a trapezoidal fifth lumbar vertebral body, iliac horns, calcified iliolumbar ligaments, an anomalous notch for the iliac artery (para-

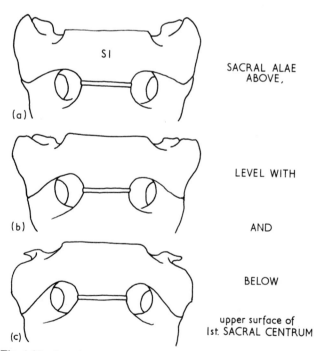

Fig. 1.37 Anterior aspect of sacrum, showing variations in relative height of sacral alae and body of S1. (After Schmorl and Junghanns, 1971.)

glenoid foramen), asymmetrical sacral facets, spina bifida occulta of the upper sacral segments and spina magna of L5, do not *per se* justify ascribing back, buttock and thigh pains to their presence.

By meticulous examination, the cause of pain should be sought in the presence of factors which may not be visible on plain X-rays, such as torsional and stress disturbances of the soft tissue of the back and sacroiliac joint;[315] although X-rays are important, of course, and anomalies cannot be excluded from the basis of assessment.

SURFACE ANATOMY

Palpation of the vertebral column and limb girdle structures is a vital part of examination for spinal joint problems; thus there should be familiarity with what underlies the surface terrain on both the dorsal and ventral aspects.

CERVICAL SPINE

The posterior tubercle of the *atlas* (C1) may be felt in the mid-line (Figs 1.1, 1.2), under the 'eaves' of the overhanging occiput, in a small proportion of people but for the most part it is an impalpable bony point, unless considerable and uncomfortable pressure is unwisely applied. Its surface mark is thus the soft-tissue sulcus between the occiput and the prominent spinous process of the axis (C2).

Unless the patient's cervical tissues are very thickened, the posterior arches of atlas (Cl) can be palpated posterolaterally immediately under the occiput. It is necessary to direct the fingertip anteromedially and slightly upward, and to ensure that there is muscle relaxation. The *lateral tip of the transverse process of the atlas* is palpable, in most people, between the angle of the jaw and the mastoid process (Figs. 1.2, 1.3). In a few, it is not easy to find, and less so when upper cervical tenderness is such as to make even the most gentle probing difficult.

The little sulcus, which is formed by the adjacent bony points of mastoid process and atlas, allows a comparison of the position of C1 in relation to the skull, and also of movement in the craniovertebral joints; 'abnormalities' are not necessarily significant.

The axis
The axis (C2) (Fig. 1.2) is marked by a large beaked spinous process; this terminates in an inverted-V which can sometimes be verified by careful palpation. While on inspection it is not as evident as that of C7, it often *feels* as large. The C2 transverse process can be identified through the soft tissues.

C3 spinous process

This is a shy little bony point (Figs 1.1, 1.2) almost concealed by the overhanging beak of C2, and may therefore be missed when palpating the neck of the prone patient from cranial to caudal (Fig. 1.38). It is most easily felt by directing the thumbtip pressure anteriorly and slightly cranially.

The remaining cervical spinous processes may be asymmetrically bifid, and may give the impression of rotation if unusually prominent on one side. Doubt about whether one is palpating C6 or C7 spinous process (which seems to arise more frequently when treating degenerative joint disease than when palpating fellow-students!) can be resolved by placing a fingertip so that it lies between the two spinous processes. On extending the subject's neck, C7 spinous process remains palpable while that of C6 glides away from the palpating finger.

C2 to C6 spinous processes

The tips of C2 to C6 spinous processes lie on the same level as the lower margin of the inferior articular facet, which is thus the lower margin of the facet-joint. Thus the tip of C4 spinous process, for example, overlies the lower margin of the C4–C5 facet-joint. Since the interarticular bony mass is marked dorsally by a little bony hump, it is quite easy to run the thumbtips down the paravertebral sulcus on either side, some 2–3 cm from the midline, and locate these humps which overlie the facet-joints. They are easiest to feel at C4 and above, and are most easily palpated with the patient in prone-lying or in side-lying.

Facetal osteophytes are usually shelf-like projections and when marked they, with their covering of thickened soft tissues, may simulate these normal bony prominences.

The lateral extremities of the transverse processes are easily located through the soft tissues on either side, although this becomes less easy below C6.

With the patient supine, the anterior aspect of the cervical transverse processes can be palpated, and unilateral or bilateral anteroposterior contact mobilising techniques employed. Locating the most comfortable point for pressure should be carefully done, with the musculature pushed to one side. Some patients may experience proximal arm pain, and some a feeling of impending syncope, if the pressure is not considerate.

C7 spinous process

The spinous process of C7 is prominent, but so is that of T1, and perhaps the term 'vertebra prominens' should be written 'vertebrae' and applied to both of them, instead of customarily to C7 (Fig. 1.1). Those of C6 and C7 are usually not bifid; further, the transverse processes of C7 extend laterally as far as those of C2, so that a paramedian perpendicular would join their tips. Those of C3 to C6 would not extend laterally to reach this perpendicular line.

C7 transverse process can be identified in front of the trapezius muscle but palpation is uncomfortable, and it is often simpler to locate it through the broad, triangular median aponeurosis of the middle fibres of trapezius.

In the prone patient, palpation of a cervical rib at C7 may require strong probing since it will lie anteriorly, i.e. deep, to the transverse process. It is much easier to compare sides when the patient is supine.

Cord segments

In the typical cervical region, the tip of the spinous process

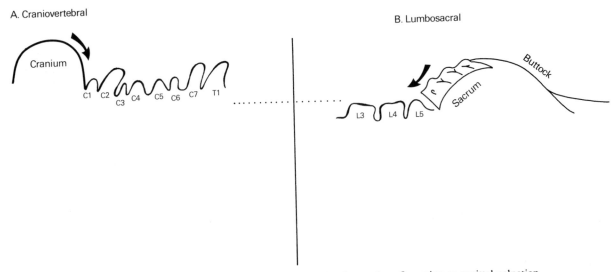

A. Craniovertebral

Cranium

C1 C2 C3 C4 C5 C6 C7 T1

B. Lumbosacral

Buttock

Sacrum

L3 L4 L5

Fig. 1.38 Similarities between craniovertebral and lumbosacral configuration on sagittal palpation.

(A) As the palpating finger moves caudally off the occiput, C1 posterior tubercle is 'the little blunt church tower at the bottom of the valley' and C2 is large and unmistakable.

(B) Similarly, as one moves cranially down the fused dorsal spines of the sacrum, L5 is 'the little blunt church tower at the bottom of the valley' and L4 is large and unmistakable.

corresponds to the level of the *succeeding* spinal cord segment, i.e. C6 spinous process is level with the C7 cord segment (Fig. 2.13).

THORACIC SPINE AND RIBS

The anterior concavity of the thoracic spine varies quite considerably between individuals. While it is obvious that the region's general configuration must conform to the patient's body type so far as sagittal curvature is concerned, there will be found a surprising variety of mid/upper thoracic curvature. Quite commonly, the interscapular region is flat and in some it will be markedly so, and this with radiographic appearance reported as 'normal'. In many, this apparent postural deviant is associated with upper thoracic and cervical joint problems (see p. 235) but by no means invariably.

Thoracic spinous processes

These characteristically 'lie down the back like the scales of a fish' so that the tip of a spinous process lies level with the subjacent vertebral body, but this does not apply to the upper two or three, and lower two or three segments, i.e. the lower margin of these spinous processes lies roughly on the same level as the lower margin of the same body.

It is seldom appreciated how variable these levels of horizontal relationship can be, and why descriptions can only be generalised; comparison of three newly articulated skeletons will make the point. In the middle seven or eight thoracic levels, the tip of the spinous process lies more or less level with the laminae of the subjacent vertebra. The tips of the spines are not bifid but slightly bulbous, and progressively become more ridge-like towards the thoracolumbar junction.

Anomalies are common, and deviation of a spine to one side or other is frequently palpable; these should not be taken as positional evidence of rotation since comparison of the relationship of the laminae will demonstrate there is no fixed rotation.

The facts that the acromioclavicular joint lies level with the C7–T1 interspace, the spine of scapula lies approximately level with T3 spinous process and its inferior angle approximately level with T7 spinous process, provide a rough guide only. For accuracy it is necessary to count downwards from T1 or upwards from L5.

A practical method of counting is to place the tips of two adjacent fingers on the interspinous depression above and below one spinous process, and to shift the two fingertips as one when transferring to the next spinous process. There can still be difficulty if the spines are very close, and virtually fixed thus by chronic segmental stiffening. Caudally, the spines become progressively more short, and project more dorsally; this shorter lever will influence the type of movement induced by transverse pressures on the side of the spinous process.

The lower parts of the thoracic laminae

These are easily felt in the paravertebral sulci as a series of flattened ridges, and it is important to remember that the ridge palpated is the dorsal aspect of the interarticular part; it overlies the lower facet-joint of that vertebra.

The first rib

The first rib articulates only with the first thoracic vertebra; the spinous and transverse processes of T1, and angles of the first rib, are on the same horizontal level. Palpation of the first rib *angle* through the trapezius muscle, which may be in some spasm, can be painful for the patient; the flat upper surface of the rib is easily felt, in the prone patient, by lifting the upper fibres of trapezius and palpating immediately beneath. By careful probing, the transverse process of T1 can also be identified.

Anteriorly, the first palpable rib below the clavicle *is* the first rib.[74] Frequently, the anterior shafts of the *2nd ribs* are unduly prominent, and simple observation from the front as well as palpation will confirm the fact.

Unilateral prominence, associated with marked local tenderness anteriorly, may occur in lesions of a second rib.

For all ribs, the intercostal spaces are somewhat wider in front than behind.[118]

On a posterior view of the trunk, the line of the *rib angles* is not vertical; that of the *8th rib* is usually furthest from the mid-line, and both above and below this level a line joining them deviates slightly inwards, more so above the 8th rib.

Grant (1958)[434] states:

Since the deep muscles of the back diminish in bulk as they ascend, it follows that the angles become progressively nearer the tubercles from below upwards, till the first rib is reached.

The important point is that generally they are nearer the tubercle more cranially, and further away more caudally.

Down to the 8th or 9th thoracic vertebra, the transverse process is level with the *upper* border of its vertebral body, and since the head of a typical rib articulates with (i) its numerically corresponding vertebral body and the one above, and (ii) the tubercle articulates with the numerically corresponding transverse process, it follows that the *rib angles* will be palpated just below, or at the same level of, the *transverse processes*.

One should be careful not to mistake a small soft-tissue nodule or fasciculus, which may be acutely tender, for 'a rib angle'; it is necessary to push the overlying soft tissues to one side to be sure one is indeed feeling an immovable bony point.

Doubts as to *which* rib angle must always be clarified by counting upwards or downwards. The single costal facet on T11 and T12 vertebral bodies is virtually level with the transverse process, but the associated rib does not articulate with it. The slight angle of the 11th rib is easily palpated at about the horizontal level of T12 spinous process, but the 12th rib, which may be 2–20 cm long, is virtually featureless and not so easy to find, especially in women.

Cord segments

In the upper thoracic region, the tip of the spinous process corresponds to the *second* succeeding segment, e.g. the spinous process of T4 overlies the T6 cord segment. In the lower thoracic spine, there is a three-segment discrepancy, i.e. T10 spinous process overlies the first lumbar cord segment. At the last two segments, T11 spinous process overlies L3 cord segment and T12 overlies the first sacral cord segment.

As with all biological measurements, there is a normal range of variation as to the precise level of caudal termination of the human spinal cord, relative to the vertebral canal.[71] The adult cord may terminate anywhere between the last thoracic and the third lumbar vertebra. Spinal cords in the female, and those of negro races, tend to be slightly longer than those of white males (Fig. 2.13).

In the newborn child, the spinal cord extends to the upper border of L3.

THE LUMBAR SPINE

The iliac crests do not invariably lie level with the L4 vertebral body, and more frequently (about 60 per cent of cases) they lie in the same plane as the L4–L5 interspace. In some 20 per cent they are level with the L5 vertebral body, and this is sometimes referred to as 'a high-riding L5'. Only in the remaining 20 per cent of cases do the iliac crests lie in the same plane as the L4 vertebral body.

For this reason, it is more accurate to localise the L4 spinous process by first finding that of L5, which in most cases can be identified by sliding the tip of finger or thumb cranially along the fused spines of the sacrum (Fig. 1.38). The blunted and often small bony point, lying at the centre of the lumbosacral depression is the fifth lumbar spinous process.

Because anomalies (in the form of transitional vertebrae and spina bifida) (p. 24) are common in this region, there may be difficulty in deciding which is the fifth lumbar spinous process. The first segment with palpable movement will decide the issue, and the vertebra immediately above the first movable joint will be the lowest lumbar vertebra, whether it is L4, L5 or 'L6'.[1180(a)]

Palpation of the prone patient's lumbosacral region can sometimes be difficult because of anomalies, and when there is the real likelihood of confusion in identifying bony points, the patient's position should be changed to that shown in Figure 14.3 (p. 455).

The important points about the lumbar spinous processes are:

1. That of L5 is surprisingly often a deep, small and blunted bony point, while that of L4 is a comparatively large and sagitally ridged eminence.

2. The ridged eminences from L4 upwards (including the lower thoracic spines) are often a little depressed at about their middles, and it is embarrassingly easy to assume that one is palpating an interspinous gap when, in fact, one's finger is in the depression which marks the middle of a quadrangular lumbar spinous process.

3. The palpable ridge of one middle or upper lumbar spinous process may be considerably broadened, giving the impression of 'osteophytosis' of the bony point; this is a normal structural variation and should not be given any special significance.

The lumbar transverse processes

These generally lie level with the interspace between the spinous processes, and they are larger in the middle of the region than at the upper and lower ends. The palpable eminences which can be detected through the soft tissues on either side are not the laminae, but are the prominent dorsal aspects of the inferior articular processes. They mark the level of the facet-joints, and lie on either side of the lower third of the spinous processes.

The facet-joints

The facet-joints lie at a depth of some 5 cm below the skin surface,[658] although this dimension is considerably reduced by firm digital pressure when palpating through the soft tissues.

THE PELVIS

Directly beneath a skin dimple on each side, the most eminent part of the *posterior superior iliac spines* lies opposite the second sacral segment, the 'spinous process' of which is not always palpable as a discrete bony point.

The posterior superior iliac spines do not invariably present with a detectable and localised eminence, but may remain simply as flatly curved bony ridges; medial to them the palpable depression is the sulcus overlying the sacroiliac joint. At this point, the synovial cavity of the joint itself lies some 3 cm or more beneath the palpating finger, this space being occupied by the massive interosseous sacroiliac ligament; yet during testing movements (see p. 334) the rhythmically changing relationship between the sacrum and the iliac spine is readily detectable in young, and many older, adults.

Some 5 or 6 cm below, and slightly laterally, the *posterior inferior iliac spines* are palpable through the upper mass of the buttock, and immediately medial to this point the lowest part of the sacroiliac joint can easily be felt.

The *sacrococcygeal joint* lies slightly higher than a horizontal line joining the upper tips of the greater trochanters; the *sacral hiatus*, lying between the cornua, is easily identified as a median depression over the apex of the sacrum.

Near the highest point of the buttock in young people, the *sacrotuberous ligaments* can be detected through the gluteal mass, and with a little practice it is not difficult to note differences in tension between them. In maturer patients, the palpation point will lie a little above the highest point of the buttock mass.

Difficulties of orientation can be resolved by identifying the *ischial tuberosities* and marking out the known attachments of the ligaments between these two eminences and the lateral borders of the sacrum.

Anteriorly, *Baer's point* (q.v.) lies a little below McBurney's point,[74] the latter being situated at the junction of the outer and middle thirds of a line joining the anterior superior iliac spine and the umbilicus. Medial to and slightly below the anterior superior iliac spine, the iliacus and psoas major muscles form a palpable longitudinal bundle, and in the medial plane the uppermost part of the sulcus formed by the symphysis pubis is easily felt.

2. Applied anatomy–general

ARTICULAR CARTILAGE OF SYNOVIAL JOINTS

INTRODUCTION

The contact-bearing surface of joints is the hyaline cartilage covering the articular surface of bone.

True articular bearing surface cartilage differs from epiphyseal growth cartilage—although adjacent, they are functionally different tissues and their fate is different.

Articular cartilage exists only in thin layers, and the two sources of nutritional fluid can only be (a) the underlying bone, and (b) the synovial fluid. Studies indicate that adult articular cartilage is primarily dependent on synovial fluid for its metabolic exchanges, albeit via the matrix.[836]

The possibility of contributions from subchondral vessels remains, but at most this nutritional route can only be of minor importance, and is probably more active during skeletal immaturity than after closure of growth regions.[1154]

The cartilage cells, or chondrocytes, occupy a firm-textured matrix, the whole forming a tough but elastic and compressible layer a few mm in thickness, enmeshed together and also bound to the underlying bone by numerous collagenous fibres. Thickness is variable at different sites of a single bearing surface.

In the deepest layer, (a) fibres are arranged as arching bundles of collagen, anchored in the calcified zone beneath and enmeshing vertical rows of closely packed oval chondrocytes. Nearer the surface, (b), cells become more horizontally disposed among fibres which are thinner, and (c) the surface layer itself is arranged of more flattened cells, with fibres thickened on the surface but with more delicate branches descending into the superficial matrix. On electron microscopy, the contact-bearing surface presents the appearance of hilly country with a matted fibrous texture.[1350] The mounds or hills are built up by groups of the thick horizontal fibres, while the intervening depressions or indentations are apparently formed by a surface layer which closely follows the contour of underlying lacunar structures, generally grouped together in pairs.[876] Around the lacunae, collagenous fibrils can be seen to anastomose and form cross-links with each other, with a 'bird's nest' appearance.

Cells are normally conceived as the source and regulators of the extra cellular material of tissues, but chondrocytes of the avascular articular cartilage are entirely dependent upon the generous matrix for their nutrition and metabolic exchanges.[1154]

Yet articular chondrocytes live in and under proper circumstances synthesise and dissolve ground substance. They may even divide, although the turnover of cells must be low, due to the relative firmness of the matrix, and this accords with the need for a bearing-surface architecture of structural stability.[836] This does not mean that cartilage is not a viable tissue capable of response to injury.

Stable collagenous tissue, the fibrous element which is the source of the tissue's tensile strength, consists of the triple helix of the tropocollagen molecule, intimately associated with, and enmeshing, the complex mucopolysaccharide molecules of cartilage, i.e. proteoglycans.[1073] Besides proteoglycans, cartilage comprises a number of solutes of much lower molecular weight.

While the collagen network is responsible for the integrity of the tissue and its mechanical strength, it is the proteoglycan–water gel[809] with its very fine pores (20–40 Å, 2–4 nM) which controls diffusion of water and salts. In health, the turnover of collagen is little, if it occurs at all, while the matrix or ground substance has a slow but steady metabolic turnover.

SYNOVIAL JOINT LUBRICATION

Investigators of lubrication processes in synovial joints have concerned themselves largely with weight-bearing joints, notably the hip and knee.

Since there is evidence[747] that the synovial plane joints of the vertebral arches, and those of the craniovertebral region,[1274] sustain considerable stress and suffer arthrotic change[508] as in the peripheral joints, the nature of synovial joint function and lubrication are of interest.[1199, 1155, 1350, 1351, 1352]

An added dimension of concern is that of the known tendency of apparently normal spinal facet-joints to become temporarily and painfully 'hitched' or 'blocked'.[1180b] The process appears to resemble the sticking of a drawer in a chest of drawers, and it is much less common in peripheral joints. Whether research in joint lubrication will elucidate the mechanism of this phenomenon remains to be seen; the function of the intra-articular synovial 'meniscoid' villi (p. 5) has recently received much attention,[677, 1093, 1230, 313] and it is possible that this research, together with studies of joint lubrication, may complete our imperfect knowledge of this ubiquitous vertebral joint problem.

Elucidation of the remarkable 'slipperiness' of synovial joints has engaged researchers in the two sciences of (a) *tribology*, the study of wear, friction and lubrication, and (b) *rheology*, the study of flow or deformation under stress, of materials and fluids.

An index of slipperiness is the *coefficient of resistance to movement* (Fig. 2.1), i.e. the shear force required to start one surface sliding upon another, divided by the normal force pressing them together.

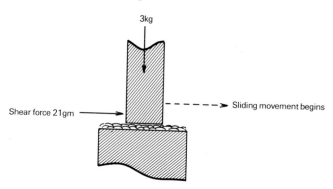

Fig. 2.1 Coefficient of resistance to movement (friction) $= \dfrac{21}{3000} = 0.007$.

The lower the coefficient, the lower the resistance to movement; synovial joints have a very low coefficient of resistance to movement. Function begets function,[851] and joint movement and loading are important for living joints. Mobility of the articular tissues and the joint fluids in response to loading appear necessary for healthy joint function. The 'cartilage/synovial fluid/synovial membrane complex' is regarded as a unit, and the health of this complex is essential to the normal function of the joint.[1199] There is normally a continuous process of microchemical removal of cartilage-surface material, with ingestion of this by the highly phagocytic synovial cells.

Synovial fluid, a dialysate of plasma, contains hyaluronic acid (mucin) which has a high molecular weight; the viscosity of synovial fluid almost entirely depends on it. Also, when hyaluronic acid is added in various propor-

tions to disaggregated proteoglycans, this interaction produces a large increase in viscosity.[501] Mucin is the distinguishing constituent of synovial fluid—without mucin, it is virtually blood plasma[827] although viscosity is not necessarily the same as lubrication effectiveness.[1352]

The viscosity of synovial fluid is variable according to the nature of the demands made upon the joint. Healthy hyaline cartilage is porous to the smaller molecules of synovial fluid secreted by the synovial cells, it is permeable and fluid-soaked, but permeability measurements show that the pore diameter of cartilage is too small to admit the synovial mucin molecules; thus analysis of the fluid squeezed out of cartilage shows that it contains no mucin.[827]

Because cartilage is not rigid, the application of load must exert pressure on the contained fluid.

Of those postulated lubrication mechanisms tabulated below, two may be briefly described:

1. *Hydrostatic or weeping lubrication.* McCutchen (1959)[825] described a mechanism by which the bearing load automatically creates in the liquid the hydrostatic pressure needed for its own support, and because load rather than motion generates the pressure,

. . . this self-pressurised hydrostatic lubrication should work at all speeds, including zero

i.e. pressure causes the weeping of liquid from within the cartilage. As the cartilage is compressed by loading, fluid is squeezed from it at a rate sufficient to keep the bearing surfaces apart (Fig. 2.2).

2. *Boundary lubrication.* Charnley (1959)[170] proposed a boundary type of lubrication (Fig. 2.3), by which hyaluronic acid molecules become adsorbed by the cartilage surfaces, and it is a molecular layer which is sheared dur-

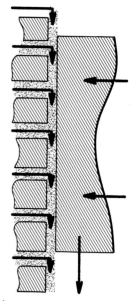

Fig. 2.2 Hydrostatic or weeping lubrication (McCutchen, 1959).

ing sliding, rather than a 'dry' contact. An active constituent of the lubricating fluid bonds itself to, or reacts chemically with, the surfaces to form strong and very slippery films.

Hyaluronic acid in synovial fluid appears to have a specific structure which allows it to interact with the soft tissue (cartilage) surfaces and act as a boundary lubricant.[1198] The film has a thickness of only a few molecules and, like the meshing of gear teeth or cams against cam-followers in a motor car, the surfaces ought to touch, yet their friction and rate of wear are so low they cannot be touching, since the molecular organisation of the hyaluronic acid chains is such as to arrange them standing up from the surface, like the cut pile of a carpet.[1199]

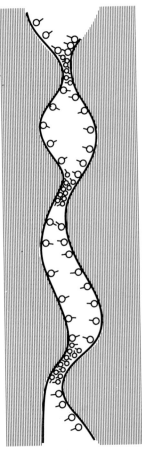

Fig. 2.3 Boundary lubrication (Charnley, 1959).

It seems logical that synovial fluid is the 'lubricating oil' of synovial joints, yet recent research indicates that hyaluronic acid may have less importance in articular lubrication than was previously thought.[1197]

Articular lubrication may be an inherent property of the articular cartilage itself, the role of synovial fluid being thus to interact with the surface, act as a bathing fluid and a lubricant of adjacent soft tissues. Yet the fact remains that when synovial fluid is present in a joint, the friction is lower than when it is absent.

A well-referenced review of the controversial physiology of synovial joint lubrication, the subject of many hypotheses, has been provided by McCutchen (1978),[827] who tabulates them as follows:

Mechanism of lubrication	Author	Year
Hydrodynamic	MacConaill	1932[781]
Mixed	Jones	1934[615]
Boundary	Charnley	1959[170]
Weeping	McCutchen	1959[825]
Floating	Barnett and Cobbold	1962[64]
Elastohydrodynamic	Dintenfass	1963[259]
Osmotic	McCutchen	1966[826]
Synovial gel	Maroudas	1967[808]
Squeeze film	Fein	1967[341]
Boosted	Walker et al.	1968[1278]
Lipid	Little et al.	1969[757]
Electrostatic	Roberts	1971[1046]

His skeleton history of joint lubrication research examines the salient methods and findings, and the bases of hypotheses; joint lubrication remains an incompletely understood function and synovial fluid is still an enigma.

We know which bearings synovial fluid can lubricate, and under what conditions. But we have only speculations about how it does this ... among boundary lubricants, synovial mucin is remarkable for its coefficient of friction ... it is concluded that ... Joints are lubricated by the complementary action of weeping[825] and boundary lubrication.[170] The weeping mechanism supplies the rubbing surfaces with fluid pressurised to nearly the full bearing pressure. The fluid carries most of the load, leaving only a small fraction to be carried out by contact of the surfaces. ... How synovial mucin accomplishes boundary lubrication is the least understood and presently the most interesting part of joint lubrication.

VERTEBRAL MOVEMENT

Observations on the movement of special segments and vertebral regions are usually included with anatomical descriptions of the joints concerned, but by reason of the prime importance of the *functional interdependence of the vertebral column*, these matters may usefully be gathered together as a single section.

Campbell and Parsons (1944)[156] provide an illustration of functional interdependence, drawing attention to balance and stabilisation of the skull on the atlas by the deep group of small suboccipital muscles comprising the anterior, lateral and posterior recti and the superior and inferior obliques, together with the ligaments and fascia of this region, but also by an external group of long hypaxial muscles, e.g. semispinalis capitis, spinalis capitis, trapezius and sternomastoid. Radiation of pain from the middle and lower cervical segments to the occipital and other cranial regions is explicable when the morphology and actions of these muscles are considered.

Irritation at any spinal segment, but the cervical ones in particular, may result in hypertonus of these long muscles and traction on their collagenous attachments to the occipital cranium ... in this way thoracic and even lumbosacral lesions such as postural malalignments and arthrosis, or myofasciitis from local or remote (visceral) causes, have been shown to produce cephalalgia and its concomitants.

(See also p. 310.)

The neurophysiological interdependence of vertebral movement is of equal importance.

The disciplines of bioengineering,[1006] biomechanics,[994, 394, 1306, 873, 968] kinematics[1307] (the study of motion of rigid bodies without consideration of the forces involved), rheology (the science and technology of deformation and flow of materials), and tribology (the science and technology of interacting surfaces in relative motion)[1007, 1351, 275] are providing a wealth of new information. New methods of stress analysis[1107, 1108] are demonstrating the effects upon vertebral structures of the forces they sustain during daily activities[30] at work and sport.[374]

Hampson and Shah[493] mention that biomaterials science, for example,

has grown up in a rather haphazard manner, it being impossible for any one specialist to encompass the whole field in sufficient depth.

The main concern of clinical therapists is the observation and detection of movement-abnormalities and postural defects of patients in pain, and workers aiming at high standards in clinical practice must somehow manage to be flexibly-minded and receptive for such new information as bears upon their practical interest, yet interpret it mainly in terms of that clinical activity. The business of getting patients better happens on the shop-floor, and the questions of 'how, and why, is this abnormal joint moving just this way?' have to be met with the means normally available in the hurly-burly of the clinical situation—hand, eye, wit, goniometer and tape-measure.

The following considerations of vertebral movement have a clinical bias.

KINEMATICS

In three-dimensional space, the spine has six degrees of freedom (Fig. 2.4)—a vertebral body can move in six different ways:

1. In the longitudinal axis of the spine, e.g. under compression or distraction effects.

2. Forwards or backwards in the sagittal plane, e.g. a degree of gliding or translation motion.

3. Laterally, in the frontal plane, by similar slight gliding motions.

4. Forwards and backwards tilt around a frontal axis, i.e. flexion and extension.

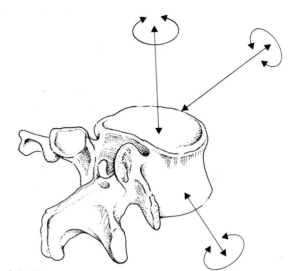

Fig. 2.4 The six degrees of freedom in vertebral kinematics, i.e. translation along the sagittal, vertical and horizontal planes, and rotation around three similar axes. Combinations of vertebral movement may involve two or more degrees of freedom simultaneously.

5. Lateral tilting, or rotation around a sagittal axis, i.e. movement in the frontal plane.

6. Rotation in the horizontal plane, around a vertical axis.

A vertebra may thus rotate about, or translate (glide) along, any of these three axes, or move in various combinations of these motions.[1306]

Coupling, i.e. two types of motion occurring at the same time, is very common in spinal function, and frequently three motions will simultaneously take place during normal physiological movement.

A consideration of cervical flexion and extension (Fig. 2.5) shows a characteristic of movement in that each typical vertebra not only tilts forward and backward (rotation about a frontal axis) but also translates forward and backwards in the median plane, making a series of steps in the anterior curved line during flexion when seen on lateral films.

Pure movement in any of the three principal planes very seldom occurs, since orientation of facet-joint surfaces does not exactly coincide with the plane of motion and therefore modifies it, to a greater or lesser extent. Tilt or rotation cannot occur at an interbody joint without some disc deflection. The axis about which the rotation and/or tilt occurs is the 'centre of rotation'. This point changes with the movement, being differently placed from one instant to another; we can therefore only speak of 'the instantaneous centre of rotation' at a moment in time; vertebral movement becomes more capable of analysis, and understandable, as the instantaneous centre of rotation becomes more completely understood. Spinal movement is complex, and the intricacies of changing relationship observed on cineradiographic and other studies are sometimes difficult to explain.

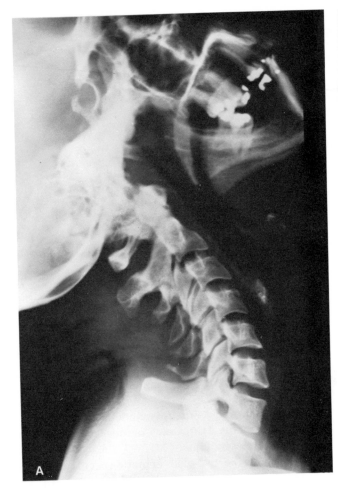
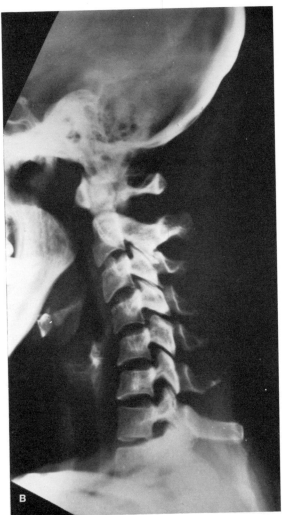

Fig. 2.5 (A) and (B) Ranges of extension (A) and flexion (B) of cervical spine in a 42-year-old female. Note that the smooth curve of an imaginary line, joining the fronts of the vertebral bodies in extension, becomes broken during flexion, and forms a series of steps, particularly evident at the C4–5 segment but also above and below it. The discs are thus horizontally distorted by these shearing effects which occur during sagittal movement of the neck. The mechanics are disturbed by C2–3 stiffness, evident on the flexion film.

Further to the observations of Campbell and Parsons,[156] this difficulty may partly be because of the unwitting tendency to visualise factors governing joint movement* in terms of localised articular and ligamentous morphology *only*, and to overlook the numerous muscular and connective tissue structures which attach at one end to either of the two moving bones but which may span several segments before attaching elsewhere. Simple examples of this guy-rope effect are (a) the tendency for elevation of the arms to impose extension on the thoracic and lumbar regions, by tension applied to latissimus dorsi and pectoralis major, and (b) the tendency for the knee to bend during straight-leg-raising because of tight hamstrings. It seems insufficiently appreciated that these factors, familar enough in the examples given, may well act in more subtle

but equally important ways during movement of a vertebral segment.

Thus far, the vertebra has been considered as a rigid body, but this is not so. The phrase 'vertebral movement' must be taken to include *deformation of the bone itself*, as well as the cartilage covering it.

Radin *et al.*[1005] subjected plugs of subchondral bone and articular cartilage to compressive tests, and demonstrated that bone is capable of deforming under pressure and thus attenuating peak dynamic forces applied; the cancellous bone is capable of making a contribution equal to that of articular cartilage. In a single vertebra the deformation must be a small proportion of 'movement' of the whole vertebral body, yet this depends on the movement. Distortion of the neural arch during rotation strains of the lumbar spine is plainly detectable[326] and the accumulation of the increments of distortion effects are obviously a factor contributing to amounts of movement of whole spinal

*Further observations are given in 'Perceiving the nature of factors limiting movement' (p. 357).

regions. Dynamic experiments on the vertebral bodies of sheep *in vivo*, and on bovine articular cartilage and subchondral bone, clearly demonstrate that bone is a structural component with plasticity, deforming under comparatively light loads. Since *in vivo* strain measurements of sheep tibiae are about the same as those recorded in human tibiae[1007] the findings have validity.

The delicacy of the skeletal response to apparently small changes in direction or magnitude of these is quite striking ... the two sides of the vertebral column seemed to be subjected to loads which differ in size or orientation.[696]

Shah[1007] refers to these experiments and reports similar differences between right and left sides, in his experimental method of brittle-coat analysis of forces applied to human vertebral bodies.

Rolander[1005] showed that with solid neural arch fusion, there is enough elasticity in the bone anterior to the pedicles to allow movement between vertebra and disc on vertical loading. While a 'solid' posterior fusion corrects gross instability, it should not be expected to completely immobilise a mobility segment.

GENERAL CONSIDERATIONS

The presence of arthrotic changes in facet-planes do not, of themselves, necessarily have any effect upon ranges of movement, neither does the presence of osteophytosis.

In general terms, the *relative amplitude of movement* available at the three regions (Figs 2.6, 2.7) is dictated by the proportion of disc height to the vertebral body height, broadly as follows:

	Cervical	Thoracic	Lumbar
Disc height	$\frac{1}{4}$	$\frac{1}{5}$	$\frac{1}{3}$
Body height	$\frac{3}{4}$	$\frac{6}{7}$	$\frac{2}{3}$

Consideration of the greatest regional range being apparent at the cervical spine must include the factors of (a) the translation occurring in sagittal movements and (b) the upper two atypical cervical segments having no disc, yet a greater range of some movements, including translation at C1–C2.

The most important factor governing the *direction* and the *nature*, and sometimes the *amplitude*, of movement between adjacent vertebrae is the orientation of facet-joint planes, e.g. the almost vertical 'set' of the thoracic facets would preclude any great degree of flexion, even without the factor of ribs crowding together anteriorly.

Regional movement characteristics are dependent upon factors which differ between regions, e.g. (a) the annulus fibrosus and longitudinal ligaments govern the amplitude of sagittal lumbar movement, (b) contact of facet-joint planes limits lumbar rotation, like the flanges on train-wheels, more so in extension, and (c) approximation of spinous and articular processes limits thoracic extension.

It is clinically useful to have a working knowledge of

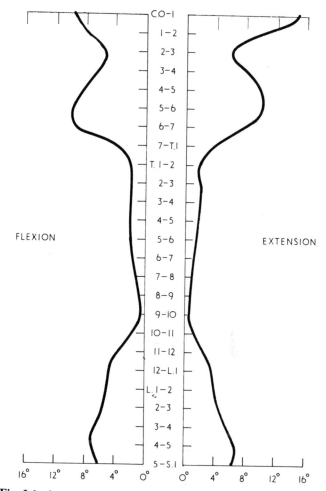

Fig. 2.6 Average ranges of segmental movement. (A general impression of *relative* segmental mobility averaged out from a variety of sources. Individuals may vary widely from the values given and the factors of age and body type should be borne in mind.)
Note: Apart from the upper cervical spine, ranges of flexion and extension depicted are average total excursions and not the excess of flexion over extension, or vice versa, at individual segments. (From Mobilisation of the Spine 3rd edn.)

relative ranges of individual segmental movements (Figs 2.6, 2.7), also of the differing factors limiting movement at the three regions and the especially important junctional areas,[437] but after the simple relative values are known, they should not be given over-much importance.

Patients will differ very widely from the values given, and concepts of 'normal' of 'average' are of minor importance.[1246]

Tables (Figs 2.6, 2.7) of ranges of movement of this kind, abstracted mean values of movement from a variety of sources,[128, 1303, 1180a, 981, 348, 90, 558, 1306, 441, 895, 769, 631] are of much less clinical usefulness than the informed and practised ability to assess the movement of a spinal segment in dynamic relationship to its immediate neighbours, and in general terms of the patient's body-type. Only in this context does the degree of movement have meaning, as when

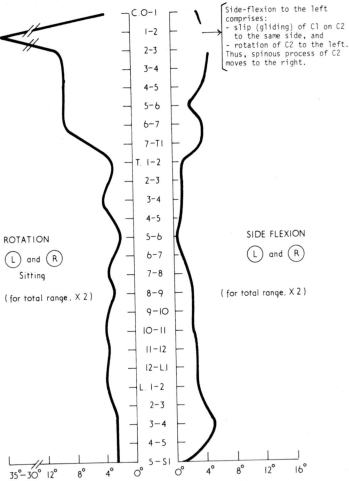

Side-flexion to the left comprises:
- slip (gliding) of C1 on C2 to the same side, and
- rotation of C2 to the left. Thus, spinous process of C2 moves to the right.

ROTATION

Ⓛ and Ⓡ

Sitting

(for total range, X 2)

SIDE FLEXION

Ⓛ and Ⓡ

(for total range, X 2)

Fig. 2.7 Average ranges of segmental movement. (A general impression of *relative* segmental mobility averaged out from a variety of sources. Individuals may vary widely from the values given and the factors of age and body type should be borne in mind.) (From Mobilisation of the Spine 3rd edn.)

assessing hip mobility in different individuals, for example.

Before description of segmental mobility and atypical combinations of movement, regional movement characteristics should be considered. Only *sagittal spinal movements* approximate to motion in one plane, assuming that no abnormal curvature exists. Pure movement in one plane perhaps does not exist.

In rotation and side-bending movements, after the first degree or two of motion, one induces a portion of the other, and they are inseparable.[1180a]

1. *Flexion* reduces side-bending and rotation ranges; it eradicates the cervical curve, usually most noticeably at segments C4–5–6, and sometimes slightly reverses the lumbar curve from the L3 segment upwards.

2. *Extension* also reduces the range of side-bending and rotation.

3. *Side-bending* restricts flexion and extension, and while the vertebral region concerned is held in the position of side-bending, the following tendencies will be noted:

a. in the cervical spine, side-bending makes rotation easier to the concavity, (i.e. to the same side) than to the convexity, whether the neck be in neutral, flexion or extension

b. in the thoracic spine below T3 and in the lumbar spine, side-bending makes rotation easier to the convexity (i.e. to the opposite side) than the concavity, when side-bending occurs in neutral or extended position. If the thoracic and lumbar spine be flexed, and then bent to one side, rotation will be easier to the concavity, as in the cervical spine.

4. *Rotation* restricts flexion and extension, and is invariably accompanied by a degree of side-bending.

Summarised, in all sagittal starting positions of the cervical spine, and in the flexed thoracic (below T3) and lumbar spines, side-bending is perforce accompanied by rotation to the same side, and vice versa; in the neutral or extended thoracic (below T3) and lumbar spines, side-bending is perforce accompanied by rotation to the opposite side.

These are the normal gross regional movement-tendencies of the vertebral column (but see below) and a useful exercise is for the experimenter to sit or stand, put the spine into the positions described and note the resistance encountered when a movement *opposite* to the physiological tendency is tried.

White[1305] reports that in the upper thoracic spine,

the direction of coupling is such that the axial rotation of the vertebral body is into the concavity of the lateral curve;

he observes that in the middle sections of the thorax this direction of coupled axial rotation still probably dominates but is neither as marked nor as consistently present, sometimes being the reverse of that described above.

It should be noted that the ribs and paraspinal muscle had been removed from his autopsy material.

Cosette, Farfan, *et al.*[206] refer to the removal of abdominal and paravertebral musculature including ligamentous structures like the lumbodorsal fascia; the effects of this automatic loss of torsional restraints should not be discounted.

There is a wide variation of normal mobility between individuals, according to body type and to age and sex, hence assessment is important during clinical examination. An initial increase in thoracic and lumbar mobility occurs, for example, during the decade 15 to 24 years, followed by a progressive decrease with advancing years, often by as much as 50 per cent.[865]

Van Adrichern and van der Korst[1262] measured lumbar flexibility in 248 healthy youngsters between 6–18 years, and reported a more marked increase of lumbar flexion range with age in boys than in girls.

After studies of a population of normal males (142) and normal females (142) between the second and ninth decade, Sturrock *et al.*[1186] reported that up to age 65, the total sagittal mobility of thoracic and lumbar spines was about 10 per cent greater in males; after 65 the position is reversed. Up to 65, men can flex about 15° more than women; after 65 women bend 5° more than men. Throughout the age range, women were able to extend more than men. This background should be borne in mind when assessing the more detailed aspects of regional movement.

Generally, male mobility exceeds female mobility in sagittal movements, and female mobility in side-flexion movements exceeds that of males. While it is well appreciated that the length of the hamstrings, and/or the degree of their tension normally existing at the time of the test, should be taken into account during assessment of lumbar flexion mobility, it is surprising how often these factors appear to be overlooked, or insufficiently noted, during examination. The occasional patient can bend to touch the floor without any appreciable change of segmental relationship in the low lumbar spine.

SEGMENTAL AND REGIONAL MOVEMENT CHARACTERISTICS

By reason of differences in the nature of their movement and thus the need for adaptation of treatment techniques, the segments are considered in the groups C0–C1 (occipitoatlantal joint), C1–C2 (atlantoaxial joint), C0–C1–C2 combined, C2–C6, C6–T3, rib movement, T3–T10, lumbar movement, T10–L3, L3–L5, L5–S1, sacroiliac joint. (For general amplitudes of movement see Figs 2.6, 2.7.)

C0–C1

The most free movement, nodding of the head, *can* occur almost alone at this joint, not necessarily accompanied by much sagittal movement of the rest of the cervical spine, unless the latter is also flexed and extended, which is commonly the case. After cineradiographic studies Fielding[348] reported that little flexion occurred, being only about 10°, and that extension was much greater at about 25°. Some side-flexion takes place at this segment and a small degree of rotation is possible, but the latter movement occurs mainly at the segment below.

Kapandji[631] gives the range of rotation as 8°–10°; other authors[981,437] consider that rotation does not occur, yet the small amplitude of movement is easily palpated (Fig. 2.11).

Sagittal movement

Cineradiographic studies indicate that the movement must be seen to be fully appreciated.[348]

Lewit and Krausova (1962),[731] Guttman (1973)[477] and Arlen (1977)[37] have analysed the immensely complex movement of the craniovertebral region; only a brief description of Guttman's analysis is given here.

During head flexion, all cervical vertebrae move simultaneously (Gutmann 1970).[475]

1. In the artificial nodding movement at the C0–C1 segment (i.e. with the rest of the cervical spine fixed, as may occur in some cases of ankylosing spondylitis or gross spondylosis or if the neck is otherwise fixed, as by voluntary muscle action), the occipital condyles *glide backwards* on the atlas; the atlas moves *forward* and somewhat cranially relative to the occiput and takes the odontoid with it so that the bony peg slightly approaches the clivus of the basiocciput. The occiput and posterior arch of atlas tend to move apart.

Only if the movement is virtually isolated to the occipitoatlantal joint, and not in the rest of the cervical spine (and in that sense is abnormal), do the posterior arch of atlas and the occiput separate, as the atlas moves ventrally in relation to the occipital condyles.[475]

2. In the more physiological flexion movement of the head and neck with all cervical segments participating, the occipital condyles *roll forward* on the atlas while the atlas itself *glides backwards* relative to the occiput, and tilts

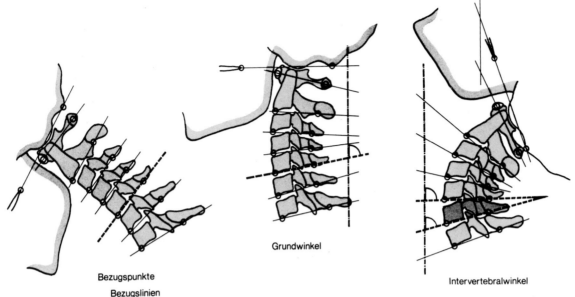

Bezugspunkte
Bezugslinien

Grundwinkel

Intervertebralwinkel

Fig. 2.8 Flexion, neutral and extension of the cervical spine. The perpendicular and other lines of reference which are drawn in on plain lateral films, and which provide the detailed parameters for diagnosis of movement-abnormalities by continental radiologists, are shown. McGregor's line is that which joins the tip of the hard palate and the external surface of the basi-occiput. (Reproduced from von Arlen A 1979 Röntgenologische Funktiondiagnostik der Halswirbelsaüle. Man. Med. 2: 24, by courtesy of the author.)

upwards, so that the posterior arch of atlas and occiput are approximated; in some cases the posterior arch of atlas appears almost to bear against the occiput (Fig. 2.8).

Arlen (1977)[37] analysed this 'paradoxical' inverse atlas tilt in 700 patients, and is in accord with Guttman, Lewit and Krausova that it is the norm, since he reports it is less frequently observed as age advances, and is significantly less frequent in patients suffering from cervical spine disorders than in those with normal spines.

In an exposition of the detailed X-ray parameters, which are adopted when employing the usual three lateral views of the cervical spine in the normal, extended and flexed positions, Arlen (1979)[38] described the reference points and reference lines which are drawn on the films. The position of the head and cervical spine, in relation to the perpendicular, is established by measurement of the angle which each reference line forms with the vertical. There are 8 such angles on each X-ray and thus a total of 24 angles. From these 'basic angles' all further parameters are derived; there is no doubt of the changes described in (2). above.

Summarising the implications of this analysis:

1. The posterior gapping of C0–C1 segment, palpated during careful passive movement tests without the weight of the head acting on the occipitoatlantal joint, and artificially localised to that segment, is normal if the rest of the cervical spine is kept still so far as possible.

2. The paradoxical inverse atlas tilt, observed on lateral radiographs of normal spines during flexion, is also regarded as physiological by the above authors so long as all segments are moving as they should.

Yet a not infrequent clinical experience is that of increasing the posterior gapping between occiput and atlas on flexion together with relief of pain on movement, by localised manipulation of the atlas; this can be demonstrated radiologically (Fig. 8.5) although in this patient lower cervical levels were also involved in his chronic neck condition.

Schmorl and Junghanns (1971)[1093] observe that:

about 50 per cent of flexion and extension take place at the craniovertebral articulations, and only part between the individual cervical vertebrae, with the lower segments between C5 to C7 showing the least mobility.

Perhaps there is no single stereotype—and there are normal differences of craniovertebral movement between individuals.

As will be seen below[611] this possibility has been investigated and its presence confirmed in other parts of the vertebral column (p. 0.00). Criteria of normality, or otherwise, cannot be applied until the cervical spine has received a comprehensive regional and segmental clinical examination.

C1–C2 sagittal movement

The total sagittal range is some 15°[1180a] but

... the range of normal movement of the cervical motor segments shows wide variations.[981]

Stoddard regards the range of this segment to be greater than at C0–C1. On lateral films, the atlantodens distance (the gap between anterior arch of atlas and odontoid) during flexion should be no more than 3 mm in the adult,[1111] and 4–5 mm in children.[128] Values above this raise the suspicion of craniovertebral instability. This is the most mobile joint of the whole vertebral column[348] although its main amplitudes of movement are exercised more during rotation and side-bending than in sagittal movement.

C0–C1–C2 combined movement in mainly frontal and horizontal planes

(Rotation at C0–C1 has been referred to above.) The atlantoaxial joint (C1–C2) allows flexion and extension, free rotation (half of the total cervical rotation range occurs here), lateral gliding and vertical approximation. Rotation is combined with side-flexion to the same side, and vice versa. Only sagittal movement approaches an approximation to movement in one plane.

A brief analysis of the complex movement is as follows:

1. *During head side-bending*, the occipital condyles glide laterally, (translate) towards the convexity, on the superior facets of the atlas.[348] The axis (C2) rotates towards the concavity, so that on anteroposterior films its spinous process is seen to move off to the convexity (see Figs 2.9, 2.10). The skull and atlas together shift laterally towards the concavity to widen the atlanto-odontoid space on the concavity side, and the considerable offset is plainly evident in open-mouth views.

Besides the lateral shift of skull and atlas together, the atlas undergoes a small lateral shift,[981] towards the concavity relative to the occipital condyles. This is in addition to the condylar translation described.[683]

Jackson[598] holds that:

lateral tilting of the head does not alter the atlanto-odontoid relationship unless there is undue relaxation of the alar ligaments

and Kapandji[631] states:

there is no movement at the atlanto-axial joint

but most authors[683, 348, 558, 981] describe the asymmetry as normal, although an excessive degree of mobility unilater-

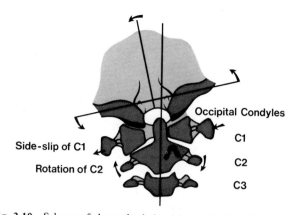

Fig. 2.10 Scheme of changed relationships of C0–C1–C2 on right-side-bending (a-p view). (See text.) (Modified from Kapandji IA 1974 The physiology of the joints. Churchill Livingstone, London, and Librairie Maloine S.A., Paris.)

ally is a factor in diagnosing instability due to ligamentous attenuation or tearing.

Fielding[348] asserts that lateral flexion of the head with the chin in sagittal plane produces more associated rotation of C2 than does head rotation.

2. *During head rotation*, e.g. to the right, the occipital condyles and the atlas initially move almost as a unit on the axis, the pivot being the odontoid (Fig. 2.11).[348] The pivot, as it lies anterior to the transverse ligament, is frontally central but eccentric sagitally, in relation to the atlantal ring. After some 25°–30° of head and atlas rotation, the axis (C2) begins to rotate right, its spinous process therefore being offset to the left.

Side-bending to the right perforce accompanies the rotation movement, and there is a degree of offset of the atlas on the axis. Near the end of the movement, the occipital condyles move reciprocally (the right condyle backward and the left forward) on the atlas for a few degrees, i.e. occipitoatlantal rotation.[1180a, 631]

The atlantoaxial shifts are produced by atlantoaxial rotation or atlantoaxial abduction, or both. These changing relationships have been analysed and pictorially demonstrated by Penning[981] and their observed extent de-

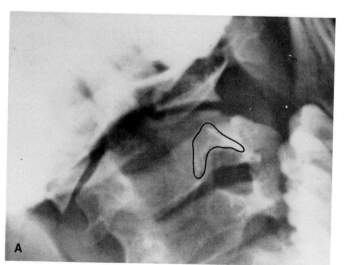

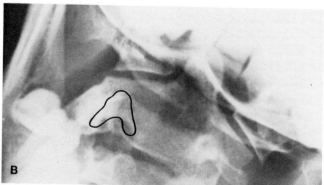

Fig. 2.9 (A) and (B) C0–C1–C2 combined movement. Right and left lateral bending views in a normal 20-year-old. Note the rotation of the axis as determined by the deviation of its spinous process, as outlined, from the midline. (Reproduced from Hohl M, Baker HR 1964 The atlanto-axial joint. Journal of Bone and Joint Surgery, 46A: 1739, by courtesy of the authors and Editor.)

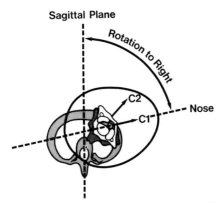

Fig. 2.11 Scheme of changed relationships of C0–C1–C2 on right rotation (plan view). (See text.) (Modified from Kapandji IA 1974 The physiology of the joints. Churchill Livingstone, London, and Librairie Maloine S.A., Paris.)

pends on the radiographic projection (Atlas AP or Axis AP). Rotatory movement and return to neutral position alternately decrease and increase the vertical height of atlas and axis; this vertical approximation is normal motion.[558] The most depressed portion of both joint surfaces are then in contact, and the approximation shows as an apparent loss of height with the head and atlas descending on the axis, and an actual decrease in the length of the neural canal in this region.

C0–C1–C2 three-dimensional combined movement

Using an X-ray photogrammetric method with computerised reduction of data, a three-dimensional analysis of the movements of C0–C1 and C1–C2 segments, in terms of the relationships between the amount of rotation, the plane of rotation and the interactions of rotation and translations with the primary rotation, has been made by Worth et al. (1978)[1345a] who also reviewed the literature.

Subjects were cadaver anatomical head and neck specimens preserved in formalin, with cervical segments down to C7 but with muscles and also mandible removed; ligaments were left intact.

Describing three-dimensional movement requires consideration of the six possible degrees of motion; i.e. rotation about any of the three cartesian axes and also translation along them.

Within the context of its experimental method, this detailed and valuable analysis provides information that:
... movement in one plane appears always to be accompanied by movements in the other two planes at both joint levels.

Movements involve patterns which are functions of the osseous geometry of the individual, and rotations around any axis will be unilaterally biased according to articular configuration, a phenomenon which has been noted by Jirout (see p. 47).

The detailed findings are exemplified by a short extract:
'*Atlanto-occipital joint.* At full extension (of 14.935°) there was a tendency toward left rotation (0.385°) and

right lateral flexion (0.375°). At full flexion (3.55°) there was a tendency to right rotation (0.248°) and left lateral flexion (0.4°). From full extension to full flexion there was a lateral translation to the left of the atlas relative to the occiput of 1.653 mm. At the same time the atlas travelled superiorly to approximate the occiput through 1.949 mm and translated posteriorly through 2.554 mm relative to the occiput.

Atlantoaxial joint. At full extension (9.13°) there was slight rotation (0.143°) and left lateral flexion (0.253°). At full flexion (4.978°) there was an increase of right rotation (2.003°) and left lateral flexion (0.4°).' Reference to the full data is strongly recommended.

The authors remark that during clinical examination the presence of *bias* during active movements, of habitual postures and of compensatory mechanisms at lower segments should be noted. Compensatory mechanisms include not only the altered geometry of lower segments, of course, due to degenerative changes in the articular configuration, but all-important soft-tissue changes too.

When describing their reasons for removing muscle, the authors repeat the assertions of previous workers that, in effect, muscle extensibility is a minor factor *limiting* movement (my italics). Yet muscle action cannot be divorced from *production* of movement nor from contributing to the *nature* of movement.

The altered extensibility of paravertebral musculature and its attachment tissues is a profoundly important 'tethering' factor in producing movement-abnormalities—and these are the lesions we treat.

C2–C6

Joint surfaces tend to separate during flexion, approximate during extension, move asymmetrically during torsion and lateral flexion. None of these movements is ever absolutely pure, especially the latter two which are always combined so that rotation is invariably accompanied by side-flexion to the same side, and vice versa (see p. 00). The configuration of the vertebral bodies and arches as well as of the discs and facet-planes governs the *amplitude* of movement (see Figs 2.5, 12.67).

The segments C4–C5–C6 are the most mobile and tend to suffer the most functional stress, at least on the basis of incidence of spondylosis.

Sagittal movements. Cervical discs appear to undergo more distortion during sagittal movement than in other spinal regions. In flexion, each vertebra tilts and translates forward on the one beneath, since the axis around which sagittal movement occurs lies within the *subjacent vertebral body*,[981] although Frankel and Burstein[373] located the instantaneous centre of rotation in the posterior part of the disc in mid-line.

In full flexion, the line joining the anterior vertebral body margins is a broken one, a series of steps (see Fig.

2.5), and the opposite occurs in extension, on a lateral view of the posterior vertebral margins.

Rotation. Assuming that the atlantoaxial segment produces about 35°–40° of total cervical rotation, the lower cervical segments each move about 8°–10° in either direction.

During rotation to the left, the left inferior articular facets glide backwards and downwards on the subjacent superior articular facets of the same side; inferior facets of the opposite side glide forwards and upwards. Thus the left side of the region is approximated, while the right becomes longer, with side-flexion to the left accompanying left rotation.[1180a] *Side-flexion* is accompanied by rotation to the same side, with backward gliding of the concave-side facets inducing rotation as described above; maintaining the chin and nose in a laterally-inclined sagittal plane requires attentive voluntary effort.

Idiosyncrasies of movement. With reference to the probable lack of a movement stereotype, Jirout[611] attempted to explain the varying positions taken up by cervical vertebrae in side-flexion. In 768 radiographic films of this movement, he observed three separate categories:

1. In which *flexion* was added to the combined side-flexion and rotation (237 examples); the more cranial the segment, the greater its degree
2. In which *extension* was added to the normal combination of movement (118 examples), and
3. In which no forward or backward tilt was added.

His analysis of the *cause* of these idiosyncrasies does not take into account all of the soft tissues which could be having a guy-rope effect, although his findings confirm the presence of individual differences in the nature of vertebral movement.

The importance of this information lies in the implication that any manipulation philosophy based on the supposed 'correctness' of this or that set movement 'logically' based on the plane of the facets, may be fallacious.

Further, he reminded his readers that if the vertebral structures showed pathological changes their dynamics were altered and the nature of added movement was different; it may therefore seem wise to allow the joints of individual patients to speak for themselves, in the prime matter of the nature and direction of the most effective therapeutic movement.

Expressed otherwise, clinical assessment of individual responses takes precedence over theories of biomechanics and theories of 'correct' techniques.

C6–T3

Flexion and extension are not great in this region, although freer than lower in the thoracic spine.

Although the caudal reduction of motion is evident, the wide differences of individual sagittal-movement ranges are manifest in the following findings of three authors:

Segment	Bhalla[90]	Penning[981]	Stodard[1180a]
C6–7	19°	15½°	12°
C7–T1	10°	8°	4°

Thus the figures *per se* are of little importance, *relative* segmental mobility being the essential factor.

All ranges quickly diminish between C6 and T3, although not in a graduated manner, and the physiological movement-combinations are the same as for the typical cervical regions, i.e. side-bending is accompanied by rotation to the same side.

White's[1305] three-dimensional analysis of the kinematic behaviour of 27 autopsy specimens of the thoracic spine, from which ribs and most of the muscle mass were dissected away, allowed the observation that the upper and lower portions of the thoracic column behave quite differently to the middle regions and have certain traits suggestive of neighbouring spinal regions.

Jirout[611] (see above) reports that added movement occurs in this region also—10 per cent of the X-rays revealing *flexion* added to side-bending and rotation and 57 per cent showing *extension* as the added movement.

Movement of ribs

The thoracic transverse processes are much stronger and stouter than in the lumbar region, since they have to buttress the ribs. Also, they are more stout, and extend more laterally, in the upper thoracic spine, diminishing in mass and length down to the lumbar region, this reflecting the need for strong attachment of powerful arm muscles.

Facets of the vertebral bodies for articulation with the heads of the ribs are not all on the body, and in the lower three or four vertebrae (T9–10–11–12) the facet has migrated backwards on to the pedicle. Facets on the transverse processes (which articulate with the tubercle of the ribs) are not uniform, and their arrangement and structure reflects the different mechanical characteristics of the corresponding rib, i.e. (a) T1–T6: the facet is concave and on the front of the transverse process, (b) T7–T10: the facet is flat, and on the upper surface of the transverse process, (c) T11–T12: transverse processes have no facet.

Each typical rib articulates with its own numerically corresponding body and its transverse process (and the body above); the heads of ribs 1, 10, 11 and 12 articulate only with the corresponding body, and not adjacent bodies.

Each rib is a curved lever which has its fulcrum immediately lateral to the costotransverse joint, and each has its own range and direction of movement, differing slightly from the others.

Active use of arms (pulling and pressing) influences the ribs directly and may well be the cause of aggravation of pain from the costospinal joints on ironing, cleaning windows, polishing a car, pushing and pulling activities.[230, 231, 232]

Respiration

The first rib, the shortest, flattest and most curved of all the ribs, has an acute angle.[437] It moves little in quiet respiration but one should not conclude, therefore, that the first and second ribs do not have an appreciable range of movement.

Second to sixth ribs: the vertebrosternal ribs are elevated, and their anterior ends take the sternum with them, moving mainly at the manubriosternal joint. This soon stops, and then the lateral part of the ribs is raised and everted.

Seventh to tenth ribs: the vertebrochondral ribs, also have their lateral parts raised and everted, but there is also some backward gliding of the neck and tubercle. This actually produces a backward movement of the anterior ends of the lower ribs.

Eleventh and twelfth ribs: because of their free anterior extremities, and lack of demifacets and intra-articular ligaments, and costotransverse joints, they can move slightly in all directions, but during respiration they are actively depressed, and fixed, by the quadratus lumborum, thereby helping to form a fixed base for the action of the diaphragm.

Sternum

In about 10 per cent of people early in the fourth decade, the manubriosternal joint is ankylosed or obliterated; later in life, the joints of the costal cartilages suffer the same fate.

T3–T10

This is the region in which the requirements of visceral function seem to take precedence over vertebral mobility. All spinal movements are very limited, rotation least so, by facet-planes, the thin discs, attachment of ribs and sternum and the configuration and proximity of spinous processes.

In terms of physiological priorities, the mobility of the costal joints and the need to avoid compressive effects upon heart, great vessels and lungs outweighs the need for a freely mobile thoracic column, although thoracic mobility-segments contribute to respiratory movement. Flexion-extension range is relatively small, and is least at the T9–10 segment (1° or 2°), while side-bending is least at the T5–6 segment (2°) where rotation is also least.

There is more flexion than extension. One can expect 2°–6° of sagittal movement per segment, 30–40 per cent of which will be extension and the rest flexion. White[1305] demonstrated that, unlike sagittal movements of the lumbar spine, the experimental removal of the neural arches in autopsy specimens significantly increases thoracic mobility in the sagittal and also horizontal planes.

(Removal of the neural arches makes no difference to the amplitudes of sagittal lumbar movement. (see Fig. 18.4.))

He also analysed the instantaneous axis of rotation in the frontal, sagittal and horizontal radiographic planes, which he found consistently located as follows:

extension	above the disc of the segment concerned
flexion	below the disc of the segment concerned
side-bending	at or near the disc and slightly to the convex side
rotation in horizontal plane	varied along a line from anterior middle point of the vertebral body to the spinal canal

Thus, axes of rotation of thoracic and lumbar vertebrae may not always depend upon the geometry of facet-plane orientation.[441]

Despite the small ranges of voluntary thoracic movement it is very easy indeed during passive tests of mobility to detect the play of movement between two spinous processes; loss of movement or increased movement of one segment is plain for even the tyro to find.

Differences between normal and reduced accessory ranges are also readily detectable with a little practice and tuition.

In neutral and extension, side-bending and rotation occur to opposite sides. In flexion, they occur to the same side, as in the cervical spine.

Lumbar movement

Bone is not brittle; on the contrary it may undergo large plastic deformations.[374]

Motion at an intervertebral joint is governed by the mechanical behaviour of its parts. During normal function, the skeletal components of joints must be capable of deforming under load.

Additional to the six degrees of freedom described (p. 39) there are certain other movements, strain deflections,[326] of small magnitude which occur in the attachment-tissues (disc, ligaments) when the joint is subjected to stress of weight-bearing and movement. Thus the small deflections occur both in the skeletal elements and the soft tissue, and each of these deformations in both the 'rigid' and soft components of the articulation provide an increment of motion which contributes to the sum of regional physiological movement, or the relative dispositions of *all* sclerous and collagenous articular tissues if frozen in an imaginary 'still' during a particularly stressful athletic activity.

While these considerations apply to all joints, the forces sustained by the lumbar spine during normal activity are great, and the additional deformations likely to be of relatively larger magnitudes, with important implications regarding the degenerative process.

A larger range of sagittal movement is possible when the discs are thick (see p. 41) as they are in the lumbar spine. Farfan (1973)[326] shows by geometrical construction that there must be deformation of the neural arches during flexion, and that in the lower lumbar spine this may be of the order of 7°. Considering the neural arches, facet-joint structures, interspinous and interlaminae ligaments *as a single segmented ligament* sustaining stress during flexion, the greatest strain will fall on the pedicles of L4 and L5, where the lumbar lordosis is most pronounced. This may partially explain fatigue fractures of the pedicles and pars interarticularis, and the occurrence of spondylolisthesis.

Lumbar rotation increases the existing level of intradiscal pressure (Troup, 1979).[1250b]

Rotational stresses also act on the pedicles. Gregersen and Lucas (1967)[441] showed that the lumbosacral joint could be rotated through 3°–13°, depending upon the subject. In his experiments on mounted segments Farfan (1973)[326] showed the neural arch to suffer considerable deformation under torque. His tests of rotation stresses on L3, for example, showed that coupling of movement occurred, the vertebra tilting forward, flexing, as it rotated. Thus the posterior annulus is stretched by tilting as well as by rotation; the instantaneous centre for flexion is close to that for rotation. The interpedicular distance is thus also increased.

The neural arch is also distorted, rotating with a magnitude of 2° towards the side to which rotation is forced. The facet-joint is compressed on the side to which rotation is forced while the contralateral facet is distracted.

The orientation of the impinged facet-joint surfaces is such that the inferior articular process is forced backward, relative to the vertebral body, effectively applying an elongation stress applied to the pars interarticularis on that side.

With regard to movement-tests of a group of mounted articulations it is possible to move most lumbar spines in the sagittal plane without inducing simultaneous rotation (although this probably depends on the presence of symmetrical facets) but it appears not possible to rotate an intervertebral joint without simultaneously inducing flexion. Side-bending without rotation or flexion seems possible only for the first degree or two of motion.

Experimental effects on mounted cadaver material may not always represent what happens in the horizontally supported spine of a living patient, all of whose connective tissues are intact.

Total range of sagittal movement of the five lumbar segments is 50°–70°, and of side-bending rather less; some movements of hip and thoracic joints make it appear more. When erect, total rotation between extremes is around 12° in sitting, and 20° in standing (surprisingly).[441]

A study of[328] 14 adult males indicates that lumbar flexion accounts for about 60° of flexion. One subject was able to flex only 54°. Further flexion from this point occurs at the hips. Extension follows the reverse order, with the pelvis tilting backward and later, extension of the lumbar spine.

Farfan (1975)[328] observes:

> As the spine flexes, it also elongates. The elongation at 60° of spinal flexion is 20 to 25 per cent at the level of the facet capsules, and more at the tips of the dorsal spines. Ligamentous tissue elsewhere in the body, when stretched in vitro, attains its ultimate tensile strength with 5 to 6 per cent elongation. We are therefore forced to conclude that the ligamentous structures remain slack for the first 20 per cent of elongation and therefore do not develop tension until only 5 to 6 per cent of the residual stretch remains in the ligaments.

T10–L3

Amplitudes of movement, especially in sagittal ranges, progressively begin to increase, as the restriction offered by the ribs, for example, begins to decrease. Pure flexion and extension, if they occur, are rocker-type movements, and normally there is no added *sagittal* translation (gliding) as in the cervical spine; although coupling occurs very frequently during the movements of daily functional activity.

While the nucleus pulposus may be held to be the axis of sagittal movement, the axis changes its position with changes in the arc of movement. During extension, for example, the axis lies immediately in front of the nucleus, and will change more posteriorly during flexion.[873]

As a rule, flexing the lumbar spine does little more than straighten the normal lumbar curve, but in younger age-groups, where the flexion movement does actually reverse it, the reversal occurs more often from L3 segment and upwards than at the two segments below it.

Farfan (1973)[326] gives the typical sagittal motions of the lumbar spine as:

	Total	*Extension*	*Flexion*
L1–2	7½°	3¼°	3¼°
L2–3	7½°	3¼°	3¼°

Charnley's (1951)[169] view that the lumbar spine never achieves a concavity is mentioned by Allbrook[18] who after a radiographic study of 25 men and 7 women, reported that in all of his subjects under 30 years, there was a definite anterior lumbar concavity in full flexion. Twenty of the 32 subjects were free of symptoms and signs referable to the back, and although the predominantly African subjects included European men and women, there were no flexibility differences associated with race or sex.

Extension engages the articular facets, and a particular feature in this region is the effect of extension on the thoracolumbar mortise joint (see p. 14). Rotation is not progressively increased caudally like other movements because the facet-planes begin to show lumbar characteristics, being orientated so as to engage face-to-face early in the rotation movement.

Side-bending progressively increases from above down in this region, and the greatest regional range occurs at the L3 segment.

Side-bending alone, or rotation alone, can occur for a few degrees only, thereafter the movement-combinations previously described begin to occur.[1180a]

L3–L5

The nucleus pulposus of the normal lumbar spine has been regarded as acting like a ball-bearing,[508] the vertebral bodies rocking forward and backward over the incompressible gel while the posterior joints guide and steady the movement like flanges on a train-wheel.

Consequent upon this view, arthrosis of facet-joints is explained as secondary to a primary disturbance of the disc tissue-system (annular tearing, rupture of hyaline cartilaginous plate or failure of the hydrophilic properties of the nuclear proteoglycans) allowing asymmetrical and distorted movement, with buffeting, grinding and other repetitive abnormal stresses upon articular cartilage. This concept of lumbar movement therefore requires a normal, healthy prestressed disc, centrifugal effects of the elastic tension exerted by a normal annulus fibrosus, the polysaccharide matrix of the nucleus retaining an 88–90 per cent volume of fluid; it also appears to require that much of functional movement should be forward and backward rocking. A moment's work-study of one's own daily activities indicates clearly that symmetrical sagittal movement of the lumbar spine is at best a very infrequent physical activity. By far the greater majority of lumbar movements are asymmetrical, even when bending—one leg is forward, one foot may be raised, the pelvis is very often a little rotated, one arm is reaching, the other not, and so on.

The dynamic stabilisation of the superincumbent half of the body weight, frequently changing its centre of gravity and the disposition of its parts (head, thorax and upper limbs), together with the handling of weights and the stresses of pulling, pushing and pressing, places very great demands upon the mid- and lower spine, and the physiological coupling of movements (see p. 39) must surely compound the nature of asymmetrical stresses and buffeting *normally* sustained by the lumbar spine.[230, 231, 232]

There is no evidence to support the contention that movement of one vertebra on its fellow is a see-saw motion with one vertebra rolling over the nucleus pulposus (Farfan[326]).

The classical notion that disc failure almost inevitably leads to secondary arthrotic failure of the posterior joints could bear some inspection; the question is relevant to the nature of lumbar movement. Lewin (1964),[727] in a detailed morphological study of the lumbar facet-joints, reported that arthrotic changes were frequently found in the posterior lumbar joints unaccompanied by either disc degeneration or lipping of the vertebral bodies.

It is now apparent that the facet-joint structures sustain considerable stress in their own right (see p. 501), and the commonly held view[870] that the first thing to go awry is the disc itself, and that seemingly associated facet-joint changes become morphologically plain some four to five years later, may need modifying.

Autopsy evidence of varying degrees of facet-joint damage is plain,[727, 326, 508] but apparently it need not be secondary to disc failure at that segment. Information regarding the nature of forces sustained by the disc is now considerable; but our knowledge regarding the magnitude and type of stresses imposed on the posterior joints is less complete, although expanding.[326]

What we *can* be sure about are the somewhat baggy posterior joint capsules, the consequent possibilities for considerable gliding movement between the facet-planes of each joint, the physiological combinations of flexion, side-flexion and rotation during most movements and the alternating and changing tendency for the joint surfaces of one side to be almost fully engaged and compressed together, while those of the opposite side are being somewhat disengaged in the plane of the facets, and gapped at right angles to that plane.

Flexion is often the freest movement[631] yet amounting in the more mature subject to no more than a partial or general eradication of the lumbar lordosis (see above). Extension may be free, or almost nil in middle age. Pure flexion and extension as such do not occur in the lumbar spine.

Farfan (1973)[326] gives the typical sagittal range of movement as:

	Total	Extension	Flexion
L3–4	18°	9°	9°
L4–5	22°	10°	12°

Side-bending decreases from about 5° either side at L3–4 to 2° at L4–5, and such combined rotation as is present will as a rule be towards the convexity; provided the region is not in flexion, when the opposite occurs.[1180a] Rotation is usually about 3° to either side, but is greater when standing than sitting.[441]

Cossette, Farfan *et al.*[206] applied torque to the L3 vertebra of fresh cadaver spinal segments (L3–L5), thus rotating the L3–4 joint; the instantaneous centre of rotation was found to be anterior to the facet-joints and in the region of posterior nucleus and annulus. The centre was found to move towards the side to which rotation was forced. Their observations on the unknown effects of dissecting away muscles etc. (p. 47) should be noted.

Mobility in this part of the lumbar column is much influenced by changes, (not necessarily or primarily of the vertebral body joints[727]) occurring at the subjacent, lowest mobility segment (L5–S1) as the years advance. It is probably more than coincidence that lumbar hypermobility syndromes have a habit of involving the L4–5 segment.

L5–S1

The wedge-shaped lowest disc and the wedge-shaped L5 vertebra, the consequent lumbosacral angle and the marked tendency for anomalies to occur at this level (see p. 24) make it difficult to describe a generalised movement-pattern applicable to most individuals.

White *et al.* (1974)[1306] give a side-flexion amplitude of 4° at L5–S1. Tanz (1953)[1205] gives the side-flexion range as diminishing from 7° during the first decade to 1° or nil during the seventh decade; presumably this amplitude might depend to an extent upon the presence of anomalies, and the orientation of facet-planes, although Lumsden and Morris (1968)[769] noted that rotation ranges were un-influenced by general orientation of lumbosacral facets, or by asymmetry of orientation between sides (Fig. 1.31). In their study of lumbosacral rotation in ten healthy, male medical students of ages 21–32 years, with no history of back problems, the above authors inserted a Steinman pin into the spinous process of the fifth lumbar vertebra, and two into the posterior superior iliac spines. No correlation was found between variations of rotation and build, height, age or weight, nor between rotation and the presence of Schmorl's nodes, disc narrowing, sclerosis of a facet, laminar defects, spina bifida of S1 and asymmetrical facet-planes. Neither could an increase or decrease in rotation ranges be correlated with radiographic evidence of lumbosacral disc degeneration. In their sample, about 6° of rotation occurred during the subject's maximum effort, when sitting straddling a bicycle seat, and standing, and about 1.6° during normal walking.

A reminder of coupling movements lies in the authors' report that rotation was always associated with flexion of the fifth lumbar vertebra on the sacrum.

Gregersen and Lucas (1967)[441] also refer to axial rotation as an integral motion of the thoracic and lumbar spine during lateral flexion, and following their study of thoracic and lumbar rotation they reported averages of around 12° in standing, and 3° in sitting, of total side-to-side rotation movement at the lumbosacral joint. There were considerable differences between individuals.

Farfan (1973)[326] observes that location by the above authors of the instantaneous centre of rotation posterior to the facet-joints would require very large deformations to occur in the neural arch, of sufficient magnitude to be detectable radiographically.

If the neural arch is not permitted to distort at the intervertebral joint, then displacements of ridiculous magnitudes are required to account for the observed rotation.

He deduces the centre of rotation to lie somewhere near the centre of the vertebral body, placing it in the midline at the posterior annulus.

White *et al.* (1974)[1306] give a sagittal (flexion/extension) range of 10° for the L5 segment, and Farfan (1973)[326] reports that approximately 18°–20° of flexion/extension occurs at the lumbosacral joint, with somewhat more (22°–25°) occurring at the L4–5 segment. The excess of flexion over extension is in the ratio of 2:1, i.e. full extension 18°, extension 6° and flexion 12°.

Among some of 28 specimens, ranging in age from 1 month to 98 years, which were carefully dissected (Heylings, 1978)[538] to determine the nature of ligamentous attachments of the lumbosacral region (p. 22), it was observed that the more caudal lumbar spinous processes separated from each other on flexion more than the cranial ones; this suggests that movement is more free at the L5–S1 segment, i.e. beyond the end of the supraspinous ligament *which terminates at the upper border of L5 spinous process* (see p. 23). Between L5 and S1 spinous processes the medial fibres of the erector spinae tendons are interwoven with fibres from the dorsal part of the interspinous ligament and the deep fibres of the lumbodorsal fascia. Heylings suggests that the substitution of a supraspinous ligament at L5–S1 by a complex of tendon, ligament and fascia would provide a more adjustable controlling mechanism of lumbosacral movement.

Allbrook (1957)[18] used the sacrum as a fixed point to measure radiographically observed flexion/extension ranges in 32 living men and women, of mixed European and African race, all under 50 except for 1, and some of whom suffered backache. A summary of his findings is as follows:

1. In healthy pain-free individuals the greatest lumbar movement occurs in the lower vertebrae and gradually becomes less in the upper segments.

2. In some the greatest movement is at the L4 segment, in some at L5, and in others the amplitudes of movement are equal at the two segments.

3. Anterior spur formation on vertebral bodies was noted at or after middle age and was always associated with movement-limitation of the segment concerned.

4. In four young patients with acute back pain but without bony abnormality, there was a general restriction of movement, not confined to a particular segment.

5. In those without pain and/or exostosis formation, ranges were from 11°–26° at L5, and 12°–27° at L4, and in those with pain and/or exostosis formation, ranges were from 0°–23° at L5 and 0°–16° at L4.

The lesson, for assessment of abnormal signs in clinical situations, is plain, i.e. while the biochemical/physical changes underlying the slow loss of normal characteristics have a predilection for the lowest lumbar segments (see p. 20) radiographically demonstrable loss of movement, with visible and palpable evidence of it at a particular segment, *may or may not have much to do with what the patient reports by way of symptoms. One is never relieved of the obligation of clinical assessment, and in this respect the factor of reproducing the patient's symptoms by regional and segmental testing movements is very frequently the vital issue.*

Nachemson *et al.* (1979)[892] examined the mechanical behaviour of 42 lumbar motion segments of fresh cadavers, to determine the influence of sex, disc level and degree of degenerative change. The normal physiological motions together with anterior, posterior and lateral shears were applied, and while differences were observed these were seldom marked. There was, however, a pronounced scatter in the behaviour of individual segments, and this often overshadowed the class differences.

Among the interesting findings were:

1. Age appeared to have no consistent effect upon the mechanical behaviour of adult segments.

2. Disc level seldom had a marked effect upon response.

3. In the six grossly degenerated specimens, no relative disc-space narrowing was observed.

Sacroiliac joint

In both sexes the normal sacroiliac joint moves. Movement in the sacroiliac joint is not *directly produced* by any muscle, however powerful may be its surrounding musculature; it is *indirectly imposed* by the action of the muscles, and movement and stress of other and adjacent body parts, the extent of its slight movement being governed by its massive ligaments and the bony configurations of its joint surfaces. To liken the minimal movements of this roughened, multiplane and massive joint, which bears stressses exceeding 50 kg during normal activity and sometimes multiples of that force, to the smooth-surfaced and freely mobile, paired and delicate occipitoatlantal joints, for example, is manifest nonsense. The craniovertebral joints are directly moved by an intricate group of small muscles which have a high innervation ratio, and are capable of rapid alterations of tension within a few milliseconds; whereas the glutei, for example, are among the coarsest muscles in the body and have one of the lowest innervation ratios.

Bourdillon (1973)[105] suggests that there are striking differences in descriptions of sacroiliac movement,[135, 992, 1301] and that the various observers were describing and measuring different types of movement, but since these various linear and angular motions have been observed and been measured, it is somewhat simplistic to attempt to resolve real difficulties by calling its main movement 'rotation'.

Meyer (1878)[855] described movement about two axes, although Fick (1911)[347] regarded these two movements as slight, and merely of a rocking type. He also described a screw movement between the sacrum and the ilia. Sashin (1930)[1082] regarded the motion as only slight at best, consisting of up-and-down gliding and slight anteroposterior movement.

By cineradiographic studies of living subjects, when changing from lying to standing, Weisl (1955)[1301] demonstrated a constant movement at the S–I joint, i.e. a ventral shift of the sacral promontory of about 5.5 mm. The axis of the movement lies about 10 cm below the sacral promontory and is variable by about 5 cm. The axis tends to be higher in puerperal women, but other than this, differences in the degree and nature of the movement cannot be correlated with height, weight, sacral curve index or sex. This 'nodding' of the sacrum also occurs during sagittal movement of the trunk; thus on assuming the standing position from lying, or on flexing the trunk, the sacral base moves forward between the ilia. On extending the trunk while standing, and on lying down, the sacral base moves backwards between the ilia (Fig. 2.12).

Clayson *et al.* (1962)[181] found that the mean maximal range of flexion/extension of the sacroiliac joint, in a radiological study of slender, young women, was 8°.

Colachis *et al.* (1963)[190] embedded Kirschner pins into the iliac spines of medical students and movements were carried out in sitting, standing trunk flexion and maximum flexion/extension scissor movements of thighs. They concluded that there certainly is movement, it is usually small but varies greatly with the individual, and shifts of 5 mm were recorded between iliac spines. There is evidence that both angular and parallel movements take place, rather than rotatory motion, and they found it difficult to accept past authors' impressions that movement occurred about a fixed mechanical axis. It is interesting to note that as the pins were being inserted into the posterior iliac spines, 50 per cent of the subjects felt a 'toothache' pain, which was localised in some but in others radiated down the posterior thigh. (See 'Referred pain', p. 189.)

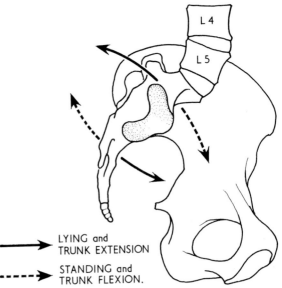

LYING and
TRUNK EXTENSION

STANDING and
TRUNK FLEXION.

Fig. 2.12 View, with right ilium removed, to show sagittal movements of base and apex of sacrum during sagittal trunk movements, and when lying and standing.

In a small group of four patients, Egund *et al.* (1978)[308b] used a stereophotogrammetric method to quantify three-dimensional movements in the sacroiliac joints; they describe, among others, a sagittal movement of 2° as rotation, mainly about a transverse axis approximating to the lower part of the iliac tuberosity. The amplitudes of observed movement in seven different body positions were smaller than those reported by other investigators.

Colachis *et al.* (1963)[190] have remarked upon the great variation of movement between individuals, when measuring the angulation of Kirschner pins embedded in the iliac spines of healthy medical students.

More recently, Frigerio *et al* (1974),[387] by a radiological technique using two X-ray beams and plates located orthogonally to one another, and by computing the data obtained, demonstrated movements on a cadaver and a living subject. Movements on the cadaver between points on sacrum and ilium ranged up to 12 mm with an average of 2.7 mm. Between the ilia themselves, ranges were up to 15.5 mm. In a male subject, *in vivo* ranges were considerably larger than those observed in the cadaver, and movements of the iliac crests relative to the sacrum, for example, ranged up to 26 mm, a little over an inch, with torsional and flexing movements of the same order. These observations provide strong support for the work, nearly 40 years ago, of Pitkin and Pheasant (1936)[992] who studied 144 male university students and among other conclusions asserted that:

1. In the standing position all motions of the trunk, with the exception of flexion and extension, normally are associated with unpaired, antagonistic movements of the ilia.

2. Rotation and lateral bending of the sacrum normally do not occur alone, but as correlated motions that are coincidental to antagonistic movements of the ilia.

3. Positions of the ilia in normal stance, as well as their relative mobility, are affected by the dominant eye and hand.

The small intrapelvic movement can be confirmed by the simple test of sitting partly on both hands on a hard seat and applying finger pressure on the sacrotuberous and sacrospinous ligaments. A slight lateral inclination of the body to the left will transfer most of the trunk weight onto the left ischial tuberosity. This produces a slight backward movement of the ilium on the sacrum, and the left sacrotuberous ligament becomes perceptibly taut, while the right sacrotuberous ligament remains relaxed. Lateral inclination to the right reverses the tensions perceived.

If perpendiculars are dropped from the centres of the hip joint anteriorly and the sacroiliac joint posteriorly, in the standing position, the horizontal distance between them is two or more inches; this small but important leverage may explain the observations of Schunke (1938),[1095] i.e. that when body weight is supported on one leg, the pubic bone of the supported side moves forward in relation to its opposite fellow of the unsupported side. He refers to this as 'rotation' of ilium at the sacroiliac joint and whatever the true nature of the movement the implications for an asymmetrical, rhythmic, shuffling-type movement occurring during walking and other functional movements of trunk and lower limbs are plain.

A consideration of the consequences of asymmetrical leg lengths cannot exclude this factor of sacroiliac movement. Further, should chronic muscle imbalance disturb the rhythmic cycle of this movement by a degree of unilateral fixation, especially in children, it may be that the stage is set for the development of diverse joint problems in the future. As patterns of referred pain vary considerably between individuals (Hockaday and Whitty 1967),[553] so patterns of sacroiliac movement tend to be equally variable. A glance at the great variety of articular configurations between individuals conforms this impression, and it behoves the need for flexibility and adaptation when using classical manipulative techniques.

SUMMARY

The complex nature of vertebral movement is still not fully understood, despite the many excellent research projects which have raised the level of our comprehension of it. White and Panjabi (1978)[1307] have commented:

The experimental techniques for precise no-risk *in vivo* measurement in the human are yet to be developed. The physiological muscle forces have not been simulated. The characteristics of the force vectors that cause *in vivo* physiological motion are not known. Studies are done to simulate vertebral motion, but it is not known whether the motion experimentally produced is the same as that which is physiologically produced *in vivo*. The vectors that should represent the existing physiological preloads are not known and at present we are not aware of published studies of kinematics that take them into consideration.

Much remains to be learnt about the movements of the spine under normal and abnormal working conditions (Troup, 1979).[1250b]

THE INTERVERTEBRAL FORAMEN

The intervertebral foramina are oval in shape when viewed laterally, with the longer vertical axis well exceeding the anteroposterior measurement. Foramina are less orifices or apertures with sharply defined edges, than ellipsoid spaces with lateral dimensions, and this is especially evident in the cervical region, where the foramen is more of a canal or gutter and commonly exceeds 1 cm in length.[117] The thoracic foramina have the shortest lateral traverse and of the three spinal regions these are most like simple openings, albeit with the sharpest though still rounded bony margins.

Thoracic movement, and consequently thoracic root disturbance by traction, are regionally the least, otherwise root sleeve fibrosis would probably be noted as predominantly a thoracic pathological change rather than a cervical one.

Since the amount of research into the nature of degenerative change in the thoracic joints is relatively small,[902, 1125] it may well be that fibrotic change at the thoracic foramina occurs fairly frequently, because of the sharper bony edges and the opportunities for chronic irritation, although little is written about it.

The lumbar foramina should perhaps be regarded as regions rather than 'portholes', with the lateral recess of the neural canal, noted on a plan view of a lumbar vertebra (see p. 28), an important part of the region; low lumbar roots are not infrequently compressed by disc material in this cubbyhole of the lateral dimensions of the neural canal (Fig. 1.32).

Root sleeve

As the ventral and dorsal roots combine to traverse the foraminal opening, they invaginate the dura and arachnoid to carry with them a separate bilaminar sleeve of these two meninges, and a short lateral continuation of the subarachnoid space (with cerebrospinal fluid) which ends at the posterior root ganglion.[437] The dural sheath ends more distally after enveloping the ganglion as a fibrous sheath, then continuing as the epineurium of the spinal nerve.

The afferent fibre population of the combined spinal nerve roots exceeds that of efferent fibres by 3:1 in the cervical region, 1.5:1 at thoracic segments and 2:1 in lumbar roots.[1193]

While the ventral and dorsal roots remain separate they can be individually and selectively trespassed upon by degenerative change.[392]

Frykholm[392] describes the different effects of stimulating, under local anaesthesia for operations on the cervical spine, (a) the dorsal root, when patients immediately experienced a pain with dermatomal distribution, and (b) the ventral root, when they reported pains in muscles which preoperatively had been painful and tender to pressure.

At the foraminal opening, the cross-sectional area occupied by the root bundle (nerve and sheath), is one-third to one-half, with the remaining half occupied by areolar connective and adipose tissue, the spinal artery and its ventral and dorsal branches, many small veins, lymphatic vessels and filaments of the sinuvertebral nerve (ramus meningeus).[1192]

Invagination of the dura and arachnoid to form the 'root sleeve' directly opposite the vertebral foramen occurs at upper cervical segments, with gradually increasing obli-

quity of successively lower segments causing greater discrepancies between rootlet formation and foraminal level Fig. 2.13). Thus the shortest cervical roots are 10 mm in length, and the longest sacral root 168 mm. This generally results in the root bundle occupying the upper part of the foramen, but at *the cervicothoracic junction* the roots may descend intradurally for some millimetres *below* the lower margin of the foramen, with consequently an acute upward angulation of the dural sleeve and a close approximation of root complex and lower foraminal bony margin. This angulation is seen in more than one-third of cases under 25 years, and between 25 and 40 years the angulation is seen in about three-quarters of cases (Fig. 2.14).

Lack of attachment to foraminal margins for the most part (see p. 62) allows roots to move about and through the foramen, and further, the relative elasticity of roots allows them to sustain a degree of lengthening which is ample provision for the normal ranges and various combinations of vertebral movement.

The elasticity nevertheless has a limit, and in the cervical spine, where the relatively free mobility may induce traction sufficient to harm the roots, two factors give a degree of protection against additional tensile stress, *viz:* (a) the attachment of roots C4–C7 to the foraminal gutter by connective tissue of the roots' epineurium (see p. 57), the prevertebral fascia and other slips from musculotendinous attachments to transverse processes (the smaller amplitudes of lumbar and thoracic movement do not hazard roots in this way and such attachments are only seen in the cervical region), and (b) the proximally wider part of the less extensible dural funnel is drawn outwards, and plugs the foramen so as to resist further lateral movement.

The relationships between facet-joint and root complex are such that the root is below and in front of the joint in the cervical region, directly in front of it in the thoracic region and in front and above it in the lumbar region.

Foraminal encroachment

While vertebral movement especially changes the *vertical* dimensions of the foramen, there is adequate room for these variations to occur without compression of the structures traversing it, which are also protected by the surrounding fat and cerebrospinal fluid, bathing the emerging root as it lies within the subarachnoid space of the sleeve.[537] A simple reduction in the height of the intervertebral disc is not usually sufficient to produce compression of roots and vessels, so long as the fat and fluid remain around the nerve roots, although reduction of the vertical foraminal dimensions can be caused by a retrolisthesis-with-extension at one segment, when the superior articular process of the vertebra below then trespasses upward and effectively reduces available space.

In the lumbar region the vertical diameter of the

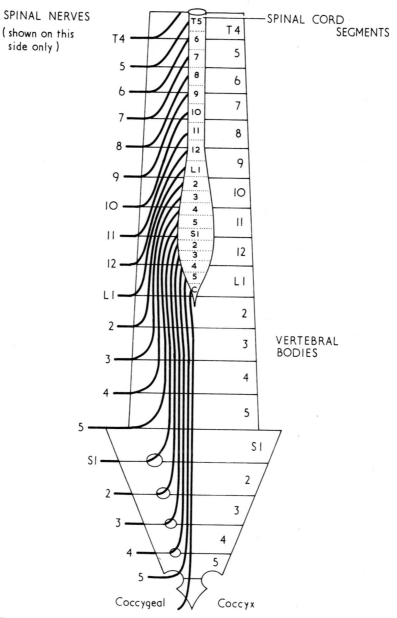

SPINAL NERVES
(shown on this
side only)

SPINAL CORD
SEGMENTS

VERTEBRAL
BODIES

Coccygeal   Coccyx

Fig. 2.13 The level of spinal cord segments in relation to vertebral levels. The spinal cord ends at L1–L2.

foramen varies between 12 and 19 mm, but the transverse diameter may be as little as 7 mm, and the opportunities for foraminal encroachment due to *horizontal* trespass are much greater.

Diminution of the *transverse diameter* is more likely to embarrass the foraminal contents, and this space-occupying effect can be due to abnormalities of the disc and facet-joints, so often the cause of acquired spinal stenosis. Nerve tissue will tolerate slow compression quite well[282, 392] and marked trespass may not give rise to much detectable disturbance of function, although repeated frictional trauma against encroaching degenerative thickening, and exostosis, may be the more likely cause of reactive changes in the nerve and consequent development of signs and symptoms.

It is a curious fact that in both the lower cervical and lower lumbar regions, where spondylotic changes are very frequently responsible for a reduction in foraminal dimensions, the foramina should be naturally smaller than in the middle and upper parts of these regions (see also 'Biomechanics of spinal cord and meninges', below).

When the transverse dimensions of the lumbar foramina appear developmentally reduced, and this is detectable on plain lateral films in the absence of acquired foraminal encroachment by spondylosis and arthrosis, a narrow neural canal (spinal stenosis) is almost certainly present.

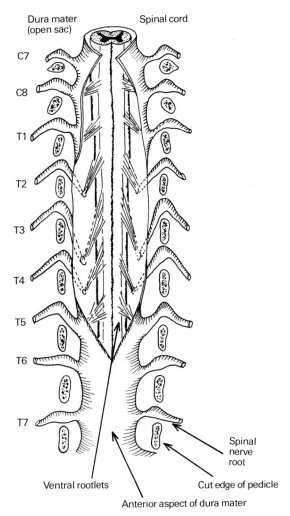

Dura mater (open sac)   Spinal cord

C7

C8

T1

T2

T3

T4

T5

T6

T7

Ventral rootlets

Spinal nerve root

Cut edge of pedicle

Anterior aspect of dura mater

Fig. 2.14 Scheme of cervicothoracic root angulations—anterior aspect (see text). (After Nathan H, Feuerstein M 1974 Angulated course of spinal nerve roots. Journal of Neurosurgery 32: 349.)

BIOMECHANICS OF SPINAL CORD AND MENINGES

In the presence of mechanical derangements such as disc prolapse, or the bony and soft tissue hypertrophy of osteoarthrosis where there is encroachment upon the dura and nerve roots, and where adhesions may follow a local irritative state, there is need to distinguish between the possible causes of pain on movement. [Troup, 1979][1250b]

In his foreword to Breig's (1978)[121b] detailed observations on adverse mechanical tension in central nervous system tissues, Verbiest remarks that the observations are of much importance not only to specialists in the neurosciences and orthopaedic surgery, but also to anaesthetists, whose activities regularly involve the positioning of defenceless patients, and last but not least to physiotherapists, for reasons which need no elaboration. Breig introduces his study in words which leave no doubt of their significance for those who treat vertebral degenerative change:

The primary source of meningeal and neural tension is the lengthening of the spinal canal on forward and lateral flexion. Normally, the soft tissues adapt freely to these skeletal movements; but in the presence of space-occupying lesions involving the spinal cord or located in the cord itself, and when there are sclerotic or fibrotic lesions that restrict the mobility or extensibility of nervous and meningeal tissues, the tension may be much increased. Even when the pathological lesion appears to be exerting an essentially compressive effect, the resulting deformation leads to a local increase in tension; it is the effects of this raised tension that appear to be of primary neurophysiological significance ... excessive tension in the cord may produce measurable changes in motor, sensory and autonomic function. These are accentuated whenever the cord is stretched, and may be reversed, and the symptoms relieved, if stretching can be eliminated and the affected tissues are kept relaxed. Even in the presence of irreversible myelopathic lesions, whether focal, sclerotic or space-occupying, the existing symptoms and neural function can be improved significantly by surgical measures designed to prevent overstretching of the cord. In the course of clinical enquiry over nearly two decades I have found that many neurological disorders in which no mechanical component has ever been suspected do in fact have their origin in tension in the nervous tissue; we are at present only just beginning to recognise the histological and neurophysiological sequelae of this tension. ... Biomechanical analyses were extended to the microscopical level. These analyses have shown that tension in the nervous tissue that gives rise to symptoms is characterised by focal deformation of its complex three-dimensional fibre network as seen in histological and microangiographical sections. It was evident that an important cause of functional disturbance both of the axis-cylinders and the blood-vessels lies in the reduction of their cross-section area resulting from tension. By slackening the nervous tissue the tension is relieved and the conductivity and circulation are restored.

Nervous tissue and the meninges have different properties and therefore show different behaviour under mechanical stress; this has important inferences when considering the effects of vertebral movement.

Nerve tissue is almost semifluid—if cut transversely it tries to flow. The sciatic nerve, for example, can stretch, it is elastic.[1036, 416] While a sudden stretch may interfere with it considerably, a slow stretching may be tolerated without undue reactive changes.

The meninges differ. The more delicate of them can stretch and enlarge circumferentially, because much of the arrangement of their fibres is around the long axis, presumably to accommodate arterial pulsation, but they cannot stretch very much along the longitudinal axis of the cord, e.g. when extended to around 5 per cent of their normal length they are taut.

STRUCTURE

The outer layer of the dura mater, basically white fibrous tissue predominating over some elastic fibres, is continuous above through the foramen magnum with the inner layer of the intracranial dura mater. The spinal canal continuation of the outer (endosteal) layer of the cranial dura mater is represented by the periosteum lining the vertebral canal. In the canal the space between the two layers is the epidural or extradural space, almost entirely occupied by fat, loose areolar tissue, and the rich plexus of vertebral veins.[437]

The caudal limit of the subdural cavity lies level with the second sacral segment, the dural tissue then extending caudally, as an increment of the filum terminale of the spinal cord, both of which structures end by blending with the periosteum on the back of the coccyx.

In addition to these cephalic and caudal attachments the spinal dura mater is attached by fibrous slips to the back of the vertebral bodies of C2 and C3,[117] and also to the posterior longitudinal ligaments of the lumbar segments.

In the lumbar region the binding of the dura is most firm along the lateral edges of the long superficial strap fibres of the posterior longitudinal ligament, with numerous cross connections of the epidural venous sinuses passing between the trabeculae of connective tissue which join the dura and ligament.[971]

Investments of dura mater are continued laterally through the intervertebral foramen (see p. 54) with the combined spinal nerve roots for a short and variable distance, as a root sleeve, or root ostia, blending with the connective tissue perineurium.

Variations occur with regard to angulation and maldevelopment and/or malformation of cervical root pouches and root sleeves.[392]

Bowden, Abdullah and Gooding (1967)[117] observe that the paired root sleeves of dura and arachnoid mater are loosely attached to the margins of the cervical foramina. These attachments increase in strength with advancing years and degenerative change.

Sunderland (1974),[1192] with regard to the remainder of the spine, describes the nerve complex as not attached to the wall of the foramen, the arrangement permitting the complex to move within and through the foramen; Hollinshead (1969)[562] reports the first sacral nerve as attached to the margins of the intervertebral foramen. On *leaving* the foramen, the 4th, 5th, 6th and 7th cervical roots are more strongly attached to the vertebral column, each lodging in the gutter of the transverse process in which it is securely bound by its epineurial sheath and by reflections of the prevertebral fascia and other slips of connective tissue.[1193]

The middle layer, of arachnoid mater, is a more delicate membrane and is separated from the dura mater by a potential space which contains a trace of serous fluid.

The arachnoid mater is continuous above with the intracranial arachnoid membrane, and ends caudally with the lower extremity of the subdural cavity at the second sacral segment. It lines the dural root sleeves, providing with the dura an investment of the ventral and dorsal spinal nerve roots but is not, like the dura, continued distally beyond the formation of the combined spinal root, i.e. it terminates by linking the adjacent layers of dura between the ventral and dorsal roots, thus contributing two laminae to the interradicular septum.

In this situation both dura and arachnoid are susceptible to the repetitive, minor, mechanical trauma of stretching, and of impingement on adjacent foraminal margins as a consequence of degenerative change altering foraminal relationships; the resulting granulation tissue frequently leads to fibrosis and scarring, with the tethering effects of root sleeve fibrosis[391] (see pp. 100, and 102).

The innermost layer, the pia mater, is a highly vascular and delicate membrane consisting of fine areolar tissue supporting numerous small blood vessels, separated from the arachnoid by the subarachnoid space, which contains the cerebrospinal fluid. The spinal membrane is altogether firmer and thicker than the intracranial pia mater, and it is intimately adherent to the spinal cord, lining the anterior median fissure and forming a sheath for the ventral and dorsal spinal roots as far distally as the interradicular septum.

It forms the ligamentum denticulatum, a series of triangular tooth-like processes lying between ventral and dorsal roots and extending laterally to attach by their points to the inner aspect of the dura mater. The 21 processes on each side begin at the level of the C1 spinal nerve root and end between the levels of exit of T12 and L1 roots. The upper 'teeth' are almost perpendicular; the uppermost and stoutest of these is attached to the dura inside the posterior cranial fossa, behind the canal for the 12th cranial nerve. The ligaments are organised to sustain a degree of tension, and when cut from their dural attachments they contract right down to the cord. The position and form of the dentate ligaments change during vertebral movement.[314]

The pia mater ends with the termination of the spinal cord, the conus medullaris, at the level of L1–L2 vertebral segments, and thereafter a fine filament of connective tissue, the filum terminale, descends from the caudal apex of the conus to attach to the dorsum of the first coccygeal segment. The roots comprising the cauda equina therefore embrace the filum terminale. Particularly in the cervical spine, the dural root sleeves are loosely attached to the margins of the intervertebral foramen.[1193]

EFFECTS OF VERTEBRAL MOVEMENT

The coverings of the spinal cord permit it to move about within the limitations imposed by connective tissue tethering, the nerve roots, cranial and caudal attachments and the ligamentum denticulatum. The dural sac changes its configuration considerably during exertion and straining. These effects are observed myelographically when the patent is asked to strain.[315]

While the spinal cord, meninges and nerve roots are affected by vertebral movement, postures and pressure differences,[119] the cord does not slide up and down the neural canal to any appreciable degree—its movement in the cervical spine, for example, is only 2–3 mm at the most, although Reid (1960)[1024] refers to higher averages. The cord and its attachments deform like an accordion as the dimensions of its protective canal change with movement.[1306] It sustains tension, and its position relative to the anterior and posterior wall of the canal is changeable. The reason why cord and dura become taut *together* appears to lie in the nature and number of ligamenta denticulata. Any small up-and-down movement of either cord or dura is quickly transmitted one to the other. Pull on nerve roots transmits its effects to the cord via the dural sheath and the dentate ligaments rather than via the rootlets. Cephalic traction on the dura is found to be equally as effective in applying tension to the cord as is caudal traction.[1024]

Injuries to the cord and nerve roots may come about as a result of loss of plasticity, ischaemia induced by either local or more remote effects, pathological displacement of vertebra, degenerative trespass by structures forming the protective neural canal and by violent traumatic distraction of nerve root attachments. After degenerative change of the cervical intervertebral discs, for example, when the vertebral bodies settle like a pile of dishes, the neural canal is shortened and the relatively inelastic dura mater will fold. Since it is tough, in certain circumstances the folds may produce lesions due to trespass upon structures within the canal.[117]

Adhesions following haemorrhages, exudes and inflammation will cause shrinkage and stiffening of the tissues and loss of elasticity of membranes. This, in turn, leads to abnormal tensions on the cord and nerve roots....

It has been suggested that the dentate ligaments hold the cervical spinal cord against the spondylotic ridges,[626] but division of these ligamentous 'teeth' does not have any effect on minimising cord pressure against the ridges.[1024]

Cervical region

Many authors have drawn attention to the discrepancy which may exist between the severity of signs and symptoms in cervical spondylosis and cervical myelopathy, and the minor nature of protrusions into the canal, or lack of evidence of cord compression. Elucidations of the factors underlying the discrepancy concentrate on the mechanical means whereby during certain movements and postures the cord may be forcedly compressed against any protrusion present, and its free mobility hampered by narrowing of the canal or by abnormal tethering of the cord in an anterior position.[120] A further and important factor is cord ischaemia due to trespass upon vessels sometimes remote from the site of its most potent effects.[656, 426]

The radicular arteries invariably lie on the anterior aspect of the nerve root. Active movements normally exert effects of tension and relaxation of the spinal cord, meninges and nerve roots.[981] Whenever the cord shortens or lengthens, its cross-sectional area increases or decreases respectively.[120] During *extension* of the cervical spine, for example, the spinal cord and roots become relatively slack,[117] and the flaccid cord deviates according to gravity towards the front or back of the spinal canal, depending upon the prone or supine position.[120] The canal is narrowed from front to back, and small ridges are raised over each disc on the anterior wall of the canal.[1024] The inelastic dura mater cockles up to a degree and the elastic ligamentum flavum bulges forward into the neural canal.

In *flexion*, the slack in cord and roots is taken up, and tension in them rises; the stretched cord is strongly applied against any spondylotic ridges or protrusions which may be present.[130]

Flexion of the cervical spine places tension on the lumbar and sacral nerve roots, as well as those of the cervical and thoracic region.[1193]

During *rotation* dorsal roots on the same side are stretched and anterior roots relaxed, and opposite effects are produced on the other side. Lateral flexion, as would be expected, shortens the neural canal on the same side and lengthens it on the opposite side. The inextensible dentate ligaments of the pia mater can, during neck movements, exert undue traction on the spinal cord when relationships have been disturbed by degenerative change. Microscopic studies show that while the longitudinal neurones of the spinal cord are straight during flexion, they assume a wavy course when the cord is relaxed during extension.[130]

On cervical flexion, extension and rotation, the spinal cord follows the shortest route through the neural canal[981] and consequently *the form* of the cord substance, its tracts and neurones and its blood vessels are modified by these tensions, distortions and relaxations.

A bony protrusion, thickened soft tissue or a ventral neoplasm of the spinal cord will deflect the cord backwards as a flat bow, during cervical flexion. Further, a localised intramedullary haemorrhage, a glial scar of demyelinating disease, intramedullary tumours and connective-tissue scars from cord injury will force the surrounding tissue into a spindle-shaped formation.[121a] The intensity of effect upon individual neurones increases with the size of the impinging structure and the degree of spinal cord tension.

In a study of 42 unselected autopsy cases, Breig, Turnbull and Hassler (1966)[120] describe deformations of the cord induced by flexion and extension movements in those with and without spondylosis. The spinal cord specimens were grooved anteriorly where it has been pulled taut over the spondylotic bars in 13 of the 17 preparations fixed in cervical flexion. The spinal cord became flattened with the A-P dimensions reduced. The flattening was frequently bilateral, although unilateral in some. The authors observe that pressure on the anterior spinal artery or arteries during cervical flexion may inhibit blood flow past a spondylotic ridge during life. Little blood would flow through the capillary network when it had been flattened by the stresses which flatten the cord opposite a spondylotic ridge during flexion. Nervous tissue is highly vulnerable to anoxia. Circulatory depletion for around 10 minutes is enough to cause injury.

Barré (1924)[68] suggested that the myelopathy of cervical spondylosis was caused by ischaemia, noting that degenerative trespass upon *radicular* arteries would impair the blood supply of the cord. Freid, Doppman and Di Chiro (1970)[384] studied the cervical cord blood supply in rhesus monkeys, and their findings indicated (a) that blood enters the cervical spinal cord mainly from the radicular arteries, and (b) it is doubtful that the vertebral arteries provide its main blood supply.

Gooding (1974)[426] draws attention to the fact that the myelopathic cord is seldom compressed when seen at operation, and even when compression is present, there is often a disappointing lack of clinical improvement when the compression is relieved.[1206]

In less than half of the patients with this condition does the level of the neurological abnormality correspond to the radiological levels of the bony lesions.[112]

There is the paradox of ischaemic myelopathy without an obvious vascular lesion. Spondylotic trespass is plain, compressive distortion of the cord's normal configuration on neck flexion is plain and local interference with its vascularity is plain. Pathological studies of spinal cord lesions[656] support the view that local ischaemia is the final step in pathogenesis of spinal myelopathy.[120] Yet *atheroma* of the spinal cord vessels, even in severe myelopathy, is very rare;[704] also, Breig observed that no *occluded* radicular artery had ever been demonstrated postmortem in cases of cervical myelopathy.

Gooding[425] comments that the radicular arteries form an important part of the cord's arterial supply[384] and mentions that since they traverse the IVF they are almost always involved in fibrotic change of the dural and arachnoid ostia of the root (Frykholm's root sleeve fibrosis, p. 102), associated with degenerative change. He observed that irritation of these vessels by trespass upon the foramina by degenerative tissue, producing *segmental vascular spasm* of the pia mater arterial network, combined with moderate cervical-cord compression, may be the twofold mechanism underlying the production of myelopathy.

Arterial spasm of the radicular and pial vessels is not uncommonly seen at operation and can be experimentally produced by trauma. In dogs, experimentally induced moderate cervical cord compression and ischaemia combined, produced more severe loss of vascular autoregulation, and more severe myelopathy, than either mechanism alone.[425]

In summary of the author's comments, degenerative change appears to remain the culprit, and possibly in the forms of spondylosis of the vertebral interbody joints *together* with fibrosis of the meningeal lamella of the root sleeve. Whether cervical flexion, by exerting tension on the contents of the intervertebral foramen, or cervical extension, by approximating the margins of the foramen, be the more potent movement or posture exacerbating the condition is probably a factor varying between individual patients, but cervical flexion would appear to be the posture responsible for the two-fold effects postulated above.

The probability that cervical myelopathy may be due to the combination of compressive and ischaemic factors is supported by the experimental findings of Hoff *et al.* (1977)[556] who discuss the multifactorial nature of the pathological changes.

When the cord is relaxed, the cord tracts and neurones are no longer subjected to pressure and distortion, and in a variety of neurological disorders a striking reduction, and even abolition, of symptoms can be achieved by surgical immobilisation of the cervical spine in a position of *slight* extension.[121a]

Cervicothoracic region

Nathan (1970)[904] observed that in a majority (76 per cent) of cases a variable number of spinal roots, more usually in the lower cervical and upper thoracic segments, followed an angulated course. Within the dura, the rootlets proceeded downwards for a variable distance and on piercing the dura were sharply angulated upwards to reach the portal of the intervertebral foramen. Since the extraforaminal course is again downwards, a handful of spinal roots (commonly occupying a junctional vertebral region prone to trespass by thickened degenerative tissues) have undergone two fairly marked angulations by the time of their emergence from the foramen. The degree of angulations may be as much as 30° and can reach 45° (Fig. 2.14). Irregular and uneven development at the dural sac has been considered as the possible cause of these angulations which may, of course, be further distorted by degenerative changes, particularly dural tethering within the neural canal and root-sleeve tethering at the foramen.

The roots affected are those between C6 and T9, with T2 and T3 most frequently and severely angulated. The angulations are increased when the neck is extended.

Thoracic spine

Reid (1960)[1024] refers to the natural elasticity of the cord and the dura, describing the degree of dorsal lift in the cadaver when the spinal canal is unroofed, but not specifying the degree of longitudinal distraction observed upon experimentally applied tension to a portion of it. Dorsal movement by free lifting, of about 1 cm, was found at the T5 level in about one-third of the cases, although in others the dura seemed rather tight; in the aged, especially, the entire dura appeared crinkled and slack. He studied cord and dura movement in 18 necropsy cases with spines normal for their ages, i.e. 11 males and 7 females between 15–57 years, with an age average of 37 years. At all levels of roots C8 to T5, for example, movement took place both in flexion and extension with a *total* range of movement of up to 1.8 cm.

It was not infrequent for the cervical dura to be quite taut in flexion, while that in the thoracic region was still loose and wrinkled, probably due to connective-tissue tethering and to a lesser extent the tethering effect of nerve roots. There were some differences between individuals. The amount of *stretching* was much less in the thoracic spine than in the neck, and the degree of compression against the anterior wall of the spinal canal varied in different areas. He reports that the amount of *movement* in man appears to be more cephalically, and most over the lowest cervical and upper three thoracic vertebrae, i.e. *movements* are minimal at the C5 root and greatest at C8–T5 approximately, and *stretch* is greatest between roots C2 and T1. Should thoracic stretch be prevented or modified by fixation of dura to disc protrusions, then the full effect of flexion must be borne by such length of cord as is isolated above the area with adhesions.

Average amplitudes during the total flexion-extension movement were as follows:

Root level	No. of observations	Average (mm)
C5	3	3.3
C6	–	—
C8	–	9.0
T1	3	12.7
T3	–	—
T5	3	6.6
T10	3	2.3

N.B. Reference should be made to the full data.[1024]

The author observes that any discussion of root direction, whether based on radiological, surgical or pathological examination, must at the same time specify the position of the head and neck relative to the trunk.

Lumbar region
Sagittal and coronal plane movements of the lumbar spine exert broadly similar effects to those in the cervical spine, on the cauda equina, but rotation movements can have little effect since they are much more limited.

Breig's (1960)[119] studies of the cadaver indicated that on extension from flexion the lumbar intervertebral canal shortens and the neural contents also become shortened

and broader. A slight posterior disc protrusion is evident at all lumbar segments, and the ligamentum flavum becomes slack and its cross-sectional area increases as the dimensions of the intervertebral foramen are reduced. The available space in the canal may be reduced to critical dimensions, this factor being more pronounced if a degree of developmental stenosis is present, together with acquired stenosis in the form of degenerative trespass by thickened sclerous and soft tissue.

On flexion, the length of the posterior wall of the lumbar canal increases by about 25 per cent, the vertebral canal lengthening by up to 7 cm.[593, 434] Meningeal tissue is unable to stretch that much, hence the need for the cord and its coverings to possess a degree of anteroposterior mobility and the roots to move in and out of the foramina to a degree.

In the cadaver, full flexion exerts traction on the dural sac, so that the roots are perforce drawn into the intervertebral foramen for varying distances, i.e.:

L1 and L2 roots	between 2–5 mm
L3 root	less than 2 mm
L4 root	negligible movement[434]

Two points should be noted:
1. Movements imposed upon the cadaver may not have the same mechanical effect on a living patient:
   a. bending forward from the neutral standing position
   b. sitting with legs dangling over the plinth edge while one knee is passively extended.
   c. sitting on a horizontal surface with legs extended and then reaching forward to the toes.
2. The straight-leg-raising test does not induce the same mechanical disturbance of the dura and nerve roots as does lumbar flexion; one essential difference is that in flexion, during clinical examination, the lumbar spine is bearing weight (as also in sitting) and the lumbar and haunch musculature are stabilising the superincumbent weight of a trunk which is being displaced somewhat outside the confines of its supporting base.

The strong stabilising contractions of powerful muscles may well add circumferential bulging of the lumbar discs, thereby inducing a space-occupying effect upon the neural canal during flexion from the standing position. Yet an important factor is, that in comparison with the straight-leg-raising test on a supine patient, the canal may well be somewhat shortened overall by the compressive effects of stabilising contractions during the lumbar flexion movement.

The essential point is the element of doubt, and therefore discrepancies between the angle at which straight-leg-raising is painfully limited, and the degree of limitation of lumbar flexion, should not immediately be ascribed to the untruthfulness of a lead-swinging patient.

The diagnosis 'plumbus oscillans' is justified when the workshy patient's real motive is legalised idleness; in the author's experience it is more frequently a superficial and insulting judgment upon a person who seeks help for pain and distress, but who has been insufficiently examined by a lazy or doctrinaire and unimaginative clinical worker.

The sciatic nerve has elasticity, the dura has little, and when considering the straight-leg-raising test and its effects, it is important to distinguish between what happens to the sciatic *nerve* and *when* it happens, and what is happening to the more proximal *roots* of the nerve.

Charnley[169] states that the nerve 'emerging from the intervertebral foramina' descends in almost a straight line through the pelvis. Goddard and Reid[416] show the roots L4,5 and S2,3 run in a sigmoid course through the foramina, i.e. there is slack to be taken up. S1 root runs most straight and direct (Fig. 2.15). The relatively long lengths of lumbosacral nerves and nerve roots attenuate peak stresses fairly efficiently,[592, 562] with the exception of S1 root which is comparatively taut and unyielding with its root sleeve attached to the margins of the first sacral foramen.

The lumbosacral cord (L4, L5) runs over a marked convexity at the ala of the sacrum, then it runs back, down and laterally to the greater sciatic notch.

During straight-leg-raising the sciatic nerve trunk is first drawn straight downwards through the greater sciatic

notch and then more anterolaterally, becoming tightly opposed to the underlying bony margins with a quite remarkable degree of pressure. Similar pressures occur between the lumbosacral cord and the ala of the sacrum, and between the roots and pedicles, i.e. the bony threshold of the foramina.

The following is the sequence of events:

1. When the heel is only 5 cm above the horizontal surface (Fig. 2.16), movement of the *nerve* at the greater sciatic notch has begun.

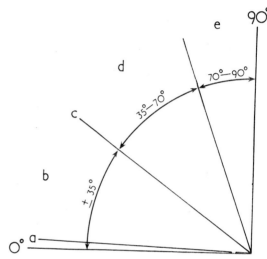

Fig. 2.16 Scheme of straight-leg raising (see text).

2. After a few more degrees the movement begins to occur more proximally as elevation continues, and the lumbosacral cord is now moving over the ala of the sacrum. The roots are still stationary.

3. At around 35° of elevation, movement of the roots now begins at the intervertebral foramen.

4. During the arc of movement from about 35°–70° the roots are moving their greatest amount.

5. Between 70°–90° there is very little *movement* at all, only the increasing development of *tension*.

Goddard and Reid[416] suggest that where downward movement is less, (a) tension in the nerve, and (b) pressure over bony prominences, is correspondingly increased.

Table of average movement (in subjects between 35–55 years) (after Goddard and Reid):

		Movement
Roots at foramina	L4	1.5 mm
	L5	3.0 mm
	S1	4.0 mm
Lumbosacral cord at ala of sacrum		4.5 mm
Nerve at sciatic notch		6.5 mm

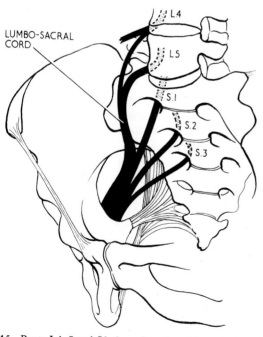

Fig. 2.15 Roots L4, 5 and S2, 3 run in a sigmoid course through the foramina—S1 root runs most straight and direct. (After: Goddard MD, Reid JM 1965 Movements induced by straight leg raising in the lumbosacral roots, nerves and plexus, and in the intrapelvic portion of the sciatic nerve. Journal of Neurology, Neurosurgery and Psychiatry 28: 12.)

Again, it will be seen that the effect on L4 is small (see also femoral nerve stretch, p. 319). A considerable increase of tension, in the sciatic nerve, is induced by holding the raised limb and then internally rotating it to the fullest extent. Straight-leg-raising produces its effects mostly ipsilaterally but can also produce contralateral effects; symptom-aggravation in the resting, painful limb of opposite side. This is said by many to occur more usually in L4–5 level joint problems.

Cailliet's[150] figures for root movement during straight-leg-raising agree broadly with those given above, but he asserts that *during bending forward in standing* the greatest root movement is at L2–3; there is less at L3–4 and none at L4, 5 and S1. This raises many interesting questions. Many people have a 5°–10° normal discrepancy between limits of left and right straight-leg-raising, and the normal full range can be anything between an angle of 75°–120°, measured between longitudinal axis of leg and horizontal surface of couch.

Throughout its course, the sciatic nerve and its roots are tethered by innumerable filmy strands of tissue to underlying fascia and periosteum of bone. In some cadavers, very dense adhesions are found between the plexus and the periosteum, at points far removed from the spinal canal. In two of the cadavers examined,[416] a convincing diagnosis of sciatica had been made before death; no disc herniation was found at post-mortem, only dense adhesions at points *distal* to the foramina. Contrary to what Charnley[169] asserts, the sciatic nerve has elastic properties and this is why movement is progressively less towards the foramina, i.e. proximally. When present, the hamstring spasm[979] which prevents full leg-raising is presumably a protective mechanism, a reflex guarding response initiated by the afferent neurones of the sinuvertebral nerve (ramus meningeus) which, together with the fibres from Stillwell's paravertebral plexus, medial branches from the posterior primary rami of lumbar roots (and autonomic fibres) is distributed to *all* the structures which could be involved in low backache of articular origin.[1354, 1361, 1362, 1177]

N.B. Pedersen *et al.*, in 1956[979] crushed vertebral joint structures in experimental animals and the standard response to artificial trauma of fascia, ligaments, capsule, muscle and periosteum was the same, *viz.* reflex spasm of mainly ipsilateral dorsal muscle and also hamstrings. They emphasise the poor localisation of pain associated with deep lesions of the lumbosacral area, and the difficulty of localising those lesions on the basis of physical findings.

Besides its well-appreciated traction effects on the sciatic nerve and lumbosacral roots, the test also tends to move, because of the lumbar-spine-flexion effect via the pelvis, *joints* which may be irritable, the joints between vertebral bodies, and also the synovial facet joints. The pelvis is tilted backwards in the sagittal plane, and also upwards in the frontal plane, i.e. a lateral tilt upwards on the tested side. The pelvis is also slightly rotated towards the untested side, all of these effects occurring towards the end of range in the normal person.

Because a clinical movement-test (or manipulation technique, for that matter) we choose may indeed move the tissue in which we are presently interested, we should not exclude from our assessment the fact that a whole family of other tissues is also being moved.

Further, the transforaminal ligament of Golub[422] may impinge upon the root as a form of partial strangulation during clinical procedures which apply tension to the root. This variable connective tissue structure is sometimes attached to the root perineurium, and the effects of its impingement may at times simulate the clinical features of disc trespass in patients with normal lumbar discs.

For those who do not enjoy easy access to dissection specimens, with opportunities to look for oneself, difficulties sometimes arise in co-ordinating the assertions of writers of more authority who have access to such facilities. For example, it is stated quite categorically that:

The nerve complex is not attached to the wall of the foramen, the arrangement permitting it to move within and through the foramen ... which allows it to adjust throughout the normal range of vertebral movements. ... the only attachment of the nerve complex to bone is in the cervical region, where the spinal nerve is adherent to the gutter of the transverse process. (Sunderland, 1975.[1193])

On the other hand, Brodal (1969)[130] refers to the nerve roots as:

... solidly fixed in the intervertebral foramina ... pain on Lasegue's test may in part be due to the ventroflexion of the spine which ensues when the leg is raised with concomitant stretching of the roots.

VENOUS DRAINAGE

The venous drainage of the vertebral column is especially rich, the internal venous plexus together with fat almost completely filling out the space between vertebral bodies and meninges, and freely anastomosing with the external vertebral plexuses; beginning an efficient transport and distributive system from the haemopoeitically active spongiosa of vertebral bodies.

The system also acts as a 'pressure-absorber' when trunk-cavity pressure rises, by virtue of its extensive communication with other veins. At the upper part of the system the cervical vertebral veins connect with the basilar plexus, the occipital sinus and cranial emissary veins, and thus with the intracranial venous sinuses.[772, 1272]

Vertebral veins in the neck, and the thoracic, lumbar and sacral vertebral venous plexuses together constitute a valveless venous pathway between the intracranial venous sinuses and the whole length of the spine, freely connected to the main venous system through the pelvic plexuses, ascending lumbar veins, the azygos system and the segmental veins at each level—the system therefore provides an alternative venous channel which can bypass one vena cava, and the cardiopulmonary or portal system. It is extensive enough to provide a venous return when a vena cava is obstructed.[338, 532, 535]

Under normal conditions, the direction of flow is quite variable and fluctuates with changes in pressure in the two systems (vertebral and caval). Further, persisting increases of vertebral venous pressure are associated with pregnancy and chronic respiratory and cardiac disease.[1362] With every rise of pressure in the trunk, as during lifting, coughing, sneezing, holding one's breath, straining, bending and twisting and during rotational trunk manipulations of any firmness, venous blood is not only prevented from entering the thoraco-abdominal cavity but is actually shunted to the vertebral system, and in many patients with low back pain these activities, which cause a rise in venous pressure, exacerbate their pain. Venous blood thus temporarily or more permanently shunted into the vertebral system, and via this the intracranial sinuses, can only be accommodated by a movement of cerebrospinal fluid from the intracranial subarachnoid space into that of the spinal column.

It has been suggested that during the lifting of weights greater than 22.5 kg (50 lb) a combination of raised intra-abdominal pressure, and the presence of the posterior longitudinal ligament together impede the rate of outflow of blood from the vertebral body, and thereby increases its crush strength (Farfan, 1975[331]). The mechanism of venous outflow impedance is thought to raise the compression strength of the vertebral body closer to that of the intervertebral disc.

The *jugular compression test* (applying firm and sustained pressure to the veins at the side of the neck) also provides an example of how the raising of pressure in the venous system can increase low back pain; sometimes paraesthesiae in the lower limbs can be produced by this manœuvre, and further aggravated by simultaneous pressure applied to the abdomen.

As elsewhere in the body the adventitia of vertebral veins and venules, as well as arteries and arterioles, are supplied with a dense plexiform arrangement of unmyelinated nerve fibres,[1362] which constitute an important part of the nociceptor system of the vertebral column, and which may be irritated in a variety of ways to give rise to pain.

The cancellous bone of vertebral bodies and their apophyses, the sacrum and ilium, the connective tissues of joints and the vertebral muscles, are all populated to a greater or lesser degree by this nociceptor network accompanying both the arterial and venous systems, and there are reasons for the view that veins act as a hollow viscus, like the gut, in which distension can be acutely painful. The adult vertebral venous system contains about 200 ml of blood, and when flow is impeded by space-occupying trespass of adjacent vertebral tissues, the resulting congestion may increase this volume to around 500 ml.[279]

As with other lesions causing spinal cord compression and obstruction in the neural canal, arthrotic and spondylotic lesions are accompanied by a dilatation of veins, both in epidural and subarachnoid spaces, and this contributes to the obstructive process. The phenomenon of pain exacerbation is also explained on the basis of temporarily engorged vertebral veins impinging on adjacent, irritable nerve roots, and again, it is seen that compression of jugular veins produces a rise in pressure of the intraspinal fluid (c.s.f.) and this in turn is likely to produce a tendency to stretching of the dura mater and thus the dural sleeve enclosing an inflamed and sensitised nerve root.

Venous engorgement and stasis has been named as one of the causes of pain in cervical spondylosis, this factor adding to the combined trespass on cervical roots.[115]

Back pain in osteoporosis may be due to the venous stasis in the spongiosa of vertebral bodies.[777]

Macnab (1977)[780] discusses the pain of osteoporosis, which is often ascribed to trabecular buckling or trabecular fractures. He observes that while the bone mass is markedly diminished, the size of the unwedged vertebral body is unchanged, so that the volume of its contents (marrow, fat and blood) must be greater. Since the fat content actually remains the same the volume of blood, and thus venous stasis, are increased.

The interosseous venous pressure of a normal vertebra is about 28 mmHg (3.73 kPa) and that of an osteoporotic vertebra is about 40 mmHg (5.33 kPa). He suggests that venous stasis in vertebral bodies may partly underlie the dull, constant pain of osteoporosis.

Where a vertebral venous plexus is already under the tension of engorgement because of space-occupying effects of disc herniations or prolapses, arachnoiditis, oedema, ligamentous flavum bulging and other modes of trespass, it is not surprising that a sudden additional increment of tension by coughing, for instance, should hurt the patient, although the precise mechanism may not be fully explained.

The venous pattern in vertebrae is similar to that in the region of the hip and knee joints,[42, 43, 44] and experimental findings point to a connection between aching pain, elevation of intraosseous pressure and impaired drainage conditions.[47]

The radiographic changes of juxtachondral bone in arthrosis of large peripheral joints seem very similar to spondylotic changes observed in the vertebral column of patients with low back disorders.

Venable and Shuck (1946)[1266] and Palazzi (1957–8)[964] observed immediate relief of pain on resecting a fragment of cortical bone from the femoral neck. Arnoldi's[43] findings, by intraosseous phlebography of 30 patients with unilateral hip arthrosis and no cardiac involvement, indicate that there is disturbed venous flow in the femoral heads of these patients, and the same findings have been noted in relation to the knee, i.e.:

1. Phlebography indicated a state of intramedullary venous engorgement in arthrosis.

2. Pressure in the femoral head of the arthrotic hip was higher than in the unaffected hip.

3. The normal channels for venous drainage were not visible in phlebographs from the arthrotic side, and the emptying of contrast material was usually delayed.

4. Phlebographs indicated that the abnormally high intraosseous pressure is caused by a high resistance to flow across the proximal part of the femur.

5. The typical aching rest pain of severe arthrosis was noted in association with femoral neck pressures above 40 mmHg.

6. The decreased difference between arterial and venous pressure is probably accompanied by nutritive disturbance.

In a later paper Arnoldi[42] describes introducing 1.4 mm-bore needles into the bone marrow of the 2nd, 4th and 5th lumbar spinous processes, and reading intramedullary pressures, in 20 patients; 10 had no radiographic evidence of disc degeneration, and 10 had radiographically evident spondylotic changes. Eight of the latter group had a history of intermittent or constant severe low back pain of long standing, and the remaining 2 had suffered severe lumbar pain together with sciatica.

1. The mean intraosseous pressure in the 'normal' group was 8.3 mmHg (1.10 kPa); pressure curves were always pulsatile, with *coughing* resulting in an immediate pressure rise and *straining* causing a more gradual rise.

2. In the spondylotic group the mean intraosseous pressure was 28.0 mmHg (3.73 kPa) and as in the controls coughing and straining were accompanied by increased pressure at all points of measurement.

The medullary cavity of spinous processes directly communicates with that of the vertebral body.

While patients with asymptomatic lumbar spondylosis were not included in the series, the findings seem to indicate that intraosseous hypertension may well be one cause of low back pain.[44]

Jones and Wise (1967)[617] experimentally induced Scheuermann's disease (p. 136) in primate animals, and attributed the changes observed to venous obstruction.

Engorgement of the epidural venous plexuses may contribute to acquired spinal stenosis ('f', p. 148).

Kéry et al. (1971)[654] produced venous stasis by tourniquets applied to rats' tails for various lengths of time, and found that lesions of bone, cartilage and spinal discs following venous stasis were more severe than those produced by arterial ischaemia of the same duration; the reparative potentiality of the tissues was also more depressed by venous stasis than by arterial ischaemia.

Vertebral venography,[772, 1272] a radiographic technique of injecting contrast medium via catheterisation of the femoral vein, has been successful in providing clear evidence of lumbar disc trespass. In 29 of 32 cases, protrusions were found at operation, when myelography indicated the trespass in only 20.

The subject is ambulant after the procedure, which can be employed on an outpatient basis. Clarke et al. (1977)[178] have drawn attention to the accuracy of ascending lumbar venography and by comparison with other investigation procedures the advantage of its fewer side effects.

AUTONOMIC NERVOUS SYSTEM

In attempting to elucidate the symptom-complexes of vertebral degenerative joint disease, autonomic nerve distribution and function, and visceral reflex activity, are of more than passing importance, e.g. in the syndrome of vertebral artery insufficiency, the dysequilibrium and nausea which often accompany upper cervical joint problems, the distressing sequelae of acceleration and deceleration trauma, the group of conditions represented by the shoulder–hand syndrome, involvement and entrapment of splanchnic nerves in anterior osteophytes of the thoracolumbar spine, and in the cold sciatic leg.

Further, serious disease of thoracic and abdominal viscera can simulate the referred pain of benign vertebral joint problems; some of these factors are discussed under 'Referred Pain'.

A glance at the intimate involvement of autonomic nerve pathways, sharing the innervation of spinal musculoskeletal tissues (Figs 1.14–1.19) with somatic nerves, will indicate the necessity of understanding this innervation and its implications.

The many descriptions of this innervation are not new. Simplified mechanical concepts, of the cause and effect of vertebral treatment techniques, are plainly an inadequate basis for discussion of treatment methods.

While the classical concept is that the autonomic nervous system regulates physiological activities at an involuntary level, below consciousness, evidence is accumulating that control of some autonomic functions can be learned, both by animals and humans.[332]

The autonomic part of the nervous system has acquired a large and steadily growing importance in neurology as well as in several other clinical disciplines ... there is good reason to believe that the autonomic nervous system is involved in producing some of the symptoms in a multitude of diseases which do not primarily affect the system itself.[130]

'Autonomic' means operating in isolation, but this is a misnomer since there is the greatest possible integration between the autonomic and the somatic system; the autonomy of the system is non-existent, but the old distinction does have some value in the sense that this division of the nervous system proceeds by itself, yet wholly and intimately related to the rich volume of afferent traffic from both the somatic and visceral receptors.

The division of the autonomic nervous system into sympathetic and parasympathetic systems rests on the anatomical, functional and pharmacological differences between them.[437]

1. ANATOMICAL

1. The sympathetic system comprises a demonstrable system of ganglionated trunks with their branches of distribution. The parasympathetic system, like a cuckoo in

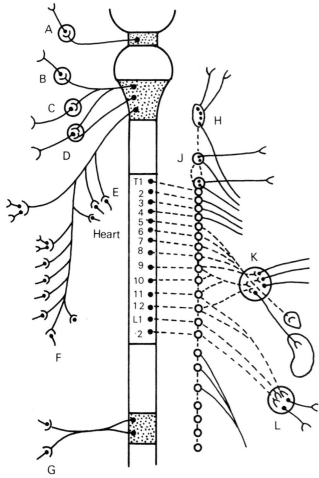

Fig. 2.17 *General plan of autonomic nervous system.* On *left:* Cranial and sacral autonomic (parasympathetic) system. Thick lines from III, VII, IX, X, and S.2, 3 are preganglionic (connector) fibres. A, ciliary ganglion; B, sphenopalatine ganglion; C, submaxillary and sublingual ganglia. D, otic ganglion; E, vagus ganglion cells in nodes of heart; F, vagus ganglion cells in wall of bowel; G, sacral autonomic ganglion cells in pelvis; thin lines beyond = postganglionic (excitor) fibres. On *right:* Sympathetic nervous system. Dotted lines from T1–12, L1, 2 are preganglionic fibres; H, superior cervical ganglion; J, middle and inferior cervical ganglia (the latter fused with the 1st thoracic ganglion to form the stellate ganglion); K, coeliac and other abdominal ganglia (note preganglionic fibres directly supplying the adrenal medulla); L, lower abdominal and pelvic sympathetic ganglia; continuous lines beyond = postganglionic fibres. (Reproduced, with legend, from Samson Wright's Applied Physiology, 1971, 12 edn, by kind permission of C. A. Keele and the Oxford University Press.)

the nest, utilises cranial and spinal nerves for its pathways, and is therefore difficult to demonstrate.

2. In classical descriptions, sympathetic fibres emerge from the central nervous system via thoracolumbar somatic nerves, i.e. segments T1–L2 (but see p. 10), while parasympathetic fibres emerge via cranial nerves III, VII, IX, X and sacral somatic nerves S234, i.e. a cranio-sacral outflow.

3. Sympathetic fibres have short preganglionic neurones, synapse in proximal paravertebral ganglia, and have long postganglionic fibres. Parasympathetic fibres have long preganglionic neurones, synapse in peripheral ganglia located close to, and often in, the viscus or organs they serve, and thus postganglionic neurones are very short (Fig. 2.17).

4. Arterioles, glands and arrectores pilorum muscle of the body surface are supplied with sympathetic nerves; the innervation of various regions of the skin of trunk and limb girdles has the same segmental representation as the splanchnic supply to large viscera. These skin areas are Head's zones of cutaneous hyperalgesia (see p. 178 and 'Referred pain').

There is no parasympathetic supply to the arterioles of skin or to musculoskeletal tissues.

2. FUNCTIONAL OR PHYSIOLOGICAL DIFFERENCES (Table 2.3)

In general terms, the sympathetic nervous system is organised to mobilise the body's resources for rapid expenditure of energy in emergencies ('fright, fight, flight'), it dilates the eye, bronchi and bronchial vessels, coronary vessels and skeletal muscle vessels, raises pulse rate and thus blood pressure and reduces blood flow for all activities which are, at that time, non-essential, i.e. peristalsis, digestive activity and blood supply to the skin, etc. Blood is therefore diverted for the vital functions. Also there is a widespread discharge of sympathetic impulses during physiological stress, such as: severe muscular work, danger, extreme temperature, asphyxia, rage, haemorrhage, fear, pain.

Conversely, the parasympathetic system is generally directed to the conservation and restoration of the energy resources of the body, and is organised as the effector for visceral motor systems and, one might say, some of the pleasures of life, distributing blood for the functions of the digestive tube, the skin, and so on.

Further, sympathetic reactions are mass responses of the whole animal, whereas parasympathetic effects are localised reactions, e.g. salivation.

3. THE PHARMACOLOGICAL DIFFERENCES ARE:

1. The chemical transmitter (except in four cases, i.e. sweat glands, muscle arterioles, the uterus, the adrenal

Table 2.1 Sympathetic

Organs supplied	Site of connector cells	Site of ganglion cells	Route of postganglionic fibres
Head and neck	T1, 2	Superior cervical ganglion	
1. Eye	,,		Along internal carotid artery
2. Face	,,		Along external carotid artery
3. Skin of head and neck	,,	,, ,,	With cervical plexus
4. Cerebral vessels	,,	Superior and inferior cervical ganglia	Along internal carotid and vertebral arteries
Thoracic viscera	T3, 4	Superior, middle and inferior cervical ganglia (man, Stellate ganglion (animals)	Cardiac branches of sympathetic
Fore limb	T5–9 (sometimes also T2–4)	Middle and inferior cervical, first and second thoracic ganglia (man) Stellate ganglion (animals)	With brachial plexus
Hind limb	T10–L2	Lumbar and sacral ganglia	With lumbosacral plexus
Abdomen 1. Viscera of abdomen proper	T6–L2 T6–12 (chiefly)	Upper abdominal ganglia (superior mesenteric, coeliac, etc.)	Along blood vessels
2. Pelvic viscera	L1, 2 (chiefly)	Inferior mesenteric ganglia (animals) Hypogastric ganglia (man)	Along blood vessels and in hypogastric nerves
Thoracic and abdominal parietes	T1–12	Ganglia of lateral sympathetic chain	With intercostal nerves

Tables 2.1–2.3 are reproduced from Samson Wright's *Applied Physiology*, 1971, 12 edn, by kind permission of C. A. Keele and the Oxford University Press.

gland itself) at postganglionic sympathetic nerve endings is noradrenalin, consequently they are 'adrenergic' endings, while that liberated by parasympathetic postganglionic endings is acetycholine, hence they are termed 'cholinergic'.[635]

2. In general, drugs which affect the sympathetic system have no effect on the parasympathetic system, and vice versa, e.g. atropine is a parasympathetic inhibitor, acting directly on the effector organs. Pilocarpine has the opposite effect, in general stimulating cholinergically innervated organs and increasing glandular secretion by inhibiting acetylcholinesterase; eserine (physostigmine) has the same general effect.

All preganglionic autonomic fibres liberate acetylcholine, whether sympathetic or parasympathetic.

The chemistry of autonomic postganglionic transmitters appears to be linked to receptor substance, and involves complex enzymatic reactions.[130]

Sympathetic fibres are very widely distributed and the number of postganglionic fibres from the paravertebral ganglia exceeds that of preganglionic fibres, e.g. at the superior cervical ganglion, the ratio of preganglionic to postganglionic is given as 1 : 196, hence the system is very diversified.[437]

So far as intra- and extracranial, and cervical, structures are concerned, interconnections with cranial nerves and somatic roots are very complex indeed. Via the three cervical sympathetic ganglia, the paravertebral ganglia and the coeliac and two mesenteric ganglia, fibres are distributed to eye, glands and arterioles of skin, and arterioles of voluntary muscle in limbs and trunk, to cardiac, respiratory and digestive system, to bladder, sphincters and genitalia, e.g. each of the five sacral nerves and the coccygeal nerve receive a grey rami communicans from the corresponding ganglion of the sympathetic trunk.

The parasympathetic system, while having a very limited origin from cranial and sacral nerves, also has a large, but less wide, distribution, e.g. the vagus (X cranial nerve) supplies the heart, bronchi, digestive tube, genitalia, bladder and sphincters, all of the neurones synapsing in

Table 2.2 Parasympathetic

Cranial nerve	Site of connector cells	Site of ganglion cells	Structures supplied
III	Cranial part of IIIrd nerve nucleus	Ciliary ganglion	Sphincter pupillae Ciliary muscle
VII	Dorsal nucleus of VIIth nerve (Superior salivary nucleus)	Sphenopalatine ganglion In salivary glands.	Lacrimal gland Submaxillary and sublingual glands
IX	Dorsal nucleus of IXth nerve (Inferior salivary nucleus)	Otic ganglion	Parotid gland
X	Dorsal nucleus of Xth nerve (Vagus)	*Heart.* Sinoatrial and atrioventricular nodes	Atrial and junctional tissue
		Bronchi. Local	Smooth muscle Mucous glands
		Alimentary canal Myenteric (Auerbach's) plexus Submucous (Meissner's) plexus	Gastric and intestinal glands Smooth muscle Pancreas: exocrine and endocrine cells
Sacral	Segments 2 and 3 of sacral cord *Nervi erigentes*	Hypogastric ganglia	Most of large intestine Bladder Prostate Blood vessels of penis

ganglia situated peripherally, many of them lying in the walls of the viscera, glands and vessels supplied, and most only microscopically visible.

Preganglionic neurones are distributed in the *cranial nerves*:

3rd (oculomotor), i.e. to the intrinsic eye muscles
7th (facial—chorda tympani branch)
9th (glossopharyngeal)
10th (vagus)

and the macroscopic parasympathetic ganglia are:

Ciliary (in orbital fat) efferent fibres to the iris and ciliary muscle of the eye
Sphenopalatine (in pterygopalatine fossa)
Submandibular (in hyoglossus muscle, just above mandibular gland)
Otic (just below the foramen ovale)

The latter three are concerned with efferent impulses to lacrimal and salivary glands.

Table 2.3 Responses of effector organs to autonomic nerve impulses

Organ	Adrenergic nerve impulses	Cholinergic nerve impulses
Eye		
Iris radial muscle	Contraction mydriasis	—
Iris circular muscle (sphincter pupillae)	—	Contraction (miosis)
Ciliary muscle	—	Contraction, accommodation for near vision
Lid smooth muscle	Lid retraction	—
Heart		
S–A Node	Tachycardia	Bradycardia. Cardiac arrest
Atria	Increased contractility and conduction velocity	Decreased contractility Increased conduction velocity
A–V Node and conduction system	Increased conduction velocity	Decreased conduction velocity. A–V block
Ventricles	Increased contractility and conduction velocity Increased irritability; extrasystoles	—
Blood vessels		
Coronary	Dilatation	?
Skin and mucosa	Constriction	—
Skeletal muscle	Constriction	Dilatation
Cerebral	Slight constriction	—
Abdominal visceral	Constriction	
Lung		
Bronchial muscle	Relaxation	Constriction
Bronchial glands	—	Stimulation of mucus secretion
Stomach		
Motility and tone	Decrease	Increase
Sphincters	Contraction	Relaxation
Secretion	Inhibition	Stimulation, especially enzymes
Intestine		
Motility and tone	Decrease	Increase
Sphincters	Contraction	Relaxation
Secretion	?	Increase
Gall-bladder	Relaxation	Contraction
Urinary bladder		
Detrusor	Relaxation	Contraction
Trigone and internal sphincter	Contraction	Relaxation
Ureter		
Motility and tone	?	
Uterus	Variable	Variable
	(responses influenced by female sex hormones and by pregnancy)	
Sex organs	Ejaculation in male	Vasodilatation and erection (penis, clitoris)
Skin		
Arrectores pili	Contraction	—
Sweat glands	—	Secretion
Adrenal medulla	—	Secretion of Ad and NA

The nuclei of the cranial nerves are more or less surrounded by *the reticular formation of the brain stem*, and have intimate functional relations with this.[129]

Sacral parasympathetic fibres emerge with sacral roots 2, 3 and 4, thus comprising the pelvic splanchnic nerves (or visceral branches of the pudendal nerve) and unite with branches of the sympathetic pelvic plexuses.

SYMPATHETIC EFFERENT NEURONES

The sympathetic system is larger than the parasympathetic system, because of its additional rich supply to the skin and to the blood vessels of voluntary muscle and the connective tissues of the locomotor system. All somatic spinal nerves have postganglionic fibres, but only a limited number of roots carry preganglionic fibres.

Over a period of 10 years, Continental anatomists (Tinel (1937),[1220] Laruelle (1940)[699], Guerrier (1944)[461], Delmas (1947)[247], have reported the cell bodies of preganglionic sympathetic neurones in the cervical segments C5–C6–C7–C8 and joining these somatic roots, although most authors give the uppermost as T1.

The French authors stated that the rami communicans from these neurones also make synaptic junctions with the small sympathetic ganglia developed around the vertebral artery in the foramen transversarium between C4 and C6.

Operative findings indicate that many individuals do not have a symmetrical arrangement to the upper limb, and it is known that prefixation and postfixation occurs, as in the somatic limb plexuses.

Swarms of fibres accompany all the vessels, and especially those accompanying the III and V cranial nerves, probably joining them in the cavernous sinus.

Further, (a) the external carotid plexus helps give fibres to the orbit, and also accompanies the lacrimal and frontal (supratrochlear) arteries and (b) the vertebral artery plexus accompanies, among others, the vascular supply to the vestibular structures, the equilibratory organs.

Some organs are innervated by one division only, i.e. most arterioles, the uterus and the adrenal medulla by sympathetic neurones (the latter organ singularly without synapses of the efferent pathway), and the glands of pancreas and stomach by parasympathetic neurones only.[635]

The arrangement whereby both autonomic and somatic efferents are supplied to muscle, as in the anal and urethral sphincters, also occurs in the diaphragm;[540] in addition to somatic fibres from phrenic and intercostal nerves, filaments of sympathetic neurones derived from the coeliac plexus ramify on the inferior surface of the muscle to supply it.

Segmental distribution (Tables 2.1, 2.2)
The salient factors of *sympathetic* fibre distribution are set out in Table 2.1, and those of *parasympathetic* distribution

in Table 2.2, although authors give slightly different values for the segmental derivation of sympathetic neurones to head and neck, upper limb and thoracic viscera, e.g.

	(Gray)[437]	(Grant)[434]
Head and neck	T1–T5	T1–T2
Upper limb	T2–T5	T(2)3–T6(7)
Thoracic viscera		
Heart	T1–T5	T1–T4(5)
Lungs	T2–T4	T2–T6(7)
Oesophagus		
(caudal part)	T5–T6	T4–T6
Lower limb	T10–L2	T10–L2

Table 2.3 sets out the responses to autonomic nerve impulses.[635]

VISCERAL AFFERENT NEURONES

Visceral afferent pathways resemble those of the somatic afferent neurones, the unipolar cells of the peripheral fibres lying in cranial and posterior root ganglia.[437]

For example, the peripheral processes (dendrites) of the vagus nerve converge on the superior and inferior vagal ganglia; other peripheral processes approach the dorsal spinal roots through autonomic plexuses or ganglia, and possibly through somatic nerve trunks, without synapse. Hence the dorsal roots of spinal nerves contain mixed somatic and visceral (so-called 'autonomic') afferent fibres, and after entering the posterior horn they and their ramifications and divisions, via synapses within the cord substance, are diversified up and down the spinal cord to numerous other segments, thereby having available a very rich potential of connector pathways.

Apart from special visceral afferents, e.g. those subserving taste, general visceral afferents form part of the vagus, glossopharyngeal and possibly other cranial nerves, of the thoracic and upper lumbar spinal nerves, and of the second, third and fourth sacral nerves. For example, sensory receptors are found at all levels in the wall of the bladder.[437] The peripheral processes may be unmyelinated or myelinated fibres of assorted diameter, and share the distribution of efferent sympathetic and parasympathetic fibres occurring in the rami communicantes and in pathways for the efferent sympathetic innervation of viscera and blood vessels, with the difference that they do not have synaptic interruptions in the autonomic ganglia.

Terminals are described, for example, in tongue, tonsils, pharynx and oesophagus, in the heart and walls of great vessels (as pressor- and chemoreceptors), pulmonary vessels, bronchial mucosa and smooth muscle, interalveolar connective tissue of lung and in the visceral pleura. Vagal afferent fibres have terminals in the stomach, intestines and digestive glands, and in the kidney, ureters and urethra. Afferent neurones of the pelvic splanchnic nerves innervate the distal colon and pelvic viscera, including the uterus and ovary, although none have been demonstrated in the testes and these may therefore reach the c.n.s. by different routes. Visceral afferent neurones have generally the same segmental arrangement as the pre- and postganglionic sympathetic fibres, ending in the same spinal cord segments giving rise to the efferent pathways to the region or viscus.

Visceral reflexes are initiated by impulses conducted along the pathways described, most not reaching consciousness, with some initiating organic visceral sensations like hunger, nausea, sexual sensation and bladder and rectal distension.

The general visceral afferent neurones entering via the dorsal roots of the thoracic and upper lumbar segments are, in the main, nociceptors, and visceral pain, produced by stretching and excessive contractions of visceral muscle (spasm), pathological changes in viscera and vascular engorgement probably also follow these afferent pathways.

The pain may be felt in the region of the organ itself–so-called 'true' visceral pain–and/or in regions of the body wall and skin, sometimes remote from the seat of initiation of pain, e.g. the pain of cardiac ischaemia is commonly presternal and also referred to left neck, jaw, occiput and inner side of left arm. Conversely, the pain of renal colic occurs more usually in the posterolateral loin of the same side, over the obstructed ureter.

Referred pain is considered on page 189.

CENTRAL AUTONOMIC CONTROL

Regulation of blood pressure, body temperature, glandular secretion and similar visceral functions are integrated at the medulla and the pons, the hypothalamus and cerebral cortex, particularly the cortical and subcortical structures which form a ring around the brain stem. Autonomically regulated responses, similar to those produced on stimulation of the hypothalamus, can be provoked by stimulation of the tegmentum of mid-brain and the periaqueductal grey matter; the three areas are anatomically so adjacent that little functional distinction can be made when stimulation effects are compared.

Autonomic ganglia are only synaptic stations and have no independent activity, yet spinal cord connector cells show a degree of tonic activity, keeping up a level of vaso-constrictor tone after complete section of the cord and thus maintaining a low but stable blood pressure.[635]

PATTERNS OF SOMATIC NERVE ROOT SUPPLY

Neat tabulations of somatic segmental nerve root supply, formulated for convenience when seeking neurological deficit during clinical examination, usually concern only dermatomes, muscles, joint movement and reflexes. It is vital to bear in mind that the *vertebral joints themselves* do not enjoy a segmentally arranged nerve supply, but receive articular nerves derived from the adjacent rostral and caudal segment, in addition to those from the segmentally related nerve root.[1177, 1361a,b, 1362, 1363]

Above the C4 segment it is wise to test muscles supplied by both a.p.r. and p.p.r. Below this, it suffices to test those supplied by a.p.r. only.

Pain referred from a single vertebral segment is not always confined to the related dermatome areas outlined below in Table 2.4 but they are a help in localising vertebral joint problems.[117, 797, 983, 1368, 1369] (See Figs 2.18–2.23.)

Table 2.4

Spinal cord segment	Dermatome	Representative muscle(s)	Joint action	Reflex
C1	—	*a.p.r. C1–2* { Rect. cap. ant. Longus capitis	Tuck chin in	
C2 + V cranial	Vertex Occiput Forehead Temple	*p.p.r. C1–2* { Rect. cap. post. maj. & minor obliques *V cranial* Mastication	Push chin up Jaw movement	— V cranial jaw jerk[953] Corneal reflex[427]
C3 + V cranial	Neck Jaw Throat Inner clav.	*a.p.r. C3–4* Scaleni *p.p.r. C3–4* Upper extensions of erector spinae	Press head and neck laterally	V cranial jaw jerk[953]

Table 2.4 (contd)

Spinal cord segment	Dermatome	Representative muscle(s)	Joint action	Reflex
C4	Clavicle Supraspinous fossa Proximal deltoid	*a.p.r. C4* Levator scap. Trapezius	Elevate shdr. girdle	—
C5	Upper trapezius Deltoid and lateral arm to wrist	Deltoid	Abduction of arm	Biceps jerk
C6	Upper trapezius Lateral arm and forearm to two lateral digits	Biceps	Elbow flexion	Biceps and brachiora-dialis jerks
C7	Midscapular Post. arm to middle three digits	Triceps	Elbow extension	Triceps jerk
C8	Scapula Inner arm to medial two digits	Thumb extensor Finger flexor	Thumb extension Finger flexion	—
T1	Lower scapular *Inner* arm to medial wrist	Intrinsic hand muscles	Finger adduction and abduction	—
T2	Inverted 'T' with limbs to inner arm, pectoral and scapular areas	—	—	—
T4	Sloping band at nipple level			
T7	Sloping band at xiphoid level	Much overlapping of adjacent dermatomes		
T10	Sloping band at umbilical level			
L1	Sloping band at inguinal level			

Table 2.4 (contd)

Spinal cord segment	Dermatome	Representative muscle(s)	Joint action	Root traction	Reflex
L2	Sloping band around upper buttock to front upper thigh	Psoas–iliacus	Hip flexion	? Femoral nerve stretch test	—
L3	Upper buttock Front thigh to inner knee and below	Quadriceps	Knee extension	Femoral nerve stretch	Knee jerk
L4	Middle buttock Outer lower thigh Shin and dorsum to great toe	Tibialis anterior	Foot dorsiflexion	? Femoral nerve stretch also straight-leg-raising	Knee jerk
L5	Mid-buttock Post. thigh Outer leg All toes (dorsum) and medial plantar	Toe extensors Tibialis posterior	Extension of big toe Inversion with plantar-flexion of foot	Straight-leg-raising	Great toe jerk[1207]
S1	Lower mid-buttock Posterior thigh, behind lateral malleolus to fifth toe and lateral plantar	a. Peronei b. Glut. max. c. Hamstrings d. Calf	a. Eversion b. Contract buttock c. Knee-flexion	Straight-leg-raising	Ankle jerk
S2	Postero-medial strip from buttock to heel	Hamstrings Calf	Knee-flexion d. Toe standing	Straight-leg-raising	—
S3–4 (somatic S2–3–4 (parasymp.)	'Saddle' area Upper inner thigh Genitals Perineum	Muscles of pelvic floor Bladder and genital function			

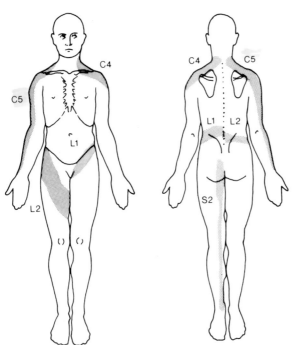

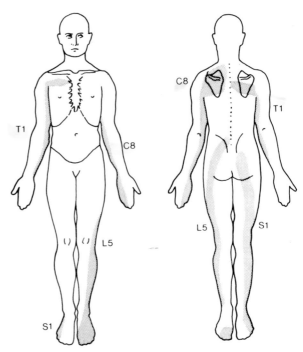

Fig. 2.18 Dermatomes. Because dermatomes are not fixed territorial or anatomical entities, but *neurophysiological* entities, whose boundaries fluctuate according to the prevailing levels of cord segment facilitation, the areas delineated above are those corresponding to body regions in which pain and other symptoms may often be partly or wholly distributed from joint problems in the general neighbourhood of associated vertebral segments. (Kirk EJ, Denny-Brown D 1970 Functional variations in dermatomes in the Macaque monkey following dorsal root lesions. Journal of Comparative Neurology 139: 307.)

Fig. 2.20 Dermatomes.

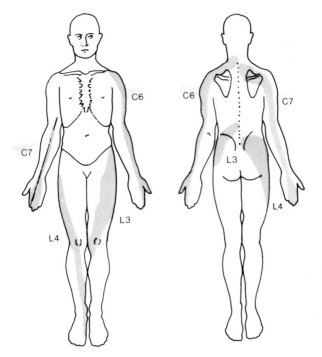

Fig. 2.19 Dermatomes.

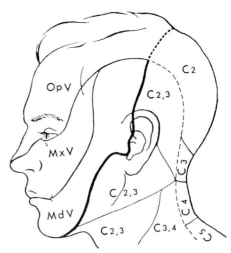

Fig. 2.21 Areas of cutaneous supply by the V cranial nerve (ophthalmic, maxillary and mandibular divisions) and the 2nd, 3rd and 4th cervical nerves. (Reproduced by kind permission of Wyke BD 1968 The neurology of facial pain, and the Editor, British Journal of Hospital Medicine.)

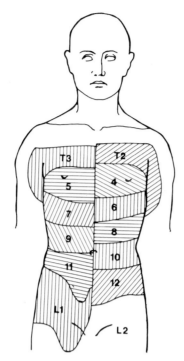

Fig. 2.22 Trunk dermatomes.

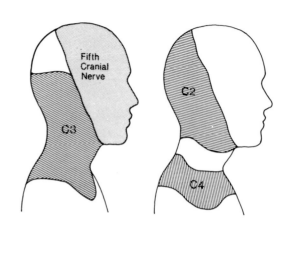

Fig. 2.23 To show extent of overlap of dermatomes.

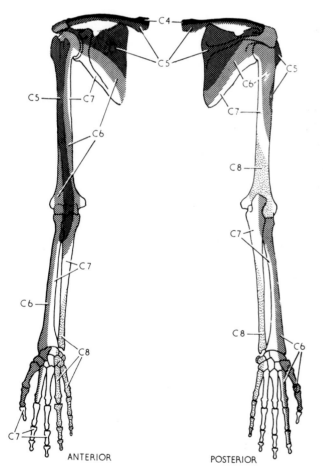

Fig. 2.24 The sclerotomes—upper limb. (After Inman VT, Saunders JB 1944 Referred pain from skeletal structures. Journal of Nervous and Mental Disorders 90: 660.)

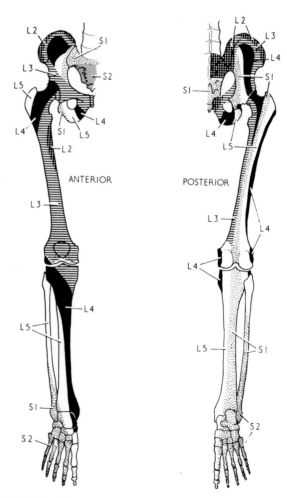

Fig. 2.25 The sclerotomes—lower limb. (After Inman VT, Saunders JB 1944 Referred paid from skeletal structures. Journal of Nervous and Mental Disorders 90: 660.)

3. Aetiology in general terms

The term 'osteoarthritis', previously used to describe degenerative joint changes (in the absence of systemic disease such as ankylosing spondylitis and rhematoid arthritis), was undesirable for two reasons:

1. The suffix 'itis' was misleading, because there is no inflammation, other than the transient episodes of so-called 'traumatic arthritis' superimposed upon an ageing joint by the stresses and accidents of living.

2. The term by definition refers to degenerative processes in *synovial* joints only.

For the non-synovial joints of the spine, we should perhaps reserve the term 'spondylosis', implying non-inflammatory degeneration of secondary cartilaginous joints (i.e. the symphyses)—the spondylosis deformans of Schmorl and Junghanns.[1093]

NB. The neurocentral joints of the uncovertebral region have a synovial membrane (see p. 5), yet share in the vertebral body joint changes because of their intimate relation to the cervical discs. Hence, degenerative change in these joints should perhaps be included in descriptions of *spondylosis*.

'*Degenerative joint disease of the spine*' therefore describes the two distinct entities, frequently combined to a greater or lesser degree,[1180b] of *osteoarthrosis* of the synovial joints, the arthrosis deformans of Schmorl and Junghanns, and *spondylosis* of the vertebral body joints (see p. 88). Despite their frequent coexistence, it is useful when planning treatment to bear the distinction in mind. The correct term for changes occurring in purely synovial occipitoatlantal, atlantoaxial and facet-joints is therefore 'osteoarthrosis',[981] but in the present-day clinical usage the umbrella terms 'cervical spondylosis', 'thoracic spondylosis' and 'lumbar spondylosis' denote unspecified degenerative changes in the vertebral regions named, unless more clarification desirably accompanies the phrase employed.

In these thoughtless, euphoric days when men talk glibly about the conquest of disease, the postponement of old age, and transplantation of the heart, it is a sobering thought that we still know practically nothing about the causation of that heterogeneous collection of aches and pains classified under the vague umbrella of rheumatism.[300]

Gradual physical change as the result of simple ageing is well manifested in joints and periarticular tissues of the body; besides the familiar visible alterations which accompany 'middle-aged spread', suppleness becomes restricted, joint tissues thicken and become stiffer, tissue elasticity is reduced and this accompanies loss of the powers of recovery. The ability to safely absorb mechanical stress diminishes, muscles become less strong, ligaments lose elasticity and joints are less well stabilised. Degeneration is characterised by slow destructive changes which are not balanced by regeneration as occurs in younger tissues.

For the most part, these changes proceed silently and need not of themselves cause symptoms; in many middle-aged people with virtually painless and functionally sound spines, the degree of degeneration fortuitously observed on X-rays taken for other reasons is sometimes quite astonishing. Yet the margin between a painless functional joint and painful disablement is now slim, and minor extra stress in the middle-aged or elderly can be the factor initiating symptoms and signs of disability out of proportion to the apparently trivial nature of the incident.

To the universal effects of ageing on the locomotor system *as a whole* are often added, in differing degrees of destructiveness according to the patient's occupation and life history, the immediate and subsequent effects on *particular joints* of undue stresses at work and play, and of trauma. The latter may be minor and repetitive, accummulating in effect as the years advance, or it may be a single violent incident in early or later life of sufficient force to fracture bones. Much of the unduly advanced secondary degenerative change in individual joints is the end-result of injury sustained months or years before, and often the traumatic incident has been forgotten by the patient, only to be recalled during the clinical examination. Injury to the cervical spine, for example, may continue to produce symptoms and signs many years later.[1274]

A radiographic examination carried out only once, and immediately after injury, yields in many cases no conclusive evidence about the changes caused by injury. Serial X-rays at different time intervals after the trauma very often uncover the true sequelae which subsequently and slowly develop.[598, 173, 1093]

For the most part, fractured bones unite and soon become strong again—by comparison with other tissues, bone forgives and forgets fairly quickly, but the debt following collagenous and cartilaginous-tissue insults is a matter of much longer-term repayment, and the retribution exacted later in terms of chronic pain and functional disablement underlies the seriousness of physical damage to joints. Joints neither forget, nor forgive.

It is useful to be reminded that *all* the mobile segments of the spine are weight-bearing segments, in whole or in part, and are always under gravitational stress when sitting, standing or walking. These joints rarely experience any natural distraction tendency such as the hanging arm exerts on the shoulder joint.

To the aetiological factors of (1) growing older, (2) getting or being too fat, (3) habitual postural strains, (4) occupational stress, and (5) trauma, there should be added (6) the tendency of some individuals to suffer degenerative changes sooner and with less apparent reason than others; probably an hereditary susceptibility to locomotor disease. Further factors are congenital defects (7) of bony or soft tissue development (Figs 1.25–1.30) and (8) pre-existent and coexistent disease.

1. Ageing gradually restricts movement (see p. 43), some becoming limited earlier than others, e.g. the symmetrical loss of cervical side-bending in the spine. This movement becomes more markedly limited than rotation and sagittal movement as the years advance.

2. Obesity adds greatly to normal stress on weight-bearing joints, especially in the lumbar region and lower limb joints. Farfan (1973)[326] suggests that obesity is not necessarily a factor in lumbar disc degeneration. The woman with heavy, pendulous breasts will tend to develop yoke area and interscapular pains due to stress on the thoracic joints, and the man with a large corpulent abdomen is more likely to suffer lumbosacral arthrotic pains by daily, forceful approximation of the more posterior lumbar joint structures, if his occupation involves much standing.

3. Asymmetrical and cumulative postural strains are likely in the neck and upper thoracic spine due to unilateral deafness or loss of vision in one eye, for example, or to the continued use of bifocal spectacles.[614]

4. Excessive kypholordosis of the upper thoracic and lower cervical regions, respectively, producing the 'dowager's hump', is more likely in those who spend a large part of the day in cramped and flexed working positions with the head held forward, and these effects would be aggravated as in (2). Postural lordotic strains in standing are a potent factor in lumbar disc degeneration as well

as in facet-joint arthrosis.[335] Lumbar degenerative changes may appear earlier in those who are sitting at work and repetitively reaching by trunk as well as arm movements, to lift weights like heavy telephone directories, for example, when the intranuclear disc pressure rises to abnormally high levels.[890]

Pathological changes aside, there are indications that low back pain episodes, for example, tend to occur with some frequency in two groups of occupations:

Group A, who are in the majority, and comprise those manual workers who are *regularly* engaged in *repetitive* handling of heavy industrial objects,[233] and

Group B, a minority, whose occupation entails a fixed posture (*any* posture) for long periods—the group would include long-distance lorry drivers and telephonists, for instance.

Singular *kinds* of occupational lumbar stress may also injure the low back. The go-go dancer rotates at the lumbo-sacral segment at a rate of 480 cycles per minute[326] but at great harm to her lumbar spine;[330] so much so that after some months, the occupation must be changed.

5a. A long period of disability, frequently extending into years, follows severe extension-deceleration or side-flexion-deceleration injuries to the neck.

The consequences of arthrosis in the upper cervical joints, for example, are usually more marked, in terms of intensity and variety of the patient's distress, than those of degenerative joint disease in other parts of the vertebral column.

b. Chronic backache may appear months after a heavy fall, or a sudden rotational strain when preventing a fall. Repetitive occupational strains combining torsion, bending and compression are especially potent in initiating the degenerative process in lumbar discs.[326]

An important mechanical factor is the size of the intervertebral body joint, the larger joint requiring more torque to produce injury. Consequently, 'heavily boned' people are less likely to sustain intervertebral joint injury.

One of the difficulties in analysing the cause of a back injury is that it can take place without pain. Evidence of old, stable fractures is common in people with no history of injury and there are innumerable cases in which the onset of pain was delayed for 24 hours or more after the injury. The reason is that neither the facets of the apophyseal joints nor the discs receive a nerve supply. Thus two of the major load-bearing tissues of the spine can be injured without pain. If these tissues are repeatedly injured, degenerative changes may set in—and this applies as much to the apophyseal joints as to the disc. What appears to be a non-accidental injury may sometimes be the culmination of a series of truly accidental, but at the same time, painless injuries. [Troup, 1979][1250b]

The incidence of low back injury due to losing one's footing, slipping on greasy surfaces and preventing a fall by sudden muscular action, being jolted by a false step, are probably much higher than is generally appreciated.

Farfan[326] holds that facet-joint orientation is an important factor in the nature of stresses developed at the intervertebral joint, and is partly responsible for the pattern of degenerative change.

c. Combined rib and vertebral fractures of the thoracic spine can produce premature degenerative changes of that region.

6. In the condition *primary nodal osteoarthrosis*,[1372] usually affecting middle-aged women, the development of painful Herbeden's nodes in the interphalangeal joints may be accompanied by pain and stiffness in the spine. The disease is probably genetically determined, and in some individuals a somewhat generalised deterioration of joint structure and function seems to occur following combined bodily and mental stress, e.g. 'the three Ws', work, worry and want

7. A tendency to secondary degenerative change may be evident at sites of minor or moderate degrees of dysplasia, and seems especially to occur in those with frank developmental defects such as a congenitally short leg producing a laterally tilted pelvis and a consequent degree of scoliosis; unequal mechanical stress on the lumbar spine and hips will predispose these structures to arthrotic change.

Hemivertebra, where a supernumerary wedge-shaped vertebral body appears on one side only, leads inevitably to an increasing scoliosis during growth, and early degenerative change.

Fused vertebrae throw an extra strain on adjacent joints (Figs. 1.26, 1.30) or adventitious joints. There may be *a developmental defect*[896] of the anterior part of a vertebral body in that it is wedge-shaped with a forward apex; and a further cause of early arthrosis may be a trapezoidal-shaped fifth lumbar vertebra.

8. *Pre-existent and co-existent disease*. The inflammatory changes of rheumatoid arthritis initiate a tendency to subsequent arthrotic and spondylotic change in the joints affected earlier than in others; examples of *metabolic diseases* producing a tendency to degenerative processes in joints are diabetes, and alkaptonuria with arthrosis, an inherited metabolic defect producing changes in the quality of discs and much consequent degeneration of vertebral body joints. Osteochondrosis of the spine (Schuermann's disease) affects the integrity of the hyaline cartilaginous plate of the vertebral body, and thus an important epiphyseal growth area, usually more pronounced in the thoracic region. Integrity of the discs is lost early in the disease, they collapse anteriorly and the extra compression falling on the front of the vertebral body joints leads to the formation of wedge-shaped bodies and marked kyphosis. Subsequent degeneration appears sooner in the affected regions.

Discs do not herniate or prolapse unless they are weakened by degeneration or by previous injury[1180b] and the commonest disease weakening the hyaline cartilaginous plate is osteochondrosis, whether its clinical presentation be obvious or subtle.

In the aetiology of degenerative change, clinically evident as craniovertebral joint problems, cervical spondylosis and brachial pain, yoke area pain, interscapular aching and chest wall pain, extra-segmental nocturnal paraesthesiae of upper limbs, cervical myelopathy, loin and groin pain from the thoracolumbar region, lumbosacral joint problems and the consequences of spinal stenosis, the factor of chance is of some significance.

The hand of cards dealt by nature to the individual at the moment of conception is an augury for good or ill, in terms of the healthy function of the musculoskeletal system. Probably ordained at that moment is the size of the neural canal, the vascular anastomosis on the surface of the spinal cord, the tendency to one or other concomitant diseases, a diathesis to connective tissue changes, perhaps a tendency to be 'proprioceptively illiterate' and a clumsy mover, to be prone to physical damage because of obsessional use of the body machinery at work or athletics and to habitually adopt particular postures.

Notwithstanding the normal accidents of life and chance environmental influences, the only early prophylactic measure seems to be care in the choice of one's parents.

(NB. More detailed consideration of aetiology is included under pathological changes of the tissues concerned.)

4. Incidence

GENERAL

With some important exceptions, the changes produced in vertebral joints by the degenerative process are usually benign, do not amount to serious disease, and can be regarded as the field of minor orthopaedics. Yet if the totality of pain in an individual's lifetime could be reviewed, it is probable that the majority of it would have been caused by degenerative changes in the musculoskeletal system, much of it vertebral and going under a bewildering host of common household names. In clinical terminology, the word 'diagnosis' tends to lose its classical meaning, in that on the one hand a frequently occurring and easily recognisable pattern of signs and symptoms may enjoy a different diagnosis for each day of the week depending upon the person examining the patient, and on the other hand the catch-all phrase 'disc lesion' might be employed in authoritarian pronouncement[780] upon *any* pain in the region of the spinal column accompanied by movement-limitation.

Our true knowledge of these conditions, as they occur in living patients, amounts to an island of certain information in a sea of embarrassing ignorance.

A very great deal of frustration, minor or more severe temporary disablement and often permanent disablement, interference with free activity, and depressing pain results from these lesions, together with a massive loss of occupational effectiveness in all walks of life.

The combined lumbar stresses of bending, torsion and compression, together with stresses associated with prolonged sitting and handling what might appear to be moderate weights, occur very frequently throughout the waking day[1338] of the average individual, as do the cervical and upper thoracic stresses of bending over work, driving, and the repetitive turning to one side, with flexion of the neck, during secretarial and administrative work.

The commonly held notion that vertebral degenerative disease is a consequence of man's 'recent' assumption of the erect posture, will not do. Lewin (1979)[725] describes the discovery that human-like (hominid) individuals clearly were walking upright as long as 3 750 000 years ago; this is more than enough time for evolutionary structural adaptations to have occurred.

Davis (1972)[234] suggests that the 'lift and carry' rate in modern times—5000 units of this activity in one day for 20th-century man—is doubtless greater than in premediaeval times, and very much greater than in preNeolithic days, when a rate of 50 lifts a day for hunter-gatherer may have been an average.

Wood (1976)[1338] proffers this as a model for the progressive increase in spinal stress following both the Neolithic age and the Industrial Revolution; presumably low back pain, and by inference pain in other vertebral regions, has increased in roughly parallel fashion; yet Horal (1969)[572] compared 212 workers reporting back pains with a similar investigation of controls. No more than 25 per cent blamed accidents for the onset of their troubles, and a similar proportion blamed lifting and handling. Among the factors causing recurrences, trauma and heavy lifting were infrequent.

The International Classification of Diseases[1345] includes a wide range of conditions, around 30 of them, which could be categorised under the generic heading of back pain. Anderson (1976)[24] observes that:

... the range of labels used in connection with back pain is a fair reflection of medical ignorance and factional interests. Furthermore, it is virtually impossible to classify statistical data on sickness absence in a meaningful way ... specific surveys are difficult to compare in the absence of agreed semantics,

and he provides a guide to the size of the problem in an analysis of vertebral and limb pain amongst 2684 male employees from a range of occupations.

The different categories were as follows:

Pain of undetermined diagnosis, 28.8 per cent, of which 11.0 per cent were limb pains, and 17.8 per cent were spinal problems, with lumbosacral pains exceeding neck-and-shoulder-girdle problems in a ratio of approximately 2:1.

Disc disease, 12.2 per cent, in which lumbar 'discs' exceeded cervical 'discs' in a ratio of approximately 3:2.

Osteoarthrosis accounted for 8.3 per cent, other rheumatic for 1.5 per cent, rheumatoid arthritis for 12 per cent, and 0.1 per cent 'unknown'. 'Negatives' were thus 47.9 per cent. Back pain was recorded in 30 per cent and low back pain as disc disease or PUD in three-quarters of these (23 per cent of sample).

Rheumatic complaints as a whole increased to age 55 and then declined somewhat, with lumbosacral pains showing a fairly steady prevalence rate between ages 25 and 65 years.

Hay (1972)[521] interviewed 3885 adults over the age of 18, comprising 85 per cent of the voter's list of an Australian electoral district, and he recorded details of those who had suffered low back pain, sciatica, or both, in the preceding 3 years.

When charting the percentage of population with symptoms at different ages, the findings were as follows (Fig. 4.1):

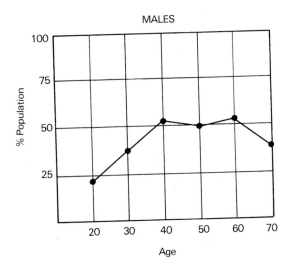

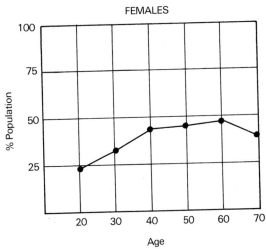

Fig. 4.1 See text. After Hay MC 1974 The incidence of low back pain in Busselton. In Symposium on low back pain. In: Twomey LT (ed.) West. Aust. Inst. Tech., Perth.

Of 2032 females, 753 or 37 per cent, had had symptoms during that time, and of 1853 males, 745 or 40 per cent, had experienced symptoms in the period, i.e:

Table 4.1

	Total	% of population	Low back pain	Sciatica	Both
Females	753	37	67 %	8 %	25 %
Males	745	40	69 %	6 %	25 %

The mode of onset is interesting, in that 'cause not known' exceeds all other stated causes, although lifting strains were higher in men:

Table 4.2

Onset	Females	Males	Total
Injury	172	190	362
Lifting strain	115	233	348
Other	138	68	206
Not known	306	239	545

The highest total of 545 of 'not known' plainly indicates that our well-worn tendency to almost *invariably* associate the aetiology of low back pain and sciatica with lifting strains may need modification.

There is little convincing evidence that the incidence and duration of low back pain have been influenced by instruction in manual handling and lifting.[412b] (See p. 503.)

Not surprisingly, moderate and sometimes more marked signs and symptoms become manifest from about the third decade onwards, and increasingly so in succeeding years.

In a group of 1137 working men[580a, 580b] between the ages of 25–54 years, the incidence of abnormal physical signs was recorded by clinical examination of the spine, and disc degeneration was recorded by radiographic examination. Less than half were engaged in light work, and the remainder were heavy workers. Attacks of stiff neck occurred in about 27 per cent of those below 30 years, and in 50 per cent of those over 45 years. Brachalgia started later than neck stiffness, only about 8 per cent of those under 30 years suffering from this and 38 per cent of those over 45 years. There was the same tendency, though less marked, for low back pain and sciatica. Neck stiffness and low back pain come first, arm pain and sciatica come later.

There was no real difference in the incidence of cervical and lumbar pain between the light and the heavy workers. The back pain of sedentary workers probably appears less often in statistics, since to a degree they can still work despite pain, as opposed to the more active industrial worker who is effectively disabled for his type of work by symptoms. There is general agreement that trauma, malalignments, and dysplasia frequently predispose the individual to degenerative disease but not the same agreement that heavy work *per se*, in the absence of injury, hastens disc disease.[157, 112, 99]

Taking the spine as a whole, some radiological evidence of degenerative change, i.e. spondylosis of vertebral body joints and/or arthrosis of facet-joints, is almost universal at 60 years, but pain and radiographic changes do not correlate in either direction in randomly selected populations.

With regard to lumbar arthrosis *per se*, Lewin's (1964)[727] analysis of autopsy findings in 104 cases showed, not surprisingly, that the frequency and degree of arthrotic changes increased with age equally in both sexes. Commonly, only minor cartilage changes were found before age 45, and after that age more advanced chondral changes such as necrosis, and other changes such as sclerosis, cyst formation and osteophytosis were very common.

Correlations between the degree of arthrosis (either demonstrated radiographically or at autopsy) and the severity or even the presence of pain is known to be sketchy.

With regard to assessments of overall incidence, figures suggest that some 20 per cent of adults suffer back pain during any one fortnight.[253]

The total number of persons afflicted with arthritis and rheumatism cannot be known for certain. Such figures as are available tend to be limited and inevitably they are rather out of date.*

Glover (1971)[412] asserts that each insured person, and there are around 26 million of them, loses on average half a day's work each year through conditions likely to be associated with back pain.

Wood and McLeish (1974)[1337] present an analysis which suggests an overall yearly loss of around 30 million man days, because of incapacity due to rheumatic complaints.

The sheer scale of the problem facing those in the front line, i.e. on the clinical shop-floor and in the community, and facing those whose responsibility is the recruitment as well as the deployment of these sketchy clinical resources, is difficult to grasp. Its magnitude has a numbing effect. One single person affected badly enough to be suffering the slow and depressing destruction of musculo-skeletal function and optimism is harrowing enough; when each of these represents a statistic making page after page grey with figures, the clinical therapist may deal with a feeling of helplessness only by working as hard as sinew and stamina will allow.

Since we do not enjoy the clinical means to deal with pain as effectively and quickly as we would wish, compassion and the powerful therapeutic effect of physically handling the painful tissues with attentive consideration and skill, are almost as important as the clinical procedures. Further, it may be that our first priority of therapeutic effectiveness does not necessarily depend upon a

* This publication, formulated to mark World Rheumatism Year 1977, is a most comprehensive *Report on Problems and Progress in Health Care for Rheumatic Disorders* (ed. P. H. N. Wood). Published by The British League Against Rheumatism.

supply of shining and expensive lumps of chromium-plated apparatus, whose cost-effectiveness perennially falls short of the expectations sometimes induced by their impressive appearance.

As dictated by the weight and the manifest emphasis of statistical evidence, the prime need, amongst a host of other needs, appears to be a sufficiently large increase in the number of clinicians and therapists skilled for specialisation in this particular work, the conservative treatment of benign joint problems. Only one in 10 000 of the population reaches the stage of myelography and operation, for example,[723] and therefore conservative treatment is of first importance.

If the manifest size of the requirement is given the immediacy it merits, every comprehensively trained and ethically responsible worker, of whatever persuasion, is a shoulder at the wheel. While the internecine war rages as to who shall have the keys of the kingdom, the patient, unconcerned about the kingdom, seeks relief from the pain.

SEGMENTAL

Spondylosis with arthrosis often exist together, and it is reasonable to expect that disc degeneration would have some effect on the movement patterns and integrity of the facet-joints of the same segment,[565] yet we find, for example, that arthrosis of the posterior *cervical* joints, most common in the upper segments, does not seem to be correlated with disc degeneration (spondylosis) at C2 and C3 segments. *There is a degree of independence of changes* in the different parts of any one segment.[1180b, 1125, 1093]

Frequently the posterior joints of the lower neck escape involvement even when the discs show marked degeneration. Studies of a primitive group compared with a civilised society produced evidence that in the latter, the incidence of disc degeneration and hypertrophic change, although rising at different rates, did so constantly throughout life, whereas in the primitive group, the incidence of hypertrophic change rose as for the civilised society but the incidence of disc narrowing (spondylosis) rose very slowly, suggesting different causes for the two types of degenerative change.[333]

At autopsy examination of 111 cervical spines, Hirsch (1967) *et al.*[548] could find no evident relationship between the degree of disc degeneration with exostosis and changes in the posterior facet-joints; according to other investigators also,[385, 976] there seems to be no correlation between changes in the discs and facet-joints.

However, in contrast, it is still unclear if an arthrosis of synovial joints, regardless of cause, may produce a secondary chondrosis of the disc, or aggravate it considerably.[1093]

Lewin[727] observed that while gross arthrotic change was commonest in the lower lumbar segments after 45 years, the initial phases of arthrosis were more frequent at the upper two lumbar segments before that age, i.e. between 26 and 45 years. After 45, about 30 per cent of subjects had upper lumbar changes, and about 60 per cent showed the changes in lower segments. In this same age section, half of the subjects had changes in three or more segments simultaneously. Intrasegmentally, arthrosis was often found in the posterior lumbar joints unaccompanied by either disc degeneration or vertebral-body lipping, age notwithstanding.

In the lower age-group, 26–45 years, spondylotic degenerative change in discs was often found as the sole pathological change, with the posterior joints unaffected, i.e. 35 per cent of the spines examined showed disc degeneration at L4–5 and L5–S1 segments and only a few showed synovial joint involvement.

After 45 years, both spondylotic and arthrotic change involved whole segments, with a frequency of about 60 per cent.

Sometimes two lumbar articular processes comprising one synovial facet-joint, i.e. enclosed in one capsule, showed marked differences in their degree of arthrotic change.

Arthrosis of the atlantodental (median atlantoaxial) joint is as common as spondylotic disease in the vertebral body joints of the rest of the cervical spine, and is surprisingly found more frequently than at the occipitoatlantal and lateral atlantoaxial joints (Fig. 4.2).[1274]

Degenerative change tends to follow an overall pattern of distribution, set out in the accompanying scheme (Table 4.3), although the pattern depicted might well

Table 4.3   Segmental incidence

	Arthrosis		Spondylosis
	Facet-joints	Costal joints	Intervertebral body joints
CERVICAL	Median atlanto-axial Upper cervical C7		Lower cervical
THORACIC	T1 T4 T5 T12	T1 T8 T9 T11 T12	Middle thoracic *
LUMBAR	L1 L2 L3 L4		L4 L5
SACRAL			S1

Ref. nos: 5, 35, 239, 117, 326, 780, 727, 902, 950, 1125, 1180b, 1274.

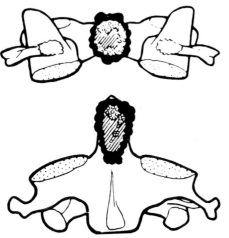

Fig. 4.2 Arthrosis of the atlantodental (median atlantoaxial) joint is as common as spondylotic disease in the intervertebral body joints of the rest of the cervical spine. It occurs more frequently than at the lateral atlantoaxial and occipitoatlantal joints. (Reproduced from Spondylosis cervicalis: a pathological and osteo-archaeological study, 1969, Munksgaard, Copenhagen, by kind permission of Dr Sager and the publishers.)

change in the future, when the amount of detailed knowledge of changes in the thoracic region approaches that already available about the cervical and lumbar regions.

Referring to arthrotic changes in the facet-joints, Shore (1935) (Fig. 4.3)[1125] mentions two peaks of especially high incidence: (a) at the cervicothoracic junction, i.e. between C7 and T1 and (b) at the facets between T4 and T5.

Acute joint problems tend to occur in the middle of vertebral regions, while chronic joint problems are more common at the junctional areas of the spine, where relatively mobile segments are related to almost immobile regions, i.e. craniovertebral, cervicothoracic, lumbosacral and, to a lesser degree, thoracolumbar. Also, the highest incidence of degenerative change, and highest segmental incidence of anatomical anomalies and dysplasias, crowd together at the junctional regions—this is more than coincidence, perhaps.

It is fundamentally important to bear in mind that: (a) *The sites of X-ray evidence of degeneration are NOT ALWAYS the site of the painful joint problem for which the patient is seeking treatment* and (b) *patients with gross X-ray changes may have no symptoms to speak of, while very frequently those with normal X-rays may suffer severely from pain, presumably due to change in radiotranslucent soft tissues only.*

It might also be mentioned that *the distribution* of joint degeneration giving rise to morphological changes seen at autopsy may well have had little relationship to the distribution of pain, type of functional disability, and vertebral

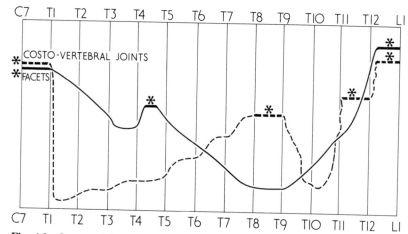

Fig. 4.3 Segmental incidence of arthrosis in vertebral synovial joints is high at cervicothoracic junction.
——— Continuous line shows findings reported by L. R. Shore. (Shore LR 1935 On OA in the dorsal intervertebral joints. British Journal of Surgery 22: 823.)
- - - - - Broken line shows findings reported by H. Nathan et al. (Nathan H et al 1964 Costovertebral joints: anatomicoclinical observations in arthritis. Arthritis and Rheumatism 7: 228.)

segments giving rise to joint problems suffered by those subjects during life.

The sites of degenerative change will differ from patient to patient, but tend overall to occur in the above pattern of distribution. Arthrosis of the lumbar spine has a tendency to occur together with spondylosis at the lower segments after the fourth decade.

It is necessary to remember, for example, that the un-common but serious thoracic disc lesions, requiring urgent surgical attention because of trespass upon the spinal cord and/or important related blood vessels, tend to occur at the junction of middle and lower thirds of the thoracic region. The factor of their dramatic presentation and seriousness does not alter the balance of overall incidence, since they *are* uncommon.

5. Pathological changes—general

The pathological changes of primary and secondary degenerative joint disease are confined to the joint(s) affected; there is no systemic or constitutional disease, although there may be hormonal changes, e.g. the menopause, associated with causing joint symptoms. Spondylosis and osteoarthrosis occur very frequently in people who are otherwise fit and constitutionally healthy. Nevertheless, localised degenerative change can produce space-occupying, as well as tethering, effects on related tissues and thereby on remote structures served by the latter; these effects can be extensive and their presentation confusing, and are particularly manifest in the central and peripheral nervous and vascular systems, by both irritation and compression of nerves and vessels.[656] Consequently, to the locally produced signs and symptoms of movement-limitation, pain, and muscle spasm, are often added the more serious effects to be detailed. When considering degenerative joint disease in the spine,

... a distinction should be made between involvement of the posterior facet-joints and the intervertebral discs, although the processes share common pathological and pathogenic features.[1154]

A. SYNOVIAL JOINTS

For many years, studies of causation of musculoskeletal pain arising from vertebral structures have concentrated overwhelmingly on changes occurring in the intervertebral discs, and it is necessary to stress that changes in the posterior joints can, and do, very frequently give rise to symptoms (Figs 1.4, 1.5, 1.25, 4.3). For this reason their degenerative changes are described in some detail. If similar changes were found in any other synovial articulation of the body, it would not be surprising if the patient complained of pain on use of the joint. The facet-joints are heir to strains, effusions, adhesion formation, cartilage fractures, loose bodies and capsular fibrosis with thickening as in other synovial joints.[508]

A radiographic, macroscopic and microscopic investigation of the lumbar spines of 104 autopsy cases—18 below 20 years, and 86 over—revealed that all of the morphological changes in lumbar facet-joints were compatible with the known picture of osteoarthrosis in synovial limb joints. The joint deformations produced by arthrosis occur partly by the disintegration and abrasions of articular cartilage, and partly by the proliferation of new osseous tissue at the base and peripheral margins of the joint surface. Whether the degenerative process as it occurs in spinal synovial joints is (a) primary osteoarthrosis, i.e. an intrinsic senescence of cartilage occurring in joints whose pre-existing anatomical configuration is normal, or (b) secondary osteoarthrosis, i.e. a consequence of abnormal mechanical stresses, however caused, be considered more of academic interest than immediate clinical importance, the frequency with which painful and disabling vertebral joint problems occur at the sites of previous trauma, impulsive occupational stress and existing anomalies is too high to be coincidental.

Murray[880] had drawn attention to an example of this highly probable cause-and-effect relationship in arthrosis of the hip joint.

The importance of detailed history-taking becomes clear. Probably primary and secondary arthrotic processes coexist in varying proportions in most spines, with a preponderance of secondary change in (a) the low lumbar region, (b) in cervical spines which have been subjected to trauma at right angles to the body axis, (c) the regions of anomalous structure, and (d) the junctional regions.

1. CARTILAGE

The pathogenesis of degenerative disease in synovial joints involves a whole family of factors,[1154] a complex of interacting mechanical and biological feedback loops. For example, the collagen of articular cartilage persists throughout life, yet it is subject to ponderously slow molecular changes which may profoundly alter the physical and architectural properties of fibres with the passage of time.

Radin et al. (1972)[1008] observed that a remarkably low coefficient of friction protects synovial joints from simply wearing away with the to-and-fro motion of repetitive physiological movement, which occurs throughout life. Cartilage is a viable tissue capable of producing mucopolysaccharide and collagen in response to injury. Many individuals complete a hard working life without manifesting degenerative disease.

The authors emphasise the clinical significance of three observations:

1. It is always movements of an impulsive nature which apply relatively high stress to joints, e.g. walking, running, getting in or out of a chair, climbing, jumping, lifting, hammering or shovelling; all of these load the joint intermittently or repetitively.[1009]

2. Longitudinal loading creates significant stress across joint structures, back and forward rubbing does not. It is highly likely that the superb lubrication mechanisms prevent the stresses of oscillation, even when under very high loads, from causing deterioration by wearing away joint surfaces.

3. In sustaining and attenuating longitudinally applied forces, especially those of high magnitude and brief intensity, the cartilage and synovial fluid play a subsidiary role to that of bone and soft tissues.

An important tissue is the subchondral bone supporting the joint structure. This was examined in patients with the earliest phase of histochemical evidence of arthrosis in cartilage, and the subchondral bone was stiffer than normal. Micrography studies, of the subchrondral bone of animals subjected to repetitive impulse loading, have demonstrated trabecular microfractures.[1009] The increased stiffness of such bone has been correlated with the healing of microfractures.

Evidence of healed or healing microfractures has also been found in the subchondral bone of patients with early degenerative disease of the hip and in the spongiosa of lumbar vertebrae of the ageing spine.[1222, 1269] As long ago as 1827 it was established that cancellous bone can act as an effective shock-absorber, and it has been shown that the remodelling of subchondral bone is a constant, active process.

Radin and his colleagues,[1008] conceiving that the arthrotic process in cartilage might represent part of the biological response to repeated impact loading, present an hypothesis as follows:

Impulse loading
↓
Trabecular microfracture
↓
Bone remodelling
↓
Resultant stiffening of subchondral bone
↓
Increased stress on articular cartilage
↓
Cartilage breakdown
↓
Degenerative joint disease

Impact loading experiments indicate that there is some justification for the hypothesis that it is only after the subchondral bone has changed, and then lost its energy-absorbing capacity, that the cartilage may begin to deteriorate,[1154] yet the cause-and-effect relationship may not be so conveniently clear-cut, because some of the experimental animals showed fibrillation changes on the cartilage surface concurrently with the subchondral bone changes.[809]

An increased incidence of trabecular microfractures in the subchondral cancellous bone is associated with the earliest ultrastructural evidence of cartilage damage. The result of the healing of these microfractures and subsequent remodelling is an increase in the stiffness of the bone. Whether the bone or cartilage changes occur first would seem to be a moot point; there appears to be an intimate relationship between the changes in the two tissues.[1010]

Radin later observed that the extreme resistance of articular cartilage to shear forces, even when exposed to abnormal synovial fluid under high loads, compares to its extreme tendency to break down under tensile fatigue.[1010]

Deterioration of the tensile strength of cartilage accompanies ageing, yet many aged people show, after a lifetime of toil, very little evidence of cartilage deterioration. Degenerative changes involve something more than ageing. Protective mechanisms appear to exist, in that load-bearing areas of all articular cartilage do not invariably wear out under the applied forces of a life's vigorous activity.

By comparing the highly uncomfortable jolt when encountering an unexpected step with our ability to jump with controlled ease from a considerable height, Radin suggests that the most obvious shock-absorbing mechanism is that of joint motion and muscular control under tension combined. This hypothesis would accord with the favourable effects of improving the function of the quadriceps muscle in degenerative change at the knee joint. Loads which are unexpected, or occur too rapidly for the appropriate neuromuscular response, are thus perhaps a serious threat to the integrity of articular cartilage.

A series of investigations have demonstrated intimate and specific relationships between the regional substructure of the collagen filaments and the distribution of polysaccharides, suggesting that all the various physical parameters of cartilage are complexly dependent upon both elements. Ageing might be resolved into two components: (1.) a loss of the self-replicating capacity of the chondrocytes[437] and (2.) the physiochemical changes taking place in the matrix independently of all functions.[1154]

1. Division of articular cartilage cells is by mitosis, but mitotic figures are infrequently seen except in the immature skeleton. It has been thought that chondrocytes of mature articular cartilage are incapable of mitotic division, and the tissue thus unable to repair itself following injury, yet clusters of chondrocytes are often seen at

the margins of fibrillation sites, and findings suggest that the failure of chondrocytes to divide ordinarily in mature cartilage is not the lack of a replicating mechanism but results from their discrete situations in a matrix which severely restricts macromolecular growth factors. A degree of matrix dissolution appears to provide the stimulus which facilitates and accelerates cell division.[1154]

2. Articular cartilage has a limited capacity for growth and repair; its somewhat stately metabolic rate begins to decline around the second to third decade and this process appears to begin around the chondrocytes. Whether it is the disintegration of collagen which comes first, or the change in the matrix, is uncertain. Chemical studies have demonstrated that the cartilage erosion is accompanied by the breakdown and release of the two principal macromolecules of cartilage matrix, proteoglycans and collagen. As for the matrix, it is clearly evident that the total proteoglycan content is reduced, and that the reduction varies directly with the severity of the process.

The perichondrocyte changes wrought in normal metabolism are probably due to a release of certain enzymes from the lysosomal granules of these cells; articular cartilage does contain catheptic and other hydrolases which can dissolve the ground substance (Fig. 5.1).

Once initiated the process is self-perpetuating, release of enzymes stimulating further release from neighbouring chondrocytes. Should the quality of cartilage begin to deteriorate, and/or be subject to undue repetitive loading or trauma, it slowly loses its characteristics by an increase in permeability of its surface layer, by becoming softer and less stiff, and by changes in the composition of the matrix (depolymerisation of proteoglycans). Surface fibrillation is also seen, with faint lines running across the normally smooth, pearly surface being visible to the naked eye.

In early fibrillation, the surface of the cartilage is partly disrupted; there is a disintegration of the pre-existing collagen fibrils at the tangential layer.

Although fibrillated cartilage has been widely equated with osteoarthrotic cartilage, it is not at present possible to recognise a *pattern of fibrillation* which is specific for progressive cartilage degeneration.[147]

The relationship between appearance of fibrillation and the essential arthrotic process (as presently understood) is not necessarily direct—fibrillation often being evident at joint surface areas not suffering the greatest stress of weight-bearing compression.

Normal lubrication mechanisms are disturbed;[949, 400, 398, 1278, 1199] since healthy cartilage is normally *impermeable* to the large molecules of hyaluronic acid, the concentration of high-viscosity fluid at load-bearing points is thereby upset, and also microscopic cartilaginous particles of a larger-than-normal size become detached. These, of the order of 100 microns or so, are not easily phagocytosed, and tend to set up chronic subsynovial reactions because

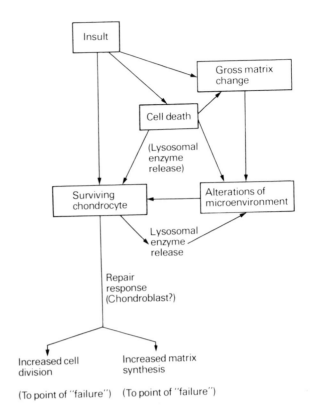

Fig. 5.1 Schematic formulation for metabolic events in the cartilage in osteoarthritis. Initiating event of unknown nature causes cell death and gross matrix disruption. There is a release of lysosomal enzymes which further degrade the matrix and produce alterations in the microenvironment. Some or all of these affect the surviving chondrocyte to release more lysosomal enzymes and also to respond by an increased rate of synthesis of matrix and cell replication. These latter events appear to keep pace with the disease up to a point where the process becomes so severe that the reparative responses fail. (By courtesy of Professor H. J. Mankin, Massachusetts General Hospital, Boston, U.S.A. and The Institute of Orthopaedics, London, W1.)

the synovium covers them with a single layer of cells and treats them as foreign bodies.

The tiny fissures allow synovial fluid to penetrate them and thus reach the deeper layers where its alkaline pH assists in further depolymerisation of the cartilage matrix. The surface becomes granular as fibrillation increases, it becomes frayed and further damage may be added by larger and macroscopic flakes forming loose bodies, which add their quota of roughening during movements. Fissures become more apparent on the surface.[194] As the lesions become more advanced, the tearing* of the collagen extends more deeply into the radial zone, sometimes later involving underlying bone in osteochondral fracture; these are often seen in lumbar facet-joints. Attempts at repair can be seen as matted aggregation of fibrous tissue on the cartilaginous surface. Intra-articular adhesions

---

* N.B 'Tearing' may not be quite correct. It has been suggested that the earliest change in arthrotic cartilage which is visible to the naked eye, i.e. fibrillation, may be the result of fatigue failure, perhaps analogous to the molecular disintegration of fatigue failure in metals.[1297]

may form,[508] from filmy strands to dense fibrosis, subsequently joining the opposed surfaces and preventing free movement, in advanced stages. In the later stages patches of complete loss of cartilage may leave bone ends exposed.

2. SYNOVIAL MEMBRANE

The low-grade inflammatory processes lead to synovial thickening, with fibrotic invasion of its connective tissue layer, some loss of vascularity, and interference with its natural secretion. It is possible that damage to this tissue can also be contributed by previous episodes of being nipped between bone ends.[677]

Intra-articular derangement, with loose bodies lying free within the joint space, or mobile but partially attached, are also found.[508, 805]

The small 'meniscoid' structures in the facet-joints (see p. 253) are apparently susceptible to temporary impaction at times, with the chronic sequelae of joint tissue damage probably adding to the natural process of senescence.

Schmorl and Junghanns (1971)[1093] observe that like any other joint, the vertebral mobility segment may become 'locked'. This is usually associated with pain, and is referred to by some as 'spinal subluxation' although 'subluxation' has not been medically proved. From recent experience, there is no doubt that the causes for such disturbances are located in the mobility segment, and the incarceration of an articular villus or 'meniscoid' structure in an apophyseal joint has been shown.[360, 1382]

A form of calcium phosphate, as crystals of hydroxyapatite normally associated with new bone formation, has been identified in the soft tissues and synovial fluid of arthrotic joints, and its presence there may be a factor in the aetiology of some forms of arthrosis.

3. CAPSULE AND LIGAMENT

Capsular and ligamentous thickening, beginning as round cell infiltration, fibrosis and later contracture of the connective tissues, accompany the intra-articular changes. Joints usually become stiffer as a consequence. Should loss of disc height accompany the posterior joint changes, capsular fibrosis may not, however, be sufficient to stabilise the now unstable segment and the resulting state is that of *hypermobility* in the presence of spondylosis and arthrosis at that segment. These chronically loose segments become subject to continual localised stress, and the products of an irritative inflammatory arthritis due to repetitive trauma are thereby added to the degenerative process. *Hypermobility and stiffness frequently occur in adjacent segments.*

Degenerative changes in particular segments are often accompanied by loss of natural characteristics in the ligaments of the vertebral arches; abnormal stresses and strains occur, there is a gradual disappearance of true liga-

mentous tissue and ruptures with cavitation lesions are frequently seen, for example, in the lower lumbar ligaments. Scars of healed tears also occur here.[1041]

The interspinous ligament never tears transversely; several studies show that the tear amounts to a separation of fibres longitudinally, secondary to translatory stress.[870]

In the thoracic spine, degenerative change later proceeding to ossification of the ligamentous structures of the costovertebral joints is not infrequent, and macroscopic evidence of arthrosis can be observed here as early as the third decade.[1093]

In the cervical spine, loss of elasticity of the ligamentum nuchae in late life deprives the neck of a degree of postural stability and flexion-controlling support.

The most important effect of fibrotic change in capsular and ligamentous tissue is that of restricting movement or making it difficult, and thus of depriving these tissues themselves, and other joint structures, of the physiological benefits of normal tissue fluid exchange, and thereby nutrition, produced by natural free movements. This effect begins with the earliest stages of degeneration, and is evident on careful palpation, when by this important method of examination, loss of movement in individual segments becomes manifest long before X-ray changes are apparent.

Autopsy findings demonstrate that complete fibrous ankylosis, and commonly bony ankylosis, may also intervene.[1093] This ankylotic bridging is remarkable in that it often does not occur uniformly by involving all the component joints of one segment, but may selectively occur at one facet-joint, or only at the symphysis between the vertebral bodies.[313] Individual pathological specimens showing the incidence of degenerative ankylosis at different parts of the same segment may represent the frozen 'still' of a stately process in time, which will sooner or later involve the whole of the segment. For practical clinical purposes of mobility-assessment, this distinction regarding ankylosis is more an academic one, because movement at the 'mobile segment' concerned will virtually be nil, and the clinical sequelae of this state of affairs is of more immediate importance than its cause.

In passing, it is wise to check radiographic appearances before employing any degree of vigour in treatment because while palpation easily detects loss of movement, it cannot always determine the *cause* of that loss. Manipulative attempts to 'improve range' at such segments will not be regarded with enthusiasm by patients.

4. BONE

The degenerative process disturbs the joint more extensively than the changes seen in cartilage only; an entire remodelling of the end-contour of bone also occurs (Fig. 5.2).[194]

Although capable of more distortion than bone, articular cartilage appears not thick enough to act alone as the sole absorber of rapidly applied shocks. The resilience of bone provides an increment of shock-absorbing capacity (see Vertebral movement, p. 40).

While some applied forces produce gross bone fracture, many produce only microfractures in trableculae, the healing of microfractures in subchondral bone then resulting in remodelling and stiffening of the bone structure.[1154, 1269]

Osteonecrosis is sometimes a feature of osteoarthrosis, possibly associated with trabecular microfractures as a focal event and therefore a secondary localised phenomenon, or possibly secondary to a discrete vascular occlusion. There is also the concept that osteoarthrosis is not primarily a cartilage disorder at all, but the con-sequences in cartilage of repetitive microfractures sustained by bone during high impact loading.[1154, 1008]

Changes first occur in the deepest calcified layer of cartilage, where subchondral bone hyperplasia begins as an irregular advance of ossification into the cartilage; it eventually becomes evident radiographically as increased density and sclerosis. This thickened subchondral base is buttressed by stout trabeculae, evidence of increased osteoblast activity beneath the degenerating cartilage. Subchondral pseudocyst formation is also seen, although this occurs far more often in fully weight-bearing joints, e.g. the hip.

At the vascular borders where cartilage, bone,

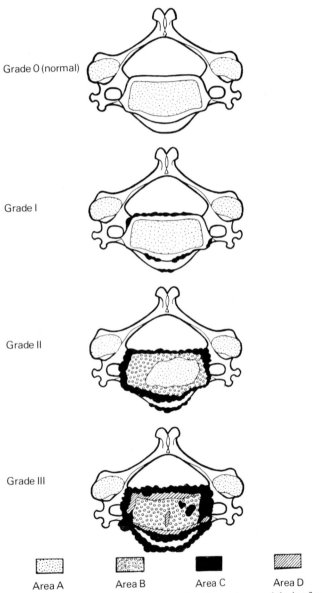

Fig. 5.2 Progressive stages of degenerative change in spondylosis of a cervical mobility segment, with degeneration of the disc. Note the extent of the trespass into the neural canal, as well as upon the intervertebral foramen. (Reproduced from Spondylosis Cervicalis: a Pathological and Osteo-archaeological Study, 1969, by kind permission of Dr Sager and the publishers.)

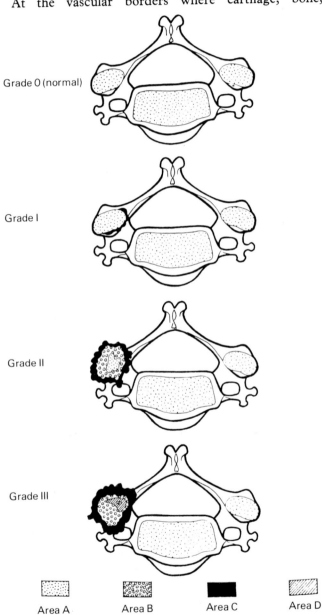

Fig. 5.3 Progressive stages of degenerative change in arthrosis of a cervical facet-joint. Note the extent of trespass upon the intervertebral foramen and the foramen transversarium. (Reproduced from Spondylosis Cervicalis: a Pathological and Osteo-archaeological Study, 1969, by kind permission of Dr Sager and the publishers.)

synovium and periosteum meet, there begins a proliferation of callus-like tissue, resulting in additional bone formation concentrated at the edges of the articular cartilage, as elevated ridges. These intra-articular but peripheral *osteophytes* grow outwards and tend to increase the lateral dimensions of the opposed bone-ends, and thus of the joint cavity and the capsule. A better term is *chondro-osteophytes*,[1180b] since they are always covered by a layer of fibrocartilage and are somewhat larger than their X-ray appearance suggests, due to the radiotranslucent covering. Marginal chondro-osteophytes usually continue the contour of the surface from which they project, and therefore in the facet-joints they are generally shelf-like extensions (Figs 1.4, 1.5, 1.25 and 5.3, 5.4, 5.5). They appear following the beginnings of articular cartilage destruction, but may precede alterations of the subchondral bone. These bony rims may add their quota of movement-restriction, and they also trespass upon related spaces. [They are relatively late manifestations of arthrosis and should *not* be confused with *vertebral body lipping*

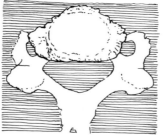
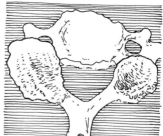

Fig. 5.5 Spondylosis of the intervertebral body joint (L) and arthrosis of the facet-joint (R). These changes frequently but not always coexist at one or more mobility segments. (By courtesy of Phillip Evans.)

(Fig. 5.6) (see p. 140) which is an exostosis of bone probably not necessarily related to the arthrotic or spondylotic process, although providing evidence of stress which has been substained.]

In advanced degeneration, eburnation of opposed bone surfaces occurs, where patches of completely exposed bone-ends are seen, the surfaces resembling polished ivory and formed of hard, compact bone, rubbing together during the very restricted movements possible at these joints. (Ankylosis has been noted under 3.)

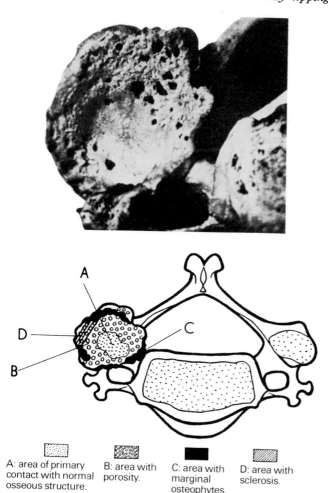

A: area of primary contact with normal osseous structure.

B: area with porosity.

C: area with marginal osteophytes.

D: area with sclerosis.

Fig. 5.4 Photograph and drawing of a facet-joint surface with moderately severe arthrotic changes. The area of the degenerated facet surface is about twice that of the normal side. (Reproduced from Spondylosis Cervicalis: a Pathological and Osteo-archaeological Study, 1969, by kind permission of Dr Sager and the publishers.)

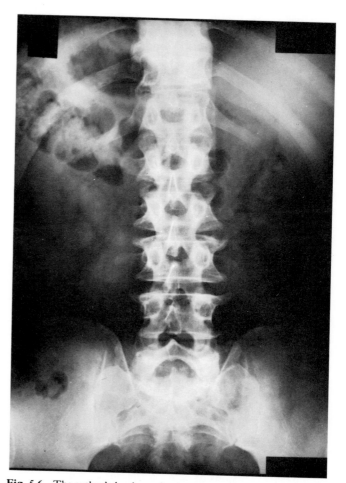

Fig. 5.6 The author's lumbar spine in 1971. 'Claw' spondylophyte on L4 and slight 'traction spurs' on the lower border of L3. There is no instability, or hypermobility, at any segment.

Arthrosis is not necessarily a progressive condition. The well-known examples of restoration of joint space after osteotomy for arthrosis of the hip, and the gradual disappearance of osteophytes after fusion of spondylotic and arthrotic lower cervical segments, testify to the fact that regression of degenerative changes will occur if stress is removed or reduced. This is of practical clinical interest to those handling musculoskeletal joint problems.

B. THE VERTEBRAL BODY JOINTS

1. UNCOVERTEBRAL ARTICULATIONS (neurocentral joints of Luschka)

While joints are primary structures, the uncovertebral clefts or joints of Luschka (see p. 5) are secondary fissures, albeit with a synovial membrane, in primarily normal cervical discs. While the presence of a synovial membrane is disputed by some, cleft-like spaces in the posterolateral aspect of cervical discs C3 to C7 can be recognised in sagittal sections during childhood,[548] and by the end of the first decade they are well established and have begun to widen and to extend horizontally from each side towards the nucleus.

Increasing disc degeneration between C2 and C7 with loss of thickness, and thus more looseness of segmental movement, increases the contact between uncinate processes of the vertebral body below and the bevelled lower edge of the vertebral body above; this process of increasing instability is often aggravated by a tendency for the horizontal fissures to extend transversely inward, and sometimes break through to meet and thus divide the cervical disc into two parts. This is seen as early as the third decade.[1229, 1230] As the junction between vertebral bodies is thus relaxed, stability of these cervical segments is now provided only by the ligaments, the muscles and the outer ring of the annulus fibrosus, which forms the small peripherally placed capsule for these joints.

The excessive movement and shearing stresses sustained by cervical movement (see p. 46) hasten degenerative thickening of the capsule by fibrosis. Increasing strain and pressure are thus placed on the bony eminences in the uncovertebral region, and under the overload, the uncinate processes are slowly forced apart, tending to become everted and smeared out to form bony excrescences (Fig. 1.4).

This bone-to-bone formation trespasses upon related spaces like a pair of enlarged lips, which enclose between them degenerated fibrocartilage and which form the posterolateral extensions of osseocartilaginous bars or bosses (see p. 86) related to accompanying changes in the associated discs.[117, 981, 1093]

2. THE INTERVERTEBRAL DISC

In the massive literature on this subject, the greater majority of contributors have concerned themselves with the lumbar discs, and because of the importance of pathological change in *all* tissues of this spinal region, the changes occurring in *thoracic* and *cervical* interbody joints are described under 'Regional variations of combined degenerative change' (pp. 125, 135).

Like other tissue, most discs degenerate to a greater or lesser degree. They:

1. Desiccate and may lose turgidity
2. May form combined osseocartilaginous bars posteriorly, with exostosis of adjacent vertebral body margins[117]
3. Develop concentric or circumferential tears between laminae of the posterolateral annulus, and radial tears beginning at the nucleus and inner annulus[326]
4. Partially disrupt their annular attachments together with portions of hyaline cartilaginous plate[780]
5. Herniate up and/or down into the spongiosa of vertebral body (microscopically and macroscopically)[1093]
6. Be themselves invaded by vascular tissue from the spongiosa[1044]
7. Undergo internal disruption or isolated resorption, and be slowly ground into rubble[211]
8. Develop a vacuum or gas within the disc[667, 668]
9. Become calcified[315]
10. Bulge into the neural canal[76, 552, 818, 820, 1371]
11. Extrude nuclear pulp into the same space either as a pedunculated mass, a sequestrum or a massive escape (burst) of nuclear contents together with rupture of the posterior longitudinal ligament.[608]

With the exception of the last-named, the relationship between these events and clinical evidence of their presence is by no means direct.

That the intervertebral disc and the vertebral bodies develop, grow and age together has been emphasised by Twomey and Furness (1978),[1256] who stress that the ageing process affects both elements. It is quite impossible to affect one of those structures alone, as the other must sooner or later also be involved, even to a lesser extent (Fig. 5.2). The phrase 'slipped disc' is unfortunate nonsense, directing lay people as well as more gullible and indolent clinical workers to consider the disc as an important interposed washer between unimportant vertebral bodies.

A clear distinction between intervertebral disc degeneration and intervertebral disc disease remains to be established, albeit our detailed knowledge of the physical and biochemical changes increases almost weekly.[4, 499, 1108, 892, 1270] The vertebral column undergoes a fairly predictable sequence of morphological changes from infancy to old age but by no means do all individuals showing these changes suffer significant spinal pain or disability.

Our essential mode of distinction, between ageing and

disease, remains that of clinical criteria, and even this distinction is blurred by the fact that an individual with demonstrable vertebral changes and painful disability is very frequently relieved of symptoms and signs while the vertebral changes persist and slowly multiply.[698]

Sciatica was first described by the early Greek and Roman physicians. However, it was not related to dysfunction of the sciatic nerve until 1764, when Domenico Cotugno of Naples published his *De Ischiade Nervosa Commentarius*. Irritation of the sciatic nerve and its component nerve roots was subsequently found to result from different underlying conditions, such as spinal arthritis, intraspinal and extraspinal neoplasms, and spondylolisthesis. More recently, it became apparent that sciatica is often caused by nerve root compression from a herniated nucleus pulposus of a lumbar intervertebral disc.[1314]

Although the first disc lesion (1893) to be described had occurred in a dog and was reported by a veterinary surgeon,[256] Nachemson (1976) observed,

. . . we have our heritage from Doctor Barr of Boston who, one Sunday morning in 1932 in the Pathology Laboratory of Massachusetts General Hospital, was the first person to understand that the material recently removed from one of his patients as chondroma was in reality a disc hernia. He solved one important part of the low-back pain problem, but, as we all know by now, it was only a minor part.[889b]

Wyke (1976)[1362] considers it should be emphasised (contrary to popular impression) that less than 5 per cent of patients with backache have prolapsed intervertebral discs; about three-quarters of the small handful afflicted in this way will have backache as the initial symptom. This leaves only the occasional patient representing that group whose pain will begin in haunch or lower limb, without backache.

Following the papers of Goldthwait,[420] Dandy,[225] and more especially Mixter and Barr[863] there has been an avalanche of published material on the intervertebral disc; an estimated 3000 papers have appeared since the war, i.e. more than 100 a year, or 2 every week. In the face of this inexorable flow, it is understandable that a senior orthopaedic surgeon should have been moved to observe,

. . . have found in the intervertebral disc not a jelly-like nucleus but a glittering nugget of gold.[924]

For a long time it has been evident that the attention of the medical profession in general has been mesmerized by the discovery of the radiologically visible gross changes in intervertebral discs associated with regional spinal disorders, in some cases to the point at which some medical men seemed to have regarded a pain in the back and the word 'disc' as synonymous. It is of course evident that there are many structures in the spine in which pain can arise.[1100]

A commonly expressed regret of orthopaedic and neurosurgeons is the wide discrepancy between much of what is said and written about the disc and what is actually observed by them during open surgical procedures. It also becomes very difficult to remember that there are other equally important articular tissues in the spinal column.[445]

. . . In the same year, Mixter and Barr published their pioneering paper in the widely read *New England Journal of Medicine* and brought to medical attention ruptured discs, which for the next decade and a half after 1934 were thought by many to explain just about everything abnormal in the lower spine.[1300]

Sunderland (1978)[1194] has summarised the changing approach to common vertebral joint problems as follows:

When investigating the problem of low back pain, one cautions against concentrating exclusively on the intervertebral disc as the site of the offending lesion lest this obscure the significance of aetiological factors originating elsewhere in the vicinity. In this respect the passage of the medial branch of the lumbar dorsal ramus and its accompanying vessels through an osseo-fibrous tunnel and the intimate relationship of this neurovascular bundle to the capsule of the apophyseal joint represents a potential site of fixation and entrapment following pathological changes involving the joint.

The observations of Arnoldi (1972)[42] are relevant,

. . . Pain in the lumbar area can originate in a number of different structural elements, and if we except the apparently clear-cut syndromes with nerve root affection caused by disc herniation we cannot say that our understanding has gained substantially from the impressive pool of detailed information.

There is no clinical sign, nor combination of signs, which prove diagnostic of a *disc* protrusion, other than the signs of a space-occupying lesion.[105] Radiographically demonstrated lumbar disc 'lesions', for example, and demonstration by epidurography that alterations in the profile of disc 'lesions' may be produced by rotatory manipulation and/or traction,[817, 1371] provide interesting corroboration of the ordinary physical changes these procedures might be expected to produce, since discs are subject to physical laws like everything else, yet this does not dispose of our difficulties of confidently ascribing the cause of clinical manifestations, with any real certainty, to changes in a particular tissue.

Barker (1977)[61] describes the incidence of back problems in a general practice with 3000 patients, and a consultation rate of about 10 000 per year; musculoskeletal and connective tissue disorders accounted for some 750 consultations annually. About one-third of these were concerned specifically with complaints of back and leg pain. Over a 2-year period, the data on all patients with back and leg pain were recorded in a standardised way, i.e. 197 cases, and it was suggested by the investigator that the intervertebral disc could account for only a small proportion of these problems.

Brown (1971)[137] reminds us that even more perplexing is the circumstance that enucleation of an intervertebral disc relieves the syndrome of low back pain and sciatica when true mechanical impingement of the nerve root is not evident during surgery.

One of the earlier (and perhaps the fullest) accounts of intervertebral disc pathology presented in British literature was that made by Beadle (1931).[76] in which he described and illustrated the now classic image of posterior or posterolateral bulges in the dorsal aspect of the longitudinal ligament, this perhaps leading to the common concept that nuclear protrusion represents a breach at about the middle of the annulus with extrusion of nuclear material through the breach. This is not necessarily correct;[780] very frequently the essential physical damage is that to the hyaline cartilage plate, a detached segment of which slides or is shifted centrifugally under traction exerted by intact annular fibres, themselves under tension of stress produced by flexion, rotation and compression forces upon a tissue-system in which concentric annular disruption has very probably already begun.

Degenerative changes (see 'Applied anatomy', p. 18) The nature of structural disturbance of the disc is more complex and varied than is sometimes conveyed by simple diagrams and by the hydrostatic theory of disc protrusion.[326]

... the word 'disc' has been used so loosely as to lose all clinical and pathological significance.[780]

The physical properties of intervertebral discs have been conceived as depending mainly upon the water-binding capacity of the nuclear pulp, the hydration of the nucleus being predominantly due to the imbibition pressure exerted by the mucopolysaccharide gel.[239] Normal function of the disc has been observed to require the presence of a fluid nuclear gel to distribute pressure evenly, together with the tensile strength and elastic properties of the pulp-retaining annulus fibrosus, which does contain elastic fibres.[139] The gel distributes the pressure put upon it in an isotropic manner.

With ageing, the soluble polymer content slowly precipitates to form a collagen matrix, and isotropy decreases with the diminution of gel viscosity.[499] Ageing is accompanied by a gradual increase in the collagen content of the pulposus and this takes place at the expense of the gel structures. The lessening of the degree of hydration from early life is progressive, a gel water-content of almost 90 per cent in children slowly decreasing to about 70 per cent in later life. There is generally a sharp rise in severity of degenerative changes in the fifth decade, among those mature people who do come to the notice of clinicians.

Degenerative changes usually become visible in the nucleus before the age of 20, but whether these are evidence of normal age involution or pathological degeneration is not certain.[326] Hirsch and Schajowicz (1953)[546] described changes recognisable as early as the 14th year, apparent as concentric cracks and fissures occurring more commonly in the posterior annulus of the lower two lumbar levels.

Splitting and cleft formation in discs are frequently the artefacts of preparation for pathological examination[1270] but these should not be compared with the macroscopic evidence of annular separations following torsional stresses applied to fresh cadaver material. Farfan (1973)[326] reported disc degeneration, presumably traumatic in origin, in an 8-year-old boy, and there are many reports of disc prolapse in children, adolescents and young adults,[77, 276, 322, 435, 929, 1066] yet Farfan also observed that normal discs may be found at autopsy in patients of 80, 90 or over. In many instances, these discs have experimentally been subjected to compression and torsional loads, and they behave in a manner indistinguishable from younger discs; injections under high pressure failed to show any annular damage or end-plate fractures.

As degenerative change proceeds:

1. The borders between pulp and annulus begin to become less definable and islands of cartilage cells begin to appear among the now more fibrous pulp. In the later stages of disc ageing the collagen of the nucleus and that of the inner annulus tend to coalesce; separation of the two elements becomes more difficult.[499]

2. The annulus progressively loses its elasticity as its cartilage content increases.

3. Degeneration of disc tissue appears to be accelerated if the disc becomes vascularised, as may happen when cartilage end-plates are damaged. Trespass into the disc by vascular tissue, through the previously closed apertures in the cartilaginous end plates, has been described by Ritchie and Farhni (1970).[1044] The more central nucleus becomes typically discoloured, 'brown degeneration', believed in the past to be due to blood pigments from small haemorrages of spongiosa vessels penetrating through minute defects in the hyaline cartilage plate. This 'brown degeneration' is usually associated with a desiccated and friable consistency of the nuclear pulp.[1270] In elderly discs, sites of previous tears are frequently occupied by fibrovascular tissue, providing evidence of previous disruption and of repair processes.[194, 195, 508]

4. Concentric or circumferential tears in the peripheral annulus, as separations of the annular laminae, notably in the posterolateral part of the disc, become evident before the more central radiating fissures begin to track outwards through the peripheral nucleus and inner laminae of the annulus.[1044] Lateral or anterior ruptures are probably rare.[1270] Fragmentation and disruption of the disc have commenced; thus the nucleus pulposus, with the retaining annulus, cannot act as a fluid suspension and shock-absorbing system with its former efficiency, and is less able to redistribute the stresses placed upon it, although nuclear herniation and protrusion do not necessarily follow because of this. The water-binding capacity is more markedly depressed in more degenerated discs; for example, when changes normally seen in the fifth decade of life occur at 40 years, degenerative joint disease, as

opposed to simple ageing, can be considered to be present. The difference between normal discs and those showing frank pathological changes are greater than when young and aged discs are compared.

5. The fissures initially affecting the deeper layers of the annulus extend later to the peripheral layers. This ageing process is frequently hastened by particular types of stress, especially rotation stress, and as a rule the posterior and posterolateral annulus are the sites most often involved in attenuation, disruption and failure, i.e. *disc prolapse*, most common in the lumbar spine. Extrusion of the nucleus pulposus seldom occurs in normal discs.

Concentric tears frequently occur without breaching the outer annulus, reducing the normal resilient stiffness of the mobile segment and allowing a certain 'sloppiness',[872] with consequently reduced ability to withstand the normal strains of movement, and the possibility of increased wear and tear on all the ligamentous and joint structures of that segment. Intervertebral joints with degenerated discs have been found to have appreciable lateral motion (lateral shear of 0.1 to 0.4 inches) at the disc when subjected to torsion; this lateral shear is not observable to any appreciable extent in joints with intact discs.[326] (See Lumbar instability, p. 139.)

Disc prolapse is frequently preceded by episodes of simple bulging, i.e. herniation, as the annulus, without actually being breached, becomes attenuated by rotational stress, and the circumferential tensile stress exerted by compression forces, acting on the nucleus pulposus and annulus.

Farfan (1973)[326] believes the hydrostatic theory of lumbar disc protrusion (i.e. that axial compression will be transmitted as hoop tension to the annulus, and increasing compression may ultimately cause rupture of it, the rupture commencing on its inner side) has many failings; when subjected to experimental proof, the predicted outcome does not occur. In compression tests, the vertebral body always collapses before the disc is damaged to any significant degree.[324] In mechanical torsional tests, of a magnitude which did not injure vertebral bone, it was demonstrated that the orientation of posterior facet-joints protected the discs from torsional stress, the resistance of isolated discs being much less than the discs of an intact lumbar segment. During testing, concentric tears appeared in the annulus, and these were similar to those occurring naturally. The change in facet-orientation at the lower lumbar spine appears to lessen the resistance to torsional stress and the development of circumferential or concentric annular tears. This would accord with the segmental incidence of annular disruption which is, of course, very much greater at the lower two levels.

An apparently logical assumption that the magnitude of weight-bearing stress is directly related to the segmental incidence, because of the higher compression loading at L4–5 and L5–S1, may not be valid. Compression loads

may cause failure of the disc in the sense that end-plate fracture may occur, but this is not failure of the annulus.

Torque strength of isolated discs is not appreciably changed by compression, but experimental torsion of intact joints with compression amounting to 50 per cent of the body weight *increased* the ability to withstand torsional stress by a similar 50 per cent. This may be because facet-joints are more approximated and provide more protection[325] by locking.

Clinicians have known for a considerable time that rotational stress figures largely in patients' descriptions of incidents causing lumbar joint problems, and Farfan readily produced annular failure, as separation of laminae, when applying torsion.

The relatively small twisting force required to injure the intervertebral joint probably occurs in everyday life; for example, using the flexed thigh as a lever to manipulate the spine, a manipulator could easily attain 1000 inch-pounds of torque by applying a 50 lb force to a femur 20 inches long. In this way, he could easily damage the intervertebral joint.[325]

The development of laminar separations in the annulus precedes that of radial perforating fissures, and the torsional stress concentration occurs mainly at the posterolateral portions of the annulus.

Farfan's[326] hypothesis of predisposing factors in degenerative change, and factors preventing the likelihood of lumbar disc damage, might be summarised as follows:

The integrity of the neural arch is a factor of immense importance for the torque strength of the lumbar vertebral segments.

Facet-joint orientation exerts an influence on stresses applied to the intervertebral joint, and is partly responsible for the pattern of degenerative change.

The initial changes of disc degeneration are the result of torsion forced beyond the normal range of motion, which is probably less than 5°.

The distortion of the annulus during experimental rotation strains is most commonly maximal at the posterior surface and especially the posterolateral angle.

Rotation also induces a forward tilt (flexion), forcing the neural arches apart and increasing the interpedicular distance. The posterolateral annulus is distracted.

When torsion is removed, the distortion largely disappears, but the disc has lost stiffness and become 'soft.'

Abnormally increased motion at a joint is usually a sign of severe degeneration, and can be observed in radiographic studies in about 15 per cent of patients with backache.[326] (Morgan and King, 1957,[872] found the incidence to be 28.6 per cent; those especially practised in evaluation of segmental mobility by palpation would probably detect a higher proportion; see p. 328.)

Lack of motion at a lumbar intervertebral joint is usually a sign of *stability* of that joint, and repeated attempts to attain 'normal' range will predictably result in sprain.

Spines with four segments will rotate less than those with five segments, and are perhaps more easily sprained. The most likely initial trauma is combined torsion, bending and compression.

When flexing in the presence of compression due to body weight, the compressive stresses anteriorly in discs are further increased, while the compressive stresses on the posterior parts are decreased, or even reversed to become tensile.

Simultaneous rotation adds an increment of tension which may rise to a critical threshold.

Forward bending of more than 20°–30° is less dangerous than extension to the same degree, thus when applying stress by loading (handling weights) it is advisable to avoid torsion, asymmetrical loading, and hyperextension (a *slightly* flexed lumbar spine is probably the optimum position).

The transverse sectional area of the vertebra is important, as the larger the area the less the stress, as load/area. Large-boned individuals enjoy a natural advantage.

Increased body-weight as such has little to do with disc damage, since the disc is relatively resistant to compression loads. The back sufferer probably gains very little by losing weight.

The orientation of the vertebral body to the line of applied vertical load, and the size of the vertebra, appear important. A small vertebra, orientated at 90° to applied load, is more likely to sustain hyaline plate damage.

A good abdominal musculature maintains the advantageous distribution of load between disc anteriorly and facets posteriorly.

Disc protrusions, though of great importance, are not always of clinical significance.

Following a radiographic and anatomical study of 182 lumbar spines obtained at autopsy, Farfan (1972)[325] concludes that,

asymmetrical articular processes lead to asymmetrical degeneration, while symmetrical processes lead to symmetrical degeneration.

Crock (1970)[211] has given one of the best descriptions of two particular types of change in the lumbar discs:

1. *Isolated disc resorption.* This occurs commonly as an isolated affection in an otherwise normal spine and it is rarely seen in patients with generalised spondylosis. Herniation, and prolapse of pulp via annular-attachment disruption, imply injuries to a still more or less recognisable tissue system, but in middle age or earlier the desiccated disc tissue can become flattened by dehydration and gross disorganisation, with fissuring of fibrocartilage and invasion by connective tissue; differentiation of pulp and annulus becomes progressively more difficult, and the once plastic, resilient and healthy disc may become a thin and hardly recognisable 'washer', an almost amorphous rubble of detached cartilage, remains of pulp, islands of calcification and patches of fibrosis. Thinning of the disc is evident radiographically as a loss of disc space, with marked sclerosis of adjacent vertebral body margins. The remains of disc tissue may be represented by little more than a low ridge of peripheral annular fibres. Often, the disc space is otherwise empty, the amount of rubble remaining depending upon the stage of resorption existing at the time of autopsy examination. It may occur both in patients who gave no history of symptoms likely to have accompanied a sudden herniation or prolapse of disc material, and also in those with a history of injury.

2. *Internal disc disruption.* This change is characterised by alterations in internal structure of the disc (specifically *excluding* escape of disc material from the confines of its space). There appear to be alterations in metabolic functions of the disc, reflected in local and often in constitutional changes. Of the pathological changes, little is known. Macroscopically, the tissue is soft, slightly yellow, and the staining properties are altered. Fibrillation of the annulus may be seen. The sympathetic trunk is seen matted to the adjacent disc, and paravertebral lymph nodes are enlarged. The density of adjacent vertebral bodies is altered, with increased vascularity and marked softening of vertebral bodies. There are three probable causes of symptoms; irritation of adjacent roots, due to abnormal vertebral movement with or without disc bulging, irritation of adjacent structures due to leaking products of disc metabolites, or leaking of protein metabolites into general circulation by vertebral vessel pathways, producing what may be an autoimmune reaction.

Lumbar disc herniation is nearly always by trespass into the extradural space. Ruptures of disc into the *intradural* space[554] are very much less common, a total of 21 cases being reported, 15 male and 6 female. These patients usually have more severe neurological deficit, and only 1 patient was neurologically normal. In 1 case, computed tomography scanning with a water-soluble contrast agent, at the L4–L5 level, revealed the intradural mass.

The importance of assessment

The salient features of disc degeneration which have been outlined may occur slowly over many decades, perhaps not proceeding to the final stages at all, or may speedily progress to practically complete obliteration of the disc as a recognisable tissue system, before the age of 40. The form and degree of degenerative change, and its consequences, are infinitely variable from patient to patient, *the available space in the neural canal being of critical importance.*[315]

Naylor (1971)[908] observes that injury should be seen only as an additional factor, and that by setting up abnormal stresses in the annulus it increases the tendency to produce annular tears. He adds:

1. All disc herniations are basically spontaneous in onset and trauma is never the sole factor.

2. Once a disc prolapse occurs some measure of defective function must remain, and predisposition to recurrence is present.

3. With the passage of time the risk of recurrence is progressively less.

The changes which occur during the life of an intervertebral disc occur in time as well as space; very frequently these changes may be advanced at one segment or minimal or absent at others. Often, an apparently similar degree of degeneration in three adjacent segments will exist in the presence of symptoms manifestly arising from only one of them, and relieved by localised treatment techniques to that single segment.

Depending upon the patient's inheritance of body-type and postural habit, work and recreation stresses, trauma, disease, psychic health, culture and temperament, the clinical presentation of pain at any particular time is frequently multifactorial, often being coloured by some underlying and transient stress which is not declared and seemingly not even fully recognised and confronted by the patient.

Neat and detailed tabulated lists, of the changes known to occur in a chronological sequence in the intervertebral body joints from childhood to old age, are useful for completeness and are aesthetically satisfying to the academician; in the hurly-burly of clinical practice, they become for the most part abstractions, having little application *of immediate clinical importance* to the effective handling of joint problems from patient to patient. Each is like no other, and therefore unique.

Expressed otherwise, it is salutary to remember not to treat the textbook, or the X-ray appearance, or the concept, but that which is an existing reality and therefore objectively verifiable, i.e. the signs presented by each individual in pain.

Retrospective examination of case histories of the subjects of autopsy examination indicates in many instances that quite marked spondylotic changes do not appear to have given rise to back pain of any severity.[1270]   There is now a shift of emphasis from the idea that disc disorders result from purely mechanical derangement, to the view that the nutrition and metabolism of the disc, and the biochemistry of degenerative change, are of equal importance.[212, 811, 908]

LaRocca (1971)[698] draws attention to three important research findings:

The first is the observation that the pH of the tissue fluid surrounding degenerate nuclear fragments is lower than the physiological pH. The second is the demonstration of the antigenicity of protein-polysaccharide from the nucleus pulposus in the same animals from which the nuclear material was obtained. A third is the combination of the laboratory demonstration of profound protein-polysaccharide disarray that occurs with intradiscal injection of chymopapain and the clinical observation that symptoms of back pain can be improved or eliminated by intradiscal chymopapain injection.

Yet among many of those concerned every day with the conservative treatment of musculoskeletal problems, there remains a tendency to regard the disc as a sort of badly packed suitcase, in that any untidy bits sticking out should ideally be stuffed back in again, or failing that lopped off, rather like a Laurel and Hardy haircut.[450]

It is interesting to note that during a series of myelographic investigations of 300 people with neither symptoms nor signs, around 37 per cent were found to have evidence of trespass into the neural canal, and in 9 per cent the changes were marked.[552]

St Clair Strange (1966)[1164] comments that the diagnosis of a prolapsed intervertebral disc, imperfectly made, has been responsible for making very many perfectly fit men and women into lifelong invalids.

N.B. There are many conditions of intervertebral discs in which degenerative processes are not the primary aetiological factor; they are not described here.

3. THE VERTEBRAL BODIES

Under the forces applied to it, the disc material tends to move centrifugally, and a frequent change, as a result of the traction by annular fibres on the periosteum of vertebral bodies, is stimulation of osteoblast activity at the edges of the bodies. This new bone formation is extended outwards as the tractive process continues, the *lipping* and *spurring* of two adjacent body margins sometimes assuming the appearance of a parrot's beak. It often occurs, in the absence of disc thinning, in the lumbar spines of men whose work or recreation involves much lifting or with the application of other forms of compressive forces, and is here probably not a truly degenerative process but the adaptation of healthy tissue to occupational stress (Fig. 5.6).

Of a group of 178 coalminers over the age of 40 years, 48 per cent had spurring of vertebral bodies without disc narrowing.[373]

When occurring with frank loss of disc substance, the vertebral lipping is accompanied by increased density of bone in the region of the hyaline cartilage plates, i.e. sclerosis of the adjacent body margins (Fig. 6.8). (See also The traction spur, p. 140.)

4. THE HYALINE CARTILAGE PLATES

Normal cartilage end-plates do not have gaps, and the protrusion of nuclear material cranially or caudally is only possible when there is a gap, or a weakness of the end-plate which predisposes to gap formation.[1270]   Defects in the plate allow small vessels from the spongiosa to penetrate the nucleus. Tiny and sometimes massive haemorrhages can therefore occur in the normally avascular nucleus. The plate degenerates and loses its tissue character, to merge with the vertebral body sclerosis, but frequently the weakened lamina of hyaline cartilage is breached by nuclear material under compression, the extent of this vertical type of protrusion trespassing into the spongiosa being outlined by its thin sclerotic bony margins; this is a very frequent X-ray appearance (see p. 262).[1093]

A further common radiographic appearance of the lumbar vertebrae is that of the plate bowing into the vertebral bodies like a cupid's bow, probably evidence of compression strains sustained by a retreat of plate into spongiosa without actual breaching. This bowing is outlined by sclerosis.

NERVE ROOT INVOLVEMENT

INTRODUCTION

An attempt to briefly summarise past and more recent work on nerve injury makes for some untidy bedfellows, because the field is a very large one and interesting developments occur neither in step with each other nor side-by-side.

Comparatively little is known about the pathophysiology of nerve root compression.[1114] Few clinical/experimental studies of root compression have been reported, most studies having concentrated on peripheral nerves, and thus the knowledge of the relative amounts of damage to myelin and axon of the nerve root is somewhat limited. Surgical biopsies of compressed roots are rarely performed. In many decompression procedures, care is taken not to incise the dura, so that the root is not even visualised.

As nerves and roots are structurally similar it seems reasonable to draw some inferences from clinical consequences of traumatic injury to peripheral nerve, and reports of experimental injury of nerves. The inferences should not be carried too far, since irritant and compressive *effects* on peripheral nerves are not quite the same as when spinal nerve roots suffer the same interference, also spinal roots themselves appear to have different *responses* to experimental compression, and to stimulation. For example:

1. During Frykholm's operations[392] on the cervical spine under local anaesthesia:
   a. the dorsal root was stimulated, and the patient reported a 'neuralgic' pain in the dermatome distribution
   b. if the ventral, motor root was stimulated, the patient reported a deep 'boring' myalgic pain, situated more proximally in the muscles which were painful and tender preoperatively.

2. In the region of the intervertebral foramen, spinal nerve roots with motor and sensory fibres of the somatic nervous system have extensive connections, via white and grey rami communicantes, with the autonomic nervous system, the whole forming Stillwell's paravertebral plexus.[1177] Peripheral nerves carry only a few autonomic nerve fibres because these have already separated to pass down the limb in the coats of the arteries. Proximal mechanical pressure on radicular nerves has a greater effect therefore on the autonomic nervous system than does distal pressure on peripheral nerve trunks.[1180b] The cold sciatic leg is much more common than similar distal temperature changes in the carpal tunnel syndrome, for example.

3. Axons compressed close to their parent neurone cell suffer a greater risk of the cell being damaged than when pressure is remote. Entrapment neuropathy at the wrist can lead to a permanent loss of power in the thenar muscles, but it is unlikely to lead to permanent damage of posterior root-ganglion cells, whereas compression at the intervertebral foramen may well cause permanent damage in the posterior ganglion cells.

4. As will be seen, there are differences in the behaviour of peripheral nerves and spinal roots subjected to the same experimental injury.[1112]

'In these matters it should be noted that damage to sensory nerve fibres is not necessarily painful' (Sunderland, 1978).[1194]

While lesions of trespass upon spinal cord and nerve roots remain the prime concern for those handling common vertebral joint problems, the study of compressive effects on peripheral nerves remains of value and interest. Sunderland's (1968)[1191] authoritative and extensive review indicates that experimental findings are sometimes contradictory, as are the interpretations of findings, e.g. the different susceptibilities of the different diameter fibres, the time needed for a complete compressive block and the most important cause of it.

Susceptibility to stress

That peripheral nerves tolerate without pain the stresses and strains of normal free active and passive movements, of a wide range, indicate that nerves enjoy *protective mechanisms*,[1194] viz:

1. With two exceptions (the ulnar nerve of the elbow and the sciatic nerve behind the hip), nerves cross the flexor aspect of joints; extension is more limited than flexion, thus tension is less likely to occur.

2. By reason of an undulating course, of the nerve trunk, of the funiculi within the perineum, of the nerve fibres within the funiculi, the nerve fibres themselves are the last to suffer tension when stretching is applied.

3. The perineurim imparts elasticity to the nerve trunk and gives it tensile strength.

4. The large amount of epineurial connective tissue,

providing a loose matrix for the funiculi, has a cushioning effect.

Nerve roots differ from peripheral nerves—the nerve fibres are arranged in parallel bundles which are loosely supported by endoneurial tissue alone; they are more vulnerable to stretch since they lack the tensile strength of peripheral nerves. Without epineurial packing they are also susceptible to compression, and the semiosseous confines of the intervertebral foramen are an added potential danger.

Traction on peripheral nerves during neck, trunk and limb movements will transmit tension to the nerve roots, and cause 'piston-like' movements of the root complex within the foramen, but a degree of protection from overstretching by transmitted forces is provided, i.e.:

1. Traction pulls the entire root/dura complex outwards, the cone-shaped dural funnel thus plugging the foramen and resisting further lateral movement.

2. Since relatively large upper limb movements are likely to greatly stress cervical nerve roots, those of C4 to C7 are firmly attached, by slips of prevertebral fascia and from musculotendinous attachments, to the 'gutter' of the cervical transverse process.

3. The elastic properties of nerve roots allow accommodation of tension to a degree, but this is limited. Nerve roots will fail under a given tension before peripheral nerves.

Conversely, there are several factors which may lower the threshold of nerve fibres for the point at which abnormal effects begin to occur, e.g.:

1. Adhesions which bind down the nerve, or reduce its mobility.

2. Changes in connective tissue which reduce its elasticity.

3. Damaged nerve fibres are more susceptible to mechanical deformation, and to ischaemia.

4. Toxic or metabolic neuropathies, and intercurrent infections, render the nerve more likely to suffer from a traumatic or ischaemic event.

Axonal transport

Those neurones with long axonal processes, which depend upon components manufactured in the cytoplasm, allow the study of traffic which moves within them.[1078]

Transfer of substances underlies trophic and other long-term influences of peripheral neurones on the metabolism, function, development and growth of the structure innervated.

Orthograde transneuronal movement of biochemical substances, proceeding from the anterior horn cell along the axon into the fibres of muscle, has been demonstrated by radioactive isotope tracing methods (Korr. 1967).[674]

The most extensively studied are the labelled proteins, some of which move slowly at about 1 mm a day (slow transport) while others move considerably more quickly (fast transport).

Ochs (1975)[946] showed that the characteristic outflow is graphically seen as a crest of advancing activity followed by a plateau, typically with less activity in it compared to the crest. The crest advances at a linear rate down the fibre, and in a large number of experiments the rate determined was 410 mm per day. The rate is independent of nerve size, i.e. diameter of myelinated fibres or unmyelinated fibres, and for a given neurone, the rate of transfer of all molecules is always the same. A range of soluble proteins, polypeptides and particulates are carried down, as are glycoproteins, glycolipids and phosphatidyl-choline, together with catecholamines and enzymes related to their synthesis.

It is common knowledge that effector cells have important influences on the innervating neurones, and Thoenen (1978)[1211] describes the evidence that retrograde axonal transport is linked to subcellular structures which are similar to those associated with orthograde transport.

Among the many experiments described were those in which transplants, preincubated in a medium containing nerve growth factor (NGF) become more densely and more rapidly innervated by adrenergic fibres than without preincubation. Preincubation in a medium containing antibodies to NGF markedly impaired the reinnervation of the transplanted tissue. These and other observations provide support for the hypothesis that NGF might act as a macromolecular messenger between effector organs and their innervating neurones.

Albuqerque *et al.* (1974)[16] have demonstrated that the important trophic action which nerves have on striated muscle is in fact related to axonal transport.

Some of the molecules delivered by axoplasmic transport are needed for transmitter metabolism and for trophic action on innervated cells. . . . With the present state of knowledge, the impact that nerve compression, stretching, angulation or other deformations may have on the neurochemistry of axonal transport is not known but can reasonably be inferred to be significant. [Samson, 1978][1078]

Sjöstrand (1978)[1141] mentions that a local supply of energy is needed to fuel the axonal transport, which is partially or completely blocked by local ischaemia or compression.

In nerves which had been subjected to local compression, an acute accumulation of labelled proteins was found in the region of the compression.

A 2-hour compression with pressures as low as 50 mmHg (6.67 kPa) caused blockage of fast transport, which was reversible within 24 hours. Reversal of transport blockage usually occurred within 3 days after compression at 200 mmHg (26.66 kPa) for 2 hours and within 7 days after compression at 400 mmHg (53.33 kPa) for 2 hours.

Sjöstrand[1141] has suggested that conduction block, transport impairment and intraneural oedema may differ in their reversibility, also that orthograde and retrograde transport may also be differentially affected by nerve injury.

Haldeman and Meyer (1970)[485] mention that the recorded study of peripheral nerve compression or constriction is more than 100 years old.

Waller (1862)[1286] described the effects of compression on the radial, median and ulnar nerves of his own arm. He did not refer to the mechanism by which these experiments disturbed nerve conduction, perhaps because it appeared self-evident that the conduction block was due to simple pressure. That this was apparently not so was demonstrated by Grundfest (1936)[460] who found that a pressure of 1000 atmospheres (101,325 kPa) was necessary to completely block nerve conduction; hence the until recently prevailing view that the clinical consequences of compression or stretching of nerves were due mainly to obliteration of the vasa nervorum.[1037]

There is a list of more than 50 reports of investigation into conduction block, ischaemia and postischaemic paraesthesiae, indicating the importance of these abnormal processes and their prime interest for clinicians. Severe and prolonged compression blocks the nerves' blood supply and produces other damage; it then loses its ability to conduct impulses. Prolonged inflammation appears to produce the same effect. Temporary compression will produce temporary loss of conduction, from minutes to days according to the degree and duration of compression. Intermittent compression or mechanical irritation may lead to inflammatory changes, with space-occupying effects produced by oedema and thus some or all of the changes and clinical features following inflammation. Traction, of insufficient force to disrupt the nerve, will cause irritation and consequent neuritis.[1180b]

Sunderland (1968)[1191] refers to the three fundamental types of peripheral nerve injury, in which:

1. There is temporary interruption of conduction without loss of axonal continuity between neurone and end-organ.

2. The axon is severed or axonal mechanisms are so disorganised that the distal axon does not survive, neither for a variable distance does the proximal axon. The endoneurial sheath is preserved unthreatened by the injury reaction and the ensuing Wallerian degeneration.

3. The fibres are severed or the wall of the endoneurial tube and its contents are so disorganised that the normal architecture of the fibre is completely destroyed.

Compressive injury to nerve results in two distinct pathological processes:[995]

1. Relatively low-intensity trauma (pressures between 150–1000 mmHg) (20–133.33 kPa) causes segmental demyelination. Electrical studies demonstrate slowing of conduction velocity (partial conduction block) in the injured segment. Distal to the injury, conduction velocity and neuromuscular function are preserved. For restoration of full normal function, only myelin resynthesis in the injured section is needed; this is ordinarily rapid and complete.

2. With more severe trauma, Wallerian degeneration occurs. Distally, the nerve becomes electrically inexcitable, and the myoneural junction and sensory end-organs degenerate. For the restoration of full function, neurones must synthesise large quantities of axonal structure proteins, axons must sprout through the distal nerve segments to re-establish synaptic contact with muscle and finally these axons must be remyelinated. This complex regenerative process is usually incomplete and unsatisfactory especially in the adult.

Denny-Brown and Brenner (1944)[249] applied compression of 170–430 g by a spring clip to a peripheral nerve for two hours, and reported intermittent loss of myelin at the nodes of Ranvier in the compressed area. There was transient paralysis of 5–18 days, but this was not associated with any gross defects of sensation, and the distal portion of the nerve did not degenerate. Despite the recovery of motor conduction within a few days, restoration of myelin was only slight at two months, and remained incomplete at six months. The authors regarded the effects of compression to be due entirely to changes produced in the axoplasm rather than due to the selective consequences of pressure on fibres of different sizes.

Barlow and Pochin (1948)[62] showed that repeated ischaemia reveals a reduction in the degree of recovery of nerve, e.g. after cuff occlusion of a human arm for 25 minutes, sensation and motor power will return to normal. For some hours afterwards, however, a second occlusion will produce earlier development of sensory and motor changes. Thus repeated pressures increase the vulnerability of peripheral nerves, although cumulative effects only appear if the periods of relief are small in comparison to the periods of occlusion.

Haldeman and Meyer (1970)[485] used different techniques to compress the frog peroneal nerve and showed that there are two mechanisms involved in the blocking of nerves by constriction and pressure. The techniques were:

1. A single loop of surgical cotton (0.25 mm) was tied loosely around the nerve, and weights which created tensions of 40, 60 and 80 g were applied to pull the cotton more tightly around the nerve.

2. A 2–3 mm wide plastic strip was placed around the nerve, and weights to effect a constriction exerting 40 g and 80 g were applied. The responses of alpha and beta fibres, to a stimulus applied at a frequency of one impulse every 4 seconds, were noted. Decreasing amplitudes of the spike potential were expressed as percentages of the maximum:

1. *With the 0.25 mm constriction*, recordings were as follows:

Table 5.1

40 g			60 g			80 g		
Time (minutes)	Alpha (% of maximum)	Beta	Time (minutes)	Alpha (% of maximum)	Beta	Time (minutes)	Alpha (% of maximum)	Beta
0	100	100	0	100	100	0	100	100
1.0	85	80				0.5	35	60
						1.0	8	0
			2	67	85	1.5	2	0
3	71	65						
			5	53	60			
6	56	35						
			8	42	40			
18	46	20						
			20	30	30			
36	44	10						
45	43	10	45	12	15			
			60	7	8			
Release			Release			Release		
5	46	35	5	10	0			
30	44	65	30	8	0	30	0	0
						60 days	0	0

At 40 g constriction the spike decreases rapidly for 15 minutes, and then much more slowly. The slow-conducting *gamma* fibres stopped conducting almost at once, within 1 minute, and are not recorded.

The *beta* spike virtually disappeared after 18 minutes. After this, the *alpha* spike continued slowly decreasing. On release, the *alpha* response was virtually unchanged at 30 minutes; the *beta* spike had increased to about half its normal amplitude, its responses being roughly similar to those of an unconstricted nerve after 75 minutes of the steadily repetitive stimulation described above.

At 60 g constriction, the amplitude of responses has diminished more quickly and to a greater degree; release of constriction had little effect. effect.

At 80 g constriction, twitching was observed as the spike potential began immediately to decrease to virtual disappearance at $1\frac{1}{2}$ minutes. Similar constriction in anaesthetised experimental animals produced paralysis which still persisted at 60 days, when the spike potential remained absent and typical Wallerian degeneration was evident distal to the constriction. There is a puzzling discrepancy between the effects of compression by a spring clip[249] and by constriction by a single, 0.25 mm wide loop of surgical cotton, and the authors refer to this when comparing their findings with those of other reports.[83, 84, 161, 1302] The second method of constriction was varied to resemble more closely the techniques of previous investigators.

2. *With the 2–3 mm constriction*, the effects were as follows:

Table 5.2

40 g			80 g		
Time (minutes)	Alpha (% of maximum)	Beta	Time (minutes)	Alpha (% of maximum)	Beta
0	100	100	0	100	100
			1	50	50
			2	25	10
3	86	50	3	13	0
			5	2	0
6	57	0			
10	21	0			
15	5	0			
Release			Release		
2	14	10			
5	28	40			
15	43	60			
30	57	70			
			45	3	0

With an 80 g compression, the spike potential reacted in much the same way as after 80 g compression with the 0.25 mm cotton. The quickly diminishing response was completely absent after 5 minutes and had not returned after 30 minutes.

With the 40 g compression, the responses were markedly different. The spike potential diminished more rapidly than with the 0.25 mm constriction at the same pressure, being completely absent after 15 minutes. On release, however, recovery started almost immediately, and continued for about 25 minutes, reaching to around 60 per cent of its original value by 30 minutes, at which time it had levelled out to remain constant. As previously, the *beta* response disappeared first. It also showed the larger recovery.

CONCLUSIONS

There appear to be two mechanisms involved in nerve block by compression:

1. The first is completely reversible and seems to leave the nerve undamaged, i.e. a reversible conduction block.

2. The second is irreversible—it disturbs nerve continuity and Wallerian degeneration follows, i.e. the irreversible conduction block.

The nature of the mechanism involved appears dependent upon the nature of compression, its duration and the degree of deformity produced by it.

1. The reversible conduction block

Depending upon the nature of the constriction, a nerve can still obtain enough oxygen, by diffusion over a distance of 5 cm, to maintain almost full activity. The usual explanation of the reversible block is anoxia, based on the knowledge that a nerve deprived of oxygen ceases to conduct in 16–35 minutes. Yet pressure may be applied to a nerve in such a way as to make it ischaemic, without impairing conduction;[83] although diffusion ceases at pressures in excess of 100 mmHg (13.33 kPa), when the nerve does become anoxic.

Cessation of oxygen diffusion is probably then due to a decrease in axoplasmic and endoneural fluid (produced by the more severe compression) through which oxygen can diffuse. If neither axons nor blood vessels are damaged during the constriction, conducting ability returns soon after compression is removed.

2. The irreversible conduction block

This is a different mechanism; the time needed to produce block with the 0.25 mm cotton stricture is longer, with the same 40 g tension. The number of fibres affected depended on the degree of constriction. Moderate constriction affected a few fibres, the others presumably being protected by the inertia of axoplasmic and endoneural fluids. With increasing stricture all fibres were blocked, and more quickly. Two months later, the nerve had not recovered conduction.

From cross-sections through the constriction it was observed that the three elements necessary for impulse conduction (intracellular fluid, extracellular fluid and an intact membrane) were all eliminated by severe constriction. The fluids had been forced out by the pressure, which had also destroyed the axolemma and myelin sheath.

Allen (1938)[19] showed that while asphyxia of a limb may cause a paralysis which is reversible, direct pressure from a tourniquet can cause permanent loss of nerve conduction. Vascular injury or irritation leading to traumatic arterial spasm may also produce an irreversible block.[485]

Alpha and *beta* fibres appear to act quite differently to compression and its consequences. In the *reversible constriction*, the beta-response disappeared long before the alpha spike was eliminated, but the beta fibres were quicker to recover and did so to a greater degree. In the *irreversible constriction*, the beta fibres were again blocked earlier, and again showed a degree of recovery. The alpha fibres showed no recovery at all.

Gelfan and Tarlov (1956)[403] found the largest fibres most susceptible to compression and the finest relatively resistant, while anoxia blocks the smaller alpha before the larger ones.

Accordingly, alpha fibres would be affected by the slight constriction itself, and would not recover conduction at release, whereas beta fibres would be affected by the anoxia occasioned by constriction, and would recover again upon diffusion of oxygen after removal of constriction. The authors make the following observations:

The latency for complete blocking in each neuronal structure is specific and irreducible in the case of anoxia, whereas in compression it varies over a wide range depending upon the magnitude of the compression force. The entire pattern of modification of neuronal responses by compression, and the postcompression recovery pattern, are distinctly different from the patterns obtained during anoxia and recovery from the latter, indicating the difference in mechanism by which (a) mechanical deformation, and (b) oxygen lack, block conduction.

Acute peripheral nerve compression

Until recently, it was held that the effects of compressing and stretching a mammalian nerve trunk, under clinical conditions, are due mainly to obliteration of vasa nervorum, i.e. an ischaemic lesion. Anatomical points of possible entrapment were viewed as localities where the nerve is especially vulnerable to focal ischaemia.[706]

Since the early 1970s there has developed the view that these are not ischaemic lesions, but are caused by the direct mechanical deformation of nerve fibres (Gilliatt, 1975).[409]

1. When a sphygmomanometer cuff is used to produce a demyelinating block in an experimental animal, the pressure needed to do this is much greater than that required to occlude blood vessels.

2. Histological examination showed most of the demyelinating lesions occurring near the edges of the compressed region, and not at its centre.

3. Physiological studies on the experimental animal confirmed that nerve damage was concentrated in those portions of the nerve under the edges of the cuff. These findings suggest mechanical distortion of nerve fibres under the edges of a cuff rather than an ischaemic process, which could be expected to be maximal under its centre.

4. Clear evidence of mechanical damage of a particular kind is observed, in single nerve fibres at the cuff edges.

The node of Ranvier, instead of being under the Schwann cell junction, had moved along the fibres ... for a distance of more than 100 microns ... the terminal loops of the myelin sheath remained attached to the axon membrane at the node, so that the whole myelin sheath had been dragged along with it, the myelin being stretched on one side of the node and invaginated on the other ... analogous to the way in which a mass protruding into the lumen of the intestine causes in intussusception ... the axoplasmic movement always occurs in opposite directions under the two edges of the cuff ... the force which moves the nodal axoplasm comes from the pressure difference between the compressed and uncompressed portions of the nerve.

It should be noted that only the *large* myelinated fibres are affected in this way, and that the nodes on the small myelinated fibres are usually normal. This perhaps explains the relative sparing of sensation, a familiar clinical feature of acute compressive lesions in man. The characteristic changes have been seen in man as well as in experimental animals. The important factor is the force per unit area, and with respect to how much pressure is needed, the results of cuff experiments in animals, and pressure by thin nylon cord, agree fairly well. Pressures of 1.5—20 kg/cm² (147.1—1961.3 kPa) are, in the baboon, sufficient to cause a block; the nerve of an unconscious patient will not be damaged if the weight of the limb is resting over a wide area, but localised pressure by external surfaces will cause the lesion.

A further important factor is the *duration* of the compression. In the baboon, both cuff and nylon cord produced a longer-duration block (with Wallerian degeneration in a proportion of the fibres) after a three-hour compression than after a two-hour compression. Wallerian degeneration was rarely found with the shorter-duration compression. It is assumed that the notable difference between a two-hour and a three-hour compression is due to direct pressure and ischaemia now acting in combination.

Chronic peripheral nerve compression

Slowly increasing compression of a nerve will initiate among other damage the vascular changes of an ischaemic lesion, and Sunderland (1978)[1194] takes the model of one funiculus (or fasciculus), in an unyielding tunnel, to describe the changes.

The only intrafunicular vessels are capillaries, since the arterioles and the venules and veins lie in the epineurium; because of their oblique course through the perineurial sheath, the nutrient vessels suffer closure when there is swelling of the bundle. Veins succumb before arteries.

The pressure gradient across the fine interrelated pressure systems in the confines of the tunnel, i.e.: (1) that in the nutrient arterioles, (2) the capillary pressure, (3) the intrafunicular pressure, (4) the pressure in epineurial veins, (5) the pressure within the unyielding tunnel, must be (1)>(2)>(3)>(4)>(5) for adequate circulation, and there is little margin of safety when the intracompartmental pressure increases. When pressure does rise, by tunnel stenosis and/or swelling of the tunnel contents, the epineurial venules succumb and initiate a series of abnormal changes, the most serious occurring within the funiculus.

First stage: Flow in capillaries is slowed, congestion occurs and intracapillary pressure rises. Intrafunicular pressure rises and a vicious circle begins. Nerve fibres are compressed and the resultant hypoxia causes the spontaneous discharges of nerve hyperexcitability. Larger myelinated fibres suffer earlier, and these changes are painful, although reversible by any procedure which relieves compression.

Second stage: Capillary flow decreases further, and the consequent anoxia damages capillary endothelium so that protein escapes and causes oedema in the tissue spaces. Protein accumulates in the endoneurial space, to add a further increment of intrafunicular pressure. Nerve fibres are now seriously at risk by severe interference with nutrition, deformation, proliferation of fibroblasts and thus extra connective tissue in the endoneurium.

The thinning nerve fibres begin to undergo segmental demyelination. Within their endoneurial sheaths, some axons are then interrupted, and these fibres degenerate. While some resistant fibres may continue normal conduction, most surviving but thinned fibres conduct at reduced velocity; a further proportion has sustained a first degree (conduction block) injury and in others the injury by deformation is followed by Wallerian degeneration. Thus at this stage the lesion is a mixed one, and as the structural changes advance, sensory and motor deficiencies in the territory supplied will reflect them.

If decompression then occurs, blood and fluid transfer is restored, oedema slowly resolves and the intrafunicular pressure subsides. The degree and duration of motor and sensory recovery depends on the extent and distribution of minor changes, and of irreversible ones.

Stage three: Continuous and long-standing compression leads to a permanent state as interference with the arterial supply is added to the existing disturbance of venous drainage.

Fibroblasts proliferate in the protein exudate, with a progressive and irreversible fibrosis constricting yet more nerve fibres. The consequence of final obliteration of the nutrient vessels is conversion of the nerve to a fibrous cord; a few fine nerve fibres may survive, within a dense and relatively avascular epineurium.

In further consideration of the *mechanical deformations* described above (p. 98), Gilliatt (1975)[409] suggests that in chronic compression 'detachment of the terminal loops of myelin from the axon at the node of Ranvier initiates a sequence of changes leading to demyelination'. Detachment allows the inner myelin layers to slip back along the axon, with first thinning of the myelin sheath and then complete demyelination of the axon at one end of the internode; redundant folds of myelin are formed at the other end.

Regarding types of trauma, longitudinal stretching may have the same effect, and it can be visualised that this could occur when a section of the nerve is tethered at the site of entrapment when other parts of the nerve are freely mobile.

This asymmetrical appearance of myelin is known to occur at entrapment sites of human median and ulnar nerves, as well as in experimental animals. Gilliatt poses the question: what part, if any, does ischaemia play in these lesions? There is good evidence that ischaemia causes the acute attacks of pain which are characteristic of the carpal tunnel syndrome. Even a short period of ischaemia can block conduction reversibly in damaged fibres, and the temporary power and sensation loss, often accompanying episodes of pain in this syndrome, is probably also caused by ischaemia.

Gilliatt also mentions that, 'the factors which determine the progression from demyelination to Wallerian degeneration within the lesions, and which cause the deposition of collagen and neuromatous thickening, are not well understood'.

Wyke (1974)[1360] has fully discussed the functional aspect of injuries to peripheral nerves as (a) the changes occurring distal to the injury, (b) those occurring proximal to the injury and (c) changes occurring in the parent cell from which the injured fibres derive. Functional changes in regenerating nerve fibres, and the phase of maturation, together with techniques of electrophysiological investigation, including skin thermography and the measurement of skin electrical resistance, are also described in detail.

Where nerve trunks pass through soft tissues such as muscle, fascia or ligament, information about local changes in lesions at these points is scanty. It is suggested that the nature of the lesion is a fibrosis secondary to mechanical irritation, but the nature of the pathology is unknown and Sunderland (1978)[1194] observes,

The biopsy specimens that I have had the opportunity of examining histologically have shown surprisingly little to account for the distressing pain associated with entrapment.

In the opinion of the writer, this may well be because the tissues examined are innocent, and a like search in the region of the associated vertebral joint, and/or foramen, might frequently reveal ample objective changes to account for the patient's distress (pp. 103, 242).

Compressive nerve root lesions

Though neural structures are at hazard in the intervertebral foramina, there is usually ample room and the root is cushioned by fatty areolar tissue; yet some roots are eccentrically placed[904] and may have a smaller margin of safety.

Remarkable degrees of deformation will be tolerated by the nerve, provided this is sufficiently slow and blood supply is not impaired. For example, Frykholm (1971)[392] has observed:

Cervical spondylosis can only be regarded as a predisposing factor for the development of nerve root symptoms. As a matter of fact, it is quite amazing to what extent a nerve root can become squeezed and deformed by a slowly growing osteophytic protrusion, without any clinical evidence of irritation or dysfunction. Reactive fibrosis may also involve the root-sheaths, and periarticular tissues, obliterating the root pouches, and yet the root may remain functionally intact. Such changes, however, always make the root extremely vulnerable to all kinds of stress and strain.

When intervertebral foraminal dimensions are significantly reduced, the veins are first to suffer and impairment of the nerve's venous return is probably the cause of the early neurological symptoms and signs (Sunderland, 1978).[1194]

Irritative nerve root lesions

Arthrotic changes in facet-joints and degenerative changes in neighbouring soft tissue may produce irregularities in the normally smooth foraminal profile, and repetitive injury to the nerve during its small movements in the foramina may be intensified by nerve root angulation over foraminal edges.[904]

The chronic irritation may initiate a friction fibrosis (p. 102), which constricts the root, interfers with its blood supply and forms adhesions which tether the root so that traction effects deform it further.

The medial branches of *posterior primary rami* traverse a fibro-osseous tunnel around the facet-joint structures as they curve backwards and medially to supply the joint and other neighbouring tissues. The little neurovascular bundle is intimately related to the facet-joint capsule, and is at risk of fixation and entrapment by degenerative changes, including capsular thickening and fibrosis, of the associated joint.

DIFFERENT RESPONSES OF SCIATIC NERVE AND SPINAL ROOT

It seems reasonable to suppose that there is a fairly close parallel between the effects of spinal root compression and peripheral nerve compression, when the factors of different effects upon ventral and dorsal roots, and the high population of autonomic fibres in the vicinity of the intervertebral foramen, are taken into account.

However, Sunderland (1978)[1194] asserts that spinal

roots yield more readily to tensile stress since they lack the perineurium and funicular plexus formations of peripheral nerves, while Gelfan and Tarlov (1956)[403] mention their impressions that spinal nerve roots are more susceptible than peripheral nerves to compression forces.

Sharpless (1975)[1112] reviewed the results of previous workers, and applied pressures of 0–180 mmHg (24 kPa) to the cat and rat sciatic nerves, and to the dorsal roots; subsequently observing, 'The single most important finding to emerge from our re-examination of this old problem is the astonishing sensitivity of spinal roots to compression.' Pressures were applied for three minutes, relieved for three minutes and higher pressures then applied in this sequence, being continued until a substantial conduction block became evident. Despite the three-minute relief periods not being enough to allow recovery at the higher pressure values, so that the cumulative effects compounded those of pressure alone (see p. 96), the difference between peripheral nerves and spinal roots was plain. A complete conduction block in the sciatic *nerve* could not be achieved with pressures of less than 150 mmHg (20 kPa), whereas *dorsal roots* were able to withstand only minute pressures, the action potentials being reduced to around half their initial values by pressures of 20–25 mmHg (2.67–3.3 kPa).

An important parameter is *duration* of compression. A transient increase of pressure will block a few fibres only, but the same pressure prolonged may produce a substantial conduction block. The consequence of *ischaemia* and *mechanical deformation* are not so easily clarified, e.g. Bentley and Schlapp (1943)[83] rendered a 4 cm length of *peripheral* nerve completely ischaemic by a pressure of 60 mmHg (8 kPa), yet it maintained conduction for many hours by diffusion of oxygen from the ends of the compressed region.

According to the observations of Gelfan and Tarlov (1956)[403] the small pressures which produced the conduction block in *dorsal roots* did so by mechanical deformation of fluids rather than by anoxia. Pressures as little as 20 mmHg (2.67 kPa) affected predominantly the rapidly conducting fibres, as a rule, though the differentiation is not always so conspicuous.

Thus dorsal roots show a differential sensitivity to unit pressure as compared with sciatic nerve, and the fast-conducting A neurones are considerably more susceptible to pressure than the slower-conducting fibres.

Sharpless (1975)[1112] summarises the phenomenon as probably due to viscosity of displaced axoplasm, and invagination of myelin. He emphasises the important point that the viscosity of displaced fluid may have an adaptive value, protecting nerve roots against *transient* fluctuations in local pressures. Thus when joints are fixed in positions which cause a significant and sustained increase in pressure, a compression block could be expected to develop. Many instances of the clinical features of idiopathic compression may be associated with occupations in which an awkward position must be maintained for some time.

Since the spinal roots are protected from small local fluctuations of pressure by their situation of floating in the bony aperture of the foramen, it may be they have not developed other mechanisms to protect themselves from more sustained forces.

Magoun's (1975)[786] extrapolation of Sharpless's observations suggest that the still smaller and slower pain fibres may be exceedingly resistant to pressure blockade, and draws attention to the dominant complaint of pain during compression of spinal nerve roots in man although as we have seen, nerve root compression is not necessarily painful, so long as it is slowly and not suddenly applied.

The 'root pain' of sciatica, for example, has for many years been ascribed to nerve root compression by discogenic trespass, and it was also assumed that the compression produced prolonged firing of the injured sensory fibres; this consequence therefore underlying the severe pain in the distal territory served by the injured nerve. Yet the neuropathy of acute peripheral nerve compression is usually painless, and experimental studies rarely show more than several seconds of repetitive firing when *nerves* or *nerve roots* are acutely compressed.

It has also been suggested that 'root pain' is actually referred pain, perceived in the limb through the activation of deep spinal and paraspinal nociceptors.

By experimentally applying minimal acute compression to normal *dorsal root ganglia*, Howe et al. (1977)[575] observed that much longer periods of repetitive firing, up to 25 minutes, were provoked.

Chronic injury produces a marked increase in sensitivity to mechanical injury, and the acute compression applied to such chronically injured sites was followed by several minutes of repetitive firing. The prolonged response could be repeatedly evoked in both slow and rapidly conducting fibres.

Thus mechanical compression of either the dorsal root ganglion or chronically injured nerve roots evokes prolonged repetitive firing in sensory neurones; the authors have concluded that 'root pain' is due to the activity of neurones directly involved in the abnormal changes, and serving the territory of perceived pain.

There remains, of course, the question of what proportion of the distal pain may be due to the mechanism postulated above, and how large is the component of pain of similar distribution, referred from the associated abnormal changes in non-neural tissues.

Wall et al. (1974)[1282] have shown that acute injury to a healthy dorsal root does not produce a sustained discharge except where there has been pre-existing minor chronic irritation or injury to the root.

Features of root involvement (see also Clinical features, p. 160).

Ventral roots comprise:
Large myelinated A-alpha neurones and a few A-beta fibres, motor efferent to the extrafusal fibres of skeletal muscle.
Small myelinated A-gamma neurones, motor efferent to intrafusal skeletal muscle fibres.
Preganglionic myelinated B fibres, sympathetic visceral motor efferent (from segments T1 to T12 inclusive, but see p. 10) and in S234 roots, preganglionic parasympathetic visceral motor efferents.

Dorsal roots comprise:
Group IA myelinated afferent fibres from primary endings in skeletal muscle spindles, and from Golgi tendon organs.
Group IIA small, medium and large myelinated afferent neurones from joints (Types I, II and III mechanoreceptors, see p. 11), afferent fibres from secondary endings in muscle spindles and from touch and pressure receptors.
Group IIIA-delta, small myelinated neurones, part of the somatic nociceptor system.
C unmyelinated fibres of both the somatic and visceral afferent nociceptor systems (the latter are not necessarily 'autonomic' afferents).

The ramus meningeus, or sinuvertebral nerve, of which there may be several filaments, has on re-entering the intervertebral foramen become a mixed nerve, and thus contains both somatic and autonomic neurones. Because the filaments of the ramus meningeus may wander up and down the neural canal for a distance of some segments before terminating in end-organs, the consequences of conduction block in these neurones may frequently involve tissues at some distance from the site of the foraminal or neural canal trespass.

The ventral and dorsal roots may be compressed individually, depending upon the nature and position of degenerative and other changes, and also the nature of root formation.

A further important consideration is the varying degree of root angulation, commonly existing as a normal anatomical feature in many individuals, occasioned by the changes in direction of spinal roots between their intradural and extradural course.

Classical anatomical descriptions present a more or less characteristic pattern for each spinal region, yet in a study of 50 dissections (adult males and females) Nathan (1970)[904, 11] observed that in a majority (76 per cent) of the cases a variable number of spinal roots, more usually in the lower cervical and upper thoracic segments, followed an angulated course.

Within the dura, the rootlets proceeded downward for a variable distance and on piercing the dura are sharply angulated upwards to reach the portal of the intervertebral foramen. Since the extraforaminal course is again down-

wards, a handful of spinal roots (commonly occupying a junctional vertebral region prone to trespass by thickened degenerative tissues) have undergone two fairly marked angulations by the time of their emergence from the foramen.

The degree of angulations may be as much as 30°, and can reach 45°. Irregular and uneven development at the dural sac has been considered as the possible cause of these angulations which may, of course, be further distorted by degenerative changes, particularly dural tethering within the neural canal and root-sleeve tethering at the foramen.

The roots affected are those between C6 and T9, with T2 and T3 most frequently and severely angulated.[11]

REGIONAL VARIATIONS

Comparatively few clinical or experimental pathological studies of nerve root compression have been reported, and postmortem descriptions of root compression are uncommon.
N.B. Only the salient features of root involvement in these regions are described here; for more generalised descriptions see under Combined degenerative change, page 125.

1. Cervical spine
The foramen allows the passage of a neurovascular bundle comprising spinal nerve root, radicular artery and small veins, contained in a firm and inelastic sleeve of the dura mater. The combined cervical root, or the dorsal root only, may be unilaterally irritated or compressed by chondro-osteophyte formation at the margins of facet-joints, and/or by the same degenerative trespass as a consequence of osseocartilaginous bar formation in spondylosis of the vertebral body joints, from the third cervical segments downwards.

Frykholm (1951)[391] ascribed the clinical features of root compression to fibrosis of the dural sleeve, and showed the characteristic thickening and opacity of the sleeve and adjacent parts of the dural sac, restriction and sometimes complete obliteration of the root ostia or funnel forming the root pouch, fibrotic thickening of the arachnoid part and sometimes a restriction and notching of the radicular nerve.

The considerable variations in formation of the lower cervical roots and root pouches are important factors, determining the nature and degree of root interference by degenerative change from patient to patient.

Wilkinson (1971)[1316] observes that disc pathology in the cervical spine is complicated, in that in addition to protrusion of the nucleus pulposus (which in this spinal region constitutes only 15 per cent of the disc volume) there is often osteophyte formation with or without root sleeve fibrosis. She describes (a) a type of dorsolateral protrusion which does not invade the intervertebral foramen but which may compress the intrameningeal rootlets against the anterior aspect of the vertebral laminae, and (b) a protrusion originating more laterally, from the uncinate region of the disc, and invading the foramina to compress the radicular nerve (or combined roots) against the articular pillar.

A notable feature of the characteristic and combined nature of cervical degenerative change is the very frequent presence of *multiple* disc change in mature patients. In 17 patients who came to autopsy, Wilkinson (1960)[1315] observed some or all of these changes in each, with an average of 3 disc lesions per subject. In 3 of them, there were 5 disc lesions. Hence the nature of discogenic root involvement in the cervical spine differs from that in the lumbar spine, where root interference more usually involves a single segment unilaterally.

The enlargement due to effusion of the capsule of the apophyseal joint may produce some root pressure.[639]

An important point is that the upper two or three cervical roots have posterior primary rami which are at least as large as the anterior primary ramus, and while the upper two cannot be involved in spondylotic processes, since the latter by definition involve the disc, they frequently appear to be vulnerable to repetitive or more sustained irritation as a secondary consequence of ligamentous insufficiency, degenerative thickening and partial disorganisation of the craniovertebral region following trauma and stress. This spinal neighbourhood is of profound clinical importance and it is wise to be alert to the possibility of segmental muscular weakness (see Patterns of Segmental Supply) and instability.

In cervical spondylosis, spinal roots can be severely damaged by protruding osteophytes. The damaged roots may contain regenerating axons proximal to the level of trespass or more commonly give rise to groups of myelinated fibres coursing through the meninges and passing along the blood vessels. The site of damage may form a neuroma at the entrance to the intervertebral foramen. In chronic states these regenerative phenomena are very common.[439]

Cuneiform areas of degeneration in the dorsal columns of the cord have also been observed, and interpreted as secondary to dorsal root damage. Histological changes, presumably due to the mechanical causes outlined, include proliferation of Schwann cells, signs of axonal myelin degeneration and an increase of connective tissue around the Schwann cells. The patchy lesions are most pronounced in mid- and lower cervical regions.

At autopsy examination of subjects older than 50 years, numerous rounded, lamellated and calcified bodies, with a hyaline central part, have been found in the sheaths covering the spinal roots and proximal peripheral nerves.[548]

The little masses are most frequently observed in epineurial and perineurial connective tissue, with a few plasma cells and lymphocytes in their neighbourhood. The masses occurred less often in the endoneurial sheath.

Cystic lesions are also found, frequently in the posterior root near the dorsal ganglion, and appear as diverticula continuous medially with the subarachnoid space containing cerebrospinal fluid. The cysts are associated with degenerative changes in related neurones.

The frequency of cysts, at the junction of posterior roots and dorsal root ganglion, varied from none in the 2nd and 3rd root to more than 10 per cent in the 6th root.[565]

At the site of pressure there is secondary swelling both of nerve and connective tissue. If the nerve traverses a confined space or tunnel, which may have been added by chronic degenerative processes, the mechanical pressure and irritation initiates oedematous changes, which further aggravate compression.[1180b] Production and absorption of oedema may account for the exacerbation and remission of symptoms.

The root may also suffer ischaemic changes due to arthrotic or spondylotic interference with the segmental radicular arteries, this also appears to be a more potent cause of cervical myelopathy.[426]

2. Thoracic spine

Aside from consideration of the thoracic-outlet group of syndromes, and such conditions as tumours of the lung apex which involve the upper thoracic nerves near their foraminal exits, reports of root compression at thoracic levels are relatively sparse, probably because it is less easy to show unilateral and obvious neurological deficit in the territory supplied by a single thoracic spinal root.

This is not to ignore the literature on thoracic disc lesions, of which Benson and Byrnes (1975)[82] have provided an excellent review, or the well-documented changes of spinal tuberculosis and thoracic neoplasms, but only that in 22 patients with surgically proven thoracic disc prolapse, intercostal muscle wasting was not seen and paraspinous muscle spasm was not seen. While weakness of the lower abdominal muscles was frequent, nearly all other neurological signs involved the lower limb (and in one-third of cases the sphincters) and thus were due to cord interference; this may be because a thoracic disc trespass usually occurs in the median plane and thus at sufficient distance from the nerve roots on either side (p. 528).

Schmorl and Junghanns (1971)[1093] remarks that several forms of intercostal neuralgia in the thoracic area have been recognised as an expression of nerve root irritation from posterior disc prolapse but, again, neuralgia is not neurological deficit.

Nathan (1959)[898] describes para-articular processes of the thoracic vertebrae, and the space-occupying effect of these structures. His observations on osteophytes of the vertebral column[900] and on arthrotic change in the costovertebral joints[902] together with his clear demonstrations of the abdominal sympathetic trunk incorporated among the degenerative outgrowths of spondylotic vertebral joints[903] provide ample reason to suppose that covert thoracic root involvement may occur more frequently than we are easily able to show, in terms of circumscribed neurological deficit.

Angulations of the upper thoracic nerve roots (*vide supra*) would certainly predispose them to the consequence of degenerative interference by surrounding structures.

That thoracic spinal root involvement occurs, is best demonstrated electromyographically. In a review describing radicular symptoms which simulate visceral disease of abdominal organs, Marinacci and Courville (1962)[806] show that diagnostic error at times leading to unnecessary abdominal surgery is easily caused by vertebral joint problems referring pain around the trunk, and through to the abdominal wall.

The resultant abdominal manifestations can usually be traced to stem from irritation of one or more thoracic spinal roots … in this group of syndromes we are concerned with the entire abdominal wall supplied by the sensory and motor roots from about T6 down to L1 level.

Epigastric pain over stomach or pancreas produced by T6–T7 irritation, gall bladder 'disease' by involvement of T7–T8, pain in the kidney region from T9 vertebral segment and 'physical disorders' of the urethra and bladder, are illustrative examples.

Radiculitis at T12–L1 roots often simulates femoral and inguinal disorders. Angiomas, disc changes, arthritic spurs of facet-joints and compression fractures are among the pathological spinal conditions referring the pains mentioned by the authors, and the five examples of root involvement confirmed by electromyography of thoracic nerves were neurofibroma at T7, neuronitis at T7, 8, 9, a central disc hernia at T9, arthrotic hyperostosis at T11 and a metastatic adenocarcinoma involving T6, T7 and T8 roots. Each patient had abdominal surgery, one had two operations and the patient with facet-joint arthrosis was submitted to three exploratory surgical procedures.

On the other hand, conventional clinical tests of oesophageal function may fail to reveal the visceral cause for thoracic pain which does originate from oesophageal disorders.[871]

3. The lumbar spine

Yates (1964)[1369] broadly classifies the causes of root interference according to their anatomical site as follows:

1. *Intraspinal*
   a. Viral radiculitis, e.g. herpes zoster
   b. Meningeal disease, e.g. malignant infiltration
   c. Extramedullary tumours.

2. *Extraspinal*
   a. Retroperitoneal, e.g. sarcoma
   b. Large pelvic tumours
   c. Sciatic nerve e.g. malignant infiltration.

3. *Spinal*
   a. Spondylolisthesis
   b. Trauma
   c. Vertebral disease, e.g. tuberculosis
   d. Intervertebral disc lesions.

A root of the lumbosacral plexus may also be compressed by impingement between the tip of a superior articular facet and the pedicle above, by the descent of a pedicle due to the unilateral collapse of a lumbar disc, by anterior trespass of thickened degenerative tissue of facet-joint arthrosis, by acquired spinal stenosis due to a combined degenerative change, and by nerve root cysts.

According to Macnab (1977),[780] backache and radicular pain of sciatic distribution, i.e. root entrapment syndromes, may result from any of the following lesions:

1. Foraminal impingement of the emerging nerve root by a subluxated posterior zygoapophyseal joint
2. Kinking of a nerve root by a pedicle, and compression of the nerve root against the pedicle by a diffuse bulging disc
3. Entrapment of the nerve root in the subarticular gutter
4. Diffuse spinal stenosis
5. Segmental spinal stenosis
6. Iatrogenic (postfusion) spinal stenosis
7. Extradural tumours
8. Lamina impingement as in spondylolisthesis
9. Extraforaminal entrapment—the corporotransverse ligament;[422] engulfment by a peripheral disc bulge.

The sites at which trespass upon lumbar nerves may occur have been summarised by Kirkaldy-Willis and Hill (1979):[662]

1. Anterior to the dura (i.e. sinuvertebral and spinal nerves at the posterior wall of the disc)
2. The medial part of the nerve canal (or beginning of the lateral recess)
3. The posterolateral part of the neural canal, by trespass of enlarged posterior joints
4. The lateral part of the nerve root canal (e.g. trespass upon the ventral and dorsal roots, root sleeve and sinuvertebral nerves, by subluxed and enlarged superior articular processes)
5. At the posterior joints, where the medial branches of the posterior primary rami may be involved.

If scoliosis is taken to include congenital or acquired curvature of the lower thoracic and lumbar spine, including those mature patients with developing rotatory curves, scoliosis alone does not cause statistically significant low back pain in patients under 60, but signs of nerve compression may appear further with ageing, because of progressive stenosis of the intervertebral foramen within the concavity of the scoliotic nerve. The narrowing is caused by the degenerative trespass of hypertrophied facet-joints, marginal vertebral osteophytes and thickening of the lamina and ligamentum flavum. Available space, particularly in the lateral recess, may be much reduced.[317, 318]

Trespass by degenerative tissue does not always occur on the concave side of abnormal lateral curvature, Wright et al. (1971)[1348] mentioning 28 cases of scoliosis, 15 of whom showed disc narrowing on the concave side and 13 presenting with changes on the opposite side.

The nature of root involvement by disc trespass may take many forms, from the detachment of a section of hyaline cartilaginous plate, already described (see p. 90), to the root being buried in a groove of bulging disc, migration of a disc fragment into the intervertebral foramen, impingement of the nerve in the lateral recess of the neural canal (see p. 28) and transforaminal lateral disc herniation.

To these should be added the restricting effects of transforaminal ligaments, which on occasions can produce a degree of entrapment in the presence of normal discs, closely simulating the neurological consequences of disc prolapse.

The lumbosacral roots descend almost vertically within the neural canal, and thus a disc protrusion at the 4th lumbar segment may impinge upon the 4th and 5th lumbar, or 1st sacral, roots and sometimes two of these. A 5th lumbar neurological deficit does not necessarily implicate the 5th lumbar disc, nor a 1st sacral deficit the 5th lumbar disc, albeit the latter combination of 1st sacral deficit and 5th lumbar joint changes occur commonly.

Brodal (1969)[130] draws attention to the descending branch of the second lumbar nerve; this filament lies in the posterior longitudinal ligament and may be involved in lesions of trespass, with consequent patterns of pain which can confuse the clinician.

Wyke (1976)[1362] describes a typical herniation of nucleus pulposus as trespassing initially on the sinuvertebral nerve, with the effects of not only interrupting mechanoreceptor afferent activity but also irritating nociceptor afferent fibres, which may give rise to pain in the lower back, in the absence of sciatica. The *selectivity* of conduction blocks would explain this sequence of events.

Further territorial aggression allows the protrusion to impinge upon the nerve roots and their dural investment after which, it is postulated, backache becomes more severe and more widely distributed, being reinforced by concomitant reflex muscle spasm.

Sensory changes as paraesthesiae and numbness, with pain in the distribution of the sciatic nerve and, it should be added, pain sometimes in the distribution of the femoral nerve, may ensue. Inconveniently, pain does not respect classical dermatome boundaries.

Wyke draws attention to the correlation between the diameter of nerve fibres and their metabolic activity, with conduction in the larger mechanoreceptor afferents in spinal nerves being interfered with earlier and more severely (by disturbance of blood flow through the vasa nervorum) than in the smaller diameter nociceptor afferents in the same nerve trunks. The consequent selective conduction loss reduces the inhibitory effects upon centripetal traffic in the nociceptor system, these changes occurring early in compressive lesions and as a result of vascular disturbance involving the vasa nervorum. He observes that as nerve root compression increases, intermittent or continuous irritation of small diameter nociceptor fibres also increases, so that backache and/or sciatica increase, and are less readily relieved by changes of posture or activity.

Nevertheless, these effects may sometimes be relieved by lying or standing, and appear to be aggravated by sitting, although the diminution or loss of the inhibitory influence of mechanoreceptor impulse traffic may render antalgic postures of partial benefit only.

The intensity of pain is an unreliable yardstick for the grading of root lesions, besides the fact that patients have differing pain tolerances.[1295]

Schaumburg (1975)[1114] was unable to discover any histopathological descriptions of acutely compressed spinal roots, although postmortem appearances of roots flattened and almost fenestrated by disc herniations have been described. There are many reports of radicular nerve and ganglion being adherent to protruded disc material, and very many descriptions of degenerative change involving nerve roots.

Lindblom and Rexed (1948)[753] suggest that root damage need not follow a massive single trauma, but may often result from repetitive small injuries. These may affect a relatively large area, and the authors describe degenerating fibres distributed in a diffuse manner over the entire root, their number being proportional to the severity and duration of the compressive injuries. In single compressed roots, they found evidence of both recent and old injuries, i.e. the presence of regenerating axons coexisting with actively degenerating axons. The resulting histological picture was a mixture of degenerating, preserved and regenerating fibres. They described nerve root compression secondary to dorsolateral disc protrusion, indicating the point of pressure to be between the distal half of the spinal ganglion and the first portion of the spinal nerve. Deformities were either a slight circumscribed flattening, or an indentation of longer stretches of nerve. Moderate and severe compression flattened both ventral root and ganglia, whereas slight pressure deformed the ventral root bundles less than the ganglia.

The dorsal root ganglia were frequently compressed so that their normal circular cross-section was distorted to a crescentic shape, and the intraganglionic, connective tissue was severely disorganised. Near the compressed margin of the ganglion, some neurones appeared flattened and atrophied, and stained abnormally, although the majority of neurones appeared normal. Microscopically, the degeneration of large myelinated fibres was more easily observed in the ventral roots, and although the dorsal root ganglia were involved as described, the dorsal roots themselves were largely spared, as confirmed by the relative absence of nerve fibre pathology, in their investigations.

If significant axonal degeneration of neurological loss *does* occur in dorsal roots, their central projections in the dorsal column also degenerate, but in many of the cases examined, there were no retrograde degenerative changes in dorsal root components, although some ventral root degenerative changes were observed extending centripetally for 1–2 cm.

Questions of (a) when, or when not, a root of the lumbosacral plexus is involved in the pathological changes underlying complaints of haunch and leg pain, with diminished straight-leg-raising, and (b) the precise nature of this involvement, are easier to pose than clarify. Much of the confident ascribing of neurological involvement with notions of root interference as the underlying cause of sciatica, and a diminished range of leg-raising, may have been misplaced.

The author has previously (Grieve, 1970)[445] drawn attention to the lack of justification for authoritarian pronouncements on this often indeterminable aspect of lumbar joint problems (since only 1 in 10 000 reach the stage of myelography and operation), and the more recent observations of Mooney and Robertson (1976)[867] when describing 'the facet syndrome' are of interest. The authors initiated a diagnostic-therapeutic procedure (facet-joint block) by injecting steroid with local anaesthetic routinely into the lower three lumbar facet-joints. As each posterior primary ramus supplies at least two facet-joints, and each facet-joint receives innervation from at least two spinal levels, the precise facet-joint accountable for abnormality could not be determined by the patient's description of pain distribution. Because of this overlap in innervation, therefore, three joints were injected. If standard radiographic views showed a unilateral single-segment degenerative change, only that joint was injected.

It is apparent to us that the localisation of pain in the low back, buttock and leg is a non-specific finding. Pain referred to those areas certainly could be developed from noxious stimuli arising at the facet-joint area. In addition, there is some question as to what constitutes a true neurologic sign. Based on this preliminary experience, we no longer consider diminished straight-leg-raising or reflex changes to necessarily implicate nerve root pressure by disc protrusion. The only true localising neurologic signs which we currently will accept are specific dermatome sensory loss, or specific motor weakness. Probably severely diminished straight-leg-raising and a crossed leg positive straight-leg-raising test are true neurological signs as well. These findings currently do suggest a ruptured intervertebral disc with nerve root involvement. All other findings of the disc syndrome may be accounted for by facet abnormality. On the other hand, the very same pain referral pattern can no doubt be caused by irritation within the spinal canal.

Patterns of referred pain from irritation of the lumbar facet-joints were found to be in the typical locations of lumbago and sciatica. For this, and other reasons, descriptions of root involvement of a mechanical nature at the lumbar and lumbosacral segments and disc changes need not, and perhaps should not, be *automatically* associated with the ubiquitous clinical problems of backache and sciatica. The two have in the past been somewhat indiscriminantly linked, and there is plainly some doubt that this is justified.[174, 552]

Following the work of Edgar and Nundy[297] the notion that extrasegmental and widely radiating back pain (in the first stages of an acute attack) may be a 'dural' sign received some reinforcement, since the anterior aspect of the dura enjoys a much greater population of nociceptors than does its posterior aspect. More than 20 years ago, Pedersen *et al.* (1956)[979] showed very clearly that *any* destructive lesion of lumbar joint structures will initiate widespread vertebral and hamstring muscle spasm; thus it may be important to remember that widely radiating protective responses including diminished straight-leg-raising need not be consequent *only* on lesions of trespass involving the cauda equina or its dural investment.

'It is apparent that causes of compression of the cauda equina and nerve roots other than simple disc protrusions are much more common than previously thought. Some authors are of the opinion that these other causes are responsible for two-thirds of the patients.'[660]

RECOVERY

In relation to peripheral nerve injuries these processes are subject to considerable variation.

Sensory recovery. Accumulated evidence[1191] tends to disprove the hypothesis that protopathic and epicritic sensibility are separate realities, as Head (1905)[525] proposed. The pattern of recovery, as regenerating axons reinnervate the skin, is but a reflection of the different stages in the maturation of new afferent processes.

The interval, between injury and the first appearance of sensory processes in the peripheral stump below the lesion, is quite variable. A guide to the recovery of sensory neurones was considered to be provided by the Hoffman–Tinel sign[557, 1219] (DTP–distal tingling on percussion).

Stewart and Eisen (1978)[1174] studied the clinical significance of the DTP sign. Fifty-one patients, who satisfied 3 or more of the following 4 criteria: (1) sensory abnormalities in the median nerve distribution, (2) thenar weakness and wasting, (3) abnormal motor latency of the median nerve, (4) abnormal sensory action potentials at the wrist, were compared with a normal matched control group.

The signs and symptoms of median nerve involvement were not secondary to local or systemic disease, or to trauma.

The DTP sign was positive in 45 per cent of the experimental group and 29 per cent of the controls; the authors concluded that the sign is of doubtful clinical significance.

While the DTP sign might be an indicator of regeneration, it is not a reliable measure of useful regeneration.

Since completely denervated muscle is insensitive to pressure, an early sign marking the arrival of immature sensory fibres at the periphery is the development of tenderness to pressure. The arrival of immature cutaneous endings is marked by a crude sensibility with distinctive characteristics. The previously insensitive area becomes unpleasantly sensitive to pinprick at high thresholds, and to extremes of temperature. The elicited sensations are abnormal, very unpleasant, radiate widely, defy localisation and lack any qualitative features.

In very general terms, the time required for the appearance of sensory recovery at the periphery varies between weeks for mild injuries and months for severe injuries (e.g. nerve suture), given the factor of distance between injury and end-organ.

The threshold to stimulation, the capacity to localise, and the remaining qualitative features associated with sensory modalities continue to improve to normal function if the pattern of innervation is re-established in every detail.

Sunderland (1968)[1191] again stresses, in relation to *motor recovery*, the variability of the process. The interval between injury and onset of motor recovery comprises three interrelated phases:

1. *The initial period*, (a) when the neurones are recovering from the retrograde changes, which increase in severity as the level of injury approaches the cell body, and are proportional to the severity of the injury, and (b) the time needed for the passage of regenerating axons to, and through, the injured zone. This interval depends upon the severity of damage, and its pathological form; some agents are more prejudicial than others to axonal advance.

2. *The intermediate period*, i.e. the time needed for regenerating axons to grow from the site of trauma to their myoneural junctions; this is dependent both on the level and the severity of the injury. The former determines the distance, and the latter the rate, of advance.

3. *The terminal period* is the time needed to effect those refinements in regenerative processes which are necessary to meet functional requirements.

With regard to motor recovery after *unilateral lumbosacral root compression*, Yates (1964)[1369] investigated by clinical and electrodiagnostic criteria the natural course of motor weakness and recovery in 48 patients. While none of the patients in this series underwent surgery, the investigator assumed that root compression was secondary to a disc lesion.

A complete motor recovery occurred in all 40 patients (see Table 5.3) in whom only 1 root (uniradicular) was affected, but in only 1 of 8 patients in whom 2 or more roots (multiradicular) were involved.

Table 5.3

Root involved	Number of patients	Percentage of total	Mean duration of weakness (in weeks)
L3	3	7.5	24
L4	1	2.5	10 (not denervated)
L5	13	32.5	28
S1	23	57.5	20
All cases	40	100	22

A typical example of *uniradicular involvement* was that of a 30-year-old woman with backache for 7 weeks and left sciatic pain to the heel for a further 3 weeks. After a further week the pain eased but the leg felt cold, numb and weak. Muscle power in the left calf and hamstrings could be overcome by moderate manual pressure and the left buttock was flabby on contraction. The left ankle-jerk was absent and sensation to pinprick was impaired on the lateral border of the foot.

On electromyography the intensity–duration ratios in both heads of gastrocnemius were normal, no spontaneous activity was detected, but the volitional patterns were reduced from normal.

Three months from the onset of sciatica, no weakness was detectable and the left ankle-jerk had returned, although the outer border of the foot was hyperaesthetic. EMG tests showed a normal volitional pattern in gastrocnemius.

An example of *multiradicular involvement* was that of a 66-year-old man with a history of lumbago and sciatica for 20 years. A further onset of lumbar pain and left sciatica, prior to attendance, began slowly to ease, leaving the leg numb and weak.

Isometric contractions of quadriceps, toe extensors, calf muscles and hamstrings could not be held against moderate manual resistance, and lighter manual pressure overcame the weak contraction of tibialis anterior. Myelographically evident small disc protrusions at L4 and L5 interspaces were assumed to be responsible for the gross muscle weakness, by L4, L5 and S1 root compression.

An EMG test three months from onset showed abnormal intensity–duration curves of partial denervation in tibialis anterior, peronei, extensor digitorum brevis and gastrocnemius, and fibrillation potentials were detected in the same muscles. Volitional activity was absent in tibialis anterior and reduced in the other muscles.

Two years later, clinical weakness and EMG findings remained unchanged and the patient perforce retired from work.

Subsequent findings in these patients are of interest:

1. In 5 uniradicular cases, not showing denervation, muscle power was recovered in a mean of 11 weeks, and the author concluded the nerve injury to be a neuropraxia. Electrodiagnosis offers a means of distinguishing the condition from more severe injury of nerve.

2. In 13 uniradicular cases with evidence of denerva-

tion, complete motor recovery occurred within a mean period of 7 months, and in 4 of these the EMG abnormalities disappeared, indicating active reinnervation.

Van Harsveld (1952)[1263] and others have shown in experimental animals that section of one lumbar nerve root is followed by complete recovery of the weakened leg muscles. This occurs by terminal branching of nerve fibres from other healthy roots supplying the muscle, the fresh peripheral axons growing down the empty endoneural tubes of degenerate fibres. The process occurs within 1 mm of the myoneural junction, beginning within two weeks of denervation and continuing for six months. Thus denervated motor units were reactivated before axonal growth from spinal root to periphery, at the rate of 1–1.5 mm per day, could complete the reinnervation of muscle.

Coërs and Woolf (1959)[185] showed definite peripheral branching, and end-plate regeneration in biopsies of muscle denervated by root compression.

3. Since complete motor recovery occurred in only one of the eight patients with multiradicular involvement, the lack of recovery may be due to the absence or reduction in number of healthy roots to supply peripheral axonal branches.

Edds and Small (1951)[292] sectioned three lumbar roots in monkeys and observed little recovery of muscle power and little evidence of peripheral branching. It has been suggested that occlusion of one radicular artery by disc trespass might occasionally cause ischaemia of several cord segments and so produce a unilateral multiradicular lesion, but with regard to effects of interference of blood supply on peripheral nerve regeneration, Bacsich and Wyburn (1945)[51] ligated regional nutrient arteries, and destroyed the longitudinal anastomoses in the epineurium over considerable lengths of the sciatic nerve of the rabbit, without adversely affecting the regeneration of nerve fibres below a crush injury.

Regional nutrient arteries have been experimentally ligated over considerable lengths of nerve trunk without affecting the structure and function of nerve fibres or their regeneration.

Muscles denervated for more than two years are unlikely to substantially recover power, and for this reason Yates (1964)[1369] suggests that cases of multiradicular involvement warrant full and prompt investigation, including myelography and electromyography to confirm the extent of denervation, with surgery urgently considered.

There is some uncertainty whether muscular paresis of unknown duration indicates surgical or conservative treatment.

Employing clinical techniques for assessing neurological deficit, Eis (1964)[309] reported complete or partial recovery of muscle power in 93 per cent of surgically treated patients, Hakelius (1970)[483b] reported complete recovery of neuromuscular function in about 50 per cent of patients

in both conservatively and surgically treated groups, and Weber (1970)[1293] showed that about 80 per cent of his patients, in the same two groups, regained normal neuromuscular function. Weber (1975)[1295] studied paresis and recovery in 280 patients suffering from sciatica, with myelographically verified disc prolapse. Following relief of pain by bed rest and analgesics for two weeks, the problem of pain inhibition reducing muscular effort was negated. The 14-day period allowed instruction and practice in the standardised muscle-testing method, which comprised fixing the foot by non-stretchable strap to a measurement beam with built-in strain gauges. The muscle functions tested were:

1. Dorsal extension of big toe
2. Dorsal extension of lateral toes
3. Dorsal extension of the whole foot
4. Eversion of the foot
5. Plantar-flexion of the foot
6. Abduction and extension of the hip
7. Flexion of the knee.

Following control experiments in 13 healthy persons, by 104 individual movements, it was evident that a difference in normal strength between the two sides could differ as much as 20 per cent, therefore in patients only the loss of strength in excess of 20 per cent was recorded as paresis. Control measurements of six patients made on several successive days showed that daily deviations in muscle power were well within a limit of 20 per cent.

1. *Conservative treatment* was bed rest, isometric back and abdominal exercise, and intensive ergonomic training.

2. *Surgical treatment* was extirpation of the prolapsed and loose disc tissue, in a prone position with hips and knees flexed.

When 128 patients, of an original 133 with paresis, attended the follow-up examination 1 year later, only a recorded difference in muscle power exceeding 20 per cent was allowed as a definitive improvement or deterioration. Patients with disc rupture at L4–5 showed a preponderance of muscle-power loss in toe and foot extensors, while disc rupture at L5–S1 included most loss of calf muscle and hamstring power.

An important and unexpected finding at both levels of disc involvement was that 30–40 per cent of *other muscle groups* were affected, in addition to the dominating weakness described above. Surprisingly, the study showed that prognosis of muscle-power recovery is no better after surgery than after conservative treatment, and tests of power of dorsal and plantar flexion of the foot and toes showed poorer results in the operated patient. Although more than 70 per cent of all pareses were partially or completely restored, significantly only 30 per cent of patients had regained full strength in all muscle groups. The findings might be interpreted in different ways, but they pose various questions regarding:

1. The root or roots involved by single disc rupture in the low back.

2. Difficulties of ascertaining the actual onset of the consequences of root compression (many patients are unaware of motor loss).

3. The difficulty in that EMG may show persistent denervation in muscles which are, on clinical testing, of normal strength. (Since slight paresis matters little for functional capability, the addition of EMG-testing to careful manual clinical examination may not be justified.)

4. Surgical indications, since the unisegmental loss of muscle strength appears insufficient reason for surgery.

5. The nature of muscle power recovery after sciatica with neurological deficit. As Weber points out that muscle function continues to improve for more than a year after root involvement in sciatica, reinnervation may include a process other than peripheral axonal sprouting although the distance to be traversed by new axonal growth would seem to require an interim of some 2 years or more. In Yates's (1964)[1369] series, motor units at varying distances from the lumbar segments recovered power during a common interval of time.

Autonomic fibre regeneration is believed to be similar to that in the cerebrospinal nervous system.[437]

Evidence has steadily accumulated over years to confirm the regeneration of postganglionic sympathetic nerve fibres[1191] although surprisingly little is known of the regenerative processes themselves. Studies suggest that the time required for restoration of function following repair of severed preganglionic fibres is less than that for postganglionic neurones.

Relatively large defects in the sympathetic trunk of experimental animals have apparently been made good by growth of fibres across a complete gap in the trunk.[520]

There is some evidence that the rate of *degeneration* differs in different regions and in different fibre-types; preganglionic *regeneration* may be influenced by the site of the lesion, and the regeneration of postganglionic neurones may include reinnervation by neighbouring intact fibres.

Adjacent healthy autonomic fibres produce axonal sprouts which form connections with the appropriate cholinergic or adrenergic endings. Murray and Thomson (1957)[879] have demonstrated that section of pre- or postganglionic fibres in the neck is succeeded by growth of sprouts from neighbouring axons, these reinnervating the denervated structures if the autonomic supply is of the same type, i.e. adrenergic or cholinergic. The stimulus for sprout formation is believed to be a humoral substance released from degenerating neurones.

SUMMARY

It is common knowledge that in aged cadavers nerves reduced to less than one-half of their normal diameter, without evidence of wasting in the regions supplied, are often encountered.[282, 392]

Peripheral nerves can be greatly reduced in diameter, without functional impairment, provided the change is a gradual one. It is possible for a peripheral nerve to be chronically elongated to something like three times its resting length,[1194] and examples of this slow kind of deformation are (a) the distortion of the facial nerve over an acoustic neuroma, and (b) an adenoma of the pituitary gland escaping from the sella turcica and trespassing under the third (oculomotor) nerve and elevating and distorting it to unrecognisability. Yet there is no detectable disturbance of function in the field of either the facial or the oculomotor nerve.

It seems reasonable, for example, to assume that the 'root pain' and signs of root involvement of sciatica are due entirely to root compression by disc herniation, but this concept could bear some inspection[1149] (see p. 93). There is a growing realisation that many features of this syndrome are difficult to understand.

Spinal nerve roots often react to compression by disturbance of function, but root pressure in spinal tuberculosis is often painless, and 30 per cent of benign spinal tumours are painless. Pressure on a peripheral nerve root does not invariably involve pain.[116, 750] Sudden, rapid compression will usually produce paraesthesiae and more or less pronounced pain, while moderate or continuous compression will produce little or no pain; for example, plaster casts pressing on the lateral popliteal nerve and osteophytes irritating the ulnar nerve.

In 1951, Lindahl[750] noticed that 7 out of 10 cases of sciatica coming to surgery had inflammatory changes in nerve roots exposed. Some of this group of patients had disc herniation, *some had not*. In 1966, he performed 20 of these operations under local anaesthesia, and while the roots were exposed, he injected 10 cc of isotonic saline rapidly around the nerve root, i.e. producing an artificial and rapid root pressure. All patients reported exacerbation of their existing sciatic pain. Fourteen had disc herniations, 6 had not.

Some surgeons have observed spinal roots to be flattened at the site of disc herniations, while others report grossly oedematous, hyperaemic roots, these being described by some as swollen to two or three times their usual size, and designated as hypertrophic neuropathy.

Brown (1971)[137] refers to those puzzling cases where removal of nuclear disc material relieves the backache and sciatica, yet at surgery there is no observable trespass upon the root. Certainly, root pain and root signs for which no adequate cause can be found at operation are common enough.[651]

Among 150 patients who had a myelogram followed by surgery, Wright *et al.* (1971)[1348] report 12 patients with positive myelograms but no disc protrusion at operation.

Bourdillon (1973)[105] reminds us,

There can be no doubt that actual protrusion and extrusion of disc material occurs in some patients and can cause physical pressure on nerve roots or on the cord itself.... Even in this connection, however, there are a number of factors which require explanation.... It is probable that some types of stimuli to the dural investment of the nerve root can cause pain but the evidence in support of this does not appear to be conclusive.

The ability of nerves to tolerate mechanical trauma without frank clinical evidence of the consequences may depend on the nature of the onset (slow or sudden) as well as the degree and duration of compression.[1295]

During foetal development many neurones degenerate and die (there is, for example, a thirteenth cranial nerve in the foetus,[129] as well as the vomeronasal nerve, both of which become rudimentary even in foetal life), this process continuing into postnatal life to senescence, when it is estimated that up to 20 per cent of the original neurone population is lost[437] but in addition to this, it may not be unreasonable to suppose that lower cervical, upper/mid-thoracic and lower lumbar nerve roots suffer some neuronal damage as a normal consequence of living, throughout maturity, and that 'the normal nerve root' in some areas of the vertebral column might always contain a large population of normal neurones, side-by-side with some degenerating and some regenerating axons. This is not impossibly the case, and might be seen as analogous to the steady incidence of microfractures, and sites of healing, in the trabeculae of bones normally stressed considerably in daily living. Clinical methods of determining the presence of neurological deficit, at least so far as they apply to limb reflexes, muscle power and sensation, are sometimes not very precise when compared to the more sophisticated procedures available, although with attentive practice and meticulous care they can be raised to a high standard of accuracy for clinical purposes.

Essentially, an all-or-none approach to the question of neurological deficit could perhaps be somewhat limited, and assessment of the consequences of vertebral joint problems might benefit from better recognition of the many degrees and form which neurological signs can take.

Our detailed knowledge of the relationship between (a) irritation and compression of spinal nerves, (b) inflammatory changes observed at operation, and (c) the clinical presentation of 'root pain' and neurological deficit, is less complete than sometimes appears. While this is widely appreciated by clinicians and therapists, it seems often to be overlooked as one of the most important factors underlying assessment, and governing the initial selection and subsequent modification of treatment programmes.

In general terms:

1. Where painful and/or limited movement is accompanied by neuromuscular function which is *moderately depressed* rather than absent, a steady recovery of muscular power, sensation and reflex activity will go hand in hand with improvement in joint range, and a lessening of pain.

2. Whereas recovery from frank uniradicular *neurological deficit* may frequently lag behind the restoration of joint range and the relief of pain, a functional degree of muscle power being restored in some 10–30 weeks, normal sensation takes a bit longer (sometimes leaving a small patch of circumscribed, objective sensory loss) and reflex response sometimes not at all. Hence, a diminished ankle-jerk, as such, is not necessarily associated with the current symptoms reported by patients, since it might well be the 'tombstone' of a past sciatic episode some 10 or 20 years before.

When severe cervical root pain and frank neurological deficit are associated, relief of pain is not always accompanied by full recovery from other symptoms and signs.

Some patients will continue indefinitely to suffer some paraesthesiae and some loss of cutaneous sensibility in fingers; there may be substantial improvement in muscle power but this may take as long as 2 years.[1316]

Electrical stimulation of nerve growth

Small electric currents can stimulate or retard the regrowth of amputated amphibial limbs, e.g. a weak electric current will encourage a frog's amputated limb to regenerate if applied in one direction; degeneration occurs if the direction is reversed.

This has prompted experiments in which electric fields have been shown to dramatically affect the growth of nerve cells in tissue cultures. Ganglia from week-old chick embryos, well supplied with nutrients and the nerve growth factor, were placed in an electric field, with the immediate effect that the clusters of nerve cells were bodily attracted to the positive pole.

When this tendency for mass migration was prevented by pinning down the centre of the ganglion, it was possible to observe the effects, upon the nerve cells themselves, of an electrical field of about 70 millivolts per millimetre.

The nerve cells growing towards the cathode elongated up to five times faster than those growing towards the anode.

The authors suggest that this may occur because the macromolecular NGF (nerve growth factor) itself carried many charged groups and it is these which are attracted to the negatively charged cathode. Thus their effect is exerted most at the tips of those nerves facing the cathode, and the findings suggest that the successful growth of regenerating nerves might be encouraged in an electric field of the right direction.[604b]

SOFT TISSUES

MUSCLE

The muscular, tendinous and aponeurotic mass which is developed in intimate relationship to the vertebral column from occiput to pelvis can be divided broadly into two functional groups: (1) phasic muscle, and (2) postural or tonic muscles, though all muscles contain differing proportions of both fast and slow twitch fibres.

1. *Small suboccipital muscles* of the craniovertebral region (Fig. 5.7) are the recti and obliques, capable of rapid alterations of tension in a few milliseconds. They have a high *innervation ratio*, that is, the number of muscle fibres per motor neurone is small, their proportion being about 3–5 fibres per neurone. Consequently, their potential rate of contraction approaches that of the extrinsic eye muscles and they are able to control head posture, and produce rapid movements, with a fine degree of precision. This

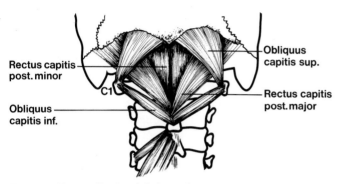

Fig. 5.7 The small suboccipital muscles.

accords functionally with the major influence of head position on body posture, and the correct correlation of orientation of the head in space with the requirements of the visual apparatus. Joint stiffness in the craniovertebral region has thus rather more extensive effects than in other regions (see p. 3).

While Basmajian (1976)[73] suggests that, 'the function of these small muscles can only be guessed at, since no direct studies have been made', implications of an important part of their function are manifest in many reports. For example, the interaction between deep neck muscle proprioceptors and optic-evoked head and eye nystagmus was remarked upon by Hinoki and Terayama (1966).[543]

2. *Sacrospinalis muscle groups* have a very much lower innervation ratio, the proportion being about 3000 muscle fibres per neurone, and so these muscle masses are characterised by slower and more sustained activity; this is a functionally important property of most stabilising muscle groups.

A further distinction may be made, in that: (a) the longer muscles of the sacrospinalis group (e.g. iliocostalis and longissimus) are regarded more as prime movers, especially during extension of the column, but (b) the shorter groups (e.g. multifides, rotatores, interspinales, intertransversarii) which arise from and insert more closely to the intervertebral joints, are important synergic muscles, stabilising and steadying the bony segments of the

column.[437] These intersegmental muscles are functionally analogous with the rotator cuff muscles of the glenohumeral joint and the short muscles grouped around the hipjoint, and their activity as possible prime movers is not so important as their dynamic stabilising function.[268]

Lifting and handling

The stresses tending to shear one vertebra upon another, applied during the lifting of a weight from the floor by stooping, are resisted not only by the strong ligamentous strapping of the joints but mainly also by the deepest, short muscles of the spine, which change the flexible column momentarily into a much more rigid though still flexible lever, the short muscles continuing to exert this effect while the longer groups and other muscles (hip extensors) extend the spine to the erect position.

The sacrospinalis (erector spinae) as a whole group has two main functions, extension of the spine and counteraction of gravitational force. The effect of the latter can rise dramatically during postures and movements which entail the centre of gravity of the trunk being displaced well beyond the perpendicular confines of its base, e.g. trunk bending or reaching movements during the lifting of weights.[890] The stress is very much more marked when reaching and lifting weights in the sitting position.

It is clinically significant that the sacrospinalis muscle group is relaxed when *full* trunk flexion is maintained, and further, during the first few degrees of trunk extension when holding a weight, the muscle remains relaxed (as shown by electromyographic quiescence[363, 364]), vigorous contraction not beginning until after the initial phase of trunk extension has been produced by the hip extensors.

Great stress is therefore placed on the posterior ligamentous structures in full trunk flexion, which is much increased when lifting, and this accords with the fact that many low back injuries sustained during the handling of awkward and heavy weights are produced during the *initial phases of extension of the trunk*. Tendons, aponeuroses and fascia are very strong, being naturally developed to withstand tensile stress (e.g. the tensile strength of healthy fascia lata is $7000\,lb/in^2$ (48 249.0 kPa), although the elasticity and recovery power diminishes after about one-third of this magnitude of stress is applied);[436] ligaments may be stretched 20 per cent to 25 per cent of their resting length before failure occurs.[373, 394, 1347]

The forces developed during the dynamic management of the mass which constitutes a human body are great, and can become of critical magnitude in many ordinary daily activities. The ability to withstand these forces safely decreases with ageing.

PARAVERTEBRAL MUSCLE

Other muscle groups, e.g. scaleni, trapezius, latissimus dorsi and abdominal wall muscles, are also intrinsically concerned in postural control, movement and protection of the spinal column. During the stress of lifting, the contraction of abdominal and other trunk muscles, together with contraction of the pelvic floor and closure of the glottis, creates an increased intrathoracic and intra-abdominal positive pressure; this mass of compressed air and fluid abdominal contents is an important flexion-resisting component and contributes a significant amount of the force needed to lift weights from the floor.[229,230,72] EMG studies indicate that the diaphragm, internal and external obliques, and the transversus abdominis contract to a much greater extent than the recti, which if contracted strongly would bring the spine into more flexion and thus increase the load upon it.[363] These findings accord with the physiological need to compress the fluid abdominal contents.

The pressures developed in abdominal and thoracic cavities are very high, and on lifting weights can go up dramatically;[229,233] during common industrial lifting activities the abdominal pressures may repetitively rise to 100 mmHg (13.33 kPa).

In the normal bimanual lift from the floor, intrathoracic and intra-abdominal pressure are at their peaks before intrinsic lumbar extension begins—intervertebral motion being delayed until maximal spinal stresses are past. (Troup, 1979.)[1250b]

So far as the internal mechanics of the trunk are concerned, there is theoretically a greater mechanical advantage of the pneumatic mechanism as compared with the erector spinae activity when the trunk is in a flexed posture; while there is some evidence in support of this theory, this is not to say that lifting in such a posture is to be preferred.[235]

While the abdominal muscles are regarded as stabilising the lumbar spine by maintaining the intra-abdominal pressure, Fairbanks and O'Brien (1980)[322a] present evidence that they also act to maintain tension, via the thoraco-lumbar fascia, in the ligamentous structures between spinous and transverse processes, thus increasing lumbar stability.

Nachemson and Lindh[887] contend that the strength of spinal and abdominal musculature is of doubtful importance for prevention of the low back pain syndrome, although they do not specify any categories of clinical presentation, other than 'localised symptoms from the lumbar region'. Tests were performed by 160 men and women, 63 of whom were suffering from low back pain. In the *male* groups, the values of muscle strength for those who had been incapacitated for less than one month were not significantly lower than for the controls, albeit pain inhibition was found to be a probable strength-reducing factor. In the *female* groups, the values for strength variables were significantly lower for patients than for controls, except for abdominal strength in older women. The abdominal muscles participate in many motor acti-

vities, including postural function, expulsion, expiration and circulation.

Like antigravity limb muscles, the abdominal musculature is well supplied with muscle spindles, and a tonic stretch reflex is easily elicited from them. In many ways, the abdominal skin reflex resembles the flexion reflex of the limbs. Contraction of the abdominal wall and simultaneous reciprocal inhibition of the antagonistic dorsal vertebral muscle serve to flex the trunk and retract the abdomen away from the noxious stimulus.[96]

The important aspect is the reciprocal action of the sacrospinalis and abdominal muscle groups—adaptive shortening of dorsal vertebral muscle, with adaptive lengthening and weakness of the abdominal wall musculature, probably constitute a dependable augury for low back problems.

The nature and periodicity of the loading applied to a disc during work are probably of considerable importance.[631] Recovery of disc thickness on removal of load is not instantaneous; if forces are applied and removed at too short intervals, or if repetitive and rhythmic loading are too prolonged, recovery is incomplete and a physical state analogous to ageing is induced.

Prolonged and heavy lifting, of lesser weights than an arbitrary maximum, might hasten the onset of degeneration,[24] the more so if rotation and asymmetrical stresses occur frequently during the activity.

By extrapolation, using the methods of stress analysis, Farfan (1973)[326] suggests an hypothesis of the degenerative process as applied to the lumbar spine, and assumes that, 'the most likely initial trauma is combined torsion, bending and compression. Of these three types of load, torsion and bending together would seem to be the most potent combination.' Thus it is wise to avoid torsion or asymmetrical loading of the lumbar spine when attempting to lift a weight; avoiding hyperextension is also wise.

Hence, we can see the importance of the anterior abdominal wall musculature which, when contracted, prevents both torsion and hyperextension ... in the absence of good abdominal musculature, the distribution of load between facet-joints posteriorly and the disc anteriorly may be affected adversely....

With regard to the widely held view that wearing a lumbar corset makes the muscles weak, Nachemson and Lindh[887] found no difference in strength between women patients with low back pain and those who had been pain-free but wearing a corset for a mean period of five years.

Walters and Norris[1290] studied the effects of spinal supports on muscular activity by EMG. There is no effect on standing and slow walking, but wearing the support *increases* muscle activity on fast walking.

Changes in resting length and tone and neuromuscular control

Troup (1979)[1250b] observes that,

When the vertebral column is stripped of its muscles it is wholly unstable. The muscles which support the spine stabilise it posturally; they control intervertebral motion during movements of the whole column in addition to being its prime movers, and they stabilise intervertebral posture during work when the spine transmits the reactions between hands and feet. All the muscles of the trunk have some supportive role: the erector spinae muscles in controlling extension, the rate of flexing under gravity, rotation and lateral flexion; the rectus abdominis in flexing the trunk against gravity and resisting extension; the oblique abdominal muscles in rotation and lateral flexion as well as flexion of the trunk; the quadratus lumborum in lateral flexion; the psoas muscles in controlling hip/trunk flexion and lumbar posture. Static tension in any of these muscles induces a reaction in the spine, equal and opposite in magnitude and direction.

In health, normal neuromuscular co-ordination is accepted as unremarkable; only in dysfunction does the underlying complexity of movement become apparent, and the disturbance of reciprocal muscle action become manifest. An explanation of the incidence of vertebral joint syndromes, and of some unsatisfactory long-term therapeutic results, might be assisted by regarding joint problems in a wider context than that of the joint alone. Much abnormality presenting, apparently simply, as joint pain may be the expression of a comprehensive underlying imbalance of the whole musculoskeletal system, i.e. articulation, ligaments, muscles, fascial planes and intermuscular septa, tendons and aponeuroses, together with defective neuromuscular control and co-ordination in the form of abnormal patterns of afferent and efferent neurone traffic.

The concept of connective-tissue tightness is not new. Mennell (1952)[851] has said,

It is very remarkable how widespread may be the symptoms caused by unduly taut fascial planes. Though it is true that the fascial bands play a principal part in the mobility of the human body, they are often conducive to binding between two joint surfaces. For obvious reasons it is of the utmost importance to restore the lost mobility in the joints, before attempting to stretch the fascial planes. On the other hand, if the mobility of these planes is not restored, recurrence of the binding in the joints is almost inevitable.

There is new evidence[305] to support the view that suppleness and flexibility of muscle and connective tissues are of prior importance. Long and continued occupational and postural stress, asymmetrically imposed upon the soft tissues, tends to cause fibroblasts to multiply more rapidly and produce more collagen. Besides occupying more space within the connective tissue elements of the muscle, the extra fibres encroach on the space normally occupied by nerves and vessels. Because of this trespass, the tissue loses elasticity, and may become painful when the muscle is required to do work in co-ordination with others. In the long term, collagen would begin to replace the active fibres of the muscle, and since collagen is fairly resistant to enzyme breakdown, these changes tend to be irreversible.

The single nerve–muscle–joint complex is not a simple mechanical entity, but one of many arthrokinetic systems which are functionally and reflexly interdependent with all others[455] (see p. 385).

Abnormal *joint* function, increasingly better examined[799] and increasingly better understood,[1270] is only one expression of motor systems impairment;[606, 607] the whole field of benign functional pathology of the motor system is as yet largely unexplored.[743]

Janda (1976)[606] observes that muscles play an important part in the pathogenesis of various back pain syndromes, and Lewit (p. 152) has drawn attention to the significance of iliopsoas spasm in the genesis of pelvic asymmetry in children.

Manifest changes in muscle are not random or incidental but follow certain typical and significant patterns. Selective tightness of some muscle groups, and lengthening with weakness of their antagonist groups, occur frequently in degenerative joint conditions of all spinal regions. A pattern emerges in which those muscles with largely a *postural* function appear to respond to pathological states by tightness, and those with mainly a *phasic* function respond by weakness and lengthening.

The differences may be broadly summarised as follows:

Postural muscle is phylogenetically older, can work for longer without fatigue, is largely concerned in the maintenance of static posture, is activated more easily and has a tendency to become shorter and tight.
Phasic muscle is phylogenetically younger, is fatigued more quickly, is primarily concerned in rapid movement and has an earlier tendency to become weak.

The distribution of the two fibre types has been examined more extensively in animals than in man, yet where investigated their relative populations have reflected the habitual nature of human muscle activity.[437] Studies indicate that intermediate types also exist, and it may be that the simple division into slow and fast mammalian muscle fibres represents two extremes of a range of fibre types.

All muscles partake in all kinds of muscular activity, and it seems reasonable that at different times the characteristics of all ranges of fibre types are required; the main difference under discussion here is therefore one of emphasis.

Other distinctions between fast and slow fibres are described.[619, 437] Muscles can be categorised in other ways, too, e.g. comparisons between 'spurt' and 'shunt' muscles;[783] those which cross one joint and those which cross two or more joints; possible correlations between muscles which tend to become tight and participate largely in flexor reflexes, and muscles which tend to weakness and to participate largely in extensor reflexes.[607]

Further, (a) muscles which tend to get tight have a shorter chronaxie than muscles which tend to get weak, and (b) the size and histochemical qualities of some muscle fibres may change due to habitual overuse, i.e. those of the athlete may differ from those of the sedentary worker.[1077]

One characteristic difference between phasic and postural muscles lies in the relative magnitude of abnormal effects, in that a small reduction of strength in a phasic muscle will initiate a disproportionately larger contracture of the antagonistic postural muscle, wheras a considerable reduction of strength in a postural muscle is not followed by an equally considerable contracture of the antagonistic phasic musculature. These characteristics are clinically evident to the most casual clinical observer, e.g. a degree of calf muscle contracture accompanies anterior tibial muscle weakness very much more frequently than even slight contracture of the anterior tibial group follows considerable calf muscle weakness.

Similarly, a glance at the cervical and cervicothoracic posture of many mature people, with a poking chin and the head carried somewhat forward of the line of gravity, will indicate the need for stretching of tightened posterior cervical structures (particularly the ligamentum nuchae) and a strengthening of prevertebral cervical musculature.

The inhibitory effect of a tight postural muscle is evidenced when weakness of the gluteus maximus accompanies tightness of the iliopsoas. Hip extension is slightly abnormal, lumbar lordosis tends to increase and abnormal loading of the lumbosacral segment initiates chronic changes which can be a cause of pain.

It is common experience that muscle imbalance tends to occur in typical patterns, e.g. as a rule, the upper trapezius, pectoralis major, lumbar sacrospinalis and hamstrings react to pain by increasing tightness, while others such as rhomboids, deltoid, abdominal muscles, glutei and anterior tibial muscles tend to show weakening and lengthening. *Yet the apparent chronological sequence of events may not be so.*

While these normal and reciprocal changes in tension and tone appear at times to be the sequelae of joint problems, clinical experience is that the genesis of many common joint conditions almost certainly lies in the habitual use of these muscle groups within a small and abnormally restricted amplitude of their available extensibility ranges, thereby slowly and covertly initiating abnormal stress patterns and chronic changes.

Changes underlying the patterns described may masquerade as the consequences of joint dysfunction, and yet in fact may largely be responsible for them. In the circumstances that musculoskeletal pain is often manifest as painful and/or limited movement of a *joint*, and is primarily investigated on the basis of seeking the nature of the *joint* abnormality, associated structural and functional defects in the whole neuromuscular–skeletal system must also be understood, and given appropriate treatment when indicated.

Those muscles which have a predominantly *postural* function, and tend to react to pain by increasing tightness are:

sternomastoid
pectoralis major (clavicular and sternal parts)
trapezius (superior part)
levator scapulae
the flexor groups of the upper extremity
quadratus lumborum
erector spinae, perhaps mainly: the longissimus dorsi and the rotatores
iliopsoas
tensor fasciae latae
rectus femoris
piriformis
pectineus
adductor longus, brevis and magnus
biceps femoris
semitendinosus
semimembranosus
gastrocnemius
soleus
tibialis posterior.

Those muscles with predominantly a *phasic* function, which tend to react to pain by weakening and lengthening are:

scaleni and the prevertebral cervical muscles
extensor groups of the upper extremity
pectoralis major, the abdominal part
trapezius, the inferior and middle part
rhomboids
serratus anterior
rectus abdominus
internal and external abdominal obliques
gluteal muscles (minimus, medius, maximus)
the vasti muscles (medialis, lateralis, intermedius)
tibialis anterior
the peroneal muscles

Janda observes that much present-day work and recreation occupations tend to favour postural muscles in getting stronger, shorter or tighter, as the phasic muscular system becomes weaker and more inhibited. More established tightness, and lengthening of antagonists, leads to chronic disturbances in functional movement patterns. By extended use, the imprint of abnormal joint function must be accompanied by abnormal imprints of neurone patterning. While muscle and other soft tissue changes (*vide infra*) frequently *accompany* joint problems, and can be seen as sequelae, e.g. muscle spasm in joint irritability (p. 197), it is clinically evident that joint problems commonly occur as a *sequel* of chronic localised postural imbalance.

The genesis of painful, degenerative joint conditions may frequently lie in more regional, and major, chronic imbalance of functional movement patterns, which place sustained and abnormal stress on joints.

While localisation of problems and their localised treatment are paramount, recognition of disproportionate tensions in prime movers, antagonists and synergic muscle groups is an important part of treatment. The connection between a craniovertebral and a lumbosacral problem, for example, may frequently be more than coincidental, although this connection more often involves vertebral regions adjacent to each other.

Abnormal patterns, unless recognised and corrected, may persist after joint mobility *per se* has been restored.

Eder (1975)[294] indicates the prime importance of perceiving and correcting muscle tension imbalance. The mobilisation and manipulation of joints without attention to the tethering effects of undue tightness leaves something to be desired; there is electromyographic evidence of improved motor co-ordination and function after therapeutic stretching of tight musculature.

A factor which bedevils one aspect of discussion of the subject, so far as the present author is concerned, is the unresolved question of whether the essential changes of tightness occur in the parenchymatous elements of muscle, or whether they chiefly involve the non-parenchymatous connective tissue of muscle, i.e. intermuscular septa and fascia.

Farfan (1975)[328] observed that when a muscle is stretched beyond its resting position, its collagenous content gives it a tensile strength which is independent of its contractile power.

Precise information on whether a chronically elongated muscle retains a full or only a reduced capacity for shortening in response to resisted exercises is not known to the author, although one's clinical impression is that treatment results make the attempts to do so very worthwhile. Farfan has also mentioned that a ligament attains its ultimate tensile length with 5–6 per cent of elongation, and if this is exceeded, it is probably unlikely that the full stabilising and tethering function of a ligament remains unimpaired. For this reason correction of muscle imbalance, and particularly a degree of selective muscle strengthening by isometric resisted exercises, is an important part of treatment. During fast and forceful movements, joint injury is prevented by fine neuromuscular co-ordination, and it is well known that as the fast movement ceases, active inhibition of antagonists changes swiftly to facilitation and contraction in order to slow the movement and avoid joint insult (see pp. 11, 83).

If these dynamic patterns of reciprocal innervation activity are disturbed or chronically defective, joint structures are at risk.

Reference has been made (p. 76) to those subjects who could be described (not unkindly) as 'proprioceptively illiterate', in whom the central nervous system regulation of motor function appears to achieve something less than the normal effectiveness of available neural machinery and functions.

An interesting field for further research presents itself on consideration of the work of Wyke (1976)[1362] (p. 10), Dee (1978)[245] (p. 11), Schmorl and Junghanns (1971)[1093] (p. 259), and Janda (1978)[607], Driver (1964)[278] and Rose (1974).[1056]

Schmorl and Junghanns[1093] referred to the specific additional stimulus which may be 'the straw to break the camel's back' and which precipitates a vertebral pain episode; there is evidence that the factors which underlie vertebral pain may embrace a very much wider field than the somewhat narrow consideration of localised mechanical changes due to localised mechanical stress or direct trauma.

Rose has considered the effects of weather on rheumatism and Driver has studied the effects of well-defined seasonal variations. Janda analysed 100 patients between 17 and 61 years who were suffering either chronic vertebral pain with little relief, or who had been admitted for rehabilitation after injury but with unsatisfactory therapeutic results. The average age was 40. In most of them, the vertebral pain began without evident cause when between 20 and 25 years old; in the otherwise uncomplicated traumatic cases, in whom a good prognosis had been made, treatment results were poor and the general musculoskeletal condition of those patients left something to be desired.

The musculoskeletal system, its nervous regulation and the psychological state in all of the patients were evaluated:

1. *Neurologically*, the patients variously exhibited increased muscle tonus and tendon reflex responses, asymmetrical hypotonia with irregular tendon reflexes, lack of co-ordination evidenced as slight dysdiaokokinesia, involuntary movements of the fingers during mental concentration, slight changes of proprioception and slight changes in discriminative sensibility.

2. *Motor efficiency and control* were studied by multichannel EMG, and almost all patients had some change in their ability for finely adjusted co-ordination, e.g. in that many more muscles were activated than were needed for the performance.

3. *Psychologically*, perceptuomotor co-ordination, visual and spatial orientation, motor memory and learning were evaluated. Fine co-ordination was poor, timing uncertain and visual analysis of length and distance, for example, was conspicuously poor. No general impairment of intellectual performance was found (many of the patients were college-educated or of high scientific standing).

It was plain that more than half of the patients appeared affected by their low tolerance to stress, appeared to live at high tension and managed the problems of daily life only with undue strain. Some appeared to *produce* stress by overreaction or overexcitability.

The overall impression given by the group was that of

lack of co-ordination of motor, sensory, and mental functioning, poor control of activation and a diminished adaptibility to, and general tolerance of, stress. In summary, given a background of chronically pre-existing muscle imbalance, of poor or defective neuromuscular co-ordination, and/or an existing but covert segmental insufficiency, the stimulus for initiation of overt vertebral pain need not be mechanical injury alone, but may be climatic, emotional or environmental stress, competitive overexcitability, endocrine dysfunction or a simple bodily movement so trivial that it is difficult to believe it responsible for the ensuing bodily distress.

These concepts are a far cry from the 'if something is "out", put it back' school of manipulation, yet they are a necessary part of any real attempt to fully understand the aetiology and nature of vertebral pain syndromes, their infinite variety of causation and presentation and our seemingly inexplicable therapeutic failures.

PALPABLE TEXTURAL CHANGES

A very tender type of tissue in the human body, so frequently a source of pain in all sorts of conditions—traumatic, 'rheumatic', postural, occupational, etc.—is the tissue of junction between muscle, tendon, intermuscular septum, or similar structure, with periosteum and bone. This of course includes joint capsules, ligaments, tendon insertions, and structures of that kind. ... a great deal of spinal pain may well be pain felt where muscle, tendon, ligament and capsule are attached to sensitive periosteum in the spine.[1100]

Palpable changes in the musculature of limb girdles, and more distal muscles, have long been associated with 'rheumatic' pains and common benign joint problems.

A host of names and phrases[1133] have been used to describe them, e.g. fibrositis, interstitial myofibrositis, muscle callus, muscle gelling or myogeloses, muscle hardening, muscular rheumatism, non-articular rheumatism, soft-part rheumatism, myofascial pain syndrome, myofasciitis, trigger points, myalgia and myalgic spots.

A landmark in the controversy over the nature of lumps, thickenings, stringiness, and palpable hard fasciculi in the muscle and other soft tissues was the paper by Copeman and Ackerman (1947)[203] in which the authors described herniations of lobulated fat, and ascribed the condition of fibrositis to their presence. The literature goes back for more than a century before this, however, and there is a rich store in German writings on the subject.

In a chapter on Examination for Sensitive Areas (Mennell, 1952)[851] the author provides a clear topographical scheme of the most common situations for the formation of sensitive deposits in the paravertebral regions and limb girdles.

During his presidential address to the Royal Society of Medicine, Glynn (1971)[414] elaborated his views on the nature of fibrositis, or non-articular rheumatism. Besides the well-recognised factors of trauma, ischaemia, toxins and exposure to extremes of temperature, he discussed the possible evidence for an origin from visceral disturbances, i.e. that visceral irritation, in which he included the nucleus pulposus of the intervertebral disc, may possibly be transmitted via autonomic neurones, and be the genesis of self-sustaining lesions within the musculature. He distinguished acute and chronic phases and observed that in the acute condition the muscular component is not responsive to treatment, but the more central lesion will respond quickly to appropriate treatment; the tender muscular areas coincide with the patient's description of pain distribution. In later, more chronic phases, he considered that only the peripheral component of the lesions responds well to therapy. The author proposed that a self-perpetuating mechanism produces the same final lesion, regardless of the nature of its genesis.

Froriep (1843)[389] mentioned 'painful hard places' in the muscles of patients with rheumatism, finding them in 148 out of 150 cases, and describing them as a 'tight stiffness' so that the muscle felt 'like a tendinous cord or wide band'. He conceived them as a connective tissue deposit and coined the term 'muscle callus'. Although most of the areas were painfully sensitive to pressure, some were not. Strauss (1898)[1184] categorised three palpable distributions of excess connective tissue, i.e. in not only the muscle but in adjacent subcutaneous tissues; involving the whole muscle only; discrete aggregations following the orientation of fibres of an individual muscle; and only the last was considered to be 'rheumatic muscle callus'. He describes excision of a firm, non-tender thickening of about the size of a walnut, in the right rectus femoris, thereby relieving the sign of radiating pain to the knee when the thickening was pressed. The histological appearance was that of degenerating muscle fibres enclosed by connective tissue. He gave further examples of pencil-sized and larger palpable thickenings within muscle, the painful thickening becoming less painful with heat and localised massage, although the bulk and texture of the 'thickenings' changed but little with this treatment.

Müller (1912)[877] described fibre 'hardenings' that may extend for the entire length of the muscle and exactly parallel to its fibres (e.g. in the medial head of gastrocnemius), together with a scattered number of thinner, hard and painful fasciculi in the rest of the muscle. Painfulness was often independent of palpation findings, but some hardenings radiated pain to distal areas when pressed; others were spontaneously painful. Confusion as to fibre direction was sometimes unavoidable when palpating multiple muscle layers.

Of special interest was Müller's description of insertion nodules in the depth of muscle near the bone of origin, and especially in the gluteus maximus of patients with low back pain. With the muscle shortened and relaxed, the small nodules feel like grains of sand or pea-sized nodules.

They may feel hard or like crystals, and are extremely sensitive to pressure. They may be found at the ilium attachments of sacrospinalis and glutei, the rectus abdominis at the xiphoid and at the aponeuroses of muscles with a scapular attachment. Although light pressure may induce a reflex contraction of the muscle concerned, strong pressure eliminates the response and reduces the pressure sensitivity.

Both kinds of nodules are seen in patients with and without musculoskeletal complaints.

In field hospitals during World War I, Schade (1919)[1086] examined rheumatic muscular hardenings at the lateral free border of the upper trapezius and the lower part of pectoralis major before, during and after anaesthesia. In all but two cases the hardness remained unchanged during anaesthesia; in two cases it softened or disappeared leaving a few firm nodules. He followed four cases through death to rigor mortis, and in these the hardenings or nodules persisted until obscured by rigor mortis. Postmortem incisions confirmed that the hardening was in the muscle, and at 3 hours postmortem direct palpation of muscle via incised skin showed that 4 cm × 1 cm cord-like hardenings in the trapezius and pectoralis major were unchanged. At 10 hours postmortem no cord was palpable in the stiff muscle. Histological examination of the previously marked cord-like hardening showed only normal muscle.

In postulating a localised and fusiform increase of muscle colloid viscosity (muscle gelling or myogelosis) the author concluded that the persistence of cord-like bands through deep anaesthesia, and in death, precluded (a) a nerve-mediated muscular contraction of individual fibre groups, and (b) a structural change such as connective tissue deposits.

Lange (1925)[692] suggested that distinction should be made between painful cutaneous areas which coincide with a hyperaesthetic area of skin;[412a] painful muscle points which are a contraction of some fibres within a muscle as a response to palpation, and muscle hardenings, which are equally tender but arise from myogelosis (*vide supra*) and are not associated with localised contractions. After several muscle biopsies, during surgical procedures for other reasons, he did not observe any great change in the muscle samples examined.

After experiments with canine muscle, Lange (1931)[693] concluded that muscle hardenings may in some way be due to a deficiency in PO_4 ions. The important German contributions in the field were added to by Ruhmann (1932),[1067] who gave a good, illustrated description of the morphology of three types of hardening:

1. Small seed-like hardenings, 3–5 mm across, which were scattered along the line of attachment of muscles.
2. Plum-sized roundish or oval masses lying within the muscle belly, and composed of aggregations of several fusiform bands.

3. Long, stringy hardenings which often extended the whole length of a muscle.

He suggested they were due to increased tension in discrete fibre bundles.

Glogowski and Wallreff (1951)[411] reported on 24 biopsies of muscle hardening, 22 samples being taken from the back muscles during surgical enucleation following disc prolapse, and 2 from the hip musculature during total hip replacement of the joint. Most of the palpable hardenings had been present in the biopsied muscle for at least 2 years. Histological examination included the use of 9 stains; in only 1 case was there a change which could have been palpated through the skin, i.e. a small connective tissue deposit.

A number of more consistent changes were disseminated among the areas of muscle hardening:

Fat infiltrations, which appeared to be filling the space vacated by degenerating and atrophied muscle fibres.
Isolated darkly staining and tightly stretched fibres with knotty swellings and a loss of striation patterns.
Isolated single fibres or groups of fibre with greatly increased nuclei, aggregated as chains both inside and outside the fibres.

There were no inflammation changes nor evidence of phagocyte increase.

An important description of the histology of muscle associated with the degenerative changes in joints was provided by Jowett and Fidler (1975).[619] Muscle dysfunction commonly accompanies degenerative joint disease, and while recognising the role of chronic muscle imbalance in initiating joint problems, it may be secondary to denervation, to reflex inhibition because of pain or secondary to stresses imposed by ligamentous failure.

The multifidus largely controls intersegmental vertebral movement, and like the limb muscles, contains populations of both 'fast' and 'slow' twitch fibres. The fibre type is neurologically determined, and differentiation is complete at birth.[600] The authors undertook biopsies of multifidus at operation in 17 patients undergoing surgery variously for disc prolapse, spondylolisthesis, lumbar instability and lumbosacral degenerative changes with neurological deficit. Results suggested that the multifidus, since its slow fibre population had increased at the expense of the fast fibres, is, with age and disabling degenerative lesions of the lumbar spine, less adapted to carrying out rapid phasic movements, and adopts an increasing postural role.

Conversely, in patients with adolescent idiopathic scoliosis, Yarom and Robin (1979)[1367b] observed that both spinal and peripheral musculature frequently showed morphological and histological abnormalities. The morphological changes were worse on the concave side of spinal curves, and suggest that there is a specific neuromuscular disorder which causes idiopathic scoliosis.

Fibrositis is the one English word most frequently employed to describe this painful muscular condition[1133] which was referred to by Adler (1900)[8] and later (1904) by Gowers.[431] Stockman's paper[1178] in the same year described cases where biopsy demonstrated nodules in the perimysium of muscles, subcutaneously, in subcutaneous fat, in fascia and in the periosteum, and he suggested that the condition was a patchy, inflammatory hyperplasia of connective tissue. He recommended that no permanent relief was possible unless massage was continued until the nodule was completely resolved.

Kraft et al. (1968)[681] defined a fibrositis syndrome with four essential features: (1) localised exquisite tenderness of muscle; (2) a palpable 'rope' in the muscle; (3) dermographia; (4) reduction of pain with ethyl chloride spray. They concluded that the 'rope' contained localised oedema, and also observed that some individuals seem to have a diathesis for the syndrome.

Smyth (1972)[1150] has summarised the clinical criteria which satisfy the diagnosis of non-articular rheumatism or the fibrositis syndrome, although the question of a pathological basis was left open. Of one clinical aspect there is no doubt whatsoever—lumps, 'rope', thickenings, hardenings and stringiness are manifestly palpable and usually, though not always, tender. Further, massage and other local attentions to these painful thickenings bring ease to patients, at least temporarily.

Travell et al. (1942)[1233] reported a study of trigger points in patients with shoulder problems and localised exquisite tenderness to pressure; the pressure induced referred pains in most of the subjects. Almost all the patients had at least one trigger point 'in the serratus posterior superior muscle', but since this is a multilayer region of the body it is probably difficult to ascertain that a trigger point lies in a specific muscle layer. Many patients had similar trigger points in the infraspinatus muscle, and pressures here consistently referred pain to the front of the shoulder and sometimes in the hand.

Experienced workers in the field of benign musculoskeletal problems of the spine are very familiar with medial periscapular muscular tenderness and spasm, and a notable paper on the subject by Cloward (1959)[184] described reference of pain to medial periscapular areas on injections for discography (under local anaesthesia) into the anterior part of cervical discs C3–4, C4–5, C5–6 and C6–7.

The painful localities were C3–4 upper fibres of trapezius; C4–5 upper scapula, medial border; C5–6 middle of medial border of scapular; C6–7 medial to inferior angle, and subsequently it has been customary for some to invariably inculpate individual cervical segments, as the cause of the pain described, on the basis of the locality of pain reference.

However, Klafta and Collis (1969)[664] analysed the pain response to 549 injections of cervical discs, and observed that the significance of the pain response is particularly indeterminate. Pain was like the presenting symptoms in 22 per cent, unlike the presenting symptoms in 67 per cent and 11 per cent of the patients had no pain at all.

Holt (1964)[564] has drawn attention to the fallacy of cervical discography. In this connection, it is a salutory exercise to carefully identify the bony prominences of the rib angles when pain involves this anatomical situation, and to observe (a) that localised pressures there can be very painful indeed, and (b) rhythmical and repetitive pressures precisely applied on the rib angles are very effective in reducing the pain.

Returning to the theme of muscular tenderness, many have noted the efficiency of inhibitory pressures, i.e. strong, sustained pressure applied directly to the tender point.

Travell (1949)[1236] noted that chronic muscular syndromes of a year or more were much less responsive to ethyl chloride spray than to injection of local anaesthetic, and suggested that an initially physiological or functional disorder in its acute stage would respond to spraying, but that later organic changes would have supervened, and needling and/or procaine were more effective than superficial application by ethyl chloride spray.

Although it is now recognised that eradications of a localised pain by localised injection certainly does not demonstrate that its source has thereby been identified, many patients are considerably relieved by localised treatment to painful trigger zones or trigger points.

Steindler and Luck (1938)[1169] reviewed 451 cases of low back pain, exhibiting referred pain to the leg on localised palpation around the lumbosacral region. In 228 of the cases, a point was located where needle contact produced local and referred pain, both of which were relieved by injection of local anaesthetic at that place. All patients achieved at least temporary relief from pain.[1133]

Travell (1968)[1241] arranged muscle biopsies under local intradermal anaesthesia; no pathological changes could be seen, and she concluded that the abnormality at trigger points must be physiological or molecular, but not cellular.

It has been repeatedly observed[1133] that injection of normal saline is almost as effective as procaine, and poking around the area with a dry needle is only slightly less effective than injecting saline. None of the three modalities are effective unless the needle produces both severe local pain at the trigger point and the typical referred pain also. The link with acupuncture is too plain to be missed, and in a review article, Melzack et al. (1977)[848] have included 42 diagrams of trigger points associated with myofascial pain syndromes. Most of their own summary of this comprehensive review is worth inclusion here:

Trigger points associated with myofascial and visceral pains often lie within areas of referred pain but many are located at a distance from them. Furthermore, brief, intense stimulation of trigger points frequently produces prolonged relief of pain. These properties of trigger points—their widespread distribution and the pain relief produced by stimulating them—resemble those of acupuncture points for the relief of pain. The purpose of this study was to determine the correlation between trigger points and acupuncture points for pain on the basis of two criteria: spatial distribution and the associated pain pattern. A remarkably high degree (71 per cent) of correspondence was found. This close correlation suggests that trigger points and acupuncture points for pain, though discovered independently and labelled differently, represent the same phenomenon and can be explained in terms of the same underlying neural mechanisms.

Levine et al. (1976)[724] reported their observations on the analgesic effects of needle puncture and suggested that in chronic, painful conditions needle puncture may be very effective in producing at least transient analgesia. Needle puncture was not helpful in the management of pain resulting from nerve involvement. It is noteworthy that they found a high score on psychometric indicators of anxiety and depression was a significant predicator of successful needle puncture analgesia in patients with chronic pain.

Puzzling exceptions[1133] to segmental reference zones may occur, in that a low thoracic sacrospinalis 'point' may refer pain to the lower buttock, while an upper lumbar 'point' may refer pain to an area over the upper buttock.

Long (1955, 1956)[761] discussed myofascial pain syndromes and allied these to the 'gelling' concept of myogeloses. He described treatment for tension headaches, trapezius syndrome, the scapulohumeral syndrome, scalenus anticus syndrome, anterior chest wall and abdominal wall syndromes, pelvic floor syndromes, and the hip adductor syndrome. He also mentions detailed criteria for diagnosis and treatment in conditions involving the piriformis, levator ani and coccygeus muscles.

In passing, the multiplicity of proper names, for various syndromes in this field, might well be reduced to everyone's advantage.

Maigne (1976)[792] has described very accurately the tender and thickened eyebrow tissues in frontal headache secondary to upper cervical joint problems, and the eradication of this manifest physical sign by accurately localised manipulative treatment to the vertebral segments concerned. With reference to the cervical spine, sensitive trigger points 'in' the sternomastoid muscle may produce severe disturbances of equilibration, the patient staggering and weaving to the side of the lesion, and having blurring and mistiness of vision ('foggy window' syndrome!), sometimes with vertigo and nystagmus. These symptoms have been relieved by treatment of the trigger point, and it is noteworthy that Langley (1945)[694] described a method of relieving typical migraine by muscle springing and stretching techniques, which included attention to the sternomastoid.

Travell (1960)[1240] discussed in detail the trigger point phenomenon as it affected the temperomandibular joint.

She gave clear illustrations of the location of trigger points within each muscle, with the area of referred pain shown in depth, and she differentiated the zone of pain reference from different parts of the pterygoid, masseter and temporalis muscles.

In temperomandibular joint problems, acute trismus of the masseter muscle[1133] which restricts jaw-opening to 1.5 cm was relieved to allow opening to 5 cm in step-like increments by four weekly injections of its trigger areas.

Simons (1976)[1133] suggests a direct neurogenic effect, rather than an indirect vascular effect, as the response to ethyl chloride spray cooling.

Travell (1954)[1239] defined a 'trigger point' as characterised by (a) circumscribed deep tenderness; (b) a localised twitch or fasciculation when pressing or pinching the muscular location of the trigger area; (c) pain referred elsewhere when the trigger point was pressed upon.

Sola and Williams (1956)[1156] concluded that the injection of normal saline produced its effect via the autonomic system, and alteration thereby of local vasomotor activity.

Brendstrup, et al. (1957)[124] provided a controlled biochemical-biopsy study of fibrositic muscle, and described an increased concentration of acid mucopolysaccharides, increased water content and chloride content and a slightly increased population of mast cells. They suggested that the 'harder' consistency of this part of the muscle was probably due to oedema.

Glynn (1971)[414] has summarised the anti-inflammatory effects of local corticosteroid injections as inhibition of collagen production; decreased population of mast cells, and of fibroblasts; lessened permeability of connective tissue; decreased metachromatic staining characteristics of connective tissue.

Simons (1976)[1133] provides a most comprehensive study of muscular pain syndromes and summarises the possible mechanism as follows:

Many patients with a painfully pressure sensitive spot in their muscles also have a palpable hardening associated with it. Other patients have the pain but not the hardening. Most German authors and the originators of the fibrositis concept concentrated on the nature of the hardening as a means of understanding the cause of the pain. Taking this approach, one can consider seven possible causes for the palpable hardness: increased fibrous connective tissue, oedema, altered viscosity of muscle, ground substance infiltrate, contracture of muscle fibres, vascular engorgement and fatty infiltration.

An extensive biopsy[857] which attempted to correlate histological changes and clinical severity failed to demonstrate changes sufficient to account for muscle hardening in cases other than chronic or in those severely affected. With chronic cases, fibroplasia was shown to be sufficient to account for palpable bands or nodules.

Subcutaneous nodules have been regarded as diagnostic of rheumatoid arthritis for a long time, yet they have been found in asymptomatic individuals without known disease, in patients with scleroderma and in another whom Zuckner and Baldassare (1976)[1381] diagnosed as fibrositis. The authors postulate that relationship to an immune mechanism, trauma and/or vasculitis seems to underlie most subcutaneous nodules.

The pathogenesis of the nodules in the cases reported above was not ascertained. Rheumatoid-like subcutaneous nodules have been described in 54 children[277] with no clinical manifestation of the disease. Apart from 1 child developing rheumatic fever, no patient in the series developed rheumatoid arthritis during a follow-up of 1 to 14 years.

Simons (1976)[1133] suggests that much of the conflicting data might now be resolved by carefully distinguishing trigger points from reference zones and acute from chronic lesions, by EMG, biochemical, histochemical and ultramicroscopic techniques. It would also be of value to correlate palpable findings of vertebral abnormality, and cineradiographic studies of vertebral movement, with palpation of trigger points.

CONNECTIVE TISSUES AND SKIN

The adaptation of structure to function is probably more common in abnormalities of the musculoskeletal system than in any other body tissues, and adaptive shortening of connective tissues with reciprocal lengthening of opposed structures occurs very frequently indeed. A tedious list of familiar examples would serve no purpose, but there are some aspects of connective-tissue changes which repay consideration.

La Rocca (1971)[698] describes the pre-employment radiographic assessment of the lumbar spine[697] and mentions the high incidence of radiographic abnormality in relation to heavy labour; yet in many cases these abnormalities were not associated with symptoms at any time. He mentions the difficulty of explaining the absence of symptoms in the presence of advanced radiological changes, and the need to postulate that the aetiology of pain lies in some peculiarity of connective tissue composition, function, or both.

Reference has been made (pp. 130, 231) to the tethering and 'guy-rope' effect of soft tissues. Epstein (1971)[315] has observed that the cause of pain in abnormalities of the lumbosacral region, for example, should be sought in the presence of factors which may not be visible on plain X-rays, such as torsional and stress disturbances of connective tissue.

The ligamentous and capsular structures of the joints have elasticity to provide certain ranges of motion and they have tensile strength to resist deforming forces. If they are subjected to a deforming force beyond their functional capacity, they do not regain their original length when the deforming force is removed.[598]

Mennell (1952)[851] observes that many joint problems are due to pathological changes in the fascial planes, and that a far greater proportion of musculoskeletal difficulties arise because of these changes than because of changes in the muscular fibres themselves. He mentions that,

... The ordinary activities of life seem to suffice to maintain a reasonable degree of flexibility in the fascial planes throughout the earlier years of existence, and the extent to which the objective is attained must vary in adult life in accordance with the requirements of different individuals.

He emphasises the importance of loss of mobility in the fascial covering of the iliopsoas muscle, and in the iliotibial band, describing stretching exercises for shortening of the latter. Janda[606, 607] and Eder[294] describe the consequences of fascial contracture involving the iliopsoas muscle, and Eder describes techniques for stretching these tight structures. Changes in fascia, fat and areolar tissue[1180b] may be secondary to changes in bone, cartilage and capsule, but are important in themselves as indicators of abnormal states.

Thickened and tender areolar tissues have been described in the eyebrow tissues (vide supra) and Stoddard (1969)[1180b] describes how the skin may be tethered more tightly in some sites than others, feels thickened and is tender. Resistance is felt when attempting to mobilise skin in the lumbar region by pinching and rolling. These changes frequently exist with chronic changes in vertebral joints, and are localised to the cutaneous area overlying the joint abnormality (see also pp. 198, 199).

Despite authoritarian pronouncements that fibrositis is a myth, probably in the pious hope that poorly understood changes represented by this unfortunate word will go away if the pronouncements are repeated often enough, and despite our somewhat better understanding of the behaviour of referred pain (p. 189), referred tenderness (p. 168), hyperaesthesia (p. 196) and muscle spasm (p. 197), we seem no nearer a scientific elucidation of the ubiquitous clinical features of changes in the texture of muscles and attachment-tissues. Although the spine is a mechanical structure and must obey physical laws, there is no method at present of direct in vivo measurement of the precise vector value of a muscle or ligament.[331]

So far as muscle is concerned, electromyographic studies show that tender areas in muscle are frequently the seat of a localised increased irritability and a continuous discharge of action potentials, which last as long as the needle remains in the muscle.[1180b] Perhaps it should not be surprising that in a tissue with a fairly exotic biochemistry and which enjoys a complex servo-system of neural control, i.e. skeletal muscle, localised and fusiform 'thickenings' are groups of fibres in a state of hypertonus which temporarily or more permanently exceeds that of the muscle as a whole.

Further, degenerative processes in joints might reasonably be expected to induce, or be accompanied by, concomitant changes in the skeletal muscle and attachment-tissues which are neurologically and embryologically linked with the functions of those joints.

It may be that objective signs of muscle abnormality, i.e. palpable nodules, bands, stringiness, seed-bodies, crepitus and the like, and the presence of muscle tenderness which is sometimes acute and surprisingly quite unknown to the asymptomatic patient until made manifest by careful localised palpation, represent external evidence in peripheral tissues of changes (whose complexity we do not yet understand) accompanying the stately progression over many years of degenerative changes in vertebral joints. Sometimes the external evidence is painful and sometimes it is not. When painful, the muscular and connective-tissue lesions tend to assume diagnostic entities, since they repeatedly occur in a singular pattern of distribution, and thus tend to be given proper names (tennis elbow, bicipital tendinitis, scapulocostal syndrome, golfer's elbow, subscapularis tendinitis, supraspinatus tendinitis (see pp. 116, 187)).

In a comprehensive survey of the autonomic nerve component in the genesis of these ubiquitous states, Ebbetts (1971)[289] refers to the vasomotor changes, produced locally in the arms by cervical degenerative change, leading to local tissue changes which probably include a low-grade collagenosis. Sometimes we come upon patients who have lived and worked through these painful episodes without therapeutic help and who are no longer in distress from them, although currently having pain from other regions.

The painless and 'fossilised' evidence is very frequently there to be found (see Palpation section, p. 352) and clinical impressions indicate very firmly that it probably represents events in the comparatively remote past of the individual's degenerative history, like the rings of a sawn tree or the strata of a seaside cliff.

The lesson seems plain—treatment of degenerative joint conditions should perhaps include treatment of the whole arthrokinetic system, as it affects that particular joint and vertebral region, i.e. abnormal movement; muscular imbalance; connective-tissue tightness or tethering; localised soft-tissue changes of a textural kind. The movement-system is more than the joint alone and we treat, in the main, abnormalities of movement.

NEOPLASMS

The classification of tumours is a comprehensive subject,[983] and of more immediate concern is the *behaviour* of new growths in the spine. As with osteoporosis (p. 247) it is unwise to rely completely on the innocence of X-ray appearances; in cadaver studies[780] radiographic changes were shown in only 25 per cent of vertebral bodies with secondary neoplasms. Large metastases can exist without visible changes in the contour or bone density of the affected vertebra; for example, an area of bone de-struction more than 1 cm diameter in the middle of a vertebral body may be present without radiographic sign of it.[315, 159]

Extensive bony metastases will often exist without symptoms referrable to the vertebrae involved; and among investigation procedures positive scans of vertebral bone occur in Paget's disease and osteomyelitis, for example, as well as in bone metastases.

Tumours in vertebral bodies may:

1. Replace bone, with some of them eventually giving rise to rarefaction on X-ray, yet often not causing symptoms.

2. Produce gradual collapse and wedging or flattening of a vertebral body, and thus deformity.

3. Produce sudden collapse of the weakened body.

4. Burst through the restraining cortex of the body, compressing nerve root and/or spinal cord, or infiltrating muscle to produce soft tissue swelling.[983]

The spine is not often *directly* involved by neoplastic spread from adjacent non-vertebral structures; when this does occur, the site most commonly affected is the upper thoracic region, from peripheral bronchial carcinoma in the lung apex.[159]

Like primary malignant tumours, benign tumours of the spine are uncommon, *most vertebral neoplasms being metastases*. These account for the great majority of cases in any representative series of vertebral tumours in adults,[1140] usually occurring via the blood stream of the systemic circulation or the vertebral venous plexuses.

The blood-borne metastases are believed to pass from the primary site as emboli into the venous system, passing via the heart and lungs to reach the vertebral bodies as arterial emboli. In primary tumours of the prostate gland, the emboli probably reach the vertebral bodies via the vertebral venous plexuses.[159] The predilection of secondary neoplasms for vertebral bodies, ribs and ilium, is most probably explained by the slower blood stream at these haemopoietic sites in the adult.

The extent of metastases to individual vertebrae is variable, there being no constant pattern of involvement by any particular type of neoplasm.[315] Metastases are sometimes classified as osteoplastic, i.e. increasing the density of bone, or osteoclastic (lytic), denoting osseous destruction, but both may coexist in the same patient and in the same vertebra. Increased bone formation with osteoplastic neoplasms has not been explained. While bone erosion by *infection*, e.g. osteomyelitis, is accompanied by early structural changes in the disc, which always becomes narrowed, the disc resists invasion by a *tumour* and is at first spared when vertebral crushing is due to metastasis. However, when the support of underlying bone is lost, the disc fragments and subsequently does become invaded by the tumour.[315, 780]

Important early radiographic appearances are a slight loss of density, associated with small changes in contour of a vertebral body, transverse process, neural arch or pedicle. Other, uncommon, changes may be a small area of increased density, or spotty areas of increased density together with translucent areas.

Asymmetrical loss of pedicle shadow on AP films makes a secondary deposit virtually certain.[780]

Although benign in the sense that of itself the nature of the tissue destruction is not malign and ultimately fatal, non-malignant new growths may often produce severe disablement by lysis of bone and by trespass on neighbouring structures.

Some benign skeletal tumours include:

1. *Chondroma*, which arises within bone, more often in the shaft of a long bone, but which may occur in scapulae, ribs and vertebrae, and composed of adult cartilage cells in a mucous stroma. When occurring in flat bones it may grow to some size before attracting attention. In the pelvis it may interfere with hip function and produce a limp.[983]

2. *An osteochondroma* forms an irregular shaggy mass and besides involving the femur, when hip movements may be affected, may occur on the surface of the scapular or pelvis. The lump is hard and not tender. The tumour increases in size until skeletal growth ceases. Some 5–10 per cent of them may become malignant after 40.

3. *Benign osteoblastoma*[604] is a tumour of osteoid tissue and atypical bone occurring in young people, and when the vertebrae are affected the lesion usually involves the neural arches, articular facets and transverse processes. There is sometimes evidence of spinal cord compression.

4. *Aneurysmal bone cysts* are uncommon, primary, benign tumours of bone and can involve the spine as well as limb bones.[1140] They occur in young people, as localised expansions of fibrous tissue honeycombed with an enormously dilated vascular bed. Radiographically they appear as localised rarefactions with bulging of the involved bone.
   Benign osteogenic tumours are all lytic, and may have caused moderate pain for a year or more before X-ray reveals the lytic lesion.[1188]

Benign non-skeletal tumours

1. *Giant-celled tumours* (osteoclastoma). There is uncertainty as to what should be regarded as a giant-cell tumour of bone.[315] It is clinically a bone neoplasm, but has a consistency like liver and microscopically resembles fibrocystic disease and osteitis deformans. Found in young adults, it occurs more often in pelvis and vertebrae. Often there is no deformity but palpation may reveal a prominent spinous process, and a kyphus may be obvious in the thoracic region when the flexed spine is viewed laterally. This is not detectable in the cervical and lumbar spines.

On X-ray a large area of rarefaction in the vertebral body may extend into the pedicles. Later, the body is wedged and flattened.

2. *A haemangioma* occurs in the vertebra and less in the long bones. The X-ray shows one vertebral body and its pedicles to be enlarged, with the shape and borders of the body unchanged. The discs are normal, but the spongiosa trabeculae are coarse and more opaque. Normally, a vertebral body angioma is regarded as an anomaly not needing treatment, unless dissolution occurs in affected bone and the local vertebral disorganisation leads to pathological spondylolisthesis and paraplegia.[983]

Malignant tumours include:

1. *Secondary carcinoma*. Bone metastases occur more frequently from tumours which do not kill quickly. The more silent the primary, the more probable are bone secondaries. Primaries may occur in kidney, thyroid, bronchus, prostate, breast. The patients are usually older women, the primary often having occurred in the breast. In men the kidney and prostate are likely sites for the primary. In less than 1 per cent of carcinoma of the stomach do secondaries occur in bone. In more than 15 per cent of bone secondaries no evidence of a primary can be found, and is sometimes not even found at postmortem. A secondary in bone may show itself many years after the primary has been removed. Secondaries may be solitary or multiple, and common sites in the adult are where red marrow persists; skull, vertebrae, pelvis, sternum, ribs and upper end of femur and humerus. A metastasis is usually osteolytic; patients may complain of pain but there may not be any symptoms until bone gives way as a result of trivial injury. X-ray may show a more or less round rarefaction in the medulla of the bone. Occasionally the presence of a secondary may stimulate osteogenesis, and this may be seen in the spine where the whole of a vertebral body may become dense.

2. *Multiple metastases*. Bone may be riddled with deposits and yet the patient may have no symptoms. Often the condition is undetected until an X-ray is taken for slight pain or a fracture. Pelvic carcinomatosis may resemble Paget's disease. Fractures often unite, and the patient may live for some time.

3. *Chordomas*. These infrequent and slowly growing malignant tumours arise from remnants of the notochord, the greater majority of them occurring either at the craniovertebral junction or between sacrum and coccyx but also arising in other regions. They are always large, encapsulated, soft and gelatinous, and eventually kill by local encroachment. The upper cervical tumour leads to a raised intracranial pressure; the sacrococcygeal tumour

may obstruct the rectum. It is not radio-sensitive and can rarely be excised.[983]

4. *Plasma-cell myeloma* (multiple myeloma). These fairly common tumours arise from the bone marrow plasma cells, and present in two forms: (a) multiple myelomatosis, and (b) solitary plasma cytoma.

5. *Myelomatosis.* Multiple foci occur in bone. Whether the growths are polyfocal or whether they are metastases is not known. They occur in middle-aged people, and are often only discovered by a radiological survey. The deposits affect the red bone marrow initially, and may exist for a considerable time without clinical signs. There are no signs unless a bone is fractured, and sometimes the disease is revealed by a paraplegia. Severe pain may suddenly be caused by pathological fracture, which is common in spine and ribs. X-rays show multiple small round translucent areas, and this multiple variety is fatal within two years.

Sarcomas (osteogenic sarcoma, Ewing's sarcoma (endothelioma of bone), parosteal sarcoma) are tumours of modified embryonic connective tissue. Aside from their histology all sarcomas present the same clinical features. The tumour spreads rapidly via the blood stream, and secondaries are found in the lungs, rarely elsewhere. Eighty per cent of primaries involve the knee, and primary bone sarcomas of the spine are uncommon.[1140]

Spinal lymphomas[315, 1040] include reticulum cell sarcoma, Hodgkin's disease (lymphadenoma) and lymphosarcoma, with common histological patterns. Lymphomas spread by direct extension from involved lymph nodes, or by lymphatics and blood vessels. Clinical features of extradural compression by intraspinal lymphomas depend upon the site of compression and the degree of involvement of cauda equina and nerve roots. Slowly growing lymphomas in the epidural space may for some time mimic the clinical features of disc disease.[1114]

Vertebral metastases are usually lytic with general demineralisation of bone, but some persistent trabeculae with increased density may show radiographically. A single vertebra or several may be involved.[315]

Reticulum-celled sarcoma presents like a Ewing's sarcoma, but the prognosis is relatively good. Metastases occur late.[983]

Hodgkin's disease and lymphosarcoma. Spinal lesions occur uncommonly, and are usually multiple when they do, being preceded by the soft-tissue lesions. Occasionally, a bone abnormality is the presenting lesion.[1140]

Intraspinal soft-tissue tumours are distinguished from vertebral tumours proper. Benign nerve-sheath tumours and

meningiomas are more common than spinal cord tumours, which include metastases of carcinoma elsewhere, glial and ependymal neoplasms, and occasionally connective-tissue tumours of uncertain origin.

Meningiomas, for example, arise from cells of the arachnoid mater, although their arachnoid attachment may be minute when they are surgically exposed.[952] The primary intraspinal neoplasms may be intradural or extradural, most occurring in the epidural space although some perforate the dura and grow both within and without the dural sleeve of the spinal cord.[1291] Tumours of the filum terminale and the cauda equina may also occur. The clinical sequelae of these neoplasms are perhaps of more immediate importance than their precise classification and nomenclature.

Cystic lesions of lumbosacral nerve roots,[1031] and cervical nerve roots,[565] have often been reported.

In the neck these small pouches, of up to 7 mm in diameter, project laterally into the dorsal root ganglion and communicate medially with the subarachnoid space. Their cavities are lined with arachnoid membrane and their walls mainly are formed by compressed tissue. They are believed to be diverticula produced by increased hydrostatic pressure of the cerebrospinal fluid. The larger cysts are invariably associated with degenerative changes in nerve roots and ganglia, and occur at the junction of dorsal root and ganglion.

A neurofibroma may be found on any nerve, from the smallest to the largest, and at any age.[983] It may occur singly, although multiple tumours are more common, i.e. neurofibromatosis, or Von Recklinghausen's disease. This is a congenital disorder of ectodermal structures characterised by pigmented areas on the skin (*café-au-lait* spots) and by intracranial and peripheral nerve tumours.[1040]

The cutaneous pigmented areas have a smooth outline, vary from a pin's head to more than 3 cm diameter and generally follow the line of the dermatomes, e.g. on the trunk they follow the course of an intercostal space. The condition is hereditary and the cutaneous lesions are present at birth. The swellings on cutaneous nerves, cranial nerves or spinal nerves are composed of a plexiform arrangement of cells resembling fibroblasts. They are smooth, sometimes nodular, growths surrounded by a fibrous capsule.[952] Because the tumours may involve any nerve the clinical sequelae may be numerous and bizarre. The swellings enlarge slowly and are rarely malignant,[983] not interfering with function unless they lie in a restrictive situation and come under pressure; thus a swelling at the intervertebral foramen will slowly enlarge the dimensions of the foramen so that this is evident on oblique radiographs. If the tumours are multiple the nerve trunks become cord-like, enlarged and tortuous. A 'dumbbell' tumour may occupy both intervertebral foramen and neural canal, thus interfering with both spinal and somatic root.

A distinctive type of dorsal kyphoscoliosis is commonly present, and next to the *café-au-lait* spots, scoliosis is the most frequent clinical and skeletal manifestation of the disease.[509] The scoliosis, which results from wedging of two or three adjacent vertebrae from a unilateral deficiency of growth, may be mild or severe. The sharply angulated and rigid curve tends to progress as the child grows, because of the persistence of growth deficiency unilaterally. The deformity is often severe and resistant to treatment.[1140]

The ends of the long bones may be misshapen in neurofibromastosis, and rarely the peripheral tumours undergo the changes of a sarcoma.[1040]

Malignant neurofibroma are uncommonly found in a somatic nerve. The single lump remains within the nerve, which must be sacrificed by excision.

Pseudotumours, or deposits, include reticulosis and xanthomatosis.[983] Of xanthomatosis—Hand-Schueller-Christian disease, oesinophilic granuloma and Gaucher's disease—the last is uncommon, with enlargements of liver, spleen and lymph nodes accompanied by areas of atrophy and radiotranslucency in vertebrae, which have an inclination to fracture.

Deposits in the body of a vertebra may mimic tuberculosis of the spine. The prognosis is good and the patient may live for 20 years.[983]

Enostoses, or bone islands of the spine, can produce sclerotic foci which will simulate mestastasis.[131]

6. Pathological changes—combined regional degenerative

CERVICAL SPINE

Because of the diversity and richness of cervical spine innervation, the nature and volume of the afferent impulse traffic from vertebral receptors in this region are also rich, and it is this traffic which contributes in large proportion to the extensive reflex effects upon muscle tone in neck, trunk and limbs (see p. 11, 'Applied anatomy').

Arthrotic degenerative change, in synovial joints of the upper cervical spine, has some clinical importance since the arthrokinetic reflexes which underlie static and dynamic posture are disturbed by these changes.

Olsson (1942)[950] reported the frequency of arthrosis in the atlantodental (median atlantoaxial) joint in 125 cases as follows:

Years	Incidence
41–50	36%
51–60	68%
61 and above	88%

and this rising frequency of arthrosis with age is much the same as the rising incidence of spondylosis in the lower cervical spine.

Von Torklus (1972)[1274] describes bilateral exostosis of the medial margin of the lateral mass of atlas, and bony outgrowths on the apex of the odontoid. Osteophytes occur typically on the upper surface of anterior arch of atlas and appear on AP films as a peridental 'halo' of sclerous tissue (Fig. 4.2). Ossification of connective-tissue attachments may also occur.

Shore's (1935)[1125] postmortem examination of 126 vertebral columns showed a 32 per cent incidence of degenerative disease at the anterior atlantoaxial joint, and in his series degenerative change was commoner here than at any other synovial joint in the spine, with the exception of the midlumbar region.

More than a hundred years ago Adams (1857)[5] drew attention to the prevalence of arthrosis at this joint,

... the atlas and the dentata have far more free movements on each other than any of the other vertebrae enjoy, a circumstance that may account for the observation that we are accustomed to see far more numerous specimens of the effects of chronic rheumatic arthritis in these vertebrae ...,

and W. Arbuthnot Lane (1886)[35] made similar observations.

Arthrosis of the atlanto-occipital and lateral atlantoaxial joints does not seem to be as common; although Schmorl and Junghanns (1971)[1093] describe the skull articulations as involved in normal ageing, together with degenerative processes causing cartilage tears, flattening, changes in the joint space and hypertrophic spur formation. Malformations and malposition in the craniovertebral region also lead to arthrosis of these joints.

Osteophytic change is common, often unilaterally, at the C2–C3 facet-joint[1242] and is often found together with obliteration of the slit-like space normally seen on lateral X-rays of the healthy cervical spine (Fig. 1.13). Surgical exposure in three patients indicated that the exostosis is more extensive than the radiological appearances would suggest, the extra bone extending medially and dorsally on to the lamina of C3. The third cervical nerve was seen curling over the thickened joint, and flattened in a groove on the osteophytic mass.

Following dissection of 50 cadavers, the author draws attention to the very constant and intimate relationship of the third occipital nerve to the C2–C3 paravertebral joint.

Lazorthes (1972)[703] has also described this constant relationship, which does not occur in quite the same way at any other cervical segment. Combined spondylotic and arthrotic trespass may take dissimilar forms at adjacent segments, with lipping of the vertebral body compressing the nerve root at the C3–C4 space and facet-joint osteophytes compressing the vertebral artery at C4–C5, for example (Fig. 5.5).[356]

After a day or two following hypertension injury or stress (e.g. decorating a ceiling), patients may develop pain referred into one or both upper limbs, and in some cases this may be due to nerve root irritation or compression by the oedema of traumatic synovitis of facet-joints, synovial effusion being the space-occupying condition.[356]

More often, this may be due to trespass by a pre-existing osteophytic spur, the sustained approximation of root and osteophyte setting up irritation and producing acute inflammatory changes in the already compromised root. The segments affected by *spondylosis*, in descending order of frequency, are: C5–6; C6–7; C3–4 and C4–5; C7–T1.[117, 239, 385] (See Fig. 6.1.)

Degenerative changes of the disc between C2 and C3 are much rarer than in middle and lower cervical segments.

Although the anatomy of the cervical and lumbar regions is fundamentally similar, the two regions are bio-mechanically and functionally dissimilar. The typical lumbar disc problem entails trespass by a soft disc substance with the consistency of crab-meat, whereas in the typical cervical disc episode space-occupying effects are more usually due to a hard osseocartilaginous spur, pro-duced by the disc together with the adjacent margins of the vertebral bodies. (Fig. 5.2). The type of posterior or posterolateral prolapse of nucleus pulposus which occurs in the lumbar region is uncommon; the nucleus comprises only 15 per cent of the disc volume and is not sufficient to produce spinal cord compression by this means, although more lateral forms of degenerative trespass frequently compress spinal nerve roots (Fig. 5.5). Vertical protrusions (Schmorl's nodes) are infrequently seen in this region.

Damage to a cervical disc sometimes occurs in the young following direct or indirect trauma or stress to the neck, when there is little or no evidence of pre-existing spondylotic change,[117] and in the more mature patients with long-standing spondylosis; similar acute disc damage may occur superimposed upon considerable degenerative change already existing (Fig. 6.1). Both of the above forms of trespass can involve root compression and the clinical signs of radiculopathy.

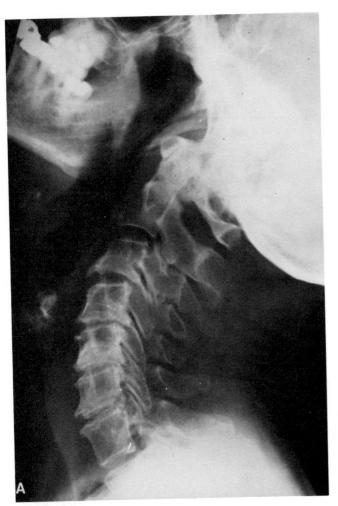

Fig. 6.1 Patient V.F.
(A) March 1973. Extension (see text).

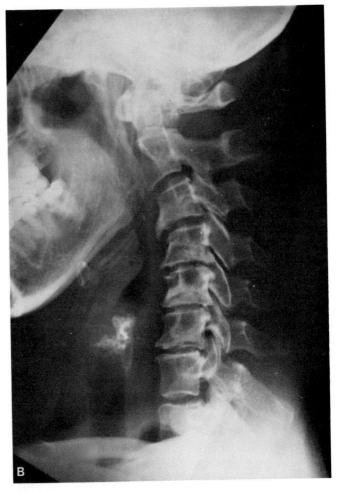

Fig. 6.1
(B) March 1973. Flexion. There is some stiffness at C0–C1 and from C4 downwards, with excessive movement at C3–C4. Loss of disc space and lipping in lower segments is shown.

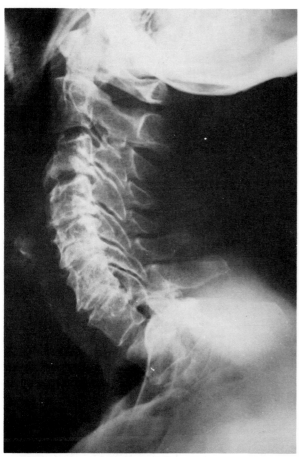

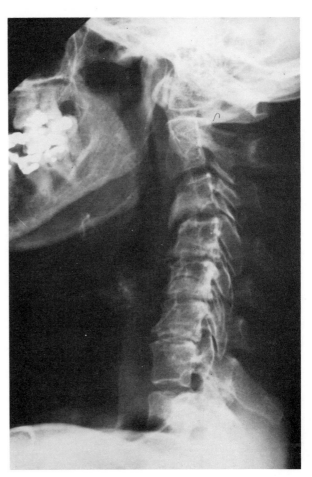

Fig. 6.1

(C) Extension, March 1974. Increased spondylotic change with further narrowing of disc spaces.

Fig. 6.1

(D) Flexion, March 1974 (cf. B). Movement is reduced throughout, with greatest movement in sagittal plane still occurring in the C3–C4 segment.

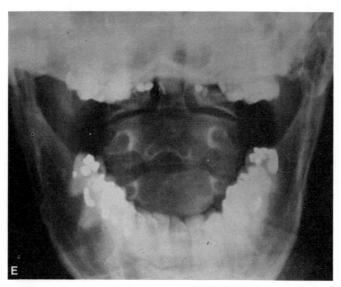

Fig. 6.1

(E) March 1974. C1–C2–C3 segments. There is little degenerative change compared with other regions of the cervical spine.

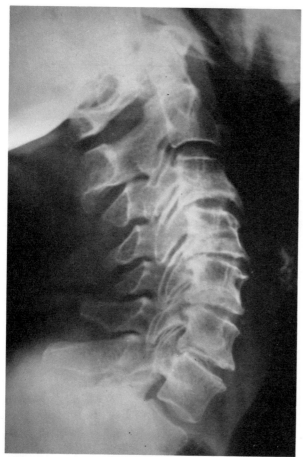

Fig. 6.1
(F) November 1974. Extension.

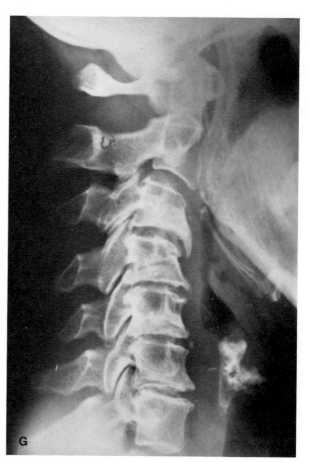

Fig. 6.1
(G) November 1974. Flexion. Increased movement is now evident in the important upper cervical levels.

More chronic forms of radiculopathy are quite common, sometimes involving more than one root, developing insidiously and causing some degree of permanent sensory disturbance and muscle wasting. The multiple nature of pathological change in cervical structures underlies the feature of ageing (Fig. 6.2). Also characteristic is the slow horizontal bisection of the disc from uncus to uncus as the slit-like spaces of the uncovertebral joints gradually extend inwards, together with nuclear material being gradually displaced along the tears in the annulus and thereby laterally into the uncovertebral joint regions.[1230] This protrusion laterally of pulp is seen only in younger individuals, before desiccation is advanced, and it occurs during the third decade; the altered, transversely split discs increasingly lose their supportive power. In later life, posterior movement of the small amount of nuclear material together with annular cartilage, freqently assumes a combined form, that of a marginal osteochondrosis, when posterior lipping of adjacent bodies, continuous at either side with the posterolateral outgrowths from the uncovertebral joints, encloses nuclear and annular material to form a hard osseocartilaginous bar which

projects into the neural canal and tends to compress the spinal cord and meninges into a series of horizontal corrugations (Figs. 6.3, 6.4).

The neural canal may also be encroached upon posteriorly, during extension of the neck, by buckling and infolding of the ligamentum flavum. This is more likely when vertebrae have settled together as a consequence of disc thinning and when fibrotic changes have occurred in the ligament.

As mentioned earlier (p. 13) the decisive factor, underlying clinical evidence of degenerative trespass upon the cervical spinal cord, is the space available in the neural canal. The clinical sequelae of cervical myelopathy are much more likely when there already exists a degree of congenital spinal stenosis.

The dura mater becomes thickened, more adherent to the posterior longitudinal ligament and adhesions are formed between dura and arachnoid. The dentate ligament of the spinal pia mater also thickens and tends to tether the cord, further restricting its normal free adaption to cervical movement.[117]

Foraminal encroachment occurs more usually by the

lateral extremities of the hard posterior ridges of osteo-chondrophytosis and these are plainly evident on oblique X-rays of the neck (Fig. 6.2(c) and (d)). Consequently, the transverse foraminal dimensions are reduced. Sometimes accompanying this are intrusions into foraminal space by chondro-osteophytosis of the facet-joints, and while changes at these joints are very common at upper cervical segments, the growth of bony spurs from facet-joints at lower levels also commonly occurs (Fig. 6.2).

The vertebral artery is frequently compressed by this means, and sometimes both artery and root together, since they are closely related here.[356] The consequences of compression may only be manifest on movements—rotation, flexion or extension.

NERVE ROOTS

The territory of the emerging spinal nerve roots is surrounded by many structures which are potential aggressors (Fig. 5.5). Thickening and exostosis of the facet-joints, osseocartilaginous ridges at the uncovertebral region, and localised bulging of posterolateral disc material are pathological changes which can lead to either transient or constant pressure upon the nerve root.[981] Local instability may produce further compression, by retrolisthesis, when the lower posterior edge of a vertebral body approaches the superior articular facet of the vertebra below, and converts the oval foraminal shape into a restricted S-shaped exit for the nerve root. The real extent of the encroachment is always greater than the radiologically evident narrowing (Figs 6.1, 6.2, 6.3, 6.4). The perineural 'safety cushion', of fat around the nerve root in the foramina, may disappear.[565]

Discs become progressively flatter with advancing degenerative change, as do the vertebral bodies, and this shortens the vertebral column. Reduction in length of the vertebral column with ageing will also produce sinuosity of the vertebral artery and a tendency to constriction of the lumen, accentuated during movements, even in the absence of atheromatous changes in the vessel wall.

Loss of disc space, radiologically evident by vertebrae appearing as dishes piled one upon another, angulates the lower cervical roots at the foraminal portal, producing a further source of irritation and inflammatory reactions in this situation (Fig. 2.14) and the first thoracic and eighth cervical roots are particularly liable to deformation in this way.[117] Localised irritation by angulation, or small haemorrhages produced by exogenous overstretching and other trauma, will initiate in the dural sleeve the familiar sequence of inflammation, granulation and fibrosis with adhesion formation, nerve root stricture and loss of elasticity and mobility, the root-sleeve fibrosis of Frykholm.[391, 392, 952, 777]

Ricard and Masson (1951)[1034] have suggested that the secondary formation of arachnoid cysts may be responsible for intradural root compression.

Among the space-occupying changes causing cervical myelopathy, posterior paravertebral ossification with calcification of the posterior longitudinal ligament has been reported,[861, 954] and unilateral facet interlocking may also reduce the dimensions of the neural canal.[106]

Keuter[656] has drawn attention to the variety of clinical features which may arise by impairment of spinal cord vascularity, particularly in those cases where the spinal tract of the trigeminal nerve shares in the ischaemic changes (Figs. 1.16, 1.17). Signs and symptoms will appear above and below the lesion, e.g. one patient showed partial analgesia and diminished temperature sense of left hemicranial area, headaches, vertigo and dysaesthesia in the C6–7–8 territory of the distal left upper limb. Radiography showed spondylotic change of the lower neck and arthrosis of uncovertebral joints in the same area. Angiography showed irregularities of the lumen of the vertebral and basilar arteries.

Other examples of bizarre and widespread clinical features are described, involving cranial and facial areas, trunk and all four limbs.

Following indirect trauma, an extraforaminal portion of protruded disc at C6 level displaced the vertebral artery on the right side, producing pain in the lower neck, hemicranial and hemifacial pain, with numbness of the right half of the face and depression of biceps and triceps jerk. Sensation was disturbed in right thumb and index finger. Radiography demonstrated disc degeneration, and angiography showed the change in the lumen of the vertebral artery on right head rotation. Surgical removal of the protrusion almost completely relieved the cranial sensory disorders.

The essential and important feature underlying clinical expression of cervical degenerative change is the enormous variability of the vertebrobasilar vascular system (Fig. 1.12).

THE CERVICOTHORACIC REGION

(Arthrotic and spondylotic changes have been described above, pages 82, 88.)

This is an important junctional area:

1. In the biomechanical sense, in that here the most mobile region of the vertebral column is physically interdependent with a region of very limited movement. Also, a number of important connective tissue structures and muscles cross the C7–T1 segment, e.g.

a. The prevertebral lamina of deep cervical fascia, covering the prevertebral muscles and continuous laterally with investments of the scalene muscles and levator scapulae; below it extends into the thorax on the front of the longus colli muscle, to blend with the anterior longitudinal ligament in the mediastinum.

b. The trapezius, scaleni, sternomastoid and longus

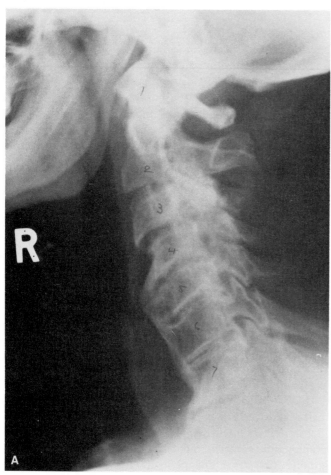

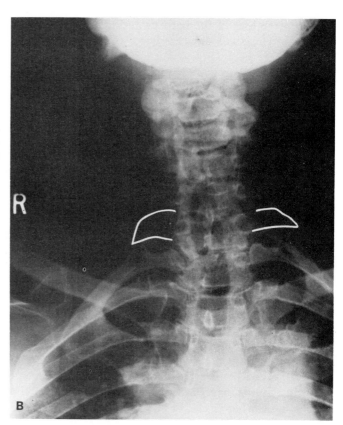

(B) There are marked arthrotic and osteophytic changes at C2-C3-C4, chronic spondylotic charges and bilateral cervical ribs (outlined).

Fig. 6.2 Patient D.C.H.
(A) Static films of advanced cervical spondylosis and arthrosis in a 79-year-old man. There is arthrosis of upper cervical joints, which is marked at C2-C3-C4, ankylosis of C4-C5-C6 and C7 with erosion of the body of C4. The patient was much more concerned about the pains of an arthrotic hip joint than the minimal symptoms in head, neck and upper limbs.

colli muscles, for example. The splenius capitis, splenius cervicis, semispinalis capitis, semispinalis cervicis, longissimus capitis, longissimus cervicis muscles all take attachment from bony apophyses of both the upper thoracic and the cervical vertebrae; the iliocostocervicalis attaches below to angles of the 3rd to 6th ribs, and above to the transverse processes of C4, C5 and C6. In descriptions of pathology underlying those clinical conditions grouped as the thoracic outlet syndrome, the possible 'guy-rope' and asymmetrical tethering effect of these structures, tightened by the consequences of chronic spasm and fibrotic change, seem not to receive the attention they might merit.

2. The region is a site of major vascular, neurological and other traffic. Many varieties of tissue with widely differing functions, and the potential for producing a variety of clinical effects remote from the site of interference, are closely packed together.

3. Junctional regions are developmentally restless and anomalies of skeletal and soft tissues are relatively common in the cervicothoracic area (Figs 6.2, 6.5D).

While signs and symptoms due to surgically proven pressure on the neurovascular bundle, as it emerges from the thoracic inlet to the arm, are well known, in non-surgical cases there is no general agreement on either the site or the mechanics of the compression,[1209, 1210] or sufficient evidence in many cases that the clinical features are due to compression at all. The poorly recognised part played by minor unilateral joint abnormalities of the upper three or four ribs, possibly often by tension of soft tissue attachments as a consequence of cervical joint irritability at higher segments, or due to the chronic sequelae of trauma, adds considerably to the confusion, because tingling in the upper limb is a very frequent symptom, and what patients are actually trying to convey by the expressions tingling, fizzling in the fingers, pins and needles, heaviness, numb feelings, etc. may not have anything to do with physical trespass upon nerve fibres or vessels, and may well be expressions of abnormal impulse traffic in autonomic as well as somatic neurones, because of facilitated cervicothoracic segments.

There can be no doubt about the clinical effects of a Pancoast tumour in the lung apex, but a causal relationship between the presence of anomalies of rib, muscle

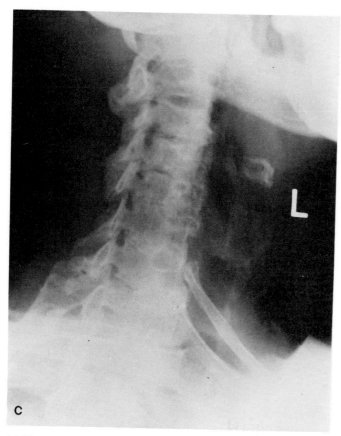

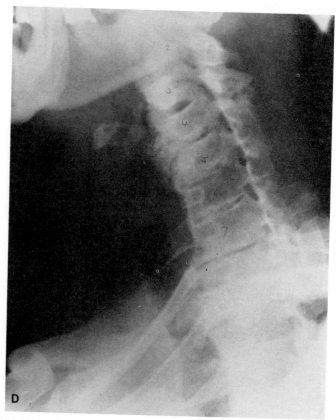

(C) Not one intervertebral foramen has escaped marked trespass by the changes of degenerative joint disease, apparent on the oblique film.

(D) The right oblique film shows similar changes, with one of the cervical ribs well shown.

attachment, plexus formation, vascular arrangement and clinical manifestations does not always exist.

Many patients complain of tingling, few (1.2 per cent)[702] have cervical ribs. Those who do seldom complain of paraesthesiae. Some have bilateral cervical ribs and paraesthesiae on one side only (Fig. 6.5), others have unilateral cervical ribs and tingling on the radiographically normal side.

True cervical ribs relate with their proximal part, head, neck and articular connections as a normal rib to the transverse process and vertebral body; false cervical ribs do not have a well-formed head but only a ligamentous connection.[1093] Occasionally, paired cervical ribs may be quite long, and be symmetrical; a single short extra rib may have a cartilaginous cap, and sometimes the anomalous rib is attached to the first rib by a synostosis or by cartilage, or by a tight fibromuscular band.

Anomalous ribs may occur as high as C4. With the extra rib at the cervicothoracic junction there may be simultaneous anomalies of the neurovascular bundle. The ribs and/or fascial bands must surely have a space-occupying effect in some of the subjects, but not all come to clinical notice because of symptoms reported. When they do, determining whether the rib is causing the patient's difficulties is not easy, as the anomalous structures vary in size, shape and relationship to the neurovascular bundle.

Causes of the thoracic outlet syndrome, some of them interrelated, have been named as:

Trauma to the head, neck and shoulder region, with haematoma formation and resultant fibrosis in the supraclavicular region.

Excessive callus after fractures of the clavicle.

Abnormality of the first thoracic rib, usually one that is unusually large or crooked, or with excess callus formation after fracture.

Abnormal size and shape of the clavicle, e.g. bifid clavicle.[764]

Inflammatory or malignant disorders in the cervical spine or shoulder girdle region.[1060]

Pancoast's tumour of the lung apex.

The scalenus anticus syndrome, 'almost always changes in the arrangement and in the course of scalenus anticus and medius are observed';[1093] connective tissue encroachments beyond the normal area of the first rib attachment are seen, being carried further forward than normal;[1209] thus the lowest plexus trunk and the artery lie not on the rib but raised by the lower apex of a V-formation of the tendinous edges of scalenus anticus and medius.

Extensive arterial thrombosis (almost 9 per cent of 120 surgical cases);[1209, 1210] in all cases a well-developed cervical rib was present, but in no case was any arterial change

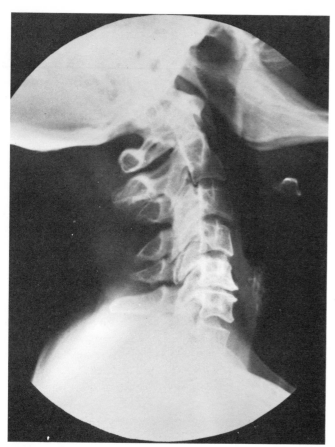

Fig. 6.3 Loss of C5–6 disc space and anterior lipping of the C5 and C6 vertebral bodies. The posterior lipping (osseus part of the 'osseocartilaginous bar') can also be seen.

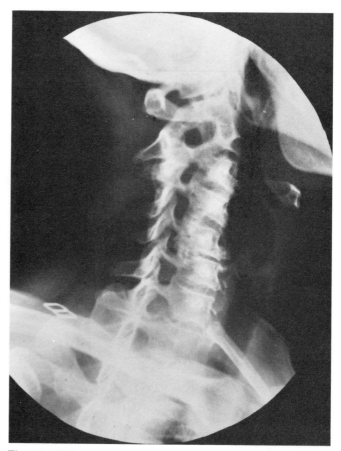

Fig. 6.4 Oblique film clearly shows loss of disc space, lipping at C5–6 vertebral margins, with foraminal encroachment at the same level. The degree of trespass upon related structures is greater than is radiologically evident, because of presence of radiotranslucent tissue.

observable where the artery lay on the rib. In 15 cases of arterial thrombi,[764] 4 had recanalised, 6 developed excellent collateral circulation but with a weak pulse and in 5 the pulse was still absent, suggesting only slight to moderate development of collateral vessels. In the absence of adequate revascularisation of distal tissues, mild trauma to the hand may result in ulceration which progressively worsens.

Aneurysmal dilatation of the third part of the subclavian artery, 1 cm distal to a cervical rib. This was present in 5 cases of a group of 120 surgical cases. Halstead (1916)[490] reported 25 cases of dilatation in a series of 525 patients. Thrombosis of the subclavian vein.[764] Swelling of the arm, heaviness and bluish discoloration of the limb may occur. While circulatory improvement from collateral vessels may sustain function and relieve symptoms, the arm rarely, if ever, returns to normal.

In 12 of 104 uncomplicated surgical cases,[1210] pressure on the lower trunk was due to a strong, taut band springing from the tip of a small cervical rib, and passing downwards and forwards in the anterior border of scalenus medius. In two young girls of 14, a large cancellous boss was situated where a well-developed cervical rib reached the first thoracic rib.

Of the above group of 104 patients 69 showed cervical ribs in various stages of development, and in almost all of them there was no naked-eye evidence that either plexus or artery had been damaged by clavicular pressure. Compression of the axillary artery by the two heads of the median nerve; experimental traction during open surgery revealed that all arterial pulsation ceased below the 'vice', but the subclavian artery was unaffected.

Sustained abduction or hyperabduction of the upper limb.

To these various causes there might be added:

Early spondylotic and arthrotic change in the upper thoracic spine and upper costospinal joints, especially when the symptoms described include heaviness of the arm, subjective numbness and paraesthesiae which tend to have a glove or extrasegmental distribution, in the absence of objective neurological signs—often only the tips of all digits are affected in this way.

Palpable and persistent elevation of the first, and often the second, ribs, due either to mild fixation following moderate trauma to the region itself, or as the consequence of increased tension in the scalene muscles. This may be an acute condition because of irritability at upper cervical segments, or the established contracture of connective-

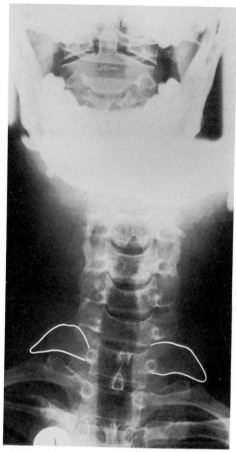

Fig. 6.5 Bilateral cervical ribs (outlined). The patient reported paraesthesiae on the right side only.

tissue elements. The unilateral combination of joint problems at the C2 and T2 segments together is well known to clinically experienced therapists.

Telford and Mottershead (1947)[1210] examined the effects, in 70 men and 50 women (240 arms), of different postures of the arms in the erect position, and among the postures were abduction, at 90° and 180°, and adduction against resistance. The results of these particular tests were as follows:

Table 6.1

	Abduction		Adduction against resistance
	90°	180°	
70 males (140 arms)			
No effect on radial pulse	131	75	18
Radial pulse diminished	6	42	38
Radial pulse absent	3	23	84
50 females (100 arms)			
No effect on radial pulse	91	35	9
Radial pulse diminished	6	35	16
Radial pulse absent	3	30	75

In passive abduction to 90° the alteration is 7.5 per cent, when the arm is adducted there is a sharp rise to 90 per cent, and plainly muscular action is now a factor; the authors offer the suggestion that pectoralis minor and subscapularis are taughtened to a degree sufficient to trespass upon the axillary artery. When describing the excellent results following surgical excision of an anomalous joint in the central portion of the first thoracic rib, Ross and Vyas (1972)[1060] include, as the most important contributory cause of the thoracic outlet syndrome, reduced tone in the muscles of the shoulder girdle, with consequent depression of the clavicle narrowing the thoracic outlet further and compressing the neurovascular bundle.

Telford and Mottershead mention that, 'it is an old observation that in certain positions of the shoulder the radial pulse is diminished or completely arrested ... it is taken for granted that the cause of this interference is costoclavicular pressure.' The authors applied downward traction to the arm in 25 bodies postmortem and report that when the shoulder girdle is depressed, the clavicle moves downwards and *forwards*; the further the clavicle is depressed the further forward it moves, *widening* the interval between clavicle and rib. At no point could the clavicle be made to impinge upon the subclavian artery. In order to press the clavicle directly backwards on to the first rib it was necessary to open and disorganise the sternoclavicular joint.

With regard to *the brachial plexus*, depression of the shoulder caused the upper and middle trunks, together with the C7 contribution to serratus anterior, to be stretched tightly over the tendinous edge of scalenus medius; the lower trunk is pulled down hard into the angle formed by the scalenus medius tendon and first rib. It was not possible by arm traction to compress the subclavian artery against either of the scaleni.

When *the shoulders were retracted*, the tendon of the subclavius muscle compressed the subclavian vein against the first rib, but the clavicle itself does not impinge upon it; the middle third of the clavicle pushes the neurovascular bundle backwards against the anterior border of scalenus medius, and in the presence of space-occupying resistance (extrafascial band, cervical rib, abnormal first thoracic rib) could compress the bundle. Sympathetic nerve fibres are present in the lower trunk.[1223, 1209] Movement of the clavicle in abduction showed no essential difference from the effects of clavicular retraction.

The authors suggest that the concept of costoclavicular compression is supposition, unsupported by anatomical evidence, and that symptoms referrable to the plexus on shoulder depression are caused by drag on the nerve cords. The plexus is stretched taut over the edge of scalenus medius, and this effect is accentuated if the attachment is carried somewhat forward on the rib. In retraction and abduction, the clavicle does impinge the plexus and vessel against scalenus medius, and this possibly explains temporary hand tingling during prolonged abduction when dressing the hair, for example, or decorating a ceiling.

In a group of 37 patients, who were treated surgically by anterior scalenotomy, after an injection of local anaesthetic into scalenus anterior had given relief of symptoms, Silversten and Christensen (1977)[1128] described the clinical features. In 21 patients no radiographic abnormality was observed; 8 had cervical ribs, 6 had a large transverse process of C7 and 3 had spondylotic changes. Neurological signs were detected in 16 patients and several patients presented with muscle atrophy, variously of the thenar, hypothenar, interosseous or upper arm muscle groups. The purpose of injection was to relax the muscle and note if symptoms were relieved. While the technique of muscle section was not described, it follows that release of the muscle and/or attachments was responsible for relief of symptoms (see Patterns of clinical presentation, p. 205). It would be of interest to have had comparisons of the degree of tension in both scalenous anterior muscles, since although expansion of the first rib attachment area is well recognised, hypertonus of the muscle itself, with its consequences on the posture of the rib, is rarely mentioned.[1180b] No one mechanical cause can explain all cases.[1210]

THORACIC SPINE

Few people have normal thoracic spines;[1180b] the presence of reduced accessory movement, localised tenderness and spreading pain on careful palpation is clinically demonstrable to a greater or lesser degree in most, and discrete areas of acute midthoracic tenderness in young women are frequent.

Group lesions are common but their precise nature and classification are not easy to decide on clinical features alone, although the combination of spondylotic change and secondary arthrotic change, particularly in the middle thoracic segments, is probably the clinical state usually responsible for the chest wall symptoms commonly simulating serious disease of thoracic viscera.[1002, 571, 433, 642, 1093, 1180b]

The precise distinction of the nature of degenerative change is probably more of academic than immediate clinical importance, because the malign and sometimes catastrophic acute thoracic disc lesion (*vide infra*) tends to occur between T7 and T10, with peak incidence at 1T9–10.[82]

1. Arthrosis
Arthrosis commonly stiffens the thoracic synovial joints, with radiographically evident peaks of incidence at C7–T1, T4–5 and the lowest thoracic segments (Fig. 4.3).[902, 1125]

The normally slight ranges of movement at the facet, costovertebral and costotransverse articulations are reduced, postmortem studies clearly demonstrating the prevalence of degenerative change at these joints. The bony rims of advanced chondro-osteophytosis of the facets tend to reduce the transverse foraminal dimensions but do not appear to cause such frank evidence of nerve root interference as is observed in the cervical and lumbar regions, although EMG testing will reveal it.[806]

When visceral disease, e.g. cardiac ischaemia, pleural and pulmonary involvement have been excluded, the back and chest wall symptoms observed in these common musculoskeletal lesions are invariably accompanied by palpable loss of movement at associated vertebral segments, and by palpable signs of joint irritability.[433]

Shore (1935)[1125] described hypertrophic changes in the posterior facet joints of 126 dried and macerated spines, and gave the peaks of incidence as C2–3–4, C7–T1, T3–4–5, T11–12–L1, rising to the greatest incidence at L2–3–4. He mentions three categories of change, in order of severity:

a. Marginal osteophytes of articulating areas
b. An intermediate zone, around the periphery of area (a), of porous bone marked by holes which vary considerably in size and depth. Some are shallow pits, some admit a pin and others penetrate the bone deeply.
c. A third and outermost zone, as a rampart of irregular osteophytes, sometimes discontinuous, of harder bone than (b) and often highly polished. The clinical effects of territorial aggression are probably due to growth of the (c) zone.

He describes as very striking the persistence of the normal contact area of the joint; though the surface of actual contact be doubled, the normal contact areas may still be recognisable. This is ascribed to the subchondral bone thickening which appears before the cartilage covering it has entirely disappeared.[361]

The rib joints often share in localised and painful loss of movement; ligamentous structures of the costovertebral articulations can degenerate to the stage of becoming ossified. These arthrotic processes have been found in 48 per cent of skeletal examinations at postmortem, and in 17 per cent of living persons, some as early as the third decade.[902]

The distribution of costovertebral degenerative change seems to show no marked difference when left and right sides are compared, but is noticeably different when comparisons are made between the superior and inferior demifacet on one vertebral body.

The upper part of each typical costovertebral joint, i.e. the inferior demifacet of the vertebral body, is more frequently affected than its fellow on the subjacent vertebral body, commonly at the joints of the 6th, 7th and 8th ribs. This higher frequency could be related to the general obliquity of the ribs, pointing medially and upward against the vertebral bodies.

The most conspicuous feature of rib joint changes is the definite overall pattern of distribution (see Fig. 4.3).

A significantly higher frequency of changes at the full facet costovertebral joints of T1, T11 and T12, in which the intervertebral disc plays no part, indicates that these single synovial plane joints are vulnerable to the functional stress and mechanical irritation of constant rib motion, which is probably less of a contributing factor in the remaining and more typical joints, where the demifacets and intervening disc, with intra-articular ligament, may effectively reduce the mechanical stresses imposed upon the articulation. Morphological criteria for the presence of rib joint arthrosis, in Nathan's (1964)[902] review of 346 spines, were first found during the third decade (20–30 years) and increased rapidly to maximal incidence during the fourth decade, but it should be stressed that a host of clinical features may be manifest in the early stages of degenerative joint disease, long before radiological and morphological criteria of abnormality have developed to the point of recognition.

Mild degrees of pre-existing but symptomless scoliosis or kyphosis can be aggravated by cramped working postures and carrying strains, and the same pattern of symptoms tends to be produced. That oedema of *interspinous ligaments* can cause referred pain has been clearly demonstrated by experiment.[269, 641, 642]

So far as macroscopic change is concerned, it is interesting that the *general* incidence of arthrosis of the thoracic synovial joints, reported by two investigators[902, 1125] widely separated in space and time, should be highest at the upper and lower ends of this vertebral district (Fig. 4.3).

2. Spondylosis

This usually occurs at the middle and lower thoracic levels, the more stately degenerative processes of the middle/upper region being rarely associated with disc prolapse, and the lower region being the site of infrequent but serious disc trespass posteriorly upon spinal cord and related structures.

In the sense of an acute tissue-trespass with pronounced clinical features, surgically proven thoracic disc lesions are very uncommon, and Epstein (1969)[315] gives the incidence as 2–3 per 1000 cases, equally frequent in men and women.

Of 2948 cases of disc prolapse, producing compression of neural canal structures, only 7 occurred in the thoracic spine, between segments T8–T12.[585]

Posterolateral thoracic disc trespass *appears* to be less eventful than cervical and lumbar lesions, probably because the foramen is larger and there is no lateral recess as in the lower lumbar spine (see Fig. 1.32), although the margins of the foramen tend to be sharper. Each thoracic root has a much smaller territory of distribution compared to those of the cervical and lumbosacral plexuses, and perhaps it is for this reason that frank evidence of root involvement is difficult to satisfactorily show. This does not mean to say that covert root compression may not frequently occur, but without EMG evidence it is less easy to prove that thoracic or intercostal 'neuralgia' actually justifies the frequent use of this nebulous word, with its vague connotations of neurological involvement.

Postmortem studies of the thoracic spine show that disc pathology is common,[1180b] and in the sense of spondylotic degenerative change, thoracic disc pathology is probably very frequent indeed. Radiologically evident narrowing of an intervertebral disc is not necessarily indicative of disc herniation, but in the event of symptoms which arouse suspicion of this, it might be a helpful hint.[315]

Most changes are less noticeable clinically, in the early stages, than the overt and relatively abrupt episodes of lumbar disc involvement. Further, the ultimate consequences of thoracic spondylosis tend to be far-reaching, and the cause of more prolonged and painful chronic disability (*vide infra*).

In terms of radiographic appearance the vertical collapse and horizontal bulging of discs tends to produce bony outgrowths in the anterior and right lateral aspects[901] of the thoracic vertebral bodies. Anatomical features (other than those mentioned below) favouring disc protrusion *giving rise to symptoms* are not present in the thoracic spine, due not only to the relative stability of the region but also to the tendency of annular disorganisation to occur on the concave side of sagittal curves. As a consequence of a general forward concavity, the radiographic changes of thoracic spondylotic degeneration are more marked anteriorly than posteriorly, since compression of weight-bearing falls most heavily on the front of bodies and discs.

The anterior lipping is sometimes quite gross in the elderly, turning these segments of the vertebral column into an almost immovable, 'fossilised' area; this is seen when a degenerate, collapsed and extruded disc allows the anterior lips of large, adjacent outgrowths to meet, and form the characteristic kissing chondro-osteophytes. The meeting of degenerative bony growths of adjacent vertebrae in this situation (and in the neck) is not necessarily a cause of pain, whereas the approximation and compression of normal bony apophyses, as in the lumbar spinous processes, because of excessive lordosis and/or disc collapse, is frequently a cause of pain. Posterior bony lippings in the thorax do occur, but they are comparatively small and may or may not give rise to symptoms.

Discs do not herniate or prolapse unless they are weakened by degeneration, stress or trauma. The commonest disease to weaken cartilage is osteochondrosis,[1180b] most evident in the lower half of the thoracic spine. Hilton *et al.* (1976)[541] reported the postmortem incidence of cartilaginous end-plate lesions in the lower thoracic region of 50 vertebral columns, in subjects between 13–96 years. The predominantly male lesions were demonstrated in 76 per cent of cases, and were most frequent in the caudal end-plate of segments, with a higher incidence and greater severity in the dorsolumbar junctional area than the lower lumbar spine. The changes seen were significantly related to disc degeneration in the T10–L1 region, but no lower.

The authors suggest that end-plate lesions developing in childhood and adolescence may predispose the segment to disc degeneration in maturity. Since end-plate changes are an essential feature of Scheuermann's disease, characteristically occurring in the lower thoracic segments of males, it may be that frank vertebral osteochondrosis is an unusually severe manifestation of a very common but often clinically occult spinal defect.

Stoddard[1180b] has repeatedly drawn attention to the causal relationship of osteochondrosis and backache due to degenerative disease. His study of the incidence of Scheuermann's disease revealed an overall population incidence of 13 per cent, with a 49 per cent incidence in patients with low back pain; the seven radiological criteria[146] are as follows:

a. Increased AP diameter of bodies.
b. Vertebral bodies wedge-shaped anteriorly.
c. Irregular and narrow disc spaces.
d. Loss of lordosis, or frank kyphosis.
e. The presence of Schmorl's nodes.
f. Flattened areas on the superior surface of bodies, near the epiphyseal ring.
g. Detached epiphyseal ring.

He regards the condition as a generalised disease of the whole vertebral column, in that the age of onset of disc protrusions is earlier in those cases with frank osteochondrosis.

In a more recent review of this ubiquitous condition, an important and largely unrecognised factor in spondylosis, Stoddard and Osborn (1979)[1183] mention that the precise aetiology of the disorder, in which the transition from cartilage to bone is irregular and patchy, remains unknown. The authors' statistical analysis showed that half the patients who seek help for backache have clinical and radiological evidence of osteochondrosis, and it is suggested that this evidence should be sought more carefully.

Vertebral osteochondrosis (idiopathic kyphosis, Scheuermann's disease)[146, 1089]

This tends to occur mainly in the second decade of life, as a consequence of changes which appear to be degenerative rather than inflammatory, involving the junction of vertebral bodies and intervertebral discs, when these structures are still in an active stage of growth and differentiation. Previously described as apophysitis,[983] the essential change is now taken to be the vertical protrusion of nuclear pulp through a defect or weakness in the hyaline cartilaginous plate.

The trespass of nuclear material may take two forms.[146] If the nuclear protrusions are small and evenly distributed, though multiple, there is no gross and localised disturbance of growth processes, and while the later onset of spondylotic changes is apparently assured thereby, there is no immediately obvious wedging and kyphosis, with the apophyseal centres little altered in appearance. On the other hand, when there is a weakening of cartilage anteriorly and a larger, more localised protrusion of nuclear material, pushing into the spongiosa of the vertebral body and passing between bone and cartilage as far forward as the anterior longitudinal ligament, there is severe disturbance of the anterior growth region; the epiphyseal zone is disrupted and the development of anterior collapse, with wedging of vertebral bodies, follows. Islands of ossification may persist anteriorly, between vertebral bodies whose anterior adjacent margins have a 'chamfered' appearance on lateral X-rays.

In passing, lumbar and cervical osteochondrosis are far from uncommon;[146] the greatest frequency of Scheuermann's disease appears to straddle the district of adjacent thoracic and lumbar vertebral segments.

Calcification of intervertebral discs can occur in the annulus, the nuclear pulposus or both, and in the cartilaginous end-plates; Sandström (1951)[1080] mentions that Luschka described the condition in 1858. Most commonly the site involved is the annulus fibrosus, and annular calcifications are the most permanent.[315]

Calcifications in adults are usually symptomless, occur in the middorsal area and as a rule do not disappear; those in children are more frequently associated with painful symptoms, and may or may not disappear on resolution of the clinical condition. They are not common, and have a tendency to involve the lower cervical or upper thoracic spine at more than one level. The condition is sometimes associated with pain, reduced movement and a raised ESR in children, but in these cases the cervical spine is more usually involved.[322, 929]

In 53 cases of disc calcification reviewed by Melnick and Silverman (1963)[840] there were 90 discs involved, and of the thoracic segments the sixth interspace was most frequently affected.

In the uncommon *thoracic disc protrusions* sufficiently severe to warrant surgery,[1116] the sequestrated material is often calcified.

In 20 surgically proven thoracic disc lesions[822] in which central protrusions predominated, calcified disc material was clearly observed in the spinal canal, with linear calcification in the adjacent disc spaces, by plain radiographs. Lateral protrusions were less frequent.

Thoracic disc trespass occurring in the lower half of the region is a lesion of potential hazard[1131] and in the past has tended to be associated with a gloomy prognosis, whether operated upon or not. In 17 cases[856] only one was markedly improved by surgery and none completely recovered. 'After the laminae are removed, the disc, under tension and now unopposed, extrudes into the spinal canal. Paraplegia may intervene.'[1116]

Shaw (1975)[1116] mentions two possibilities of pathological change: (a) simple local or circumferential compression, and (b) pressure upon the anterior spinal artery with concomitant disturbance of blood supply to the cord. The condition of thoracic spinal canal narrowing between T4 and T9, corresponding to a cord region whose blood supply is somewhat hand-to-mouth, contributes to the potential hazard of these lesions and the possibility of infarction of the cord.

Besides often being calcified, the usually cherry-sized disc material is often adherent to the dura, and may pierce it.[315]

Comparatively small protrusions may have disproportionate effects, since the extradural space is limited. The extruded material can vary from a soft swelling to a bone-hard excrescence, and there may be irreparable damage by erosion of the dura, erosion of the spinal cord,[1029] and bruising with a blue discolouration of the cord.

The consequences may be an acute onset of signs and symptoms, or the gradually progressive development of bizarre clinical features. Benson and Byrnes (1975)[82] described the clinical course of 22 patients, and stressed the important radiographic finding of disc calcification.

Gout

Gout involves the spine as well as peripheral joints. Acute episodes of sacroiliac or spinal pain, with intense muscle guarding and severe limitation of movement, may accompany acute episodes in peripheral joints, although the classical signs of a red, hot, swollen and tender joint are not so evident in spinal involvement. The acute symptoms may subside in a few days. A severe manifestation of gout may occur as paravertebral muscular irritability, any movement setting up acute muscular pains—passive testing is usually precluded by the irritability of muscle,[1180b] as is any unnecessary movement.

In some gouty patients, tophaceous invasion of the spine may occur which can result in erosive lesions, and by their physical presence cause painful reactions.[1220a]

The erosive and destructive lesions may alter the mechanical supporting structures of the spine. Gouty osteophytosis in the thoracic spine tends to involve the right more than the left; Nathan and Schwartz (1962)[901] ascribed the almost invariable right-sidedness of thoracic outgrowths in normal subjects to the effects of aortic pulsation discouraging bone formation beneath it, and this also appears to influence the thoracic spinal changes of gout.

Advanced and marked spinal osteophytosis, exceeding the normal spondylotic exostosis at joint margins, is described as having a pronounced relationship to gout and diabetes, these patients sharing similar constitutional features.

In Tkach's review (1970)[1220a] of 100 subjects with gouty arthritis, more than 55 per cent, 32 women and 23 men, gave a history of significant pain in the thoracic region in addition to pain in other vertebral regions, and he men-

tions pronounced osteophytosis and bridging of paravertebral structures being present in patients with gouty arthritis and hyperuricaemia; and also suggests the possibility that the clinical expressions of gout and diabetes may be interchangeable, giving examples to suggest this. From the data he presents, 'it would appear that the presence of primary osteoarthritis coexisting with gouty arthritis is a potent factor in causing spinal pain'. As most of the women in his series were menopausal, osteoporosis may have compounded the increase in thoracic spinal pain.

Spinal osteoporosis

In spinal osteoporosis there is preservation of the vertical trabeculae of vertebral bodies and a tendency to disappearance of the more horizontal ones, and this may be an explanation of healing microfractures observed in the vertical trabeculae of osteoporotic lumbar vertebrae by Vernon-Roberts and Pirie (1973).[1269] The authors determined a statistically significant correlation between the number of trabecular lesions and age, and a direct relationship to the degree of osteoporosis. Very few nodules of woven bone callus formation were found on horizontal trabeculae.

The question of whether trabecular fractures can be a cause of back pain is not yet determined, but the authors make the point that a structure with cross-ties, i.e. horizontal trabeculae, is more vulnerable to load if the cross-ties are removed. Thus the structure will buckle under one-quarter of the original load required, and for 'load' one might also read 'vertebral manipulation'.

It is worth remembering that the most prominent manifestations of osteoporosis,[1099] in terms of vertebral collapse, are usually localised to the thoracic and upper lumbar region with pain usually referred[896] diffusely to the low back; ribs are especially vulnerable to fractures.

Acute fixations of rib joints (see p. 233)

These occur commonly, most usually in the upper half of the thoracic region, and show all the usual characteristics of synovial joint locking.[315] Articular discs or little 'menisci' of synovial tissue are found in these costal joints as in almost all other synovial articulations of the spinal column.[312]

Schmorl and Junghanns (1971)[1093] mention that the probable incarceration of an articular villus or meniscus in vertebral synovial joints is common, and that there is no doubt that the causes for such disturbances are located in mobility segments, the locking causing pain in capsules and ligaments, and painful reflex muscular tensions. The temporary and palpable fixation may also be due to roughened articular surfaces.

So far as the upper two ribs are concerned, fixation in somewhat elevated positions may be due to spasm of scalene muscles, secondary to an irritative lesion involving their segments of origin.

Developmental *spinal stenosis* in the thoracic region (p. 16) appears to be uncommon. Acquired stenosis due to Paget's disease[39] has been described, the tomographic appearance showing a reduction in vertical height and an increase in the anteroposterior diameter of the diseased bone. Osteitis deformans can occur in any vertebra from the atlas to sacrum, the lumbosacral region being most frequently involved.

Acute and chronic costochondrosis (Tietze's disease)[1015,1217]

Acute and chronic costochondrosis of the costal cartilages may simulate disease of the thoracic viscera, or mimic the anterior reference of pain from vertebral joint problems. The small, localised and painful swelling, of two or more costal cartilages on one side, appear to have no relation to the vertebral joints. Specimens obtained by excision or needle biopsies are usually unrevealing, but may nevertheless represent a traumatic or low-grade inflammatory response at the costochondral junctions. Their main importance lies in the recognition of their innocence, although they are a frequent cause of anxiety to patients and can be severely painful.

Slipping rib-tip

A slipping rib-tip may produce acute, localised pain at the costal margin, and is attributed to increased mobility of the cartilaginous tip of the 8th, 9th or 10th rib.[823] The somewhat fragile anterior attachments, normally by loose fibrous tissue, allow increased mobility, and moderate trauma to the infrasternal region may force a cartilaginous tip upwards and inwards in close relationship to the intercostal nerve. The nature of the condition lies in the fact that surgical excision of the anterior 4 cm of rib completely relieves it.

Scapulocostal crepitus

Subscapular crepitus is not infrequent. Apparently harmless aggregations or stringy thickenings of soft tissue can be palpated in many areas adjacent to the spinal column and iliac crest; it is reasonable that they might occur in the subscapular soft tissues also, and be the more evident to patient and clinician in the bony compartment between ribs and shoulder blade.

The 'roughening of the posterior thoracic wall' may sometimes, on meticulous examination, be found to consist of a mild postural fixation of one to three ribs, forming a slight elevation of their angles which disturbs the normal upper posterolateral thoracic contour. The fault thus may lie at the costal joints.

LUMBAR SPINE

Narrowing of disc space, spondylolisthesis (p. 143) and transitional vertebrae tend to apply abnormal stresses to the posterior joint structures;[317] conversely, dysplasia of lumbosacral facet structures, or gross degenerative change in facet-joints (Fig. 1.25), can be the cause of spondylolisthesis.[923]

Degenerative loss of normal resilient stiffness in low lumbar discs can usher in a group of changes, of which facet-joint damage may be one, although arthrosis does not inevitably follow spondylotic change. Arthrosis of posterior joints is common in the mid and lower lumbar regions, and it is at the lumbosacral articulation that degenerative change of both synovial and vertebral body joints seem to occur most often.

The lumbosacral segment is the lowest truly mobile one of the spine, sustaining heavy forces and suffering great stress; also, anomalies are frequent and these factors may tend to hasten degeneration (Figs 1.27, 1.28, 1.29). The incidence of arthrosis and spondylosis at one lumbar vertebral segment is age-related, with spondylotic and arthrotic change involving whole segments in about 60 per cent of subjects over 45.[727]

The degree of damage commonly sustained by the articular processes and facet-joint surfaces is often severe; chip fractures, fissure fractures, facet overriding and marginal bony ridges produced by traumatic grinding of surfaces are not infrequent, and what appears clinically as episodes of osteoarthrotic locking of lumbosacral facets can occur.[508] Yet the presence of macroscopic changes at autopsy may not be an index of the pain and disability suffered by these subjects during life, and it is known that the correlation between radiographic[552] and morphological[392] changes, and clinical features, for example, tends to be imprecise. When *severe* structural changes are found in the low lumbar discs of young persons, they may often be associated with correspondingly severe change in the posterior synovial joints.

Degenerative disc changes may produce irregular movement and sometimes *instability*,[508] the facet-joint structures being buffeted and injured by the traumatic distortion and intensification of their normal movement stresses.

Instability is sometimes a source of chronic symptoms, because of excessive movement at the hypermobile segment (see p. 143) and tends to involve the L4–5 segment.

Ligamentous strain[1180b] will occur as a consequence of segmental hypermobility, but is also often due to defective posture, increased lumbar lordosis being a common cause. This is often seen in multiparous women and corpulent men. The added forward shearing stresses when standing or walking tends to throw extra compression on the vertebral arches and facet-joint structures, and excessive stress on the ligaments in the two forms of (a) nipping between bony apophyses (e.g. the interspinous ligament), and (b) traction stress (e.g. the iliolumbar ligaments).[852, 983] This latter effect is increased if the inferior articular processes of the fifth lumbar vertebra are poorly developed and do not form an efficient bony hook.

Thus the cause of arthrosis and ligamentous stress here can be (a) segmental hypermobility and instability alone, (b) lordotic postural stress alone, and (c) both. Increased lordosis with disc collapse may lead eventually to the state of 'kissing spines' (Baarstrup's syndrome)[49] when bone-to-bone compression of the spinous processes occurs, and gives rise to an unpleasant localised pain occurring especially on extension.

Sclerosis of the adjacent bone surfaces of an adventitious joint between spinous processes is sometimes evident on X-ray.

Ligamentous strain may also possibly arise as a result of habitual postural slumping in young people, yet joint pain in juniors may not always have this attractively simple explanation.

Disc narrowing is not always accompanied by instability. On occasions the gradual loss of disc height is accompanied by slow concomitant shortening of collagenous tissue in annulus fibrosus, interspinous ligaments and facet-joint capsules; patients who tend to overprotect their backs for years on end may then suffer a generalised ache from segmental stiffness as a consequence of adaptive shortening.

Lumbar instability

Intervertebral instability—a loosening of the mobility segment—is the most common form of insufficient performance in the mobile space between two vertebrae. This applies from the anatomo-pathological standpoint as well as from the clinical one.[1093]

Knuttson (1942)[667] observed 'the vacuum phenomenon', radiotranslucent streaks at the lumbosacral disc space, usually associated with marked narrowing of the disc, and more apparent on lateral films taken during extension, since widening of the space increases the radiotranslucent area. Both Knuttson and Gershon-Cohen (1946)[404] attributed the change to degeneration of the nuclear pulposus. Marr (1953)[810] found gas in the lumbar discs of 2.026 per cent of 2419 radiographs, most occurring at the lumbosacral space and associated with loss of disc space, marginal osteophytosis and eburnation of bony surfaces. Some do not accept the presence of a radiotranslucent space as indicative of instability, but do regard it as a stress phenomenon. Gas in the disc is occasionally seen in the lower cervical spine, and the same change has been observed in the symphysis pubis during and immediately after pregnancy,[315] when the pelvic articulations have been loosened by hormonal changes. According to the literature, radiographic evidence of the incidence of gas in the disc is very much exceeded by the incidence of abnormal motion of low lumbar segments.

Knuttson (1944)[668] states that the first radiological sign of disc disease is abnormal motion on flexion from the neutral position. He established the important significance of this lumbar vertebral instability by the routine use of lateral X-rays at the extremes of flexion and extension. Macnab (1969)[773] describes other abnormal movements, and ascribes them to annular tears and fracture of the hyaline cartilage plate.

Hadley (1936)[479] reported apophyseal subluxation as a disturbance of lumbar segment mechanics. Morgan and King (1957)[872] assert that 'primary' instability of lumbar vertebrae is the commonest cause of low back pain, and report the clinical and radiographic features of the condition among a group of 500 consecutive cases of lumbosacral pain. The incidence of instability was 28.6 per cent (143 patients). The authors refer to the work of many earlier writers who had repeatedly observed the coexistence of lumbar instability and the presence of concentric separations of the annular laminae, together with radial tears of the annulus.[508, 382, 383, 752]

Friberg (1948)[382] examined 500 intervertebral discs, obtaining postmortem radiographs of full flexion and extension, and then cutting the discs horizontally. In all the spines which showed radiographic evidence of instability, he found fairly widespread incomplete radial tears or crescentic fissures between the annular laminae. Only a minority of patients with low back pain have a bony discontinuity, such as isthmic (Group II) spondylolysis or spondylolisthesis, which can be shown radiographically.

The abnormal motion, as a lumbar listhesis, was described by Junghanns (1930)[624] and labelled 'pseudospondylolisthesis', since there is no neural arch defect. This degenerative spondylolisthesis occurs more frequently in women and involves the L4–5 segment.

Rosenberg's (1975)[1058] study of 20 skeletons and 200 patients with Group III (degenerative) spondylolisthesis (Fig. 1.25), included descriptions of the markedly degenerated small joints in the anatomical specimens. The slipped vertebra and subjacent vertebra always showed profound changes in their articular processes. Rarely was there the remnant of an articular process, or evidence of residual subchondral cortex to delineate where an articular process might have been. The 'articulation' was much broader than the area originally covered by the articular process on each side, these having worn away so that the 'joint' existing was formed by the front aspect of the remains of L4 inferior articular processes, for example, abutting onto the entire posterior surface of L5 superior process. In only one case was there a spontaneous fusion of articular processes in the slipped position.

Advanced degeneration of posterior joints often occurs without degenerative spondylolisthesis, but the latter cannot occur without prior degenerative changes in the facet-joints; occasionally slipping is detectable before facet-joint changes can be demonstrated radiographically. Whether the dominant cause of Group III spondylolisthesis is disc degeneration or facet degeneration is uncertain.

Rosenberg offers the explanation that degenerative changes in the fourth and fifth lumbar articular processes are due to the relative instability of the L4–5 segment compared to the stability of the L5–S1 interspace. Among the 200 patients, all body types were represented but none predominated. Physical findings were unimpressive in the majority. The most constant physical finding was the ease with which these patients could touch their toes without bending their knees or obliterating the lumbar lordosis.

In 90 per cent of cadavers over 40 years, Rissanen[1043] noted that the interspinous ligaments between L4 and L5 had degenerated or completely ruptured. Because he considered an unstable spine to be one of the commonest causes of an unsatisfactory result after operation for nuclear prolapse, Barr (1951)[67] advocated spinal fusion as an additional procedure during these operations.

Morgan and King (1957)[872] excluded the 'secondary' form (i.e. that deriving from nuclear prolapse) of instability from their series of 143 patients, and their observations concern only the one form of primary instability that occurs in the absence of any other radiological abnormality of the discs or vertebrae, except anteroposterior sliding.

Observing that nuclear prolapse into the neural canal is an important cause of acute lumbosacral pain and sciatica, they assert that lumbar instability, presumably caused by structural annular defects, appeared to be the commoner and consequently more important cause of a milder type of lumbosacral pain and sciatic neuritis, and this accords with Farfan's observations (p. 91 in Pathology section) that:

1. The loss of normal disc stiffness or turgidity after experimental rotation strains is probably akin to the soft, or loose, segment in the living, and

2. abnormally increased motion at a joint is usually a sign of severe degeneration.

Macnab (1977)[780] describes some stages of this degenerative process, in that excessive degrees of extension and flexion are permitted and a certain amount of backward and forward gliding movement occurs as well. Symptoms are produced by ligamentous strains, and posterior joint strains. A further stage is segmental hyperextension, when loss of elasticity in anterior annular fibres allows excessive approximation of posterior structures, aggravated by a lax abdominal wall and/or a tight tensor fascia lata. On lateral films, the tip of the subjacent superior articular process is seen to rise above the level of the lower margin of the vertebral body above, and this trespass converts the normal ovoid outline of the intervertebral foramen into a 'lazy-S' silhouette. He also

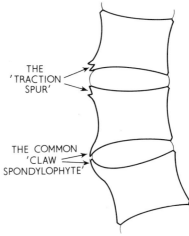

Fig. 6.6 The 'traction spur' and the 'claw-type osteophyte' or spondylophyte. Macnab (1977) regards the traction spur as radiological evidence of segmental instability, and the spondylophyte as cupping the disc, growing around it during the degenerative process, but not associated with instability. Cyriax (1969) views the latter osteophyte formation as a beneficial process, limiting mobility and thus hindering further disc protrusion.

describes the traction spur[774] (Fig. 6.6), a characteristic exostosis of the vertebral body, projecting horizontally about 2 mm away from the discal border of the vertebra. This is ascribed to an excessive strain applied to the outermost annular fibres (see p. 18), the small traction spur being clinically significant and probably indicating current instability. The large traction spur probably indicates that the segment has been unstable in the past but is now stable because of fibrotic changes occurring within the disc. He gives the telltale radiographic signs of degeneration in the stage of segmental instability as the Knuttson phenomenon (see above), abnormal movement and the traction spur.

The presence of osteophytes or traction spurs need not necessarily signify an unstable joint (Farfan, 1973).[326]

Radiographic changes may at times help in assessment, and at times confuse it (Figs 5.6, 6.6, 6.7).

Mooney (1977)[870] equates segmental lumbar instability with facet arthropathy.

Howes and Isdale (1971)[576] reported a prospective study of 102 cases of backache with particular reference to the presence of ligamentous laxity. Neurological signs were invariably absent, and of the 59 men and 43 women between 16 to 70 years, nearly all the men had varying features of spondylosis or spondylitis, while only half of the 43 women could be diagnosed as suffering from these conditions, the majority of the remainder exhibiting hypermobility. *The authors suggest that the clinical features of the loose-back syndrome are an important differential diagnosis of backache in women.*

Newman (1952)[920] described a distinct group of patients with backache from mechanical causes, comprising 20 per cent of those seen in a year. The patient is more commonly a female between ages 15 and 35, and the onset is often associated with a fall or blow on the back, a lifting strain, childbirth, violent activity or horseplay during adolescence. Many are young housewives, nurses or young men doing occasional or unaccustomed heavy manual work. There is no evidence of neurological involvement. The nature of the stress or violence, when of sufficient force, is to tear the supraspinous and interspinous ligaments, the capsules of the posterior joints, and occasionally the posterior longitudinal ligament and posterior annulus. The ligamentum flavum stretches but does not rupture. The affected spinal region is often the junctional area where the mobile spine meets the relatively immobile pelvis, and damage to or laxity of the supraspinous ligament may be evident by a depression at the L4–5 or L5–S1 interspace, markedly contrasting with the resistance of an intact ligament at adjacent and other levels. Lateral radiographic views in extremes of flexion and extension may show mechanical instability, and on injection of a local anaesthetic there is first an increase of pain due to tension, followed by temporary relief of pain.

Bremmer (1958)[122] asserts that this type of case forms a fairly typical clinical group of large dimensions and in the early stages the condition is essentially an instability with associated ligamentous strain. In some cases there seems to be an insidious primary degeneration of the disc whereas in others a traumatic incident may be the cause. In his series of 250 consecutive cases diagnosed (not ideally, he allows, because of the state of our ignorance) as 'lumbosacral strain', those presenting with nerveroot involvement or generalised lumbar spondylosis were excluded from the group; a distinguishing feature was the paucity of physical signs. It would have been of interest to know the palpation findings in each of these patients.

Armstrong (1965)[40] refers to the occasional rupture of the interspinous ligaments which may be produced by sudden flexion injuries, without fracture or intervertebral disc injuries, and Dehner (1971)[246] describes the serious injury to the spine which can be caused by an abrupt deceleration crash, when the car occupants are wearing lap seat belts.[1054] Severe flexion of the torso can cause tear-

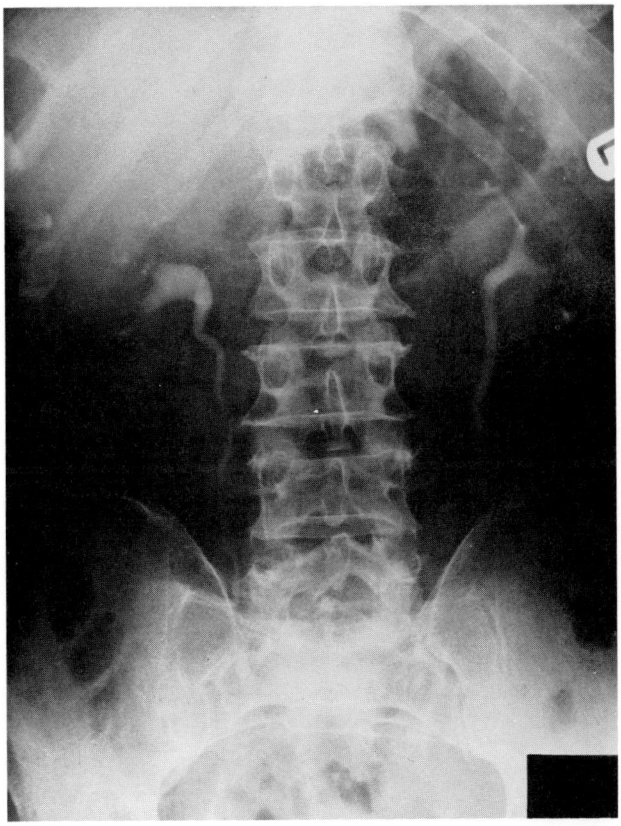

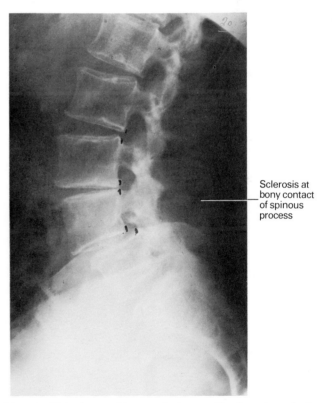

Sclerosis at bony contact of spinous process

Fig. 6.7 Two examples of 'traction spurs' and 'claw spondylophytes' existing at the same segment (viz. L2–L3 and L3–L4) in a 67-year-old man. For severe bilateral limb pains on standing and walking, and severe leg restlessness at night, he had received prolonged treatment for 'osteoarthrosis of knees and ankles'. On careful clinical examination, both L3–L4 and L4–L5 were hypermobile; the L2–L3 segment was much less mobile, despite the presence of a 'traction spur'. His clinical features of spinal stenosis cleared up almost entirely with a few treatments of lumbar traction combined with abdominal strengthening exercises and a temporary corset.

Fig. 6.8 This 72-year-old woman had severe burning pain at the low back and both buttocks after being up for 2½ hours in the morning. Whether her pains were due to the lordosis as such, or the lumbosacral problem (so far as radiographic appearance is concerned), or the group III spondylolisthesis at L4–L5, or her bony approximation at L3–L4 (Baarstrup's syndrome), is anybody's guess. Other than diminished movement there were no significant signs, and little further information derived from palpation. She improved considerably on traction in a well-flexed position, bilateral hip and knee flexion exercises, and isometric abdominal exercises, although it is still not known precisely why.

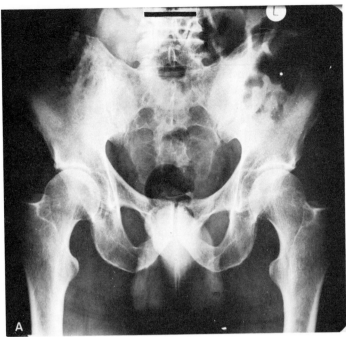

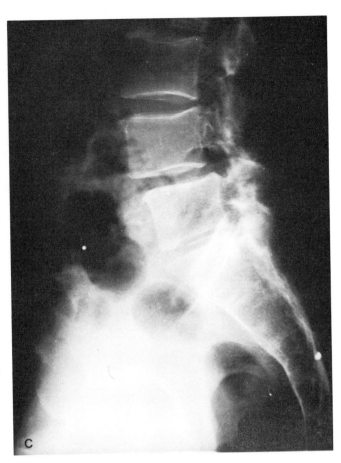

Fig. 6.9 (A) The a-p view of low lumbar spine and pelvis shows the anomalous facet-plane at L4–L5 on the left, and radiographic evidence of arthrotic changes there. (See Fig. 1.25)

(C) The lateral *standing erect* film reveals the effects of gravitational stress at the L4–L5 segment, i.e. a 1st degree group III (degenerative) spondylolisthesis. Clinical features suggested that his left haunch and thigh pain were emanating more from an early arthrosis of the left hip joint, than from the changes at L4–L5, although there may have been a degree of root irritation of the articular nerves to the hip. There were no neurological signs.

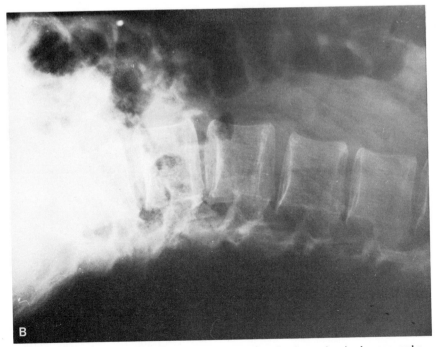

(B) The lateral *lying* view of lumbar spine reveals the low lumbar arthrotic changes, and a degree of backward slip of L2 on L3. There is no change in relationship between the vertebral bodies L4 and L5.

ing of the posterior elements, with or without injuries to the vertebral bodies.

Occasional non-union of vertebral bodies, after fracture at the thoracolumbar junction, have been reported, the unstable segment showing persisting mobility of about 20° on dynamic radiography.[1063]

Leaving aside the more obvious causes of unstable segments in the lower half of the spine, i.e. some of those mentioned above, the spondylolysis with or without spondylolisthesis (see p. 145), Newman's[926] observations are of special importance. He defines instability as a loss of integrity of soft-tissue intersegmental control, causing potential weakness and liability to yield under stress. The most common level is the L4–5 segment. His general comments[924] summarise the present situation:

There are clinical syndromes associated with compression injuries and with encroachment of tissue into the spinal or intervertebral canals which are comparatively common and well recognised. There are other syndromes which are probably more common, but far less well understood, which are associated with tension strain and breakdown of the extension mechanism both of the long lever and of the individual segments. The pain is often very persistent and the clinical signs, apart from tenderness, non-existent. There is a tendency to label the syndrome with a functional element. This is often a harmful step, psychologically.

During manipulative treatment, with or without anaesthesia, the most common error is failure to recognise the hypermobile lumbar vertebral segment.[279]

Herbert *et al.* (1975)[534] have observed that considerable amounts of new collagen are synthesised in discs next above those most involved in degenerative change, and it may be that this is some form of compensation for a degree of loss of function in the lower disc.

Spondylotic degenerative change in the intervertebral body joints, with some of its consequences, has been described in general terms (p. 88), and it remains to describe some salient characteristics of this process in the lumbar disc.

A common injury occurring as a consequence of a sudden cough while bending, or a flexion-rotation strain, or extending the spine from a flexed and rotated position, appears to be that of an immediate strain, possibly a tear of the annular fibres or of the annular attachment to the hyaline cartilaginous plate of the vertebral body (see p. 256).*

Depending upon the extent and depth of the traumatic tear, and the presence and degree of radiating internal fissures already present as part of the degenerative process, the injury may remain as a peripheral and partial breach of annulus attachments or may be accompanied by rupture of the posterior longitudinal ligament and associated annulus, with a massive extrusion posteriorly of nucleus pulposus.

Alternatively, the clinical course of events may accord

* Information on this aspect of disc pathology is immense, and only an outline is given.

with the concept of nuclear pulp slowly tracking through the breached annulus, or annular attachment, usually posterolaterally or posteriorly, over some hours following the injury.

Ruptures may occur following mechanical stress as described, but spontaneous ruptures also occur, when there is no history of any precipitating event. There may not even be any gross breach of the annulus; the semifluid material appearing at times to escape by dissecting its way through the annulus fibres.[896]

Radiographically demonstrated disc-bulging can commonly be present without manifesting its presence to the patient in the forms of signs and symptoms. In a series of 300 healthy asymptomatic persons,[552] approximately one-third were found to show myelographic evidence of trespass into the neural canal, in some cases grossly so. Conversely, nerve root involvement, with neurological signs in the root distribution, may occur in the absence of observable mechanical interference (see p. 89). Frequently the disc prolapse itself is but part of a family of changes at the segment (*vide infra*).[750, 775, 508]

The trespass may remain as a central, backward protrusion, bulging and stretching the still intact posterior longitudinal ligament into the extradural space, and compressing structures to a greater or lesser degree, but it frequently extrudes (either initially or, more commonly, afterwards) in a posterolateral direction.

Presumably the factor of internal radiating ruptures and concentric tears already present has a bearing on the direction of nucleus pulposus movement from patient to patient. The extrusion often takes the form of a small nipple-like tumour pressing against the dura mater (to which it tends to adhere later when organisation and reactive fibrosis occur), and tending to lie not only to one side of the mid-line, but often a little above or below the central horizontal plane of the disc.

The incidence is very much greater at the lower two lumbar segments; of 2948 cases of disc prolapse involving cord or nerve root compression at lower cervical, lower thoracic and lumbar segments, the incidence[585] in the latter was L1–2 segment (6), L2–3 segment (14), L3–4 segment (135), L4–5 segment (1667), L5–S1 segment (1098); thus indicating the frequency of low lumbar disc pathology giving rise to symptoms and severe enough to compress structures in the neural canal. Prolapse of nuclear pulp can presumably only occur in more or less undesiccated discs, but there can occur shifts of generally desiccated and amorphous disc substance in more mature people.

TYPES OF DISC TRESPASS

Disturbances in the anatomical configuration of the annulus are manifold;[174, 552, 780, 817, 1371] there is little general agreement on the classification, hence reports of treatment whether conservative or surgical lose much of their significance.[780]

Vertical protrusions are described on pages 88, 93.

Massive posterior prolapse may severely injure the cauda equina (both the intrathecal and extrathecal roots), producing signs which indicate a serious degree of interference with conduction in a number of roots and with the articular mechanics of the vertebral segment (see p. 150).

Less severe posterior protrusions disturb the mechanics of the joint, producing signs of articular derangement, but may not manifest signs of nerve root compression. A factor of critical importance is the size of the neural canal; a disc trespass of given extent will produce the more serious clinical features in the patient with a less roomy canal.

Posterolateral protrusions are commonest, the combination of degenerative change and disc prolapse being associated with much unilateral sciatic pain; the lumbosacral roots, passing downwards to reach their foraminal exits, are closely related to the posterior and posterolateral aspects of the lumbar discs, and a very frequent consequence of posterior and posterolateral nuclear extrusion is compression of nerve roots and their meningeal sleeves.

Root compression, squashing and distortion is not necessarily the sole cause of sciatic pain[174, 282, 392, 416, 750, 777, 811, 908] (see p. 110) accompanying these events, although it may certainly exacerbate their effects; there appear to be irritative biochemical reactions accompanying extrusion of the pulp and producing the nerve root inflammation frequently observed. Compression would further irritate the sensitised root. Depending upon the degree of nerve root damage by mechanical and biochemical factors, signs of loss of conduction will appear distally in the territory of the involved neurones. Sometimes the proximal changes involve two adjacent roots, so great is their obliquity in the low lumbar region, e.g. the 4th lumbar disc can compress the 4th lumbar and/or the 5th lumbar root, depending upon the size of the protrusion and its relationship to each of the two roots, since both lie closely to the disc on their passage to the foraminal exits. Prolapse at the 5th segment can likewise impinge upon the 5th lumbar root, the 1st sacral, or both. Shifting disc material may possibly occlude a radicular artery, producing ischaemic changes in more than one root; this may preclude a beneficial muscle-power recovery process which requires the presence of adjacent healthy roots.

In 40 cases with *single root involvement*, the muscle weakness recovered spontaneously in about 24 weeks, by peripheral axonal sprouting from adjacent healthy roots.[1368, 1369]

In a minority of cases with *multiradicular involvement*, spontaneous recovery of muscle power did not occur, and

in four of these patients the weakness remained two years later.

Macnab (1977)[780] observes that it is unusual at operation to find disc herniation consisting solely of nuclear material exuding through a defect in the annulus. The displaced material almost invariably consists of varying amounts of nucleus, annulus and cartilage plates.

Sylvest, Hentzer and Kobayasi (1977)[1203] obtained the prolapsed tissue and interspace contents during hemilaminectomy from 6 patients of ages 31 to 70 years, and studied the ultrastructure of the tissues removed from the L4 and L5 interspaces.

According to surgical findings, 5 patients had a protruded disc, and 1 disc was ruptured. Division of material into *annulus fibrosus* and *nucleus pulposus* proved inaccurate; chondrocytes were always the predominant cell type, and could be divided into three categories, (1) healthy cells, (2) a chondrocyte arrangement showing cloning cells and evidence of increased secretion, and (3) a type characterising a stage of cell death. Necrotic chondrocytes are also found in cartilage from arthrotic peripheral joints. Surrounding the necrotic cell remnants were matrix vesicles, and these seemed to be the products of disintegrated chondrocytes. The intercellular substance showed degraded collagen fibrils, and a dense amorphous material was also found, which seemed to be a glycoprotein and which was interspersed with collagen fibrils.

A few elastic fibres were also found, mainly at what appeared to be the borderline between annulus and nucleus; there was no evidence of severe degeneration of those fibres.

Macnab (1977)[780] suggests the classification:

Type I
Peripheral annular bulge — The annulus protrudes circumferentially beyond the peripheral rims of the vertebral bodies, and does not commonly give rise to serious root compression

Type II
Localised annular bulge — A discrete eminence; when producing clinical signs to warrant operation, the myelographic defect is unilateral. The annular fibres themselves remain intact, and on incision the nucleus does not extrude

Disc herniation and prolapse

Disruption of annular fibres allows prolapse, with a portion of annulus displaced posteriorly. The nucleus follows the displaced segment of annulus and some nuclear material may be forced through the break in the annular attachments.

Type I
Prolapsed intervertebral disc — Displaced nuclear material is confined solely by a few strands of annulus, and on incision of these the nucleus spontaneously extrudes

Type II
Extruded intervertebral disc — The nuclear material displaced has already burst through the restraining annulus and lies under cover of the posterior longitudinal ligament

Type III
Sequestrated intervertebral disc — Extruded nuclear material lies free in the spinal canal. It may remain trapped between nerve root and disc, or may migrate to lie behind the vertebral body in the nerve root 'axilla', in the intervertebral foramen or in the mid-line just anterior to the dural sac

Massive central sequestration involving several roots of the cauda equina, with sphincter paralysis, is more commonly seen at L4–5 level.[780] Unexpected root involvement may occur with pre- and postfixation of the sciatic plexus, and bizarre clinical pictures may result when anomalies of root emergence are present.

Posterolateral protrusions extending into the intervertebral foramina are the type which usually produce the characteristic clinical picture of discogenic sciatica.

Combined changes[315, 508, 618, 755, 963a]
Some patients present with a combination of severe arthrosis in facet-joints, an unstable lumbosacral segment with loss of disc space, backward and downward collapse of the body of L4 so that it encroaches from above upon the L4–5 intervertebral foramen, advanced overriding of facets, a thickened and buckled ligamentum flavum and an L5 nerve root which has been severely squashed and distorted.

This acquired stenosis of the neural canal tends to produce characteristic symptoms which simulate peripheral vascular disease, i.e. intermittent claudication, and more

easily so if there is already a degree of congenital stenosis (see p. 28).

The multiple variety of degenerative changes in the lumbar region is well illustrated in an analysis of 227 patients whose pains and disabilities were sufficient to warrant surgery: only 70 had a simple prolapse of nucleus pulposus; 65 had lumbar spondylosis; 5 had spinal stenosis. The remainder had combinations of two or more of these conditions, observed at myelography and confirmed at operation.

Spondylolisthesis[927]
Spondylolisthesis was first described in 1782 by the obstetrician Herbinaux,[921] who mentioned it as a cause of obstruction in labour, although (*vide infra*) surprisingly it seldom interferes with normal labour. The term by itself denotes a mechanical consequence, and not a precise diagnosis of cause as well as effect; the forward slip (olisthesis) of a vertebral body on its subjacent fellow being secondary to congenital defect, stress, degenerative change, trauma or disease. The condition is a not uncommon radiological finding, is frequently unknown to the patient and is often symptomless. It is not possible to give an accurate estimate of the percentage of all cases that do experience pain.

On the basis of the changes observed in 319 cases, Newman (1963)[923] categorised spondylolisthesis into five groups; this essentially remains, with some changes, the method[1329] of grouping the condition:

I. Dysplasic (congenital)
II. Isthmic
   a. Lytic—fatigue fracture of the pars interarticularis
   b. Elongated pars interarticularis, without bony discontinuity
   c. Acute fracture of the pars interarticularis
III. Degenerative
IV. Traumatic—acute fracture in other areas of the bony hook
V. Pathological
   a. General ⎫
   b. Local ⎬ General or local bone disease

(The category IIc is not accepted by all authorities.)

Male and female patients in the five groups of 319 patients were disposed as follows:

Group	Males	Females	Totals
I	20	46	66
II	93	71	164
III	22	58	80
IV	3	0	3
V	4	2	6
	142	177	319

In this group of patients the descending order of frequency was therefore: isthmic (group II) 164; degenerative (group III) 80; dysplasic (group I) 66; pathological (group V) 6; traumatic (group IV) 3.

The severity of slip, or olisthesis, is usually expressed in quarters of the AP dimension of the vertebral body,[849] i.e. a slip equal to half the sagittal diameter is a second-degree listhesis, and a forward displacement equalling three-quarters of it is a third-degree slip. Extreme examples of vertebral body slip are termed spondyloptosis.[915]

Because of the normal lumbar lordosis, gravitational force tends continually to shear one vertebral body forward upon the body below, and the integrity of the bony hook mechanism,[927] i.e. the pedicle, the interarticular portion of the neural arch and the inferior facet, may be disturbed as briefly described above.

I. *Dysplasic or congenital spondylolisthesis* occurs at the L5–S1 segment, and may cause secondary degenerative change.

Minor forms of spinal dysraphism,[605] as spina bifida occulta, have an incidence of about 10 per cent, and the defects of fusion of the neural arch of the upper sacral vertebra may be accompanied by a poorly developed upper sacral facet or neural arch of L5, which do not provide sufficient resistance to withstand the forward thrust at the lumbosacral segment.[927] The condition frequently becomes apparent during the adolescent growth spurt (girls 12–14 and boys 14–16) when the developing spine is subject to the combination of increasing body-weight and increasing stress. The pars interarticularis may remain unchanged, but usually either elongates or comes apart.[1329]

Adolescents with a severe degree of slip will show increased lordosis, a prominent sacrum and bilateral loin creases. Neurological symptoms may occur due to stretching of the cauda equina or nerve roots.

Normal birth occurred in 28 cases of adult patients with the dysplastic type, there being no maternal or foetal death. Slightly delayed birth occurred in two cases and greater delay in another.[927]

This category rests on the first sacral and/or fifth lumbar vertebra having congenital changes of such a nature as to make the joint incapable of withstanding the forward thrust of the body-weight above. The L5 vertebra may also show wide spina bifida. The condition appears to be about twice as common in girls as in boys.

II *Isthmic (spondylolytic) spondylolisthesis* is the commonest type, and the basic lesion, the intrinsic defect, is in the pars interarticularis; possible secondary changes in the shape of L5 vertebral body are not fundamental to its aetiology. The fifth lumbar segment is most commonly affected[927] and the fourth and third less so. Upper lumbar segments may occasionally show the defect of spondylolysis, but seldom the forward slip.

Subtype (a). The spondylolysis is a mechanical failure in a seemingly normal isthmus (Fig. 1.29C) and that the failure is a discontinuity, rather than a congenital defect, is no longer questioned.[1250] Sometimes the fracture heals. There is a strong hereditary component in the aetiology of this subtype.[1329] Friberg (1939)[381] reported on three generations of the descendants of 1 man with spondylolisthesis, and in 66 individuals found 15 cases. The incidence varies between races, from an average of 5 per cent in the skeletons in North American anatomy departments[509] to nearly 40 per cent in Alaskan Eskimos.[1175] While a familial and racial susceptibility is well established, there is no evidence of structural differences to account for these predispositions. The isthmus, of two layers of cortical bone joined by thick, parallel trabeculae, is undoubtedly very strong.

The factor of heavy and repeated occupational stress during particular postures may be considerably important in causing spondylolysis; the fast bowler, the trampoline jumper and the ballet dancer, for example, are at risk. Fatigue fractures of the neural arch were common in World War II, especially in recruits undergoing strenuous training; the neural arches were overloaded by the carrying of heavy packs, which shifted the line of weight-bearing posteriorly.[922, 747, 1108]

The child's spine is particularly susceptible to fracture between the ages of $5\frac{1}{2}$ to $6\frac{1}{2}$ years.

After the age of 20, it is rare for the olisthesis at the lumbosacral level to increase, probably because of the stout transverse processes and sturdy iliolumbar and lumbosacral ligaments. In adults, lytic lesions at L4 and L3 are likely to show further slip, more especially if L5 is sacralised, when movement stresses are added to the segments above; also, the L4–5 region is normally the most mobile, especially in the sagittal plane.

The smaller anteroposterior dimensions of the neural canal at L2, L3 and L4 are a factor in the increased incidence of spinal stenosis, and consequent cauda equina compression.[597]

Not all cases of spondylolysis lead to spondylolisthesis;[970] the shear strength of the intervertebral disc provides a major resistance to olisthesis in these cases of neural arch fracture, although this effect may vary with posture. In the usual bilaminar defect, a single unit of spinous process, laminae and inferior articular processes remains quite loose in the vertebral column; at operation it can be grasped with forceps and rattled about freely, hence is called by some surgeons 'the rattler'.[213]

Farfan *et al.* (1976)[329] suggest that there are three mechanisms which may result in failure of the neural arch with or without displacement of the body of the pathological vertebra, i.e. flexion overload, unbalanced shear force, forced rotation.

Subtype (b). An isthmic type where there is initially no bony discontinuity, but the pars interarticularis gradually elongates as the vertebral body slips forward. The distinguishing feature is that the slip occurs, and may be advanced, before a break in either one or both interarticular parts appears. The degree of elongation may be marked.[224]

It is secondary to repeated microfractures which heal in a somewhat elongated position as the L5 vertebral body moves anteriorly.

Subtype (c). The category rests on the presence of a *pars interarticularis* fracture secondary to severe trauma,[1329] although the inclusion of this type is not universally accepted, since it completely resembles the common stress fracture.

III *Degenerative spondylolisthesis*, more common in females, occurs very frequently at the L4–L5 level, and is the type most often associated with nerve root involvement (Figs 6.8, 6.9C). In a study of 200 patients with group III spondylolisthesis,[1058] and 20 skeletons, the condition was four times more frequent in females and four times more frequent when L5 was sacralised. In this series, the slipping never exceeded the equivalent of a third of the vertebral body, i.e. a second-degree slip.

While the annular wall of the lumbar disc retains a surprising degree of elastic resilience and stiffness after fenestration and enucleation procedures,[807] it is important to remember that degenerative change can, without herniation or protrusion, proceed to a stage where the nucleus becomes a fibrillated system of collagen, mucopolysaccharides and denatured non-collagenous proteins suspended in a low-viscosity fluid,[499] with a consequent decrease in normal stiffness.

An unstable and 'sloppy' intervertebral body joint (see 'Instability', p. 139) can produce severe changes in the posterior elements. Ligaments become unduly stressed by irregular movement and their ability to sustain tension is reduced; under the combined reduction of disc stiffness and ligamentous strength, additional strain may cause grinding away and disorganisation of the facet-joint structures, of such degree as to allow the whole intact vertebra to shift forward, without any neural arch defect occurring.

Farfan (1975)[327, 329] postulates that there are multiple small compression fractures of the inferior articular process of the olisthetic vertebra. There is remodelling of the articular processes at the level of involvement, and as the slip progresses the articular processes become more horizontal. When the lesion is at L4, the L5 vertebra is more stable than average. The defect can occur in men at the level of an anomalous facet-joint (Fig. 6.9); its genesis may also lie in rotational stress[329] or a combination of factors.

Together with changes in the intervertebral disc, the posterior joint changes may markedly narrow the intervertebral foramen in its transverse dimensions.

This form of instability also profoundly affects the neural canal structures, even though the amount of shift is radiographically minor.[970] Dural constriction is aggravated by the shape of the neural canal, especially a restricted lateral recess, and further aggravated by loss of disc height and the arthrotic trespass of degenerative changes in facet-joints. The degree of transient compression which can occur during certain postures and movements is best demonstrated by lateral films taken during flexion and extension in the erect position.[970]

Flexion while standing allows the upper vertebra to slip forward on the subjacent vertebral body; in extension the degree of slip is reduced but the intervertebral foramen shows a marked reduction in size.

The same mechanical influences probably do not occur during flexion in lying, i.e. when hips and knees are flexed onto chest, since the direction and magnitude of gravitational stress upon the spine is then considerably changed, and flexion is occurring from below upwards, as it were.

IV *Traumatic spondylolisthesis* is rare. Severe trauma causes a fracture of some part of the bony hook other than the pars, which permits gradual displacement to occur; fractures have been reported in the pedicles of lumbar vertebrae which permit the forward slip to occur.

The distinguishing feature of this category is the *locality* of the traumatic discontinuity of bone.

V *Pathological spondylolisthesis* is secondary to the weakening or disruption of bone structure by disease. This may be a general condition such as osteogenesis imperfecta or local infective or neoplastic disease.

Spondylolysis acquisita is regarded by some writers as a form of pathological spondylolysis.[780] It occurs following posterior spinal fusions and is seen in the pars interarticularis of the lamina at the cranial end of the fusion. Thus pain, now from a different source, may recur following the successful fusion of a vertebral defect.

In summary, spondylolisthesis is due to lumbar instability.[921] The characteristic lesion of the pars interarticularis is by no means always present. When occurring it is secondary to instability, and is caused by attenuation or fatigue or a combination of both. It is not the *cause* of the spondylolisthesis although its presence may permit an additional degree of slip.

Spinal stenosis

This term tends to be used for description of both (1) developmental narrowing of the neural canal, and (2) acquired narrowing, due either to degenerative trespass, or as the sequelae of dysplasic (group I) spondylolisthesis, for example. It is also used to denote the clinical syndrome caused by the narrowing.[956]

Cervical and thoracic stenosis have been referred to (pp. 13 and 16) and it remains to consider some pathological changes occurring in the lumbar spine (Figs. 1.32, 1.33).

The lumbar spinal canal is an obscure region of the body, yet the pathological events that occur within it have an important bearing on low back pain and nerve root compression syndromes.[52]

A plan view of the lower lumbar vertebral canal presents a triangle, with anterior base and posterior apex. The two sides are formed by the pedicles and laminae, with the ligamentum flavum closing the interlaminar space. The bony *lateral recess* is formed on each side by the junction of side and base of the triangle.

In the developmentally narrow and therefore stenotic canal, the AP dimensions of the triangular space are reduced, from above 20 mm in the normal to less than 15 mm for example.[956] The laminae and pedicles are thicker and shorter, and the facets are larger, encroaching upon the posterolateral portions of the triangular space and contributing to reduction of room in the lateral recess. The altered configuration is such that the canal begins to resemble a trefoil shape, or even a shallow inverted T. At myelography, an AP diameter of less than 14 mm is suggestive of stenosis.[956]

A formula for recognising the congenitally narrow canal on plain radiographs, by relating the dimensions of the canal to those of the adjacent vertebral body, has been described.[618] The product of interpedicular distance and anteroposterior diameter of the canal (body to spinous process base) is related to the product of AP and transverse diameters of the vertebral body. The relation is expressed as a ratio, the normal range being 1 : 2 to 1 : 4.5. In a series of 20 cases,[1292] developmentally narrow canals had ratios ranging from 1 : 4 to 1 : 8.

In a number of pathological states the existing structural variations may play an important part in the incongruity between contents and capacity of the canal.

Degenerative disease occurs in a wide variety of forms in the lumbar spine, and if *acquired* stenosis is defined as a degree of trespass into the neural canal by virtue of abnormal changes, it must be very common indeed; in one study[552] of abnormal myelographic appearances of 300 *asymptomatic* subjects, a greater or lesser degree of discogenic trespass was demonstrated in 37 per cent. It is common knowledge that provided the canal is roomy enough, the clinical features of an episode of single disc protrusion, and subsequent recovery after surgical enucleation, indicate that the clinical course is related to that single abnormality and no other, i.e. the episode is not complicated by existing congenital anomalies.

Conversely, even a small disc herniation may cause severe trauma to the cauda equina if the available space in the neural canal is already restricted by developmental stenosis.

Because degenerative changes in the lumbar spine are ubiquitous, *the decisive factor in production of symptoms and signs is the available space*, and very frequently this factor is of more importance than the precise nature of the degenerative trespass.

Developmental stenosis may be due to:

1. Congenital narrowing of the neural canal[52] (associated with the changes described on p. 28).
2. Achondroplasia,[956, 1292] which may affect the whole spinal canal
3. Spina bifida.[605]

Acquired stenosis may be the result of:

1. Degenerative change
   a. posterior and posterolateral disc herniation and prolapse
   b. massive central disc protrusion
   c. ligamentum flavum thickening[1292, 52, 315]
   d. posterior vertebral lipping[315]
   e. thickening of the neural arches[315]
   f. facet-joint arthrosis[317, 618]
   g. degenerative (group III) spondylolisthesis[926, 1329, 1058]
   h. isolated disc resorption[211, 214]
2. Dysplasic (group I) and isthmic (group II) spondylolisthesis[1326]
3. Space-occupying new growths[315]
4. Paget's disease[177, 515]
5. Iatrogenic disease following surgery[1088, 1292]
6. Venous congestion.[1292]

1. Degenerative change. Some authorities refer to restrictive changes causing unilateral sciatica, and localised to the lateral recess, as lateral stenosis; and that associated with neurogenic claudication and myelographic block as central stenosis. In the former, the nerve root may be virtually buried as it lies in a groove of a laterally bulging disc.[780]

Discogenic trespass into the neural canal is described on page 144. The space-occupying effect of massive disc extrusions, with rupture of the posterior longitudinal ligament, is such as to produce complete spinal canal obstruction, with the entire degenerated disc and a rim of fibrocartilage being extruded into the epidural space. The characteristic myelographic appearance is that of a complete block.[315]

Posterior spondylotic ridging or lipping and thickening of the laminae and ligamentum flavum freqently produce compressive effects, the myelographic appearance of indentations into the dural sac being enhanced by thickening of the neural arches.

The ligamentum flavum sometimes undergoes necrosis and becomes oedematous in association with disc degeneration. The process is thus degenerative rather than hypertrophic (as it is sometimes described), with fragmented elastic fibres in a brown, semifluid matrix. The swollen ligamenta flava trespass upon the spinal cord posteriorly, and on occasions these are the only changes found on surgery for sciatic pain. Posterior and lateral indents can be observed on myelography, and on spinal extension may be observed at every segment, the swelling being a contributory factor in both spinal stenosis due to a narrow canal and sciatic syndromes in those with a developmentally normal canal.[1300]

In a group of 12 patients with lumbar nerve root compression by facet-arthrosis, Epstein (1973),[317] congenital vertebral anomalies and stenosis of the spinal canal were contributory factors. This trespass by thickened facet-joint structures is more pronounced in the lateral recess. Narrowing of the spinal canal produced by buckling of the ligamentum flavum, overlapping of the laminae, and disc collapse with a diffuse annular bulge, may be more pronounced when there is also subluxation of the posterior facet-joints, and enlargement of the opposed joint surfaces by osteophytosis. The nerve root,[780] as it loops around the pedicle and emerges at the intervertebral foramen, may be trapped in a constricting subarticular 'gutter' formed by excess bone.

The neural canal restriction in degenerative spondylolisthesis (group III)[1058] may be due to several factors, and occurs four times more frequently in women and five to six times more frequently at the fourth lumbar level than at the third (see p. 147) (Figs 6.8, 6.9C).

Neurological symptoms may develop; these are caused by compression of the 5th lumbar roots and rarely by constriction of the theca.[927]

The maximum slipping in Rosenberg's[1058] series was 30 per cent, the forward movement of L4 vertebra being halted when the isthmus abutted on the upper margin of the superior articular process of the 5th lumbar verbebra (see also p. 145). Isolated disc resorption,[214] which is characterised by gross narrowing of a single disc space and commonly occurs in an otherwise normal lumbar spine, may present with the disc space reduced to 3 mm, and marked sclerosis of the adjacent vertebral body margins.

Although marginal osteophyte formation is minimal, a thin layer of annulus remnant may cover the ridge of bone projecting into the neural canal. When established resorption of the lumbosacral disc is present, the S1 root is predominantly affected by the nerve root canal stenosis, and becomes impinged between the inner margin of the superior facet and the buckled flaval ligament behind, and in front by the bony ridge covered by remaining annular fibres.

2. *Dysplasic (group I) and isthmic (group II) spondylolisthesis.* In group I, luxation at the lumbosacral joint occurs as the 5th lumbar vertebra grinds its way over the top of the sacrum with a glacier-like action;

... the inferior facets become worn and grooved, and the neural arch attenuated and sometimes broken. At the outset, the spinous process slips forward with the rest of the vertebra, but later it stabilises itself on the fibrous roof of the sacrum and the vertebral body, continuing to slip, leaves it behind.[921]

Removal of the neural arch may reveal that the 1st sacral roots, or the whole cauda equina, are compressed.

If the pars interarticularis remains completely unchanged the degree of slip cannot exceed more than 25 per cent.[1329]

The basic lesion in group II spondylolisthesis is in the pars interarticularis (Fig. 1.29C); there may be separation of the pars or elongation without separation. Usually, the degree of displacement is not severe, but is inclined to be greater if spondylolysis is present in childhood.[927]

3. *Neoplasms* (see p. 121).

4. *Paget's disease* (osteitis deformans) is characterised by destruction of bone followed by reparative changes. The destructive phase may predominate but most frequently there is a combination of destruction and repair, with expansion of bone. When involving the vertebral body, it extends backwards to involve the neural arches.

The disease affects the vertebral column, especially in the lumbosacral region, more commonly than any other part of the skeleton.

Collins (1959)[195] found the disease in 76 per cent of 46 cases in which full necropsies were made.

Lesions are not confined to the lower spine and may occur in any vertebra from the atlas downwards, although the lumbar vertebrae and sacrum seem to be involved in at least three out of every four cases. Enlargement and deformity of the vertebral laminae may occasionally lead to objective neurological signs from compression of the spinal cord.

This ancient disease has been identified in Egyptian tomb skeletons and in those of Saxon times.[39]

5. *Iatrogenic stenosis.* Neural canal constriction following spinal fusion is not rare, and iatrogenic stenosis may follow both a successful and also an unsuccessful fusion.[1292] A dowel graft may intrude into the canal, or the trespass may be due to bone hypertrophy associated with a pseudarthrosis (more correctly an adventitious joint) resulting from unsuccessful posterior fusion. After a successful fusion on a patient with a marginally narrow canal, degenerative changes of the mobile segment above may be sufficient to initiate the clinical features of stenosis. Iatrogenic stenosis may also occur due to scarring after laminectomy with fusion procedures.[1088] Removal of the ligamentum flavum on both sides will result in a scar which may constrict the contents of the neural canal.[326]

6. *Venous congestion.* Weber and De Klerk (1973)[1292] describe the presence at operation of congested, widened and often tortuous epidural veins, such as to simulate intradural vascular anomaly.

Changes in posture, straining and coughing will also

alter the room available for the cauda equina because of engorgement of the epidural venous plexuses.[315]

Kirkaldy-Willis *et al.* (1978)[661a] have presented a spectrum of the progressive pathological changes of lumbar spondylosis and stenosis, based on the dissection of 50 lumbar spines obtained at autopsy and supplemented by observations made during the course of laminectomies in 161 patients.

It was evident to the authors that the progressive degenerative changes described sometimes lead to narrowing of the central spinal canal and lateral nerve canals, hence spinal stenosis is not a separate entity but is part and parcel of the degenerative process.

'Starting with repeated minor trauma, the degenerative process continues over many years until gross spondylosis is observed . . . the whole spectrum of degenerative change is shown below.'

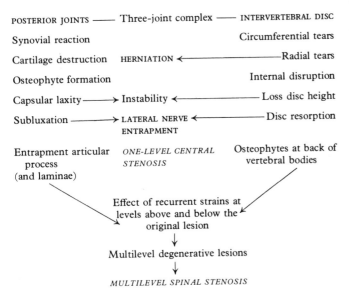

The exposition is accompanied by 25 illustrations of wonderful clarity; the authors remind us that entrapment of nerve in the lateral recess was described by Williams (1932),[1320] a year or so before the now classic paper by Mixter and Barr (1934)[863] on herniation of the disc.

SPHINCTER DISTURBANCE

Sphincter control is not usually disturbed in *cervical* myelopathy.[117] Spondylotic change in the *thoracic* spine is frequent, but not usually associated with alterations in the sagittal diameter of the neural canal, or with spondylotic spurs which intrude sufficiently to compress the spinal cord.[315]

A case of thoracic stenosis has been described,[430] but the clinical description makes no reference to sphincter disturbance. Shaw (1975)[1116] mentions that bladder func-

tion is sometimes impaired in prolapse of the thoracic intervertebral disc and in a series of 22 patients Benson and Byrnes (1975)[82] found that two-thirds of the patients had no urinary or bowel symptoms, only three of the group presenting with retention of urine. One patient had faecal incontinence. Most of the minority with urinary symptoms reported either hesitancy, urgency or a sense of incomplete evacuation.

A review[45] of 95 cases from the literature mentions that two-thirds of the cases showed abnormality of sphincters.

Lumbar spondylotic lesions of trespass into the neural canal are more likely to cause disturbance of voiding when they are multiple, and also when the prolapse is a massive central protrusion which completely blocks the canal,[1062] although sphincter disturbance does not necessarily follow (*vide infra*). High lesions are more likely to produce severe bladder dysfunction. Involvement of a single nerve root is unlikely to cause bladder problems.

Reports of patients with bladder symptoms, and little or no back pain or sciatica, have appeared in the literature during recent years, [766, 610, 1268] and Sharr *et al.* (1976)[1113] observe that because definite abnormal neurological signs are often absent, the diagnosis may remain obscure for many years. Among 73 patients with chronic urinary symptoms, the authors found incontinence to be one of the commonest problems, the clinical diagnosis of *neuropathic* incontinence depending particularly on the patient's unawareness of bladder filling, emptying and urethral flow. Six of their patients, with minor myelographic irregularities commonly accepted as normal, were treated surgically because they fulfilled other diagnostic criteria, and were found at operation to have significant lumbar spondylosis.

Emmett and Love (1971)[311] also mention that in some of their worst cases the myelographic appearances were either negative or equivocal. Jennett (1956)[610] describes a patient admitted with complete double sphincter paralysis and a useless, numb right leg. The history included backache and left-sided sciatica 20 years before, and during the 18 months before admission a further three or four bouts of right-sided sciatica, with a single attack of bilateral sciatica four months before admission. Paralysis of the right leg was total below the knee and there was distal wasting and weakness in the left leg. He had retention of urine with infection and a flaccid anal sphincter. After the patient's death from uraemia before operation, a small disc protrusion was found compressing the L3 root, but within the theca a dense and discrete band of arachnoid adhesions was observed exactly opposite the protrusion, firmly embedding the roots of the cauda equina, which could only be separated by sharp dissection.

Among the 25 cases of compression of the cauda equina by prolapsed intervetebral disc, Jennett mentions 4 cases whose onset of paralysis occurred while resting in bed. Also described is the subsequent history of a patient with right-sided sciatica, for which she was manipulated under anaesthesia. On recovery from the anaesthetic she was unable to empty the bladder and both legs were numb and weak. At subsequent operation a large disc protrusion at the lumbosacral level was removed. The author also describes 2 patients in his series who had very little pain, i.e. the type in which diagnosis may be very difficult.

Following myelography after some years of stress incontinence, a 52-year-old man was operated on for an obstruction opposite the second lumbar disc. Only a small, calcified portion of the L2 disc was seen, until examination of the intrathecal space revealed a dense band of fibrous arachnoid thickening, thick and opaque enough to conceal the cauda equina. In 11 of these cases there was profound paralysis, usually of anterior tibial, peroneal and calf muscles. Objective sensory loss of all modalities, typically in the whole sacral region, was present in 24 of the patients, but some had not noticed this until called to their attention by careful sensory testing.

Some degree of paralysis of the urethral and anal sphincters occurred in all but 2 of the patients and in 14 of them it was complete, with retention of urine and faecal incontinence.

Complete sphincter loss was always accompanied by complete bilateral sensory loss in the saddle area, often in the whole sacral distribution. In 17 cases there was a massive, loose fragment largely filling the vertebral canal, behaving like an extradural tumour. In the remaining 8 cases the protrusion was no larger than that in uncomplicated sciatica but focal thickening of the arachnoid was seen in each.

Jennett makes the important observation that while the persistence of a myelographic abnormality after surgery may be due to arachnoid adhesions, the possibility of there being two lesions must be borne in mind.

Love and Emmett (1967)[766] report three cases of urinary retention who had no evidence of radiculopathy on physical and neurological examination, although all were obese women and had been bed-wetters in their youth. The authors comment that this suggests their bladder innervation may have been abnormal or their cauda equinae unusually vulnerable, or both. At operation one had a cauda compressed by a 4th lumbar disc, and a congenitally short cul-de-sac. The second patient had protrusions of the 4th and 5th lumbar discs, and the third a 4th lumbar protrusion. Two of the patients had been previously referred for a psychiatric opinion.

Ross and Jamieson (1971)[1062] observe that large, central lumbar protrusions are likely to give rise to a lower motor neurone type of bladder paresis, whereas protrusions at higher spinal levels may compress the cord and produce upper motor neurone dysfunction.

Aho, et al. (1969)[12] reported their findings in 19 patients, of whom 18 were operated on. The cauda equina syndrome began acutely without earlier sciatica in only one patient.

The disc trespass occurred at L5–S1 in 11 cases, at L4–5 in 6 and at L3–4 in one. The protruded material excised was larger than 1.5 by 1 cm in 12 of the patients, and was centrally situated in 15 of them. The lesion was accompanied by rupture of the posterior longitudinal ligament in 11 cases. Severe disturbance of urethral function occurred in three patients with saddle anaesthesia on one side only.

As in sciatica unaccompanied by sphincter paralysis, it appears that *the size of the neural canal* remains the crucial factor. Small or lateral prolapses can produce cauda equina lesions when there is congenital stenosis, and the size alone of the prolapse does not dictate the degree of cauda equina compression. Even massive lumbar disc prolapse need not produce cauda equina pressure.[1050]

The authors mention that the incidence of degenerative changes on X-ray in their patients was no higher than the general incidence for patients with lumbar discs or a normal population.

While surgical opinion should be urgently sought in all cases of sphincter disturbance and saddle anaesthesia, a case is reported[1062] where acute lumbar pain, with right-sided loss of ankle-jerk and a weak knee-jerk, accompanied by perianal anaesthesia and painless urinary retention, recovered full bladder function during a week of bedrest with traction and catheterisation. Six months later micturition remained normal.

Sharr, et al. (1976)[1113] mention that 39 of their 73 patients have not been treated surgically because of age, lack of progressive worsening and lack of clear diagnosis, but there has been improvement in some by conservative measures such as bedrest and lumbar support.

Jennett (1956)[610] stressed the incompleteness of recovery after operation '... recovery from cauda equina lesions is slow, but it is doubtful if it is realised just how unsatisfactory it can be'. Sphincter paralysis is the most serious factor, and although ambulant, pain-free and not inconvenienced by sensory loss a patient may have residual defective sphincter control. It may be three or four years before the end state of sphincter control is reached.

Aho, et al. (1969)[12] reported that the majority of their 18 patients, i.e. 11, still showed abnormal bladder function on cystometry at follow-up examination, and their review of the literature indicates that only a small proportion of patients show signs of clearing of bladder symptoms.

THE PELVIS

It is gratifying to note the slowly increasing number of descriptions of pathological changes due to stress in the pelvic joints,[284, 993, 1081, 1036, 1157, 506, 505] particularly so since many erroneously believe that musculoskeletal abnormalities of these joints, unassociated with pregnancy and violent direct trauma, are virtually non-existent.

The pathological or radiological changes of, for example, tuberculosis, ankylosing spondylitis, rheumatoid arthritis or Paget's disease of the articulations are well documented, but since physical treatment directed specifically to the joint is most unlikely to be indicated in these clinical situations, there is little point in dwelling here on their pathology, other than in general terms and for completeness of information. It is more difficult to describe the pathology of common, painful and disabling musculoskeletal disorders of the pelvis, largely because of the comparative lack of reports providing surgical and necropsy evidence of joint changes acceptable as abnormalities probably underlying clinical features during the patient's lifetime.

For example, although there is more than one type of pathology underlying the condition of 'tennis elbow', it is universal clinical experience that a very common type of this malady has clear-cut signs, symptoms and functional restrictions, and responds very well to local injection of hydrocortisone or triamcinolone and/or mobilisation and manipulation; yet an X-ray of the joint reveals nothing and the customarily tested ranges of movement are often normal. Although the upper limb is fruitful territory for pain referred from more proximal joint changes, confidence is justified that the site of that particular abnormality of the elbow region has been identified, it has been correctly diagnosed and on a localised basis has been adequately treated.

Precisely the same criteria of examination by a process of exclusion, identification of the site of the lesion causing the patient's current complaint, and localised treatment governs the management of common sacroiliac joint problems.

The former does not excite comment; the latter seems to create unnecessary difficulties, and as the perennial subject of academic debate, the sacroiliac joint seems born to trouble as the sparks fly upwards. By virtue of a now reasonably large body of evidence,[451] a basis for description may be summarised as follows:

1. The joint is a movable, weight-bearing, part synovial/part fibrous one, and thus heir to the troubles which plague other synovial joints, viz:
   a. A hindrance to movement (usually reversible) at some point on its limited range of motion
   b. Fixation (not always reversible), sometimes at the extreme of possible range
   c. Irritability, sometimes severe
   d. A tendency to hypermobility when adjacent articulations become stiff or ankylosed
   e. Arthritis and arthrosis
   f. Involvement in disease of adjacent bone
   g. Instability due to ligamentous insufficiency.

2. While bearing in mind its special characteristics, there is no good reason for doing other than dealing with its abnormalities according to the principles underlying the treatment of all other joints.

Because the sacroiliac joint is not immobile; it very frequently bears multiples of the whole body-weight during functional activities; it is the first weight-bearing joint between vertebral column and lower limb; manifest asymmetry of the two joints is not uncommon, considerations of postural asymmetry on an AP view, and their possible genesis, are of fundamental importance.

Postural asymmetry of the pelvis

This may reasonably be assumed present when, in the absence or presence of frank lateral pelvic tilt, there is apparent torsion of one ilium in relation to the other, so that for example the left anterior superior iliac spine is higher than the right, and the left posterior superior iliac spine is lower than its fellow.

On the basis of these findings, Lewit (1970)[736] observed the condition in almost 40 per cent of 450 schoolchildren. In a further group of 72 children aged 6–7, the findings were as follows: pelvic torsions (28), slight scoliosis (13), difference in leg lengths (5). All of the latter group (72) were re-examined after a year. Not a single pelvic torsion had disappeared, and a 29th had developed. Of the slight scolioses, 2 had recovered and 3 new cases appeared; leg length differences had disappeared in three children.

The children were arranged as statistical twins; one of each twin was treated, leaving the other as a control. After 7 years, the results were: Of 15 cases given gentle manipulative treatment, 3 relapsed, 1 of whom recovered spontaneously. Of 14 untreated cases, 4 made a spontaneous recovery, 2 of these during the last year, and in both of these cases spasm of the iliacus muscle was still present. Two of this group were lost to the trial. Four new cases developed during the period, 1 during the first year which was treated, and 2 others which recovered spontaneously. The fourth appeared too late for inclusion.

Lewit makes the following interesting observations:

1. The iliac crests themselves remained at the same horizontal level.

2. There was little correlation between scoliosis and pelvic torsion in his material.

3. Effective treatment of the asymmetry did not affect the development of scoliosis.

4. Sacroiliac asymmetry (or torsional fixation) is an extremely constant lesion.

5. There is increasing evidence that the asymmetry, however effectively treated by gentle manipulative procedures, is due mainly to muscle spasm.

6. If this iliacus spasm can be abolished by procaine, preferably to the sacroiliac joint itself, the pelvis straightens just as permanently as after manipulation.

These observations pose some important questions:

1. What is the importance of psoas as well as iliacus spasm in the production of these torsional states?

2. What may initiate it; does it arise because of some irritative condition of the growing spine or in the growing sacroiliac joint?

3. How far into the future may this asymmetry be prolonged, unrecognised or ignored, by chronic unilateral muscle spasm?

4. Might reversible torsion, in the plane joints of the child's pelvis, be slowly 'frozen' after puberty, into later irreversibility by articular ridges and furrows as the physical stress of weight-bearing activity stimulates their development?

5. Bearing in mind the functional interdependence of the vertebral column, what are the long-term prospects for cervical, thoracic, lumbar, lumbosacral, sacroiliac and hip-joint involvement in these children?

6. In terms of degernative joint disease is the child, as in other respects, father to the man?

There is in medicine a natural law . . . that any single pathological event is bound to project itself into a number of different clinical manifestations (Steindler, 1962).[1171]

Cramer[209] has provided an analysis (Fig. 6.10) of distortion in the adult. *If the great variation of joint configuration between individuals is borne in mind, it is probable that there is no one type or degree of asymmetry.* Certainly, the abnormality illustrated seems to require a maniuplative correction of heroic complexity, should one believe correction feasible and choose to attack it so.

The aetiology of pelvic asymmetry in the adult is not easy to decide. Figure 6.11(A) 16 January 1967, (B) 13 June 1969, and (C) 9 June 1975, shows the radiological appearances of a woman 39 years old in 1975 who at the age of 5 was admitted to her local hospital for trouble with her right hip. While under more recent surgical care for the secondary osteoarthrosis which developed, the condition was retrospectively assessed as probably due to non-articular Still's disease or possibly a synovial tuberculous infection; Perthe's disease was considered unlikely. She had had several hospital admissions in the past, and at one time had the hip in plaster for 9 months. The notes at the time of her first admission 24 years before were unhelpful, and X-rays were not available. The original diagnosis and subsequent surgical care of her hip condition need not concern us further, but the radiologically evident pelvic asymmetry, there when she presented in 1967, and still persisting, is of interest. Wasting of the right buttock may well have disturbed her pelvic posture when lying on the X-ray table, but this factor could not be responsible for the appearance of pelvic asymmetry. When did this asymmetry begin? Why is it there? Is it a fairly long-standing iatrogenic consequence, or was it there in early childhood?

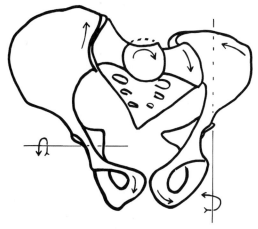

Fig. 6.10 A scheme of altered positional relationships in pelvic distortion or asymmetry. (After: Cramer A, quoted in Lewit K 1969 The course of impaired function in the spinal column and its possible prevention. Proceedings of the Faculty of Medical Hygiene. Charles University, Prague.)

A 46-year-old man (Fig. 6.12) presented on 30 April 1973 with pain in and around the left hip. There was a vague history of 'paralysis' as a child, but no definite details; also pulmonary tuberculosis 12 years ago, now clear and under routine observation. He attributed a three-month history of the ache around the left hip area to a fall on that side three years previously. Retrospective radiological opinion was 'old Perthe's and early osteoarthrosis of the hip'. Confining our attention to the pelvic asymmetry, i.e. obturator foramen shadow, levels of pubis, width of ilia, etc., is this entirely due to an off-centre view? Why is it there? How long has it been there? Was it produced by the fall?

Leg lengths (see p. 282)

Pregnancy

The hormonal influences resulting in softening and relaxation of the pelvic girdle and lumbar joints in pregnancy also occur to a lesser degree during menstruation and the menopause (Colachis, *et al.*, 1963).[190] A number of postmortem specimens in various stages of pregnancy showed clearly that the increased range of movement is easily recognisable by the fourth month, and that at full term the range increased by about two-and-a-half times. In one subject, the anterior margins of the joint could be separated by almost 2 cm (Brooke, 1924).[135]

The normal 4 mm width at the symphysis pubis increases more than twofold to 9 mm.

Obstetric and gynaecological surgery

Sacroiliac strains sometimes follow gynaecological and obstetric operations (Grieve, 1976).[451] The lithotomy position is not above suspicion in causing some of these strains (Bankart, 1932).[57] Among 63 cases of backache in an average gynaecological service, there were 22 classed

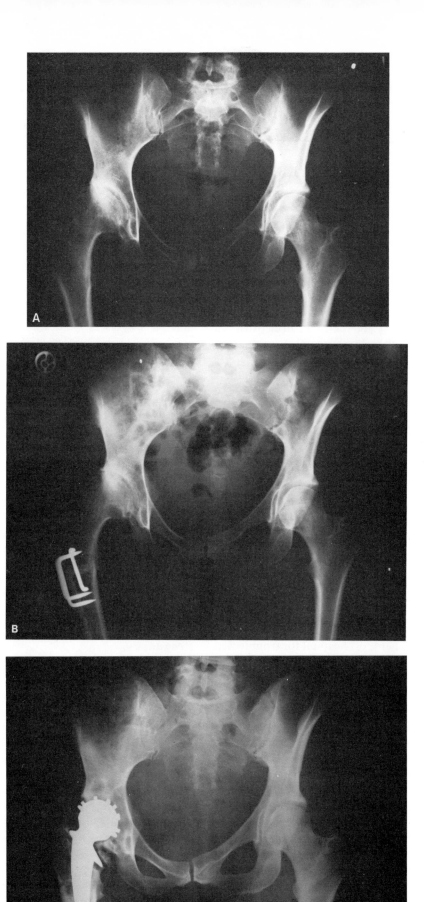

Fig. 6.11 (A, B and C) Anteroposterior pelvic views of a 39-year-old lady with right hip involvement from the age of 5. (A) 16.1.67, (B) 13.6.69, (C) 9.6.75. The asymmetry of symphysis pubis remains unaltered. (See text.)

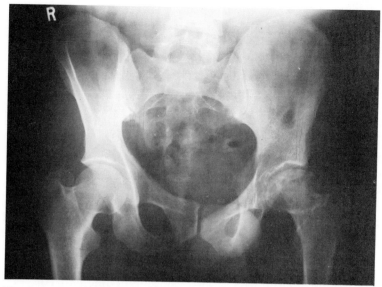

Fig. 6.12 Anteroposterior pelvic view of a 46-year-old man with an osteoarthrotic (L) hip. (see text.)

as 'traumatic'. All of these had received a general anaesthetic while in the lithotomy position and first suffered backache on discharge from hospital (Shafiroff and Sava, 1935).[1106]

In the course of two years, every woman who underwent major gynaecological surgery at the Prague Clinic and subsequently complained of postoperative sacral area and neck pain was examined for musculoskeletal abnormalities (Novotny and Dvorak, 1971).[940] The results were:

Table 6.2

Operations	Number	Sacroiliac disturbances	Cervical spine disturbances
Abdominal	449	52 (11.6%)	33 (7.3%)
Vaginal	539	51 (9.4%)	23 (4.2%)
Total	988	103 (10.4%)	56 (5.6%)

Ankylosis or surgical fusion, and adjacent hypermobility

Continuing evidence of the functional interdependence of the vertebral column is provided by the frequency with which ankylosis or fusion of joints results in compensatory increase of movement in adjacent articulations. Brooke (1924)[135] considers that the sacroiliac joint is incorporated in the movement of the spine as a whole and shares in the maintenance of general flexibility and free motion from occiput to coccyx. It is difficult adequately to stress the fundamental importance of this concept, now increasingly recognised as the proper basis for understanding the symptoms and signs of movement-abnormalities in any part of the vertebral column.

A direct relationship was observed between movements of sacroiliac and lumbar joints. Of 38 ankylosed sacroiliac joints examined postmortem or in the dissecting room, 81 per cent showed a very free range of movement much in excess of normal at the lumbosacral junction. The remaining 19 per cent showed ankylosis at both sacroiliac and lumbosacral joints, yet with compensatory increased mobility at the lumbar spine. One specimen, with a restricted tuberculous hip, had an unusual degree of compensatory laxity at the sacroiliac joint.

Trauma and stress

The pelvis is an architectural entity in which the bony and connective tissue elements are structurally and functionally interdependent.

Pauwels (1965)[975] calculated the relative magnitude and direction of the forces which affect sacroiliac and pubic joints in one- and two-legged support. Resultant forces cause a preponderance of tensile stress in the symphysis during weight-bearing on both legs. During rhythmic one-legged support in walking, strong shearing forces are acting vertically in opposite directions on the symphysis; the contribution of an intact symphysis pubis to pelvic stability has been well assayed.

The flying buttresses of Notre-Dame cathedral are no more wonderful than the flying buttresses formed by the superior and inferior rami of the pubis, a reminder that function governs structure. The importance of the pubic joint and the interpubic ligaments is evident if they are divided, when the strong sacroiliac ligaments offer little resistance to an unfolding of the pelvis.

Lichtblau's (1962)[745] interesting case report, of a 33-year-old woman whose persistent non-union of a fractured radius and ulna was treated by grafting with bone from the left iliac crest, emphasises the interdependence of pelvic joints. Two-and-a-half months after operation, the patient reported left low back pain, radiating to left sacroiliac area and right groin. X-rays then revealed marked left sacroiliac joint dislocation with stress fractures of both right pubic rami and subluxation of symphysis pubis. Review of earlier X-rays revealed sacroiliac subluxation with slight displacement at the symphysis, *before* the pubic fractures. The actual strength of the interpubic ligaments is also demonstrated, since persistent stress initially resulted in rami fractures rather than further attenuation and stretching of these ligaments.

Harris and Murray (1974)[506] made a radiological study of the pubic symphysis in 37 athletes (26 footballers and 11 others) and 156 young men as controls. Changes similar to osteitis pubis were found in 19 (76 per cent) of the footballers and 9 (81 per cent) of the other athletes, and in 70 (45 per cent) of the controls. The authors conclude that repeated minor trauma is the primary aetiological factor, and although the radiological appearance may resemble osteitis pubis, there was in their series no evidence that the lesion observed was caused by infection.

Durey and Rodineau (1976)[284a] also described lesions of the symphysis pubis in athletes, a pubic arthropathy encountered among those engaged in football, rugby, athletics and fencing.

Degenerative joint diseases

The normal life-history of the sacro-iliac joint conforms essentially to the same pattern of degenerative change that occurs in peripheral joints (Newton, 1957).[928]

Radiographs of 88 patients without known joint disease were surveyed and approximately 30 per cent had radiological changes of erosion, condensation, or both. Six per cent were under 50 years. The incidence was higher among males (Cohen, 1967).[186]

Sashin (1930)[1082] examined both joints of 257 cadavers and found osteophyte formation distributed as follows:

Age	Females	Males
40–49	50%	85%
50–59	85%	100%

In the older age-group, 60 per cent of male joints were ankylosed, but only 14 per cent of females.

Newton (1957)[928] observes that after the third decade there is usually an irregular loss of superficial cartilage, with fibrillation, later leading to erosions of varying size. The opposed surfaces may be firmly fixed together by debris, as if glued together, or because connective tissue extensively replaces areas of degenerated cartilage. In either case the X-ray appearances are normal. Because of the joint configurations, a firm fibrous ankylosis is probably as efficient, in limiting movement, as a bony one. The presence of a mobile painful joint in a man over 50 or a woman over 60 may be something more serious than a benign musculoskeletal problem.

Sacroiliitis

It is certain that the joint is lined by synovial membrane, and that it can be affected by traumatic, inflammatory and infectious diseases in the same manner as other articulations.[186] The joint is invariably involved in ankylosing spondylitis, and may share in the changes of gout, ulcerative colitis, regional ileitis (Crohn's disease), rheumatoid arthritis, Reiter's disease and tuberculosis. The pain of sacroiliitis is usually unrelated to position (Sashin, 1930).[1082]

The natural history and treatment of rheumatoid arthritis and ankylosing spondylitis are different, although the conditions share many similarities. Fallet, *et al.* (1976)[323] report 9 patients who fulfilled the diagnostic criteria for both conditions, and in 8 of the 9, the histocompatibility antigen HLA-27 was present. The authors mention that if chance association is not the explanation, basic concepts of differential diagnosis should be reconsidered.

Bickel and Romness (1957)[93] describe a case of true diastasis of the sacroiliac joints with hypermobility; radiographic examination showed diastasis of both joints with measurable superior subluxation of both ilia. Retrospective analysis led to the conclusion that the condition was an unusual and early finding in rheumatoid spondylitis, and may have been caused by rheumatoid granulomatous nodules.

Tuberculosis of the joint also occurs in young adults, usually between the ages of 20 and 40,[1153] and is commonly associated with tuberculosis in other parts of the body. Pain, as sciatica or lumbar or hip pain, is the most common presenting feature.

Early radiographic signs are haziness or loss of definition of the joint line, followed by irregularity of the articular surfaces with areas of erosion. Later changes are those of bony ankylosis of the joint.

Osteomyelitis of the joint may occur in 5–10 per cent of patients with acute haematogenous osteomyelitis; Trauner and Connor (1975)[1232] report two cases in which the initial X-rays were interpreted as normal but a radioactive bone scan revealed abnormalities.

Sacroiliac joint abnormalities, with radiological changes, accompany several rather uncommon disorders, e.g. alkaptonuria (ochronosis), multicentric reticulohistiocytosis (lipoid dermoarthritis), familial Mediterranean fever and relapsing polychondritis.[1028a]

Bone disease and metastasis

Three out of every four patients with *Paget's disease* present with lumbar spine and/or pelvis affected, and the X-ray should be seen before using any degree of vigour during treatment of mature patients (Collins 1959).[195] The same naturally applies to *osteoporosis*.

Sullivan (1976)[1188] mentions that *osteomalacia* occurs in two main groups, i.e. young and vegetarian Asian women, and elderly women who live on bread and tea. The softness and flexibility of osseous structures leads to change in the shape of the pelvis which is plain on X-ray.[315]

Primary neoplasms in breast, bronchus, prostate, kidney, thyroid and suprarenal glands may give rise to secondary deposits in the lumbar spine and pelvis; it is wise to enquire about persistent night pain and a possible history of previous illness when examining the joint.

THE COCCYX

Transitional vertebrae at the sacrococcygeal junction are not rare, and the incidence varies from 5 to 14 per cent.[315] There are many variations of anomaly and while this is not of great practical significance, anomalies in the region may tend to confuse palpation findings; this is particularly so when coccydynia is of recent traumatic origin, and the coccyx has in fact been deviated backwards, forwards or sideways since childhood. When the coccyx is deviated anteriorly by trauma, lateral radiographs may show an angulation of as much as 90°. In one of the author's patients, this traumatic deviation predated pregnancy by more than a year, but gave rise to no apparent difficulties during subsequent labour.

Referred pain, and referred diffuse tenderness, frequently occur in the coccygeal region from joint problems at the lumbosacral segment and in ankylosing spondylitis. Strain of its soft-tissue attachments may occur during childbirth.

An acute traumatic periostitis occurs when force is directly applied to the bone-tip, and it may or may not be accompanied by forcible subluxation of the sacrococcygeal joint. Exquisite tenderness is very accurately localised to the tip. In about 6 per cent of all pelvic fractures there is an associated coccygeal fracture.

The fractures can cause difficulties in differential diagnosis, since congenital variations of the coccyx are manifold.

Developmental deviations of the coccygeal axis may cause discomfort after long periods of sitting.

SERIOUS PATHOLOGY SIMULATING MUSCULOSKELETAL PAIN

Bourdillon (1973)[105] describes a patient in his mid-thirties who, after exhaustive clinical and X-ray examination had proved negative, was labelled a neurotic and discharged, despite his consistent complaints of low back pain; three months later he died of leukaemia.

Vertebral causes of spinal pain, and those visceral and other diseases which may produce clinical features simulating benign musculoskeletal pain, have been summarised by Brewerton (1977).[126]

There are no copper-bottomed guarantees that one is invariably dealing with a benign joint problem, simply because the patient may describe a pain which seemingly accords very closely with the therapist's experience of hundreds of others with just such a pain which was more or less satisfactorily cleared up by the appropriate physical treatment (see p. 159). Suspicion is aroused when pain cannot be provoked or modified by postural changes or by movement of the vertebral region concerned, yet the fact that pain *can* be provoked by spinal movement is no guarantee that conditions other than a benign musculoskeletal problem can therefore be discounted (p. 301). For example, the pains of *hiatus hernia* may be worsened by lying, bending or putting on socks and shoes. In *Bornholm disease*, a benign condition probably due to a virus infection, pain at the costal margin or upper abdomen is the striking feature, and pain provocation occurs on coughing, deep breathing, and on thoracic movement, as well as when yawning or laughing. The condition occurs in small epidemics but sporadic cases also occur. The neck and 'yoke' area pain of *epidemic cervical myalgia* may also be aggravated by movement, with the accompanying stiffness simulating a cervical joint condition.[918] The severe pain of 'dry' *tuberculosis pleurisy* over the nipple, axilla of scapula, is intensified by every movement and inspiration.[1040] In *upper urinary-tract* lesions, loin pain is provoked by movement or exercise and relieved by rest.

When the clinical features are not very marked, and only mild or vague symptoms are described, it is wise always to bear in mind the infinite range of biological plasticity of response, and the infinite capacity of the occasional patient to say what he or she believes the clinician wants to hear.

Wilkinson (1975)[1317] has mentioned differentiation of lumbar disc lesions from other disorders such as secondary carcinomas, tuberculous osteitis, myelomatosis and osteitis deformans.

Morgan and Hill (1964)[871] remark that the character, distribution and duration of oesophageal pain are very similar to those of cardiac origin, and that differentiation may be difficult. Also, conventional clinical tests of the oesophagus often fail to yield positive results when the thoracic pain *is* of oesophageal origin. At times, both may simulate the pain of spinal joint problems, of course.

Fulminating neck pain of sudden onset, with cervical rigidity and dysphagia, may be due to thickening of the cervical prevertebral soft tissues and an amorphous deposit of calcium in front of the C1 and C2 segments. The patient's distress is rapidly relieved with phenylbutazone. Mobilisation is not indicated and neither immobilisation nor surgery are necessary, as the calcium deposit begins diminishing within days.[89]

Without vigilance, the highly subjective exchange of history-taking can lead to a facile assumption of easy familiarity with the supposed nature of 'a simple joint problem,' when in fact one may be looking at the tip of a very different kind of iceberg.[1130]

If there is reasonable doubt, it is unwise to go on with physical examination procedures which may include stressing vertebral joints and neural canal structures; the suitability of physical treatment should be confirmed before doing this.

7. Clinical features

THE CONSEQUENCES OF DEGENERATIVE AND OTHER JOINT CHANGES

The clinical features of degenerative and other joint diseases[21, 91, 117, 202, 242, 285, 391, 392, 555, 656, 704, 707, 777, 919, 981, 1079, 1173, 1277, 1281, 1341] are described under (1) those *subjective* abnormalities which are reported by the patient but are not always detectable by the observer, although they may be assessed, and (2) those *objective* changes which are observable, whose degree can be measured, or estimated.

Symptoms can sometimes be likened to a strong breeze, in that while the air-movement itself cannot be seen, its effects can be observed. Similarly, a patient in severe or chronic pain will manifest it plainly by facial expression and other behaviour, which is observable. Often, the manner of relating symptoms also assists the process of assessment.

Symptoms reported by patients are:

Pain, including head and face pain, in a great variety of characteristics and presentation.

Feelings of stiffness and difficult movement, until 'warmed up'.

Variability of symptoms (notably joint pains) with weather changes.

Frustrations by restriction of daily activities in varying degree (e.g. head movements, free use of arm, or fine intrinsic movement of fingers).

Paraesthesiae (abnormalities of sensation as smarting, tingling, 'pins and needles', skin areas of 'hot feelings', 'burning sensations' and 'cold feelings', 'heaviness' of a limb, feelings of 'fullness' and 'puffiness') e.g. 'the cold sciatic leg'.

Hyperaesthesia (increased sensitivity of skin).

Dysaesthesia (diminished sensibility, numbness. N.B. Often the area outlined is not numb, but only *feels* numb).

Localised anaesthesia (sensation loss in a circumscribed cutaneous area, which can be objectively confirmed).

Dysequilibrium (feelings of giddiness and instability).

Momentary blackouts.

Head heaviness.

Scalp tension.

Nausea (sometimes preceding actual vomiting).

Dysphagia (feelings of a lump in the throat or difficulty in swallowing).

Depression and other psychic symptoms, e.g. the feeling of a weight on the head.

Suboccipital and nuchal crepitus.

Difficulties of concentrating and remembering.

Feelings of pressure behind the eyes.

Foggy or blurred vision, and photophobia.

Feelings of chest constriction, or precordial distress.

Interferences (uncommonly) with bladder and bowel function and control.

N.B. Many of these symptoms, while being familiar and frequent manifestations of degenerative joint disease and its consequences, are often the indications of more serious pathology, such as neoplastic, vascular and neurological disease which are beyond the scope of physical treatment directed to the pathological changes as such. Nevertheless, they cannot be excluded from description, because when some of them form part of the disturbed function due to arthrosis and spondylosis for which such treatment is indicated, they provide data upon which to base ASSESSMENT, both of the extent of the joint problem which the therapist is handling, and of the efficiency of the treatment procedures.

Signs frequently observed are:

Limitation of movement, abnormally increased movement and distorted movement.

Palpable swelling, and periarticular thickening.

Palpable changes in the texture of muscles.

Localised changes in skin texture, and of pliability of subcutaneous tissues.

Joint irritability.

Muscle spasm.

Muscle and inert tissue contracture.

Muscle weakness and wasting.

Changes in tendon reflex responses.

Undue tenderness of bony points and soft tissues.

Palpable crepitus.

Changes of contour and attitude (deformity).
Aphonia and dysphonia (loss of voice and difficult, hoarse speech).
Vasomotor and sudomotor changes (blanching or flushing, or sweating).
Unilateral pupillary changes.
Spastic weakness of lower limb.
Ankle clonus.
Exaggeration and inversion of tendon jerks.
Extensor (Babinski) response. } in cervical myelopathy

The following factors require consideration before examination, assessment and treatment can be discussed:

1. Neurological changes.
2. Pain and tenderness.
3. Autonomic involvement in pain syndromes.
4. Referred pain.
5. Abnormalities of feeling.
6. Changes in muscle and soft tissues.
7. Deformity.
8. Functional disablement.
9. Psychological aspects of vertebral pain.

Abnormalities of movement are discussed under Tests of movement (p. 312) and palpation in assessment (p. 628).

NEUROLOGICAL CHANGES

(See also Root pain, p. 175, Pathological changes, p. 94, and Assessment in examination, p. 350, and in Treatment p. 444.)

The salient clinical features of root pressure, spinal cord involvement and cauda equina involvement are described in outline below in order that these important sequelae of degenerative change may be held in mind.

(a) Signs and symptoms of root pressure

When spinal nerve root involvement, by irritation, or intermittent or sustained compression by physical trespass, is sufficient to produce interference with normal conduction, *signs* will be manifest in the tissues supplied by the root, as muscle weakness, muscle wasting, and diminution or loss of reflex response; reflex changes may alone be caused by painful facet-joint changes (see p. 250).

Symptoms are pain (so-called root pain, although root pressure as such is not necessarily painful and the appellation does not mean the production of root pain is understood, or that there is any certainty of the root being mechanically involved), and paraesthesiae, hyperaesthesia or dysaesthesia, sometimes leading to circumscribed loss of sensation, usually in more distal parts of the root distribution. Thus the changes are those of a lower motor neurone lesion, although the complete clinical syndrome is seen less frequently than partly developed examples of it, in various combinations from patient to patient. The pain frequently does not respect classical dermatome boundaries and may be felt in the *myotome* and *sclerotome* of the nerve root, or adjacent roots.

Paraesthesiae, hyperaesthesia and dysaesthesia will usually but not invariably be associated with the relevant *dermatome*; their distribution, especially distally, may often assist in identification of the root involved, in uniradicular lesions. Anomalies of peripheral innervation should be borne in mind (see pp. 12, 194).

Surgical decompression of an entrapped nerve root relieves symptoms due to autonomic neurone involvement as well as those due to somatic neurone compression; relief of these symptoms signifies the presence of sympathetic nerve fibres, although other than the ramus meningeus (of mixed somatic and sympathetic neurones) all sympathetic nerves are *extra*foraminal. There may be an unexplained reflex mechanism to account for this phenomenon.[149]

(b) Signs and symptoms of spinal cord involvement
(see also Cervical spondylosis section)

Cord involvement is possible due to changes occurring at any vertebral level, but is far more frequent in the cervical spine (cervical myelopathy) than in other regions;[2, 117, 1079] thoracic disc protrusions occur rarely, and involvement of the neural canal structures in the lumbar region is more likely to occur below the vertebral level of termination of the cord, i.e. L1–L2 (see Cauda equina). Cervical myelopathy, the most common spinal cord disease after the age of 50, can be due to pressures by single or multiple osseo-cartilaginous bars (see p. 126), to localised tensions arising from changes induced in the meningeal ligaments (see p. 57) and from ischaemia due to local or more distal interferences with vascular supply (see p. 6). The pressures, tension or ischaemia may be constant and unremitting, or intermittent, e.g. only during certain movements. Consequently, the extent and distribution of damage to grey and white matter are most variable, particularly so when they are of an ischaemic nature (see p. 226), and the presenting signs and symptoms correspondingly differ from patient to patient. The condition commonly takes the form of a slowly progressive spastic paraplegia. There may be dysaesthesia in the hands, with clumsiness and weakness of hand movements, spastic weakness of the lower limbs with slight general wasting, and exaggerated knee- and ankle-jerks. There may be limb pain. Inversion of tendon jerks may be observed, the triceps jerk being obtained on testing for the biceps jerk, or a finger-flexion jerk being obtained on testing for the supinator response (brachioradialis). Ankle clonus is sometimes present and the plantar reflexes are likely to be extensor. The patient will often report difficulties of walking. Sphincter control is not usually affected. Thus the clinical presentation can be that of a partial or complete *lower motor neurone lesion*, of involved cervical roots at the level of the causative lesion, e.g. when compression is the cause, and that of an *upper motor neurone lesion* (usually partial and patchy) below the cervical level. Generally, physical treatment of its cause is either contraindicated, or pointless, although careful cervical traction avoiding overmuch flexion and a supporting collar may be of value pending other measures.

(c) Cauda equina involvement

The clinical features of involvement of a single root of the lumbosacral plexus, commonly by a prolapsed intervertebral disc, represent a partial cauda equina lesion, in the sense that one of its roots on one side is affected, but the term by general use refers to the more serious and more extensive paralysis which accompanies interference with the *lower sacral* roots especially, together with others.

Although the cause of these uncommon and extensive root lesions[1062] is at times a massive protrusion of the disc (see p. 150), which occupies all available room in the neural canal, there also occurs a band of dense intrathecal adhesions which produce a similar clinical syndrome by strangling the roots of the cauda equina, the accompanying disc prolapse being insufficient in terms of magnitude and trespass to produce the symptoms and extensive signs observed. The dense fibrous thickening of the arachnoiditis is observed to be firmly embedding the intrathecal roots (p. 534). Involvement of the cauda equina in the changes of ischaemia may occur by physical interference with its vascular supply.

The clinical picture is usually that of multisegmental interference, frequently bilaterally, with much more extensive paralysis than in single unilateral root lesions, and marked especially by symptoms about the anus, perineum, genitals and inner upper thighs. There may be pain in the perineum, with paraesthesiae in the 'saddle area' and localised patches of numbness. Some degree of paralysis of anal and urethral sphincters occurs in most cases, with retention of urine (see p. 150). There may be a complete unilateral foot-drop, or a total distal paralysis. The saddle paraesthesiae and sphincter disturbances are referrable to interference with the 3rd and 4th sacral nerves with their autonomic components, and although other roots are affected, the S3 and S4 damage contributes the main hazard to the patient, which is that of permanent sphincter paralysis.

The onset of micturition difficulties and 'saddle-area' symptoms may be sudden, but can be insidious. Examinations of patients with back pain and sciatica must *always* include an enquiry about saddle paraesthesiae and function of sphincters; the condition requires prompt surgical attention, delay is dangerous, and physical treatment procedures almost always contraindicated.

However promptly the surgical attention is received, recovery from sphincter disturbance is likely to be prolonged.

PAIN AND TENDERNESS

A. INTRODUCTION

It is when attempts are made to verbalise feelings and sensations that inadequacies of language are most apparent. The characteristic quality and intensity of musculoskeletal pain, the nature and degree of bodily and mental distress produced by it, are hard for patients to convey, and equally hard for therapists to perceive; yet its *behaviour* related to time, posture and movement can provide a clear basis for assessment. Pain is our universal inheritance and, as therapists, our perennial headache. From antiquity to our own time, the phenomenon of pain has prompted philosophers, physicians and others to describe it, categorise it, so that common ground of conception might serve progress in the understanding and mastery of this most elemental human condition.

The description of pain as a disturbance of neurological function[1355] does not mean, of course, that neurological disturbances cannot occur without causing pain (e.g. Adie's pupil); similarly, 'a disorder of the affect', scientifically in keeping with physiological criteria, provides the bone, yet somehow the meat of pain remains absent. Pain has been described as 'a linguistic abstraction for a rich variety of emotional experiences',[842] substitute the word 'love' for 'pain' and equally the description fits like a glove. Add our further universal experience, that love can very frequently cause psychic pain and suffering, and that bodily pain cannot but involve things which lie behind our defences, our feelings and our emotions, and we soon confront the major difficulty of subjecting pain to inspection and analysis:

> The constant effort ... to separate the purely physiological from the purely psychological, and to label symptoms as either organic or functional, has a certain futility about it ... clinical impression that probably 50 per cent of all psychiatric referrals in a general hospital can be classified as pain syndromes.[356]

Clearly, pain has dual aspects, i.e. the perception of pain and the reaction to it.

Perception of pain may be evaluated in terms of quality and intensity, while *reaction* to pain is manifested by tachycardia, anxiety, fear, panic and prostration.

The former may be termed as the pain sensation, which in some patients can largely be kept isolated as merely an unpleasant and unwelcome visitor in a body part, while the latter, the pain experience, may involve some patients in emotional and physiological effects which can be extensive.[512, 1245] Some of the changes have been noted (see p. 115).

Although pain does not always arise entirely from

organic causes, it is real, it is there, it is necessary and protective in terms of giving notice, providing warning that something is amiss.

Yet 'anyone who has suffered prolonged, severe pain would regard it as an evil, punishing affliction that is harmful in its own right'.[846] Patients are not imagining pain that they are actually feeling (or feel they are feeling) although by tension, anxiety and unco-ordinated use of their own bodies, may involuntarily be creating part of the difficulties they report. Some appear to have poorly developed kinaesthetic appreciation of their own locomotor apparatus; they are awkward movers and when in greater or lesser pain from joint problems, they generate a disproportionately large amount of spasm (see p. 351) by way of protective response, although this in itself may not be adding to pain, and this tends to include spinal segments unusually remote from those involved by changes. They are difficult to teach exercises to and may be said without disparagement to be, by nature, physically illiterate. Concerning this, the assumption that proprioception is entirely a matter of afferent impulse traffic may not be correct. Observations suggest that awareness of limb position and movement depends to a degree on *efferent* impulse traffic.[847]

In contradistinction there are the few patients who for some kind of gain are manifestly pretending that pain is more severe than it is. With experience, it becomes less difficult to decide in which category a patient may belong, but this is never easy, and it is prudent to be more hesitant than not in labelling anything as imaginary. After examination of a joint, the conclusion, 'There are no signs to be found' and the unspoken inference that the patient 'is not on the level' or 'a phoney' can sometimes mean that the examination has been less thorough, or has been conducted with less compassion, than it should.

B. PERIPHERAL EVENTS

The immense amount of experimental and clinical work on pain has often been concerned with cutaneous sensibility and, less frequently, with the deeper musculoskeletal tissues, although accounts of the latter have been of much significance.[640, 641, 642, 342, 343, 1149]

The work of Lewis (1942)[730] and of Keele and Armstrong (1964)[634] have been concerned with the quality of pain associated with the different pain-sensitive structures of the body. The pain experienced depends not only on groups and sizes of afferent fibres, but also on the arrangement of fibres in a tissue, the particular layer of the tissue and the actual structure stimulated. Pain due to cutaneous stimulation differs from that due to stimulation of the periosteum, or the muscles, for example.

On the basis of their findings, Keele and Armstrong assert, 'The stratification hypothesis should be taken into account in all studies of the sensory accompaniment of noxious stimulation', and report experiments in which stimulation of three different strata in the skin produced three different types of pain.

Because it is not at all easy to specify in which of the family of musculoskeletal tissues a particular 'joint' pain is arising (although pain from the deepest structures, bone and periosteum, tends to remain localised) it is probably wisest to trust that in our present state of knowledge clinical effectiveness in this field of work will best be served by paying particular attention to the *behaviour* of pain related to time, posture and movement, rather than basing clinical procedures on questions of which specific tissue, however important and necessary it is that these questions be answered as our means of doing so become available.

The distribution and nature of nociceptor endings in *musculoskeletal and associated tissues* has been outlined (p. 10), i.e. free nerve endings in ligaments; in all other tissues supplied with nociceptors a plexiform unmyelinated network weaves through the matrix and between cells and fibres of the part.

Normally, this receptor system is relatively inactive, yet takes some part in the general functions of somatic sensibility, e.g. the cornea of the eye, while sensitive to the four modalities cold, touch, warmth and pain, is supplied with only one type of end-organ, i.e. free nerve endings.[437, 907] It must be added that there are fibres which are totally inactive[1212] in normal circumstances and which begin generating the afferent impulses of nociception only when their endings of fibres are depolarised by the noxious agents described below. They remain high-threshold to all other than noxious stimuli, only becoming sensitised, and thus low-threshold, by stimuli which can cause the pain experience.

The question of stimulus-specificity of afferent endings[907] is important, and while the majority of non-myelinated fibres are polymodal, and can be excited by many sorts of stimuli, as has been implied above, they are stimulus-specific in the sense that they are the nociceptors, the small fibre system of the gate-control theory (*vide infra*) and thus are excited by stimuli which have the potentiality to cause the pain experience.

Afferent impulse traffic from these nociceptors in musculoskeletal tissues is markedly increased when the unmyelinated fibres are depolarised by (i) mechanical forces sufficient to damage or deform them,[1362] i.e. pressure or distraction, and (ii) the presence in their tissue-fluid environment, in sufficient concentration, of irritating chemical substances.

Substances which modulate or stimulate nerve ending sensitivity include:

calcium ions	lactic acid
potassium ions	5-hydroxytryptamine, bradykinin
hydrogen ions	and other polypeptide kinins
noradrenaline	histamine
acetylcholine	prostaglandins

Prostaglandins E occur in low concentrations in all inflammatory exudates and have the effect of sensitising nerve endings to both mechanical stimuli and chemical mediators. They are a factor in the production of tenderness, and actually produce pain and cutaneous sensitivity to pain when given in concentrated dosages.[496, 1138]

Acetylsalicylic acid (aspirin) inhibits the biosynthesis of prostaglandins and it is upon this enzyme-blocking action that some of the analgesic and anti-inflammatory effects of aspirin depend.

The extravasion of blood in a bruise, for example, and the tissue-destruction accompanying it, entail a breakdown through the stages of protein—polypeptide—peptide—amino-acids products which can be violently irritating, and not all of which are yet known.

These peripheral events, depolarising a sufficient population of nociceptors in musculoskeletal tissue and thus generating a volume of afferent impulse activity to reach a critical threshold, are not in themselves sufficient to result in pain, because its intrusion upon consciousness appears to rest on the activity of a series of steps of neural censorship, of modulation.

Clinical work and experimental findings suggest that, other factors given, the intensity of pain experienced by patients is not directly related to the degree of tissue damage itself, but depends upon mechanisms of convergence, summation and modulation at spinal and supraspinal levels.[842, 907, 1285]

C. CENTRIPETAL TRANSMISSION TO SPINAL CORD

The velocity of impulses conducted in nerve fibres is related to the fibre diameter; the thicker the fibre the faster the conduction velocity.[401] In large myelinated fibres the impulses are propagated with a speed of some 75–100 m per second; in the finest unmyelinated fibres the velocity is only 1.5–0.3 m per second. There is no clear correlation between fibre size and sensory modalities perceived.[841, 589]

Nerve fibres are subdivided into three groups, A, B, and C. The myelinated A fibres fall into four groups, partly overlapping, alpha, beta, gamma, delta—with decreasing conduction velocities and diameters. The B group covers myelinated preganglionic autonomic fibres, and the C group unmyelinated fibres which are postganglionic efferent autonomic fibres, and somatic and visceral afferent fibres.[437] In myelinated fibres the conduction velocity as measured in metres per second is approximately the figure obtained when the diameter of the fibre is multiplied by six.[582]

In all peripheral nerves, fibres of sympathetic origin are also present. Environmental changes affecting fibres may include anaesthetic solutions, compression and traction,[392] ischaemia, anoxia and electrical stimulation.

(i) *Local analgesia.* All nerve fibres are susceptible to modifications of their activity by analgesic drugs; this was believed to be directly related to size with the smaller fibres affected first and the larger fibres last, depending upon concentration of solutions. In practice, a handful of large fibres react as do the small ones, and effects of local anaesthesia should not be conceived on the basis of fibres as homogeneous material with resistance to analgesia exhibited on the basis of thickness only; their mode of action is also a factor.[905] In general terms, the conduction in smaller fibres is more easily blocked by dilute solutions, the larger diameter fibres requiring stronger concentrations.

(ii) *Compression.* Sustained compression blocks conduction in larger diameter afferent fibres earlier and more severely than in smaller fibres,[1362] although temporary constriction need not interfere with conduction.[485] Pressure may be applied locally to produce ischaemia but oxygen can diffuse along a nerve over a distance of 5 cm to maintain almost full activity, although the diffusion ceases when pressure is increased above 100 mmHg (13.33 kPa). Provided there is no damage to axons or blood vessels during constriction, conduction ability returns within about 18–35 minutes after pressure is released and circulation restored.

In general, compression will block nerve conduction in the order of fibres A–B–C and anoxia will do so in the order of B–A–C.

(iii) *Electrical stimulation.* Large fibres respond more quickly to stimulation than do smaller fibres.

Nociceptor impulse transmission

Impulses subserving pain are not transmitted centrally by small diameter fibres only. There is evidence that noxious stimuli tend to excite receptor-fibre units across the full diameter range and because painful stimuli are usually intense, they generally fire many low-threshold as well as high-threshold fibre units.[196]

In general, the number of fibres activated by a stimulus tends to increase with the intensity of stimulus, as does the frequency of impulse volleys.[906]

Thus the pain-production-potential of a noxious peripheral event may depend as much on the total *number* of fibres activated, and their frequency of impulse volleys, as on the particular fibre-diameter groups recruited.

In summary, experiments indicate that the 'traffic for pain' (hereinafter 'the input') is conveyed centripetally by:

Large fibres. A beta neurones, diameter 5–12 μm, myelinated, conduction speed $\pm$ 30 m/s.

Lowest threshold for noxious stimuli.
Low 'electrical stimulation' threshold.

High threshold to chemicals, e.g. anaesthetic.
Sensitive to conduction block by transient compression, and recovers slowly.

Inhibitory to input transmission at the region of the substantia gelatinosa (see below).

Small fibres. A delta neurones, diameter 2–5 μm, unmyelinated, conduction speed 12–30 m/s.
C neurones, diameter 0.5–1 μm, unmyelinated, conduction speed 3–6 m/s.

Higher threshold for noxious stimuli.
High 'electrical stimulation' threshold.
Low threshold to chemicals, e.g. local anaesthesia.
Less sensitive to conduction block by transient compression, and recovers earlier.

Facilitatory to input transmission at the region of the substantia gelatinosa (see below).[1325]

Clinical evidence suggests that types of pain may be ascribed to types of fibre, e.g. following a blow, we experience both a 'fast' pain and later a 'slow', a second pain.

Fast pain. Immediate, crisp, localised pain. Large fibres with their lower threshold have picked it up quickly.

Slow pain. Developing a second or two later—spreading, diffuse, nasty. Small fibres pick it up a bit later and transmit more slowly.

Recent experimental evidence shows that the properties and behaviour of afferent fibres themselves are at least as complex as their receptor end-organs.[985, 986] It is doubtful if nociceptors can become adapted or fatigued, and experimental results are contradictory—reason suggests that adaption should not occur if pain is to serve its presumed purpose as a warning system.[1138]

D. MODULATION

Though many sensations may readily be placed into broad categories labelled touch, pain, warmth and cold, the vocabulary of even the most articulate is clearly inadequate to describe the innumerable gradations of sensation which fail to fall into these somewhat convenient but arbitrary ... pigeonholes. [Calne and Pallis (1966).][155]

What is perceived by the mind in normal life is not the stimulus of a single receptor or frequently not only a single type of receptor; the individual experiences a complex impression resulting from the spatial and temporal summation of stimuli of different kinds.[130] The central nervous system has a dynamic plasticity whereby sensory input from any part of the nervous system can be accepted or ignored, accentuated or diminished, or ascend directly to consciousness. (In some chronic pain states, the input seems to become hopelessly short-circuited in a vicious circle of self-perpetuating activity within the complex of short-chain interinternuncial neurones. See Fig. 7.1.)[518]

Thus, although the overall volume of input is a relevant stimulus parameter,[846] the intensity and volume of afferent impulses do not produce equivalent magnitudes of effect. Radiographic evidence of advanced degenerative change, in spines which are functional and painless despite being stressed considerably each day, seems to bear this out.

Three features of the input have much significance, i.e.:
(i) The somatosensory basal or background afferent activity preceding and accompanying the stimulus, and especially that of mechanoreceptors.
(ii) The stimulus-evoked activity.
(iii) The relative intensity in large versus small fibres.[842]

In (i), mechanoreceptor afferent impulses from joints, periarticular tissues, neuromuscular spindles and cutaneous receptors, with the rich volume of impulses from visceral afferent neurones, comprise the normal centripetal flood of neural activity, and transaction, upon which nociceptor excitation is superimposed, and by which its ultimate fate may partly be influenced, i.e. at spinal cord level, nociceptor information impinges upon a hornet's nest of steady neural activity already existing, resulting from the spatial and temporal patterns of traffic, and summation of stimuli, of many different kinds.

Cells intrinsic to the substantia gelatinosa in the dorsal horn of the spinal cord (s.g. cells) can control, and thus organise by a system of 'gating', the amount of sensory input allowed onward transmission to higher centres by the transmission cells (T cells).[842] Gating, in electronic engineering, is a technical term to describe the electronic equivalent of raising or lowering a lock-gate—thus influencing the flow of electrons. The old thermionic valve, and the modern transistor, are methods of gating.

Briefly, large A fibre input, and the input of the larger myelinated mechanoreceptor afferents, tend to inhibit onward transmission by closing the gate, while the small A and C fibre input tends to facilitate transmission. Pain will be experienced, and the variety of responses to it activated, when the output of T cells reaches or exceeds a critical level.

Excessive pain, or pain reasonably out of proportion to the degree of stimulus by tissue damage, may occur because converging impulses *summate* to overcome the gate-control mechanism; and it is in this context that the basal activity existing, particularly of visceral receptors, may provide the increments necessary for summation to occur, and further, may be the mechanism whereby the normally trivial nature and small amplitude of a movement, setting up a disproportionately severe exacerbation of pain from an already irritable and highly reactive joint, is enough to trigger summation mechanisms.[1281]

The substantia gelatinosa gate comprises groups of small cells in Lamina V (Rexed),[1030] forming a closely packed functional unit which extends the length of the spinal cord (Lissauer's tract). Collateral branches of the larger mechanoreceptor afferents, after traversing synaptic junctions in Rexed Lamina II, ascend and descend in Lissauer's tract before terminating by axoaxonic synapses on the nociceptor afferents in Lamina V, exerting their inhibitory influence on the transmission of nociceptor excitation. Thus awareness of pain is also inversely related to the existing volume of non-nociceptive afferent activity of mechanoreceptors, and this is an important factor in the segmental modulation system.

E. PERIPHERAL MODULATION[845, 637, 1362]

By rhythmic movement of the body, or a body part, and by cutaneous contact and soft-tissue compression, i.e. stroking, holding, pressing, rocking and by rhythmic manual or mechanical mobilisation techniques, the large-diameter (6–12 μm and 13–17 μm) mechanoreceptors are stimulated, and there is unequivocal evidence that the afferent impulse activity so generated has an inhibitory and thus modulatory effect upon the first synaptic relays of small-fibre nociceptors in the substantia gelatinosa. Thus, also, the soothing effects of radiant heat applied to the body surface, and the effect of a hot water bottle resting on the body part, are similar in so far as heat is applied, but markedly different in that the latter involves mechanoreceptor stimulation by body contact, while heat applied by radiation does not.

The spinal segmental modulation mechanism outlined above is not fully autonomous; it is more a modulation-effector and besides mediating mechanoreceptor influence from the periphery, the dorsal root modulating mechanism itself is governed by descending impulses from supraspinal centres (see below).

Chemical modulation also occurs at the substantia gelatinosa[215] and a long-known peptide (Substance P), with the properties of a vasodilator, has now been recognised as a neurotransmitter or modulator; it occurs in the C fibres as they enter the substantia gelatinosa and could be the important factor in initial perception of pain since in tiny concentrations it facilitates neurone activity.

The substance is found in other central nervous system regions, e.g. the ventral horns of the spinal cord, the central grey matter of the cord and the hypothalamus.

Hannington-Kiff (1977)[496] neatly describes its possible roles as the 'hinge-oil on the gate' in the substantia gelatinosa which allows access to the spinothalamic tract, as the transmitter substance in the multisynaptic ascending system and the chemical activator of the flexor withdrawal reflex from painful stimuli.

F. ASCENDING TRACTS

Traditionally, the spinothalamic tracts are regarded as the spinal cord pathway for rostral transmission, from cord segments and the medulla to the thalamus, of impulses subserving pain.

The lateral spinothalamic tract is a recent evolutionary acquisition, and even in man it only contains something like 1500–2000 fibres which, in terms of total neuronal population, is but a meagre handful.

Clinical and experimental evidence indicates that only a proportion (perhaps no more than 25 per cent) of the neurones conveying nociceptor excitation, for onward transmission by the T cells, ascend directly to thalamic nuclei, and these comprise the larger, fast-conducting neurones; while most of these larger neurones cross the grey matter of the cord to ascend in the contralateral side, some ascend ipsilaterally.[1138, 1362]

The greater majority of fibres in the tract are unmyelinated and small and do not even reach the thalamus other than by many synapses. Most of them terminate on the reticular formation in the brain stem, and others ascend for varying distances to make synaptic connections with internuncial neurones within the grey matter of the cord.

The *pathway for pain* is a complex system of many routes, some of them ascending for a few segments only before beginning what may be called a 'synaptic stepladder' in their rostral direction.

Thus there are pathways of varying lengths, some of fast-conducting long neurones with few synapses, and many short slow-conducting neurones making plentiful synapses.

Further, some tracts are phylogenetically older than others.

Ascending pathways. It is probably unnecessary to distinguish an anterior spinothalamic tract. Classical descriptions of the ascending tracts gave little attention to unmyelinated, multisynaptic pathways, which modern histological techniques have demonstrated more fully and which are of considerable size. Recognition of their importance is associated with recognition of the significance of the reticular system. Two ascending systems are described,[496] according to whether they are *oligosynaptic* or *multisynaptic*.

(i) *The oligosynaptic ascending system* includes the exteroceptive fibres of the dorsal tracts as well as the lateral spinothalamic tract. The latter receives the axons of the dorsal horn T cells, after these neurones have crossed over the white commissure to the opposite side of the spinal cord. The spinothalamic pathway is a composite traffic system and includes at least spinotectal, spinovestibular, spinorubral and spinoreticular neurones.

(ii) *The multisynaptic ascending system* comprises (a) the spinal reticular core of the fasciculi proprii and (b) Lissauer's tracts.

a. Neurones of the fasciculi proprii originate at the margins of the whole central grey matter, and extend upwards as chains of neurones to reach the brain-stem reticular formation. Synapses lie within the grey matter, the axons traversing several segments in either direction.

b. Lissauer's tract comprises the neurones of substantia gelatinosa cells, the axons traversing one or two segments in either direction before synapsing again in the substantia gelatinosa with other cells. Where the spinal cord becomes continuous with the medulla, the substantia gelatinosa is continuous with the spinal tract of the 5th cranial nerve. Spinal reticular core fibres reach the palaeothalamus and those of Lissauer's tract the neothalamus.

Via the oligosynaptic ascending system accurate information about the *locality* and nature of potentially painful stimuli is quickly transmitted to ventral nuclei of the thalamus; both components of the multisynaptic system lack a somatotopical arrangement.

Recognition of the categories of fast and slow pain mentioned above (p. 164), and the existence of fast- and slow-conducting peripheral and central transmission pathways, invites the obvious hypothesis.[1360]

G. PROJECTIONS IN BRAIN STEM AND CORTEX

The concept of a single pain centre in the brain is totally inadequate to account for the complexities of pain.[846, 906]

Clinical and research experience indicates that pain requires a critical level of activity in several thalamic nuclei, this being dependent upon:

(i) the overall volume of afferent nociceptor impulses (i.e. total number of fibres activated, the frequency of impulse volleys, the particular fibre-diameter groups recruited)

(ii) modulation, by segmental dorsal horn mechanisms, in the thalamus itself and by descending influences, from supraspinal centres, mediated via the segmental dorsal horn mechanisms

and the concurrent participation and influence of cortical and hypothalamic nuclei.

Thus the following localised regions of the cortex and the hypothalamus are specifically concerned with separate factors of the pain experience:

Via the thalamocortical radiation[1355] in the posterior limb of the internal capsule, a pathway to the superior paracentral region of the same-side cortex subserves *perceptual* recognition of a somatosensory experience, i.e. the *existence* of tissue abnormality, of its *site* and of its *nature*, but not the experience of 'hurt'. This perceptual capability appears to depend more upon mechanoreceptor rather than nociceptor excitation.

In the anterior limb of the internal capsule, the large projections from thalamic nuclei to the orbitofrontal and cingulate areas of the cortex are specially significant in experiencing the 'hurt', the *unpleasant emotional affective component* of the pain experience. The surgical procedure of orbitofrontal leucotomy relieves the emotional distress, the 'hurt' of pain, while the perceptual awareness of the site and nature of the tissue-abnormality remains.[380]

Thalamocortical projections, to the temporal lobe on each side, are linked by association-fibres with the other cortical regions mentioned above, and it is in the temporal lobe that recent and longer-term *memory* of past painful experience appears to reside. Nociceptor and mechanoreceptor impulses reach the temporal cortex from the medial thalamic nuclei and the pulvinar; in this long-term storage system, seniority of storage residence, and recall, of painful experiences appears to depend not so much on *intensity* of the experience as its *duration* and *frequency of occurrence*.[1362]

Together with projections from the thalamus, the subjacent hypothalamic nuclei receive projections from the reticular and other systems. Since sympathetic and parasympathetic efferent activity to all body regions is effected by the neurone pools of hypothalamic nuclei, it will be evident that *visceral and hormonal effects* of nociceptor excitation will be mediated through the projections mentioned; examples of the effects are cardiovascular changes such as cutaneous vasoconstriction, increase in heart rate, rise in BP, etc.; pupillary changes; nausea and vomiting; sweating.

The *degree* and comprehensiveness of efferent autonomic vasomotor and secretomotor activity is not a reliable parameter of the intensity of a pain experience; the former are reflex effects and not directly related in terms of magnitude to the stimulus.

There is no correlation between the intensity of the subjective emotional change, and observable changes such as palpitation, spasm of muscle and other reflex responses.

H. CENTRAL MODULATION

Patients vary considerably in their responses to the state of perforce having to give hospitality to the (almost always) unwelcome guest of pain, and thus also vary considerably in their degree of suffering.

Psychological and experimental evidence supports the concept of pain as a private and personal experience, whose quality and intensity are influenced by: the unique past history of the individual;[846] the meaning or significance which the 'pain-situation' has for the person; the person's cultural and environmental background; to a greater or lesser degree, the placebo effect, or power of suggestion; the person's state of mind at the material time.

Thus, pain becomes a function of the whole individual, including thoughts, preoccupations, anxieties, obsessions (if there be so) and hopes, and all of these factors influence the actual patterns of nerve impulses within the brain and the spinal cord, as do various metabolic and hormonal influences, and the pharmacology of day-to-day intake of food and drink such as tea, coffee and alcohol.

Various parts of the brain, and their activities, have different evolutionary ages, and the significance of pain for the individual depends upon the activity of our most recent cerebral development.

Nathan's[906] observations on vision, 'one may exaggerate a little and say that the older parts of the brain are for looking, and the most recently developed part is for seeing', may be paraphrased by substituting 'perceiving' and 'suffering' respectively—this broadly encapsulates the processes of higher centres in central modulation.

The higher central nervous system processes of awareness, knowing, attention and anticipation can influence nociceptor transmission at spinal segmental levels, and the modulation is exercised through several systems. The *mid-brain reticular nuclei* exert a powerful inhibitory control over spinal transmission cell activity by reticulospinal pathways and exert facilitation effects on the cortex by alerting activity in reticulocortical projections, yet are themselves subject to modulatory fibre systems projecting on to them from the whole cortex and particularly the frontal cortex, as follows:

(i) *At dorsal horn level*, modulatory impulses are impinged continuously but at variable frequency via the reticulospinal tract;[1279, 1359] this inhibitory effect is enhanced by distraction, or concentration of attention elsewhere, by emotional excitement, by hypnosis and by stimulation of other body parts. Conversely, this reticular blockade is reduced by sudden intense stimuli, by direction of attention to the site of damaged tissue, and by barbiturate drugs.[843]

(ii) Reticular modulatory influences are themselves driven or governed by neuronal activity in corticofugal projections, from the paracentral and frontal regions, to the *reticular formation*; some of these augment the reticular blockade and some have the opposite effect.[130, 1279]

(iii) Other corticofugal projections from the paracentral region descend directly (in the contralateral corticospinal tract) to the *spinal cord internuncial synaptic relay systems*, and may inhibit or facilitate the onward transmission of nociceptor impulse traffic. The latter effect may be mediated via presynaptic and inhibitory axoaxonic synapses on the large diameter mechanoreceptor collaterals, thus reducing the modulatory effects normally exerted by the latter.[26, 346] Thus the paracentral cortex, subserving perceptual awareness of the existence, site and nature of pain (yet not the factor of 'hurt'), projects both positive and negative feedback influences upon the magnitude of central

transmission, exercising these influences at spinal level.

(iv) Modulation is also exercised at supraspinal level, i.e. on the *thalamic relay nuclei*, via corticothalamic projections from the paracentral, frontal, parietal and temporal sections of the cortex,[941] which produce long-lasting postsynaptic inhibitory effects upon thalmic traffic.

(v) Originating in the mid-brain reticular nuclei and in some thalamic neurones, a facilitatory stream of impulses of varying magnitude is transmitted in *reticulocortical projections*,[1359] perpetually cascading upon those areas which receive the thalamocortical projections, and continuously modulating the intensity of consciousness of all sensory awareness and of affective emotional experience. Overall, nociceptor activity thus impinges upon a fluctuant degree of awareness and attention, and the response of the whole person to pain has much to do with the existing bias, or concurrent excitability levels, of the mesencephalic reticular nuclei.

(vi) The activity of *periaqueductal grey matter (p.a.g.) in the mesencephalon* is of interest. Neurones project into the medulla, and via the median raphe nuclei down to the segmental dorsal horn cells. Stimulation of these mid-brain neurones, by indwelling electrodes in patients with chronic pain, produces behavioural analgesia continuing long after the time of implant. Morphine also stimulates p.a.g. activity, and experiments have demonstrated that an endogenous protein narcotic substance is produced by normal brain metabolism, the substance having a predilection for p.a.g. neurone cell bodies. Electrical stimulation apparently enhances the effects of the endogenously produced narcotics, which appear to be serotonin-based.

Thus biochemical modulation within the central nervous system must also be considered, and there are concentrations of *opiate receptor cells* in the periaqueductal grey matter, the amygdala, the thalamus, the head of the caudate nucleus, the hypothalamus, the putamen and the prefrontal cortex.

The notably limbic distribution of these receptors suggests the link between anxiety and pain.[496] There are also opiate receptors in the central grey matter of the spinal cord, and the activity of natural opiate-like transmitters may have a function at the first synapses of nociceptor pathways.

Returning to intracranial endogenous narcotic substances, there is *enkephalin*, a five amino-acid peptide, which is present in nerve terminals closely related to the opiate receptors, and *endorphin*, occurring mainly in the pituitary gland.[1152]

A substance comprising part of the pituitary hormone,

subsequently named beta-endorphin, proved to be much more potent than morphine, and like morphine was counteracted by naxolene.

Knowledge of endogenous neuropeptides with opiate properties is advancing and changing at bewildering speed, and while Bishop (1980)[96a] discusses the biochemistry and neurophysiological effects of two of these substances, together with a tabulation comparing their properties, more than 20 of these 'neuro-active' peptides, including a third form of enkephalin, have now been found in various regions of the central nervous system. While their number continues to increase almost weekly, there is little point in attempting a meaningful summary of current research findings.

When the present furore of discovery has settled somewhat, yesterday's physiology may well be transformed into a network of interactions:

... as intricate and ineffable as a spider's web. [Wingerson (1980)[1330a].]

It has been mentioned elsewhere (p. 487) that internal opiate activity may also be stimulated by the technique of acupuncture.

Hannington-Kiff (1977)[496] has suggested that:

... the ideal method of pain relief must always be prevention of the ingress of noxious stimuli rather than an attempt to suppress intense neural activity already in the central nervous system.

In summary, complex processes of modulation are mediated through many pathways.

The interactions ... may occur at successive synapses at any level of the central nervous system in the course of filtering the sensory input. Similarly, the influence of central activities on the sensory input may take place at a series of levels. The gate-control system may be set and reset a number of times as the temporal and spatial patterning of the input is analysed and acted upon by the brain.[842]

By the time the patient feels pain, a highly integrated and complex series of events has already taken place, and it should be emphasised that a simple stop-go conception, of pre- and postsynaptic inhibition of input at posterior root levels, is not sufficient to account for observed pain phenomena and experimental findings.

Whatever role dorsal horn synaptic inhibition does play, it is much more complex than some current hypotheses may account for, and its role is not that of solely determining whether an input will cause pain or not.[907]

Wall (1978)[1285] has restated the gate-control theory of pain mechanisms as follows:

1. Information about the presence of injury is transmitted to the central nervous system by peripheral nerves. Certain small diameter fibres (A delta and C) respond only to injury while others with lower thresholds increase their discharge frequency if the stimulus reaches noxious levels.

2. Cells in the spinal cord or fifth nerve nucleus which are excited by these injury signals are also facilitated or inhibited by other peripheral nerve fibres which carry information about innocuous events.

3. Descending control systems originating in the brain modulate the excitability of the cells which transmit information about injury. Therefore the brain receives messages about injury by way of a gate-controlled system which is influenced by (1) injury signals, (2) other types of afferent impulse and (3) descending control.

He mentions that it appeared to some that the entire theory rested on the simplified diagrammatic mechanism, essentially only a cartoon of the theory, as was made clear in the text. More recent work is summarised; for example, it is known now that loss of large fibres is not necessarily followed by pain, and the cause of pain in neuropathies remains as speculative as it was in 1965. Further work[250] has supported the theory that Lissauer's tract and the substantia gelatinosa are involved in the regulation of afferent impulses.

All the work since 1965 shows that cord cells responding to injury are subject to inhibitions of peripheral origin but the mechanism remains obscure ... that a gate-control exists is no longer open to doubt but its functional role and its detailed mechanism remain open for speculation and for experiment. [Wall, 1978.]

I. TENDERNESS

The concept of a spinal dorsal horn gate or filter for sensory input, itself yet subject to modulation by other very complex nervous system activities, both peripheral and central, and also to summation effects whereby the critical levels of excitation may exceed current 'gate settings', goes some way to improving understanding of some clinical features in vertebral pain syndromes. It is puzzling that an ordinarily innocuous stimulus, usually designated as touch or pressure, should become painful and sometimes exquisitely so, e.g. tender spinous and transverse processes in the region of vertebral joint problems, tender rib angles associated with lesions at thoracic levels, and tender posterior superior iliac spines in degenerative changes of the low lumbar segments.

Further, cutaneous areas of the trunk and limb girdles (Head's zones of cutaneous hyperalgesia, see p. 178) whose *somatic* innervation is segmentally equivalent to the *autonomic* innervation of a viscus, also become tender during abnormal states of the viscus concerned.[986, 1065] Though there are some differences between joints and between species there are reasons for the assumption that conditions are essentially the same in the cat and in man.[130, 998]

Electrical activity, originating in the cat spinal cord, was observed passing antidromically along posterior roots, beyond the ganglia, to the periphery in muscular and cutaneous nerves.[816] This dorsal root reflex, together with the dorsal root potential[69, 70] which was shown to be due to impulses arriving 'by the same rootlet or by neighbouring ipsilateral or contralateral roots', are factors integral to the gate-control theory.

An important feature of somatic sensibility is that any single spot on the trunk is innervated by fibres which run into many neighbouring posterior roots. In this context the observations of Sunderland (1968)[1191] are noteworthy:

The nature of the fibre branching in human cutaneous nerve trunks is such that, though the individual branches of a single fibre cannot be traced to their destination, there is justification for the belief that the territory served by a posterior root ganglion neuron is greater than is generally acknowledged to be the case, and that, as suspected by Walshe, it assumes macroscopic proportions. [Lavarack et al., 1951.]

The T cells of dorsal horn Lamina V normally have a restricted field of reception,[250] which governs the degree of their basal activity, so that the arrival of diffuse afferent traffic from the territory of several neighbouring segments is inhibited and effectively negated.[842] Full, normal sensibility,[907] and especially adequate spatial sensibility, depends on this great overlap of fibres from posterior roots, and at the primary posterior horn synapses of afferent fibres, there is convergence of input from these neighbouring roots. The threshold of T cells is not reached by input arriving in only one root; there has to be 'a background polysynaptic facilitation derived from stimulation of the same sensory field arriving via two or more roots'.[250]

Should inhibitory mechanisms be overcome by tissue abnormalities, initiating summation of afferent input exceeding the T cell threshold, two things have happened:

(i) Any single dorsal horn, and perhaps more than one, is 'receiving' through a gate which freely transmits stimuli from a wider region.

(ii) The area of neighbouring roots, including their distal extent, is effectively in a state of what may be conceived as peripheral facilitation, whereby the innocuous mechanical stimuli of touch and pressure, in the absence of normal inhibition, now become pain. The degree or intensity of these events will depend upon modulation activity described previously.

Thus tenderness may extend far distally, in the so-called 'innervation territory' of the segment(s) concerned, e.g. the subcutaneous head of the fibula in sciatica (but see below).

Should disease or abnormality of a viscus excite sufficient input traffic, via visceral afferents, to summate and exceed T cell thresholds, the segmentally linked cutaneous area will also be tender, faithfully reflecting the facilitated state of cord segments now indiscriminately, to a greater or lesser degree, allowing unimpeded and uninhibited traffic; some frank nociceptor impulses, some the normal ongoing basal activity of afferent traffic, but all enhancing facilitated T cell transmission levels.

N.B. A single important consideration requires emphasis, i.e. that if, in an experimental animal, many neighbouring dorsal roots are sectioned either side of a single root left intact, and the normal T cell inhibition of the intact root is removed by giving a subconvulsive dose of strychnine, the now facilitated single dorsal horn remaining will effectively transmit nociceptor stimuli from a wide area of supposedly denervated territory of neighbouring segments. Thus, dermatomes are not immutably fixed anatomical entities, but neurophysiological entities, their size and boundaries at a particular instant being an expression of the rising and falling levels of facilitation, and thus efficiency of sensory transmission, in the dorsal horns of spinal segments.[659] It is upon this basis that tenderness might reasonably be explained.

Bearing in mind the known phenomenon of referred abdominal tenderness, particularly manifest in vertebral joint problems at the thoracolumbar junction, the upper, middle and lower lumbar region and the sacroiliac joint, the coexistence of anterior spinal tenderness in low back pain syndromes should not be surprising (pp. 241, 251).

When palpating the region of the lumbosacral promontory, via the abdominal wall, O'Brien (1979)[945] found tenderness in more than three-quarters of patients with low back pain. Of a control group of 50 asymptomatic individuals, only 2 exhibited tenderness and both had experienced back pain during the previous three months.

Available evidence suggests that the sign of tenderness is not specific to particular levels, but generally indicative of lumbar abnormality.

J. VARIATIONS IN RELATIVE DENSITY, AND EFFECTS, OF DIFFERENT FIBRE POPULATIONS

Knowledge of the characteristics of mechanoreceptor and nociceptor fibres of different diameters, and of the extent to which pathological processes may upset relative population densities, provides the partial explanation of a number of painful states, and also the possibilities of selectively enhancing inhibitory-neurone activity by artificial stimulation.[653]

Mechanoreceptors. The process of ageing, as it succeeds physical maturity, is associated with progressive, selective degeneration of the larger-diameter, myelinated, afferent, mechanoreceptor neurones in all peripheral nerves, while the smaller-diameter unmyelinated fibres remain less affected by the degenerative process.[41]

It has been suggested that the diminished pain tolerance of elderly people may be due to the consequent loss of inhibitory effects exerted by afferent mechanoreceptor impulses on the dorsal horn gate mechanism.[1362] Further, the group II large-diameter fibres convey afferent impulses from touch and pressure receptors, and these fast-conducting fibres share in the degenerative depopulation of large neurones, helping to weight the relative numbers of fibres on the side of the small unmyelinated gate-facilitation neurones.

Wyke[1362] refers to a mechanism of mechanoreceptor depletion underlying the paravertebral zones of cutaneous hyperaesthesia which Glover[412(a)] observed in patients with backache, and these observations could be equated with the phenomenon of tenderness (above).

It is also suggested[933] that the intense cutaneous hyperalgesia in postherpetic neuralgia may be due to selective viral damage to the posterior root ganglion cells of large-diameter mechanoreceptor afferent neurones in the peripheral nerves, although this explanation may equally be applied to the large nociceptor afferents, and loss of their inhibitory effects.

Yet in four cases of postherpetic neuralgia, Weddell[907] compared affected and non-affected nerves, and found an *increase* in non-myelinated nerve fibres. Further, it has been observed[1378] that the individual large-fibre degeneration is followed by small-fibre degeneration. There are also neuropathies in which there is a decrease in the number of small fibres and yet there is a lot of pain.[907]

Nathan gives further examples of observations on ratios of nerve fibre degeneration in pathological states which do not support the concepts of Wall and Melzack.

Nevertheless, sufficiently encouraging successes (p. 487) have been achieved in the treatment of chronic, severe pain by the introduction of electrical excitation of large fibres (p. 488), either peripherally (p. 489) or by indwelling electrodes.[847, 27, 1117, 1280, 1311] The effectiveness and degree of analgesia produced appears to depend upon:

(i) The frequency of stimulation—a high frequency being more effective than a low frequency, and
(ii) The nature of the pain—a burning superficial pain being easier to deal with than a deep cramp-like pain.

This major step forward in the understanding and management of pain provides a significant basis for further development.

Encouraging results have been reported (Rutkowski, *et al.*, 1977)[1069] of the use of electrical stimulation in 367 unselected patients with chronic low back pain. All had been treated unsuccessfully by conventional methods and the lengths of history ranged from 6 months to 20 years.

Sterile hypodermic or acupuncture needles were used and the best results were obtained with the following parameters:

Shape of current	Sine wave
Frequency	1–2.5 Hz
Intensity	300–600 A
Voltage	5–15 V

The mean number of treatments was 11.

Effects were categorised as:

Relief		No. patients
100%	(no pain)	76
75%	(slight pain occasionally)	121
50%	(appreciable alleviation)	99
25%	(slight reduction in pain)	39
0%	(no effect)	32
		367

208 patients could be followed up for 6–36 months and, of these, 70 per cent asserted that relief of pain was similar to that at the end of treatment sessions.

K. TYPES OF PAIN

Some generalisations may be made about *common characteristics of pain associated with vertebral joint problems.* (More specific regional descriptions are given under Syndromes, p. 205.)

Introduction

A scientific and comprehensive attack on the problems of joint pain is increasingly evident in the expanding literature on:

pain and its neurophysiological basis[1285]
biochemistry and the ultrastructure of
    polysaccharides[4, 499]
the physical characteristics of intervertebral discs[807]
facet-joints and the natural history of
    cartilage[1155, 1008, 1009, 1010]
the genesis of degenerative processes[808, 1008]
biomechanics, stress analysis and ergonomics[1107, 1108, 231, 234]
the dynamic anatomy of neural canal
    structures,[119, 120, 121(a), 121(b)] and the conservative[1180(b)] and
    surgical[926] treatment and epidemiology[1338] of vertebral
    joint conditions.

It is an exciting time to be working in this field, and stimulating for those who have wearied of authoritarian pronouncements as a substitute for demonstrable clinical fact.

A rational approach to the problem of vertebral pain is to list[1062] and classify all of the structures from which pain *could* be arising, and among these of course are the ubiquitous connective-tissue structures, in their various forms. In the near or more distant future, it may well be that our clinical method will be precise enough to enable confident identification of the tissue(s) responsible for the patient's complaint. Having achieved this, our concurrent or next step is the improvement of methods of influencing the abnormal state of the tissue(s) concerned.

We shall probably remain bedevilled by the tendency of vertebral changes to involve a whole family of different tissues, by the complexity of the pain experience itself and by the clinically familiar situation of coping with long-standing abnormalities which have engendered a host of secondary changes.

Pending the desirable amount of information, a better awareness of the need for prompt attention to aches and pains persisting for more than a few days, and a clinical environment which encourages the best deployment of treatment skills, we can probably work to the greatest effect by emphasising, and basing treatment on, what is objectively verifiable, i.e. the signs and symptoms in themselves, rather than basing treatment on speculative concepts about them, or about what we feel *ought* to be producing them.

For these reasons, the priorities in this text are *the signs and symptoms per se*, which are objectively verifiable in the presence of the patient.

(i) Joint pain

In the absence of a clear history of trauma, or frank vertebral stress, which by their nature often clarify treatment indications, and in the absence of any radiological changes, especially those showing serious disease or significant mechanical defect, a dull, deep or nagging ache is typically reported in what are probably the early stages of degenerative joint disease; and which, in a general way, we term arthrosis and spondylosis.

The ache also characterises hypermobility syndromes of the low back, and can become severe, but in these cases there is often a history of trauma, especially in young people. Its distribution is not always easy for the patient to describe by outlining it on the body surface. The changes producing it appear to be confined to a joint and its periarticular structures, without physical involvement of the spinal cord or peripheral nerves. In the reasonable assumption, rather than the absolute and substantiated knowledge in all clinical situations, that this type of pain is caused by mechanical and biochemical irritation of nociceptors in synovial joint capsules, with the innervated connective tissue (see p. 10) of symphyseal joints probably concurrently involved (especially in the low lumbar and lumbosacral segments), treatment procedures which are likely to improve the fluid exchange in connective tissues are indicated, together with the removal of mechanical causes of nociceptor stimulation.

The proposed special characteristics of *arthrotic* pain, and those of *spondylotic* pain, are discussed on page 205 and it will thus be evident that treatment methods will need a general bias according to the behaviour of symptoms to achieve the best results; albeit individual assessment of the patient's needs should always have priority over theories.

In peripheral joints the area of pain or ache is described as 'an ache all round the joint', and in vertebral joint problems the description may be 'all across my back/shoulder blades/neck' but is frequently unilateral, or worse uni-

laterally, and the pain commonly spreads laterally and distally to limb girdle area when provoked.

Miller and Kasahara[860] have described small myelinated and unmyelinated fibres entering the numerous foramina of the epiphyseal and metaphyseal regions of long bones, traversing the thin cortex and supplying the interior of bone. Small unmyelinated fibres wind about the trabeculae of the spongiosa or spread out on the undersurface of the articular cartilage. It is tempting to ascribe the dull background ache of arthrosis to compressive effects impinging upon these plexuses, and they may well be involved in the production of joint pain, particularly since subchondral bone changes form part of the pathomorphology of degenerative change; yet it is difficult to equate this hypothesis with relief of symptoms by intra-articular hydrocortisone injections.

Reiman and Christensen (1977)[1025] have also demonstrated unmyelinated nerve fibres in the subchondral bone marrow of osteoarthrotic femoral heads; the nerves exceeded those found in normal control specimens, since they were related to the increased amount of vessels subchondrally in the bone marrow, in the granulation tissue and into the calcified layer of articular cartilage.

Whether the same occurs in vertebral degenerative disease, and might be a factor in vertebral pain, remains to be seen.

There is evidence[43,44,772] that the factor of engorgement, in the subchondral bone of arthrotic joints and in the spondylotic neural canal, should be borne in mind as a possible contributory factor in vertebral pain syndromes of this type. (See p. 62, Venous engorgement.)

Intraosseous vessels are richly supplied by adrenergic vessels.[281]

(ii) Ligamentous pain

The pain of oedematous connective-tissue joint structures, due to additional stress superimposed on a degenerative joint, may probably be the same as that encountered in peripheral joints, i.e. it is more usually a dull ache, worse after immobility or rest and aggravated by local tension. In hypermobility conditions, e.g. the 'loose back' syndrome, sustained tension on ligaments is probably the cause of localised pain provocation, albeit with a latency period of some 5 to 30 seconds, when testing positions of extension, side-flexion or flexion are statically held to observe their effect.

This holding of position is a useful assessment procedure, as in assessing root pain; with the difference that hypermobility pain is localised to the region of the joint but root pain spreads distally into a limb. The patient can usually locate the source of ligamentous pain in a peripheral joint with a fair degree of accuracy, and tests applying local tension assist in identifying it. For example, the patient can sometimes indicate with some precision the site of unilateral cervical pain which is only aggravated by active or passive movements applying tension to that aspect, but not by those which relax it.

It is tempting to regard this as an example of cervical ligament pain; the tension is applied to periosteal attachments of muscle, tendons and to musculotendinous junctions as well as to facet-joint capsules and ligaments, to dural root sleeves and other meningeal structures; yet resisted isometric contraction of the same muscles commonly does not hurt. Since one very short treatment session very frequently clears up this example of localised pain (when there are no other signs), and some three to six treatments may be required for what appear to be similar ligamentous problems at peripheral joints, the precise nature of the vertebral lesion is probably different; the presence of interbody and neurocentral joints as well as the foraminal structures cannot be discounted. It is this factor of multiple articulations, and many different types of specialised structural arrangement, which bedevils any attempt to accurately diagnose the site and nature of the lesion in benign vertebral joint problems.

For example, there are 97 synovial joints,[315] including rib and sacroiliac joints, 23 symphyseal joints and 10 neurocentral joints associated with the vertebral column, each synovial and neurocentral joint with its separate capsule and synovial system.

The number of ligaments between adjacent bones thus well exceeds 200, hence the futility and pointlessness of attempting specific diagnosis as in the minor strains of peripheral joints. It is particularly in this context that:

a. Junghann's[1093] concept of 'the mobile segment' and
b. the approach[797] of emphasising meticulous examination and informed assessment together with treatment procedures based on the signs and symptoms in themselves rather than on the diagnosis, are of fundamental clinical importance.

This is not tantamount to saying that diagnosis is unimportant, which would be foolish, but only that after an initial sorting procedure has allowed the conclusion that the painful condition is a benign musculoskeletal problem, an informed 'indications' examination by the person treating the patient will be much more productive and useful if it emphasises the *manner* in which the problem is manifesting itself, rather than becoming a perhaps interesting but nevertheless sterile exercise of intelligent guesswork as to which ligament is involved.

A burning ache is often reported when connective tissues appear to have been unduly stretched for periods; moderately sustained neck flexion produces a typical 'yoke' distribution of similar pain across the shoulders, and patients with lumbosacral instability describe a lumbar ache of this type after having had to stand, and sometimes to sit, for long periods. It can also be produced in treatment at suboccipital and yoke regions by badly adjusted sustained, and less frequently, rhythmic, traction to the neck.

The same type of pain occurs as a result of sustained stress on ligaments during habitually poor posture and sustained occupational stress, and seems very much as described in the tarsal, and long and short plantar, ligaments of the foot when the ache of foot strain is reported. The sprains or strains of moderate traumatic stress on the spine, as in clumsy lifting techniques, horseplay and minor accidents, may involve excessive tension on spinal aponeuroses and musculature, probably underlying a type of periosteal-attachment pain, seen peripherally in one type of tennis elbow, as part of the symptoms reported by the patient.

(iii) Muscle pain
In addition to the tension on vertebral muscle and its various arrangements of attachment-tissues, a prolonged increase of tone (see p. 196) in muscle overlying the lesion may add to the quota of pain reported by the patient, yet quite commonly, patients present with obvious hypertonus of muscle overlying joint problems but do not draw attention to the spasm as causing their pain, even when questioned specifically.

Also, asymptomatic individuals may for some days show obvious spasm of vertebral muscle groups, often unilaterally, and remain unaware of its presence until indicated to them.

The high nociceptor population of skeletal muscle, distributed as a plexiform network round all vessels except capillaries, is stimulated by environmental chemical changes; an accumulation of abnormal metabolites in muscle, notably lactic acid, 5-hydroxytryptamine (serotin), bradykinin and histamine, probably underlies some of the localised painful muscular aches which accompany joint problems. Again, prolonged enlargement of muscle vessels may, by mechanical distension of the vessel, depolarise its plexiform nociceptor membranes and also set up a contribution to muscular pain.[1362]

In normal individuals, muscles soon hurt if they are subjected to prolonged isometric contraction, or contraction in shortened positions, and more so if the individual is untrained or unaccustomed to this type of effort. These effects are more pronounced if the muscles are not 'warmed up' beforehand, or if the subject is elderly.[1362] The muscles will also become tender.

Muscles may also be painful and tender in irritative lesions involving segmentally related viscera.

The characteristic of vertebral and limb girdle muscle pain, which at times appears to be secondary to spinal joint problems, is more usually an oppressive weary ache and is most unlike the severe cramp pains commonly experienced, e.g. in the calf, from other causes.

Patients with no history of trauma to the soft tissues, and no evidence of infection, may initially report a median or slightly paramedian spinal pain, which after the interval of a day or longer spreads more laterally to overlie a large muscle group, which is obviously hypertonic and also tender.

Our difficulty is that the pain, tenderness and spasm, which we assume to have a common genesis (i.e. the joint abnormality), may be mediated via different mechanisms, e.g. the pain may be referred and not necessarily due to the accumulation of metabolites in the muscle (if metabolites do invariably accumulate). Further, the tenderness may also be referred (see p. 169). The hypertonus is reflexly provoked, without doubt, yet the association of pain with spasm may not necessarily be direct (see p. 196).

The muscular fatigue, and ache, which follow abnormal and prolonged postural stress, may not necessarily be the same as reflexogenic paravertebral spasm in muscles *not* being subjected to postural stress, and only related segmentally to the spinal abnormality.

Further, a common clinical experience is that of markedly diminishing or completely relieving pain overlying hypertonic paravertebral muscle, e.g. the trapezius or glutei, with one mobilisation technique and within 45 seconds, although complete eradication of the more median pain may require further mobilisation techniques or another treatment session. It seems unlikely that accumulated metabolites could be washed out of intercellular spaces of large muscle groups in that short duration. The relationship of spasm and pain may be more complex than we tend to assume (see p. 197).

(iv) 'Remembered' pain

In general terms, the amount of pain referred distally into a limb from vertebral joint problems governs the duration of treatment needed for its relief, and the further distal the pain the longer will be the treatment. Assessment of a patient's treatment needs may be inaccurate if history-taking is not sufficiently thorough.

Patients with a history of previous shingles, boils and carbuncles in the limb girdle regions and especially painful lacerations, sprains or fractures of limbs, may present with excessive pain, or pain reasonably out of proportion with coexisting signs, proximally or more distally in the associated limb.

It is important to note that the site of a previous and painful limb injury will be disproportionately painful if referred pain of vertebral degenerative disease later invades that limb. The central nervous system appears to retain a memory for previously well-trodden neurone pathways, and pain at the old site is easily rekindled in later years, even if the limb subsequently be amputated for other reasons.[906]

A common clinical observation is that weather changes affect symptoms more than signs. Climatic influences could affect the human body by various mechanisms; these include stimulation of thermoreceptors resulting in changes in dermal blood-flow and sweat secretion, disturbances of biological circadian rhythms and changes in the viscosity of the blood. The low-threshold Type I mechanoreceptors in joint capsules are very sensitive to *changes* of capsular stress, including that initiated by changes of atmospheric pressure.[1357] The same phenomenon of remembered pain frequently occurs during particular combinations of barometric pressure and prevailing weather, e.g. on an especially cold day a patient may report unexpectedly severe pain at the site of a previously painful fracture, the clinical presentation thus very closely simulating pain referred from a coexisting but actually well-localised vertebral joint condition. It is tempting to dwell on theories of 'storage of latent-facilitation in the computer-programme memory of the c.n.s.', and this may be speculative, yet there is plainly the registration of an experience, its storage and then its recall by the neural mechanisms underlying the pain experience.

(v) Night pain

'Pain and stiffness at night and early in the morning play a major part in the suffering caused by chronic rheumatic ... and painful musculoskeletal disorders.'[511]

Night pain is probably multifactorial, e.g.

a. The intellectual, occupational and/or emotional preoccupations of normal waking hours being reduced, cerebral modulation effects (p. 166) are likewise reduced, with the tendency and time for attention to brood over the injured part, and for the pain to intrude more forcefully upon consciousness. These effects may be enhanced if the patient is depressed, or is currently suffering a degree of emotional distress or feeling resentment about a marital, social or occupational injustice, real or supposed.

b. Lying down considerably reduces compressive effects on vertebral joints, with associated structures, and modifies the nature of physiological stress they normally sustain. Although usually the other way about, some patients will report quite severe midthoracic joint pain and lumbar pain at night, which is quickly relieved on sitting up or standing up. The intimate and regular association of posture and effect is too frequent to be coincidental, and on occasions this pain may be ligamentous (*vide supra*), and thus due to lateral translation stress on an abnormal joint, not possible when under the compression of standing.

The release of weight and traction effects on neurovascular bundles on lying down may also explain the onset of extrasegmental paraesthesiae in the upper limb, but this occurrence may also be due to the compressive effect on the upper lateral thorax when lying on the side, thereby 'shuffling' costovertebral and costotransverse joints whose plane is practically vertical on recumbency in side-lying. Clinical experience indicates that the upper thoracic joints are frequently involved in production of paraesthesiae without accompanying neurological signs, although the nature of the phenomenon remains unexplained. Simple compression often aggravates joint problems, as relief of it reduces pain.

c. It is characteristic of degenerative joint disease that pain and stiffness are increased after prolonged immobility, or rest, and this may wake the patient after some hours.

d. It is also characteristic of benign joint problems that particular movements and postures provoke symptoms; patients have their favourite ways of lying, but also turn and shift during the night, and these movements may light up the pain.

e. Bone pain in a limb due to a Brodie's abscess, or other staphylococcal or tuberculous infection, is characteristically worse at night, with a deep, constant, throbbing intensity causing most distress in the small hours of the morning (see blow).

f. Inexorable night pain, regardless of body position, raises the suspicion of neoplastic disease, inflammatory arthritis or osteitis, and psychogenic problems. NIP is a very useful mnemonic, and during history-taking the mandatory questions (p. 305) must not be forgotten, although it is wise to be hesitant in labelling any pain as psychogenic.

(vi) Throbbing pain

The rhythmic, pulsatile wave of arterial pressure is associated with the temporal quality of throbbing, beating and pounding pain. This characteristic quality may be mediated via the activity of Type II mechanoreceptors. These rapidly adapting low-threshold endorgans only fire off at the beginning and end of movement (or stress), and, of course, vascular pulsation is movement.

The vascular congestion accompanying inflammatory processes in vertebral joints, whether involving the capsules and ligaments of facet structures and/or the trespass of disc material and thus also the posterior longitudinal ligament and anterior aspect of the meningeal sleeve, undoubtedly contributes to the factors underlying the type of pain reported by the patient, i.e. mechanical depolarisation of nociceptors in capsule and ligament; biochemical stimulus of nociceptors, by the irritative polypeptide kinins of tissue breakdown; depolarisation of plexiform receptors in engorged venules and arterioles; stimulation of the local mechanoreceptor population as described.

The temporal quality of rhythmic surging, being superimposed upon the pain, may be due to the peripheral facilitation postulated in tenderness (on p. 168), in that normally unperceived mechanical stress in tissues are perceived as pain, or add increments to pain.

These pain states may be accompanied by obvious and palpable muscle spasm, and may not.

(vii) Bone pain

Congestion is usually painful, and when within the confines of an enclosed space, with rigid or semirigid boundaries, can be excruciating. Throbbing (above) is characteristic, but not all pain arising in sclerous tissue has this quality.

Pain may arise from a number of causes, e.g. (a) primary, but much more frequently secondary, neoplasm (see p. 121, (b) venous engorgement of vertebral veins of cancellous bone, and more especially the subchondral and juxtachondral bone abutting onto an arthrotic joint,[42, 43] (c) in osteoporosis of the lower thoracic spine, when the aching pain is very commonly referred to the lumbar area, and frequently but not always when stress fractures have occurred (it is wise to recall that 30–40 per cent of bone salts must be lost before osteoporosis is radiologically evident, and that 50 per cent of all thoracolumbar vertebral body fractures are pathological stress fractures), (d) in osteitis,[647] osteomyelitis, and (e) Paget's disease.[195]

Wyke[1362] draws attention to the particularly intense pain occasioned when the periosteum becomes involved in the changes occurring.

(viii) The 'irritable joint'

A not infrequent clinical experience, which becomes less frequent with awareness and recognition of its likelihood through careful history-taking, is that of a small and seemingly innocuous amplitude of joint movement, in testing procedures, treatment procedures or the activities of daily life, lighting up a disproportionate amount of intense pain; the severe exacerbation may last for many hours or more before pain settles to its pre-existing level.

The salient factor is the *unusually high reactive nature* of the joint condition, and this may be evident in (a) pain exacerbation immediately following a particular movement, and (b) the onset of severely increased pain being delayed, sometimes by some hours, and lasting sometimes more than a day.

In (a) it is probably reasonable to assume that the normally trivial nature of the movement or stress has been superimposed upon existing marked facilitation of substantia gelatinosa T cell transmission of nociceptor impulses to supraspinal centres (see p. 164), which state we probably express when we use the word 'irritability'. As a small splinter piercing the skin of the lateral shin is as nothing compared to the pain of the same splinter being driven into the nail-bed of a finger, so the trivial movement of a vertebral joint may be enough to provoke an increment of nociceptor activity which summates with existing and already facilitated traffic to produce pain out of all proportion to what might be expected. In (b) vascular congestion may be the dominant factor. If the nature of the lesion is such that a degree of tissue destruction has occurred (as opposed to the pain of tissues placed on tension by physical trespass of neighbouring structures) inflammatory changes will be present, with vascular stasis in the area.

Even a small amount of movement may be enough to locally mobilise inflammatory exudates with high concentrations of irritative products and/or add to the tissue damage with the further production of exudate over some hours, aggravating the vascular stasis which prevents normal fluid exchange between tissues and also provoking the further stimulation of plexiform nociceptors in vessels of the part.

States of irritability probably combine both of the factors postulated, in varying degree.

Mechanical analysis of acute exacerbations of pain should probably include several factors, e.g. (a) the biomechanical forces involved—bending over a basin with a supporting hand on the basin is very different from bending over a basin with both hands to the face. The difference in compressive forces on lower lumbar discs may be as much as 200–300 lb (90–135 kg). (b) The nature of the movement-abnormality—elevation and abduction of a shoulder may be difficult and painful, but not excruciatingly so, whereas internal rotation may be the exquisitely painful movement, and an unguarded reach for a hip pocket or waistband severely provokes the reactive joint. (c) The speed of the movement (as above)—the same movement performed more cautiously is often far less provoking. (d) One movement may apply tension to irritable structures, while all others do not disturb it or tend to relax the tension.

(ix) Root pain

Compression of spinal nerve roots, and peripheral nerves, does *not* necessarily cause pain;[116, 392, 750, 1194] the one is not an inevitable consequence of the other. Similarly, so far as the phenomenon of pain reference is concerned, the view that the referred pain and tenderness of root involvement is somehow different from referred pain of non-root involvement appears to have no demonstrable basis, although from clinical experience and experimental findings we know that when a nerve root *is* involved together with musculoskeletal changes, the pain will have a typical intensity and quality, and usually a more distal distribution. Put more succinctly, all root pain is referred pain, but not all referred pain is root pain. Further, the amount of pain referred distally into a limb need not be due solely to the inclusion of the nerve root in the changes which have occurred because joint problems, in the absence of root changes, also refer pain distally into a limb, and the two frequently coexist.

Pain with the qualities of 'severe, sickening toothache' in the arm or leg and with a distribution more readily outlined by the patient, may be secondary to root irritation and compression, though the cause-and-effect relationship is not necessarily direct (see p. 106).

The term *root pain* is probably justified when:

a. The pain has some of the unpleasantly malicious and severe qualities described

b. It is more severe in a limb than in proximal vertebral regions

c. It lies in the general distribution of a nerve root, with accompanying paraesthesiae being most pronounced in the distal territory of the dermatome

d. Exacerbation of the pain and/or painful paraesthesiae surging distally into the limb by vertebral movement begins after *a latent period* of a few seconds, sometimes longer, rather than simultaneously as occurs more commonly with musculoskeletal pain not apparently due to root involvement.

The pain may or may not be accompanied by neurological signs.

Limited spinal movement does not always accompany root pain syndromes, neither is foraminal encroachment always radiographically evident; even when evident at the vertebral segment related to the limb territory innervated by that root, the causal relationship is not thereby established. Patients often describe a sickening quality to this type of pain and it should be treated with care, since it is a clear manifestation of irritability and probably root irritability (although the mere appellation does not clarify why) and is easily stirred up by careless handling during examination and treatment.

Explanation of the noticeably delayed provocation of root pain and paraesthesiae, during and/or following a sustained testing movement, may possibly lie in that:

a. The selective effects of transient compression on nerve fibres of different diameters, and their selective rates of conduction recovery and thus nociceptor impulse reactivity; yet clinical observations are that existing and intense root pain in a limb is not suddenly *eradicated* by a testing movement, or during a position, which reduces the vertical dimensions of an intervertebral foramen—only that *added* pain is provoked after a latent period. This may well be done to small fibre activity, but the mechanism seems not fully understood. It might also be explained—

b. On the basis of a humoral mechanism, i.e. the dispersal and peripheral spread of the irritative exudates of root inflammation. Not all testing movements do invariably compress inflamed roots, but depending upon the degree of degenerative trespass existing, movements or postures may possibly displace exudate into surrounding tissues, with the effects of further reactive chemical depolarisation of nociceptors being somewhat delayed by the duration of return seepage of exudate. It may also be that the hydrodynamic buffer of chronic vascular congestion and stasis of the region may have a slight delaying effect upon the speed of mechanical end-organ depolarisation due to the movement itself.

Although staphylococcal infection is not the same as root irritation, those who have experienced the somewhat delayed onset of intense nauseating pain, lasting some hours, following accidental compression of a fulminating boil or carbuncle, will very well appreciate the latent exacerbation of an irritable and provoked nerve root. Presumably, both mechanical and humoral effects are often combined in varying degree.

(x) Other common examples of pain exacerbation are:

The severe 'shooting' pain provoked in a lower limb by a cough or sneeze, and added to existing sciatic pain, is probably often due to the sudden distension of vertebral veins directly caused by the rise in intrathoracic and intra-abdominal pressure. It may also possibly be due to mechanical depolarisation of nociceptors as the posterior annulus at the longitudinal ligament sustains the violent increase in tensile stress applied to the annulus fibrosus when the pelvis and thorax are approximated by the trunk musculature.

A momentary *localised* 'catch' or 'jab' of pain during a vertebral movement is reasonably associated with a disturbance of joint mechanics occurring at that point on the range, either due to a joint derangement or to instability of a segment, or both.

While 'burning' pain is produced by chemical irritation, a steadily increasing but localised burning ache in certain postures, or on sustained testing movements of cervical and lumbar regions, may possibly be stretch pain due to overmuch tension on ligaments, since it frequently accompanies syndromes of manifest hypermobility.

THE AUTONOMIC NERVOUS SYSTEM IN VERTEBRAL PAIN SYNDROMES

Under this heading it is convenient to discuss briefly one aspect of the question of what the *purpose* of manipulative and allied treatment is held to be; and by reason of the subject-matter this discussion is not as irrelevant as it may seem. Reference is often erroneously made to 'autonomic afferent neurones'; while the neurones of the visceral motor system are clearly distinguished, on morphological and physiological grounds, from the efferent somatic neurones supplying skeletal muscle, the appellation 'autonomic afferents' to visceral afferent neurones, and especially to those conveying impulses subserving visceral pain, has no valid basis as the autonomic system is entirely efferent. Certainly pain evoked by visceral afferents often has a subjective quality that distinguishes its experience from that of pain of somatic origin, but it is not autonomic pain and should be designated for what it is—namely, visceral pain.

Several factors might be considered:

a. The morphology of visceral afferent neurones resembles that of somatic afferent neurones (see p. 68).[437]

b. The dorsal spinal roots convey afferent traffic from the soma and viscera alike, and the dorsal spinal ganglia contain the nerve cell bodies of visceral as well as somatic afferents.

c. It has been shown[999] that the small-fibre nociceptive afferents from both somatic tissues and viscera converge on the Lamina V s.g. cells (p. 178) and the somatic and visceral afferent fibres, conveying nociceptive impulses, have the same histological appearance, being mainly unmyelinated neurones with diameters of 0.2 μm–1.5 μm[437] (although some somatic nociceptive afferents may be up to 5.0 μm in diameter).

d. Irritation of spinal joint nociceptors simultaneously evokes a large number of reflex alterations, including paravertebral muscle spasm and alterations in cardiovascular, respiratory and endocrine function.[1356]

e. Feinstein *et al.*[342, 343] by 6 per cent saline injections into thoracic paravertebral muscle tissues, induced referred pain together with pallor, sweating, bradycardia, fall in blood pressure, subjective 'faintness' and nausea.

f. Pain *unaccompanied* by a greater or lesser degree of visceral reflex activity, e.g. one or more of changes in pulse rate, blood pressure, vasomotor and temperature changes, sudomotor activity and pupillary diameter, never occurs.

Experimental evidence has been quoted to provide some support for a concept of 'autonomic pain'. Gross (1974)[459a] describes electrical and mechanical stimulation of the cervical sympathetic trunk during surgery under local anaesthesia—pronounced pain and much-increased anxiety were produced, the painful regions not corresponding to spinal somatic nerve distribution. Direct stimulation of the upper cervical ganglion produced severe pain in the ipsilateral mandibular teeth and postauricular area. Pinching the adventitia of the common carotid artery produced the same effect.

During complete lumbar anaesthesia, cutting of the splanchnic nerves induced cries of pain from the patient.

Gross further recounts how a topographically well-defined pain, such as a neuralgia of the ulnar nerve, may be successfully affected by local anaesthesia of the sympathetic nervous system. He suggests that in vascular pain (*vide supra*) the topography of vascular zones has the same significance for the analysis of such disorders as does the (vertebral) segment for the identification of diseases of the spinal cord and its roots.

Since:

(i) the concept of a dermatome, as *a fixed anatomical territory*, is fallacious, anyway
(ii) somatic roots also carry autonomic efferent neurones
(iii) the so-called 'autonomic' pain, produced by the experiments described, assuredly also evoked objective somatic changes such as muscle spasm and cutaneous hyperalgesia
(iv) it is axiomatic that pain as such invariably involves both soma and viscera

the insistence on such an entity as 'autonomic pain', pure and simple, requires gymnastics of logic which become a little unrealistic.

Thus there may be difficulty in deciding which words of the patient's description allow confident identification of a visceral contribution to the pain reported on every occasion. Therefore, it is suggested that autonomic pain is a term that should be dropped, as it is meaningless.

In *all* pain states, the somatic and autonomic nervous systems are activated, in a variety of manifestations and degree.

Considerations of spinal pain, and of referred pain (p. 189) in spinal conditions, should include attention to visceral reflex phenomena also. Musculoskeletal pain cannot be adequately considered in isolation from the associated changes in the efferent autonomic nervous system. There are similarities between the two systems in that: there is evidence that axon reflexes can be elicited at terminals of autonomic postganglionic fibres;[437] the phenomenon of 'peripheral axonal sprouting' occurs in sympathetic nerve fibres as in somatic nerves;[1105] degenerative changes in the autonomic system are the same as in the somatic system.[437]

Descriptions of pain

Melzack and Torgensen[844] arranged over 100 words, commonly used by patients to describe pain, into a kind of Roget's *Thesaurus* of adjectives and pointed out that to specify pain in terms of *intensity* only was not enough. The *quality* of pain may also have a meaning, e.g.

Causalgic pain	burning, searing (yet occasionally this results from badly administered cervical traction)
Visceral pain	stabbing, cramping (yet this also occurs in joint problems)
Vascular congestion	throbbing, pounding pain
Rheumatism and arthritis	gnawing, nagging pain
Menstrual pain	cramping, heavy, drawing
Haemorrhoidal pain	smarting, itching.

Among the oft-employed adjectives (many of a sensory nature in terms of temporal, spatial, penetrative, pressure and thermal qualities, and of an evaluative nature ranging from 'mild' to 'unbearable') were those describing affective qualities and visceral properties, like 'exhausting, fatiguing, nagging, heavy, tiring, choking, nauseating, sickening, suffocating, wretched'. The authors make the point, however, that the multiplicity of words to describe the experience of pain lends support to the view that it is a label representing a myriad of different experiences, refuting the traditional concept that pain is a single modality with one or two qualities only. Words with the affective qualities mentioned above, among the rich variety of expressions employed to convey the particular nature of their suffering, are very frequently used by patients with degenerative joint conditions of the spine, and the circumstance that we suspect a proportion of these pains may, for instance, be arising from venous engorgement (p. 63) is perhaps insufficient justification for asserting that this or that proportion is visceral (in this case, vascular) pain, and the rest is just 'ordinary' pain, because the vascular afferents from the spine are somatic afferents.

Having experienced more than one short, sharp bout of renal colic, as well as acute unilateral lumbar joint pain which was relieved by specific mobilising techniques, the author's own experience is that there was not a great deal to choose between them in terms of quality, although the difference in intensity was marked. Both occupied the identical body region, and in both the whole animal was involved.

Neuwirth (1952)[916] describes autonomic pain as dull, deep-seated pain; lancinating, throbbing, smarting, burning; associated with formication, numbness, chilliness, hyperaesthesia; tingling, fullness and puffiness; and further, the pain is not confined to dermatome boundaries.

While some of these adjectives are mutually exclusive, making recognition of so-called autonomic pain difficult, and while a somewhat inflexible reliance upon the significance of whether a pain lies in the territory of a 'dermatome' or not is shown to be misleading, an increased awareness of involvement of autonomic neurones in all vertebral pain syndromes[518, 571, 598, 917, 1168, 1342] can do nothing but good, increasing our understanding of the comprehensive nature of musculoskeletal pain, and thankfully putting yet further behind us the clinical encounters during which the physician or therapist demonstrates to the patient, with the aid of diagrams, that they cannot possibly be suffering from the pain and other symptoms for which they have sought help, simply because the clinical features do not accord with a particular concept.

Suggesting that associated changes in the efferent autonomic system are part of *all* painful states is not to say that (a) some vertebral joint problems, particularly in the cervical spine, do not exhibit an array of symptoms and signs which appear to involve the sympathetic and parasympathetic systems as responsible for the more distressing aspects of the patient's condition, nor (b) that peripheral injuries such as fractures may not involve the vertebral and upper costospinal articulations in secondary changes associated with limb symptoms of a particularly prolonged and disabling degree (see p. 185), nor (c) that irritative conditions of a viscus may not be reflected in manifest vertebral changes, with alterations of cutaneous sensibility in segmentally related somatic areas.

There is evidence that the same visceral afferent fibres subserve both normal visceral sensation and also pain.[588] Nathan[906,907] observed, 'one can suggest that the signalling of events from the viscera is simple, because there are only simple events to report; but the events occurring to the outside of the body are of many kinds and they may require a more complicated system to report them'.

The simple events affecting viscera and amounting to noxious stimuli are mainly distension and traction; yet these are non-nociceptive (i.e. mechanoreceptor) visceral afferents. Cutting or burning the bowel, for instance, does not cause pain, although ischaemia of cardiac muscle is intensely painful.

In animals visceral afferent fibres are slightly activated by passive disturbances of a viscus, and more intensely activated by active contraction. Intense contractions of these viscera in man, e.g. the stomach, causes pain[907] One may hypothesise that, in comparison to the cutaneous ability to register the wealth and variety of changes in man's external environment, the three main categories of events (with their consequences) likely to occur in the deeper musculoskeletal tissues are (a) mechanical trauma, distraction or trespass by related tissues, (b) infectious invasion, and (c) non-infectious but noxious changes in their biochemical environment. If this notion is correct, the degree of organisation and sophistication of the locomotor tissue nociceptors together with their peripheral connections is possibly somewhere between those of skin and viscera, although both appear to share an enormous wealth of spinal and supraspinal synaptic pathways.

Visceral and somatic convergence

The principle of metameric segmentation, linking vertebral segment to the spinal cord segment, spinal roots and sympathetic trunk, includes the innervation of internal organs.[686]

Thus, general visceral afferent fibres occur in the vagus, glossopharyngeal and possibly other cranial nerves, and in the second, third and fourth sacral nerves, i.e. the *parasympathetic pathways*. In general, the afferent fibres occupying the pre- and postganglionic pathways of the *sympathetic system* from soma and viscera have a segmental arrangement[437] as follows:

Head and neck	T 1–5
Upper limb	T 2–5
Lower limb	T10–L2
Heart	T 1–5

Bronchi and lung	T 2–4
Oesophagus (caudal part)	T 5–6
Stomach	T 6–10
Small intestine	T 9–10
Large intestine as far as splenic flexure	T11–L1
Splenic flexure to sigmoid colon and rectum	L 1–2
Liver and gall bladder	T 7–9
Spleen	T 6–10
Pancreas	T 6–10
Kidney	T10–L1
Ureter	T11–L2
Suprarenal	T 8–L1
Testis and ovary	T10–11
Epididymis, ductus deferens and seminal vessels	T11–12
Urinary bladder	T11–L2
Prostate and prostatic urethra	T11–L1
Uterus	T12–L1
Uterine tube	T10–L1

Lamina V cells of the substantia gelatinosa receive multiple inputs.[846] The relation between input at the posterior horns from soma and viscera was reported by Kostyuk (1968),[680] who demonstrated that afferents from the viscera can cause presynaptic inhibition upon somatic afferent impulse traffic, and also exert postsynaptic inhibition which is under supraspinal modulatory control from the bulbar reticular formation. It was also shown[999] that visceral afferents inhibit the effect of converging afferent impulse traffic from the skin, and conversely, stimuli to the skin can cause inhibition of Lamina V neurones on which visceral afferents terminate.

There was the same mutual inhibition exhibited by group III afferents from skeletal muscles and skin.

Expressed briefly, Hinsey and Phillips (1940)[544] postulated, as had, in effect, Sturge (1883),[1185] Ross (1888)[1061] and McKenzie (1909)[832] that both visceral and somatic afferents are capable of acting on common spinal cord pools of neurones, which are subject to summation, facilitation and inhibition effects, and this view is supported by more recent experimental findings.[272]

Thus in disease of a viscus, the patient will very frequently experience cutaneous pain; this painful skin area will often be acutely tender and cutaneous vasoconstriction may also be evident. Further, the underlying muscle will show a greater or lesser degree of hypertonus, i.e. spasm.[635] The skin areas of the body wall which have the same segmental innervation as a particular viscus, one somatic, the other autonomic, and which show the changes mentioned in visceral disease, are termed 'zones of secondary hyperalgesia'.

As Head[526] discovered in his studies of herpes zoster these zones or segments are garland-shaped zones of skin. The zones of secondary hyperalgesia of Head, Kappis-Lawen and Lemaire[686] are tabulated in Table 7.1 and if

Table 7.1

	Head	Kappis-Lawen	Lemaire
Heart	C3–C4. T1–T8	—	C3–C4. T1–T5
Descending aorta and aortic arch	C3–C4. T1–T3	—	C3–C4. T1–T3
Thoracic aorta	—	—	T4–T7
Pleura	—	—	T2–T12
Oesophagus	(T5)–T8	T5–T6	T1–T5–T8
Stomach	C3–C4. (T6) T7–T8	T6–T8 (T9)	(T5) T6–T9
Liver and biliary tract	C3–C4. T7–T10	T9–T10	(T5) T6–T9 (T10)
Pancreas	—	T8	T6–T9
Intestine	T9–T12	—	—
Small intestine	—	T9–T10	T9–T11
Large intestine	—	T11–T12	—
Transverse colon	—	—	T9–T10
Descending colon	—	—	T11–T12
Rectum	S2–S4	—	—
Kidneys and ureters	T10–L1 (L2)	T11	T1–L1
Adnexa	T11–L1	T12–L1	—
Peritoneum	—	—	T5–T12

these are compared with each other and also with Tables 2.1 and 2.2[635] and with Figure 2.23 it will be evident that (a) the zones roughly accord with the trunk dermatomes, and (b) there is considerable variation within a broadly generalised pattern.

Kunert[686] observed that hyperalgesic zones are more commonly found in acute and subacute visceral disease than in the more chronic disorders.

Somatovisceral and viscerosomatic reflexes

Kuntz[688] has observed that,

... reflex responses of viscera, including splanchnic blood vessels, elicited by localised stimulation of segmentally related skin areas, are common physiological events. The efficacy of cold and warm applications in the treatment of visceral disease undoubtedly depends upon the reflex responses elicited through cutaneous stimulation.

Conversely, Elbe[310] has demonstrated that stimulation of a viscus produced spasm of spinal muscles in two or three segments on the same side of the vertebral column, and innervated by the same segments. If the stimulus is intense more vertebral segments show motor irritability, and sometimes this irritability will spread to the contralateral side. Renal colic (uroliathis) is a good example of an irritative lesion of a viscus inducing spasm of vertebral muscle in the loin, tenderness of skin and pain—the question of whether the pain is 'in the muscle' or 'over the ureter region' is not as simple as it looks[1062] (see Referred pain, p. 189).

Sato[1083] has clearly shown that noxious cutaneous stimulation will decrease the frequency of pyloric contractions, and that this cutaneogastric reflex is mediated at spinal segmental level. He also describes cutaneocardiac and cutaneovesical reflexes, and in the latter showed that perineal stimulation can reflexly affect bladder function, in either an excitatory or an inhibitory way depending upon whether the bladder is resting or not.

Kennard and Haugen (1955)[650] report an investigation of patients with cardiac disease and a familiar reference of pain to shoulder, pectoral area and medial arm. These patients have the well-known pectoral and periscapular 'trigger spots' which when firmly pressed will severely exacerbate existing pain for many hours. Further, injection of local anaesthetic into these trigger spots will considerably reduce local tenderness and pain, and also the retrosternal pain over the diseased viscus. The pain may even disappear permanently.[1235]

This has important implications for the field of diagnostic local anaesthesia, and it is for these reasons that it is wise to note that the eradication of local pain of musculoskeletal origin also, by injection of a local anaesthetic in limb girdle areas, does not necessarily indicate that its source has been thereby demonstrated, e.g. bicipital tendinitis. Less tender but similar small, localised and pressure-sensitive areas in normal subjects will produce marked discomfort when pressure is applied, and these normally sensitive regions should be well known to anyone experienced in the field of benign joint problems.

Stoddard[1180a] draws attention to medical opinion, of some 25 years ago, which observed that, 'the sharp distinction which is customarily drawn between the autonomic and somatic nervous systems, though useful for purposes of description, is to a considerable extent misleading'.

It would not be difficult to gather together a tediously long list of somatovisceral and viscerosomatic reflex behaviour, but the essential point is that disease/abnormality of viscera or somatic vertebral structures is an abnormality of the whole animal, and will involve the whole animal in the pain experience, with all its associated phenomena.

This two-way traffic, of cause/effect/cause, all traversing the related cord segment(s) (and also initiating a two-way traffic up and down between the cord segments, and with the 'master ganglion'[1123] of the autonomic system, the hypothalamus, and the nociceptor pathways, outlined on p. 165) provides not only the basis of autonomic neurone involvement in spinal pain syndromes, but also the explanation of why osteopaths and chiropractors set so much store by an understanding of the neurophysiology of autonomic nervous systems and of which viscus is innervated by which spinal segments, in the expectation that certain visceral conditions may be influenced to a degree by spinal manipulative treatment.

The osteopathic concept[1180b] is that the focus of this viscerosomatic and somatovisceral activity is the 'facilitated spinal cord segment(s)', and that the principle of osteopathic treatment is the disintegration of the disease-producing pattern by the appropriate manual or mechanical 'adjustive' technique applied to the vertebral column.[1180a]

For those who are not osteopaths or chiropractors, yet informed and experienced in manipulative work, knowledge of the foregoing examples of the intimate link between soma and viscera does not mean that manual treatment of the vertebral column necessarily implies acceptance of the notion that one of its purposes is to influence visceral disease. Since treatment without indication is a speculation, and since ordinary, workaday clinical competence to recognise and assess comprehensive indications in the whole field of thoracic and visceral disease would require the combined skills of physician, and abdominal and thoracic surgeon, it is probably unwise to profess, or imply, this as part of the basis of physical treatment of the spinal column.

All those experienced in manipulation can report numerous examples of migrainous headaches, dysequilibrium (vertigo), subjective visual disturbances, feelings of retro-orbital pressure, dysphagia, dysphonia, heaviness of a limb, extrasegmental paraesthesiae, restriction of respiratory excursion, abdominal nausea and the cold sciatic leg being relieved by manual or mechanical treatment of the vertebral column, but while these effects are noted,[687] and the underlying mechanisms investigated with the purpose of understanding better what we do, they are insufficient reason to put the cart before the horse.

In other words, the prime impulse for physical treatment of the vertebral column is properly vertebral column disorder, and not visceral disorder. This is not to say that the comprehensively trained non-medical manipulator is not a skilled and well-informed professional but only that those who have not undergone this type of training do well not to profess the basis of it; because it will add no more arrows to their quiver, and the posture is unnecessary.

Further, this question is entirely separate from manipulative work itself, which is a prerogative shared by many disciplines and which in the last decade or two has seen significant developments by other than osteopaths and chiropractors.[797, 798, 445, 451, 835, 627, 48]

The following case-history[686] *illustrates important points:*

A 46-year-old woman slipped when doing her housework and, in an attempt to prevent herself from falling, twisted the upper part of her body. She immediately felt a violent pain beneath her left shoulder blade, accompanied by sweating and shortness of breath. For days afterwards she had the impression of a 'respiratory block', especially when she breathed in. The doctor called in to see the case thought, quite reasonably, that the patient may have suffered a spontaneous pneumothorax, but this could not be confirmed by either physical or radiological examination. Acute pleurisy was also considered, especially as the left half of the thorax seemed to lag behind a little during respiration. Coronary thrombosis was likewise regarded as a possibility, but further tests failed to provide any supportive evidence. The X-ray picture, however, showed slight thoracic kyphosis, Schmorl's nodes, and narrowing of the intervertebral discs from T3 to T5; the patient was suspected of having had Scheuermann's disease at some time in the past.

A final diagnosis was only established by careful palpation of the thorax, the thoracic spine, and the region of costovertebral attachments; it was here, in fact, that the source of intense neuralgic pain was located, the patient reporting violent pain in response to pressure exerted on the spinous processes of T3 and T4, as well as on a point three fingerwidths to the left of this area.

Depending upon one's standpoint, these events may be viewed as:

a. Evidence of somatic joint changes influencing the function of a major viscus (the lung) by somatovisceral reflex behaviour; the sudomotor changes of increased sweating, incidentally, providing ample evidence of autonomic involvement in pain syndromes, or
b. Reflexly induced severe spasm of intercostal and diaphragmatic musculature mediated by nociceptor and mechanoreceptor stimulation, coupled with voluntary muscle guarding against any movement likely to exacerbate a severely painful and acute costovertebral joint condition.[1357]

Any experienced manipulative therapist faced with this history and the manifest clinical features would have carefully examined the thoracic joints as the prior emphasis of investigation, and drawn the obvious conclusions as to treatment, once serious visceral disease had been excluded. Examples of this kind are very common[571] and Kellgren[642] refers to the manner in which pain from somatic structures may closely simulate visceral disease, faithfully reproducing the character and distribution of visceral pain, of angina with breathlessness, abdominal pains with nausea and vomiting, the flatulence of choleocystitis and the frequency of renal disease; additionally, visceral signs such as abdominal tenderness and abdominal rigidity are often produced.

In many of these cases back movements were painless, and it was not until the spine was examined *segment by segment* that the pain was provoked.

In summary, perhaps the fairest comment on these matters is that of Kunert,[686]

... the diagnostic importance of spinal lesions must not be overestimated, as it so frequently is, and that, in particular, the origin of disorders of the internal organs should be sought in such lesions only when all other possible explanations have been examined and discarded. Nothing can discredit the inherent diagnostic value of the relationship between the spine and the internal organs more than to insist on finding such a connection where none exists and to seek corroboration in threadbare hypotheses. *We have no evidence that lesions of the spinal column can cause genuine organic disorders.* They are, however, perfectly capable of simulating, accentuating, or making a major contribution to such disorders. There can, in fact, be no doubt that the state of the spinal column does have a bearing on the functional status of the internal organs.

Stoddard (1969)[1180b] observes, 'To claim that mechanical lesions are the only aetiological factors in disease is, of course, ludicrous. They are rarely if ever totally responsible, but they cannot *or should not be discounted in any disease.*'

N.B. The poor localisation of visceral pain, the reactions of viscera to noxious stimuli and observations on so-called 'true' visceral pain are under Referred pain (p. 194).

Further examples of autonomic involvement require consideration; and these are very commonly seen in degenerative and traumatic conditions of the craniovertebral, cervical and cervicothoracic regions.

The neck has been aptly described as 'a triumph of packaging'; a great variety of structures and specialised tissues is contained in a region which bears the weight of the head, transmits and protects vital parts of the vascular, respiratory, digestive and nervous systems and yet is the most mobile part of the spinal column.

Inevitably, there is little room for trespass by one tissue upon the territory of another, and most of the more serious effects of degenerative change in the cervical spine are due to this circumstance, since it is common that cervical structures with widely differing and important functions are closely packed side by side.

A host of facial and cranial symptoms, including headache, together with disturbances of vision, hearing and equilibration, can arise from benign abnormalities of the craniovertebral joints and associated structures; abdominal queasiness or nausea, and vomiting, may also be encountered. The salient facts of anatomy, and of articular, vascular and neural function require consideration, with special emphasis on the atypical articulations of the upper two segments, upon mechanoreceptor function of the upper cervical joints, on the great variability of the mode of vascular supply and venous drainage (pp. 2, 6, 7) and the many links between somatic roots, cervical sympathetic ganglia and postganglionic branches, and the ninth and tenth cranial nerves.

The variety of signs and symptoms presented by patients need not all be *primarily* due to autonomic nerve involvement, yet it is probably infrequent for this not to be underlying a greater or lesser proportion of the clinical features, by reason of sharing in the changes essentially brought about by trespass, oedema and inflammation.

With reference to degenerative change, Campbell and Parsons,[156] Neuwirth[916, 917] and Cailliet[149] refer to additional symptoms and signs, which are not limited to somatic root distribution and which do not seem to be due to involvement of the somatic sensory or motor fibres of cervical nerve roots. Those most frequently encountered may be listed as follows:

Equilibration	giddiness, listing
Vascular system	pulse and BP alterations, pallor, facial flushing, feelings of fullness and puffiness of the face, sensations of hot and cold in the fingers, puffiness of fingers, facial sweating
Hearing	tinnitus, roaring in the ears
Pain	precordial distress, facial pain, cranial pain, pain in or behind the eyeball, auricular pain
Vision	decreased visual acuity ('foggy window' syndrome), tingling *in* the eyeball, retro-orbital pressure, ptosis[1052]
Sensibility	dysaesthesia in the face, tightness and tingling of the scalp, formication of neck and face, numbness of facial areas, pharyngeal paraesthesiae such as tickling in the throat, 'a lump in the throat', dysphagia.

Changes of pupillary diameter, and frank dysphonia or aphonia are also seen.[1105, 242]

HEADACHE

The pathogenesis of face and head pain is a complex subject[1355] and despite a great deal of research which has provided new information, much about its causation remains unclarified.

The smooth muscle of blood vessels can give rise to pain, apparently similar in mechanism to that when spasm occurs in the smooth muscle of internal organs.[518]

There *is* vascular sensibility—clinical evidence substantiates that blood vessels have sensory nerves, like other visceral afferents.[130] Neuwirth[916] considers that the vascular pains in facial areas supplied by the branches of the external carotid artery are produced by vasoconstriction, because of irritation of the sympathetic nerves in the artery. While not all would agree with the discogenic origin of symptoms, or call the pains sympathetic, his observations of 25 years ago are as relevant today:

Facial pain in cervical discopathy may appear in such diversified forms that they are apt to baffle even a skilful diagnostician if he is not acquainted with the bizarre characteristics of sympathetic pain. Often the pains are erroneously assumed to originate in the structures where they are felt, for instance in the eyes, the ears, the tongue, the gums and the lips (orolingual paraesthesiae). In the effort to discover the underlying cause of the craniofacial pains, dentists, otolaryngologists, ophthalmologists and other specialists are consulted; the skull, the sinuses, the orbits, the jaws and the teeth are X-rayed, and many types of treatment are employed, including surgery, but to no avail. Eventually some patients, despairing of relief, become neurotic and resort to narcotic drugs to alleviate their sufferings.[295, 296] Finally, physicians, unable to discover signs of organic pathology, make an ultimate diagnosis of psychosomatic pains. Such a mistake may be serious, with harmful consequences.

Unilateral occipitofrontal headache, so often the dominant feature of craniovertebral joint problems and so often relieved by accurately localised mobilisation of these joints, is frequently described by patients as 'my migraine', although the term has tended to become a portmanteau word covering any and every type of headache, with the consequence that some confine the term to classical migraine and others employ it for all headache, in the milder to most severe forms.

It has been stated that classical migraine occurs in approximately 10 per cent of patients with migraine,[386] and this aptly describes 'the tail wagging the dog' state of affairs with regard to the terminology of headache.

Much migraine is attributed to arterial dilatation, and during the headache phase of an attack of classical migraine there is dilatation of the arteries of the scalp and an increase in cerebral blood-flow. The question of why some patients with migraine should experience unilateral headache is not understood; there is both clinical and experimental evidence to suggest that the vascular changes in migraine are bilateral, and yet the pain remains predominantly unilateral.

The suggestion that serotonin (5–HT) might play some role in the normal regulation of the tone of the cranial arteries, and that a sudden lowering of the blood serotonin levels might lead to a loss of constrictor effect, resulting in arterial dilatation and, clinically, an attack of migraine, has been a central hypothesis for some years, yet the evidence supporting the regulatory effects of serotonin is scanty.[1158]

Clinical experience leads to the conclusion that whatever the mechanism may be, much headache is very closely linked with movement-abnormalities of the upper cervical joints[1242] and sometimes with degeneration changes at joints of the lower cervical[285] and upper thoracic regions. An important anatomical feature is the distribution of the meningeal branches, of the spinal nerves C1, C2 and C3, to the floor of the posterior cranial fossa. Some of the nerves cross the mid-line.[657]

With regard to autonomic neurone involvement in the genesis of headache, Sheldon (1967)[1120] has suggested that the precise nature of the trespass upon nerve roots is less important than the fact of irritation of the sympathetic nerve component in cervical nerve roots. He regards this irritation as initiating the abnormal vasomotor responses, the resultant headache, and the sometimes bizarre but nevertheless explicable associated symptomatology.

Degenerative and traumatic conditions of the cervical spine can simulate so many of the clinical features of migraine, trigeminal neuralgia and vertigo; one is led to the conclusion that any such diagnosis reached *without* a comprehensive and competent examination of the cervical spine, including careful palpation, may be based upon findings which are incomplete.[202]

With reference to trauma of the neck and/or head, and the chronic, bizarre symptoms characterising these injuries, there is from research findings a gratifying increase in objective evidence which substantiates the patient's complaints.[205, 260, 598, 679, 919, 967, 985, 1224, 1225, 1226, 1231, 1257, 1363]

At the time of sustaining forces of deceleration or acceleration, symptoms akin to cerebral concussion may be experienced, with momentary lapse of consciousness or an intracranial blinding, explosive sensation. This is followed by headache, restlessness, mood changes, insomnia and vasomotor instability.[149]

The syndrome is described because it is similar to the kind of clinical picture seen in many cases of degenerative joint disease of the neck and upper thorax, although perhaps less dramatically and less distressingly. Seventy-two patients who had sustained this type of trauma were examined by tests of vestibular function, audiometry and electronystagmography.[1224] Bearing in mind that cerebral concussion, gross haemorrhage and contusion of the brain can be produced by 'whiplash' injuries, and that acute flexion and extension of the neck can also produce transient ischaemia or haemorrhage in the labyrinth, the investigators sought objective evidence of the vertigo—an hallucination of rotatory movement; dysequilibrium—sensations of instability without rotatory movement; roaring, hissing, ringing noises in one or both ears; hearing loss; difficulty in understanding speech, reported by these patients.

These are not purely disturbances of the autonomic system as such, but with these complaints they had pain, of course, and neuropsychiatric symptoms. We recall the numerous connector pathways between hypothalamus and cortex. Some tend to attribute these symptoms to emotional factors, but the investigators produced objective evidence that over two-thirds of the patients showed specific abnormalities underlying their complaints. Most of the pathology was subtle, and not immediately apparent on cursory examination.

An incidental finding was that vestibular abnormalities were more common than auditory abnormalities.

Kosay and Glassman[679] note that patients with cervical spine trauma frequently present symptoms apparently out of proportion to objective findings, and by further audio-vestibular evaluation revealed tangible abnormalities in about 50 per cent of their cases. They observed tinnitus, high-frequency sensorineural loss, semicircular canal weakness and positional nystagmus; and assert that the nystagmus may be vascular, neurogenic or neuromuscular in origin. Thus a number of factors[657, 1145, 598, 586, 587, 94, 118] may be contributing to the patient's distress, and prominent among these is emotional disturbance.

This extract from Wolf,[1333] indicates the tenuous and sometimes unjustifiable basis for pronouncing that these patients are imagining their difficulties:

The frequent association of manifestations of physiological dysfunction with overt emotional disturbance has led to the widely accepted but confusing proposition that emotions are the cause of bodily reactions. The confusion is further compounded by the difficulty of defining an emotion ... the old concepts of autonomic organization are being revised, qualified, and elaborated. In place of the automatic, sympathetic–parasympathetic balance theory there has emerged evidence for an almost unbelievably complex system of excitatory and inhibitory neurons and of enzymes and enzyme-inhibitors that provide elegant regulatory checks and balances through their effects on membranes. These effects are now known to be discrete and purposeful as they play their part in everyday adjustment, while they are generalised and 'shotgun-like' only under catastrophic circumstances.

The complicated cause-and-effect relationship of trauma to sensitive structures and upset to delicately balanced functions, the depression caused by this and sometimes by therapists' ill-concealed disbelief when bizarre symptoms are reported, together with disappointment at lack of progress and sometimes gradual loss of interest by therapists handling the patient, bedevil the lives of these unfortunate people. It should not be surprising that some cannot stand up to this prolonged onslaught upon themselves from within and without, and begin conveniently to develop and exhibit the very neurotic traits wished upon them by trauma and occasionally by unimaginative handling, but which were not there previously—the cycle is thus complete, and sometimes its inexorable progression has all the elements of Greek tragedy.

Theories of causation
The precise nature of the disordered function responsible for these symptoms and signs is not easy to clarify, and it is important to remember that two or more factors may be operating at the same time in one patient, e.g.

1. It has been determined that interfering with afferent impulse traffic from upper cervical joints in experimental animals produces nystagmus and disturbance of equilibrium,[238, 94] and the somewhat alarming dysequilibrium of patients can be due to the disordered and abnormal patterns of afferent impulse traffic from the mechanoreceptor

endings in the upper cervical synovial joints, because of the effects of degenerative change, and trauma, suffered by these soft tissues.[598, 1363] The veering, weaving types of dizziness (vertigo) often reported, and the 'listing' seen in patients, may have this basis. We recall that the upper neck joints are prime organs of equilibration.

2. There may be vertebrobasilar ischaemia, due either to atheroma of the vertebral artery, or because of trespass by osteophytes or thickenings of adjacent soft tissues. This trespass may, for example, be transient, occurring only on certain movements.[981]

3. There may be vertebrobasilar ischaemia due to *spasm* of the artery, following irritation of the accompanying plexus by the same vertebral joint changes.[242]

4. Mechanical trespass upon the vertebral artery is frequently demonstrated by vertebral angiograms, yet in 15 cases of poor progress after cervical trauma,[1257] only 1 patient was shown to have mechanical obstruction on head rotation—though the investigators agreed that transient arterial constriction could be present in more subtle or functional ways. They report that in these patients there are many disorders such as cold extremities, excessive sweating and oversensitivity to environmental stimuli; and by mecholyl, temperature and e.e.g. tests conclude that there is much to support the suggestion[1257] that a suitable term for many aspects of this clinical state might be 'autonomic nervous system concussion'.

5. Direct mechanical irritation of sympathetic and parasympathetic neurones may underlie some of the distressing concomitant symptoms like disturbances of visual acuity, nausea, vomiting, voice disturbances and difficulties with swallowing.[242]

6. Maigne[792] postulates a vasculosympathetic mechanism for unilateral supraorbital headache, on the anatomical basis that (a) the sympathetic plexus around the internal carotid artery is continued into the cranial cavity and accompanies the arterial branches, thus also emerging via the supraorbital foramen with the supraorbital artery, and (b) the superior cervical ganglion communicates with spinal nerve roots C1, C2 and C3. Thus a somatic–autonomic–vascular link exists, between the somatic cervical structures and the region of the eyebrow.

7. The trigeminal nerve is accompanied by both sympathetic and parasympathetic neurones. The ophthalmic and maxillary branches are primarily involved with sympathetic fibre activity, and these ramify peripherally accompanying somatosensory neurones, the blood vessels and as free nerve endings. The third mandibular branch is primarily associated with parasympathetic fibre activity.[684] It is known that some afferent neurones from the face descend in the sympathetic trunk down to upper thoracic levels, in addition to the great volume of afferent impulse traffic (Fig. 1.16) descending to synapse at the lower part of the spinal tract of the V cranial, and pain in the face can be produced by stimulating the superior

cervical ganglion, and likewise by stimulating the *proximal* cut ends of these sympathetic neurones.[1145]

8. Since the spinal tract of the V cranial nerve, at C1–C2 level, lies at the boundary areas between the territories of (a) the anterior and posterior spinal arteries, and (b) the peripheral and central supply and it is a cord area likely to suffer from vertebrobasilar ischaemia,[656] the distressing facial symptoms accompanying degenerative joint disease in the neck have been attributed to this. Ischaemia affecting the brain stem may very occasionally be sufficient to produce 'drop' attacks, sudden transient episodes of quadriparesis when the patient falls to the ground without losing consciousness.

9. The spinal tract of the V cranial nerve[1355] may also be involved in the spread of excitation when those cord segments are subject to summation effects and facilitation by an increased volume of normally subliminal impulses from the nociceptor endings in upper cervical connective and other tissues.

10. Trauma and degenerative change can produce adhesions of the spinal meninges, which bind down or tether the dura mater, so that on movements of the neck an undue amount of traction and distortion is sustained by the soft spinal cord. This alternative mechanism can produce localised ischaemia in certain segments and associated tissues, and the resulting symptoms will depend largely on the particular pattern of end-artery supply of the cord substance.[120, 121a, 656, 704]

11. Hard, posterior, horizontal ridges of combined disc- and-vertebral body margins very frequently result from degenerative change lower down in the neck. These unyielding ridges project backwards and trespass onto the arterial anastomoses of the surface of the spinal cord. Again, the particular pattern of arterial supply may underlie the cranial and facial symptoms resulting, especially on certain movements, notably flexion.[117, 130]

12. The last type of aetiology differs from the flexion-headache sometimes suffered by schoolchildren.[737, 477] This occurs when the transverse ligament of the atlas has been attenuated and loosened by a retropharyngeal spread of throat infections. Other tissues besides ligaments may be involved by the physical trespass of oedema. These young necks are unstable, and certainly should not be mobilised.

This brief survey of some hypotheses serves only to suggest the nature of many changes underlying the clinical features described. The field is a complex one, and the single subject of a monograph which treats it on a more extended basis.[242]

THORACIC SPINE

The splanchnic nerves and paravertebral ganglia lie on the heads of the ribs, close to the vertebral column, and

Nathan[903] has very clearly demonstrated splanchnic nerve trunks severely distorted by anterior and anterolateral osteophytic trespass, and incorporated into the overgrowth of degenerative, thickened tissues. Compression and irritation must be a matter of course, but whether this has any effect on the normal function of viscera innervated by these fibres, and how this may be manifested, is a matter of conjecture; clinical descriptions in the literature are very scanty, although the mechanisms and pathways of thoracic spinal pain have been well elucidated by Wyke (1970)[1356] and some observations on thoracic nerve root involvement are given on pages 103 and 241.

Lewit (1978)[743] discuss vertebrovisceral and viscerovertebral reflex mechanisms, and suggests that when vertebral lesions of specific segments appear to be linked with visceral abnormalities, there are never any signs of true root involvement. He also suggests that the influence of spinal lesions on visceral function is largely hypothetical, but mentions evidence of the effects of visceral lesions on vertebral mobility segments.

With his colleagues, he was able to establish a so-called spinal pattern of vertebral lesions, in which particular thoracic segments tended to exhibit abnormalities of movement as a result, rather than the cause, of disease in segmentally associated viscera, e.g. peptic ulcer and cardiac disease.

LUMBAR SPINE

Cassese and Aliperta[148] reported on findings by oscillograms, rheograms and photoplethysmograms of 38 patients with discogenic disease, and concluded that in cases of lumbar hernia sympathetic neurones were included in the compressive lesions, and further, that secondary pain of a vegetative nature was a possibility.

Hakelius et al.[483a] describe the cold sciatic leg. Nearly all patients state that they suffer from cold in the lower leg and foot of the affected side. Twenty-eight patients, 14 males and 14 females, with a mean age of 35.5 years (range 19–52 years) were examined by thermocouple tests of skin temperature, distal plethysmography and other tests. In all but one of the cases the diagnosis of discogenic trespass was confirmed myelographically. The basal skin temperature was generally lower on the affected leg and patients with signs of S1 root involvement had a lower skin temperature than those with an L5 involvement.

Following operation, the previous differences in skin temperature between affected and unaffected limbs was substantially reduced.

The authors demonstrated by associated tests that the difference is conditioned by a regionally enhanced vasoconstrictor activity in cutaneous blood vessels, and recall the work of other investigators[6] which supports the observations that increased activity in sympathetic vasoconstrictor tone can be reflexly excited by pain. Pain in visceral organs can also elicit vasoconstriction in the corresponding dermatome, as a result of reflexly increased flow of impulses in the vasoconstrictor fibres.

A reduced skin circulation in the sciatic leg is particularly noticed in its distal extent, where autonomic innervation is extensive. The findings seem to be corroborated by the normalisation of low skin temperature with the cessation of pain, regardless of whether this has occurred after conservative treatment or surgical removal of pressure on the nerve roots.

The cauda equina should be mentioned here—when this is compressed there is always great pain in the leg.

The reason for intermittent claudication symptoms is quite probably local vascular changes in the nerve roots. Exercise (i.e. walking) increases the blood-flow to the cauda equina, and this little extra fluid congestion, or engorgement, is enough to aggravate the root pain. But simple pressure, because of stenosis, comes into it as well, because this pain does not go when the patient stops walking, i.e. just stands still (as it does in peripheral vascular disease); the patient must sit, thus flexing the spine and thereby making more room in the stenotic neural canal, which is somewhat reduced in diameter during extension movements and the extension posture of standing.

STATES OF CHRONIC PAIN WITH DYSTROPHY

Some severely neuralgic states, more often of the upper limb, together with phantom limb pains and causalgic pains, appear to have in common an underlying neural mechanism of self-perpetuation.

This is assumed to be an activity of self-exciting reverberating circuits in neural pools of the spinal cord, whereby normally non-painful stimuli easily trigger summation mechanisms to maintain and increase the painful state (Fig. 7.1). A characteristic feature is dystrophy, to a greater or lesser degree, and pain continuing for weeks and months long after its biological usefulness has passed.[846]

'Causalgia' is not a diagnosis, it only means 'severe burning pain', the numerous clinical forms of the state described have been given various names:[1166, 320, 1342]

Causalgia
Phantom limb
Shoulder–hand syndrome
Reflex sympathetic dystrophy
Sudek's atrophy[1187]
Sudek–Leriche syndrome
Posttraumatic osteoporosis
Babinski–Froment syndrome
Algoneurodystrophy
Changes in paretic limbs of hemiplegics

Swollen atrophic hand with cervical osteoarthritis
Acute bone atrophy
Minor causalgia
Posttraumatic arteriospasm
Posttraumatic oedema
Posttraumatic spreading neuralgia
Posttraumatic sympathalgia
Posttraumatic trophoneurosis
Posttraumatic vasomotor

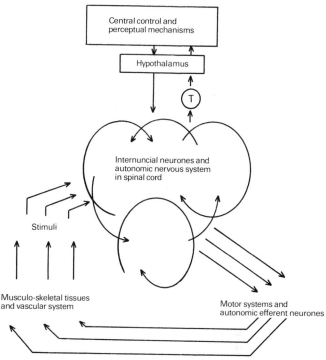

Fig. 7.1 Scheme of abnormal and self-perpetuating excitatory activity in internuncial neurone circuits of spinal cord.

Neurotrophic rheumatism syndrome
Painful disability of the shoulder and hand after coronary occlusion
Postinfection sclerodactylia
Reflex dystrophy
Reflex hyperaemic deossification
Sympathetic trophoneurosis

There are only general, rather than rigid, patterns to the course of the condition, and so many variations in the clinical features that no stereotype exists.

Steinbrocker (1947),[1166] the first to describe the shoulder–hand syndrome, reported a group of over 200 patients, among whom were 6 idiopathic cases. He reported[1167] the precipitating factor in 146 cases, and it is interesting to note that 75 per cent of the cases were idiopathic, postinfarctional, cervicodiscogenic or intraforaminal spurring and trauma; although the radiological appearance of foraminal encroachment need not, of itself, be a cause of pain or disability.

In a further group of 139 patients with the syndrome, 23 per cent of the cases were ascribed to cervical arthrosis or discogenic disease.

A principal feature is that the manifestations can be reduced and often relieved by interfering with the autonomic nervous system, by sympathetic block and sympathectomy, and this together with the obvious trophic changes indicate the intrinsic role of sympathetic nerves. They appear to develop a 'sick' physiology, and probably a 'sick' pharmacology too.

The self-perpetuating facilitation in cord segments may be likened to a stuck needle on a record (Fig. 7.1).

Table 7.2 Precipitating factors in 146 cases of the shoulder–hand syndrome

Idiopathic	33	23%
Postinfarctional	30	20%
Cervical-discogenic or intraforaminal spurring	29	20%
Posttraumatic	15	10%
Multiple inconclusive	16	11%
Posthemiplegic	9	6%
Miscellaneous	14	10%
Postherpes zoster	3	
Calcific tendinitis of the shoulder	2	
Pancoast type tumours	2	
Diffuse vasculitis	2	
Brain tumour	2	
Febrile panniculitis	1	
Gonococcal arthritis	1	

Three important features are (1) pain which is chronic and severe (on occasion this is much less evident in comparison with the other features), (2) dystrophic changes, (3) neurological involvement.

In the shoulder–hand syndrome the signs in the upper limb are painful disability; swelling of hand and fingers; changes in skin colour and temperature; hyperidrosis or anhidrosis; glossiness of skin, with atrophy of subcutaneous tissues; stiffness of joints, and of normally soft pliable tissue; radiologically, a patchy cottonwool appearance of bone trabeculae.

NEUROLOGICAL CHANGES

Muscle weakness is most evident, but it is difficult to assess power accurately because the patient frequently finds strong resisted movements painful.

LOCAL CHANGES

Vasomotor activity produces spasm of arterioles,[320] and the venule end of capillary loops, thus the capillary is blocked and the filtration pressure increased.

There is oedema and thus swelling, adding a further difficulty to already painful movement. Cyanosis and anoxaemia, by their production of metabolites, further increase capillary permeability and thus added oedema, establishing the vicious circle.

Arteriolar smooth-muscle spasm contributes to pain, as presumably does the skeletal muscle contraction, a spasm which appears unlike that induced by joint problems unaccompanied by the dystrophy syndrome.

The three phases are:

1. Shoulder pain and disability of the limb, diffuse swelling, exquisite tenderness and vasomotor changes in the hand—the radiological 'cottonwool-cloud' appearance is evident. This phase lasts 3–6 months and may disappear spontaneously.

2. Pain and disability, and swelling of hand and fingers, tends to recede, and may indicate spontaneous recession.

In some, vasomotor changes and tenderness may remain. Atrophy of nails, skin and muscles occur, with thickening of the palmar fascia in a few. Fingers and wrist movement begins to be limited by contracture.

3. Vasomotor changes and tenderness are absent. Muscle weakness, flexion contracture of the hand and sometimes shoulder become established, and may be irreversible.

All of these findings may precede, accompany or follow a painful disease, usually in later life, or accompanying an injury to the limb, and the severity of the syndrome is unrelated to the extent of the precipitating cause. The syndrome is not associated with any particular occupation, nationality or race, and there is bilateral involvement in about 25 per cent of cases.

With the exception of the postinfarction group, women are affected more than men.

Steinbrocker[1168] asserts that the shoulder–hand syndrome occurs much more frequently than is reported, either in complete or partial forms (see p. 185). Since spontaneous recovery of milder forms frequently occurs, many signs of the early phases of the syndrome are probably overlooked. Individuals doing light work seem as prone to the disability as those doing heavy work, and he states that if a patient has had neck pain and limited cervical movement over a considerable period, subsequent complaints regarding the limb may well be related to arthrosis of the cervical spine.

Bourdillon's[105] observations strongly suggest that following an injury persistent pain may have a spinal origin. This can be seen following minor and simple injuries but also after fractures, commonly about the wrist, although the persistent pain may remain localised to the trauma site or involve the whole limb and limb girdle.

The several possibilities are (a) injury to normal vertebral structures at the time of trauma, (b) injury activating a pre-existing chronic or subclinical vertebral joint problem, and (c) the nociceptor impulse activity itself being responsible in certain situations for setting up or triggering the bizarre and chronic facilitated state of neurone pools, and of 'sympathetic perversion'.[320] (Fig. 7.1).

From what has been said about the convergence of somatic and visceral afferents at the posterior horns of the spinal cord, the vagaries of referred pain (p. 192), the inextricably linked activity of somatic and autonomic neurone activity, and the marked tendency for abnormalities of the cervical and upper/middle thoracic spines to induce many diverse symptoms in the upper limb, all cases of what may be called 'reflex sympathetic dystrophy' should be examined for vertebral abnormalities, and treated for these in addition to local measures for the affected limb (see Syndromes, p. 205).

Bourdillon[105] describes four cases in which a marked improvement was admitted by the patients, *before* the outstanding compensation claims were settled.

In times recently past, traumatic injuries of the wrist and forearm received mainly local attention to the more manifest injury, and the embarrassing development of posttraumatic capsular contracture of the glenohumeral joint prompted therapists to be awake for the phenomenon of 'the stubbed shoulder',[850] and to include prophylactic shoulder mobilisation as a routine measure in these injuries. Likewise, direct violence to the side of the head is also a 'whiplash' (acceleration) injury to the neck, and a fall on the outstretched hand also produces lateral acceleration and deceleration forces to the cervical and thoracic spines and upper costospinal joints.

There is much to be said for including a search for vertebral abnormalities in all cases of both upper and lower limb injuries. The spinal changes uncovered may not always be recent, or significant, yet very frequently indeed they are, and should be given the benefit of any doubt and treated.

ASSOCIATED CHANGES IN PERIPHERAL JOINTS WITHOUT FRANK DYSTROPHY

Steinbrocker's observations (p. 185) may be the clue to ultimate elucidation of clinical features familiar to many, i.e. that joints situated in shoulder and pelvic girdle, and more distal areas, to which the pain of vertebral joint problems is frequently referred, themselves begin to undergo secondary changes which add a further quota to the painful and restricted movement uncovered by detailed examination. These more peripheral associated changes, for example in the shoulder and elbow regions, can very frequently be eradicated by mobilisation and manipulation of the vertebral joints, the restoration of pain-free movement in the peripheral joint occurring together with improvement of the spinal joint abnormality. This is not always the case; a common clinical experience is that the more chronic are the associated changes in the vertebral and peripheral joints, the more frequently is it necessary to attend to both spinal and peripheral joint changes.[797, 289, 466]

Common examples are capsulitis of the glenohumeral joint, bicipital tendinitis, supraspinatus tendinitis, lateral epicondylitis (tennis elbow), etc., associated with C5–C6, and often T2–T3–T4 joint problems. Likewise, medial epicondylitis (golfer's elbow) associated with C5–C6–C7–T1 vertebral joints, and painful restrictions of hip-joint mobility associated with L3–L4 segment abnormalities. Further, the association of painful temperomandibular joint conditions (in the absence of defects of dental occlusion) and upper cervical joint changes, may be more than coincidence.

Maigne[792] refers to the thickening and loss of suppleness of the eyebrow which occurs in unilateral supraorbital headache in referred pain from the C2–C3 segment of the same side. Within minutes of an injection of local anaesthetic into the C2–3 facet-joint, the eyebrow thickening is diminished and its suppleness becomes the same as the normal side. This was observed in 86 per cent of 50 cases of unilateral supraorbital headache of cervical origin, i.e. 43 of the cases were relieved of the headache by injection and/or manipulation.

Most experienced workers are familiar with the fact that eradication of a local pain by injection does not necessarily mean that its localised origin has thereby been demonstrated.[780]

Authors have expressed this vertebral–peripheral link in various ways,

Pain in or about the shoulder joint from irritation of cervical nerve roots may give rise to reflex sympathetic dystrophy with resulting changes in capsule and tendons. Similar changes may occur at elbow, wrist and fingers.[598]

Tendinitis around peripheral joints, fibrosis of tendon sheaths and of palmar fascia, and swelling of the fingers, are frequently associated with cervical spine disorders. Fibrotic nodules and contracture of the palmar fascia are seen following injuries of the cervical spine.[598] The phenomenon of peripheral joint changes associated with vertebral syndromes is well documented by French as well as German authors,[242] and Maigne[789] describes these 'cellulo-tendinomyalgic' syndromes in the upper limb accompanying C6 joint problems, and in the lower limb associated with S1 lesions, both with and without frank spinal root involvement. 'In certain sciaticas there occurs ... a true tibioperoneal (superior tibiofibular) periarthritis.'

As the palpable sulcus between the radial head and the lateral epicondyle is less evident on palpation of a 'tennis elbow' side compared to the normal elbow, so the many carpal articulations of a 'carpal-tunnel syndrome' side may feel thickened and much less flexible to careful, uniarticular testing movements, in comparison to the normal side.

The fact that a unilateral release operation in carpal-tunnel stenosis sometimes relieves bilateral paraesthesiae perhaps indicates that the genesis of these states may lie more proximally.[289]

Clinical observations indicate that reflex sympathetic dystrophy and its synonyms, the shoulder–hand syndrome, the ubiquitous low-grade collagenosis postulated on page 188, the frozen shoulder and chronic capsulitis of the shoulder, carpal-tunnel syndrome, etc., may on many occasions be manifestations, *to a greater or lesser degree*, of the same malign, self-inflicted wound of chronic facilitatory states of lower cervical and upper thoracic cord segments, as a consequence of trauma to limb girdle and/or silent, degenerative spondylotic change, inducing connective-tissue changes in the limb.

In rheumatoid arthritis, osteoarthritis, capsulitis, posttraumatic restriction of shoulder movement and pulmonary arthropathy the humeral head is carried high and forward on the glenoid—this classical postural abnormality of the articulation need not *always* be a *sequel*, and can frequently be observed in its milder forms in painful cervical joint problems before the patient has begun to report shoulder symptoms.

Peripheral joint movement-restriction, when recent, and particularly at the shoulder, need not be entirely due to connective-tissue changes, of course, e.g. its almost immediate eradication *during* traction to the cervical spine[340] may indicate the relaxation of spasm in muscles of the rotator cuff; yet muscle spasm can have little to do with the demonstrable tightness of connective tissue in more distal joints, and later its frank development at the shoulder joint is soon clinically evident as the main factor restricting movement.

The stiff (frozen) shoulder, freezing arthritis, periarthritis, etc., are frequently employed as general terms for pain which apparently arises from a number of conditions, and these states of arthropathy are not always clinically distinguishable; some believe capsulitis to be a doubtful pathological entity.[583]

The pain of cardiac ischaemia is a well-documented cause of the stiff shoulder, and shoulder–hand syndrome; temperature changes in the left arm of these patients suggest that there is abnormal sympathetic activity.[1316]

Hypertrophic pulmonary osteoarthropathy, occurring in middle-aged males, may be associated with abdominal conditions such as dysentery as well as the lung conditions of carcinoma, tuberculosis, chronic empyema and bronchiectasis. In neoplastic disease the peripheral limb changes may develop in a matter of weeks. Significantly, pneumonectomy for bronchial carcinoma may be followed by objective evidence of peripheral improvement within a matter of hours.[1040]

These considerations of shoulder pain, restricted movement and pain on resisted movement are, of course, bedevilled by *degenerative conditions of the rotator cuff*, a very common clinical state.

Spasm of rotator cuff musculature, and other limb girdle muscle groups innervated largely by segments C5 and C6, may 'hitch up' the head of humerus in the glenoid cavity by a few millimetres and thus disturb the synergic co-ordination of normal humeroscapular movement; this chronic state of mild hypertonus may itself be a potent factor in the genesis of degenerative rotator cuff lesions, although the repetitive trauma of shoulder overuse cannot be discounted.

Supraspinatus tendinitis seems the most common of these diagnoses about the shoulder, and it seems significant that this tendon and the subdeltoid bursa, best situated to suffer trauma against the unyielding acromion during daily use, attract the most attention in the great volume of literature on this subject.

While a diagnosis of supraspinatus tendinitis may sometimes have a demonstrable basis of local tissue change,[776] the genesis of these changes may well lie more proximally.

In a personal series of 138 consecutive cases of shoulder pain Richardson[1039] found that 90 per cent belonged to the rotator cuff syndrome/capsulitis group of lesions and observed a greater response to injections of methylprednisolone acetate plus oral indocid in those with pain on resisted movement, although the clinical features described included pain on resisted abduction and external rotation, and he refers to the confused terminology of the subject.

In what may be called adhesive capsulitis, and by some, frozen shoulder, it is commonly asserted[1316] that the condition gets well of itself in 18–24 months without treatment, yet Richardson[1039] asserts that even after two years full function may not be restored; and in a group of patients with painfully restricted movement 42 per cent of those affected had marked loss of mobility 6 years after onset of the original disability.[176] Our handling of these shoulders could surely be improved.

Gunn and Milbrandt[466] studied 50 patients who were resistant to four weeks of conservative local treatment to their 'tennis elbows', and their findings suggest that in this group, the underlying condition may have been a reflex localisation of pain from radiculopathy of the cervical spine. Treatment directed to the cervical spine appeared to give relief in the majority of patients. All were right-handed but 3 had only left-side complaints. Eleven had lateral epicondylar symptoms on both sides, 12 had concurrent medial epicondylar symptoms and 7 had bilateral medial and lateral epicondylar involvement.

They conclude from their findings that the condition of tennis elbow is related to cervical spine disorders; when local treatment failed, neck treatment was tried and consisted of mobilisation (Maitland's techniques), cervical traction, isometric cervical exercises and heat or ultrasound. Results were good—of the 47 patients who responded 44 were assessed at 3 and 6 months, and had remained symptom-free. The authors suggest that their report challenges some current concepts.

The extensive literature, on what may well be a ubiquitous low-grade collagenosis, has been well reviewed by Ebbetts,[289] whose discussion of autonomic involvement in vertebral pain syndromes is accompanied by a full bibliography. In his view,

each syndrome is progressive, the primary autonomic disturbance leading to local tissue change so that the condition created is eventually locally autonomous ... and beyond a certain point is not reversible by cervical manipulation alone.

With reference to the observations on migraine, trigeminal neuralgia and vertigo (p. 181) a covert mechanism of efferent autonomic neurone effects in vertebral joint abnormalities should perhaps be borne in mind when treating conditions such as carpal-tunnel syndrome, subscapularis tendinitis, infraspinatus tendinitis and the like.

Without a comprehensive examination of the neck and upper thorax, including competent segmental palpation, treatment procedures may be based on findings which are incomplete.

The importance of cervical investigation in any patient with head, neck, chest, shoulder and arm pain cannot be over-emphasised. The usual diagnosis of arthritis, bursitis, neuritis, muscular rheumatism, fibrositis, fasciitis, tendinitis, pseudoangina, migraine, etc. should not be made until cervical nerve root irritation has been ruled out entirely, if that is possible.[598]

REFERRED PAIN

The phenomenon of referred or projected pain, i.e. that felt at a greater or lesser distance from the lesion producing it, is well recognised but not fully understood. It is a frequent source of difficulty, in identification of the vertebral segments involved and therefore in the correct localisation of treatment.[116, 553, 356, 592b, 598, 640, 641, 642, 797]

Serious visceral disease can produce spinal pain which mimics that of relatively innocent vertebral joint problems[686, 806] and conversely, pain referred around the chest wall from vertebral and rib joint involvement can very easily simulate the pains of visceral disease such as pleurisy and cardiac ischaemia.[907]

This confusing problem may have an element of our own making. As infants we quickly learn that painful trauma to digits of hand or foot hurts precisely 'where the action is', so to speak, and very early in life perhaps unwittingly develop the unspoken expectation that this will apply to the whole body.

The logic of structural anatomy (a heart is a heart and not a limb, the scapula is not a liver) plainly does not apply to where damage will hurt. Pain behaviour sometimes becomes unnecessarily difficult to understand, perhaps because we may lean too heavily on the expectation that organs and deep body parts *ought* to, or *should*, hurt where the damage is. We find it singular that they may not, and term examples of this surprisingly undisciplined behaviour 'referred' or 'projected' pain.

With hindsight, it appears that much of our clinical confusion might have been avoided if we had earlier recognised our subconscious tendency to link the organisation of pain with the organisation of structural anatomy, and so far as its characteristic and natural behaviour are concerned, had allowed the body to speak for itself.

In a recent review[1325] of the problem, the sentence, '... cardiac pain may be felt in the arm' illustrates the unspoken expectation very clearly, and the covert assertion, almost, that this behaviour is illogical. Perhaps it is not cardiac pain, but chest, neck and arm pain perceived because of cardiac abnormality. The subtle difference is important. Further, a source of confusion is added by the notion of 'true visceral pain' (see p. 194) which invites the questions of what is 'untrue' visceral pain, and what is the difference.

A degree of unreality intrudes when referred or projected pain is designated as an error of cortical perception, i.e. that visceral and deep musculoskeletal pain, by not being where we feel they *should* be, so transgress the bounds of order, logic and anatomy as to merit the definition of misguidedness!

Lesions of the body surface, of its distal extremities, of bone and of muscle usually hurt in the region of the damage—lesions of more proximal, and of other deeper structures hurt elsewhere too. Accompanying the spread of pain to other places are referred tenderness (see p. 169), muscle hypertonus and sometimes cutaneous vasoconstriction or flushing, and sweating.

The complaint of pain and the demonstration of local tenderness may obscure the fact that the offending pathologic lesion is centrally placed, and may lead the clinician to believe, erroneously, that the disease process underlies the site of the patient's complaint. This erroneous belief may be apparently confirmed by the temporary relief of pain by the injection of local anaesthetic. Such pain relief may be maintained for a surprisingly long period of time. These points must be borne in mind when considering soft tissue lesions.[780]

Referred pain may or may not be accompanied by secondary hyperalgesia ... injection of procaine into the superficial or deep hyperalgesic structures will reduce the amount of pain. When cutaneous hyperalgesia is marked, pain originating from deep structures may be greatly relieved by spraying ethyl chloride coolant on the affected area. Spread of excitation in the central nervous system may produce widespread painful contractions of skeletal muscle remote from the noxious stimulus. Procaine injected into the affected muscles abolishes this type of pain.[635]

That pain of proximal origin may be reduced by injection at its site of reference is a decided advantage, and has many clinical applications, but it is basically important to increase our understanding of the mechanisms underlying these phenomena, because their nature is not yet fully elucidated. Familiar examples of pain perceived at a distance from the site of tissue damage are:

Upper limb pain in neck and also shoulder lesions.
Headache from cervical joint problems.
Pectoral and costochondral pain from thoracic joint conditions.
Pain in the epigastrium, and/or posterior body wall, in gallbladder disease (see also p. 194).
Groin pain from joint problems at the thoracolumbar junction.
Low backache in osteoporosis of the lower thoracic spine.
Pain in posterior thigh and upper calf from sacroiliitis.
Pain referred to the foot from lumbar intervertebral disc disease.
Thigh and knee pain in arthrosis or tuberculosis of the hip.

The upper thoracic nerves also contribute sensory fibres and the distribution of pain down the medial border of the arm, forearm and hand and radiation up in the neck towards the lobe of the left ear suggests that there are communications between the sympathetic nerves and somatic afferent fibres at the levels of the superior, middle and inferior cervical sympathetic ganglia.[117]

Clinical experience, of shoulder and arm symptoms being relieved by mobilisation of thoracic segments as low as T8, is not rare. The injection of hypertonic saline into the lumbosacral supraspinous ligament may give pain radiating down the leg as far as the calf. It may also be associated with tender points commonly situated over the sacroiliac joint and the upper outer quadrant of the buttock.[780]

SEGMENTATION

Considerations of pain reference or projection need to include some reference to *dermatomes* (Figs 2.18–2.23), *myotomes* (pp. 69–71) and *sclerotomes* (Figs 2.24–2.25), i.e. the regional distribution and innervation of musculoskeletal and associated tissues evolved from the three primitive germ-layers of the embryo. Throughout differentiation, growth and existence they retain the parenthood of their source connections (a) with the embryonic mesodermal somites and (b) the ectodermal spinal cord segments and cranial nerve nuclei. The three embryonic germ-layers with, among others, the tissues derived from them, are:

Ectoderm
Epithelium of epidermis, of body cavities, and of mouth and anus; c.n.s. and p.n.s.

Entoderm
Structure and epithelium of digestive tube (except each end of it) and associated viscera and of the respiratory system

Mesoderm
Whole cardiovascular and lymphatic systems
Epithelium of synovia and bursae, and of pleura, pericardium and peritoneum
The corium or true skin
Muscle tissue of all kinds
All connective and sclerous tissues.

In the first weeks of intrauterine life, the central longitudinal *notochord* develops around it a flexible rod of mesodermal cells which will ultimately form the primitive vertebral column. By the fourth week, a series of transverse grooves has divided the mesoderm into 42–44 mesodermal somites, the most caudal few of which are fated to become the coccyx while the upper 4–5 undergo atypical development to become the face and cranium. The bulk of them develop to become the foetal vertebral segments, each somite forming the adjacent halves of two vertebral bodies and the enclosed disc, the nucleus of which will contain some remaining cells of the primitive notochord.

Concurrently, the ectodermal neural tube begins the formation at its upper end of the intracranial part of the c.n.s., and in the rest of its extent the intravertebral part of the c.n.s., i.e. the spinal cord.

In general terms, the ectodermal cord segments, and the future nerve root associated with them, retain their first family associations with the mesodermal somites, which by the fifth week of intrauterine life have begun to develop the limb buds. Lateral growth and differentiation of the limbs convey with them the somatic nerve roots with their sister autonomic neurones, and the different regions of skin with underlying muscle, fascia, joint, periosteum, bone and blood vessel have thus immutably fixed their innervation by the corresponding somatic segmental nerves, but also by others (see p. 169) and autonomic neurones, although the latter are derived from a greater 'spread' of segments (see p. 178).

A *dermatome* (Figs 2.18–2.23) is thus the longitudinal band of skin *mainly* innervated by a spinal nerve root, and a *myotome* is the mass of muscle tissue innervated by one root—more correctly, the total population of motor units supplied by one root since L3 root, for example, will supply parts of many muscles although one root is not necessarily a segmental entity (see p. 13). Thus most muscles help to form more than one myotome, e.g. flexor digitorum profundus is supplied by C8 and T1; and, of course, may be supplied by several distinct anatomical nerves, e.g. f.d.p. is supplied by both median and ulnar nerves, conveying neurones derived mainly from the two segments above.

The *sclerotome* (Figs 2.24, 2.25) forms the embryonic tissue from which the axial skeleton will ultimately be derived, but the term is also taken to include the bone and cartilage of the appendicular skeleton, too; one fully developed adult sclerotome being that skeletal tissue with the parenthood of one mesodermal somite.

Dermatomes generally overlie myotomes, e.g. the skin innervated by segments L2-3-4 (via the lateral, intermediate and medial cutaneous nerves) broadly overlies the muscle supplied by L234, and both correspond roughly to the L2, 3 and 4 sclerotomes; but there are several body regions where innervation of skin differs from that of deeper structures, and among them are: the face, pectoral region, heart and diaphragm, scapular region, thenar eminence and buttock. They are evident on comparison of a classical dermatome chart with myotomes, the segmental innervation of muscles. For example, the skin of the face is innervated by the 5th cranial nerve, and the muscles of expression by the 7th cranial; the intrinsic scapular muscles are supplied by C5-6, and the skin covering the region is innervated by T234, the heart is derived from the T123 somites, the diaphragm from C345, and the trunk dermatomes covering the region are derived from somites T5678. The important point is that superficial tissue and the underlying structures have broadly the same innervation in some places; in other places they do not, and it happens that the latter body regions are those frequently involved in vertebral pain syndromes.

THEORIES OF REFERRED PAIN

Doran[272] summarises the following points:

1. Localisation of *cutaneous* sensation to a particular area has been shown to be determined by the cells of the cortical postcentral gyrus to which the skin area is linked.
2. The dermatomes are represented as a mosaic on the postcentral gyrus with an overlap corresponding to the overlap of dermatome boundaries.
3. If a localised area of postcentral gyrus is stimulated, a sensation occurs in the related area of the body surface, and conversely, if a local area of skin is stimulated, cortical electrodes will register activity in the related area of the postcentral gyrus.

Because the faculty of localising noxious stimuli *to the skin surface* is highly developed and very accurate, and that of perceiving the locality of deeper lesions is considerably less developed, the physiology of cutaneous sensation is of less help when considering the clinical presentation of musculoskeletal tissue damage and visceral conditions.

Descriptions of the behaviour of referred pain tend to rest on a segmental theory, i.e. that should a lesion occur within the mass of tissue originally derived from particular embryonic segments, the pain is likely to be felt somewhere within that family of tissues sharing the same origin, irrespective of their distal migration and subsequent development into the structures of mature adult anatomy.

Thus a lesion in the heart will be painful in segmentally related tissues, a subphrenic abscess will hurt at the point of a shoulder, and an arthrotic or tuberculous hip joint (which began life as, largely, the L3 and L4 mesodermal somites) will hurt down the thigh and especially at the knee—tissues which also started life as part of the same somite 'family'. Thus maps or charts of dermatomes (Fig. 2.18) and a knowledge of the myotomes, with a grasp of sclerotome distribution, become important as reference data when ascribing tissue damage to a particular locality on the basis of the body territory occupied by pain, i.e. the segmental theory.

From the assumption that the symptoms of low back pain only occur when and if the degenerative trespass impinges upon pain-sensitive structures and nerve roots, Gunn and Milbrandt (1978)[472] suggest that the confusing combination of types of dysfunction is due to a mixture of interference with afferent, efferent, sensory, motor and autonomic neurones. The authors suggest that:

... referred pain into the *dermatome* is felt as paraesthesiae ('numbness', 'deadness', or 'tingling'), in the *myotome* as muscle pain and tenderness, and in the *sclerotome* as a dull, aching or boring, deep pain which is characteristically difficult to localise as it has a tendency to radiate either proximally or distally. To confuse the picture, atypical distributions of sensory disorders conforming to vasal topography may occur in autonomic dysfunction.

Difficulties arise because:

1. Pain distribution of a known segmental origin often appears quite wayward, by transgressing the expected dermatome boundaries, and
2. While myotomes are anatomical entities, dermatome boundaries are not. They have been likened to 16th-century maps of the globe, and there is a great deal of dermatome overlap.[434, 437]

They can be experimentally plotted by observing *the areas of vasodilatation* when a dorsal root is stimulated, or by plotting *the area of remaining sensibility* in animals after cutting *three roots above* and *three roots below* a given root; the modalities employed can be sensibility to pain; thermal sensibility; tactile sensibility,[434] and if the latter is employed the dermatome boundaries tend to be rather larger and thus overlap more.

Clinical observation of sensibility defects in patients with established root lesions has also contributed some information to the formulation of charts.[117]

Kirk and Denny-Brown (1970)[659] used the 'remaining sensibility' method when investigating the dermatomes of the macaque monkey.

Section of dorsal roots *proximal* to their ganglia produced patterns of dermatomes observed previously by Sherrington in 1893,[1122] but if in other animals the roots were sectioned *distal* to their ganglia the dermatome immediately became twice the size, with skin sensitivity increased; and it stayed increased.

Resectioning the same dorsal roots proximal to the ganglia reduced the dermatomes to their conventional or 'classical' size, but not immediately, and only after a delay of three or four days.

Injection of small doses of strychnine sulphate (to depress inhibition and thus increase facilitation at synapses in the spinal cord) produced an enormous expansion of an isolated dermatome area, irrespective of where its dorsal root had been sectioned. The conclusion is that the experimentally observed size of an isolated dermatome is a variable quantity, and at any one moment is more of an index of the efficiency of sensory transmission in the same and neighbouring segments of the spinal cord, than a fixed cutaneous territory.

Denny-Brown, *et al.* (1973)[250] have further shown that, in the behavioural reaction to cutaneous stimulation of the dermatome area subserved by an isolated dorsal root, the dermatome territory is considerably expanded when Lissauer's tract is sectioned. The simple proposition, that the receptive field of an isolated dermatome can be much widened by an adjacent *destructive* lesion, is a clear reminder that the concept of dermatomes as numbered and finite territories is akin to describing an iceberg while looking only at its tip.

Briefly, dermatomes seem not so much anatomical entities as *neurophysiological entities*, whose boundaries fluctuate according to the prevailing levels of facilitation of cord segments.

As we have already seen (p. 169), the painful state *is* a state of cord segment facilitation, and thus it follows that a dermatome of normal subjects is likely to be smaller than the same dermatome territory in a patient whose pain is currently being referred around the trunk wall or into a limb, *the pain mechanism itself inducing an enlarged spread of distal reference*, and not necessarily into one dermatome. Figures 2.18–2.23 therefore depict, not fixed segmental surface territories, but somewhat changeable cutaneous areas, roughly corresponding to body regions in which pain and other symptoms may often be partly or wholly distributed from joint problems in the general neighbourhood of associated vertebral segments.

For example,[342] Feinstein and others injected the musculotendinous interspinous tissue of normal subjects at each level from occiput to sacrum with a 6 per cent saline solution. One hundred and forty individual observations were made in 5 subjects. All described the local and referred pain as 'deep' and 'aching'; the word 'area' did not seem appropriate for expressing the essentially three-dimensional character of the pain. Individuals added descriptions of 'gripping', 'boring', 'heavy', 'crampy' or 'lumpy', and the pains were frequently accompanied by acutely unpleasant autonomic reactions.

Of interest is the distribution of pain—referral into the shoulder was observed following stimulation as high as C3 level. Following stimulation of C6 segment, pain was referred into the arm and forearm of two subjects. On both C7 and C8 stimulation, pain was provoked in the ulnar side of arm and forearm. Referral to radial side of forearm and hand occurred in none of the subjects. Pain was referred to the buttock and posterior and anterior aspects of thigh, following injections at segments L4, L5, S1 and S2. The pain reported by patients need not be arising from vertebral changes, and may be originating in tissue damage of underlying or neighbouring peripheral structures.

Similarly, pain may be referred to the ear from the cervical plexus (C2 and C3),[652] and from the temperomandibular joint.

Neurological deficit will be manifest in the structures supplied by the involved spinal nerve root (see Patterns of segmental supply) or peripheral nerves, yet specifying the level of abnormalities solely on the basis of distribution of signs in the limb is unreliable. While the nerve supply of muscle is fixed, spinal roots are not segmental entities; soon after emergence of rootlets from the spinal cord, communicating branches pass between adjacent segments, and single rootlets may each contribute to adjacent segmental nerves.[117, 598] Thus, the clinical localisation of a lesion producing radicular pain is not always certain, e.g. the neurological findings may be identical irrespective of whether discogenic trespass is located at L3–4 or L4–5.[1348]

In a series of 560 patients, surgically treated for disc disease, correct preoperative clinical localisation was achieved in only 39.2 per cent.[695]

Because conservative treatment precludes myelographic and surgical corroboration of the segmental level to be treated, a clear grasp of the vagaries of pain distribution is necessary, and explanations of referred pain, based on concepts of anatomically fixed segmental boundaries of cutaneous sensibility, may not suffice to elucidate all the clinical features of pain in joint problems. The factor, among others, of facilitated cord segments must also be incorporated, and this appears to apply to root involvement also.

There are many clinical observations concerning the variability of pain reference:

1. Pain is not always distributed to the expected dermatomes, but may spread over a wider area.[130]
2. Pain of cervical spondylosis may be felt in myotome areas and not necessarily in dermatomes.[1079]
3. Pain referred from deep somatic tissues differs in location from the conventional dermatome.[342]
4. Pain caused by irritation of one spinal nerve root may extend in some cases more widely than the recognised distribution.[116]
5. Referred pains are not invariably of segmental root distribution. They may miss out a segment and then spread into two adjacent segments.[553]

Convergence and summation of afferent impulse traffic (see p. 178) may be the mechanism underlying reference of pain at times, in that the spread of excitation among neighbouring neurone pools and cord segments produces radiation of pain to uninvolved distant regions.[635] Referred pain may induce *chronic peripheral effects*, and joints which lie in areas to which pain is commonly referred often undergo secondary change with painful stiffening, thereby adding to difficulties reported by the patient. Further, pain may be due to:

Vascular engorgement (p. 63) or vasospasm, and may represent a vascular distribution.

Ischaemia of cord segments by remote trespass (p. 6) upon blood vessels supplying them.[426]

Irritation of afferent nerve fibres by physical trespass at some point on their pathway which is remote from the situation occupied by their nociceptors (p. 23).

Physical irritation, or involvement in the neuronal spread of pain, of autonomic neurones (p. 183).

Because of these considerations, it is wise to be flexible in deciding where the pain of a particular distribution or segmental territory *ought* to be coming from. That its localisation depends upon c.n.s. mechanisms and not on impulses travelling down peripheral nerves, is demonstrated by the fact that when the skin of a transposed end of a pedicle graft is injured, the pain is perceived at the original site, and not in the position to which the graft has been moved.[136]

Thus, 'the nerves don't know where they go', and pain happens *within* the central nervous system, not residing 'in' the damaged locality, though it may be perceived so.

Pains do not really happen in hands or feet or heads; they happen in the images of heads and feet and hands (Miller, 1978).[859]

Pain is not referred or projected down nerves to the site of reference:

1. Cases are reported of anginal pain being referred to a phantom upper limb.[187]
2. Anginal pain referred to the left arm is not abolished by a complete brachial plexus block with local anaesthesia.[504]
3. Harman[503] succeeded in provoking *pain* and *paraesthesiae* in phantom limbs by saline injection.
4. Referred pain to the tip of the shoulder, initiated by phrenic nerve irritation, occurs just the same when all the cutaneous nerves to the shoulder-tip have been excised.[271]
5. Referred pain was experimentally evoked in areas previously anaesthetised by regional nerve block.[342]

We should bear in mind, when the severe pain of a vertebral joint problem is referred to a limb, and meticulous examination of the limb fails to reveal any evidence of neurological signs, that we really have no demonstrable basis for assuming as a matter of course that the pain is due to root involvement, even if there is radiological evidence of foraminal encroachment at the segment we believe concerned.

In many cases, but by no means all, neurological signs may begin to appear, and we then of course have evidence of root involvement, although we are still not in a position to describe the nature of it.

Clinical procedures are governed by the needs of individual patients, the level of pain and irritability being the prime and immediate indications, and our criteria for the pain of suspected root involvement might well be *the temporal nature of pain behaviour during testing movements* (see p. 175), rather than assuming by rule of thumb that because the pain is bad it must be due to root compression and/or inflammation.

If this is acceptable, we are in difficulties regarding theories of referred pain of root and nonroot involvement, because roughly only 1 person in 10 000[723] gets as far as myelographic and surgical corroboration of radiculopathy; without this corroboration, or signs of neurological deficit, we are theorising very much in the dark, since it is not possible to be absolutely certain that a particular pain is due only to nerve root involvement.

Perhaps all root pain is referred pain, but not all referred pain is root pain, i.e. *any* pain not localised to the site of tissue damage can be held as 'referred'.

In sentences such as, 'If there is evidence of referred pain or sciatic pain, exploration ... is recommended',[912] a difference between the two is implied yet what are the grounds for the unspoken implication that sciatic pain is not also referred pain?

A classification of the mechanisms believed to underlie pain distribution might be as follows:

A. *Local pain* is pain perceived at the site of tissue damage, and as we have seen, this occurs most frequently at the body surface or when damage involves the distal extremities. Referred pain may coexist, of course.

B. *Referred pain of root involvement* is pain experienced in tissues (a) which are not the site of primary tissue-damage, but (b) are generally innervated by neurones involved in the tissue-damage and the distinction can be made more certainly only when neurological deficit is apparent, e.g. the root symptoms and signs of cervical and lumbar degenerative change (see p. 0 0). As we have seen, root pain is not necessarily confined to the innervation territory of the involved root, and may well be accompanied by pain referred from the joint problem in its own right, as well as from the root.

C. *Referred pain without root involvement* is pain experienced in tissues which are (a) not the site of tissue damage, and (b) whose afferent or efferent neurones are not physically involved in any way, e.g. the non-root pain of musculoskeletal origin, the pectoral and upper limb pain in cardiac ischaemia and body-wall pain in gall bladder disease.

It is this type of referred pain which is often explained on the basis of the segmental theory, i.e. referred to related dermatome territory or into tissues embryologically linked with the viscus or tissue suffering the pathological change. We should consider this a little further, because serious visceral disease often simulates the pain of benign joint problems.

The pain from viscera is essentially similar to that arising from deep (somatic) structures such as muscles, ligaments, joints and periosteum (Appenzeller, 1978).[34]

If the site of referred pain is experimentally anaesthetised, referred effects due to stimulation of deep structures may often be abolished. Thus we are concerned with Head's zones of cutaneous hyperalgesia (p. 178), representing the spinal cord segments containing groups of cells upon which terminate both the visceral afferents of the viscus and the somatic afferents from the body wall and limbs (see p. 179).

Doran's[272] clinical findings on the pattern of pain reference in 56 patients who, after cholycystectomy, had the balloon of a Foley catheter left in the common bile duct are interesting. The balloon was inflated on the 12th postoperative day, when the patients had recovered sufficiently from the operation, were well orientated and able to report the pain experienced on artificial distension of the bile duct. Reference of pain was as follows:

No. of patients	Areas of pain	
20	Pain in epigastrium region	(T6–T10)
10	Pain in (R) hypochondrium	(T7–T11)
6	Pain in epigastrium *and* across back	(T6–T10)
5	Pain *only* in back but on one side	(T7–T9)
11	Had no pain at all	
56		

His authoritative account includes an interesting and extended discussion of visceral pain being referred to areas of the body wall which are segmentally linked with the diseased viscus by embryological derivation. The fact that 11 (about 20 per cent) patients experienced no pain at all might be due to a complete absence of visceral afferents from their common bile ducts, or might not. This is also of interest when considering the concept of true visceral pain,[437,272] i.e. defined as pain felt *in the organ*—the logical implications of this notion are that the 11 patients did not have a bile duct in which to feel the pain!

According to Brain and Wilkinson[117] the *gall bladder* is innervated by the phrenic nerve and pain is referred to the cutaneous distribution of the 3rd, 4th and 5th cervical segments over the point of the shoulder, but in none of these patients with an artificial *bile duct* stimulus was the pain referred in this way.

Two facts emerge of much importance to those handling spinal problems:

1. Pain in the posterior trunk may have nothing to do with primary spinal joint conditions.
2. With a standard lesion, 56 patients produced widely differing references of pain, and some had no pain.

Mechanisms concerned in the localisation of pain are ill-understood (Kellgren, 1977),[647] and at a given time in one individual the experience of pain is influenced by many factors, including that of its distribution being influenced by pre-existing pains in other localities.

This tendency for individuals to differ, by showing an idiosyncrasy in their patterns of pain reference, has also been reported by Hockaday and Whitty,[553] who repeated the experiments of Kellgren,[641] Sinclair and others,[1139] Travell and Bigelow,[1243] etc., and injected 6 per cent saline into the interspinous ligaments of normal subjects. A response involving referred effects of some sort occurred

after 94 per cent of injections. They found that while an individual's response remained consistent there was a definite and sometimes marked variation from person to person.

They concluded that because the site of reference of pain from connective-tissue lesions is quite variable between individuals, this does not support the concept of an anatomically fixed segmental reference like dermatomes.

Further information that individual idiosyncrasy might be a factor in pain reference was provided by Klafta and Collis (1969),[664] who performed 549 cervical disc injections over a 10-year period, while investigating the diagnostic usefulness of evaluating pain associated with discography. Pain produced was like the presenting symptom in 121 patients (22 per cent); pain was dissimilar to the presenting symptom in 369 patients (67 per cent) and there was no pain in response to disc injections in 59 patients (11 per cent). There were normal discs, degenerated discs and disc protrusions among all these groups.

Patterns of root innervation of muscles are also subject to variations from orthodox tabulations (p. 13).

Brendler (1968)[123] electrically stimulated 56 anterior cervical roots, at open operation, in 32 patients, and examples of the patterns of innervation, on the basis of motor responses, were:

Trapezius supplied by C1, 2, 3 and 4
Deltoid supplied by C3, 4, 5, 6 and 7
Biceps supplied by C5, 6 and 7.

It now remains to consider in more detail the characteristics of referred pain of non-root musculoskeletal origin, and to suggest a method of clinical examination which reduces the possibilities of confusion. Important investigations in this field were the reports by Inman and Saunders (1944)[592b] and Campbell and Parsons (1944)[156] on clinical and experimental findings of referred pain in category (C) (p. 193), i.e. pain experienced in tissues which are not the site of pathology, and whose afferent neurones are not involved in any way. The authors described their findings thus: referred pain is an obscure pain associated with traumatic and inflammatory lesions involving bony ligaments, tendons, fascia and other mesodermal structures of the body. Characteristics are a dull, aching, boring quality, difficult to describe; it lies deep ('in the bone', as patients sometimes say); it radiates for considerable distances; the area outlined by the patient does not correspond to peripheral nerve distribution or spinal nerve root distribution.

The radiation of pain is accompanied by concomitant symptoms and signs and these are feelings of deadness and numbness, although there is no objective numbness; feelings of heaviness; soreness of muscle (cramp); tenderness of muscle, and muscle spasm at times; tenderness of bony prominences; secretomotor and vasomotor changes (blanching, sweating).

In upper cervical joint problems the following may be encountered: nausea and giddiness; otalgia and migraine; tingling of the scalp; visual symptoms; pulse alterations.

These referred pains in experimental subjects were produced by scratching the deep tissues; drilling; injecting irritants like formic acid, and the site and nature of the pains were compared with extensive clinical observation of patients.

The site of the 'lesions' in patients and of the tissue damage artificially produced in models, together with the referred symptoms resulting, correlated very well. The pain appeared to be segmental in character yet did not correspond to dermatome or myotome distribution. The authors postulated that the pains were referred according to a *sclerotome* distribution (see Figs 2.24–2.25).

In these experiments the following observations were made:

The area of reference becomes painful only when the initial pain at the focus has lasted for some time (i.e. minutes or hours).

The referred pain may persist after the local pain has vanished.

The pain is not always distributed to the expected dermatomes, but may spread over a wider area.

Referred deep pain is most common, with skin hyperalgesia less so, and muscle spasm least.

The order of sensitivity found was:

periosteum (with the lowest threshold)
ligaments
fibrous joint capsule
tendons
fascia
muscle (this was least sensitive).

So far as ligaments and capsule were concerned, those parts in the neighbourhood of bony attachments were especially sensitive.

Classifications into local and referred pains cannot be applied consistently, and instead pain is described as (i) moderately well localised, and (ii) diffuse pain which is poorly localised, but that from deeper periosteum is more diffuse and referred.

In summary therefore:

1. The area occupied by category (B) pain, distal paraesthesiae and neurological deficit is sometimes but not always a helpful clue as to which root is probably involved.
2. The description of referred pain in gall bladder experiments (p. 194) explains pain of the third category (C) on the basis of reference in to dermatomes.
3. The two reports above also describe (C) category

pain, but this time from musculoskeletal tissues and explained as referred into a sclerotome distribution.

4. The area occupied by referred pain of non-root origin can be a help in deciding where to look for the more proximal joint problem (when such exists) but it is wise to make a wide search.

Clinical observations[797] indicate that:

1. Pain arising from lesions in skeletal muscle, bone and superficial periosteum is generally localised to the area surrounding the tissue damage.
2. Pain from lesions of synovial joints and their immediate periarticular structures may be (a) localised, (b) localised and also referred, and (c) referred only. Examples are: (a) pain felt at the T6 segment, (b) pain felt here and also spreading laterally around the lower scapular and subaxillary area, and (c) pain reported anteriorly at the costochondral and sternal area only, although careful tests of thoracic movement and localised palpation tests will often provoke the anterior pain.
3. The pain of an intervertebral disc lesion, not involving neighbouring tissues, may also be localised and referred, with the most pain being felt proximally.[184]
4. Root pain (category B), resulting from nerve root compression or other involvement by degenerative change, by disc trespass or foraminal encroachment by other tissues, is usually more severe in its distal extent, although some pain may be felt locally. Hence root pain is also referred, but not all referred pain is root pain.
5. The spread of pain from combined lesions, which occur at cervical as well as low lumbar segments, may be extensive and not easy to ascribe to particular segments without detailed examination.[916, 1180b, 1281]
6. Proximal vertebral lesions tend to refer pain to more distal areas; elbow- and knee-joint problems can refer pain both proximally and distally, and wrist and ankle conditions may refer pain proximally.

A remarkable property of referred pain is that it can appear to be exactly the same, when produced by either of two (or more) separate sources[105]

and experienced manual therapists will be familiar with the phenomenon of relieving what appears to be an identical, unilateral 'yoke' area pain by mobilising, on the painful side, in one patient the C1–C2 segment, in another the C4–C5 segment, in another the joints of the first rib, while in some, any two or all three sites must have attention before signs and symptoms are relieved.

Similarly, while pain from low lumbar disc changes tends to have a sciatic distribution, i.e. buttock, posterior thigh and calf, the distribution of pain on injection, under fluoroscopy control, of irritant saline into low lumbar facet-joints has a like distribution. This has been described by the experimenter Mooney (1977),[870] who had his own joint cavities injected as well as injecting those of other normal subjects and patients.

Conclusions

Deciding, by a process of Sherlock Holmes detection, that the lesion lies here or there because that is where it *ought* to be, without careful and systematic vertebral palpation, is not enough.

It is a profound mistake to arbitrarily apply conventional anatomical description to all individuals, whilst holding 'all is based on simple anatomy'. Anatomy is not simple, it is very complicated and so are the neurophysiological mechanisms underlying it. Our understanding of them is far from complete. There are so many considerations and variables:

1. The wandering of the sinuvertebral nerve, up and down the neural canal before terminating in receptors.
2. The variability of dermatomes.
3. The 'untidiness' of sclerotomes.
4. Pre- and postfixation of plexuses.
5. Differing myotomes—deltoid, for example, may be supplied by C3, C4 or C7, and not necessarily by C5–6.[123]
6. Differing pain tolerances.
7. The nature of the lesion, about which we can often only make an intelligent guess.
8. The fact that individual responses vary quite widely.
9. The somewhat fulsome descriptions given by patients.

Three-quarters of the emphasis, in assessing where to work in mobilising or manipulating the vertebral column, should perhaps rest on what is found by palpation, following regional active, and passive segmental, tests of movement.

During examination (see p. 303) *therefore, a standard clinical method might include these basic principles:*

1. The suspension of disbelief while listening to the patient.
2. Examination by a process of exclusion from proximal to distal.
3. The inclusion of all tissues and structures from which pain *could* be arising.
4. Allowances for the odd fact which does not fit in.
5. A careful search over several segments to either side of the suspected level, by detailed palpation.

The findings of referred cutaneous sensation in most subjects suggest that sensory disturbances which are not confined to dermatomal distributions should not be glibly dismissed as hysterical.[34]

ABNORMALITIES OF FEELING

The nature of abnormalities is difficult adequately to convey. 'Tingling', 'prickling', 'pins and needles', 'electric feelings', 'fizzling in the skin', probably only approximate to what the patient wishes to describe and few patients are analytical about precise distribution unless assisted to be

so. Paraesthesiae can occur from many causes, some vertebral or in the region of the axial skeleton, e.g. cervical rib, and some peripheral, e.g. entrapment neuropathies such as carpal-tunnel syndrome, but the concern of the therapist is to seek aid in localising spinal joint problems, if the cause be so, and thus when the distribution of paraesthesiae, especially distally, is roughly similar to the territory of a spinal nerve root, it may be a help in identifying the vertebral segment probably responsible, and with greater certainty when they accompany so-called root pain and signs of neurological deficit in the myotome of that segment. The distribution of paraesthesiae may be extrasegmental, i.e. involving more than one root, and on occasions when 'glove' paraesthesiae of the lower forearm and hand are reported, together with statements that the arm generally feels heavy and numb, examination-planning should include the upper and midthoracic spine and associated rib movements. It is important to distinguish between *feelings* of numbness and actual sensory loss, because frequently an objective test of sensation is negative, and objective muscle weakness cannot be detected in the arm. It should be remembered that paraesthesiae can also be painful. A localised patch of unilateral, paravertebral *hyperaesthesia*[412a] can very often be detected on palpation adjacent to the site of lumbar joint problems, but it is often not reported during history-taking. A similar but much more intense disturbance of sensation may be described by patients as lying bilaterally over the cervicothoracic region.[839] In the latter situation the hyperaesthesia or hyperpathia sometimes reaches an intensity which is more distressing to the patient than pain. This change might be due to mechanical interference with peripheral nerves, but it appears unlike the paraesthesiae usually associated with root interference.

When paraesthesiae is described in part of a limb, it is wise to check that other limbs are normal in this respect; patients sometimes unwittingly withhold information because specific enquiry is not made. Bilateral paraesthesiae and particularly their distribution are of significance since they may contraindicate certain treatments.

Persisting small localised areas of complete loss of sensation in a limb can be an unnecessary source of anxiety to patients, but are not disabling unless the distal parts of the fingers are involved, when burns during cooking, ironing and smoking can occur.

CHANGES IN MUSCLE AND SOFT TISSUES

Spasm

Tone in striated muscle is due to three sets of influences: elastic tension of the collagenous tissue elements; interdigitation of the actin and myosin elements; the number of motor units active at any one moment.

Most of the tone in normal muscle is of reflex origin, and is maintained by afferent impulses.[130] Together with the neuromuscular spindle afferents, the Type I and Type II articular mechanoreceptors (see p. 11) govern the degree and distribution of tone; although supraspinal influences are also important and these will differ from person to person, also in the same individual in different circumstances.

The clinical features of spasm, tenderness of muscle and muscular aches are without doubt interrelated, although the traditional concept that spasm of muscle inevitably causes its own contribution to pain may not necessarily be correct.

Intrinsic muscle spasm manifested in clinical states *directly involving the muscle itself*, such as trauma (avulsion of periosteal attachments, rupture of muscle fibres and tearing of connective-tissue elements), strain, haemorrhage, metabolic disturbances, inflammation, tender nodules, Bornholm disease and new growths, are a direct cause of local muscle spasm, and pain.[622]

The genesis of the spasm may possibly lie partly within the muscle parenchyma, if damaged, and be due to the biochemical changes of electrolyte imbalance, and is probably reflex also.

In reflex muscle spasm, secondary to nociceptor irritation in joints and associated structures and in which no changes have taken place within the muscle itself, other than spasm, ordinary clinical observation shows: (i) that these muscles can commonly be neither tender nor painful, despite a degree of spasm which is virtually board-like and persists over some days, and (ii) the 'spastic' muscle may at times be tender, and be included in the locality indicated by the patient as the site of pain, often in cervical and cervicothoracic problems.

The concept that constant mild cervical traction is necessary to 'overcome muscle spasm for *the relief of pain*' is questionable.[622] When the paraspinal muscles overlying a cervical joint problem are in spasm, compressing the spine by pressure on the crown shortens the muscle but increases the pain. Similarly, tilting the head towards the painful side should relax the muscle, yet it sharply increases the pain.

A clinical state very frequently observed by physiotherapists is that of the deviated or 'windswept' vertebral column, secondary to a lumbar joint problem in a patient with equal leg lengths and a level pelvis, held in postural asymmetry by obvious and palpably severe spasm. Movements are limited and distorted, yet although restricted the patient is in no pain and neither is the 'spastic' vertebral muscle tender. Many of these patients have no sciatica and no neurological signs.

In spasmodic torticollis due to basal ganglia disease, marked muscle contraction may take place, yet the patients do not inevitably complain of pain, only of tightness and a pulling sensation.

In the so-called muscle-tension headache, pain is believed due to spasm of neck and scalp muscles. In several patients who were particularly susceptible to tension headache, Judovitch[622] electrically induced hypertonus in the upper cervical and scalp muscles, and maintained this 'spasm' for 20 minutes during the time they complained of headache. In spite of the fact that 'spasm' was greater in degree than that usually observed during an attack, no symptoms were provoked and patients reported that their pain was alleviated.

He asserts that in many joint problems, reflex skeletal muscle spasm may have little to do with producing pain, or as is commonly believed, the establishment of a vicious pain cycle.

Clinical observations suggest that although muscle spasm is common the causal relationship between it and *pain* is not yet fully elucidated, neither is the frequent absence of clinically detectable postural spasm in low lumbar hypermobility syndromes in young women, causing a chronic ache of depressing persistence, with no limitation of movement and no neurological signs; although reactive spasm may be provoked in response to heavy-handed palpation.

Nevertheless, experimental injury of anaesthetised animals provides clear evidence that hypertonous *per se* will follow damage of acute onset to musculoskeletal tissues.

Wyke[1356] gives unequivocal demonstrations that Type IV joint receptors in joint capsule, fat pads and ligaments, when subject to sufficient irritation, will provoke intense non-adapting motor-unit responses simultaneously in all muscles related to the joint, as well in more remote muscles elsewhere in the body.

It is suggested that the arthrokinetic pathway is polysynaptic and that it projects to *gamma* fusimotor rather than to *alpha* motoneurones. The hypertonus (spasm) in musculature overlying the lesion in low back pain is also suggested[472] as due to denervation supersensitivity of the 'gamma–alpha loop', and therefore an early sign of irritation.

The precise nature of acute derangement of a cervical, thoracic or lumbar joint, or precise result of trauma which may injure it without derangement, is not always clear, but its effects are plain:

1. If there is intra-articular derangement[508] of the facet-joint (see p. 253) the discharge of Type IV nociceptors in joint capsule and fat pads will evoke intense motor response, the ensuing muscle spasm 'locking the joint like a mouse-trap.'

2. Assuming that on occasions the joint will have suffered tearing of tissues, the combination of synovial effusion, hyperaemia and possibly extravasation of blood will combine to produce physical trespass by fluid. Swelling tends to bulge anteriorly, where the capsule is thinner, and there may be capsular tearing. Spinal root irritation might be expected to occur, since the root lies immediately

anterior to the synovial joint capsule (except in the upper two cervical segments).

Whether the degree of reactive muscle spasm would be much greater when tissue tearing occurs, when root irritation might also be a factor, probably depends as much on the temperament of the person in whom it occurs, and their emotional state at the time, as upon the magnitude and nature of the damage. Since a proportion of a joint's nociceptor fibres course *through* the paravertebral muscles related to that joint, it is proposed[1356] that continued muscle spasm allows accumulation of metabolites which will irritate (a) the plexiform network of nociceptors within the walls of the blood vessels, as well as (b) the joint nociceptors traversing muscle, thereby adding pain of muscular origin to that generated by the nociceptor system of the injured joint itself.

It is likely that the applied stress need not involve the actual articulation at all; the junctional attachment-tissues of intermuscular septa, ligament, muscle, tendon, aponeurosis, capsule and periosteal insertion can be a fruitful source of pain,[143, 1100] and injury to these junctional tissues is likely to be as potent a source of reflex muscle spasm as any other. Their importance in the production of spinal pain syndromes is being increasingly recognised (p. 250).

The distribution of *spasm* from spinal joint problems, when it exists, does not necessarily allow precise identification of the tissue damage causing it. For example,[979] in anaesthetised experimental animals, lesions were mechanically produced by successively crushing lumbar and sacral structures, i.e. joints, fascia, ligament, muscle and skin. Also, hypertonic saline was injected into these tissues to produce irritative lesions. The increased hypertonus in lumbodorsal muscle and hamstrings was recorded electromyographically, and results indicated that stimulus of *any* deep structure caused non-specific widespread spasm in the experimental animals.

In this connection, the poor localisation of the patient's pain, associated with deep lesions of the lumbosacral area, is emphasised by the authors as is the difficulty of localising the precise tissue-changes in many of these lesions on the basis of physical findings such as the distribution of spasm.

The protective response of spasm will often involve a whole vertebral region, yet can sometimes be much more localised so that it seems to splint or stabilise two or three segments only, whose lack of participation in normal active movements of the whole region can only be detected by close observation during the movement and *by careful and systematic palpation*.

At times it is clinically obvious that a proportion of deformities, which disappear quickly on successful treatment, are due to an asymmetrical distribution of spasm, maintaining an injured and irritable joint in the least painful, or antalgic, posture.

Common examples are the loss of normal lordosis at the neck and low back; the cervical problem is generally much easier to deal with than the loss of lumbar lordosis (sometimes to the extent of a slight kyphosis) seen associated with severe spasm fixing the patient in a degree of flexion, often combined with side-flexion either towards or away from the painful side. On other occasions a more symmetrical distribution of increased muscle tone is obvious, yet there is no gross change in attitude, movements are not markedly restricted and following reduction of pain on movement this more generalised spasm disappears.

Other soft tissue changes[1133, 1134]

Tender, nodular changes can be palpated in large masses like the gluteus maximus, with stringy and equally tender fasciculi occurring especially in sacrospinalis, trapezius and other muscle groups of the neck. They seem to occur both with, and in the absence of, detectable joint problems. Localised areas of *thickening*, of deep periarticular soft tissue, can readily be palpated overlying the facet-joint area of painful segments of the cervical spine; similar thickening can be felt unilaterally over painful thoracic and lumbar segments but is not quite so readily detectable. More superficially, subcutaneous areolar tissue is often perceived to be thickened and bound down over the dorsal and lumbar sites of chronic joint lesions.

Changes in skin texture, in the form of slight but definite resistance to stroking when compared with neighbouring areas, are frequently associated with localised regions of tenderness and thickening overlying joint abnormalities. They presumably indicate a disturbance of sudomotor activity in the associated area of segmental skin supply; the changes may be due to involvement of postganglionic sympathetic afferent neurones in somatic root irritation and compression, or are more probably mediated via preganglionic efferent neurones sharing in the heightened impulse activity of facilitated cord segments.[1180b]

Early and subtle signs in low back pain have been described by Gunn and Milbrandt (1978).[472] Skin, connective tissue and muscle may share in sensory disorders which may be due to irritation of autonomic neurones, and these detectable changes may be confusing in that their atypical or unexpected distribution conforms more to a vasal rather than a neural topography. They are ascribed to early and reversible neuropathy, rather than late and severe denervation, and it is suggested that,

... localisation of the level of injury lies in detecting abnormalities in different structures belonging to the same segment but receiving their ultimate segmental innervation through different peripheral nerves.

The signs are as follows:

1. As the patient undresses and cool air plays on exposed skin, there is a brief *pilomotor effect* ('*goose flesh*') in the dermatomes of the affected segment.

2. Vasoconstrictor disturbances due to denervation sensitivity produce a combination of pallor and cyanosis, as *mottling of the skin* in the affected region.

3. A sudomotor reflex, evidenced as *increased sweating*. This may be spontaneous or because of the stress of pain or of the examination procedure, or both; its distribution indicates a central rather than a segmental effect.

4. *Myalgic and cutaneous hyperaesthesia*—acutely tender motor points occur in the affected segments, with the degree of tenderness and the number of tender points related to the severity of the patient's condition. The authors refer to the tendency of clinicians to attribute a tender gluteus medius motor point to 'gluteal bursitis'. Glover (1960)[412a] has well described this feature.

5. Partial denervation is mentioned as the cause of *cutaneous trophoedema*. There is gradual fibrosis of the subcutaneous tissue, and the overlying skin tends to be fissured and prone to folds, with a baggy, inelastic texture—the *peau d'orange* effect previously described by Stoddard (1962).[1180a] There is pitting oedema to small localised pressure and this lasts longer than in normal skin.

The authors found one or more of these early and subtle signs of nerve irritability (including muscle hypertonus) in all of 30 patients with low back pain; the signs were largely resolved when the patients were pain-free. Some of the signs were also found in about half of control groups; the implications of these findings are discussed by the authors.

DEFORMITY

Muscle spasm, secondary to joint derangement or irritability, does not lead to contracture of soft tissues in young people, but in middle-aged and elderly people when persistent muscle spasm has produced both long-standing changes of attitude and palpable changes in the texture of muscle tissue, a degree of shortening by tissue contracture is usually present. The main changes are probably in connective-tissue elements within the muscle, as well as in the fascial planes between the muscle-groups.

Similar changes of shortening will develop in the periarticular connective tissues, on one aspect of the joint, together with adaptive lengthening of the structures on the opposite aspect which are maintained in a lengthened state. Contracted inert structures on one side will induce a degree of fixed side-flexion to the same side, often with slight rotation. Conversely, degenerative processes can add unilaterally to the bulk of joint tissues and induce a tilt *away* from that side. Secondary changes of shortening need not be due to spasm, however, but are often noted, e.g. in the dorsal lumbar connective tissues of patients whose pain is due to chronic changes brought about by excessive lordosis (see p. 267) and spasm is not a feature.

Congenital and acquired deformities tend to produce asymmetrical stress on joint structures and thus predispose them to early degenerative change (see p. 274). Conversely, degenerative joint conditions frequently produce changes of body contour and attitude, e.g.:

Cervical spine

In patients who present with head, neck and shoulder pain, deformity of neck posture is often evident as a slight lateral tilt, or slight rotation. These deviations may be towards the side of a unilateral pain, or more usually away from it. Rotatory atlantoaxial fixation may be evident as asymmetry of cervical rotation, palpable on careful examination and visible on anteroposterior films of the craniovertebral region.[208, 1346] Sometimes a changed contour is the appearance of a muscle-group in spasm (see p. 196) but can also be due to a chronic disturbance, at one segment, of joint mechanics which has induced a slight postural compensation. Spasm is not always detectable, but palpable loss of segmental movement is manifest.

Cervicothoracic region

1. Habitual flexion of the cervicothoracic junction tends to produce chronic overstretching of the posterior muscles and joint structures of the upper thoracic spine, with adaptive shortening of anterior ligaments and muscles, especially the pectoral group. The movement of extending the head and neck then occurs as an overaccentuation of the normal degree of cervical lordosis, but with little cervical movement.

2. The appearance of a slightly elevated shoulder girdle may be due to unilateral spasm of scalenus and trapezius muscles; additionally, the first rib may be slightly elevated and thus more easily palpated on the affected side; thus the deformity has two contributory factors.

3. The fibroelastic ligamentum nuchae helps to resist the constant tendency for the head to droop forward, and its degenerative loss of elasticity in advanced age is one of the reasons for the progressive lowering of the head in the elderly, when standing and sitting.

Thoracic spine

1. Osteochondrosis producing kyphosis in this region has been noted and similarly, congenital or long-standing acquired scoliosis will predispose the affected regions to early degenerative change.

2. On occasions, a loss of normal kyphosis is evident in the region between T3 and T7, the spinal section presenting a perfectly flat interscapular area which changes little on movement; frequently combined with this is a normal and sometimes increased prominence of C7–T2 spinous processes, and a tendency to neck and head pain.

Lumbar spine

During examination of patients in whom backache and sciatica coexist with lateral curvature of the spine, it is important to distinguish between cause and effect. When well-compensated pre-existing lateral curvature underlies the secondary lumbar pain and sciatica for which the patient seeks treatment, a plumbline held at the external occipital protuberance will usually be in line with the gluteal cleft, whereas in lateral deviation or listing which is secondary to joint abnormalities in a previously straight spine, the plumbline tends to fall across one buttock (Fig. 8.6).

1. A short leg, whether congenital or acquired during childhood, predictably can have long-term effects. These patients may suffer in early adult life from back pain and sciatica, arising from changes due to continual one-sided stretching and attenuation of the annulus fibrosus of a low lumbar disc on the side of the *shorter* leg, and from localised arthrotic and spondylotic change, when middle-aged, due to the extra unilateral compression strains on vertebral bodies, discs and facet-joint structures on the side of the *longer* leg. A similar tendency is produced by a tilted upper surface of the sacrum.

2. Conversely, lateral deviation of the spine is frequently the *result* of an acute lumbar derangement,[241b] sometimes but by no means always secondary to disc protrusion and root compression.

Some common root and protrusion relationships are recognised by surgeons[239] at operation for this condition: protrusion lateral to the root; protrusion directly beneath the root; protrusion medial to the root; protrusion lying in the angle of the junction of the theca and the dural sheath of the root, i.e. the root 'axilla'.

It is postulated that these relationships may dictate the direction and degree of the listing or deviation of the spine towards, or away from, the painful side which is often seen, but there are other considerations. For example, nuclear material may shift to produce an annular bulge and become trapped between adjacent vertebral body margins, effectively jamming and distorting the joint (see p. 264) or the unilateral exit of material from between the vertebral bodies may be sufficiently complete to allow a vertebral body tilt towards the same side. Listing, to one side or another, may be accompanied by a fixed and accentuated lordosis or a fixed lumbar kyphosis,[797] these postural abnormalities primarily indicating the disturbance of the joint produced by the derangement, and perhaps by involuntary adoption of the least painful posture and its maintenance at times by postural spasm. Listing or lateral deviation *away* from the painful side is said to occur more frequently in L5 sciaticas when caused by 4th lumbar disc involvement, and listing *towards* the painful side to occur mostly in S1 sciaticas, due to 5th lumbar prolapse.

Yet similar lateral distortion of the normal lumbar posture to one or other side frequently occurs in the absence of both detectable nerve root involvement and sciatica, when the cause is presumably a joint derangement not involving nerve root interference.

In a series of 500 patients with low back pain and/or sciatica, and listing secondary to joint derangement, 479 deviated *away* from the painful side and the remainder deviated *towards* it. Clinical impressions suggest that in 70 per cent of cases the derangement was at the L5–S1 segment, and in the remaining 30 per cent at the L4–5 segment.[833]

SEGMENTAL DEFORMITIES

Palpation will often reveal what appears to be undue spaces between spinous processes, undue bony prominences, apparently deviated spinous processes especially in the thoracic spine, asymmetrical bulk of the bifid cervical processes and irregularity of posterior superior iliac spines. These apparent and sometimes real bony abnormalities are very frequently of no significance but can on occasions assume importance.

FUNCTIONAL DISABLEMENT

Degenerative processes and their consequences interfere with normal function in a variety of ways; on occasions the disablement is severe and serious, examples already described being: the neurological consequences of cervical myelopathy; sphincter paralysis associated with cauda equina lesions; the sudden 'drop' attacks of vertebrobasilar ischaemia.

The degree of restriction usually amounts to less serious but annoying and sometimes severely frustrating difficulty in performing an everyday movement, working or sleeping in a particular posture and the free enjoyment of leisure; apart from the mental distress which is frequently noted accompanying upper cervical joint problems, prolonged physical frustration of any kind is sufficient cause for depression, as is chronic tiredness for want of restful sleep.

Posture

Symptoms arising from degenerating joints are characteristically aggravated by certain positions, and partially or completely relieved by other positions. These differ from patient to patient (see below).

Pain

Disturbance of sleep by aches arising while lying in various positions are very commonly reported. Much sciatica and brachalgia are at their worst at night, and aside from this frequent characteristic of joint problems, the situation is often aggravated by unsuitable pillows, mattresses and beds.

It is important to know that severe and inexorable night pain may be evidence of more serious joint pathology, for which physical treatment is contraindicated.[91]

Daily activity can be restricted in a number of ways:

Head and facial pain will interfere with concentration, disturb social life and often require periods of bedrest during attacks.

Cervical rotation often produces jabs of pain, and a painful neck can make reversing a car hazardous; pain on neck flexion precludes activities like sewing, reading and gardening. Playing wind instruments and the violin become especially difficult. Many patients suffer more severely from cervical degenerative change if they do not avoid prolonged extension movements; decorating a ceiling can initiate weeks of extra pain and inconvenience.

Pain on jarring the neck may prevent walking, and driving a car, and severe limb pain can be exacerbated when the spine is jarred on clumsily negotiating the edge of a pavement.

Root pain in a limb may be severe enough to render it functionally useless.

The yoke area pain of cervicothoracic joint problems is especially likely to prevent activities like lawnmowing, cleaning windows, decorating and jobs which require the ability to push or press with the hand.

Carrying luggage or heavy shopping will aggravate symptoms arising from upper thoracic segments, and sleeping is often impossible while lying on the side of a unilateral scapular area pain.

The pain of midthoracic joint problems may interfere with free respiration and prevent ordinary housework, working with the arms forward or elevated anteriorly, and carrying. Painful neck, thoracic and lumbar joint conditions will interfere with dressing.

Lumbar discogenic pain will be aggravated by sitting in chair, car seat, bath or bed, and any activity requiring bending; lifting, vacuum cleaning and gardening frequently aggravate low-back-joint problems.

The patient with lumbar disc herniation is usually more comfortable standing or lying, and in acute discomfort when sitting, since it is in the latter posture that the intradiscal pressure is highest (see p. 22). Conversely, pain on standing, because of arthrotic changes due to an increased lumbosacral lordosis, is relieved on sitting, because the lordosis is then less accentuated and painful stress diminished.

The pain of spondylolisthesis often tends to be aggravated on standing, and relieved to a degree by sitting, for the same mechanical reasons.

Combined spondylosis and arthrosis of low lumbar segments sometimes gives rise to intermittent claudication on walking (see p. 276).

Painful lumbar joint problems can effectively preclude coitus, although many patients are naturally loth to report this particular frustration; yet it can be a guide for assessment of treatment.

Where the main factor responsible for chronic pain appears to be that of gravitational compression, pain may steadily increase from a relatively pain-free early morning to a regularly pain-wracked evening. Evening leisure activities are correspondingly restricted, the pain being relieved after a night's rest.

Sensation changes causing functional disablement

Paraesthesiae in the hand are often worse in the small hours and for an hour or so after rising; handling utensils and cookers, and preparing food, may be difficult and occasionally dangerous during this period if utensils are heavy and hot. Sometimes the symptoms are aggravated during the day if anything is handled and any fine work with the fingers is then effectively halted. It is interesting that symptoms occurring distally but due to vertebral changes, can be aggravated by the local stimulus of cutaneous and mechanoreceptors in the hand.

The patchy dysaesthesia which occurs in some elderly patients may involve almost all the digits and make attempted use of the hands very frustrating, since it is usually associated with some wasting of intrinsic muscle and also stiffness.

Acutely tender thoracic spinous processes sometimes prevent complete rest in a high-backed chair.

Paraesthesiae accompanying sciatic pain do not appear to have severe disabling effects on patients, but some are distressed by these symptoms and 'saddle anaesthesia' accompanies other changes (q.v.) which are certainly disabling.

Disabling stiffness

Joint symptoms, especially stiffness, are usually intermittent or their degree tends to vary with time. Often, painful stiffness is more noticeable after periods of rest, and some patients are most comfortable if they keep lightly on the move and do not remain still for long periods. Stiffness may be at its worst on rising in the morning, easing on moving around and on increased activity and then building up again in the evening; this often characterises *arthrotic* joints. The similar rhythmic behaviour of symptoms due more to *spondylosis* is usually in terms of weeks or months, rather than diurnally, and these examples of variability of symptoms should be borne in mind during assessment and the formulation of treatment programmes.

Sustained flexion of a vertebral region often increases stiffening, which can be overcome only slowly on extension; it occurs in each of the vertebral regions.

Rising from a chair may be momentarily painful but the patient is frequently more concerned with painful *stiffness*, and it may be minutes before the fully upright posture is reached. At times this may probably be due to the slow shift of disc material as the posture of the lumbar curve is altered from the relative flexion of sitting to the normal lordosis of standing, but this characteristic difficulty of movement after rest is also reported in arthrosis of the peripheral joints. The inability to move joints at will, quickly and painlessly, is disability enough.

Motor weakness

Compared to pain and stiffness, muscle weakness is less commonly a cause of interference with activities, but involvement of the triceps, small muscles of the thumb, dorsiflexors of the foot and calf muscles can create difficulties for the patient. The more serious motor disabilities, including sphincter disturbance, have been mentioned previously.

Concomitant symptoms and signs

Vertigo (dysequilibrium) is sometimes severely disabling, the patient being afraid to go out without a companion. Rotation and extension of the neck are performed very cautiously or not at all, and general changes of trunk and head postures made slowly. Hence, rising in the morning must often be done by little stages. The distress occasioned by difficulties of concentration and remembering, nausea and vomiting, speech difficulties, has been noted.

THE PSYCHOLOGICAL ASPECT OF VERTEBRAL PAIN

There is now a unified medicopsychosocial or multifactorial concept of all diseases, where research into the psychological aspects of disease is closely linked with advancement of the clinical sciences.

At a relatively unscientific level, the reaffirmation of the 'whole man' approach to medicine has enabled many practitioners to regain a dimension of their practice that seemed in danger of being lost.... Apart from the purely humanitarian aspect of this total approach, it represents sound medical practice.[878]

While manual therapists should not aspire to be psychiatrists, we cannot escape confrontation with patients whose clinical presentation is at first puzzling, and whose handling and treatment may make considerable demands on our perception and capacity to understand.

Phrases like 'psychological overlay' and 'a large functional element' have no precise meaning, and the word 'psychosomatic' is merely shorthand recognition of what is common knowledge, viz: there is no pain which is exclusively organic; yet these words may carry a connotation that the patient is 'not quite on the level'.

The phrases seem too frequently used to describe patients who may be exhausted by chronic pain, or

frightened, anxious, timid or diffident because of the overwhelming nature of the circumstance in which they find themselves. Not infrequently, these states may have been produced by genuine misunderstanding between patient and clinical worker; sometimes they may have been nurtured by resentment at having been given a hasty and inadequate clinical hearing in the first instance, and occasionally by indifferent or unimaginative handling.

Use of the phrases in clinical records may at times be unjustified, taking little account of many of those in pain who are, in fact, putting in some quiet and unsung heroism in a difficult domestic background, the true extent of which is unlikely to be entirely revealed by naturally reticent people to bluff, hearty and bossy clinicians.

The fact that medical and/or surgical findings are negative, or are insufficient to explain the pain on an organic basis, does not justify a diagnosis of psychogenic pain. Such a diagnosis requires positive psychiatric findings.[813]

Phillips, E. L. (1964)[989] has suggested that,

... the vastly different circumstances under which persons live and work can ... be assumed to complicate any initially clear relationship between personality variables on the one hand and physical illness or disease on the other ...

A surprising number of lay people have very fixed ideas about the causes and nature of joint and muscle pains, the ideas being derived for the most part from patent medicine advertisements. It is not always easy to explain to patients, in their own terms, what the nature of the problem is—more especially, when we are not too sure ourselves! The factor of certainty about its benign and self-limiting nature is not always much comfort to the overimaginative patient suffering painful, bizarre and distressing symptoms. It is not always easy to give explanations which are 'true', brief, adequately descriptive and satisfying to the patient. Overuse of the words 'arthritis' and 'disease' is also unjustified and harmful. *It is better to spend some of the time trying to 'read' the patient than spending all of the time trying to understand the joint problem.*

Emotional reactions to illness

Rees (1970),[1018] remarking on the types of attitudes and emotional reactions to physical illness, observes that clinicians no longer tend to seek a single cause for a particular disorder, but regard illness as the resultant of interaction between many forces in the individual and his environment.

Certain mental changes tend to occur in all ill people, whether normal or abnormal personalities—regression, denial, depression, withdrawal, anxiety, anger and hostility may be encountered. There is a vast range of reaction to low back pain, for example; difficulty is encountered when the patient's reaction seems more extreme than normal and the pain seems to have a significance and importance far beyond the obvious disruption caused by the joint problem.[1334]

It is likely that a trace of each or most of the attitudes mentioned, to differing degrees and in different combinations, occur in the majority of patients; and further, that most people are probably aware of their particular tendencies or traits and try to cope with them, with variable success. Rees mentions the following types:

The very dependent and overdemanding person badly needs others to bolster feelings of acceptance and security, tending to welcome illness as a return to a childhood state of secure, happy dependency. When the hopeful expectation of unlimited care is not altogether fulfilled, the patient may be hurt, resentful and depressed. When limits have to be imposed, they are best introduced as steps to regaining independence.

The obsessional person has excellent self-discipline, being neat, meticulous and excessively conscientious. Illness is untidy and thus represents a threat to self-control, so that redoubled efforts to be responsible and orderly may lead to these individuals becoming inflexible and opinionated. Their wish to co-operate fully and with the utmost responsibility can be encouraged to their advantage.

The suspicious, guarded, querulous (paranoid) person is quarrelsome, watchful of others and tends to blame misfortunes upon others. They harbour grievances and deep sense of hurt, and of having been let down. Therapists should listen but not get too involved; argument is useless and results in loss of co-operation.

Withdrawn, introverted (schizoid) persons are uncommunicative and tend to remain uninvolved in daily events and others' concerns. They are unsociable, with minimal emotional reactions.

Cyclothymic people swing between elation and depression, their outlook reflecting their prevailing mood.

Overanxious people tend to meet dangers halfway, and when ill tend to detect sinister import in ordinary symptoms.

Hypochondriacal individuals make excessive demands for minor complaints, sometimes giving the impression of believing they have at best only a precarious hold on physical health.

The hysterical personality seeks attention, and these individuals tend to manipulate people and situations to their advantage. Their eager, warm and personal response carries with it an expectation that the clinician will reciprocate in a personal way. Their seemingly vivid emotional responses are in fact shallow, and they respond best to firmness laced with sympathetic interest. Walshe (1951)[1288] reminds us:

There is, indeed, no symptom-complex of somatic illness that may not have its hysterical 'double'. Symptoms referrable to almost any of the viscera or to the skeletal structures may dominate the clinical picture, and thus in every field of medicine and surgery the clinician is called upon to differentiate between physically and psychologically determined symptoms.

Yet true conversion hysteria (when anxiety engendered by an overwhelming conflict is converted into a physical symptom) is a rare condition, the disorder usually occurring in the less sophisticated members of society.[1334]

A diagnosis of hysteria is made with caution, since follow-up studies of such patients have demonstrated a high incidence of severe physical or mental illness.[1335]

Alexithymia Sometimes, patients are encountered who seem not to have any words for their feelings.[914] These alexithymic persons lack the ability to experience psychological states such as sadness or anxiety, and they tend to somatize a mental conflict, in that their thought processes are preoccupied with the minute details of external happenings such as bodily dysfunctions. They are likely, under stress, to produce a back pain, for example. This process is not the same as conversion hysteria, when the subject is more likely to express the conflict in complex psychological terms in addition to the 'lesion'.

Depression can complicate the clinical picture in any physical illness, and when severe will produce its own effects such as sleep disturbance, loss of weight and of appetite, fatigue and reduction of powers of concentration.[1018]

Forrest and Wolkind (1974)[368] reviewed the outcome of treatment for low back pain in 50 male patients, and suggested that there are two distinct populations among low-back-pain patients. The 'poor responder' group was characterised by a depressive syndrome described principally in somatic terms, and in these patients depression was masked and unrecognised. The authors suggest that it is rare to find patients with a depressive illness without somatic symptoms.

After mentioning the substantial evidence that anxiety, emotional conflict, stress and personality changes are important factors causing or producing pain, Merskey and Boyd (1978)[854] report examining the life experience of 141 chronic pain patients, in terms of disturbed upbringing, neurotic traits and personality problems, both currently and premorbidly. Significantly fewer of the three factors were reported in those patients with an organic cause for their pain; those without organic cause for their pain showed a higher incidence of family disturbance, personality problems and neurotic traits. *Their data provided support for the view that a significant proportion of the emotional disturbance associated with chronic pain is a secondary effect;*

... the common sense view is that not only does pain follow from psychological illness but that lesions which cause chronic pain tend to produce psychiatric disturbances.

Gilchrist (1976)[407] found, among 1499 patients attending general practitioners over a period of six years, that while those with a history of low back pain were more likely to have had a diagnosis of anxiety than those without back pain, there was no significant difference in the incidence of depression between those with and those without back pain.

These findings suggest that while depression does not necessarily predispose a patient to complain of back pain, chronic low back pain can be a cause of psychiatric disturbance, including depression. The depressed patient is subjectively sad and miserable, seeing everything in the worst possible light. While antidepressant medication and simple psychotherapy can be very effective,[1334] experienced manual therapists are very familiar with the simple antidepressant effect of relieving the pain which has engendered the depression.

The common-sense approach has been well summarised by Thompson (1980):[1213a]

Backache associated with hysteria or malingering is rare, and usually suspected on the basis of other features in the presentation. Some cases of coccydynia (coccygodynia) in women are clearly related to emotional disturbance. Many patients with musculoskeletal lesions may react adversely to continued pain, and some may exaggerate or prolong the effects of a mild spinal disability to suit their own purpose, but this should not prevent accurate diagnosis and management of the organic component of their illness. Indeed, the relief of that part of the complaint attributable to organic causes is an essential prerequisite to resolution of the emotional component.

Accident and compensation neurosis

While it would be foolish to state that such a condition does not exist, it would be equally misleading to label all psychiatric problems associated with injury as being of this type.[1171]

Wolkind (1974)[1334] suggests that injury and feelings about possible compensation disturb a person's psychological adjustment and that a combined approach is required so that physical and emotional balance is regained. It has recently been suggested (Maruta and Swanson, 1977)[813] that it may be best to conceptualise and to treat chronic pain patients as simultaneously having both emotional difficulty and chronic pain, without implying any priority; the term 'chronic pain behaviour' thus serves as a diagnosis, in that it encompasses *all* of the patient's behaviour related to pain.

It is a medical fallacy that all patients whose symptoms are related to litigation will recover rapidly once recompense has been made; frequently, this does not occur. Parker (1977)[972] strongly emphasises that the usual case of accident neurosis can rarely be explained in terms of a single aetiology (p. 186).

'Functional' backache

Back pain can be of considerable value to an inadequate personality, and is most unlikely to be relinquished easily.

Tegner (1959)[1208] remarks that,

... the diagnosis of psychogenic backache is fraught with danger. These sufferers are not malingerers. They do experience backache and they do not fall into the traps set for malingerers ... it is not justifiable to diagnose 'functional' troubles because examination and investigation reveal no sign of organic disease. This is a refuge for the diagnostically destitute. The diagnosis ... can only be made if there is good evidence of emotional instability and after meticulous weighing of the evidence.

He describes a patient for whom aspirin (by synonym) was prescribed by her despairing doctor. She reported next day that the tablets had upset her so much that she had to take two aspirins to relieve the symptoms.

These patients are remarkably successful in achieving their ends through their illness. As a group, they receive extraordinary care and comfort from friends and relatives. They are surprisingly selfish ... the patient with organic backache will be filled with pity and sympathy for the patient with psychogenic pain ... nothing is going to help these patients, for their symptoms are too valuable ... they exhaust the general practitioners, consultants, psychiatrists and physiotherapists ... they will always be with us, and the burden must be shared in turn by all the team.

8. Common patterns of clinical presentation

Since the consequences of degenerative joint disease can present in a bewildering variety of sign-and-symptom combinations, description of some common patterns may usefully begin with summarising some distinction between spondylosis and arthrosis.

ARTHROSIS AND SPONDYLOSIS

Distinctions are clearest in the cervical region; the two conditions coexist most frequently in late maturity at the lower lumbar region.[1180b]

Group lesions are more common than lesions of a single segment, the great majority of patients presenting with (i) a dominant problem, and (ii) one or more associated problems at other segments.

The dominant problem is not always the aspect requiring the most attention, although it may be troubling the patient most.

The subdivision of clinical presentation is justified by the fact that each can occur separately, though more often they may be combined in varying degrees. Many of these clinical presentations can be treated more specifically when segmental palpation accurately localises the site of the problem.

Common vertebral joint abnormalities have a potential for presenting in a variety of clinical forms which far exceeds that of any list of syndromes, and this multiplicity will be more apparent when examination is comprehensive, and the 'mileage' of patients treated has been considerable. The notion of syndromes represents an attempt to package the unpackageable, to facilitate assimilation, but the attempt can be counter-productive.

There is in medicine a natural law that any single manifestation, subjective or objective, may have behind it a multiplicity of organic causes, just as any single pathological event is bound to project itself into a number of clinical manifestations (Steindler[1171]).

If taught *only* in textbook syndromes, the unimaginative tyro begins to think only in syndromes, and may even-

Table 8.1 Comparisons between spondylosis and arthrosis

	Spondylosis	Arthrosis
General incidence	Common, most people have it	Less common
Segmental incidence	Lower cervical Midthoracic Lower lumbar	Upper cervical Upper and lowest thoracic Lower lumbar
Symptoms	May be asymptomatic and not requiring treatment or characterised by periodic episodes of symptoms	Almost always causes symptoms and needs treatment; never completely free of pain
Position	Pain related to position is important	Posture makes little difference to pain, except in low lumbar spine
Stiffness	Episodic, and variability is over period of many weeks	Stiffness varies diurnally, easing after activity
Crepitus	None	Commonly present
Nerve root involvement	Nerve root and cord pressure is common, due to disc degeneration, osseocartilaginous bars, disc prolapse	Sustained root pressure is less common, but root irritation may occur on certain movements
Pathological changes	Primarily in disc and vertebral bodies: disc degeneration lipping and irregularity of vertebral bodies Facet-joints may be approximated where discs are narrowed	Discs and vertebral bodies normal, with changes similar to other synovial joints: cartilage destruction loss of joint space chondro-osteophyte formation at edges of facets
X-ray appearance	Common	Less common

Note: After X-ray has excluded serious disease or significant mechanical defect, the presence or absence of radiological evidence of degeneration is of little significance; for example, foraminal encroachment by exostosis at a particular segment does not necessarily indicate that signs and symptoms are present because of it.

tually reach the stage where a supposed confidence, in ability to retain flexibility of approach, becomes slowly and inexorably misplaced as hardening of unexamined ideas and concepts proceeds unwittingly almost to the stage of fossilisation. The author speaks from personal experience.

Unless the cerebral organisation of ideas is daily subjected to test on the proving-ground of the clinical shop-floor, there tends to come a time when clinical presentations which do not fit fairly neatly into this or that list of syndromes are regarded with the beginnings of disapproval and suspicion, and the patient too easily labelled difficult, a fool or neurotic. Informed flexibility flies out of the window; both clinical examination and treatment degenerate into boring and ineffective stereotypes. Like clinical workers themselves, patients *are* at times difficult, occasionally fools and now and again neurotic, but the population of patients too frequently and conveniently labelled as such is much too high.

The factor of biological plasticity will guarantee an infinite variety of clinical presentation from patient to patient; there is always the inconvenient sign or symptom which does not easily fit into the arbitrary concept, always an element of untidiness of clinical feature which negates the neat theory, the facile exposition and the 'logic' of authoritarian pronouncements about what changes *ought* to be underlying the patient's complaint. It is folly, and unimaginative, for the clinical therapist to go through professional life looking only for textbook syndromes; there is no black or white on the clinical shopfloor.

For example, prompted by the knowledge that a neonate with HLA-B27 is 300 times more likely to have ankylosing spondylitis than someone without this antigen, the heredity of many rheumatic syndromes has been re-examined;[713] the consequence is that the diseases under consideration will require redefinition.

Patients with HLA-B27 may have uveitis or peripheral arthritis without sacroiliitis or the clinical features of spondylitis; the arbitrary categorising of spondylitis, Reiter's disease, psoriasis, ulcerative colitis and Crohn's disease now requires modification—genetic analysis indicates that they are all part of an interrelated mixture of disease processes and clinical features.

According to estimates,[153] some 2 per cent of the UK population suffer symptoms related to minor forms of ankylosing spondylitis; apart from the hard core of patients with stiff spines and X-ray evidence of sacroiliitis, there is a large constellation of milder forms of spondylitis, with widespread minor aches including chronic backache, but without radiographic abnormality. Frank spondylitis is commoner in men, but milder symptoms occur almost equally in the sexes. Some 10 per cent of adults with ankylosing spondylitis have a history of rheumatic disease early in the second decade, the symptoms subsiding until spondylitic episodes occur again in young adulthood. Much more frequent and more covert involvement almost certainly exists.

The occurrence of milder spondylitis should be considered when chronic backache, thoracic ache and cervical pains begin insidiously in a patient under 40 and have been present for more than three months. Morning and evening stiffness relieved by movement, and a clear-cut response to anti-inflammatory drugs, indicate the possibility of mild spondylitis.

Among the constantly growing host of clinical specialities, the field of vertebral musculoskeletal pain is singular, in that (a) the features of benign spinal joint problems frequently mimic the features of a very wide variety of more serious conditions; (b) spinal musculoskeletal pain, at one time or another, is our almost universal inheritance and, in sum, is probably responsible for more restriction of free physical activity than any other medical or surgical condition.

There is a reason for everything—it is no accident that, of all lay practitioners, the overwhelming majority are largely concerned in treating, by one method or another, common aches and pains from the spinal locomotor apparatus. Thus the massive extent of the market dictates the extent of the service, however variegated the service may be. However well qualified as a basis, the would-be specialist in this field requires much experienced help before the *meaning* of different groups of signs and symptoms begins to become clarified.

For these reasons, any course of instruction by lecture, demonstration, discussion period, seminar, symposium, recommended reading of papers, books (such as presently occupies the reader) and practice among classmates, however inspired, is bound eventually to wither somewhat, to be less than the sum of its parts, *unless the instruction be substantiated by a sufficiently long and adequately supervised period of clinical work on patients.*

It is during this important stage of clinical training that the student will experience the untidy reality underlying classroom and book teaching, which perforce begins as an artificially neat package of salient and indispensable information, but which for ultimately effective use should have built into it the seeds of its own obsolescence, so that flexibility might remain the most important factor.

Although library and operating theatre are complementary, the surgeon does the ultimate learning of his craft at the operating table, not in the library.

TRAUMATIC 'BLOCK' OR 'LOCK' OF THE OCCIPITOATLANTAL JOINT

Like any other joint, the vertebral mobility-segment may become locked, and this is usually associated with pain (Fig. 8.1).[1092]

The patient, frequently a young adult, often has had some trauma to the head, sometimes the neck, or both, during horseplay, skylarking or wrestling; lateral trauma during a right-angle road traffic accident; a knock on the vertex when going over a hump in a car at speed; falling from a moped or bicycle; a bang on the head during body-contact sports.

Some patients, many of them alert and competent witnesses, can recall no past or recent trauma, but give a clear

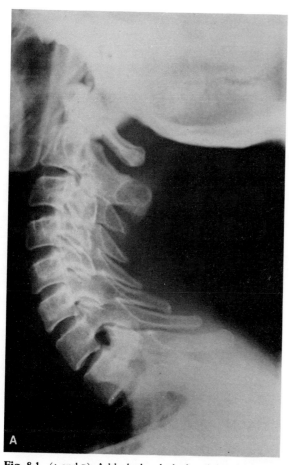 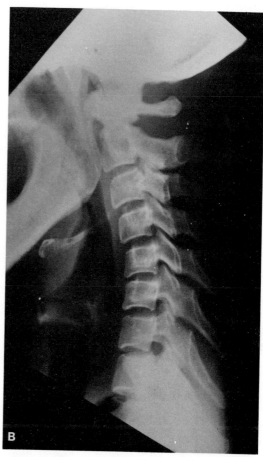

Fig. 8.1 (A and B). A blocked or locked occipitoatlantal joint. There is no change in C0–C1 relationships between (A) extension and (B) flexion.

history of a head or neck movement, or transient body posture, from which the symptoms began. There is usually suboccipital pain on one side; this may or may not spread to the frontal area but most often does not involve the whole hemicranium (Fig. 8.2).

On examination, the head may be held perfectly straight (Fig. 8.3), but spasm of upper cervical muscle frequently produces an abnormal suboccipital contour, which may not be obvious on cursory inspection. Rotation and side flexion to the painful side are limited, by pain as well as block in varying proportions, and the opposite movements feel tethered and elicit a milder pull of the painful side. There are no neurological signs, or interference with limb girdle joints, and on palpation the lateral mass of the atlas is often prominent posteriorly, with the overlying soft tissues thickened on the painful side. It is also tender.

The spinous process of C2 often remains centralised on AP X-ray films, but may be deviated to the opposite side, and sometimes (i) the atlas is asymmetrically placed in relation to the odontoid, and (ii) there is an asymmetry of the C1–C2 joint space.

'It has to be kept in mind that there is no strict interdependence between clinical symptoms and radiological pathology in the cranio-vertebral region.'[1274]

While the radiographic appearance is not pathognomonic of this type of joint problem, and when present it may persist following relief of symptoms, the restoration of acceptably normal relationships with relief of pain and limitation simultaneously occur often enough to justify a probable link between the X-ray signs and clinical features.[1092]

The description of this clinical state is confidently derived from the fact that mobilisation or manipulation specifically applied to the C0–C1 joint on the painful side frequently relieves all the signs and symptoms of it; yet the clinical presentation is not always as clear-cut, and when passive testing movement of the *opposite* craniovertebral joint elicits more of the characteristic pain than testing the joint on the painful side, movement of the contralateral joint should take precedence in early stages of treatment. The incarceration of an articular villus or synovial meniscus in an apophyseal joint may produce locking, which has been shown by Zuchschwerdt,[1382] and it is reasonable to suppose that the same may occur at the craniovertebral joint, although at times the signs appear to be those of a purely *functional* block, with the opposite craniovertebral joint appearing to move quite normally on passive physiological-movement testing.

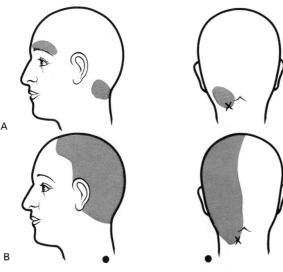

Fig. 8.2 (A) A common unilateral occipitofrontal distribution of pain when the headache is due to a block of the occipitoatlantal joint on the same side. It may begin in the supraorbital region, with the occipital component mentioned only in passing.

(B) Unilateral occipital pain, spreading to the vertex, and sometimes the whole hemicranium to include the supraorbital region, is more likely when the segments caudal to C0–C1 are responsible for it, i.e. C1–C2, C2–C3. When the segments C2–C3 and/or C3–C4 are the most tender, thickened and irritable to palpation, the distribution of pain often includes auricular, mandibular and anterolateral throat areas.

If the use of passive-movement techniques is governed by conclusions about the precise nature of postural asymmetry, and by assessment of the precise pattern of movement-limitation, mobilisation or manipulation treatment must needs follow a pattern set by these findings; frequently, simple localised mobilisation of one or other joint by the most convenient method, and guided by initial responses, relieves the condition.

Three important aspects need emphasis:

1. Occipitoatlantal block often exists together with the clinical sequelae of traumatic injury to the neck (Fig. 8.4) or shoulder girdle as a whole, and it is important to be alert for this circumstance when assessing patients whose pain and paraesthesiae, from lower cervical segments, might tend to dominate planning of a treatment. A surprising degree of relief, from seemingly nebulous complaints, will accompany adequate examination and mobilisation of the craniovertebral joint, together with treatment for the more caudal lesions. For example:

Patient R.S., 27 Years (Fig. 8.5A–E). This heavily built man suffered a broken nose during a football match in 1968, and five months later began to get paraesthesiae of C8–T1 distribution in his right hand. A whiplash injury in 1971 further exacerbated his condition, and after two years of occipital headaches, recurrent right-sided attacks of acute torticollis, a constant right scapular pain and a more severe but periodic right supraspinous fossa pain, with continuing paraesthesiae as above, he was unable to use his arm to any extent and had to reduce his daily activity to essentials.

Examination. Extension, right-side-flexion and right rotation were all reduced, provoking the supraspinous fossa pain and if

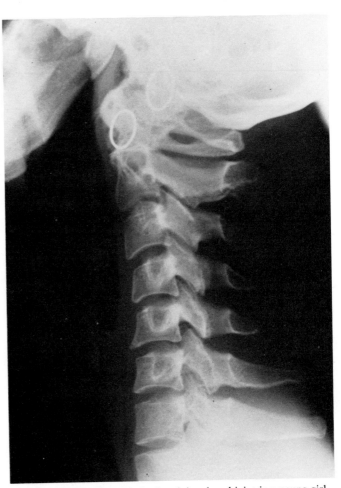

Fig. 8.3 Patient M.A. Block of occipitoatlantal joint in a young girl, following trauma to the neck. Postural spasm has eradicated the normal cervical lordosis. Relieved by mobilisation of atlas.

sustained for a few seconds, the forearm paraesthesiae. His right biceps muscle was weak. The general distribution of palpation findings is shown in Fig. 8.5C. Stiffness of the craniovertebral joints and the persistent hypermobility of the C6–C7–T1 region are evident from the films of 21 August 1973 (Fig. 8.5A and B).

Treatment. Heat, traction and a night collar had helped somewhat in the past, but the benefit had evaporated. He was asked to continue with the collar, and a regime of localised mobilising to segments C0–C1–C2, and more gently to C6–C7 on the right side, with resisted exercises to stabilise the cervicothoracic region, reduced his symptoms within four treatments. By that time his paraesthesiae were only sporadic, biceps power was normal and his neck movements no longer provoked arm symptoms. Four further treatments cleared his symptoms. When seen some months afterwards, he was playing football again and only occasionally troubled by neck pain. He had had no further episodes of acute cervical joint problems. Fig. 8.5D and E (22 October 1973) depict a better range of craniovertebral and C1–C2 movement.

2. *It is particularly important to be aware of the dangers of traumatic tearing or attenuation of craniovertebral ligaments.*[353] On examination there may be some slight general weakness due to pain inhibition when neck flexion and

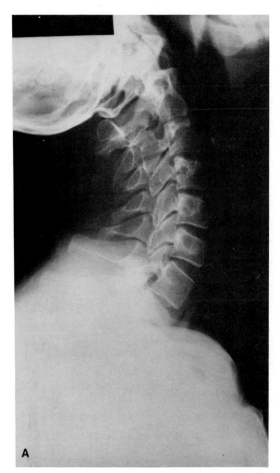
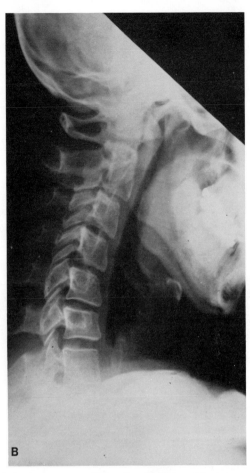

Fig. 8.4 (A and B) Slightly abnormal change of joint relationship in the upper cervical region on flexion. There is increased lateral tilt of the atlas, evidenced by the changed image of the neural arch of atlas compared to the extension film, and there is some forward slip of C2 on C3. There is also some slight lateral tilt of C2.

extension are resisted, but marked inability to push the chin up or press it down against resistance should raise the suspicion of craniovertebral instability, and the need for extra care in handling. A complaint of occipital numbness or paraesthesiae denotes the need for caution, since there is the possibility of tearing of atlantoaxial ligaments with joint derangement and trespass upon the C2 nerve root. Diminished sensation to pinprick in the occipital region innervated by the greater occipital nerve (posterior primary ramus of C2) should alert the therapist.[1165] Mobilisation is contraindicated until the suitability of physical treatment has been confirmed.

3. It is important to distinguish between (i) the patients who report cervical and head pain but are not aware that symptoms are arising from a blocked C0–C1 joint, until localised treatment relieves it, and (ii) those patients whose upper neck and head pain is clearly perceived by them as centred on a very tender and highly irritable C0–C1 joint; any movement of it other than the most careful and considerate is likely to add to their pain and intensify the degree of muscle guarding.

CRANIOVERTEBRAL HYPERMOBILITY IN CHILDREN (GRISEL'S SYNDROME)[1274]

'Flexion-headache' is frequently observed in children and is sometimes associated with acute wry-neck or torticollis.

Wry-neck may be the first sign of rheumatoid disease in a child, and the initial attack involving the occipito-cervical joints may go unrecognised for what it is, in the absence of clinical changes in the limb joints. Other articular presentations may occur in which the head is held in the mid-line, with all movements severely restricted.

Atlantoaxial dislocation, observed on lateral films of the region, may be evident as an increase of the dens/anterior atlas arch distance up to 6 mm or more, and this instability occurs because of inflammatory attenuation of the transverse ligament of atlas. Forward dislocation may be combined with pathological rotation of the atlas, seen on AP tomograms which may give the appearance of unilateral destruction of the atlas but in fact is the appearance of gross atlas rotation. Distension of surrounding soft tissue adds to the local disturbance by acute synovitis and the ligamentous laxity.

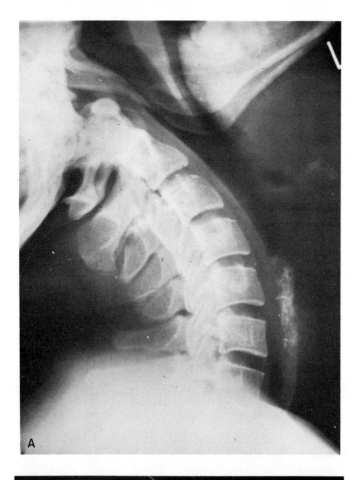

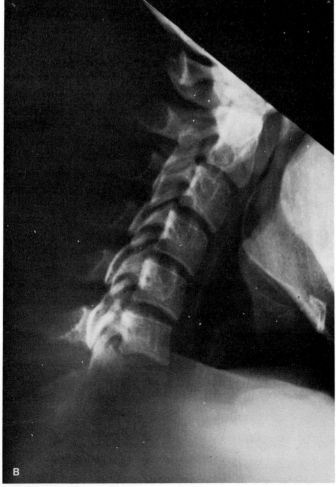

Palpation Findings

○ Tender	X Stiff Segment	⊛ Prominent
● Sore	‖‖ Thickened (deep)	E Early
p Pain	⇕ Elicited Spasm	M Middle
ps Paraesthesiae	⋁⋀⋀ Hypermobile Segment	L Late

C

Fig. 8.5 Patient R.S.

(A) Extension (see text).

(B) Flexion. C0–C1 and C1–C2 segments are stiff. C6–C7 is hypermobile.

(C) August 21. Palpation findings. The point on the range of accessory intervertebral movement at which the findings were encountered is not depicted (see text).

(D) Extension.

(E) Flexion. C0–C1 and C1–C2 segments are less stiff. C6–C7 is still hypermobile.

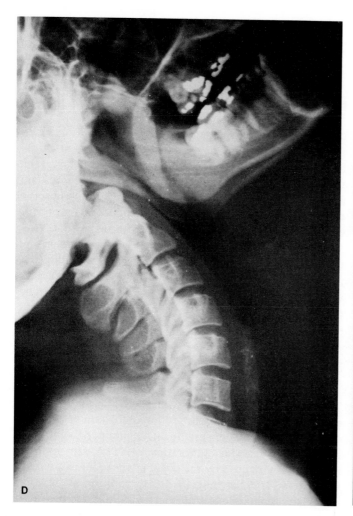

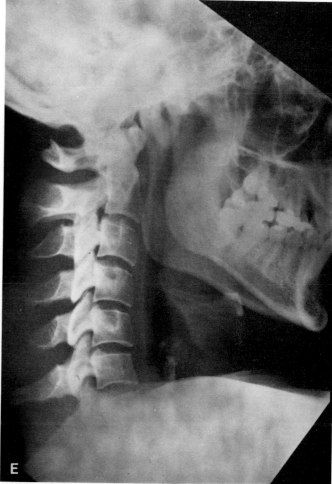

Von Torklus (1972)[1274] observes that it is likely that some cases of chronic atlantoaxial derangement may have their origin in an early rheumatoid arthritis.

Grisel (1930)[458] described the same clinical presentation in children and adolescents with upper respiratory tract infection, e.g. tonsillitis and other pharyngeal infections, which appear to produce the same inflammatory attenuation of the craniovertebral ligaments. Just a century before, *Bell* (1830)[80] described C1–C2 subluxation as a complication of throat infection. Acute wry-neck occurs and is accompanied by the same atlantoaxial dislocation.

In every one of a group of these cases, *Gutmann* (1970)[475] radiographically found an insufficiency of the transverse ligament of atlas, so that in flexion (e.g. bending over school books, reading and writing) the odontoid process does not stay in close contact with the anterior arch of atlas, but on the contrary, the arch moves forward and the odontoid moves backward. This movement abnormality always occurred together with a blocking of the occipitoatlantal joint in the frontal or transverse plane.

The ligamentous insufficiency is temporary, and is apparently a sequel to the pharyngeal inflammation, a much increased retropharyngeal space shadow being apparent on lateral films, e.g. enlarged from a normal 6–7 mm to over 20 mm.

The articular signs and abnormal radiographic appearances settle with support and appropriate medical treatment. Movement-techniques are contraindicated, and therefore acute torticollis in juniors requires careful investigation before it is regarded simply as a transient and innocent joint derangement.

THE ADULT 'RHEUMATOID NECK'

Involvement of the cervical spine is common in rheumatoid arthritis, and occurs in some 40 per cent of cases,[1111] although only a smaller proportion show serious instability of the craniovertebral joints; this appears more often in patients with sero-positive disease, a chronically raised ESR, nodular involvement and a history of medication with steroids.

The incidence of atlantoaxial subluxation in rheumatoid patients has been reported as around 25 per cent,[198, 818] taking as the positive sign an anterior odontoid/atlas separation of more than 3 mm on lateral films of cervical flexion. Rana *et al.* (1973)[1012] studied 41 rheumatoid patients with atlantoaxial subluxation—40 were seroposi-tive, and the mean duration of rheumatoid arthritis, at the time of diagnosis of subluxation, was 16 years (range 4–39 years); 36 of the patients were taking corticosteroids.

Ball and Sharp (1971)[55] described the morbid anatomy of the condition; weakening of the transverse ligament allows the subluxation, and this is accompanied by undue loading of other joints and ligaments of the occipitoatlan-toaxial complex. The transverse ligament may be atrophied or completely destroyed by rheumatoid granu-lation tissue, but may remain surprisingly healthy in a few cases of severe subluxation; the posterior aspect of the odontoid may be eroded by granulation tissue between it and the transverse ligament.

In a further study by Rana, et al. (1973)[1013] 8 of the 41 patients (vide supra) were observed to have the tip of the dens displaced upwards above McGregor's baseline (a plane between the upper posterior edge of hard palate to the most caudal point of occiput) by 10 mm or more, i.e. more than twice the normal of 4.5 mm. This upward translocation of the odontoid is another feature of upper cervical invovement in which a mixture of erosion, sclerosis and osteoporosis of bony elements accompanies the soft tissue changes.

Disorganisation of cervical joints is not confined to the upper neck; for example, Whaley and Dick (1968)[1304] reported fatal dislocation of C4 on C5 in a woman of 62 with a 15-year history of rheumatoid arthritis.

The clinical features do not appear to be related on a one-to-one basis with pathological changes. Most patients report pain in the upper cervical and/or suboccipital areas, spreading to mastoid, temporal or frontal areas. The pre-sence of pain does not necessarily imply any abnormality of the central nervous system, and patients without head and neck pain may present with abnormal neurological signs.

Neurological signs may be a sequel of occlusion of ver-tebral arteries, intrinsic vascular disease, compressive lesions by rheumatoid inflammatory tissue or a combina-tion of these. Clinical features may include trigeminal nerve involvement as facial sensory loss and a transiently depressed corneal reflex; vertigo on head extension, paraesthesiae of hands and/or legs, transient heaviness and uselessness of upper limbs, difficulties in walking, urgency of micturition and transient loss of consciousness may occur.

Upward translocation of the odontoid in the eight patients mentioned above was unaccompanied by neuro-logical signs in two of them, but in the remaining six con-siderable neurological involvement included hyperalgesia or sensory loss in the trigeminal distribution, patchy sen-sory loss in upper and lower limbs and trunk, upper and/or lower limb spasticity, limb weakness, clonus and extensor plantar responses.

The degree of derangement is not related to the signs

and symptoms;[210] a gratifying recession of abnormal signs often occurs when the neck is supported in a firm and com-fortable polythene collar, and there is a good case for con-servative treatment in these patients.

Surgery is indicated when the neurological signs are progressive.[1012]

Swinson, et al. (1972)[1201] described three cases of verti-cal subluxation of the axis, all of whom had advanced rheumatoid disease with destructive peripheral arthritis. Two of the patients were managed conservatively, and the third improved after foramen magnum decompression and immobilisation in a rigid collar. The authors observe that serious neurological changes do not necessarily occur even with extreme degrees of vertical translocation.

Physical treatment by movement has no place in the management of the rheumatoid cervical spine, unless the possibility of precarious joint stability has been radiologic-ally excluded, and even then the neck should be handled prudently, and the responses to cautious early treatment carefully monitored.

ROTATORY FIXATION OF THE ATLANTO-AXIAL JOINT

The term 'rotatory fixation' is employed because the out-standing radiological feature is that of fixation of the *atlas* on the axis in a relationship normally attained to a greater or lesser degree during rotation.[1346] The axis itself is rotated, as evidenced by the offset of the spinous process. Coutts (1934)[208] has described the condition as 'fixation in a position possible to a normal neck', and it is probably correct to avoid indiscriminate use of the term 'subluxa-tion', which implies partial derangement; this is not always present. When present, 'subluxation' is justified.

Fielding and Hawkins (1977)[354b] observe that rotatory deformities of the atlantoaxial joint are usually short-lived and easily correctable, and that only rarely do they persist causing a torticollis which is resistant to treatment. The authors were describing their findings in seventeen patients with irreducible atlantoaxial subluxation (fixa-tion), who were aged 7 to 68 years, with an average of 20.6 years. Thirteen of the patients were treated by atlantoaxial arthrodesis.

Experienced manual therapists who for many years have routinely employed careful segmental palpation, as part of the comprehensive examination of the craniover-tebral region in patients for whom surgery is not indicated, would probably agree that the incidence of mild and per-sisting rotatory atlantoaxial fixation is very much higher than supposed, being revealed by this examination method in a fair proportion of adult patients with symp-toms about the neck and cranium and signs of a degree of rotatory limitation. The greater majority of this group present with a normal posture on cursory inspection; their symptoms, and restricted motion, can very often be considerably improved without recourse to vigorous techniques or extreme head/neck positions during treatment.

It is important to bear in mind that full-range cervical rotation is not without the possibilities of serious damage and sometimes catastrophe. Coutts[208] observed that when the transverse ligament is intact, complete bilateral dislocation of the atlantoaxial articular processes can occur at about 65 degrees of rotation at that segment, and where there is a transverse ligament deficiency allowing some 5 mm of anterior displacement of atlas, complete unilateral dislocation can occur at 45 degrees of rotation.

Excessive rotation, combined with anterior shift of the atlas, can severely compromise the vertebral arteries, and brain-stem and cerebellar infarction have occurred due to excessive head rotation.

'The importance of recognising atlantoaxial rotatory deformity lies in the fact that it may indicate a compromised atlantoaxial complex with the potential to cause neural damage or even death.'[354b]

The patient may present: (1) with normal symmetry of head and neck, or (2) with the head tilted to one side and rotated to the other, i.e. the 'cock-robin' deformity.

1. With head and neck in normal posture the clinical features may be:

a. *Positional fixation of C2 in rotation without X-ray evidence of arthrosis*, in which case it may be simply a functional block and fairly easily dealt with, or it may be part of a recent traumatic block of the occipitoatlantal joint following mild injury, in which case release of the craniovertebral block will frequently also release the atlantoaxial fixation. Many patients give no history of trauma.

b. *Positional fixation of some years' standing*, in which case there has been adaptive shortening of ligaments and therefore strain on adjacent joints. There may be no arthrotic changes visible on X-ray, but this does not preclude the presence of chronic soft-tissue changes, or the likelihood of untreated but resolved ligamentous tearing or attenuation by trauma, or of a block following an unguarded movement, in times past. It is not possible, radiologically, to differentiate between spontaneous and traumatic rotation-fixation,[1274] or between recent changes and those of some years' standing, without taking account of both history and clinical findings.

The characteristic 'end-feel' of a firm and virtually painless resistance, limiting one or other movement on examination with over-pressure favours an established fixation. (Tests should be more cautious if there is a history of recent trauma or spontaneous locking during an unguarded movement; the patient presents with tilt and rotation of the head and is unable to correct it.)

c. *Positional fixation with X-ray evidence of arthrotic changes*. It is important to remember that patients with clear X-ray evidence of rotational fixation (i.e. the spinous process shadow of C2 being offset to one side, on AP open-mouth views) may present with the clinical features of spondylotic changes lower in the spine, and with no symptoms referrable to the upper neck, adaption to the asymmetry presumably having occurred years before. A good clue, that head and upper cervical symptoms may be associated with radiographic appearances, is that rotation is limited to the same side as the C2 spinous process offset from the mid-line.

2. *Those few patients who present with a postural tilt to one side and rotation to the other* have a diminished range of movement, in that they cannot overcorrect either the side-flexion or rotatory component of the deformity, although they may be able to actively adopt the neutral posture for a short period. Typically, the side-flexion is held at some 10 to 20 degrees, as is the rotation, and extension is also limited. The sternomastoid muscle on the side *opposite* to the tilt is often in some spasm, as if trying to correct it.

If the abnormal position persists and spontaneous reduction is not possible, soft-tissue contracture develops and causes fixation. Some will have facial asymmetry, in the form of unilateral flattening.

When there is associated anterior displacement of the atlas on the axis, there may be a compensatory 'swan-neck' deformity of the lower cervical spine.

Aetiology

Inco-ordinated movement while stirring in sleep, during functional activities while working in confined spaces and during athletics, may lead to spontaneous blocking, even in childhood.[1274] It is a condition of its own, apart from spondylosis.

When patients present with normal head and neck posture but X-ray evidence of segmental rotatory fixation the genesis of the condition may probably lie in the physiological necessity to normalise the head position, and thus the visual and equilibratory apparatus, in correct orientation to the verticals and horizontals of one's environment. The intrinsic lesion (traumatic or functional block or fixation) probably affects the C0–C1 (see p. 206) or C1–C2 segment rather than C2–C3, and a consequence of this is a tendency for head orientation to be disturbed, in that rotation of the skull and C1 *together* might be induced. Reflexly, this abnormal tendency is negated by normalisation of the head and atlas, provided ligamentous integrity allows it, thereby inducing C2 perforce to become rotated beneath the atlas. Thus the C2–C3 segment is also strained as a consequence.

The onset of the 'cock-robin' deformity may be spontaneous, particularly in children, or may be associated with an upper respiratory tract infection (Grizel's syndrome[458]).

The cause may also be minor or major trauma, usually to the head, and occasionally the onset may date from surgical procedures to the mouth or pharynx.

A typical case[354b] emphasises the delay in diagnosis:

... A 7-year-old girl who began to have torticollis two weeks following an ear infection. Traction, physiotherapy, a Minerva jacket, neck manipulation, a halo cast, and finally a Milwaukee brace had failed to correct the deformity. She had been seen by many doctors, including a psychiatrist, and all the while she had an unrecognised atlantoaxial rotatory fixation. Cineroentgenography 25 months after onset confirmed the diagnosis, and after partial reduction by skull traction atlantoaxial arthrodesis was performed because of the lesions' resistance to reduction.

Rotational fixation may be the consequence of an inflammatory process, as in acute cervical arthritis in juniors, but in these cases there is often an accompanying increase of the atlantodens distance during flexion.[1274]

It is important to remember that torticollis may be congenital and caused by bony anomalies—the skeletal wryneck—and in 40 per cent of these cases there is a history of breech presentation; almost 70 per cent show basilar impression.[354c] Congenital torticollis is not considered here.

Clinical features

Fielding and Hawkins[354b] mention that an important finding which differentiates spasmodic torticollis (wry-neck) from atlantoaxial rotatory fixation is that in the former a shortened sternomastoid is the deforming force and is in spasm, whereas in the latter the elongated sternomastoid is in spasm.

Some patients give a history of recent minor trauma to the head, others report an unguarded movement. When trauma to the head and/or neck has been in any way severe, the probability of tearing of atlantoaxial ligaments is present (see above) and handling should be prudent. Not all patients hold the head in the neutral position, and some may present with painful and restricted rotation to the side of the head tilt. This latter group require much care in handling.

Symptoms are variable, but usually include occipital and hemicranial pain, face pain and paraesthesiae sometimes, and a feeling of restriction of the upper neck. Headache may be diffuse and not unilateral.

N.B. 'Persistent asymmetry of the odontoid, in its relation to the articular masses of the atlas on open-mouth AP views, with this asymmetry not being correctable by rotation, forms the basic radiological criteria for diagnosis.'[1346]

Surprisingly, this appearance may persist after symptoms have been cleared, and the signs have regressed, at least on examination of gross movements. This distinguishes the condition from fixation due to muscle spasm,

and from acute torticollis, which is usually a lesion of the C2–C3 segment (see p. 216).

Wortzman and Dewar (1968)[1346] infiltrated, with local anaesthetic, the lateral atlantoaxial joints under fluoroscopic control in four patients, completely but temporarily relieving discomfort and movement-limitation. Films taken after infiltration showed a persistent rotational deformity. Two cases of acute torticollis received the same injection, with no relief of symptoms or movement-restriction.

The hypothesis of functional block in some cases is of interest in the light of observations of the above authors:

... rotational atlanto-axial fixation is due to damage of an unknown nature at the atlanto-axial joint itself. The lesion cannot be reproduced by the sectioning of alar and/or transverse ligaments. The relief of pain and freedom of movement following injection of local anaesthetic into the joint itself also indicates that one is dealing with disease localised to this joint ... still unexplained is the cause of the fixation.

Fielding and Reddy (1969)[351] ascribe the condition to loss of ligamentous integrity, but mention that the mechanism of rotatory locking is poorly understood; they describe the case of a 65-year-old woman who awoke, yawned and twisted her neck, with immediate sharp pain. Her head remained rotated left and tilted right, which she could not correct. After 10 days of cervical traction she turned her head to the left, increasing the deformity, and died. Necropsy revealed that the atlas was displaced forward and rotated across the canal of the axis, damaging the cord.

A total of 11 fatal instances of rotatory atlantoaxial deformity have been described from 1908.

These findings indicate the prime need for awareness of the possible mechanisms underlying postural asymmetry of head and neck and radiographic evidence of rotatory fixation.

Diagnostic mistakes are possible if the head is not in the mid-line on AP films, or if there are pre-existing anomalies (or asymmetries, *vide supra*) of atlas, axis or occipital condyles. Similarly, their presence may predispose the patient to rotation-fixation on trauma or functional stress.[1274]

In summary, when the head *is* normalised, it *may* be a functional block. When the head is not normalised the condition may be more serious and testing movements are best conducted with care; physical treatment, if indicated, should in the early stages be restricted to gentle traction and support.

Fielding et al. (1978)[354c] suggest that manipulation of these fixed deformities is unwise, because of the inherent dangers. The authors probably refer to hazardous gross movements of the head and neck.

It is a mistake to assume that acute and transient torticollis in children is necessarily due to the common

C2–C3 segment derangement which occurs in adults. 'Atlantoaxial rotatory displacement is a common cause of torticollis in childhood, and almost all patients recover spontaneously from the condition even without treatment'. (Fielding *et al.*, 1976.)[354]

'Persisting torticollis in young patients, particularly after trauma or an upper respiratory tract infection, suggests a diagnosis of atlantoaxial rotatory fixation.'[354b]

ARTHROSIS OF UPPER CERVICAL SEGMENTS

Hadley (1936)[479] and Wright (1944)[1349] have provided an analysis of the aetiology of facet-arthrosis (see also p. 125). The segments affected may include the atlantodental (median atlantoaxial), occipitoatlantal and atlantoaxial joints and the C2–C3 (Fig. 2.5) and C3–C4 segments or any combination of these (Figs 1.5, 4.2, 5.3, 5.5).

In a table of segmental incidence of upper cervical arthrosis, unilateral involvement of a C2–C3 facet-joint would perhaps be highest together with the median atlantoaxial joint, and frequently the only radiographic change easily evident is that of C2–C3 arthrosis;[1242] atlantodental arthrosis is sometimes seen, albeit less easy to visualise on X-rays.[1274]

Like arthrotic changes in the hip-joint, painful symptoms and manifest signs may be present years before X-ray evidence of degenerative change becomes apparent.

Bearing in mind that vertebrobasilar ischaemia may arise from spondylotic interference with vessels in the mid- and lower cervical spine, upper cervical symptoms are possibly due more to arthrotic changes of synovial joints than to spondylosis of C2 to C4 vertebral body joints, and a common pattern is as follows: patients are usually adult, mature or middle-aged, and apart from a slight general lowering forward of the head in more mature patients, and the beginnings of a dowager's hump, there is usually no lateral or rotation asymmetry of head and neck alignment. Symptoms have often been present for months or years, steadily becoming chronic.

Some patients, frequently women, have accepted their 'migraine' as one of the facts of life; they present with neck pain and are mildly surprised when examination seeks a possible link between the two. Often past or more recent trauma is recalled but sometimes there is no recent history of injury, although after the first treatment session it is common for people to have been reminded by near relatives of recent traumatic stress they had forgotten. Headache is a very common symptom; it often spreads to forehead and eyes, and is accompanied by feelings of retro-orbital pressure. It is nagging and wearing in character, often present on rising, and may worsen as the day goes on, depending on activity. Working with the head bent forward often aggravates headache. When bilateral it may be worse on one side; headache which is solely occipital usually accompanies occipitoatlantal joint problems. Head extension commonly provokes or increases the headache, and often provokes dizziness; the upper neck pain may be aggravated by extension and, in unilateral pain, by side-flexion or rotation to the painless side. Bilateral pain is usually worsened by all neck movements but not symmetrically so. The postural spasm of neck muscles may disappear on lying down.

Some will appreciate that their so-called 'migraine' (but not the concomitant symptoms) is coming from the upper neck (see p. 218). On palpation the suboccipital soft tissues are unduly tender and frequently thickened, and chondro-osteophytes at facet-joint margins are palpable in some. The patient is frequently worried about the nuchal crepitus, and may need reassuring that it is harmless. Headache is accompanied by one or more of a host of concomitant symptoms and signs:

Vertigo (dysequilibrium or instability)
Momentary vagueness, more rarely 'drop' attacks
Nausea, and sometimes vomiting
Dysphagia
Dysphonia
Foggy or blurred vision
Retro-orbital pressure
Depression or other psychic distress (cf. weeping fits)
Suboccipital and nuchal crepitus
Vasomotor and sudomotor changes
Constriction of pupil

The frequency with which dysphonia and dysphagia accompany joint problems at the C3 segment may be more than coincidence.

Symptoms may have a bizarre quality, such as 'my eyeballs are tingling', or 'I feel as if I am wearing a helmet of headache'.

The production of signs and symptoms has been investigated, among many others, by Campbell and Parsons (1944)[156] who injected capsular, fascial and muscular structures with irritant solutions, and scratched with a fine needle the periosteum of upper cervical vertebrae and the periarticular structures of 40 subjects, half of whom were hospital staff and half were patients suffering head pain.

The cranial and facial symptoms provoked in normal subjects resembled the symptomatic pain of clinical cases very accurately. Pain was predominantly frontal and periorbital from the occipital condyle and basiocciput region, together with forehead reference. Pain from irritation of cervical interspinous connective tissue between C2 and C5 was referred to occipital and upper cervical areas, and occasionally to frontal regions.

Concomitant signs and symptoms were provoked by stimulation of basal, suboccipital and interspinous tissues, and included giddiness, listing, pallor, sweating, pulse alterations, nausea, ptosis and occasionally tinnitus. There was a marked resemblance between these effects and the clinical features of the 'post-traumatic head' syndrome, and also a strong resemblance to non-traumatic neuralgias and myalgias of the occipito-cervical-facial regions (see pp. 181–184).

The authors mention the tendencies to which these patients may be prone, observing that,

Morphological, physiological and psychological stresses form a field of reciprocal relations ... feelings of inadequacy and inability to cope with life in terms of previous capacities, altered social relationships in familial and occupational fields ... prolonged ill-health which often has too few objective signs to make it legitimate in the eyes of others ... problems of compensation. (See p. 183.)[205, 295, 296]

Objective evidence of covert but important physiological and pathological changes is no longer lacking.[1242, 1224, 260] Electronystagmography and cupulometry studies have established a physical basis for the bizarre and distressing symptoms reported by patients.[243]

The spinal tract of the 5th cranial nerve (p. 11) and the morphology of the bulbothalamic pathways (p. 165) are of importance when assessing the production of these clinical states. Patients often report that nasal breathing is freer, and their 'sinusitis' is better, after localised attention to upper cervical joint problems. It is sometimes forgotten that the trigeminal nerve innervates the mucous membranes of the nasal and oral cavities and the maxillary and frontal sinuses.[130]

Another important feature is the profuse interconnections between somatic cervical nerve roots, the 7th, 8th, 9th, 10th, 11th and 12th cranial nerves and the superior cervical sympathetic ganglion.[156, 1105] (Possible mechanisms of symptom production are tabulated on p. 183.)

The justification for assembling these clinical features under arthrosis lies in their very frequent occurrence when the upper two segments with their purely synovial joints are the ones mainly involved, although spondylotic changes between segments C2 and C7 can and do produce occipital headache, for example.[285]

Patients with advanced degenerative change of lower cervical interbody joints (spondylosis) often present with the clinical features of upper cervical facet-arthrosis, and following localised treatment to the upper segments are sign and symptom free, i.e. the spondylotic lower segments are plainly having no *current part* in production of symptoms reported; yet the functional interdependence of the spine should not be forgotten (see p. 38).

If one accepts the general proposition that joints never forgive and never forget a traumatic insult, it follows that, in upper cervical arthrosis, the previous history may well include episodes outlined on pages 206 and 212; further, there need not be any detectable radiographic changes accompanying severe symptoms from vertebral facet-joints.

Wing and Hargrave-Wilson (1974)[1330] suggest that the association of upper cervical joint strain with giddiness has been neglected. The combination of abnormal electronystagmographic recordings with neck movement, together with normal routine audiological and vestibular findings, is specifically diagnostic of true cervical vertigo. They described the clinical, audiological, vestibular and radiographic findings in 80 patients with cervical vertigo, also reporting electronystagmographic findings both before and after manipulation of the cervical and upper thoracic spine.

Electronystagmography after manipulation recorded significant improvement in 73 per cent of the patients; 53 per cent were completely relieved to the stage where medication was not required and they returned to normal activities.

Pains and other symptoms of obscure origin have been grouped together as Costen's syndrome,[495] i.e.

Neuralgia of the second or third divisions of the V nerve
Pain in and around the ears
Stuffy sensation in the ears
Pain up the back of the head and down the side of the neck
Headaches
Sinus pains
Impaired hearing
Tinnitus
Altered sensation in the tongue and throat.

These are usually included in consideration of temperomandibular joint problems; experienced manual therapists are aware that some of these patients can be completely or considerably relieved of some of the components of their distress by localised mobilisation of the upper cervical segments, when there is little or no clinically detectable change in temperomandibular joint function.

ACUTE TORTICOLLIS OR WRY-NECK

A segment between C2 and C7,[1162, 165] more usually C2–3, is the site of a usually transient but acutely painful unilateral joint condition, often manifest on rising in the morning and characterised by an antalgic posture of slight flexion and side-flexion away from the painful side.

The varieties of combined movement in normal cervical and upper thoracic spines (p. 47), differences in the tolerance to pain, variations of body type and musculature, normal mobility existing and the level of the lesion are probably some of the factors deciding (i) which antalgic neck posture will be assumed, and (ii) its degree of fixity by postural spasm of muscle.

Further, we suspect but do not know precisely what the

lesion is, and the abnormality may not be the same from patient to patient.

Full elevation of the painful-side arm may be neither possible nor pain-free. Movements towards the side of pain are very restricted or impossible, as is full extension, and attempts provoke a severe jab of pain; early in the day the provoked pain can usually be localised to the upper neck on the convex side of the deformity, but as the day wears on a generalised ache is superimposed upon the local pain and unguarded movements will elicit jabs of pain spreading to the upper trapezius and shoulder area. The patient is then less able to accurately localise its source; Spisak (1972)[1162] reported a group of 103 patients among which 80 per cent were unable to localise the pain.

In his series *the onset* was variable, 3 per cent reporting mild trauma to the head, 8 per cent reporting the onset of pain on head rotation, 31 per cent on waking in the morning and 23 per cent describing pain coming on over 1–2 hours without apparent cause. Others mentioned irritation by cold ('sleeping in a draught', 'had the window open').

The condition occurs more frequently in children and young adults. Some subjects seem surprisingly active during sleep, e.g. powerful tooth-grinding (bruxism), fist-clenching and back-scratching; the neck may be powerfully twisted during sleep. Conversely, during heavy sleep one aspect of the neck may suffer the prolonged stretching of a strained posture which would be intolerable for more than 15–20 minutes if the subject were awake. Possible mechanisms are:

1. The prolonged stretch, probably in the posture of the fixed tendency, induces slight oedema which congests and thickens a meniscoid synovial villus (see p. 5), inducing it to remain as an impacted synovial inclusion on subsequent change of neck posture during the night.

2. The prolonged stretch initiates oedematous thickening of the particularly tight joint structures of the C2–3 segment, with periarticular congestion and consequently a localised irritability, but with no inclusion.

3. The slow shift of cervical disc substance during a strained posture during sleep.

The high frequency of C2–C3 involvement may be associated with the unique anatomical and functional position of that segment. It is the first mobility-segment with a disc, the upper component functionally belonging to the craniovertebral complex and the lower component forming the first typically cervical vertebral joint; it is thus a transitional region.

Colachis and Strohm (1966)[193] demonstrated its uniqueness in that traction produces here the least separation of all the typical cervical segments, and Spisak mentions that its ligaments are stronger than in the other typical segments.

Most cases respond to localised mobilisation and support by a significant lessening of pain within 24 hours, many clear up spontaneously with a comfortable support in a few days; some may not be clear of pain for 10 days or more. Probably it is wise to avoid the immediate use of Grade V thrust techniques of manipulation in these cases unless the symptoms are minor, the therapist can have confidence that they are innocuous and the responsible segment has been localised.

A frequent clinical presentation of this syndrome is that of a roughly similar neck deformity occurring together with two broad types of pain behaviour, and a further difference between the two so far as history and the indicated treatment are concerned.

Deformity

Patients tend to hold the neck slightly side-flexed and rotated away from the side of pain, and a little flexed. Movements which increase the deformity are much easier than those which correct it, and in type ii below, the flexion component may be somewhat greater.

Onset

Type i is sudden and associated with a particular movement. The abnormal neck posture is necessarily imposed, by pain, from that instant. The onset may be on waking, during the night or at any time during the day.

Type ii. A common pattern is that the patient retires normally at night and wakes with a stiff and painful neck.

Pain

Type i. This is unilaterally localised to the pillar of the neck, and commonly does not spread to the yoke area, the scapula, shoulder or arm. Attempts to correct the deformity are accompanied by sharp jabs of pain localised to the neck.

Type ii. The pain tends to occupy one side of the base of the neck, and spreads unilaterally to the yoke area and the middle region of the scapula, and spreads down the outer or posterior arm, sometimes as far as the elbow. Careful and considerate attempts to correct the deformity meet with a very painful resistance which has the firm, springy quality of a cartilage injury at the knee. The provoked pain may spread distally.

Regarding the probable nature of the underlying joint derangement, it seems reasonable to speculate that the type i condition might be due to impaction of a synovial villus (meniscoid structure) between the surfaces of a cervical facet-joint, and that type ii may be a result of the slow shift of cervical disc substance.

The best distinction lies in the circumstance that type i is, as a rule, easily relieved in a single treatment by localised mobilisation or manipulation, whereas type ii can often be badly provoked by these techniques, and requires instead sustained traction in flexion, and/or rotational distraction manœuvres which also need to be sustained; it will also take longer to relieve, particularly if the flexion deformity is marked.

A handful of cases presenting in this way may defy the most careful attempts with heat, support and gentle mobilisation to alleviate the pain and the clinical state proceeds, seemingly inexorably, to a manifest low cervical root involvement with neurological signs. It is difficult in these few cases to avoid the conclusion that a slow shift of cervical disc material has impinged upon the neighbouring nerve root.

It is important to distinguish the condition from epidemic cervical myalgia and the conditions previously described (pp. 157, 212).

Mehta (1973)[839] draws attention to the value of nerve block at C2 and C3 in resistant cases.

It is useful to remember that, uncommonly, vertebra plana and oesinophilic granuloma of the cervical spine may be present, in children, with sudden onset of neck pain and torticollis, usually without a history of significant trauma.[1121]

Vertebral involvement occurs in a descending order of frequency in the lumbar, dorsal and cervical spines.

HEADACHE (see p. 181)

While pain in cranial and facial regions is a frequent complaint in cervical spine disorders[598] headache may be the presenting symptom of disorder not involving the musculoskeletal tissues, e.g. dental malocclusion with consequent temperomandibular joint irritability, which commonly refers pain to the temporal regions.[937] Conversely, facial pain mistakenly believed to be due to disorders of the jaw joint may be referred from the cervical spine.

In a series of 951 patients referred primarily for temperomandibular joint disorders, 23 cases were experiencing the referred pains of cervical spondylosis;[375] it is a common clinical experience that face pain, other than in the auricular and temporal area, may arise from cervical joint problems.

The phenomena of referred pain occur frequently in the trigeminal system, because the mechanism for such reference appears to be very highly developed in this neurone complex[273] and this adds to the difficulties of localisation[1355] (Figs 1.16, 8.2).

Stating the obvious, headaches may also present as the dominant clinical feature of serious intracranial conditions[417] such as space-occupying vascular and neoplastic disease or meningitis.

Chusid (1973)[175] classifies headache under the categories summarised below:

Vascular headache of migrainous type

Recurrent attacks are widely varied in intensity, frequency and duration, commonly unilateral in onset and sometimes associated with nausea and vomiting. Cranial arterial dilatation occurs in the painful phase but causes no permanent change in the vessels (see p. 182).

1. Classical migraine—vascular headache with transient visual and other prodroma (see p. 181).
2. Common migraine—vascular headache without focal aura and less often unilateral; frequently termed a 'sick headache', 'atypical migraine', 'premenstrual headache', etc.
3. Cluster headache—a type of migraine occurring in cyclic groupings of headache which last 30–60 minutes each, perhaps three or four times a day, and then disappear for a period of weeks, months or years before the next 'cluster' begins.
4. Hemiplegic migraine and ophthalmoplegic migraine, in which sensory and motor phenomena persist during and after the headache.[111]
5. Lower face headache—occurring typically in the region implied, possibly of vascular origin and including atypical facial neuralgia, etc.

Muscle-contraction headache

This is characterised by aching sensations of tightening or pressure in the suboccipital and cervical musculature. More commonly bilateral, it is often associated by both patient and clinician with sustained contraction of skeletal muscle, and goes by generalised terms as that above, or tension headache. There is evidence (see p. 197) that the tension may not be the cause so much as one of the manifestations of a non-muscular abnormality.

Sheldon (1967)[1120] observes that the easy labelling of headaches in innumerable patients as tension headache is unrealistic. Although it may be known that tension exists, careful analysis shows that tension is *not* the prime agent in nearly as many headaches as is commonly stated (see p. 198).

Similarly, many patients with the presenting symptom of headache are diagnosed as 'migraine' when organic pathology, later uncovered, had no true relationship to the description of so-called migrainous complexes. Sheldon tabulated the findings in 109 patients who had been diagnosed as migraine, and the ultimate findings, in descending numerical order were:

1. Cervicooccipital syndrome 67
   (with convulsive disorder) (4)
2. Intracranial aneurysm 15
3. Brain tumour 11
4. Cerebrovascular disease 4
5. Hypertensive disease only 3
6. Aneurysm plus cervicooccipital syndrome 2
7. Aneurysm, cervicooccipital syndrome, myasthenia gravis; subdural haematoma; neck tumour, posterior fibroma 3

Combined migrainous and tension headache, with both features co-existing

Other categories include headache due to nasal vasomotor reactions, glaucoma, hypochondriacal states, dilatation of cranial arteries due to infections, poisons and foreign-protein reactions, or to essential hypertension; neoplasms, subarachnoid haemorrhage, cranial neuritides and cranial neuralgias and headaches due to other disease of ocular, aural, nasal, dental structures and sinuses—the list is formidable.

Lance (1969)[691] among others, has also classified headache, and the preponderance of inverted commas in any list of the nomenclature of head pain reveals the degree of uncertainty regarding this ubiquitous clinical feature.

Mehta (1973)[839] observes that the aetiology of many cases of headache remains unknown and treatment remains empirical.

Magora, *et al.* (1974)[785] studied the involvement of the cervical spine in 57 patients suffering from headache, and mentioned the constellation of clinical features as occipital pain, hemicranialgia or more widespread pain, vertigo, difficulty in swallowing, tinnitus, nystagmus, contracted neck musculature and limitation of head movements. As such the features may *mimic* tension, ophthalmological headache or migraine, and be superimposed upon them. By X-ray of the whole neck and electromyography of the semispinalis muscle, the authors studied the various clinical presentations. A major striking finding was the high incidence of e.m.g. evidence of nerve involvement in the headache syndrome. No correlation between X-ray and e.m.g. abnormalities was observed.

While its pathogenesis is still not fully understood, headache is a common symptom of cervical spondylosis, and it may occur both with spondylotic changes of the lower neck as well as that due to synovial joint changes in the upper neck.

This symptom is less often related to disc degeneration than to arthrosis of the upper cervical apophyseal joints. These joints tend to be neglected because X-ray films need to be taken at a special angle to show them well.[1097]

The justification for stressing the importance of cervical joint problems in the genesis of headache lies in an analysis of 5500 cases of cervical spine disorder, in which more than 85 per cent were the result of trauma and in which headache was one of the most frequent complaints.[599]

Frykholm (1971)[392] stated,

In my experience cervical migraine is the type of headache most frequently seen in general practice and also the type most frequently misinterpreted. It is usually erroneously diagnosed as classic migraine, tension headache, vascular headache, hypertensive encephalopathy or post-traumatic encephalopathy. Such patients have usually received an inadequate treatment and have often become neurotic and drug-dependent. (See Arthrosis of upper cervical segments, p. 215.)

Possible underlying mechanisms have been discussed elsewhere (pp. 183, 184).

A particular and common type of headache is described (Lewit, 1977)[742] in which the pain is considered to be arising from the posterior arch of the atlas. The basic and common finding is unilateral tenderness of that structure on carefully localised palpation, and movement-restriction (blockage) of the occipitoatlantal joint (Figs 8.1, 8.3, 8.4). Frequently, the pain is increased on head extension. The presence of cranioicrtebral joint restriction is elicited by springing the occiput against the stabilised atlas, i.e. producing a dorsal shift of the head, or by extending the rotated head on the atlas while the atlantoaxial joint is held stabilised. Thus, the classical occipital neuralgia, previously considered due to irritation of the greater occipital nerve at its point of emergence through fascial planes of the neck, is most likely to be referred pain from an abnormal craniovertebral joint (see also p. 100).

The definitive treatment is localised mobilisation or manipulation, and failing this, needling of the posterior arch with acupuncture needles. Segmental exercises may also be indicated.

Lewit suggests that the diagnosis of occipital neuralgia is, as a rule, as little justified as that of intercostal neuralgia.

TEMPEROMANDIBULAR JOINT

This is a highly specialised articulation, and because of the interposed disc between temporal bone and mandibular condyle it may best be described as a hinge joint with a movable socket.[495]

Movements of the mandible are *coupled* by the bilateral articulation, in which the bearing surfaces are avascular fibrous tissue and not hyaline cartilage.[86]

The commonest complaints affecting the joint are the consequences of stress, trauma and muscular tension or trismus. As in other joints, clinical features can exist before positive evidence of degenerative changes can be demonstrated, and if these are treated on the correct aetiological basis, the majority can be cured. Transpharyngeal X-rays can provide clear evidence of existing arthrotic erosion.[1227]

Joint problems may present[937] with any combination of the following features:

Pain in or around the ear
Pain on jaw movement
Tender muscles of mastication
Clicking, popping or snapping on joint movement
Grating, grinding and less obvious crepitus
Limitation of movement
Ear symptoms, including subjective hearing loss, a feeling of 'fullness' and tinnitus
Scalp soreness

Tender or painful teeth
Throat pain on swallowing, or throat soreness
'Burning' pain on the side of the neck
Upper trapezius pain spreading out to the point of the shoulder
Head pain in known 'jaw clinchers'.

Many tense patients grind their jaws, and have jaw-pressure symptoms which must be distinguished from meniscal injuries.[1126]

Hankey (1954)[495] described the features of 150 cases, in which women were affected three times as often as men. Twenty-three of the cases complained of trigeminal neuralgia without any other symptoms, and these caused great difficulty in diagnosis. Fifty-seven per cent of the cases developed the symptoms between adolescence and 30 years. Few had symptoms which were severe at the onset but most sought help within 6 months. Most had a gradual onset and only 37 per cent started suddenly.

Extrinsic trauma was more common in men, and could occur after a blow to the side of the face or axially on the chin, and included extraction of lower molar teeth, which may strain the joint ligaments. *Intrinsic* trauma could be laughing, yawning or eating.

Painless unilateral or bilateral clicking, which is not the same as crepitus, occurred in 30 per cent of the cases, and in 27 per cent clicking was painful. The remaining 43 per cent had no clicking, but a variety of other symptoms more or less localised to the joint, among which movement-restriction was common.

Movement, wide opening or mastication usually provoked the pain, which would be either sharp and stabbing but transient, or a steady dull neuralgia or gnawing soreness. Only nine patients complained of deafness, tinnitus or lingual symptoms. Some had occasional locking, or recurrent subluxation; early or initial restriction may be self-reduced at first, but leaves a synovitis with tenderness and stiffness.

Repeated intrinsic trauma may initiate degenerative changes with capsular looseness, clicking and poor apposition of disc to condyle.

Hankey[495] observed that trismus, either reflex or mechanical, is a common cause and anything which upsets the delicate muscle balance between the two joints (which really comprise a single joint with a bicondylar arrangement[437]) may initiate symptoms. In 20 of his cases the underlying factor was an impacted third molar or carious tooth.

The most frequent aetiological factor initiating degenerative change is the cumulative effect of altered stresses and strains imposed by *malocclusion*, the aetiology of which is a subject in itself. Among the causes, teeth-grinding (bruxism) is often a sign of anxiety, and the teeth may be worn away to the extent that malocclusion occurs.

While psychogenic factors may be contributory in that they may initiate habitual tooth-grinding. Kirveskari (1978)[663] suggests that an underlying morphological change must be present before teeth-grinding can cause the 'pain-dysfunction' syndrome.

Copland (1954)[204] observes that the rest position is almost permanently abolished; joints are always compressed and muscles are always tensed, so that pain is caused for this reason alone.

Changes in the occlusal relationship of the teeth lead to small degrees of remodelling of the articular surfaces of the joint.[437]

Malocclusal displacement may account for no more than a 1–2 mm shift, and yet produce extreme pain. Ballard (1956)[56] suggests that a high percentage of 'derangement of the temperomandibular joint' are, in fact, reflex disturbances of the basic co-ordinating patterns of mandibular movement. While malocclusion can be the cause of obscure facial pain, pain is also dependent upon the psychological factors and the pain tolerance of the individual.

Rocabado (1977)[1053] has done much to clarify the functional interdependence of the cervical and temperomandibular joints, the relationship between neck and jaw movement, the interrelations of muscular activity of neck and jaw, and movements of the mandible in relation to the position of the head and the rest of the body. The normal functions of opening and closing the mouth, biting and chewing, swallowing, speech, yawning and respiration are bio-mechanically linked, and not surprisingly therefore the author has been able to emphasise the constantly recurring link between jaw, neck, yoke, shoulder and craniofacial pain.

Chronic abnormalities of dentition, of occlusal articulation of the joints of the jaw and of the craniovertebral region, and of the masticatory and suboccipital muscles, are likely to affect one or other member of this interdependent family, with persistent effects often spreading further afield.

It is suggested that one of the many causes of tinnitus might be an abnormal functional relationship of the temperomandibular joint, induced by chronic hypertonus of the temporalis and masseter muscles. This would tend to maintain an habitual approximation, upwards and backwards, of the mandibular condyle towards the middle ear, possibly disturbing the normal pressure relationships in the region of the tegmen tympani and tympanic plate.

Twigs from the auriculotemporal branch of the mandibular nerve (V cranial) supply the joint—it is not possible for this nerve to be compressed against the tympanic plate by a retruded condyle.[495]

While the *stapedius* muscle is supplied by the 7th cranial (facial) nerve, the *tensor tympani* muscle is supplied by a branch of the nerve to the *medial pterygoid*;[437] the latter two branches are from the mandibular nerve, a division of the 5th cranial, and it is conceivable that associated temperomandibular and craniovertebral joint abnormalities may induce auditory disturbances in more than one way, i.e. (i) chronic approximation of the mandible in the condylar fossa and (ii) increased nociceptor and mechanoreceptor afferent traffic from vertebral joints activating a degree of facilitation in the spinal tract of the 5th cranial nerve.

In this connection, the observations of Travell (1960)[1240] (p. 119) on the trigger points of jaw musculature, and the successive relief of restricted jaw-opening by weekly injections at trigger points, are of both clinical and aetiological interest.

Patients with hyperactivity of the masticatory muscles may develop simultaneous hyperactivity of the sternomastoid muscle, initiating an abnormal loss of the natural cervical lordosis with, in some patients, an anteposition of the head. The craniovertebral posture and suboccipital musculature are then disturbed, with the chronic effects of pain being referred to cranial and cervical regions not normally associated with the temperomandibular joint.

As a therapist working with orthodontic and dental groups, Rocabado has described some clinical presentations:

1. Headache and temporal pain, overactivity of the jaw musculature with an unconscious habit of teeth-grinding, a postural tendency to side-flexion and rotation of the head with a painful unilateral scalenus anticus syndrome and a tendency to raise the shoulder of that side.

2. Antepositioned posture of the neck with a flat cervical spine, referred occipital pain and malocclusion, the last being the dominant factor and taking priority in treatment.

3. A lady with posterior capsulitis of the temperomandibular joint, the pain of which was acutely exacerbated each time she cleansed her ears by partially inserting an index finger during washing. Her pains were referred to the upper and midcervical area, and upper chest, and she tended to adopt an abnormal head and neck posture when in pain.

4. Orthodontic problems in a child of 10 years, a mouth breather, with an anteposition of the head and a hyperactive sternomastoid muscle acting as an accessory muscle of respiration.

More than 60 per cent of the patients attending this specialised clinic were women between the ages of 25 and 55 and most of the patients who were assessed as concurrently having a cervical joint and temperomandibular joint condition exhibited hypermobility of the jaw joint.

Investigation

Diagnostic local anaesthesia may be required; among the most important investigations are bite analysis and joint radiography.

The clinical and radiographic features of 130 cases were reported by Toller (1973)[1227] and radiographic changes of the surface of the mandibular condyle were present in all of the cases, although not always detectable at first attendance. Pain, X-ray changes, crepitus and limitation of jaw movement were all present in most cases. The condition affected mostly women, being commonest in the fifth decade. Transpharyngeal radiographs showed the anterior part of the condyle to be more frequently affected, from early loss of lamina dura to shallow and more severe erosions of condylar bone.

Rocabado[1053] suggests that when seeking to analyse the genesis of pain in the jaw region its functional context should also be considered. The *whole masticatory system*, i.e. dentition, occlusion, the temperomandibular joint, the masticatory and facial musculature, the postural relationships of head, neck and upper thorax, and the state of related musculature and soft tissues, should be systematically examined.

Apart from the necessity for specialist attention to dentition and occlusal correction, many patients may exhibit one or more of other important clinical features which will need correction, e.g. stiffness or laxity of the temperomandibular joint, abnormal movement patterns of the mandible, coexisting craniovertebral and cervical joint problems, abnormal head and neck posture, asymmetrical muscle tightness from occupational and/or psychological stress and a restricted range of head, neck, shoulder girdle and arm movement. The author suggests a simple experiment to demonstrate by palpation the intimate structural relationship, as distraction and compression effects, between the capsule of the jaw joint and the auditory meatus—the tip of an index finger is held within the auditory meatus while the mouth is fully opened and closed.

The attachments of the trapezius muscle, the platysma, the sternomastoid, the digastric and supra- and infrahyoid musculature, the longus capitis, the ramifications of the deep cervical fascia and the intimate functional relationship between opening of the jaw and extension at the craniovertebral joint, suggest the rational link of these concepts with those of Janda (p. 113).

Rocabado mentions that the important *lateral pterygoid muscle*, with its bicipital arrangement of one attachment to the joint meniscus and one to an anterior depression just below the head of the mandible, may function abnormally in hypermobility of the joint, and that imbalance between the two heads may occur.

Management

The condition may require injection of hyalase, hydrocortisone or local anaesthetic, dental as well as orthodontal attention, and surgical attention in the form of menisectomy or condylectomy.

A single intra-articular injection of corticosteroid can successfully relieve intractable pain, but is more successful in patients over the age of 30 years; the older the patient, the greater the likelihood of clinical improvement.[1228]

Physiotherapy may be indicated, as the only treatment or in conjunction with biofeedback relaxation techniques and those mentioned above.

Trott and Goss (1978)[1243] analysed 34 patients treated by physiotherapy techniques. Physical and e.m.g. tests revealed that temperomandibular joint function was abnormal in all cases with minimal muscle involvement. Nineteen patients (56 per cent) had pain referred from the cervical spine. Physiotherapy treatment for restoring full painless joint range was successful in 6 of 10 patients. Biofeedback relaxation therapy was successful in 19 of 24 patients; there were significant psychiatric factors in the remaining 5 of this latter group.

Patients with or without upper cervical joint problems may have cheek, ear, temporal and postauricular pain, and the distinction between pains of cervical origin and those arising from temperomandibular joint abnormalities is usually not difficult.

At times the distinction is not easy. (i) Postauricular and face pain may be referred[375] from the neck, and often from the craniovertebral region (i.e. segments C0–C1–C2–C3), and attention to the cervical problem alone will relieve these pains. (ii) Painful temperomandibular joint movement on occasions exists *together* with craniovertebral joint problems, and treatment of the latter may reduce lateral face pain and the pain on jaw movement, although not be sufficient to completely relieve it.

The type of patient frequently referred for treatment is a fairly slim woman of a little over 30, or older, who has a tendency to preoccupation with the pressures of life and family demands, and who habitually clenches the jaw. Cervical joint problems frequently coexist, and the patient often has a stiffish neck, chronic neck muscle hypertonus and often a slightly elevated 1st rib on the side of the most affected temperomandibular joint. There may be some joint-clicking on the most painful side of the face, and tenderness of mastication muscles on both sides. The amount of movement-limitation may not be severe, but can be painfully limited to the extent that the patient's index and middle finger cannot be freely inserted between the teeth. Lateral mandibular movement away from the most painful side may be the most *painful* movement, although opening is the most *limited* movement. The complex of signs and symptoms may have been compounded by the removal of a molar tooth.

When the patient is to be treated by mobilisation techniques for both cervical and jaw pain, it is for obvious reasons wise to first note the effects of attending to *either* the jaw or the neck before combining the treatment of both causative lesions.

The initial use of cervical traction for the neck problem may by aggravating temperomandibular soreness invalidate the assessment findings. Crepitus may still remain in some, many years after the patient is pain-free, with good jaw movement and adequate function.[1228]

ACCELERATION AND DECELERATION TRAUMA ('whiplash' injury)

Injury to the cervical spine is almost without exception due to indirect violence,[1274] the force being applied to head or rump and the neck sustaining a considerable proportion of it.

The direction of the force, the position and relationship of the head and spine, and the state of tension of the neck muscles determine the localisation of stress. When injury has been severe, these patients suffer what might be regarded as multiple 'sprained ankles' in the neck, with all the added complications of nerve root and plexus traction injuries; meningeal traction; tearing of ligaments and probably muscle; trauma to blood vessels and lymphatics; upset to sensitive structures and delicately balanced functions.

Ray and Wolff (1940),[1016] when discussing the pain-sensitive structures probably contributing to headache, mentioned the scalp arteries and the narrow zones of dura along the large arterial trunks (e.g. the meningeal and cranial base arteries) as especially sensitive. These structures are frequently involved in whiplash injury, the effects of which are compounded if direct trauma to the head is sustained at the same time. Conversely, in the presence of direct head injury alone, the potential additional injury to the cervical spine must always be remembered. Occasionally, neurological signs of upper cervical cord or lower brainstem injury may be present.

In general, hyperextension will injure the upper, and hyperflexion the lower cervical spine ... in the presence of head injury, the potential additional injury to the cervical spine must always be remembered.[1274]

Chusid (1973)[175] mentions that so-called chronic post-traumatic headache may arise from one of several mechanisms. The 'post-concussional syndrome'[205] may not be entirely due to intracranical changes and further, a moment's thought may show that a sideways fall on the outstretched hand can produce a lateral whiplash effect on the cervical spine besides a Colles fracture. Patients need not have been in a motor-car to have suffered acceleration or deceleration trauma to the neck, many of these injuries occurring during athletics or on the sports field.

In a group of patients described by Roca (1972)[1052] one developed the acute traumatic cervical syndrome after a fall in a shower.

The inflammatory reaction to injury includes space-occupying oedema, and if this persists and becomes indurated, fibrotic hyperplasia of connective tissue adds to the chronic trespass upon nerve roots, arteries, veins and lymphatics, besides interfering with the normal free adaptation of cervical soft tissues to functional movements and postures of the neck. Bleeding, between normally mobile planes of delicate intraspinal and extraspinal soft tissues, tends to become organised and to add to tethering effects by adhesions.

Tearing or attenuation of ligaments and capsules, accompanied later by patchy areas of firm fibrosis, may eventually produce a residual pattern of chronic stiffness and instability in adjacent segments.

Because of the chronic disturbance of normal tissue-fluid exchange in collagenous structures and muscles, the normal biochemical environment of nociceptor and mechanoreceptor endings is almost certainly disturbed, adding chronic irritative effects to nociceptor endings besides upset to the important afferent traffic from joint and muscle receptors, upon which equilibration depends.

Stoddard (1969)[1180b] observes that pure flexion/extension injuries do not normally involve the facet-joints, and that there needs to be some element of side-bending and/or rotation to involve the *capsules* of these joints. A glance at the posterior surface of neural arches at C6, C7, T1 and T2 indicates that forcible extension (of a flexible structure carrying a 3.5–4.5 kg weight, i.e. the head) will violently engage the lower edges of the inferior facets on the narrow horizontal bony ledge marking the base of the superior facets below. A multiple acute traumatic periostitis at facet-joint margins is probably one of the family of lesions sustained in a severe extension-acceleration injury.

Stoddard also regards a tear of the anterior longitudinal ligament to be more important than posterior ligamentous tears, partly because they are sometimes undetected but also because these ligaments provide the only anterior support for cervical vertebral bodies.

The upset to delicately balanced functions is briefly discussed on page 183.

Depending upon the nature and magnitude of the violence applied, these cases present with one or more of the following:

Suboccipital, neck and yoke area pains, unilaterally or bilaterally, with bouts of frontal headache which may be periodic and transient or remain as a dull and constant background ache
Facial and anterolateral throat pain
Patches of subjective facial numbness
Otalgia
Retro-orbital pain—sometimes paraesthesiae 'in' the eye
Subjective laryngeal disturbances, with compulsive clearing of the throat
Upper pectoral area and axillary pain
Feelings of instability or dysequilibrium, with sometimes a tendency to list to one side
Disturbances of hearing and/or vision
Depression, and feelings of fatigue

A belief that they are becoming neurotic and 'should pull themselves together.'
Irritability, insomnia and light-headedness.

They tend to move the neck cautiously and apprehensively, and are glad to return to a neutral position in which they feel most comfortable.

Bilateral muscle spasm is common, and is not always superficial. Referred pain, without neurological signs, tend to spread to upper limbs, and paraesthesiae with subjective numbness begin to occur in the arm, either with a patchy and changing distribution, or distally and more or less confined to the territory of a single root, with later objective numbness.

Roca (1972)[1052] described 15 patients with ocular manifestations after whiplash injury, mentioning that blurred vision, strain, fatigue, diplopia, photophobia and inability to read may occur, with anxiety and a degree of depression soon to follow. Among the clinical features were included amaurotic episodes, decreased accommodation and convergence, anisocoria, possible vitreous detachment, hyperphoria, hypertropia, ptosis and inability to focus.

N.B. The most important clinical aspect is that of a highly reactive 'brittleness' of condition during the early stages. It is quite different to the irritability of a single peripheral joint, for example, where unwisely energetic handling may stir up severe pain for hours or days. If the badly injured whiplash patient is handled vigorously with careless movement, the exacerbation can be very severe, with headache of hideous intensity, bizarre visual upset, psychic distress amounting to abject misery, and cervical pain of frightening viciousness. The 'brittle' stage may last for a week or for two to three months, and may return for a few days during the following months if the patient stumbles, is badly jolted or is given unnecessarily vigorous treatment.

A retrospective analysis[559] of 146 patients, after 5 years, indicated that there was a statistically significant correlation between poor treatment results and the following findings soon after injury:

Numbness or pain, or both, in an upper limb
A sharp reversal of cervical lordosis visible on X-ray
Restricted motion at one segment on 'bending' films
The need for a collar for more than three months
The need to resume physiotherapy more than once because of a recurrence of symptoms.

CERVICAL SPONDYLOSIS

The lower cervical region is especially prone to spondylosis (see pp. 126, 205), radiographically evident in the majority of middle-aged people and certainly symptomless in many (Figs. 5.2, 5.5, 6.1, 6.2, 6.3, 6.4).

Because of the complex anatomy and biomechanics of neck structures, the whole system is vulnerable. A simple experiment which will give an idea of the stresses imposed on the neck in a working day is to grasp a 3.5–4.5 kg weight in the hand, resting the elbow on a table with the forearm vertically under the weight. Twist the forearm, lower the weight a little to one side or another, raise it again; continue this for two minutes. The weight represents a head, and the wrist represents a neck. The cervical vertebrae with associated ligaments and muscles are stronger than similar structures of the wrist, of course, but this simple experiment will give a good idea of why they need to be, and of the work they are doing. Should the vertical forearm now be given an unexpected and forceful lateral push, the experimenter has experienced something like the stresses imposed during an acceleration or deceleration (whiplash) injury to the neck.

Cervical spondylosis, so often the late retribution (see p. 75) exacted by cervical structures in response to physical stress, seems less a precise diagnosis than a statement drawing attention to the coexistence of head, neck, yoke and arm pain, in the presence of some loss of normal neck movement, sometimes with upper limb neurological abnormality and frequently some radiographic change in the lower cervical region. None of the the four factors need have any frank relationship to the other three; they may or may not be clinically associated in the great variety of presentation of neck pain considered to be due to spondylosis of the lower cervical spine. Myelopathy is discussed below.)

The diagnosis may also include patients with associated peripheral changes in the upper limb; these may go by proper names such as periarthritis, bicipital tendinitis, lateral epicondylitis and medial epicondylitis, etc.[340] (See pp. 116, 187).

The radiological appearance of compression of a cervical articular process is a not uncommon finding, even though some patients may not be able to recall a recent traumatic incident. When its nature can be ascertained or strongly suspected, the trauma is usually a combination of hyperextension with compression injury; Smith *et al.* (1976)[1146] suggests that attention to this possibility is warranted when patients report persistent neck pain.

The forms of presentation are many; cervical spondylosis embraces changes of multiple genesis. They may include changes masquerading as cervical when the upper thoracic region, or more distal tissues, may largely be responsible for the clinical features.

For example, paraesthesiae which are worse at night, and not provoked by neck movements, may be caused by first thoracic root compression or by median nerve impingement in the carpal tunnel—either may occur in association with cervical spondylosis[1370] and can be difficult to separate clinically, although electrodiagnosis will assist in detecting carpal tunnel compression.

Frykholm (1971)[392] mentions the consequences of a painful condition which need affect only one of the many neck joints; spasm of neck muscles and a significant impairment of normal mobility may occur. A similar effect is produced by trauma, which may affect one or several of the joints and their ligaments.

Pain and muscle spasm initiate vascular spasm, causing additional pain. In those cases with some spondylosis existing, or with structural anomalies predisposing certain segments to nerve root trespass, there is always the risk of radicular irritation.

Nathan (1970)[904] observed that in a majority (76 per cent) of cases a variable number of spinal roots, more usually in the lower cervical and upper thoracic segments, followed an angulated course. Within the dura, the rootlets proceed downwards for a variable distance and on piercing the dura were sharply angulated upwards to reach the portal of the intervertebral foramen. Since the extraforaminal course is again downwards, a handful of spinal roots (commonly occupying a junctional vertebral region prone to trespass by thickened degenerative tissues) have undergone two fairly marked angulations by the time of their emergence from the foramen. The degree of angulations may be as much as 30° and can reach 45°. Irregular and uneven development at the dural sac has been considered as the possible cause of these angulations which may, of course, be further distorted by degenerative changes, particularly dural tethering within the neural canal and root-sleeve tethering at the foramen.

The roots affected are those between C6 and T9, with T2 and T3 most frequently and severely angulated. *The angulations are increased when the neck is extended.*

The previously silent progression of degenerative change may be stirred up by some slight trauma or stress, or the onset is insidious. The causative stress may be an unusually long car journey, decorating a ceiling, hanging curtains, horseplay with children or a night in an uncomfortable hotel bed. Frequently the stress is trivial, such as minor trauma to the head, neck or arm, e.g. the tugging of a dog on a lead, or an hour's reading, knitting or sewing with the head bent forward. Commonly, the episode begins as vague neck pain and slight stiffness, with pain later spreading from the base of the neck to upper trapezius and upper scapular areas, over the deltoid and down the lateral or posterolateral arm on the same side. It may begin as an upper scapular region ache, and arm pain may also involve the posterior axillary boundary, sometimes involving the upper pectoral area.

The dull aching pain is commonly unilateral but can be bilateral and is aggravated by movement of the neck towards the most painful side, as well as by extension and/or flexion. Movement of the shoulder on the same side is slightly limited and often hurts near the extreme of range; this sign may be missed during cursory examination. Patients often report pain along the lateral forearm muscles on functional movements involving wrist extension or wrist flexion (see p. 188). The pain and/or restricted neck movements may wax and wane over a period of weeks or months, to reappear some months later and trouble the patient more severely, or then to regress for years. Paraesthesiae may develop, for example, in the thumb and index finger (C6 root), the middle three digits (C7) or the medial two (C8) and this together with weakness in the myotome (representative muscles being, respectively, those producing elbow flexion, elbow extension, and extension of distal phalanx of thumb) *may* (see below) indicate involvement of the appropriate spinal nerve root (see p. 160). The C6 or C7 tendon reflex may become depressed or be absent. Alternatively, paraesthesiae may be the first symptom noted, sometimes but not always to be followed soon after by 'root' pain of a particularly unpleasant nature in the arm. Sustained holding of an extreme neck movement will then exacerbate the arm pain and paraesthesiae, after a latent period of some seconds. In the presence of severe 'root' pain, neck movements may not be markedly limited. The C7 root is the one most often affected, with weakness of the triceps muscle.

Although it seems that the greater majority of patients with cervical spondylosis have pain which is not due to root involvement it is common experience that those with signs of currently developing root changes suffer a particularly severe and 'sickening' type of distress.

Frykholm[392] has emphasised the vulnerability of the root complex and his observations, which have a mechanical bias, are summarised as follows:

1. A nerve-root angulated and fixed at its exit point (be it from dural sheath and/or intervertebral foramen) cannot tolerate too much of the stretching which occurs when the neck is flexed and tension is applied to all of the rootlets. The angulations at dural exit are increased on *extension* (see p. 224).

2. If the tolerance of a root-complex be exceeded the nerve will suffer acute damage, followed by intra- and periradicular oedema, in a situation very probably already crowded by chronic degenerative thickening and fibrotic change.

The root symptoms usually develop gradually during some days or weeks. Brain and Wilkinson (1967)[117] describe several types of clinical presentation of root involvement:

1. Acute radiculopathy, due to dorsolateral disc protrusions, in relatively young patients with no evidence of spondylotic changes (see pp. 126, 217).

2. Acute radiculopathy, due to acute disc trespass or exacerbation of a pre-existing trespass in patients with radiographic evidence of established spondylosis.

3. Acute or subacute root involvement, in patients who are known to have spondylosis and episodes of neck pain. There is nothing in the recent history to suggest acute disc trauma.

4. Symptoms of chronic root involvement develop insidiously, or an acute radiculopathy does not subside but leaves some permanent sensory disturbance.

They mention that any of neck pain, radicular symptoms, cervical myelopathy, headache and the symptoms of vertebrobasilar ischaemia may occur, either singly or in any combination; and with regard to myelopathy, the changes in the spinal cord are produced in a complex fashion by the pressures and tensions to which it is subjected.

It is now some 12 years since a report appeared on the Multi-Centre Trial of Physiotherapy for Pain in the Neck and Arm,[127] when it was observed that, 'this study is a reminder of how little is known of the natural history of this common syndrome'. While understanding has been enlarged[1, 2, 3, 120, 344, 392, 981, 988, 1316] it remains difficult in any particular case to account confidently for the production of all the symptoms and signs, and to be as precise as we would like about forecasting the response to treatment.

Patients admitted to the trial satisfied one of the following sets of criteria:

1. Pain in the neck and arm (with or without paraesthesiae), the symptoms having a root distribution and being associated with limited and painful movements of the neck.

2. Pain in the neck and arm of full root-distribution with paraesthesiae but without clinical evidence of abnormality in the neck.

3. Pain or paraesthesiae in the neck and arm of partial root-distribution but with definite evidence of clinical abnormality in the neck.

With *regard to neurological signs*, 40 per cent of the 493 patients in the trial had abnormal neurological signs in the upper limb, usually a diminished triceps reflex, weak elbow-extension and minor sensory loss in the fingers. It is not always easy to be sure, on clinical grounds alone, that pain and limitation currently troubling a patient are necessarily associated with neurological signs, of which the patient may be unaware and which can be the 'tombstone' of past episodes, remaining unaltered after current pain and restriction are completely relieved.

Bearing in mind the authors' comment that only limited conclusions could be drawn from a study of this kind, it is of interest to quote from their findings:

There was no significant difference in the rate of improvement in patients with abnormal neurological signs when compared with those having no such signs; and patients with abnormal neurological signs responded equally well in the five treatment groups.

With regard to *effects of restriction of neck movement* on prognosis:

There was no significant difference in response to treatment of 36 patients who had no restriction of neck movements in any direction when compared with patients who did have restriction of neck movement, and their rate of improvement was the same.

It is striking that the words 'root-distribution' appear in each of the three categories for entry, perhaps implying a conclusion that pain in the neck and arm must inevitably concern the nerve-root, and further that this pain should be wholly or partially in the territory of a nerve root. (See Referred pain, p. 189.)

The authors mention that some of the findings do not fit well with the concept of a steadily progressive degenerative disorder, and Sandifer[1079] (quoting Lees and Aldren Turner, 1963) observes that, 'static disability for long periods is the rule and progressive deterioration is exceptional'.

The correlation between X-ray findings and *gross anatomical findings* on inspection is between 68 per cent and 86 per cent, depending upon whether the changes are moderate or severe, respectively.[344]

When foraminal encroachment is detected by X-ray, the actual degree of trespass, including that by radiotranslucent soft tissues, will be considerably greater. Yet many patients with very severe changes on X-ray are entirely asymptomatic; the correlation between X-ray signs and *clinical features* is very low, and the value of radiographs in assessing the degree of clinical involvement remains in doubt.

Radiographs will often demonstrate severe degenerative change at one or more levels, while a relatively normal-looking segment above or below will be hypermobile and be the cause of the patient's distress.

The complex innervation of the neck and its vascular arrangements have been mentioned (pp. 6–12) and there are three aspects of radiculopathy and myelopathy which require emphasis:

1. *Angulation of roots at the cervicothoracic region.* Radioculopathy need not be due to spondylotic trespass by disc material; a violent extension movement, or a sustained extension posture (decorating a ceiling) can probably exert sufficient traction at the point of angulation (p. 224) to initiate the changes of a localised traumatic neuritis.

2. *Localisation.* Foraminal encroachment by exostosis, evident on X-ray, may have little to do with causation of neurological signs. Phillips (1975)[988] observes:

Analysis of 200 cases reveals that the two neurological syndromes, brachial neuritis and myelopathy, associated with cervical spondylosis are distinct with very little overlap. While upper limb motor and sensory loss are doubtless due to nerve root compression in cases of 'pure' brachial neuritis, they are more likely to be due to cord damage in cases with myelopathy (with spastic paralysis of lower limbs). In either group of cases, neurological features in the upper limbs are not very helpful in localising the level of significant intervertebral disc pathology.

Further;

... we early came to the conclusion, reinforced by long experience, that contrary to the statements of many physicians on this topic—but in agreement with Brain *et al.* (1952)[114]—neurological findings are of extremely limited use in assessment of the precise level of cord and root involvement, and may be misleading.

3. *Disturbance of blood supply* (see also p. 59). Many authors have drawn attention to the discrepancy which may exist between the severity of signs and symptoms in cervical spondylosis and cervical myelopathy, and the minor nature of protrusions into the canal, or lack of evidence of cord compression;[426, 1254, 942] an important factor is cord ischaemia due to trespass upon vessels sometimes remote from the site of its most potent effects.[656] The normal spinal cord does not enjoy reserves of blood supply. 'Man has just as much nervous system as he can supply with oxygen and no more.'[1343] Turnbull *et. al.* (1966)[1254] could find no arterial anastomoses within the substance of the spinal cord.

Following injury to the vascular supply, survival or death of spinal tissue must depend upon adequacy of remaining intact channels; there is little possibility of effective collateral circulation.

Dutton and Riley (1969)[285] describe intractable occipital headache of four years duration, accompanied by giddiness, aural disturbances and facial numbness, which were relieved for a further four years by removal of a bony spur between the 6th and 7th cervical vertebrae.

One essential and important feature underlying clinical expression of cervical degenerative change is the great variability of the vertebrobasilar vascular system (Fig. 1.12); the way patients present often depends very largely on the hand of cards nature has dealt them by way of arrangement of the intrinsic and extrinsic spinal cord blood supply. In a microscopic and microangiographic analysis of 43 cervical spinal cords, the anterior radicular arteries varied from 1 to 6, and the posterior radicular arteries from none to 8. It seems the only prophylactic measure is care in the choice of one's parents.

Patients with cervical spondylosis may present as follows:

1. A localised and chronic midcervical pain, without yoke area or arm pain, arising from overstressed midcervical segments because cervicothoracic segments are stiff. Pain is relieved by localised mobilisation of the lower segments.

2. Chronic and advanced spondylotic changes of the low cervical spine, which has irredeemably stiffened, have imposed undue stress on upper segments, and the juxtaposition of hypermobility and hypomobility is plain (Fig. 6.1).

3. A 'monk's cowl' of symmetrical neck and yoke area pain, steadily worsening during the day, aggravated by driving moderate distances, reading or sewing for more than an hour and characterised by an unpleasant burning quality. The spinous processes of C7 and T1 are promi-

nent, making a small localised 'bison's hump', and are very tender to pressure. The paravertebral soft tissues are palpably thickened and sore, and on examination accessory movement is difficult to produce. The pain is aggravated by flexion, and extension is achieved mainly by mid-upper cervical movement. Both rotations may be limited, as are side-flexion movements, with the junctional region taking little part in these movements. Both shoulders are stiff, with arm elevation especially limited. If treated during the early stages the localised pains are readily relieved, but the condition may become chronic and a more extensive fixed-flexion deformity established. Consequently, the head is carried now somewhat forward of the line of gravity in the average, entailing increased work for the posterior neck and suboccipital muscles to maintain the normal orientation of the head, and thus the visual and equilibratory apparatus. This produces undue approximation and painful compression of the facet-joint surfaces; secondary contractures occur in the posterior cervical and suboccipital structures and the combination of stiffening joints and overworking muscles produces extensive head, neck and 'yoke' pain which may require prolonged treatment.

4. Unilateral occipital and neck pain, together with pain spreading down the preaxial border of the arm to the wrist, all of which are relieved by mobilisation of a single segment, C4.

5. Painful and restricted left cervical rotation and right-side-flexion, with no other articular sign, relieved by mobilising the C6–7 mobility segment on the left.

6. The upper and middle trapezius, and the scapulae, are prominent; a localised 'dowager's hump' or 'bison' at C7–T1 coexists with an adjacent pronounced flattening of the upper thoracic spine. *At times the latter appears almost concave posteriorly.* The lower cervical segments are stiff and there is left unilateral headache, bilateral neck pain, pain in the left upper arm and over the left upper rib posteriorly. Apart from some spondylotic changes, the X-ray appearances are usually reported as unexceptional.

7. Thickening and stiffening of segments C5–C6–C7–T1 unilaterally are limiting neck movements towards the painful side, and tethering those to the opposite side. Elevation and external rotation of the painful side arm are limited, but internal rotation exceeds that of the painless shoulder. The first, second and third rib angles of the affected side are acutely tender.

Since cervical spondylosis is a disease like chronic bronchitis, in the sense of existing in time as well as space, more emphasis should be given to the frequency with which clinical features can present as a mixture of old and newly acquired.

In none of these examples of clinical presentation were there any neurological signs; patients without radiculopathy frequently suffer chronic and disabling pain. Should neurological signs be present, the character and

behaviour of the pain can often provide a clue that the signs are 'old and cold', and have little to do with the patient's current complaint. In the majority of cases spondylosis is not associated with neurological disability[1204] associated with the current episode.

When neurological signs are appearing or have recently developed, the associated root pain is not invariably severe, and even when severe pain *is* manifest, it is untrue that there is no point in trying to relieve it by active physical treatment. The gratifying results of mild and skilfully applied traction, governed by watchful assessment, show that many of these patients can be given early and effective help.

When root involvement *is* producing current neurological signs in an upper limb, the full hand of cards (root pain, paraesthesiae, objective numbness, muscle weakness and a depressed or absent reflex) is not often present. Most patients with distal evidence of root changes have one or other or some of these, but not all. The behaviour of root pain is variable, and it may regress and disappear between 2 to 12 weeks after onset.

This process can be hastened:

8. A fit and athletic 39-year-old man began to be aware of an upper scapular ache during badminton 14 days previously. The pain spread distally to index finger in a day, with objective numbness of its lateral border the day after. Sustained side-flexion to the right for six seconds provoked more pain spreading down the arm. Resisted extension of the right wrist produced a sharp pain down the lateral upper forearm. The right triceps was weak and the triceps jerk was diminished. The intensity of arm pain was moderate.

9. A 40-year-old field-sports enthusiast woke with yoke, scapular, arm and left index finger pain five days previously; the intensity was described as 'a dull painful ache', not sufficient to warrent interference with his love of a day's rough shooting. Paraesthesiae were confined to the index finger, and sensibility was not impaired. There was no muscle weakness and the reflexes were normal. Central vertebral pressures on C6 provoked the distal paraesthesiae.

The root pain in both these instances began significantly to recede after the third treatment by careful traction.

10. A 50-year-old clerical worker developed left scapular tingling and right scapular pain after carrying a fireside chair in front of her three weeks previously. The pain rapidly spread distally 'inside' the arm and forearm, and was described as a searing and nauseatingly severe pain. There were no cervical articular signs other than aggravation of the right arm pain, after a latent period of several seconds, when extension and right-side-flexion combined were sustained. The right triceps was weak, but there was no other neurological deficit. Gentle rotational mobilisation had no effect, but 3.5 kg of cervical traction for 5

minutes reduced the arm pain, which continued steadily to recede to mild discomfort over the next 7 days.

As classical migraine (p. 182) occurs in about 10 per cent of patients with headache, so 'typical' cervical spondylosis is more of a *rara avis* than a common thing, when measured against the very large group of patients who do not fit conveniently into textbook patterns.

Except in C8 root lesions muscle power commonly recovers in around four to six months from the onset of neurological signs; muscles innervated by the C8 root may take twice as long to recover power. Where a reflex response and muscle strength are only slightly depressed and sensation changes are minimal, they will often steadily recover during treatment, as pain also diminishes and neck movements, if manifestly limited, are restored. An absent reflex jerk may remain so for the rest of the patient's life, and the loss of bulk due to pronounced muscle wasting may also remain, if the onset of palsy occurs in late middle age or after.

Some may lose their pain but continue to be troubled by some lack of cutaneous sensibility and by paraesthesiae in the fingers.

Brief case history

Patient VF, 56 years. This woman recalled no trauma or stress to her neck. She suffered frontal and temporal headache, dizziness (dysequilibrium) on head movements of any amplitude and on changing the position of her trunk. She had neckache which came on with considerable force after late morning, and an oppressive 'yoke' pain and paraesthesiae in all right-hand digits after using her arms for housework. She changed her trunk position with care and on rising in the morning preferred to stabilise her head with a hand until upright. Neck flexion for more than a few minutes provoked dizziness, 'blood rushing to the head' and neckache. She was unable to go out to work. Her problem was compounded by an arthrodesed hip and a chronic backache. Increasing degenerative change and loss of movement are evident between March 1973 (Figs 6.1A and B) and March 1974 (Figs 6.1C and D).

Some occipitoatlantal movement occurred in the earlier films but a year later there was very little; movement between C1–C2–C3 had also diminished.

Although extension was fairly free, flexion was chronically and markedly reduced from C4 downwards, degenerative change having produced the familiar mixture of hypermobility and stiffness with the C3–4 segment bearing the brunt of available sagittal movement.

Examination. All neck movements were reduced and had a jerky, precarious quality. Palpation determined that rotation at the C1-2 segment (Fig. 6.1E) was not excessively limited, and that the low cervical stiffness extended to the upper thoracic spine and rib joints. There were no neurological signs.

Treatment. It is mandatory in this situation to localise movement-techniques carefully and accordingly C1 and C2 were mobilised, to the patient's tolerance, in the side-lying position and with the segments C3 downwards being kept undisturbed during this part of treatment; she could not relax when lying prone. Careful mobilisation localised to the lower cervical and upper thoracic spine also had to be done in this position. The upper ribs were mobilised in crook lying. A collar at night, and for times of stress during the day, helped to ease the more distressing symptoms. Progress was naturally moderate yet she would derive more benefit from a stabilisation procedure if the stiff segments were carefully mobilised. After weekly treatment sessions spread over a three-month period, because her tolerance of both travelling and mobilisation was low, the segments C0–C1 and C1–C2 were moving more freely, and this was achieved without disturbing the already mobile C3–C4 segment (Figs 6.1F and G).

Cervical spondylotic myelopathy[942]

This presents in three clinical forms:

1. A symmetrical quadriplegia with little weakness but marked spasticity, and intense paraesthesiae in the hands; there is dysdiaokokinesia but objective sensory changes are minimal
2. Spasticity and weakness affecting one arm and leg more than the other, with a contralateral reduced pain and temperature sense and a sensory level on the trunk
3. A denervation atrophy of some upper limb muscles combined with spastic paraparesis of lower limbs (see p. 160).

Since spondylosis is common it may often coexist with other disorders of the spinal cord.

Acute brachial neuritis (neuralgic amyotrophy)

This painful disorder is characterised by brachialgia and usually an extrasegmental distribution of paralysis of muscle, e.g. shoulder, shoulder girdle and arm muscles.[1079]

There may be paralysis of spinatii, serratus anterior, deltoid and triceps in varying degrees.

Often there is no demonstrable cervical or upper thoracic joint change to account for the neurological deficit or the considerable pain,[1180b] and the cause remains uncertain.

The symptoms may develop a few days after an infection or operation, or may be precipitated by an inoculation for prophylaxis, or administration of serum.

Pain begins in the root of the neck or in the scapular region, spreads over the shoulder and down the lateral arm to upper forearm. Both arms may be involved. The duration of pain may be a few days or some weeks; the amount of paralysis is at first concealed because the limb is kept still.

Recovery occurs in a matter of weeks but the paresis may not recover within a year. Physical treatment is restricted to treatment of the sequelae; both stiffened joints and weakened muscles should receive attention.

THE THORACIC OUTLET (OR INLET) (see Cervicothoracic region, p. 129)

Patients with clinical features suggesting changes of trespass at the thoracic outlet present with a multitude of signs and/or symptoms, which may be grouped somewhat artificially as follows:

1. *Predominantly vascular features* (sometimes denoting interference with subclavian vessels, and/or distribution of sympathetic vasomotor fibres, see p. 176):

Diminished pulsation in radial and ulnar arteries
Obliteration of radial pulse when the shoulder is abducted and extended, and on Adson's test (*vide infra*)
Attacks of Raynaud's phenomenon
Puffiness of the hand
Swelling of the limb and feelings of heaviness
Bluish discoloration of the hand
Local peripheral symptoms with 'dead' fingers
Pains of cramp in hand and fingers
A pulsating lump above the clavicle
The limb may develop claudication and become gangrenous with ulceration of digits.[702]

The circulatory disturbances are sometimes but not always increased by carrying heavy suitcases and shopping or wearing a heavy overcoat, and surprisingly can be exacerbated by repetitive stamping actions such as occupy Post Office clerks.

A moment's thought indicates how very many structures of the upper thorax may be included in the slight postural changes induced by 'hanging a weight from the shoulders', and how this would also disturb cervical mechanics, the tone of cervical musculature and the posture of the head.

Adson's test[175] may be positive on the affected side. The subject sits with hands on thighs and takes a deep inspiration. While holding it he extends his head and rotates as far as possible to one side, then the other. Obliteration of the radial pulse on one side is said to be significant. The difficulty is that Adson's test may be positive in a person who is asymptomatic.

2. *Predominantly neurological features* (in some cases due to trespass upon nerves of the brachial plexus or associated autonomic neurones):

Paraesthesiae, in the distal territory of a single nerve root, usually C8 or T1, but often extrasegmental, often worse in the small hours and often bilateral; sometimes symmetrically so and sometimes not
Muscle weakness, and muscle wasting, usually T1 distribution
Objective numbness
More often, subjective numbness with no actual sensory loss
A tendency to drop things, and to be clumsy
Disturbance of stereognosis
Inability to do up buttons, thread needles or perform small repetitive finger movements like winding a watch
Pain in the hand, forearm and arm
Spasmodic hypertonus of finger flexors ('flexor cramp')
Horner's syndrome may sometimes be observed.

The clinical course may show considerable variations between patients, and frequent remission, or slow progression, may occur.

The subdivision is artificial because patients frequently complain of symptoms, and may exhibit signs, which may have both a neural and a vascular basis, with a preponderance of one or other in most instances. In non-surgical cases there is often no general agreement on either the site or the mechanics of compression, or sufficient evidence in many cases that the clinical features are due to compression at all.

The cause has been ascribed to loss of tone in shoulder girdle muscles, poor posture or excessive stress to those parts by lifting and straining, yet a surreptitious inspection of any group of mature people at a party, or of lifetime agricultural labourers, will indicate many with poor shoulder girdle posture but who, on enquiry, have no upper limb problems.

Other causes are said to be pregnancy, operations, obesity and the altered stance of middle age.[1040]

Differential diagnosis is concerned with excluding causes such as cervical spondylosis, syringomyelia, Pancoast tumour, shoulder arthropathy, ulnar tunnel syndrome and carpal tunnel syndrome, etc.

Menopausal women may develop bilateral acroparaesthesiae which disturbs sleep;[267] this can be due to hormonal imbalance increasing the fluid content of tissues and thus trespass upon the median nerve in the carpal tunnel. When the signs of motor and sensory paralysis are present, a diagnosis of nerve involvement follows; the change may be that of a pseudo-ganglion or fusiform enlargement of the nerve where a hard structure or unyielding stenotic passage impinges on it.[706, 222]

Non-paralytic entrapment may occur, and this may be made manifest by increased conduction time on e.m.g. testing, or prolonged evoked potentials; relief of symptoms on resting the limb, or by injecting corticosteroids at the entrapment point; immediate relief after surgical decompression.

On the other hand, operative treatment is not uniformly successful, and 25 per cent of e.m.g. examinations in cases of carpal tunnel syndrome, for example, yield normal results.[222]

Clinical experience is that many patients with extrasegmental paraesthesiae and digital clumsiness present the features of cervical spondylosis, poor posture of the shoulder girdle, and some slight restriction of the shoulder joint on that side.

Thoracic inlet and carpal tunnel syndromes often simulate the features of cervical spondylosis.

The sensory symptoms do not by themselves form the basis for a diagnosis of entrapment neuropathy without other diagnostic criteria.[706]

Excluding peripheral causes, clinical experience suggests we may be mistaken if we try *invariably* to interpret upper limb acroparaesthesiae only in terms of physical trespass upon structures of the neurovascular bundle itself. We have already seen (p. 6) that vagaries of cervical spinal cord blood supply may give rise to hand muscle wasting when the lesion is at the foramen magnum, and that osteophytes at C6–C7 can produce occipital headache (p. 129). Keuter (1970)[656] has emphasised the importance of a wider view, and of holding in mind the reasonable likelihood of vascular changes sometimes occurring at sites remote from where they might be expected.

Nathan[903] has shown how the sympathetic trunks may be embedded in thickened, degenerative soft tissue of the thoracolumbar region, but whether this also occurs at the stellate ganglion or in the upper thoracic sympathetic trunks and might be a factor in producing symptoms, is uncertain. Bilateral extrasegmental paraesthesiae, in the absence of neurological signs, can sometimes be relieved by mobilisation localised to segments T3, 4 and 5.

A variety of the modes of trespass is set out on page 131, most of them verified at open operation, although the number of patients who come to surgery is small compared to those who are treated conservatively, and in whom the cause is not always satisfactorily established.

The majority of patients do not develop symptoms until middle age, and vascular symptoms tend to predominate over the neurological symptoms, although both are present to varying degrees.

If there are bilateral but asymmetrical cervical ribs, the smaller and shorter of the two tends to produce the more symptoms, possibly because a supernumary fibrous band is attached to the smaller tip.

Common presentations are as follows:

Cervical rib (Figs 6.2, 6.5). The proportion of cervical ribs confirmed as the cause of trespass upon the brachial plexus is small.[222] The features are:

Pain, proximally localised at first, begins to spread down the arm, usually on the medial side, but sometimes laterally. Pain tends to migrate distally if repetitive actions such as stamping documents or cleaning shop front windows are continued. Sometimes pain is negligible but wasting and weakness of the hand is more noticeable.[983] Paraesthesiae may initiate the hand symptoms, or may follow pain as the first symptom.

The *position* of the limb may not always influence the pain although *use* of the hand may aggravate both pain

and paraesthesiae; both are frequently worse at night, although in some, nocturnal paraesthesiae do not occur. Similarly, elevation of the shoulder girdle will exacerbate the paraesthesiae in some, but not in others.

Sensibility changes may be patchy, e.g. there may be hyperaesthesia confined to the index and middle finger, and dysaesthesia in the ring and little fingers.

At times the fingers may become icy cold and numb, at room temperature.[983]

Weakness of grip, and later atrophy of the small hand muscles, may follow, if they have not been the initial and only feature. For example:

A 72-year-old man, whose X-ray showed a rudimentary right cervical rib, began two months previously to feel pain in the right forearm, with dorsal pain and paraesthesiae in the right middle three fingers. His left middle and ring fingers had 'tingled for years'. He achieved only three hours sleep a night, and nocturnally relieved his distal symptoms to an extent by hanging his arms downward. He found difficulty in doing up buttons. The right hand was at all times warmer than the left, and the fingers were always fatter. Cervical movements were surprisingly good, as were combined movements, and none provoked his symptoms. Arm elevation temporarily *reduced* his pain and paraesthesiae during the day. There were no neurological signs, and no signs on cervical and upper thoracic palpation, other than undue stiffness. X-ray revealed 'severe spondylotic changes from C3 to C7, with large osteophytes and considerably reduced spaces at C5–C6–C7. The osteophytes encroach upon the spinal cord.'

Rhythmic cervical traction of 9 kg for 15 minutes relieved the right hand pain at each pull/phase of two minutes. Five successive tractions, slowly progressed to a firm and sustained pull, steadily relieved the temperature difference, the ache of right hand and forearm ache and the disturbance of sleep.

Tingling appeared at the tip of the thumb, and remained at the lateral three fingers of the right hand, and the middle two of the left. The forearm and hand ache were completely relieved.

Five weeks after treatment ceased the left hand paraesthesiae and the right forearm ache remained completely relieved, but the ache in the right hand has worsened. He was referred for surgical opinion. The correct analysis is probably that the left symptoms were spondylotic and the right due to the cervical rib, and that a surgical opinion was indicated.

Scalenus anticus syndrome (Naffziger's syndrome)

Dan (1976)[222] refers to the importance of dividing the scalenus medius when excising an anomalous rib, while Silvertsen and Christensen (1977)[1128] describe the clinical features and operative results after the scalenus anterior had been divided *without* excision of a cervical rib, if present. Section of the scalenus anterior muscle, in 37 patients who complained of pain and/or paraesthesiae in the upper limbs and tenderness over the muscle, was preceded by injection of local anaesthetic into the muscle; following the diagnostic injection, all of the patients experienced relief of pain.

On the 37 patients 38 scalenectomies were performed. Radiological signs were:

Normal	21
Cervical rib	8
Cervical spondylosis	3
Large transverse process of C7	6

The patients had had symptoms for an average of $2\frac{1}{2}$ years. Diffuse pain or paraesthesiae occurred in 19, ulnar radicular pain in 12, radial radicular pain in 2, and both diffuse and radicular pain in 5.

The criteria for assuming pain as radicular, rather than referred pain without root involvement, were not given.

Neurological signs were found in 16 patients; 8 patients had a weak handshake, 2 had atrophy of the thenar muscles and one had hypothenar muscle atrophy.

Patients with neurological signs seemed to be relieved more often than those without, but there was no difference in the efficacy of operation between those with or without cervical rib.

A postoperative questionnaire after some months revealed that 5 had no symptoms, 19 had negligible symptoms, 12 were unchanged and 2 were worse.

Several points for discussion arise, e.g.

1. What might be the effects on cervical mechanics of division of an important guy-rope muscle like the scalenus anterior? Might the mechanics of the first rib also be disturbed?
2. Bearing in mind the phenomenon of *referred* tenderness, what might be the mechanism responsible for tenderness of this muscle?
3. Is there an unelucidated 'acupuncture' effect on injection of local anaesthetic? (See p. 118.)

It has been suggested that there may be a link between the scalenus syndrome and headache,[33] which is not unreasonable in view of the muscles' attachments.

When the well-worn paths of nerve compression or entrapment, and vascular trespass, have been trodden, and the certain cases with these changes excluded, it is salutary to bear in mind that a number of important muscles and connective-tissue structures link the lower cervical and upper thoracic vertebrae; the factors mentioned under (3) (p. 130) should perhaps be included in any clinical assessment of the genesis of acroparaesthesiae, when signs of trespass upon nerves or vessels are absent. *Important factors* in analyses of the frequency of extrasegmental paraesthesiae are:

1. The distal segmental territory of a spinal nerve appears to be more of a flexible dimension than may always be recognised[659] and thus the basis for confident appellations of 'extrasegmental' may not be justified.
2. Many of these patients never reach the stage of surgical consultation or are entered as a statistic in retrospective surgical analyses, having been relieved of their distress by simple physical means.

As an example of the means, distressing bilateral glove paraesthesiae in mature people may not infrequently be relieved by mobilising the upper three or four thoracic segments, and seems more effectively relieved when treatment combines adequate stretching of the pectoral structures and improvement of the range of shoulder elevation.

THE CLAVICULAR JOINTS

The factor of changes in the shoulder joint which often appear to be secondary, and allied, to cervical and upper thoracic joint problems has been discussed (p. 187); in this connection the clavicular joints must also be mentioned, since possible changes in either need to be excluded during examination for spinal problems.

(a) Sternoclavicular joint

Pain over the upper lateral pectoral area may be referred forward from lower cervical and/or upper thoracic vertebral joints, and lower paramedian thoracic pain is frequently referred from upper thoracic segments.[456] Upper medial pectoral pain is more likely to arise from the sternoclavicular joint, surprisingly overlooked at times during an otherwise exemplary examination of the cervicothoracic region and associated peripheral structures. Early arthrosis of the medial clavicular joint may simulate referred vertebrogenic pain, particularly from the upper and middle neck. The joint is an important component of the shoulder mechanism, the sternal end of clavicle moving downwards through some 30°–60° during shoulder elevation, also during which the clavicle rotates axially backward through some 50°.[1021]

When pain is provoked or aggravated in this region on overpressure to cervical rotation towards the painful side, the effect on the joint of sternomastoid and scalene muscle traction should not be forgotten. Minor subluxation here will present as an 'enlargement' of the sternal end of clavicle, and if this is suspected, the effects of testing the full range of scapular mobility should be noted before the joint is palpated.

Advanced arthrosis, and traumatic attenuation of fibrous capsule and costoclavicular ligament, present with manifest changes of contour and attitude, and are easy to identify.

In a follow-up of cases of traumatic dislocation, Savastano and Stutz (1978)[1085] concluded that stability of the sternoclavicular joint was not necessary for normal function of limb and did not interfere with arm movement.

(b) Acromioclavicular joint

This weak and poorly stabilised articulation is an intrinsic component of the shoulder mechanism; as the scapular begins rotating outward early in the movement of shoulder elevation, the coracoclavicular ligament is tightened and there is a range of about 15° of rotatory gliding in the joint.[1021] After about 135° of elevation, a further 15° of gliding occurs between the lateral end of clavicle and the acromion—this 30° of movement provides an increment of mobility for functional use of the arm.

The true incidence of acromioclavicular joint pathology contributing to shoulder pain is unknown. Zanca (1971)[1379] analysed 1000 cases of shoulder pain, among which 12.7 per cent of the patients presented with radiographic abnormalities of the acromioclavicular joint, and by the same criteria, 20 per cent with glenohumeral abnormalities such as calcified deposits in tendons of the rotator cuff.

Degenerative change in this articulation, as a cause of shoulder pain and disability, is frequently overlooked.[1344]

In the absence of radiographic changes the incidence of pain from the joint, more commonly because of minor subluxation, and the early changes of arthrosis, is probably very much higher.

The joint should be tested whenever the neck and forequarter is examined. Even minor degrees of subluxation or laxity may be painful; pain is usually localised to the joint but may be referred as far as the lateral forearm.[1379]

There is little or no change in the apparent range of scapulohumeral movement, but full elevation hurts at the joint, especially if overpressure is applied. Likewise, the extremes of functional glenohumeral movement, and accessory movements of the clavicular joints, are also painful when passively tested. Active shoulder shrugging often hurts. The cardinal signs of acromioclavicular joint changes are (i) acute tenderness accurately localised to the superior aspect of the joint, (ii) severe provocation of pain on gently forced traction across the chest,[983] and (iii) localised pain on passive tests of a-p gliding movement. Subluxation shows an unduly prominent clavicle, with an upward 'step' just medial to the acromion.

CONDITIONS OF THE THORACIC INTERVERTEBRAL JOINTS, THE COSTAL JOINTS AND SCAPULOCOSTAL JOINT

Grant and Keegan (1968)[433] refer to the ominous significance, until otherwise explained, of chest pain and observe that a more general recognition of musculoskeletal chest wall pain might save unnecessary worry and invalidism.

They comment:

We recognise our diagnosis is a clinical one lacking technological confirmation, a fact which may partly explain both its neglect and the confusion in the nomenclature ... X-ray films of the rib insertions do not seem to be helpful ... our experience would be in keeping with the idea that many cases of pain in the chest wall are due to anatomical misalignment of a rib. This need only be of slight degree to produce discomfort and disturb the equilibrium of the musculoskeletal structures of the thorax.

Radiographic appearances are almost invariably reported as normal, although the condition can at times be manifest on a-p views of the upper thorax.[1180b] Their report of the distribution of thoracic tenderness in 41 patients allowed a grouping into costal and vertebrocostal syndromes:

Table 8.2 Sites of tenderness in the vertical plane

	Right	Left	Bilateral
Costal syndrome: 31 cases			
Single ribs tender: 20 cases			
2 or 3	1	1	–
4 or 5 or 6	3	7	–
7 or 8 or 9 or 10	1	3	–
11 or 12	3	1	–
Multiple ribs tender: 11 cases			
2/3	1	1	–
3/4 or 3/4/5 or 4/5 or 5/6	2	3	–
6/7/8	–	1	–
10/11 or 11/12	2	1	–
	13	18	–
Vertebrocostal syndrome: 10 cases			
Single spines tender: 7 cases			
T3	3	–	1	2
T4	2	–	–	2
T7	1	–	–	1
T8	1	–	–	1
Multiple spines tender: 3 cases			
3/4	1	–	1	–
3/4/5	1	–	–	1
5/6	1	1	–	–
	1	2	7

Table 8.3 Sites of tenderness in the horizontal plane

No. of cases	Costochondral Jn	Rib shaft	Costovertebral Jt	Dorsal spine
3 ⎫	+	+	–	–
9 ⎬ Costal	–	+	+	–
1 ⎪ syndrome	–	–	+	–
18 ⎭	+	+	+	–
2 ⎫ Vertebro	–	–	+	–
⎬ Costal				
8 ⎭ syndrome	+	+	+	+

While the authors suggest a fairly detailed nomenclature of costal and vertebrocostal pain, it may be preferable to avoid proper names where possible, pending more general agreement on the clinical entities and their forms of presentation. Also, it is clinically useful to emphasise the behaviour and distribution of changes rather than give them names, other than in the case of those classical thoracic conditions which need no full description here.

The lesions, some of them of acute onset and some chronically established, tend to occur in patterns which can be discerned and workers with much experience of these cases might group some of them as under, besides adding syndromes from their own clinical experience. For example, craniovertebral joint problems are accompanied surprisingly frequently by lesions of the third rib, on the side of the hemicranial pain.

In all of the upper thoracic conditions, the shoulder girdle and glenohumeral joints should be carefully examined, because arm movement is very often restricted and painful; frequently a proportion of the upper limb symptoms reported are in fact attributable to abnormalities of the clavicular and/or glenohumeral joints.

Patterns of presentation are as follows:

Acute or chronic elevation of first and/or second rib
Chronic unilateral lesions of upper rib joints
Flattened upper thoracic region
The so-called scapulocostal syndrome
Chronic generalised upper thoracic stiffening
Polymyalgia rheumatica
Upper/mid-thoracic spondylosis with stiffness
Upper/mid-thoracic spondylosis with hypermobility
Tietze's disease
The rib-tip syndrome
Acute hemithoracic pain
Chronic anterior chest wall pain
Abdominal pain of spinal origin
Scheuermann's disease
Ankylosing spondylitis
Lesions of lowest ribs
Acute lumbar pain of thoracic origin
Osteoporosis
Erosion of ribs in rheumatoid arthritis
Thoracic disc lesions.

Acute or chronic elevation of first and/or second rib

The fixation of synovial joints of the craniovertebral region 'in a position possible to a normal neck' has been recognised for more than 40 years (Coutts, 1934);[208] this fixation within the normal range of movement is more likely to occur when the joint(s) concerned lie within and belong to a movement-complex of many other joints, such as occurs in the spine, the carpus and the tarsus.

One of these is the first rib; although it moves very little in quiet respiration[482] its costotransverse and costovertebral joints appear more mobile than expected, and the clinical state of being painfully 'hitched' upward is common.

Among complex articulations a degree of fixation of one joint component is much more likely to remain undetected by cursory examination, although the fact of something causing pain and a greater or lesser degree of difficult movement is known well enough to the patient. These abnormalities, usually covert[1180b] until detected by careful

clinical and sometimes radiological examination, occur much less frequently in single large articulations like the glenohumeral or knee joints, and when they do are much more likely to be due to relatively gross intra-articular derangement.

The clinical features which usually accompany the painful, unilateral fixed elevation of an upper rib justify separating it from the 'thoracic outlet' group of conditions, since the distribution of pain typically includes the lower neck more often than the upper limb beyond the shoulder girdle. Upper cervical and suboccipital pain, on the same side, often accompany the detectable, unilateral change in the resting attitude of the 'yoke' region.

A common antalgic attitude adopted by the patient is that of slight side-flexion towards the painful side, while reaching across to rest the fingers of the opposite hand over the unilaterally painful 'yoke' area. The patient reports an oppressive, dull, nagging ache, at times accompanied by a burning feeling over the upper trapezius on the side of the pain and occasionally by a degree of unilateral hyperaesthesia which can be far more troublesome than pain.

On observation, the upper trapezius fibres are in some spasm, and palpation quickly reveals increased tenderness of the muscle mass. Cervical rotation towards the painful side is restricted, as side-flexion to the opposite side feels tethered. Extension hurts the painful side and flexion elicits a pulling pain over the yoke area unilaterally. Movement of the shoulder on that side may be moderately painful at extremes of range. There are no neurological signs.

By careful and gentle palpation which avoids causing further reflex spasm or voluntary muscle guarding, the positions of the angles of first ribs can be compared.

Postural deformities including scoliosis and kyphoscoliosis, or a pronounced 'dowager's hump' are excluded from this description. It is more common before 50, and appears to occur more frequently in young adults. The condition may exist as a localised entity, but more often tends to involve a degree of fixation at the second rib also and be allied to a region of upper cervical tenderness at the C2–C3 segments.

Since the scalenus muscles take origin from the apophyses of C2 vertebra and downwards, it is tempting to explain the rib elevation as due to chronic hypertonus of the scaleni muscles secondary to upper cervical irritability, but the aetiology may not be as attractively simple as this.

Very commonly, the cervical musculature is tensed during exertions involving the upper limbs; to the writer's knowledge there appears to exist no cineradiographic study of the mechanical influences on the upper two ribs during pulling and pushing activities of the upper limb. The scalene group comprise powerful muscles, and the intercostals, serratus anterior and subclavius, all of which attach to the first rib (as do the clavipectoral fascia and intercostal membranes) may transmit forces which induce fixation.

Certainly, the condition is sharply aggravated by pulling activities such as hoeing, raking and sweeping leaves. It is also tempting to speculate that many mature people, with more chronic unilateral fixation of cervicothoracic joints, with chronic arm pain and restricted neck movement but no neurological signs, are in fact presenting with the chronic sequelae of untreated upper rib fixation in times past.

Chronic unilateral lesions of upper rib joints

Costal joint lesions are much more frequent than is generally accepted, and only rarely do they spontaneously resolve. Where not adequately treated they may lead to chronic symptoms.[164]

The table of segmental incidence of degenerative change (p. 80) has been derived as far as possible from descriptions of the process observed in joints at autopsy, and from skeletal changes seen after maceration of bone.

This does not preclude the frequent occurrence of painful joint problems during life at sites other than those mentioned; among these are commonly the upper three or four rib articulations on one side, often presenting as a small family of involvement.

The basis for ascribing the changes to costotransverse and costovertebral joints is given below; meanwhile, it is useful to recall the distribution of upper thoracic spinal nerves.

1. *Anterior primary rami.* T1 root supplies a large branch to the brachial plexus, and a much smaller branch (the first intercostal nerve) passes forward in the intercostal space to end on the front of the chest as an anterior cutaneous nerve of the thorax; it also supplies the axillary skin. The C4 root supplies the skin overlying the clavicle.

T2 root supplies a lateral cutaneous branch (the intercostobrachial nerve) to the brachial plexus; it joins the medial cutaneous nerve of the arm, and also the posterior brachial cutaneous branch of the radial nerve. It supplies axillary skin and the posterior arm.

T3 intercostal nerve frequently gives off a second intercostobrachial nerve, which supplies axillary skin and medial arm.[437]

Succeeding anterior primary rami of upper thoracic spinal nerves end by piercing the pectoralis major and supplying the skin of the upper thorax. The lateral cutaneous branches supply the axillary region. Intercostal nerves 4, 5 and 6 innervate the mammary region.

2. *Posterior primary rami.* The lateral branches of the dorsal rami pierce the deep structures more or less in line with the angles of the ribs;[788] that of T2 may descend to the level of T6 before ascending again to terminate on the back of the scapula near the acromion process.[789]

While referred pain often lies within the peripheral distribution of individual spinal nerves, just as frequently (p. 192) it is less tidily referred; upper limb pain commonly arises from lesions in the upper thoracic spine, as well as from the lower cervical region and the shoulder itself. The referred pain is often accompanied by concomitant symptoms, the patient reporting heaviness and uselessness of the arm, and numb feelings in the limb, although there is no objective numbness and very frequently no neurological deficit.

When the upper three or four costal joints are involved, the patient reports a mid- or lower-scapular area of pain, as an oppressive dull ache.

When contour changes due to kyphosis or kyphoscoliosis have been excluded, the overlying upper thoracic region will often appear to be slightly more eminent posteriorly than that of the opposite side. At other times, a single rib and sometimes a pair of ribs are palpably more eminent than their adjacent fellows and those of the opposite side.

Cervical extension and flexion provoke the pain, and movements towards the painful side do likewise. Movements away from it feel tethered. There may be upper pectoral pain on the same side and sometimes mammary pain. Elevation, external rotation and abduction of the shoulder may be limited by some 5° or so, the nature of the limitation being pain and 'tightness' combined. The internal rotation range may paradoxically be freer than that of the uninvolved shoulder. Pulling clothes over the head is sometimes difficult, as is reversing a car.

Pain commonly involves the axillary region and spreads into the upper limb; the whole forequarter may have a feeling of frustrating uselessness. There may be extrasegmental paraesthesiae, or the patient may report the limb as feeling 'not quite right'.

Palpation of spinous processes T1 to T4 may elicit no greater tenderness, but palpation in the paravertebral sulcus and more especially of the upper three or four rib angles themselves elicits marked tenderness, and provokes acute pain localised to the upper thorax on that side.

Localised mobilisation by central vertebral pressure on the spinous processes is usually less effective than posteroanterior unilateral movements on the side of pain combined with mobilisation of the affected ribs; the sternocostal joints of which are also more tender than on the unaffected side.

'Chapman's point'[164] refers to the tenderness of associated sternocostal joints—the referral of pain and tenderness anteriorly is said to follow the anterior cutaneous branch of the intercostal nerve.

The distinction[1180b] between lesions of ribs fixed in inspiration or fixed in expiration may be more of academic than clinical importance, and seems not to have much bearing on results provided the costal joints are adequately mobilised.

N.B. The distinction between the condition above when acute, and acute elevation of the first or second ribs, rests on the ease with which the former may be relieved by a single thrust manipulation applied to the rib angle, compared to the need for several treatments of persuasive, rhythmic mobilisation of the rib joints in the latter.

The second rib syndrome

A distinctive localised contour change of the pectoral region tends to occur when the second rib appears to have sustained stress more than its adjacent structures. The cause is invariably trauma or strain, which may take the form of a jolt when carrying a heavy weight on the shoulder, the sudden taking of a severe strain when handling a weight above the level of the shoulders, being banged about in a road traffic accident or prolonged pulling and hauling stresses at work.

There are no neurological signs or symptoms and the subjective changes reported are those of a useless or heavy limb, the patient feeling unable to grip efficiently or to use the arm in housework, for example, for very long at a time.

There may be associated upper cervical joint problems, referring the pain to the head; the glenohumeral and clavicular joints are usually unaffected but shoulder pain may be reported.

Careful inspection and comparison of the upper pectoral area will reveal an individually eminent second rib anteriorly on the affected side, and surprisingly, the angle of that rib may also feel more prominent posteriorly, giving the impression that the head and neck of the rib are 'stuck' at the extreme lateral extent of their small accessory movement range.

Rotations of the neck are the least affected movements, with flexion and extension provoking the existing unilateral pectoral pain, 'like a hot horseshoe' straddling the yoke area on the affected side. Side-flexions to either side are abruptly halted and produce a stabbing pain over the upper pectoral area.

The affected rib is acutely tender anteriorly and posteriorly, and the distinctive feature is that gentle mobilisation of the rib provokes the bulk of symptoms reported; palpatory testing procedures at the first and third rib do not.

When the condition has become chronic, the acute pain on movement disappears, sometimes to be replaced by a steady ache in the upper limb, with 'heaviness' and 'uselessness'.

If the shoulder girdle is held a little elevated, which may relieve the arm symptoms, an upper pectoral ache then appears on that side, and the patient has perforce to choose between one or other symptom. In the writer's experience one of these patients had, when in acute pain 18 months previously, been diagnosed as pleurisy and given a course of antibiotics; together with the prominent second rib, the spinous process of this patient's T2 was markedly depressed.

In all cases of trauma to the neck, yoke and shoulder girdle region it is wise to bear in mind the possibility of traumatic disturbance of the architecture of upper rib articulations. Long after the root pain in upper limb, and the cervical discomfort, have been cleared up, there not infrequently remains a tendency for the upper limb to become heavy and uselss after moderate activity, and on occasions the patient's persistent complaints may unfortunately raise a suspicion of malingering.

A careful examination of the upper three ribs may reveal abnormalities which have been missed during conventional procedures for the root pain and the neurological deficit.

Flattened upper thoracic region

This has been mentioned ((f), p. 227), but is described again here because painful stiffening of the lower cervical spine appears to be linked with the upper thoracic changes.

The flattened, and at times apparently lordotic, upper/midthoracic spine has long been recognised as a postural change which augurs difficulty; it was described in a chiropractic text by *Smith, Langworthy and Paxson* in 1906. While many middle-aged people with upper thoracic stiffening and a 'dowager's hump' are free of joint pains, notwithstanding clear X-ray evidence of considerable degenerative change, the flat interscapular area very frequently goes with intractable head, neck, shoulder girdle, arm and rib-joint pains, and grumbling, chronic disability.

On palpation there is general stiffness of a particularly unnatural kind, marked by a lack of resilience which gives an impression not unlike that of the stiff, 'burned-out' rheumatoid joint.

The author's impression is that an apparently high incidence of 'true frozen shoulder' (for want of a better term), among patients who also exhibit this peculiar postural change, may be more than coincidence. Cavaziel (1974)[164] mentions that joint problems affecting ribs very seldom cause any extra tension of vertebral musculature, and indeed there may be little palpable evidence of paravertebral muscle spasm; while costal joints presumably *could* escape the consequences of this apparent postural abnormality, the upper rib angles on one or another side are frequently tender, the C7–T1 segment is frequently very stiff as well as appearing prominent, the lower cervical segments sometimes feel 'board-like' to accessory-movement tests and there is the combination of unilateral (sometimes contralateral) cervical headache, neck pain, an asymmetrical pattern of neck-movement limitation, restriction of shoulder movement, and upper thoracic or hemithoracic pain. Pain of a non-radicular distribution may spread into the arm, and a frozen shoulder may coexist. It is probably coincidence that the determination of histocompatibility antigens in 38 patients with frozen shoulder, and 216 normal blood-donors, established that HLA–B27 was significantly more common in patients with frozen shoulder (42 per cent) than in the controls (10 per cent)[140] (see also p. 206).

Without invoking chronic muscle spasm, it is difficult to explain the 'fixation' of a vertebral region in what appears to be an abnormal posture; the possibility that one is observing a variant of normal posture should not be discounted.

The so-called scapulocostal syndrome

Descriptions of the symptoms said to indicate this condition include many clinical features which could be shown to be present because of other lesions, yet when these have been excluded there remains a small group of patients in whom firm palpation of soft-tissue attachments to the medial scapular border will reproduce the scapular and arm pain reported. Pain can be referred to this region from the lower cervical segments (see p. 118); and the presence of referred tenderness from low cervical lesions, overlying an area of innocuous fasciculi in the soft tissues of the scapular border, cannot always be ruled out.

Yet again, the pain reported can at times be directly overlying the site of *costal* joint abnormalities giving rise to it (see p. 234).

Pain unilaterally along the medial periscapular border is common, as is the finding of tender nodules and fasciculi in the periscapular soft tissues in patients who are otherwise asymptomatic.

If, in some who report periscapular pain but whose cervical and thoracic movement tests are normal, the medial border of the bone is elevated and its under surface explored by palpation, the scapular attachment of serratus anterior may be found painfully tender.[217]

Sometimes, the medial border cannot be elevated or distracted from the chest wall as easily as that of the non-painful side, and an association between this difficulty and the patient's localised symptoms may then reasonably be made, provided other causes have been excluded.

Attention is naturally directed to the trapezius, rhomboids, levator scapulae and deeper layers comprising the cervicis muscles (longissimus, semispinalis, and iliocostalis); while postural spasm of the painful side trapezius can often be seen as well as palpated in some lower cervical joint problems, statements about 'palpable loss of tone' in the trapezius are easier to make than to substantiate, and acute tenderness of the trapezius is very common indeed. Probably a more acceptable test is flat-handed resistance to isometric contraction of the scapular retractors while the trunk is well stabilised.

This test will sometimes reveal lack of power (or inhibition of a good contraction) of the trapezius, coexisting with difficulty in passively distracting the scapula from the chest wall.

Scapulothoracic crepitus on active or passive movement of the shoulder girdle may be fine or coarse, and occasionally be that of a dull, snapping sound. The crepitus may be attributed to a roughened posterior thoracic wall, misalignment of subscapular ribs or projections such as soft-tissue nodules or fasciculi in the subscapularis muscle.

The possible existence of congenital soft-tissue subscapular anomalies should not be ruled out.

The most consistent features seem to be:

Pain along the medial scapular border
Tenderness in parascapular and medial subscapular soft tissues
Palpably fine crepitus, and fasciculi or nodules, apparently within the soft-tissue attachments (see p. 116)
Reproduction of arm and scapular pain on firm palpation of its medial perimeter
Unexceptional cervical and thoracic spine movement tests
Scapular pain on use of arm
Discomfort on extremes of scapular gliding movement when passively tested
Difficulty in distracting the scapula from the chest wall.

The cause of scapulothoracic crepitus remains in doubt; many subjects have noisy movement but are otherwise sign and symptom free. Whether these subjects will eventually develop pain and other problems is undetermined. In others, crepitus coexists with scapular pain and some of the other features mentioned.

When testing the condition of soft-tissue attachments at the medial border of the scapula, it is convenient to stand behind the seated patient, whose ipsilateral wrist is drawn medially across the lumbar region by the therapist's contralateral hand.

The medial scapular border can then be palpated by the therapist's thumb of that side. The patient may also be lying prone, of course.

Chronic generalised upper thoracic stiffening

An example of clinical presentation described above [(3) in Cervical spondylosis, p. 226] may present with the most prominent features in the upper half of the thorax and with less obvious spondylotic changes in the lower cervical spine.

The changes are quite characteristic, with noticeably rounded shoulders comprising a generally stiff, hardened and forward-curved upper thoracic region; the vertebral body joints and all the upper rib joints share in the regional fixation by a smooth rounded kyphosis.

From around the T6 segment upwards, the whole region is tender, board-like to palpation and sore. The forward upper thoracic curve ends at the base of the neck, as though the neck were a separate structure with completely different curve characteristics.

The patient, usually a middle-aged woman, describes a constant, oppressive dull ache across the yoke area and upper back, with painful stiffening of both shoulder joints and marked inability to reach up for things on a shelf or to hang curtains, for example.

Abduction and external rotation of the shoulders are very restricted, as is internal rotation. The pectoral structures are plainly tight and normal shoulder girdle retraction is not possible.

Extension of the head and neck is also very restricted, because the low cervical/upper thoracic segments seem virtually 'fossilised'.

The line of the throat, seen laterally, does not even approach the vertical on extension, let alone go beyond it as is normal in some. Other cervical movements are likewise restricted—the whole carriage of the upper thorax appears shifted forwards. Symptoms include aching and heaviness of the arms, with extrasegmental paraesthesiae and early morning stiffness. The arms feel imprisoned to other than comfortable functional use in front of the body below 100° elevation.

Polymyalgia rheumatica

This organic condition, which affects females much more than males, has to be distinguished from other causes of vague aches and pains, in middle-aged people, with little or nothing in the way of abnormal physical signs.[263]

When a woman over 60 reports severe early morning stiffness and pain in the upper and lower limb girdles its likelihood should be suspected. In a well-referenced description of the condition, Plotz and Spiera (1978)[997] suggest the following criteria:

Shoulder and/or pelvic girdle pain which is primarily muscular, rather than arthritic or tendinous, in the absence of true muscle weakness
Patient is over 60
No evidence of rheumatoid or other inflammatory arthritis
Marked elevation of ESR is the most uniform laboratory finding, and is associated with moderate anaemia, mild fever, fatigue, lethargy, anorexia and weight loss. The plasma viscosity is raised
Absence of objective signs of muscle disease
Prompt response to systemic corticosteroid.

The *onset* is more often acute and the patient may be able to pinpoint the onset within an hour.

Stiffness is worst after resting and can severely but temporarily paralyse the patient, who may initially need help to get out of bed and move about. The arms are tender to pressure and very painful to move; there may be generalised swelling of the hands.

Low back pain may radiate to buttocks and posterior thighs, and the pressure on painful thighs by a chair or toilet seat may be hard to bear; driving is difficult for the same reason. Electromyogram studies reveal nothing. The syndrome is not normally associated with any other condition and its cause is obscure, but may be a form of arteritis. Giant cell arteritis occurs in temporal arteritis and also in polymyalgia rheumatica, and it is probable that the two diseases[583] are different manifestations of a single underlying pathological process. Its distinction from the other syndromes described and the indications for management by a rheumatologist must always be borne in mind, since prompt treatment with corticosteroids may be a matter of urgency.

The condition has a natural course of 6 months to 10 years, and most patients recover completely.[263]

Coexistent joint problems

The likelihood of a coexisting, localised and innocent joint problem, unconnected with the medical condition and amenable to localised treatment, should not be forgotten.

So long as the examination findings are unassailable, and treatment is moderate and governed by careful assessment, the localised problem will respond in the normal way. For example:

In 1976 a 58-year-old housewife developed polymyalgia rheumatica, with an ESR of 100 mm/hr. She began improving at once on steroids. In February 1979 she was preparing food and felt sudden right neck pain, which improved on use of a home vibrator. In May, during a long bout of watching television, the acute pain returned and she began to get an ache over the right yoke area and also the occasional frontal headache. She presented in July 1979 with the symptoms as described, together with a bruised feeling in the right upper trapezius on movement of the right shoulder girdle. The referring letter from her physician mentioned her medical condition, its treatment by steroids and the probability that her neck pain might respond to local treatment.

Her constant, unilateral background ache, unilaterally provoked by neck movements or using her right arm, together with the mode of onset on two occasions and easily distinguishable by her from her regular 'rising a.m. stiffness', taken together with the articular pattern of limitation and pain provocation, and the palpation signs, were sufficient to indicate a joint problem in its own right.

Of her movements, left side-flexion felt tethered on the right side and provoked a C4 level pain there. Left rotation was similarly a little restricted. Right side-flexion was normal but right rotation was reduced by some 10 degrees and hurt more severely at mid-neck on the right side. She had a small hard kyphus at C7–T1, some contracture of the ligamentum nuchae, with sore, thickened and stiff segments between C2 and C5 on the right, the most tender and limited of which was the C3–C4 segment. The three upper right ribs were a little prominent posteriorly and both the associated vertebral transverse processes and the rib angles were sore to palpation, with reduced and painful accessory movement. Her right shoulder was painfully limited, by a few degrees, in elevation and internal rotation. There was no neurological deficit, and her pain and articular signs were cleared in three treatments of localised mobilisation to neck, upper thorax and right shoulder joint, and gentle stretching of the ligamentum nuchae, since when she has remained trouble-free, although still taking a diminished dose of steroids.

Upper/midthoracic spondylosis with stiffness

Discussion. In a lecture delivered to the International Society for Manipulative Medicine, Maigne and le Corre (1969)[788] stressed the frequent *cervical* origin of median or paramedian upper thoracic 'dorsalgias', and showed that thumb pressure on the anterolateral part of the lower cervical spine (at the level of the emergence of the nerve roots) will often elicit interscapular pain.

Maigne (1972)[789] mentioned subsequently that the special sensitivity of one cervical segment will be noted, that this pressure will elicit or aggravate a pain radiating into the arm, and that in the majority of cases of interscapular dorsalgia it will provoke the habitual dorsal pain. Further, they demonstrated a particular point of remarkable fixity of painful tenderness which lies 2 cm lateral to the line of the spinous processes at the level of T5–T6. Pressure on the cervical 'sonnette' (bell) point 'rings the bell' of thoracic dorsalgia.

Others (p. 118) have drawn attention to this common phenomenon of pain reference.

Maigne and le Corre observe that attentive examination of superficial soft tissues overlying the paramedian levels of T3–T6 often reveals great sensitivity to skin pinching and rolling, and that this sensitivity extends obliquely outward and downward, as a band several centimetres in height following the line of the ribs. They note its frequency after minor cervical injuries, in neualgias of the typical cervicobrachial type and its frequency after badly performed manipulations.

Concerning the possible mechanisms of pathogenesis, the authors found that the consistent paramedian 'T5/T6 point' coincided exactly with the superficial emergence of the lateral branch of the posterior primary rami of T2 spinal nerve. This branch has a more extensive cutaneous distribution than its fellows, since having descended to T6 level it then climbs up and outward to the level of the acromion process of scapula, sometimes giving branches to rhomboids and trapezius which it perforates (Fig. 1.20).

Infiltration of this nerve with Novocaine at its exit between T2 and T3 immediately eradicated the dorsal pain, the pain provoked by paramedian pressure at T2–T3, the cutaneous sensitivity to manipulations of soft tissues and the provocation of dorsal pain (ringing the bell) by cervical pressure. The sensitivity of the low anterolateral cervical region remained unaltered.

The authors postulate an anastomosis between the posterior primary rami of lower cervical and upper thoracic nerves—especially the second thoracic. For those handling daily some 20 or more cases of musculoskeletal problems, it will be common experience that cervical movements can provoke interscapular pain, and that localised cervical treatment will eradicate it. The functional interdependence of the vertebral column has been emphasised (p. 38).

Possibly we should not make too much of this, because just as commonly upper/midthoracic pain is produced by local changes in the thoracic segments and the relief of symptoms by localised *central* vertebral pressures infers that the underlying changes are those of early spondylosis. The changes may be characterised by (i) palpable stiffness, or may present as (ii) a mixture of segmental stiffness and hypermobility, or (iii) a site of hypermobility only, sometimes at a single segment and sometimes comprising two or three, to make a palpably 'loose' region in the interscapular area.

As an example of the first (i), a fit and athletically inclined man of 36 complained of increasingly frequent bouts of symmetrical bilateral aching situated paravertebrally at the horizontal levels of T8–T9–T10. The bouts occurred every two months or so, lasting some days, and when severe necessitated a day or two in bed; milder attacks were sufficiently severe to prevent any physical activity and work was not possible. There was no pain radiation to neck, upper limbs or low back, nor any neurological signs or symptoms. Cervical and thoracic movements were symmetrical and painless, although the midthoracic region was observed to move almost *en bloc*. Straight-leg-raising combined with passive neck flexion did not provoke the thoracic pain.

The patient speculated that a road traffic accident 15 years before may have initiated the slow development of stiffness.

Cervical palpation revealed nothing exceptional, but the thoracic region between T3 and T6 was palpably stiffened, with a much diminished range of accessory movement; the spinous processes of T3–T6 were markedly tender to central pressures as were the transverse processes bilaterally. Symmetrical and localised mobilisation techniques to the named region relieved the symptoms, the freedom from restriction and pain lasting to date for some nine months; the relief also depending, no doubt, on the segmental exercises the patient was shown.

A further, not uncommon, variant of this grouping of clinical features is that of unilateral or bilateral glove paraesthesiae of upper limbs, and a tendency to generalised headache accompanied by palpable joint abnormalities in the T2–T3–T4–T5–T6 region. More often than not, the joint problem is at the junction of the upper and middle thirds of the thoracic spine, i.e. T4–T5.

One of the interspaces will feel unusually tight, and an adjacent spinous process (usually the caudal one) will be palpably depressed and a little more mobile than its fellow; both will be sore to palpation. The patient may be wakened from sleep by the troublesome paraesthesiae, or may wake with symptoms present at the normal time.

Unusually, the patient may recall some trauma or physical stress from which the symptoms may be dated, but more often the onset is insidious, beginning with mild paraesthesiae and mild headache; having become established, there is little variation in the clinical features and it is not always possible to provoke or relieve them by physical movement tests. There are no neurological signs.

While the palpation signs described can be detected in asymptomatic people, the syndrome is distinguished by the fact that both the paraesthesiae and the headache can routinely be relieved by accurately localised mobilisation to the segments concerned.

It is difficult to avoid concluding that aberrant sympathetic neurone traffic underlies the clinical presentation.

Upper/midthoracic spondylosis with hypermobility

Movement-abnormalities due to spondylotic change can be manifest as stiffness, and also as looseness, of a segment. Hypermobility and stiffness occur very frequently in adjacent segments, the one possibly being a consequence of the other.

This occurs in the cervical spine (Figs 6.1, 8.4) and in the lumbar spine (p. 139); it also plainly occurs in the thoracic spine, and on occasions the degree of looseness is such as to defy conservative treatment and to require surgical fusion.[721]

The comparative lack of movement in thoracic vertebrae (p. 48) seems not to preclude it suffering segmental hypermobility, within the context of its relatively reduced range of movement. In the instance of surgical fusion outlined above, the patient had suffered frustrating restrictions of activities because of interscapular pain for some considerable time, and after the failure of conservative treatment to relieve him, had remained free of the trouble two years after the fusion. The fact that he began to develop cervical problems after that period in no way nullifies the presence, and surgical relief of, his segmental thoracic hypermobility.

Examples are:

1. Patients often present with midthoracic pain, frequently provoked by thoracic testing movements but sometimes curiously not, and with no other problems in the neck, arms, rest of the trunk or lower limbs. Segments T1–T2–T3, for example, may be palpably stiffened, and somewhat tender, but T4 and T5 have a decidedly 'boggy' feel on posteroanterior central vertebral pressures and this provokes a sharp, voluntary muscle-guarding response by the patient.

If the palpation is rough or too vigorous, the presenting pain is severely aggravated for many hours afterwards. Segments T6, T7 and below may be a little tender but are otherwise negligibly involved and are neither stiff nor more mobile.

2. A single segment, and more commonly a group of two or three segments, can be found to be palpably loose in relation to the comparatively small but normal accessory-movement range of their neighbours.

Grant and Keegan (1968)[433] described certain fairly consistent features of musculoskeletal pain in the chest wall, i.e. reasonably accurate localisation; accentuation by movements of the thoracic spine—twisting, bending or turning in bed; exacerbation by breathing, coughing and straining; association with posture and position; a history of twist or muscular stress, sometimes requiring questioning to elicit.

Most people have very little real conception of the enormous forces (p. 499) developed by co-ordinated muscle action during activities such as wrestling, pulling, dragging, bending and lifting, pushing a motor-car or digging and shovelling clay; nor of the applied violence of car accidents. Patients should be questioned with care about stresses of this kind, because very frequently they give little account to some 'ordinary' physical stress which in fact may have severely strained vertebral structures.

Very frequently a history of this kind of stress predates the onset of midthoracic pain, yet it is circumspect not to be too enthusiastic in ascribing pain to a particular event. However, when violent retching and vomiting necessitates a flexed position of the trunk, and thoracic pain of acute onset coincides with it, there is no doubt of the relationship between cause and effect.

There also seems little doubt that excessive applied stress can strain and attenuate the soft tissues of thoracic segments in precisely the same way as occurs at all other synovial joints.

A 32-year-old man developed interscapular pain after a strenuous pulling episode on an oil rig two years before. Two episodes of acute thoracic pain occurred in the interim. Thoracic extension provoked the worst pain; other movements did less so. There were no neurological signs and no pain radiation, although there was *right* occipitofrontal headache and a painfully tender and thickened *left* occipitoatlantal joint. Cervical palpation revealed nothing of note other than changes at the left C0–C1 segment, but T4–T5–T6 were all noticeably 'soggy' on central vertebral pressures, which provoked a sickening pain locally. The same gently applied techniques relieved it.

Tietze's disease

Tietze's disease was described by him in 1921;[1217] the changes and clinical presentations are briefly described on page 138. The cause of the painful cartilage is still unproven, but Rawlings (1962)[1015] mentioned a usual history of repetitive or acute overloading or stress of the rib cage. A painful, tender mass overlies the costosternal junction, and there is no other evidence of abnormality. In about 50 per cent of patients the mass is at the second rib; there is no heat or redness. The histology may be that of perichondrial swelling with round cell infiltration.

Cavaziel (1974)[164] asserts that the condition denotes torsion of a rib. Hydrocortisone injection appears to be the definitive treatment.

The rib-tip syndrome

The rib-tip syndrome (p. 138) is characterised by bouts of severe lancinating pain localised to the costal margin unilaterally at the anterior ends of the 8th, 9th or 10th rib. The pain can be confused with pleurisy, coronary thrombosis and gall-bladder disease, to the extent that laparotomy may be performed.

The pain may be associated with hyperaesthesia in the territory of the related intercostal nerve. Diagnosis can be confirmed by hooking flexed fingers under the imprisoned rib(s) and pulling anteriorly, when the characteristic and localised pain is provoked.[529]

A popping or clicking sensation on deep respiration or sudden thoracic stress may be accompanied by stabbing local pains, which in some may radiate around the flank to the back. The author has recently seen a woman whose recurrent episodes of thoracic distress were so severe as to render her speechless, almost afraid to breathe and completely unable to make love with her husband for fear of precipitating an attack of pain. Having experienced this once, she felt, 'I dare not risk it again'.

Some typical histories include direct trauma to the costal margin. In the patient mentioned above, vigorous thrust manipulations had recently been repetitively applied to the interscapular dorsal spine while she was in the prone position; she could recall no other direct or indirect trauma to her thorax.

Acute hemithoracic pain

This condition is distinguished from that above by the wider area of pain and by the usual lack of direct violence in the history, in which a trunk twisting or reaching episode is more usually associated with the acute onset of pain. A representative description of clinical features has been given (p. 180) and Kellgren (p. 194) has described many examples of it.

In many cases, the cause appears to be a mechanical or functional block of a costal joint or, as Grant and Keegan (1968)[433] have expressed it, 'anatomical misalignment' of a rib. The authors have drawn attention to the unhelpfulness of X-rays, and it may be unreasonable for us to expect that derangements of the costotransverse and costovertebral joints would be detectable radiographically.

'Changes to the costovertebral articulations cause intercostal pain which may be relieved by manual therapy.' [*Schmorl and Junghanns* (1972).[1093]]

Swezey and Silverman (1971)[1200] have demonstrated that overriding of vertebral facets, of the order of 3 mm at the C5–C6 segment and 3.5 mm at the L5–S1 segment, is not detectable on routine X-rays. Since these segments are a great deal more mobile than the thoracic joints (Figs 2.6, 2.7) it seems pointless to wait for X-ray evidence before accepting the existence of costal joint derangement. (See also Thoracic disc lesions, p. 248.)

The clinical picture can be quite dramatic, and because the features can simulate acute visceral conditions it is understandable that a simple benign, musculoskeletal cause is not thought of initially.

After an acute onset, chronic pain may persist for months or years if treatment is not given. Grant and Keegan[433] give an illustrative case history which includes a description of axillary and arm pain associated with upper thoracic joint problems of acute onset:

A small frail 45-year-old woman had been engaged in nursing her invalid father; work which involved shifting him around the bed. She complained of an 'agonising' pain in the left side of the chest over three months and had been investigated elsewhere— X-ray chest, cardiograph, blood count and sedimentation rate being described as normal, but the cervical spine X-ray showed degenerative changes of C4–C5 disc. Referred to clinic as possible angina for further opinion. She was unable to remember the exact commencement of her discomfort but on questioning localised the pain as being 'gripping' over the 3rd and 4th left costochondral cartilages going through to the back in the left scapular area and axilla. She had also pain down her arm at night and felt depressed and very worried about her heart. On examination, radiology of the chest, thoracic spine and ribs was normal and the cardiograph again negative. Twisting her back was painful. She was tender over the 3rd–5th cartilages anteriorly, the shaft of the 3rd rib along its course to the axilla and the costovertebral joints of the 3rd, 4th and 5th ribs.

Chronic anterior chest wall pain

Anterior chest pain may persist for months, or years, and tends to occur in patients over 45 who develop the condition some six or more months after an attack of coronary artery occlusion.

Prinzmetal and Massumi (1955)[1002] point out that the patient with cardiac insufficiency may suffer musculoskeletal chest wall pain just as frequently as anybody else. Further, that 'fibrositic' lesions of the chest wall are very common accompaniments of coronary disease.

The patient begins to complain of pain in the anterior chest wall, usually continuous and with no radiation to neck, jaw or arms, but usually most severe in the sternal region. Patients are quite often able to differentiate between it and the previous cardiac pain. There are no vasomotor changes such as salivation or perspiration.

Exacerbations may be acute because of some sudden body movement, the most frequent being flexion, extension, or rotation of the trunk, rotation of the neck or elevation of the arms. The authors suggest that in the differential diagnosis between this symptom-complex and other conditions such as coronary disease, the following major differences will be revealed by patient questioning and careful physical examination:

1. The pain of angina pectoris is paroxysmal, and precipitated by physical exertion and emotional tension—anterior chest wall pain tends to be continuous with acute exacerbations.
2. Pain radiation in angina pectoris is characteristic, while pain of the chest wall does not usually radiate outside the boundaries of the thoracic cage.
3. The vasomotor accompaniments of angina pectoris are absent in chest wall pain.
4. Musculoskeletal pain is not accompanied by systemic or cardiac symptoms. Temperature, ESR and blood counts remain normal.
5. The electrocardiograms taken during exacerbations of coronary arterial disease show features which are absent in the chest wall syndrome.
6. The pain of angina pectoris is relieved by glyceryl trinitrate, while chest wall pain fails to respond to this drug.
7. While some tenderness of the chest wall may be present in angina pectoris, it is mild and tends to disappear after an attack. The tenderness of chest wall pain is exquisite and persistent.
8. The prompt improvement in chest wall pain after corticotropin therapy does not occur in angina pectoris.

Other authors[291, 20, 308a] have drawn attention to examples of chronic soreness of the anterior chest wall unaccompanied by the signs and symptoms of coronary artery disease or pericarditis. The patient's general health is usually very good.

There appears to be a viscerosomatic interrelation, in that visceral changes can give rise to somatic changes in adjacent musculoskeletal structures. The examples of pulmonary arthropathy and the shoulder-hand syndrome (p. 185) provide a basis for the notion that, '. . . it is entirely possible that somatic anterior chest wall pain is pathogenically analagous to the shoulder-hand syndrome'.[1002]

The symptom-complex is often misdiagnosed as coronary heart disease and treated accordingly; this may give rise to the anxiety and depression associated with convictions about incurable heart disease.

Among a group of 18 patients who were referred to hospital for suspected myocardial ischaemia, and who were found to have painful rib lesions, 3 had had a previously confirmed episode of heart disease, although no evidence of recurrence was found.

Kunert (1975)[687] discussed the condition from a somewhat different aspect, suggesting that there may be a causal link between vertebral column changes and cardiac factors causing chest and heart pain.

Abdominal pain of spinal origin

Those who spend most of their working day dealing with vertebral joint conditions become aware of the frequency with which lower thoracic, upper lumbar (and sacroiliac) joint problems can refer pain to the abdominal wall.

Spinal root or referred pain often arise synchronously and in the same segments as visceral abnormalities either because of summation or through visceroparietal reflexes. The latter are occasionally so marked that the visceral source of trouble is obscured. Conversely parietal pain can cause reflex visceral symptoms. . . . An acute abdomen may be simulated by aching from skeletal structures in febrile illnesses.[46]

Marinacci and Courville (1962)[806] in a description of radicular syndromes which simulated intra-abdominal surgical conditions, mentioned the most common cause of *radiculopathy* as virus infection, neoplastic lesions, arthritic spurs, ruptured intervertebral disc, compression fractures and vascular tumours (p. 103).

They describe the potentials for pain referral, e.g. T6–T7 root irritation producing epigastric pain, T7–T8 irritation simulating gall-bladder disease, pain in the kidney region from T9 root irritation, and T10–T11 root irritation suggesting disorders of urethra and bladder. They suggest that in these cases the clinician is dealing with a 'counterfeit' symptomatology.

Since reflex muscle spasm and tenderness may accompany both visceral disease and abdominal pain referred from the spine, it has been suggested that the physical signs may be unhelpful in resolving this diagnostic dilemma.[712]

Ashby's (1977)[46] prospective study of 73 patients presenting in one year indicates the following criteria for audit of the diagnosis of abdominal pain of spinal origin:

The diagnosis was regarded as confirmed if *both* the following criteria were met:
1. *Either* (a) the clinical features were *typical*, for example, cutaneous pain or marked postural aggravation,
   or (b) the clinical features were *compatible* and there was a sustained remission of pain for an arbitrary 3 months after intercostal block; *and*
2. No visceral or abdominal wall lesions manifested over an arbitrary year of follow-up.

It was considered that root or peripheral nerve irritation was suggested by descriptive qualities like 'pricking', 'burning', or 'sore', and referred pain from descriptions like 'nagging', 'toothache', and 'difficult to describe'. The objective criteria for distinguishing root irritation pain from referred pain, and the basis for not also describing the former as referred, are not given.

'Tenderness near the tip of a vertebral transverse process was a particularly valuable sign as it indicated nerves to inject.'
Ashby considered that:

. . . pain may arise through one or more mechanisms: (1) primary root pain; (2) referred pain from structures of the vertebral axis; (3) secondary effects, (a) referred pain due to excessive reflexes provoking high-threshold receptors in joints and muscles, or (b) root pain due to compression by reflex muscle spasm.

It is of interest that in the papers quoted, the authors' concern with spinal nerve roots and peripheral nerves is manifest; there appears an undue preoccupation with nerves, and insufficient emphasis given to the possibility that very many examples of pain referred to the abdominal wall need not concern irritation or compression of nerves at all, as thigh and knee pain in arthrosis of the hip does not concern physical involvement of nerve trunks. Further, that referred pains in the abdominal wall are more often of quite innocuous origin, their genesis being everyday sprains and traumatic stresses of vertebral joints, or early degenerative changes of localised soft tissue and thickening which do not show up on X-ray. The basis for this assertion is the frequency with which referred abdominal pains can be relieved, by specific spinal mobilising techniques which, because of their gentleness, could not by any stretch of imagination be 'putting discs back' or 'taking osteophytes off nerve roots' (or vice versa).

We have referred (p. 239) to commonly limited conceptions of the *magnitude* of forces acting upon thoracic joints.[230, 231, 232] The neck, shoulder and scapular muscles, the diaphragm, abdominal wall muscles and the quadratus lumborum all exert great forces which stress thoracic structures. Heavy functional use of arms and shoulders transmits stress to the thorax; the rise in intrathoracic pressure and distortion of the rib cage under stress are considerable.

Pulling, as opposed to pushing with the arms, considerably alters thoracic capacity and thoracic stress patterns. Joint strains, particularly habitual ones, are likely to initiate slow degenerative changes,[902] and since this notion is acceptable as the basis for much of cervical and lumbar degenerative change, why not for the thoracic spine, too? The fact that radiological changes are difficult to demonstrate is not of great consequence, since it is well known that clinically evident joint abnormalities, with painful movement and referred symptoms, correlate poorly with X-ray changes.

Entrapment neuropathy of lower thoracic nerves must be considered. Abdominal wall pain because of entrapment neuropathy at or near an operation scar[1048] is real enough, as is its relief by local infiltration of anaesthetic solutions and corticosteroid, yet in many cases without operation scars the provocation of pain by pressure on the trigger site is probably analogous to pressure on a tender trapezius muscle in cervical joint problems; provocation of pain by coughing, straining or tensing the abdominal muscles by raising head and shoulders off the pillow[839] employs manœuvres which also markedly stress thoracic joints. The basis for a diagnosis of entrapment neuropathy may sometimes be fallacious.[1194]

Eradication of a local pain by local injection does not necessarily mean that its source has been thereby demonstrated. The factors of 'needling' and effects of acupuncture cannot be dissociated from assessment of injection effects; three phenomena are involved: the actions of the substance employed, effects of its physical mass and cutaneous puncture by needle. Perhaps this phenomenon should not be relied upon, willy-nilly, as a basic tenet of diagnosis in musculoskeletal problems.

It is my experience that 'the need for a routine and deliberate search for tenderness localised to the anterior abdominal wall'[1048] is balanced by the need for a careful vertebral examination which includes meticulous spinal and paraspinal palpation. The general standard of examination of the spine seems not as high as it might be, nor does the phenomenon of referred tenderness appear to receive the appreciation it should. Perhaps the diagnosis of entrapment neuropathy at the abdominal wall in patients who also exhibit spinal problems should not be made until the vertebral column, thoracic and pelvic joints have been comprehensively examined; the simple business of rattling through the spinal movements, testing for neurological signs and taking anteroposterior and lateral X-rays does not amount to a comprehensive examination.[452]

Abdominal and anterior chest pain from posterior thoracic joints may exist in the absence of lateral or posterior thoracic pain; as has been mentioned (p. 195), pain from synovial joints may be localised to the joint region, localised and referred or referred only, as commonly occurs in arthrosis of the hip.

Scheuermann's disease (vertebral osteochondrosis)

This is the commonest spinal disease and cause of back pain in adolescents. It is twice as common in boys as in girls.

Although mentioned here under thoracic conditions, vertebral osteochondrosis is a process which may affect any part of the spine: '... we must free ourselves from the conception that it is a condition particularly affecting the thoracic spine ...'.[146] Any thoracic or lumbar level may be affected.[1180b]

Lumbar osteochondrosis is far from uncommon[1093] and may well be as common as the thoracic form (p. 136), cervical osteochondrosis in the active stage is often symptomless but may be the cause of recurrent discomfort in the neck and cervicoscapular region.[146]

While the association between the deformity of adolescent kyphosis and thoracic osteochondrosis is plain, there is a tendency to overlook the fact that for every single gross postural example of this association of cause and effect, there are a great many cases where kyphosis is not a marked feature of the condition, yet the principal symptoms for which the patient seeks help are ascribable to radiological and clinical evidence of thoracic or upper lumbar stiffening due to osteochondrosis.

Alternatively, a frank kyphosis produced by Scheuermann's disease may be quite painless.

It is important to remember that thoracic kyphosis per se may be secondary to tight hamstrings and not due to vertebral pathology.[983] If the positions of the anterior superior iliac spine and the greater trochanters, in the normal standing posture, are marked and the subject then bends forward, the two marks are virtually horizontal when the toes are reached by the fingers. If they are not, the thoracic spine is constantly undergoing flexion stress, not only in stopping but in sitting on the floor with the legs straight.

When due to the changes of Scheuermann's disease the kyphosis, onset of which is never observed, begins early in the second decade before there is any chronic spinal pain, although occasionally young people may have 'growing pains' during the first decade and then a period of quiescence until they begin to work during the second decade.

The kyphosis is often discovered during a routine school medical examination. The curve is smooth and appears as an exaggeration of the normal posture. It is accentuated in flexion. The lumbar and cervical curves are increased in compensation.[1313]

The biomechanical effects upon neural canal structures can be altered by the kyphosis, since the resting length of the canal has increased. Extremes of head and neck flexion, and of lumbar and hip flexion with the knees straight, will have the potential of provoking earlier than normal pain which may be due to tension effects. This potential is increased if the canal is congenitally stenotic.

In the absence of treatment and supervision over some years, the deformity progresses until ossification completes itself at about 22 years.[983, 1180b]

Pain starts some years after the deformity begins to be manifest, often on beginning work which involves stress to the spinal structures. The pain is sometimes localised to the mid- and lower thoracic region, but more usually is localised and also spreading to upper lumbar regions. The pain is not only stress-dependent but also time-dependent, in that it tends to build up towards the end of the day, or at the end of a period of work or athletic activity.

The pain during adolescence ceases when growth is complete, but begins again during adult maturity, when the stresses occasioned by a region of stiffness begin to make themselves felt in adjacent regions, often the lumbar spine.

The usual clinical picture is that the onset of pain is insidious, it is never really severe, there is no systemic illness and the main complaints are of backache and fatigue.[1180b]

There are variations:

1. A patient may report quite localised backache in the junctional region *between* the radiologically affected segments and those with normal appearances. Treatment directed only to the junctional region relieves the ache, while the deformity remains, of course.

2. Less commonly the patient, usually a young adult woman, shows no marked postural kyphosis but has severe radiological changes, several segments showing blurring and fuzziness of the disc–vertebral body interface, and not always with wedging. The symptoms are those of a chronic dull background ache, upon which is superimposed severe jabs of localised thoracic pain, more noticeably during rotation movements. The clinical presentation appears to be that of a thoracic column whose architecture has been disturbed by disc degeneration to the point of initiating repetitive small joint derangements—in themselves harmless and not threatening nerve roots or the spinal cord but amounting to a severe functional restriction, the cause of chronic problems.

Since this section on types of presentation has a clinical bias, it is no transgression to mention the important effects of the same condition occurring lower in the vertebral column.

Lower thoracic and upper lumbar osteochondrosis (p. 136) may remain undetected until the patient, usually a male, is in the late 20's or early 30's, when chronic stress on adjacent and normally mobile segments begins to declare itself.

A common presentation among men around the 30-year-old age group is that of lumbosacral area pain manifestly arising from a tender and midly irritable L5 (and less often L4) segment, passive movement of which stirs up the local pain. From L4 upwards the lumbar and often the lower thoracic spine is flat, stiff and sometimes feels quite solid to accessory-movement tests. In more chronic cases, small areas of light brown cutaneous discoloration overlie the mid and upper lumbar spinous processes, indicating sites of chronic pressures on the prominent bony points by the backs of chairs.

The most striking features of this very common presentation are the extraordinary stiffness of the affected midlumbar region; the tendency for the *painful* segment to lie next below the stiff region; the way this regional stiffness may remain concealed despite so-called comprehensive examination; an apparent general lack of awareness of this ubiquitous clinical finding.

'Covert lumbar osteochondrosis' is probably the correct diagnosis in much backache of young adult males, when more frank causes have been excluded. A generalised lumbosacral ache, worse after a day's work or recreational stress, underlies short sharp episodes of more acute pain after digging, bending and lifting episodes or sudden rotational strains.

It seems, in effect, that the lowest lumbar segment is being repetitively sprained or strained, due to the stress imposed by the immediately adjacent stiff spinal neighbourhood. The principle of treatment will be plain—settle lower segment irritability and improve mobility of the stiff region.

Ankylosing spondylitis

'This disorder may be *underdiagnosed* by a factor of about 80 in females and 10 in males.'[153]

The complex interrelationship between a large group of rheumatic conditions is slowly becoming better understood (see p. 206).

The antigen HLA-27 is among several which can be identified on cell surfaces; among the human leucocyte antigens, HLA-27 is usually present in 4–5 per cent of the population, but was found in 72 of 75 patients with classical ankylosing spondylitis,[125] and in only 3 of 75 controls.

Brewerton *et al.* (1973) observe that the diagnosis of ankylosing spondylitis has previously tended to be provisional for a number of years, e.g. 7 patients had not developed radiological evidence of sacroiliitis until more than 5 years after the original clinical diagnosis,[1366] and it is now feasible that identification of this and other rheumatic disorders will be considerably hastened.

'From the viewpoint of genetic analysis they are all part of an overlapping mixture of clinical features and diseases.'[713, 893]

The disease is more common among the relatives of patients known to be suffering from it;[780] clinical investigation of first-degree relatives of spondylitic patients reveals features of the condition in 15 per cent or more of them.[713]

Several factors mark the difference between rheumatoid arthritis and ankylosing spondylitis:

1. The majority of cases occur in young men
2. Asymmetrical joint involvement, usually of lower limbs, occurs often
3. Restricted chest expansion, due to costovertebral joint involvement, is common
4. Radiography reveals sacroiliitis sooner or later
5. The rheumatoid factor is negative[1264]
6. Bone scanning techniques may be helpful.[700]

Although manifest spondylitis is common in men, milder symptoms are found almost equally in both sexes. Calin and Fries (1975)[153] succinctly discuss the sex incidence of the disease:

The reason for male predominance in diagnosed cases is more difficult to analyse. Many young women complaining of chronic low-back pain may not be investigated because it is common to blame the female pelvic organs for any untoward symptoms. There is also a reluctance to subject young women to pelvic radiation. Frequent statements that ankylosing spondylitis is rare in women further decrease the chance that correct diagnosis will be made. It seems possible that young men in physically more active occupations are more likely to find back pain and stiffness a limiting factor in their daily life and are thus more likely to consult

their physicians. The fact that women tend to have more peripheral joint involvement than men may mean that some cases in women have been misdiagnosed as rheumatoid arthritis. It remains possible that the disease is more severe in males, on the average, than in females.

Resnick *et al.* (1976)[1028] studied the clinical and radiographic differences between men and women (98 patients) with the disease. In the 18 female patients there was a later onset, a higher incidence of peripheral joint involvement, more frequent involvement of the cervical spine and a generally milder course.

Radiographic differences in the women were a high incidence of cervical spine changes, a combination of cervical and sacroiliac changes with normal lumbar and thoracic spines and frequently a severe osteitis pubis.

More frequently than not, the patient is an otherwise healthy, strong and athletically minded man—certainly no shrinking violet. A small percentage of patients give a history of rheumatic disease, or flitting joint pains in the lower limbs, during the 10th–15th year, after which pain disappears. Mild spondylitic symptoms begin insiduously in late adolescence or early manhood, and most often take the form of low back pain, with severe morning stiffness. Some, but not all, report alternating sciatica, sometimes spreading to lower thigh. Stiffness may also disturb sleep, and there may be chest as well as lumbar pain. The stiffness is relieved by exercise and aggravated by rest. In around 5 per cent of patients the disease may start in the thoracic spine and in some 13 per cent the condition originates in the cervical spine.[780]

Typically, the backache and stiffness wax and wane for periods of some weeks or months; after a trouble-free interim the pain is noticed to have migrated up the spine, and is more pronounced in the upper lumbar and lower thoracic regions. Respiration may feel less free, and while the low back no longer hurts its movement may feel limited, although surprisingly often patients remain unaware of their manifest lumbar restriction.

Patients rarely seek advice merely because the spine is stiffer than it used to be.[1180b] The writer recalls a patient over 50 who was referred for the neck pains of cervical spondylosis, and in whom the whole vertebral column, other than the upper neck, was virtually fossilised. He vaguely recalled low back pains and alternating sciatica while in the Army many years ago, but the condition had not been diagnosed.

A consistent clinical finding in spondylitis is marked restriction of side-flexion, and this sign should always arouse suspicion of inflammatory vertebral disease.

The patient's general condition is often better than in rheumatoid arthritis, but this does depend on the amount of pain which has to be borne and the severity of the condition. A common feature is that of increasing and frustrating weariness, and it may be noticed that the patient finds difficulty in leaning forward when asked to sit on a plinth for examination of the chest.[1040] The spinous processes, ischial tuberosities and calcanei may show marked tenderness.

Some of the patients who present annually with acute anterior uveitis have identifiable rheumatic disease,[713] and iritis is present in about 25 per cent of patients with ankylosing spondylitis.

Typically there are no symptoms suggesting nerve root or peripheral root involvement. The course and manifestations of the disease are seldom dramatic, and marked stiffness with spinal ankylosis can occur without appreciable symptoms for many years.[153]

Chest expansion is reduced to less than 5 cm. Shoulders and hips are affected in 40 per cent and more peripheral joints in 25 per cent, the knees accounting for 15 per cent of peripheral joint involvement.[583] Atlantoaxial subluxation, and erosion of the sternoclavicular joint, may also occur.[970]

On occasions a rapidly progressive form involves the larger peripheral joints as well as the spine, producing unusually severe disablement. In the few cases with severely advanced disease, the vertebral column is fixed in a flexion curve, increasingly pronounced from the flattened lumbar spine upwards, save the craniovertebral region which is hyperextended and may excape fixation. Involvement of both hips adds considerably to the difficulties of progression.

Sacroiliitis. The sacroiliac joint is usually the first to be involved, and there is early clinical, and later radiological, evidence of this. Manual gapping or approximation of the ilia, and pressure over the sacrum, sharply provoke localised pain. Other tests, such as resisted, static isometric contractions of the hip abductors and adductors, may do likewise. Since the earliest signs of the condition are manifest on these tests for sacroiliac joint irritability, they should never be left out in any examination for thoracic and lumbar pain.

The radiological appearances of the joint are characteristic, beginning with irregular definition,[780] a 'motheaten' character of the joint margins; oblique views initially show widening of the joint space by inflammatory destruction of bone. Subchondral sclerosis is later evident on both sides of the joint, this appearance distinguishing the condition from osteitis condensans ilii (q.v.). Multiple erosions and a patchy sclerosis may be seen, and in some the sclerosis may be linear rather than broad.[189] Eventually the joint is obliterated.

The ischial tuberosities appear roughened and the outline of the symphysis pubis may be blurred.[583]

Ankylosis. Ossification of connective tissue structures occurs somewhat late in the disease, and gives a typical 'bamboo' spine appearance.[780] This is preceded by a 'squaring' of the vertebral bodies, evident on lateral views

taken early in the disease. The sternal joints also become fixed.

Systemic illness is revealed by a tendency to lose weight, by a raised ESR in 80 per cent, anaemia and sometimes pyrexia. The level of the ESR is not a good guide to the degree of activity of the condition.[1040]

Somewhat similar clinical features are seen in Reiter's disease, psoriasis, ulcerative colitis and regional ileitis (Crohn's disease).[828] In a series of 80 cases of Crohn's disease, Deshayes *et al.* (1977),[254] 6 cases of asymptomatic sacroiliitis were observed (see p. 156).

Other factors occasionally associated with ankylosing spondylitis are cardiovascular changes and pulmonary fibrosis.[780]

The condition is very uncommon in the Negro races.[75]

Rarely, the vertebrae may be involved in destructive lesions,[539] and fractures can occur through the indirect violence of stumbling and falling or because of sudden violent movements of the arms.[434]

Hollin *et al.* (1965)[561] reviewed the incidence of cervical fractures, most often at C5–C6.

Resnick (1974)[1026] found involvement of the temperomandibular joint in 32 per cent of 25 consecutive cases of long-standing ankylosing spondylitis.

The muscle tissue of patients with ankylosing spondylitis has been studied histologically, histochemically and by electron microscopy, and has been shown to be grossly abnormal. The changes probably have a neuropathic basis.[88]

Prognosis. Spontaneous resolution occurs sooner or later, and in general terms the sooner the onset the more severe the disablement. Women do better than men. An onset in the late teens is not a good augury for the future, in either sex, but if clinical features do not appear until the end of the third decade the degree and rate of involvement is correspondingly less.

Since limited respiratory movement endangers general health more than does vertebral fixation *per se*,[1180b] the maintenance of thoracic mobility is important. An active regime suits the spondylitic patient better than a restful regime—while allowing for the periods of acute flare-up.

Lesions of the lowest ribs
The single costal facet on T11 and T12 vertebral bodies is virtually level with the transverse process, but the associated rib does not articulate with it. The slight angle of the 11th rib is easily palpated at about the horizontal level of T12 spinous process, but the 12th rib, which may be 2.5–20 cm long, is virtually featureless and not so easy to find, especially in women.

As a cervical rib is the most common variant at the cervicothoracic junction, the presence of a lumbar rib[1093] is the most common thoracolumbar region variant, having the radiographic appearance on AP films of articulating end-to-end with the transverse process of L1 vertebra. It occurs two or three times more often in men, who are more exposed to direct violence at work and play, and its presence may cause difficulties in that direct injury to the loin, as sometimes occurs in boxers, may be misdiagnosed as a fracture of T12 transverse process.

Evidence of these functional stresses imposed on musculoskeletal structures at the thoracolumbar junction is not lacking. Nathan (1964)[902] observed the changes of costovertebral arthritis in 168 (48 per cent) of 346 skeletons, the highest frequency of arthritic change occurring at the single costovertebral joint of T11 and T12. The intervertebral disc need play no part in this degenerative change. Nathan suggests that this type of single joint, being that of a floating rib, is more vulnerable to the mechanical irritation of constant rib motion.

Nathan's (1959)[898] description of the para-articular processes of the thoracic vertebrae, bony spicules springing from the upper and lower attachments of the ligamentum flavum,[1092] gives the highest incidence of these spicules at the T9–T10–T11 thoracic segments. While their genesis remains in doubt, their segmental incidence may be significant.

Shore (1935)[1125] described the incidence of facet-joint arthrosis as highest at the T12–L1 segment. Nathan's (1962)[900] analysis of spinal osteophytosis in 400 vertebral columns revealed the highest incidence of 4th degree (fused) osteophytosis to be at the T8–T9, T9–T10 and T10–T11 segments. Plainly, the region is no stranger to stress, and is a common site for degenerative change.

The attachments of the 12th rib, although short, include the quadratus lumborum, the diaphragm, the serratus posterior inferior, part of the sacrospinalis group, the latissimus dorsi and the external abdominal oblique muscles. It also gives attachment to the middle layer of the lumbodorsal fascia.

The lowest ribs are considered to have only a poor range of movement,[1180a] and are regarded as subject only to stresses imposed by quadratus lumborum spasm, or to secondary involvement in T11 and T12 intervertebral joint lesions. Yet the many attachments of powerful muscles to the 12th rib, the unequivocal evidence of degenerative changes in the two lower ribs and their situation at a junctional region subject to powerful forces indicate that covert joint problems here may be much more frequent than we have supposed.

Among 41 patients with rib pain, the criterion of which was tenderness along the length of the rib, Grant and Keegan[433] found that one of the most common complaints was tenderness of the right lower three ribs. Seven patients localised it to the 11th and 12th rib only, the tenderness being over the costovertebral joint as well as the short shaft. Among the suggested diagnoses on referral to hospital were renal calculus, cholecystitis and peptic ulcer.

Cough fractures of a rib (at least 200 cases have been reported) are not rare, and are known to chest physicians; but these fractures occur as a rule between the 4th and 9th ribs.

Descriptions of stress fractures of the lower ribs are uncommon, since only about 30 have been reported; Horner (1964)[573] described 4 more cases in which violent exertion produced a more or less identical set of clinical features which included radiographic confirmation of fracture of the 11th and/or 12th rib. The features were a sense of thoracic constriction, severe pain on trunk movements, painful inhibition of deep respiration, prounced loin area soreness which may last for a week or two and severe tenderness over the fracture sites. Horner compared the applications of force probably underlying cough fractures with those producing stress fractures of lower ribs, where the external abdominal oblique is not now interdigitating with serratus anterior, as in the typical ribs, but with the latissimus dorsi. This may explain why ribs 11 and 12 are more often fractured by strong use of the arms and trunk when handling heavy loads, and not by the stress of coughing. He reported four other cases of muscular exertion producing clinical features identical to the fracture cases (see above) but with no fractures evident on X-ray; these patients may have had muscle tears rather than fractures.

Kleiner (1924)[665] has suggested that the subject with superior muscular development is more likely to fracture a rib, whereas those with weaker musculature are more liable to overstress the muscle attachment, and presumably the rib-joint, during a given physical exertion.

Macnab (1977)[780] takes the opposite view, and it may be that other factors, such as a degree of osteoporosis, the precise nature of the stress and the state of the tissues (i.e. whether warmed up or not) at the time of injury will govern the nature of it.

The injury resulting from *externally applied* violence may produce a different clinical picture, in that breathing is not restricted by pain and not all trunk movements hurt. Common examples of this are represented by that of a 32-year-old lift maintenance engineer, who described chronic hemithoracic pain over the left lower ribs, and knife-like abdominal pains localised to a point on the left linea semilunaris, following a road traffic accident almost two years before. His lap seat belt restrained the pelvis while his trunk was thrown forward and to the right. The abdominal area was tender, and the pain was aggravated on activities involving pulling with the arms. Left side-flexion and left rotation of the trunk aggravated the pain; respiration did not. Left unilateral pressures on transverse processes of T9 and T10, and transverse vertebral pressures towards the left side, on spinous processes T9 and T10, uncovered pronounced local soreness. Pressures on the left 11th rib angle reproduced the stabbing abdominal pain. The same techniques relieved the hemithoracic pain and the abdominal tenderness.

Horner[573] makes the important point that pain on respiration, when associated with low back or loin pain, is a significant finding.

Cavaziel (1974)[164] asserts that lesions of the 12th rib may produce an 'inguinalgia' or simulate the pain of periarthrosis of the hip.

In connection with suspected lesions of the lower ribs, it is important to remember the phenomenon of referred tenderness, and the fact that the lateral branch of T7 posterior primary ramus innervates the superficial loin structures at the horizontal level of vertebral segments T11 and T12.

Acute lumbar pain of thoracic origin

Lateral branches of the posterior primary rami of spinal roots T12, L1 and L2 innervate the skin and superficial structures of the upper posterolateral buttock and the posterior iliac crest (Fig. 1.20).

Maigne (1972)[791] observes that rotational stress can produce the changes of acute traumatic lesions in the facet-joints of segments T9–L2, and has demonstrated that these lesions can refer pain unilaterally to the low back and upper buttock region. More chronic lesions can also occur. The facet-joint changes are said to irritate the posterior rami which are intimately related to the joint.

Transverse pressures, on the spinous processes of the named region, towards the side of pain, and unilateral posteroanterior pressures on the same side, will elicit local pain and sometimes the referred pain. Palpation will also elicit marked tenderness over the iliac crest at the point where distal nerve filaments of the lateral branches cross the iliac crest. According to the author, these changes represent 60 per cent of acute and chronic backache generally considered due to lumbar or sacroiliac joint changes; this type of pain referral may also coexist with pain of lumbosacral origin in about 20 per cent of cases.

Positive signs only assume full significance when they are balanced by the appropriate negative findings, thus the thoracolumbar region signs will have less weight if a careful search reveals equally frank lumbar or lumbosacral abnormalities on testing articular signs, and on palpation.

Thoracolumbar junction joint problems frequently refer pain to the anterolateral abdominal wall too, and the presence of this symptom often provides a clue as to the probable site of the lesion, or one of them. Some patients with lumbar pain from these junctional region changes will experience provocation of pain on both trunk rotations; in others the pain reported is provoked only on rotation towards the painful side.

Osteoporosis

Vertebral bone is by far the most interesting bony territory in the body ... it is almost wholly cancellous. Having, through its trabecular structure, a huge area of endosteal surface it can display great cellular activity. It can resorb, regenerate and remodel itself quickly and, like the cancellous bone in the epiphyses of the long bones, it has a much more rapid metabolic turnover than compact bone. Degenerative processes such as osteoporosis therefore become manifest first and foremost in the vertebral column. [Collins, 1959.[195]]

There is a reduction of the mineral content of bone with diminution in size of the bone mass. The marrow elements of the cancellous bone are unaffected.

The term osteoporosis has a precise meaning—'a quiet atrophy of bone due to failure of regeneration rather than to an accelerated rate of destruction'. (Collins, 1949.[194]) Normal catabolism outstrips anabolism until there is insufficient osteoid tissue capable of normal calcification, thus there is a less dense X-ray appearance.[195]

A degree of general osteoporosis is a normal accompaniment of sexual involution and ageing, but a more severe degree of senile osteoporosis particularly affects the spongiosa of the vertebral column, causing characteristic radiographic appearances and clinical symptoms. If the vertebral spongiosa of normal and osteoporotic bone are macerated, the normal architectural strength provided by a myriad of little bony plates is seen to be reduced to a delicate web of thin struts. Healthy vertebral spongy bone will resist a crushing force of 600–800 lb/in^2 (4136.88–5515.20kPa); porotic vertebrae are able to withstand 300 lb/in^2 (2068.44kPa) or less.[200]

Briefly, the maintenance of normal mature bone requires muscular and gravitational stress; dietary protein, calcium, phosphorus and vitamins C and D; parathyroid hormones, and the sex hormones oestrogen and androgen, and it will be evident that there can be, and are, a multitude of causes other than ageing which underlie the loss of bone mass.

The disease is five times more common in women, and commonest in postmenopausal women, although an idiopathic type may be present in women under the age of 30.[897]

The aetiology of secondary osteoporosis, and of that different condition osteomalacia, are not considered in detail here; of more immediate concern are the important points in the history, and the clinical features.

The age of the patient, the duration of symptoms and a history of immobilisation are important. Osteoporosis may occur in malnutrition, vitamin deficiencies, immobilisation, the postmenopausal phase, Cushing's syndrome, thyroid gland disease, acromegaly, ovarian and testicular maldevelopment, following total or partial gastrectomy and after operations on the urinary tract or pelvic structures.[897]

Idiopathic osteoporosis has been mentioned, and Macnab (1977)[780] states that it is more common in men around the age of 40.

Treatment by corticosteroids may have produced the side-effect of osteoporosis; the different condition osteomalacia may be induced by prolonged use of laxatives or aluminium hydroxide.[583]

X-ray changes. Some 35 per cent of bone salts can be lost before osteoporosis becomes radiologically evident—this is a somewhat conservative estimate. X-ray appearances are non-specific, being common to the various causes of the condition. When clinical features suggest the changes of osteoporosis it is probably unwise to rely on innocuous X-ray appearances as being conclusive.

The fish-vertebra deformity arises from expansion of the vertebral discs compressing the porotic vertebral bodies into a biconcave form;[195] this does not always occur since it depends upon disc turgescence being retained. Often the vertebrae become porotic after the discs have already become degeneratively narrowed. Farfan (1973)[326] states that the adjacent vertebrae become osteoporotic concurrently with degenerative changes in the disc.

Macnab (1977)[780] discusses the cause of pain and observes that since the blood content of the vertebral body spongiosa must increase *pari passu* with the diminution of bone mass, there is a relative increase in the volume of the blood pool. The marrow fat content does not increase in osteoporosis. Venous pressure in normal vertebrae is about 28 mmHg and that of osteoporotic vertebrae is around 40 mmHg—venous stasis is thus implied.

Clinical features. Pronounced osteoporosis of the spine can be symptomless.[897] The persistent aching pain of spinal osteoporosis is felt in the low thoracic area, sometimes with girdle pain; there is frequently low back pain which may radiate to buttocks and upper thighs, and backache is most often the presenting symptom.[780] A gradual onset of pain may be sharply punctuated by the feeling of something 'giving' in the middle back, as a consequence of a trivial jolt or minor stress, although crush fractures of a vertebral body can occur without the sudden stress of stepping from a kerb, coughing, sneezing or straining. These are less painful in the middle or upper thoracic spine, but can cause severe pain when occurring at the low thoracic and upper lumbar spine. Some 50 per cent of vertebral body fractures at the thoracolumbar region are due to this cause, i.e. they are pathological fractures. The persistent aching pain is somewhat relieved by lying down; both prolonged standing and sitting tend to make it worse, as does walking.

Some degree of kyphosis usually occurs; this may be a rounded kyphosis or more sharply angulated at the site of vertebral collapse. There is an overall loss of height in severe cases, with the lower ribs settling on the iliac crests and folds of abdominal tissue becoming evident. There are no abnormal neurological signs as a rule and cord compression is not common.

The progressive kyphosis may lead to chronic ligamentous strain and muscular fatigue, adding a further increment of weary aching to the patient's distress. Unless fractures have occurred, there is commonly no pronounced bony tenderness, and the lack of this sign should not mislead the clinical therapist.

Backache associated with osteoporosis is common. A radiological technique for diagnosing osteoporosis was employed in a survey of 481 patients with backache, 31 per cent of whom were found to have spinal osteoporosis.[255]

Erosion of ribs in rheumatoid arthritis
Rheumatoid disease, together with poliomyelitis, hyper-parathyroidism[612] and scleroderma, may be the underlying cause of erosive lesions in ribs.

Anderson *et al.* (1972)[23] report the clinical features in 18 cases, all of them satisfying the classical diagnostic criteria for rheumatoid arthritis. All 18 patients also showed atlantoaxial joint changes; most had a dorsal kyphosis and erosive changes in the glenohumeral joint were also common. Two forms of erosion were seen: (i) a localised rounded 'scalloped' defect involving five ribs (2 to 6 inclusive), occurring symmetrically at the external surface of the rib angles, at the point of attachment of the costocervicalis muscle; (ii) a more diffuse lesion involving the superior margin of the rib.

Erosion of vertebral bone by the rheumatoid process is well recognised; Schmorl and Junghanns (1971)[1093] mention erosion of the tips of spinous processes.

Thoracic disc lesions
A proportion of those concerned with the conservative and especially manipulative treatment of common vertebral joint conditions plainly give the impression, at least, that the phrase disc lesion has immediately triggered a concept of the disc being likened to an overpacked suitcase, whose contents have bulged the sides of the suitcase or have burst it and in one way or another are trespassing upon adjacent territory and structures.

This notion is an unfortunate inheritance if unwitting adherence to it, as the only important disc change, precludes a more comprehensive grasp of the multitude of possible changes in the disc.

For example, the presentations described on pages 238 and 239 are also disc lesions, so far as we can know. Scheuermann's disease (p. 242) is decidedly a lesion of discs, and a very important one, yet it is uncommon for the clinical features of any kind of *trespass* to be part of the signs and symptoms of this disease.

Nathan's (1968)[903] elegant exposition of the spondylotic changes in thoracic and upper lumbar intervertebral body joints, incorporating sympathetic trunks in the overgrowth of degenerative tissues in 78.4 per cent of 195 cadavers, is also describing disc lesions.

The description of gross, anterior thoracic vertebral lipping in the elderly (p. 135) is of disc lesions.

1. *Minor lesions.* The known tendency for arthrotic facet-joints (p. 134)[1125] to trespass upon related structures and

the space-occupying effects of para-articular processes (p. 103)[898] of thoracic vertebrae are two factors which must be borne in mind when ascribing clinical features to thoracic disc lesions in the absence of more obvious signs that this is indeed the cause.[82]

The demonstration of thoracic root involvement by e.m.g.[806] (p. 104) is one step, but there remains un-answered the question, '*What* is the nature of trespass?' The question may well be of academic rather than of clini-cal importance to some, but it is of much interest to the clinical therapist.

Postmortem studies show that in general terms thoracic disc pathology is common, and the nature of this has been discussed (pp. 135, 136).

A clinical rule-of-thumb adopted by many clinical therapists is as follows:

a. If the patient describes the thoracic pain as 'shooting directly through' the thorax from back to front, the cause is likely to be a lesion of disc trespass.
b. If the pain is referred horizontally around the chest wall, this denotes mainly a synovial joint problem and does not involve the disc to any extent.
c. If the pain is clearly referred down and around the chest wall in the plane of the ribs and intercostal spaces, this is referred root pain due to root involvement (pre-cise nature undetermined).

The writer must confess that he just does not know.

Stoddard (1969)[1180b] observes that:

Thoracic pain, especially when accompanied by girdle pain, which has a sudden onset for no apparent reason and for which no pathological explanation can be found, is *probably* due to a disc protrusion. The pain may be intense and any movement—even breathing—can be enough to accentuate the pain. Certainly coughing and sneezing accentuate it. The pain of pleurisy is accentuated by breathing, but in these cases breathing is checked at a certain phase of inspiration; the breathing 'catches' and the pain suddenly stops further inspiration. The reverse holds for a disc protrusion because full inspiration, so long as it is smooth and gentle, can be achieved without pain; but when the breathing is hurried or accompanied by thoracic movement then pain is pro-voked.... The clinical distinction between those patients who have nerve root pressure and those who have none is as useful in the thoracic spine as it is in the lumbar and cervical spines because treatment of the two is different. With the thoracic and milder cases ... we make an *assumption* of herniation rather than full prolapse of the disc ... [My italics.]

The examples of acute hemithoracic pain (p. 240) may indeed at times be due to painful though minor thoracic disc lesions amounting to a localised joint derangement, as might the example given on page 238. Should these pre-sumed disc lesions be successfully treated by a single dis-traction, or thrust manipulation, this again does not pro-vide certain evidence that 'the disc has been put back', since each thoracic vertebra takes part in 10 joints (count-ing both demifacets on one side as a single joint) and among those are the costal and facet-joints; intra-articular synovial fringes—meniscoid structures—in the latter are found almost universally, and the opportunities for impaction of a meniscoid structure are obvious. For the writer, the question remains open.

2. *Lesions urgently requiring a surgical opinion*[1131] (see p. 136). These lesions had acquired an unfortunate reputa-tion (now more optimistic) and although infrequent, the serious consequences of immoderately vigorous handling during examination and/or treatment, or of delay in seek-ing a surgical opinion, require that no thoracic spinal ex-amination be thought complete without a thorough in-vestigation for neurological symptoms and signs in lower limbs.

Most of the younger patients describe recent forceful injury, i.e. heavy falls on the buttocks or heels by para-troopers, weight-lifters and acrobats, or a rotational stress on the trunk. Some more mature patients develop symp-toms insidiously, and in these cases there is often evidence of degenerative change, which may inculpate trespass by the ligamentum flavum as well as exostosis. Benson and Byrnes (1975)[82] describe one patient whose onset was sudden and catastrophic on simply rising from a bed.

The history may span seven days to many years, with an average of two-and-a-half years.[158] Pain is a very com-mon complaint, and may be felt in the posterior thoracic region with a radicular distribution anteriorly, or may ini-tially be in the lumbar region, the pelvis and legs;[1131] girdle pain may accompany leg pain.[1116] The pain may be sharply increased during a cough or a sneeze, and when the neck is flexed. The quality of pain is variable—it may be constant and dull, spasmodic, cramping, 'burning' or lancinating. Pronounced 'heavy-leg' feelings, and numb-ness of extrasegmental distribution below the lesion, are accompanied by marked sensations of a particularly un-pleasant and disagreeable kind.[158]

While the pain may fluctuate weakness is progressive; leg weakness is a constant complaint. Some may not be able to walk, even with support.

There may be loss of temperature sense in one foot, for example, or both feet may feel cold. Lower motor neurone signs may be seen in lower thoracic disc disease but more common are the upper motor neurone signs of spastic weakness, clonus, exaggerated tendon jerks and an extensor response on plantar stroking.

Bladder function is not always impaired;[1116] sphincter disturbances existing can take various forms—there may be retention of urine, hesitancy, urgency, or a sense of in-complete evacuation. Faecal incontinence appears to be uncommon.

In a review of 22 patients,[82] half of whom were in the 40–50 year age group, paraspinous muscle spasm was not seen. Muscle power was impaired in all but two, the loss ranging from mild paresis of one leg to complete para-plegia. Weakness of the lower abdominal muscles was common, as was foot-drop.

The radiographs of 10 patients showed disc calcifica-tion. The causative lesion was most commonly at the 9th segment, with the majority of lesions occurring at either T7, T8 or T9.

LUMBAR SPINE AND PELVIS

Haldeman (1977)[486] lists some 26 causes of low back pain, as a few examples of the many factors which may underlie this ubiquitous complaint. He makes the point that 'any therapeutic procedure aimed at a single aetiological factor, in an unselected population of patients with low back pain, could not be expected to help more than a small percent-age of these patients'.

In combining types of backache, the principal tissues involved and the nature of the cause, Wyke (1976)[1362] lists some 20 categories of low back pain.

Anderson (1977)[24] discusses methods of classification under the main headings of site, system, severity, structure and syndrome, after suggesting that 'the low back' lies between the lower costal margins and the gluteal folds. Among his observations he mentions:

... this field is perhaps richer than any other in what can be de-scribed as the syndrome phenomenon. The situation arises from the fact that practitioners specialising in low back pain form an opinion over a long period of observation and therapy that, when a specific group of symptoms and signs are found to coexist, then treatment along certain lines is associated with a high degree of recovery. The details of the syndrome are seldom tested in terms of inter- or intra-observer error, nor is the therapy likely to be the subject of a randomly controlled trial. After all, it has taken years of careful observation to evolve the syndrome, so no disciple can ever achieve the same diagnostic expertise as the originating master, and if the treatment is 'obviously successful' it would be unethical to withhold it from any sufferer.

The muster of items, in any classification, depends to an extent on the degree of subdivision intended, of course, but also depends upon how common the classifier believes *multifactorial* backache and sciatica to be (see p. 263). The difficulties are compounded by the fact that almost every pathological change,[1248] and lumbosacral anomaly,[1327] to which back pain has been attributed has subsequently been demonstrated in the symptom-free population.

A spinal mobility-segment comprises two synovial facet-joints besides the single intervertebral body joint; one lumbar vertebra takes part in six articulations and four of these are facet-joints. The synovial joint structures con-tain a more varied and much richer population of mechanoreceptors than do the intervertebral body joints or their ligaments (see p. 10); the population of nocicep-tors is also much richer.

Clinical workers, for example Ghormley (1933),[406] Hadley (1936),[479] Badgley (1941),[53] Kraft and Levinthal (1951),[682] Epstein *et al* (1973),[317] Shealy (1974),[1118] and Mooney and Robertson (1976)[867] hold the view that facet-joint changes might be responsible for much of the low back pain and sciatica so often ascribed to disc lesions.

There is a gratifying increase in the recognition of the probable part played by abnormalities of neural arch structures in production of low back pain and proximal sciatic pain.[302]

Stereovision radiography techniques provide a better evaluation method of the probable cause of some cases of low back pain, in that damage to facet-joint structures is visualized more easily. In seven patients, paired stereo-scopic radiographs identified fractures in the neural arch structures in all, whereas standard X-ray views revealed the fractures in only two of the patients.[1136]

In a survey of anatomy, biomechanics, investigation procedures and diagnosis, Hazleman and Bulgen (1979)[522] observe that 'few patients with back pain have disc pro-lapse, and it is frequently over-diagnosed'.

The experiments reported by Mooney and Robertson (1976)[867] indicate that categorisation of the more common and benign lumbar pain syndromes may need much re-apraisal. Electromyogram studies on the hamstring muscles were performed on two patients, while the L4–L5 and L5–S1 facet-joints were being injected with hypertonic saline; the precise location of the needle was confirmed by arthrogram. In 15 seconds increased myo-electric activity appeared in the hamstrings, reducing straight-leg-raising to 70°; these effects could be obli-terated by introducing 1 per cent xylocaine into the facet-joint cavity.

All of a group of six patients with a straight-leg-raising below 70° had a normal SLR test within five minutes of facetal block.

On the basis of their findings (p. 318) the authors observe that localisation of pain in the low back, buttock, and leg are non-specific clinical features—many of the previous criteria of the 'disc syndrome' can be accounted for by facet abnormality, or may be caused by irritation within the spinal canal. Their studies confirm the position that, lacking *definitive* neurological signs, it is impossible by pain complaints alone to specifically localise the precise site of abnormality, and the precise nature of the change. What should constitute definitive neurological signs is arguable, since reflex changes, too, can be caused by pain-ful conditions of lumbar facet-joints (see p. 252). This par-ticular sign may not be conclusive evidence of physical trespass upon nerve roots, leaving aside consideration of the *nature* of the trespass, which need not be discogenic.[317]

The authors suggest that the only true neurological localising signs are perhaps specific dermatome sensory loss, or specific motor weakness. *Severely* limited straight-leg-raising and a crossed-leg positive SLR may be others.

Since dermatomes are hardly specific territorial entities (p. 169), the need for reappraisal of commonly accepted neurological criteria is plain.

Major orthopaedic surgical procedures and the management of trauma, can be based on sound diagnostic principles; the treatment of benign and minor orthopaedic problems must needs be to a large extent empirical. Positive signs, which are reasonably assumed to identify a particular lesion or involvement of a particular segment, only acquire full significance in the presence of negative signs elsewhere; joint problems do not always present so neatly, however, and in many cases one has to proceed initially on the basis of the greatest weight of likelihood rather than a clear-cut diagnosis. Continuous reassessment during treatment provides guidance and correction.

Thus there is a dilemma of classification, when the clinical field is one in which, however many facts are gathered by examination, certain and precise diagnosis cannot often be made. It follows that any arrangement of syndromes must be unsatisfactory, either because the dilemma is, seemingly, overcome by authoritarian pronouncements on the nature of pathological change,[514] or better, that certain spheres of ignorance are accepted and the truth 'we do not know' is plainly implied or stated.

The upper lumbar region

Lewis and Kellgren (1939)[729] observed that all the essential features of renal colic, pain diffused from loin to scrotum, iliac and testicular tenderness and cremasteric retraction, can be provoked by a stimulus confined to the somatic structures of the spine. The stimulus was injection of spinal ligaments with hypertonic saline.

Kirkaldy-Willis and Hill (1979)[662] mention that lower abdominal and scrotal pain, from upper lumbar disc herniations, is not infrequently confused with renal or ureteric disorders.

Patterns of referred pain from experimental injection of interspinous tissues at the L1 and L2 segments[343] indicate that unilateral loin pain is likely to be more frequent than groin pain, but that the latter will certainly occur.

Since the first lumbar root provides branches for the iliohypogastric and ilioinguinal nerves, and together with the second lumbar root forms the genitofemoral nerve, a loin and groin pattern of referred pain and tenderness from lesions at the upper lumbar segments may be expected to occur in some.[718]

Sunderland (1975)[1193] mentions that:

In the case of the 12th thoracic and upper three lumbar nerves the lateral branch (of the dorsal rami) descends through muscle to pierce the lumbodorsal fascia just above the iliac crest before descending vertically across the crest to innervate the skin of the buttock as far down as the greater trochanter.

The clinical entity rests on the findings that pressure on the spinous processes and over the facet-joints of L1 and/or L2 elicits marked tenderness, and sometimes reproduces the loin and groin pain; pressures on the low thoracic vertebrae and ribs elicit neither tenderness nor pain reproduction.

Paige (1959)[962] classified a group of 41 such patients, who over a 2-year period comprised 10 per cent of 403 patients with lumbar spine disorders.

The group was subclassified as follows:

Group 1. Patients with pain radiating from L1 to the area above the area of the iliac crest (15 patients).
Group 2. Patients with pain referred to the iliac fossa (12 patients).
Group 3. Patients with pain referred to the genital or suprapubic area (4 patients).
Group 4. Patients whose pain in one of these areas was initiated or aggravated by menstrual periods (10 patients).

This type of problem appears to be more frequent in women during the fourth and fifth decade, and the pain often has two sites, (i) the posterolateral loin and (ii) the iliac fossa and inguinal region. Some patients in this group will have pain over the lumbosacral area as well as the groin, and a proportion of these will also have palpable signs at the L5–S1 segment, thus presenting with two problems.

The common features of low back are present, in that sitting on a hard dining chair is more comfortable than a soft easy chair, coughing and sneezing may hurt, sleep is disturbed by turning over in bed and there is painful stiffness on rising in the morning. Some may dislike walking up and down stairs. The most characteristic feature in unilateral lesions is aggravation of loin and groin pain by bending to the opposite side; in bilateral pain the same bilateral pattern emerges. Extension also provokes it but flexion and straight-leg-raising need not, although there may be an arc of pain on flexion in some. There are no neurological signs *and no disturbance of pelvic organs or functions, or sensibility changes of skin supplied by sacral nerves.* In men there may be a testicular ache which may wax and wane with the loin and high lumbar pain. The important point is that the ache is linked to the loin and groin pain.

Loin pain may be the feature of an upper-urinary-tract lesion in women. Of 100 consecutive female patients referred to a urology clinic with loin pain, 22 per cent had upper-urinary-tract lesions. In the 53 per cent of cases where the pain was provoked by movement or exercise and relieved by rest, a urinary-tract lesion was found in 21 per cent of them.

Hence the prior exclusion of visceral disease is a necessity.[371]

N.B. Careful history-taking is mandatory, and any report of groin, testicular or labial pain or ache should alert the therapist to possible involvement of the low sacral roots by discogenic or other trespass, a serious lesion in which physical treatment is absolutely contraindicated. Perineal, anal or genital pain, with numbness and/or paraesthesiae, and disturbance of sphincter function such as defective control of micturition, amount to an urgent indication for surgical opinion (see p. 150).

When lumbar and/or buttock pain is referred from the upper lumbar segments (p. 251), rotations are often painful. When loin and groin pains are more dominant, side-flexion to the painless side is often the most provocative movement.

There is a smaller group, usually tall young people (often men) in the early twenties, who stand with a characteristic sway-back posture and do not complain of loin and groin pain, but of a low and midlumbar 'background' ache, which on physical activity becomes more pronounced and migrates upwards to overlie the L1–L2 region. There is often a history of an episode of severe stress, or of habitual occupational stress. While lumbar movements are of good range and virtually painless, there is plainly a localised 'hinge' or angulation at the upper lumbar spine on extension. There are no other signs, articular or neurological, except that on palpation the L1–L2 segment is grossly hypermobile.

Young adults may present with the vertebral column listed to one or other side, or a straight spine with momentary deviation on flexion, and a history of recurrent back trouble—this immediately triggers the concept of an L4–L5, or L5–S1, shift of nucleus pulposus within an intact annulus (p. 254).

These segments are found to be innocent, and the listing corrected by localised attention to L1–L2, or L2–L3, as the case may be. Frank hypermobility at high lumbar segments is not rare in mature agricultural labourers.

The upper/midlumbar region

Lumbar osteochondrosis (Scheuermann's disease) has been mentioned (p. 242). The spread of pain from lesions of segments L2 and L3 includes the low outer loin, the upper outer buttock, outer haunch area, lateral and anterior thigh, and sometimes anterolateral leg as far as the ankle. Lesions of the L3 segment frequently refer pain to the anteromedial thigh, and those of L4 to the shin and dorsum of foot to the great toe. Pain in an oblique band across the upper posterolateral haunch and the upper anterior thigh is observed *alike* in lesions considered due to third lumbar disc trespass and in experimental injections of hypertonic saline into the interspinous tissues[343] of segments L2, L3 and L4.

Kellgren (1938)[640] and Hirsch (1963)[551] have also demonstrated that hypertonic saline injections into the intersegmental soft tissues and facet-joints, respectively, produce a sclerotome pattern of pain spreading to posterolateral haunch and limb. Patients with palpable and localised irritability of the 3rd lumbar segment (and no other)

may report pain in this distribution and also reaching as far as the lower shin.

Mooney and Robertson (1976)[867] describe their clinical experience which indicates that the intervertebral disc does not explain all low back and leg complaints. The authors injected, under fluoroscopic control, the facet-joints of 5 normal subjects and 15 patients with low back pain and sciatica, and observed that the pain referral pattern from irritation of the lumbar facet-joint is in the typical locations of lumbago and sciatica; the L3–L4 facet-joints usually produced pain down a slightly more lateral aspect of the leg.

The findings of previous investigators (p. 198) indicate that the presence of pain in this distribution does not necessarily indicate a disc lesion; changes in any or all of the structures comprising a mobility-segment may be causing the pain.

In 465 patients treated *surgically* for low back and lower limb disability,[523] almost 10 per cent had femoral rather than sciatic distribution of pain. In these 45 patients, 'it was common to find minimal restriction of straight-leg-raising, weakness of the quadriceps, diminution or absence of the knee jerk, and sensory abnormality of the anterior thigh'.

Hazlett (1975)[523] observes that *in patients who come to surgery*, the most frequent cause of femoral neuropathy associated with lumbar spine abnormality is related to discogenic or facet-joint changes affecting the L4 nerve root at the L4–L5 intervertebral foramen, and this was more common than more central changes at the L3–L4 disc level. The 'full hand of cards', i.e. all of the signs comprising a segmental neurological deficit, is not always present in all patients.

Depressed deep tendon reflexes need not invariably be taken to indicate spinal nerve root involvement.[867] Three patients with this neurological deficit had it abolished following local anaesthetic injection of lumbar facet-joints.

The possibility that diminished reflex responses may be due to segmental central nervous system disturbances, as well as to physical trespass upon nerve roots, is strongly suggested by a report[315] of four patients with bilaterally diminished ankle-jerks, in whom the verified unilateral disc lesion did not approach the opposite nerve root.

Prone-knee-bending with hip extension may exacerbate the symptoms, but back pain provoked by this test is not reliable evidence of a particular type of lesion since so many musculoskeletal structures are disturbed by it (p. 319).

Benign midlumbar joint problems tend to present in characteristic ways, with pain in the distribution described, often aggravated by extension and sometimes no other lumbar movement, and pain in the anterior thigh on straight-leg-raising; standing for too long is disliked, as is a bed which is too firm. Spondylosis and/or arthrosis of the L3 and L4 segments seems to occur together with early arthrosis of a hip rather more often than might be explained by coincidence (Fig. 6.9).

Joint problems at L3, for example, may take the form of facet-joint arthrosis, spondylosis without root involvement, lesions of disc trespass, and acquired hypermobility secondary to surgical fusion of L4–L5–S1 segments.

Hazlett[523] observes that low back pain with femoral neuropathy is not uncommon five or more years after an L4–L5–S1 two-level fusion; the cause can be an L3–L4 disc trespass but can also be a reflex disturbance from neural arch structures, which is evidenced by the fusion mass, facet-joint or spinous process overgrowth and associated inflammatory changes in soft tissue.

Anterior thigh pain and numbness, or paraesthesiae, may be considered secondary to entrapment of the lateral cutaneous nerve of thigh as it emerges through the fascia lata, or by the inguinal ligament (meralgia paraesthetica); some of these cases also have a lordotic posture and plainly a coexisting irritable, and sometimes a stiff, L2–L3 or L3–L4 segment, adequate mobilisation of which relieves the meralgia paraesthetica (p. 100).

Psoas weakness may be present in L1 and L2 lesions, and it is important to remember that spinal metastases have a predilection for the L2 vertebral body, similarly, 'meralgia paraesthetica' may be the symptom of retroperitoneal malignant tumour.[365]

Laminectomies (for want of a better term in more general use) at the L3 segment amount to around 5–10 per cent of all operations for lumbar discs—this does not mean that L3 joint problems are rare, only that *disc trespass* severe enough to need surgery is uncommon.

Pain and tenderness can often be elicited by palpation at the L3 segment when similar findings are manifest at one sacroiliac joint, in the absence of inflammatory arthropathy like ankylosing spondylitis, for example.

Sudden backache

The many problems related to the treatment of low back pain illustrate how very thin and unsubstantial are theories, with experience alone being tangible. [Finneson, 1977[356]]

Like other terms tending to have an umbrella use, e.g. frozen shoulder, sciatica and migraine, acute lumbago has no meaning more precise than sudden pain in the back. Most workers can be succinct about the essential clinical features of this event, but there is often some disparity between the histories described.

Pain developing over a few hours, and sudden backache, may present from a variety of causes (some of them visceral, like renal colic), and patients of varying age-groups will relate a variety of histories.

Farfan (1973)[326] argues that since the facet articulations are part of the intervertebral mobility-segment, 'it is not possible to distinguish with any degree of certainty between facet derangement and derangement of the whole

joint', yet while the difficulty may remain, its ultimate elucidation is not likely to be furthered much by restricting conceptions of underlying changes to derangement only. Articulations do not need to be deranged before they cause pain and other symptoms.

Since it is frequently not possible to *know*, the following classification of some examples of sudden musculoskeletal back pain must be speculative, yet may serve as a guide when planning the first moves in treatment. *The headings are suggestions for the nature of changes believed to have occurred.*

Impacted synovial meniscoid villus

Lumbar joint hypermobility may be induced by many causes, including hormonal activity in the premenstrual state and in pregnancy. Hypermobility (p. 258) is very frequently a consequence of lifting, straining, or applied trauma, and the stresses sustained by the lumbar spine are sufficient to attenuate ligaments of the intervertebral body joint and to result in circumferential tears or separation of the annular laminae (see p. 256). The resulting loss or diminution of disc turgidity, while not immediately producing any lesion of trespass, is sufficient to disturb mechanics of the facet-joints, and to allow undue gapping of these articulations during normal body movements.

The patient with sudden backache due to presumed locking of a facet-joint is usually a young female but may be a young man, and there is often a degree of hypermobility. They often excel at athletics or ballet dancing, and during some activity which may be reaching up to open a window or adjust curtains, a lumbar synovial joint locks. No outside force is applied, the condition being consequent upon a body movement involving reaching or stretching. It is reasonable to suppose that the opposed joint faces of the hypermobile segment come apart more easily than usual, and the normally slight negative pressure within the joint cavity is further lowered by the greater distraction. A villus of synovial tissue is presumably 'sucked in and nipped', and thus the meniscoid structure is impacted between joint surfaces. On resumption of normal posture the pain of impaction induces reactive muscle spasm, fixing the articulation rigidly to produce a locked joint.

Burnell (1974)[143] is of the opinion that muscle spasm, either due to primary injury or as a secondary protective response, can be a cause of very severe pain. 'Muscles in spasm around the joint cause that joint to become painful.' His view appears to lay stress on the increments of *joint* pain added by muscle spasm, and not that the muscle spasm *per se* need be the main cause of pain, at least in acute lesions (see p. 197). Extension and side-flexion towards the pain may be nearly full with pain near the extreme of range, with side-flexion to the painless side restricted early in the range and hurting more. Flexion is cautious and limited. Straight-leg-raising is limited by pain with the movement of the painless-side leg equally restricted.

There are no neurological signs. It is feasible that effusion into the joint cavity may follow, and this may assist in releasing the impacted synovial fringe, if such has occurred. The joint is sore for some days, but most appear to settle down as does an acute torticollis (p. 217).

'Locking' of arthrotic facet-joint

The patient is usually middle-aged or elderly and somewhat fat, and a degree of degenerative change of both disc and facet-joints is presupposed. The history is that of a simple non-stressful daily activity such as bending down to pick up something, adjust a shoe or get out of a bath. Sudden pain in the low lumbar region to one side fixes the patient in the flexed posture, and they regain the vertical with some difficulty.

It may be that muscular inco-ordination, slowly increasing in step with degenerative changes in vertebral joints, permits undue stress or joint-surface angulation to occur during a badly performed and impulsive bending movement of the trunk.

Pain is unilateral and paravertebral; extension, and side-flexion away from the side of pain, appear to hurt the patient most. Flexion may not appear to be very limited, but often provokes a jab of localised lumbosacral pain when tested by overpressure. In others, fairly painless flexion is performed with the lumbar spine fixed in lordosis which disappears immediately on restoration of normal freedom of lumbosacral movement by localised techniques.

There are no neurological signs and straight-leg-raising may not be limited very much, although there may be a localised shoot of pain at the extreme of leg-raising on the painful side; depending upon the patient's 'normal' there is increasing resistance to passive raising of this leg after about 45°, although another 30° or so can be traversed.

Shift of nucleus pulposus within a presumably intact annulus fibrosus

Patients with a leg-length discrepancy and thus an established mild scoliosis, secondary to a permanent lateral pelvic tilt (p. 270), show that compensation has occurred because (i) a perpendicular dropped from the external occipital protuberance would pass through the gluteal cleft, and (ii) rotation of the vertebral bodies has occurred in some (see p. 265).

While this primary postural asymmetry may give rise to secondary joint problems of particular kinds, *we are concerned here only with those patients whose pelvis is level, but whose spine is secondarily deviated, or listed, to one or other side as a consequence of the primary joint problem*; a perpendicular dropped as above would now lie across the gluteal mass on the side to which the patient is deviated or listed (Fig. 8.6). Thus a patient whose trunk appeared as 'windswept' to the left side would carry the head vertically over the left buttock, or at times over the left greater trochanter.

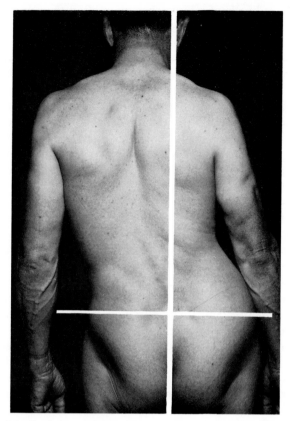

Fig. 8.6 Deviation, or listing, of the lumbar spine to the left side. Below the horizontal line, which joins both posterior superior iliac spines, the buttock contours are symmetrical and indicate a level pelvis. This deformity was secondary to joint derangement, but listing need not always be so. (Reproduced from: Bianco AJ 1968 Low back pain and sciatica: diagnosis and treatment. Journal of Bone and Joint Surgery 50A: 170, by kind permission of the author and the Editor.)

The lateral listing is sometimes compounded by a degree of postural flexion, too, or may show a component of pelvic rotation when active flexion is attempted, but the essential feature is the lateral list of the spine on a level pelvis.

Among the factors distinguishing lateral listing secondary to joint problems from fixed compensated postural scoliosis are that in the former, (i) lateral deviation is not compensated; (ii) there is usually no vertebral rotation component (see p. 265), and (iii) the iliac crests lie on the same horizontal plane.

This does not mean to say that patients with a mild leg discrepancy may not also suffer a further list which is secondary to a primary joint problem, yet the salient difference between the two conditions is plain. The coexistence of lateral list and pain does not necessarily indicate that the list is solely secondary to the pain; what it does mean is that both factors are secondary to joint derangement. The list and the pain can vary independently.[794] Pain may be completely relieved while the list remains, and presumably this reflects the continuing presence of a mechanical disturbance, or at least some tissue-abnormality which has a mechanical effect on vertebral carriage. Similarly, the list can be eradicated and the pain remain.

The term sciatic scoliosis[833] is often indiscriminately applied to the coexistence of back pain, *with or without sciatica*, but with associated secondary lateral listing of the vertebral column. This umbrella use of the phrase tends to obscure the real incidence of a large group of patients whose acute onset of backache is accompanied by either a contralateral or an ipsilateral secondary spinal list, *but who have no buttock pain to speak of, no sciatica,*[794] *no neurological symptoms nor signs, and whose straight-leg-raising is unaffected.* When sciatica, and often neurological changes, too, *are* caused by a lumbar joint derangement which induces secondary lateral listing to one or other side, the onset is usually gradual and insidious,[40] and these patients are not being considered here (see p. 264).

Since few indeed (1 : 10 000) of the population come to myelography and subsequent surgical procedures,[723] during which nerve-root-and-disc-protrusion relationships can be directly scrutinised, observations on the surgical nature of cause-and-effect between disc trespass, nerve root and spinal deviation are thus based on an incidence of 0.0001 per cent.

Because a considerable number of patients with backache and listing of the spine are successfully managed conservatively, and on follow-up over many months remain sign- and symptom-free, it is reasonable to suppose that root and disc relationships in many cases may have little to do with inducing these postural deviations. Radial cracks or fissures of the inner margins of the annulus are common during the long process of disc degeneration, and posterolateral movement of the nuclear gel may occur within an intact outer annulus[791] (p. 145), tending to force the joint open on that side. Sustained and persuasive lateral correction procedures[833] are very often successful, and it is difficult to believe that a disc *protrusion* has been 'pushed back' or 'pushed further out' by these manœuvres.

Trespass into the foraminal territory by bony articular facets has also been mentioned as a possibility.[1170]

It may be that the mechanism of derangement is other than those suggested and that on occasions the simple physical trespass of oedema, or synovial effusion, is sufficient to induce the secondary and antalgic postural deviation.

Males are affected in the ratio of 2 : 1, mainly between the ages of 25 and 50. Prolonged work in postures of lumbar flexion is a frequent factor in the history, e.g. farm tractor drivers whose work involves long hours of sitting and twisting to look behind, sales representatives who drive long distances and telephone operators who sit for long periods, are among the groups who seem prone. The precipitating episode is usually trivial, perhaps shifting a dining chair or reaching to a low bookshelf. The pain is unilateral and over the lumbosacral junction; the patient usually lists away from the painful side, and less frequently towards the painful side. It is uncommon but certainly not rare for a patient with only unilateral pain and a contralateral list to have this change under treatment to an ipsilateral list, or vice versa; the patient is unable to hold the normal posture, but tends to be comfortable when the spine is deviated to one or other side.

The lumbar spine may be flat, with the sacrospinalis musculature prominent but this is not invariably so and some have no obvious spasm.

Extension is difficult and if side-bending to the painful side be attempted it amounts to no more than a partial straightening of the list. Side-bending into the list is almost full and often painless. Flexion may be restricted and painful, but in some patients is surprisingly free and virtually painless. There may be a short arc of flexion during which the spine momentarily deviates before continuing further in the initial plane of movement. If this flexion deviation is manually prevented by the examiner,[794] a formerly painless movement may become painful at that point on the range of movement. If manual prevention does not provoke pain, the small arc of deviation is likely not to be related to the back pain episode, although this does raise the possibility of adhesions from past episodes, or some bone or soft-tissue anomaly. Straight-leg-raising is often normal and there are no neurological symptoms or signs. The segment involved may be L5–S1, or L4–L5, with the possibility that on occasions both segments may be contributing to the lateral spinal deviation. An alternating list and the more gross deviations are said to be more likely when derangement involves the L4–L5 segment, since the iliolumbar ligament stabilises the fifth lumbar segment.[218]

McKenzie (1972)[833] observed that in two-thirds of 500 such patients the responsible segment was considered to be L5–S1 and in the remainder, L4–L5. Intrapelvic asymmetry in young people, consequent upon sacroiliac joint problems, may need to be included among the factors to be assessed, since it is not rare for lumbar discogenic problems and sacroiliac joint abnormalities to coexist (see pp. 265–6).

Traumatic disc distension

Concepts and things must be given names, and the clinical features mentioned below are sometimes described by the phrase disc 'glaucoma', because this term borrowed from ophthalmology aptly describes the changes of disc congestion which are believed to have occurred.

In the healthy young disc, the imbibition function of mucopolysaccharides is so efficient that these molecules of high weight can exert a hydrophilic attraction to an amount of water nine times their own mass.[971]

Young adults of either sex report a jolt, such as landing heavily on the bottom on a hard surface or being on the wooden seat of a light van travelling on a rutted road. The sudden compression trauma to the disc may produce the vascular response of swelling, so that by taking up more fluid than normal it slightly expands in all directions, placing more tension on the annular fibres, and also the upper and lower hyaline cartilaginous plates. It is possible that small lesions of bursting may occur in the hyaline plate.

There is central or bilateral low back pain which comes on over some hours; there may be a spread of pain to both buttocks. Movements are 'globally' limited by rising pain, since any trunk movement tends to increase intradiscal tension. Similarly, a rise in trunk cavity pressures by coughing, sneezing or straining will also severely exacerbate the pain.

Sitting, which normally causes an increase in intradiscal presssure, will also exacerbate the pain, and the patient is most comfortable when lying down. There is neither sciatica nor neurological signs, but straight-leg-raising may be bilaterally and equally reduced by hamstring spasm.

Macnab (1977)[780] in briefly discussing the hydrodynamics of fluid transfer between disc and vertebral body, mentions that sudden severe loading of the spine may produce a rise of fluid pressure within *the vertebral body*, great enough to produce a 'bursting' fracture.

Presumed tear of annular laminae (Fig. 8.7)

Acute injuries of an intervertebral disc may be due to the magnitude of a single stress applied to a previously healthy disc, or to a minor but final increment of stress suffered by a previously attenuated annulus. The former is more likely to occur in young people while the latter is probably more common in mature patients.

Annular tears can occur with or without nuclear prolapse, though there may be herniation in the sense that nuclear material may bulge posterolaterally at the point of attenuation and weakening of the annular wall.

The immediate cause may be rotational bending stress;

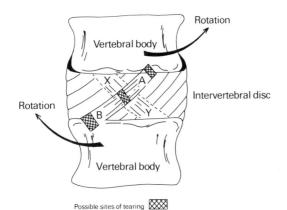

Fig. 8.7 Scheme of possible mechanism of partial annular tear by rotational stress in flexion.

Arrows indicate direction of vertebral rotation, which applies tension to fibres A–B but relaxes fibres X–Y, since attachments of the latter are approximated. The lesion could not be as neat as depicted, and probably need not be visible externally. A partial detachment of some annular fibres from the vertebral body may also possibly occur.

overcoming the inertia of a weight being lifted; a cough or sneeze while bending; a sudden jolt while carrying.

Hence the annulus gives way (i) because of a purely compressive stress, without rotation, which is transferred as sudden hoop or circumferential tension applied to the annular wall, or (ii) because of rotational tension falling heavily upon those fibrous laminae which are so disposed as to have their attachments most forcefully drawn apart by the trunk movement. This effect is more pronounced when the lumbar spine is flexed, since the facet-planes are less engaged and rotational movement is likely to be greater. Thus the common factor is excessive annular tension.

There is frequently an element of combined trunk flexion and rotation when the force is sustained. The patient is more often a young man who may both feel and hear something 'give' in the back during the traumatic incident. Immediate acute pain in the low lumbar region may very soon be felt over most of the posterior trunk, and the patient may need to be helped from the floor; it may not be possible for him to stand at all for some little while. This spread of pain has been ascribed to the tendency of the well-innervated anterior dura mater to refer pain very widely,[218] but could equally be due to the known propensity[659] for facilitated cord segments to considerably expand the pain-receptive territory of a single dermatome. A sudden and marked increase in nociceptor impulse traffic is the facilitating agent!

Depending upon the extent of annular disruption, the pre-existing state of the disc and the size of the neural canal, the subsequent events may follow several courses:

1. Provided the annular damage is not such as to completely breach it, or completely detach the annular attachment to the vertebral body, the patient may be able to stand and walk, although painfully. The pain may have spread to both buttocks.

On examination, all movements are restricted by pain but frequently one rotation will hurt very severely whereas the other will not be so painful. What is probably happening is that the most painful rotation repeats the rotation trauma and tends to gap the tear still further, while the opposite movement relaxes the torn fibres and relieves the painful tension. Hence *the history of the incident* is vitally important.

Straight-leg-raising is painfully limited on both sides, but the restriction settles to one side only when the lumbar pain is becoming more localised. Neck flexion will also hurt in the low back. There is neither sciatica nor any neurological signs, either immediately after the injury or later.

2. At the time of injury, or within hours or three or four days of the event, pain begins to spread into one buttock more than the other, and continues distally to invade the posterior thigh, calf or anterolateral leg, and ankle and foot. The neurological symptoms and signs of unilateral nerve

root involvement become apparent (pp. 160, 175) and it is presumed that disc prolapse has occurred (p. 143).

3. The posterior longitudinal ligament is ruptured and a massive extrusion of disc substance impinges upon the cauda equina. The patient lies still on the floor, apprehensive of the least movement of limbs, head or trunk, and may report numbness and/or paraesthesiae in both lower limbs. Attempts to flex the neck or test the straight-leg-raising, or even the move the patient onto a stretcher, alarm and frighten the patient. Saddle paraesthesiae or anaesthesia are evident, and urethral sphincter disturbance soon declares itself. *Surgical opinion is urgently indicated.*

The adolescent 'acute back'

The most rapid growth increase during adolescence—between 12–14 years in girls and 14–16 years in boys—tends to coincide with an increased incidence of back problems, not all of which could be labelled as 'acute'. Backache among boys appears to be on the increase; in a school population with an annual intake of 150 boys a year, the incidence rose from 6 per cent in 1969/70 to 13 per cent in 1974/75 (Grantham, 1977).[435]

Of the pupils reporting back pain the greatest number of new cases (31.2 per cent) occurred during the 15th year, and the greatest number of recurrent backaches (36.2 per cent) occurred in the 14-year-olds. Among 58 pupils (records of 11 were unavailable) with recurrent backache, the radiological findings in 47 of them indicated a prolapsed disc in 12, and spondylolisthesis in 12. Eleven boys had no positive X-ray features and in the remaining 12 there were vertebral fractures (3), marked scoliosis (3), incomplete neural arch (2), osteochondrosis (3) and ankylosing spondylitis (1).

In 36 surgically documented lumbar disc protrusions in children and adolescents,[108] the incidence in the 12–16 age bracket among male juniors was about three times as high as that of female juniors.

Children are healthier and larger than in times past, and because the whole spectrum of school athletics is increased, more games are played more intensely and to a far higher standard than before;[435] this applies equally to girls and boys, and other writers[880, 146] have drawn attention to the increased risk of joint problems when young people are encouraged to prolong and intensify physical effort at games, athletics or agricultural work, for example.

In relation to the onset of disc prolapse, Bradford and Garcia (1971)[108] noted a high incidence of trauma in their 36 cases; the fact that boys are more likely than girls to sustain a traumatic injury seems significant. Among a total of 173 patients (Turner and Bianco, 1971)[1255] under 19 years, with spondylolysis or spondylolisthesis, 74 were boys and 31 per cent had a history of low-back trauma at the time of onset of symptoms (see p. 268). In juniors there is a similarity between the signs and symptoms of disc pro-

lapse and those of disc space infection, in which there is frequently a history of trauma; this factor of trauma has also been noted in relation to cervical disc calcification in young people[322,929] and narrowing of the lumbar intervertebral disc spaces in children.[276]

Bradford and Garcia (1971)[108] suggest it is possible that some cases of disc infection in children may actually be herniations of the intervertebral disc.

In summary, acute low back pain in adolescents may indicate:

1. Disc space infection
2. Spondylolysis or spondylolisthesis (see p. 268)
3. Other lesions
4. Herniated or prolapsed lumbar disc.

Beks and ter Weeme (1975)[77] remark, as do others,[1296] that the clinical features of lumbar disc lesions in adolescents and children are essentially the same as in the adult. Significant trauma is associated in some 30–60 per cent.

A feature of the juvenile disc lesion is the severity of signs.[1066] In contrast to adults, their complaints are minimal, but objective signs are dominant. Loss of lordosis, combined with lateral curvature, is typical of adult lesions, but these changes in juniors are more pronounced. Straight-leg-raising is more diminished, and their walking and sitting difficulties are more manifest. There is usually back pain and unilateral sciatica, but this may be bilateral, and some present with sciatic pain without backache. The child has difficulty in walking because of the inability to put one foot in front of the other. There is often considerable spasm, a loss of lordosis combined with a contralateral tilt and a most marked inability to bend forward; many cannot reach the patellae. Other movements are also severely limited. Among 43 patients,[77] 39 had a mild scoliosis. Paravertebral muscle spasm was present in 37 patients. Pain is aggravated by sitting, coughing and sneezing, and relieved in a particular lying position which is not the same from patient to patient.

Straight-leg-raising is limited to below 30° on the affected side, and to between 45°–65° of the contralateral limb. Motor deficit may occur, from mild degrees of weakness to complete foot-drop.[1296] In the group of 43 patients mentioned above, 31 had absent or depressed ankle-jerks and 7 had decreased knee-jerks. Only 5 had normal deep tendon reflexes. On myelography, 39 of these children had defects indicating one or more lesions of disc trespass, and four were normal.

At operation, one or more disc herniations were found in 42 cases. The levels of the lesions were:

L3–L4	1
L4–L5	20
L5–S1	18
L3–L4 and L4–L5	1

L4–L5 and L5–S1	2
L3–L4 and L5–S1	1
	43

Among this group of young patients, there was an approximate 50 per cent correlation between trauma and disc lesions.

Traumatic tension-lesions of ligaments and of muscles with their attachment-tissues

'It would seem reasonable to assume that many of the acute and temporarily painful episodes (of the low back) are due to acute muscular, ligamentous or capsular strains.'[91]

Wyke (1976)[1362] mentions that much minor trauma to body tissues, including those of the lumbar spine, does not normally give rise to pain because the mechanical stimulus activates mechanoreceptors at the same time as nociceptors are irritated (see p. 162), and inhibitory effects upon nociceptor impulse traffic are therefore simultaneously generated.

Acute or unremitting muscular strain producing partial tears of muscle-attachment tissue is a young man's injury, where strong muscles are guarding a healthy spine,[780] but traumatic ligamentous strain may also occur in people who are less fit, and this may include traumatic flexion strains which exceed the elastic limits of the supraspinous ligament, for example. The writer has suffered one such; besides producing possibly strained and oedematous posterior longitudinal and interspinous ligaments, the supraspinous ligament overlying the insulted segment was extremely tender and very sore, exhibiting a roughening not palpable at segments above and below. The interspinous ligaments are commonly involved in hyperflexion or hyperextension injuries.[143]

Muscle attachments. Stretching or tearing of spinal muscle attachments, unassociated with other injury and due to abnormal muscle contraction associated with unbalanced or involuntary convulsive movement, does occur.[1251] Violent twisting stress, such as missing a ball at golf, or the vigorous gyrations of fast bowlers, may strain or tear some of the sacrospinalis attachments to the iliac crest. There is always a history of specific stress.[780]

Similar stress in an older man with weaker muscles and less resilient joint structures, is likely to produce strains of the synovial facet-joints or stress fractures of the lower ribs (see p. 246). (That severe and convulsive muscular exertion can be sufficient to produce fracture is manifested in the occurrence of the 'clay-shoveller's fracture', when a low cervical spinous process is fractured by the pull of muscle.[982]) There is tenderness and sometimes visible bruising over the region of the iliolumbar ligament, and the site of most acute tenderness is always paramedian. The injury is usually at or close to one attachment of the muscle, or at the point where the fleshy fibres joint a tendon or an aponeurosis.[1251]

The most provocation of pain occurs when the specific stress is repeated as a testing movement, either as resisted muscle contraction or as passively applied tension.

This having been said, it sometimes happens that the signs of an assumed muscle-attachment tear, secondary to some positional stress or body movement, may be quite considerably abated during a treatment session by joint mobilisation with repetitive and gentle persuasive techniques. A history of either producing or sustaining specific violent force is important for the decision that a tension-injury has occurred.

LUMBAR SPONDYLOSIS

In the sense that many low back problems are not of acute onset (although there may be acute episodes in the continuing history), 'lumbar spondylosis' seems the appropriate generic term for a representative list of these chronic states.

Lumbar instability (p. 139)

'The spine acts as a supporting column and provides flexibility. To do this it cannot be limp. In addition to its flexibility and elasticity, its expansile turgescence gives it stability, and internal resistance to movement like a loaded spring.'*

The notion that an intervertebral body joint may be unstable, or less stable than it should be, by reason, e.g. of an excessive degree of *translation* movement being added to sagittal plane movements seems unacceptable to some, despite clear evidence[872] that this occurs, that it hurts and where indicated surgical fusion of the unstable or 'sloppy' segment can relieve the symptoms and signs of it.[720]

The successive crossed fibrous laminae of the annulus (Fig. 1.22) can be likened to layered sections of flat coiled springs, which lie one inside the other and act as if the springs were under a distraction force, thus tending to approximate the vertebral bodies and their hyaline plates against the resilient resistance of the nucleus.[508] Gravitational compression tends to reduce the height of the nucleus pulposus and enlarge it circumferentially; annular elasticity provides restraint. Disc turgidity, or turgescence, is probably entirely due to the elasticity of the fibres of the annulus fibrosus which encompasses the nucleus, and not to an inherent expansile property of the nucleus pulposus itself. This hypothesis has been experimentally tested,[508] the results strongly suggesting that it is correct. Thus 'expansile turgescence' refers to a healthy disc system in which the nucleus is at all times under a varying degree of restraint, and that if this restraint is reduced by failure of either the annular restriction or the integrity of the hyaline cartilaginous plate, or both, the

* With acknowledgement to the unknown author.

balance of forces and biomechanical properties are disturbed; the resilient stiffness of the disc system of that mobile segment is diminished, with the consequent sequelae of additional and progressive ligamentous strain.

Lumbar instability is defined as 'a loss of integrity of controlling intersegmental soft tissues, and of the balance of restraint against disc expansion'.[926]

The condition has no relationship to the generalised ligamentous laxity in inherited diseases of connective tissue like Marfan's syndrome or the Ehlers–Danlos syndrome.[705, 1365]

A physical mass, i.e. the human body and its component parts, must obey physical laws; it cannot do otherwise. Yet also subject to physical laws are muscle tension, tissue fluid content, vascular flow and venous engorgement; the changes in these factors are governed by spinal segmental reflex systems, themselves under the influence of higher centres, i.e. brain-stem hypothalamus and cerebral cortex.

Intervertebral instability—'the most common form of insufficient performance in the mobile space between two vertebrae'[1093]—will manifest itself earlier or later according not only to a given ergonomic circumstance but according to other factors too, which are equally important but which are not given enough recognition by those who conceive the spine only in terms of a mechanical engineer.

Latent instability, the initial stage of loosening of the motor segment, may through specific influences or additional stimuli be transferred into overt conditions, with typical symptoms and signs.

The probable mechanisms of loosening have been outlined (p. 139). In the early stages, loosening can be compensated by muscles, the mechanoreceptors initiating spontaneous reflex controlling mechanisms. Repetitive overstress finally leads to insufficiency of the compensating mechanisms, and the cause for this is usually a specific event, which Schmorl and Junghanns (1971)[1093] call 'the additional stimulus'. 'Through this stimulus, a quiescent insufficiency is transferred into a recognisable performance-weakness, meaning disease symptoms.' This is mostly a mechanical stimulus, but it can also be allergic, thermal, toxic, climatic, endocrine or even psychic. 'The more attention a physician pays to *the changing nature* [my italics] of vertebral complaints, the more he will become convinced of the significance of the additional stimulus.' Exciting causes, which may make manifest a previously covert mobility-segment insufficiency, are coughing, sneezing, compression, unfavourable body torsion, vibration, percussion (motor-cycle, motor-car, horse riding), straightening after bending (with or without added weight), sitting in constrained positions, getting out of bed, bathing, stepping awkwardly off a kerb or bending to scratch a knee.

The non-mechanical stimuli mentioned above have an unfavourable effect, e.g. cold and dampness may have a negative effect on blood vessels and nerves and may cause muscular tension. 'As far as allergic, toxic, climatic and endocrine influences on muscles are concerned, they may be considered as similar influences upon the motor segment—in the end, a mechanical influence.'

The psychic influence is also mechanical in its end-result, the psychically unstable patient frequently transferring his personal difficulties into a physical ailment. With the appearance of slight lumbar pain, 'the patient is in a stage of fearful, tense expectation that a new attack of pain will occur. With the slightest indication the complaints, the wrong movement or spasm induce muscular changes which provide the "missing additional mechanical stimulus".' The stimulus initiates a new attack with all its consequences (p. 115).

Types of patient: (a) *The tall young man* (see p. 252); (b) *the young nurse/housewife*
The patient is in the late teens or early twenties, and relates a history of a sudden jolt while under load, i.e. lifting a patient, or a hyperextension injury when hitting the water from a high diving board. There may have been the sensation of feeling something 'go' in the back. Because the pain is not too bad the patient continues working, but is aware of a chronic, persistent ache across the low lumbar region, sometimes spreading to buttocks and upper thighs. The ache is aggravated in the 'slouch-sit' position, premenstrually and when tired. The foetal position when sleeping aggravates pain, and the patient may wake in the small hours with pain severe enough to necessitate getting up (with some difficulty) and walking about to relieve it.

The nagging low backache is constant or nearly so, and may savagely remind the patient of its presence on any attempt to reach for a child or working tool, drive or walk any distance, or attempt a normal amount of housework. Standing or sitting for an hour or so may become a burden. Sooner or later the patient finds she can do whatever she wants to, e.g. stand, sit, shop, bend, but for no longer than about 15 minutes. The patient often gives a history of prolonged conservative treatment of various kinds, and because of her failure to respond to therapy begins to doubt that there is anything *physically* wrong with her, and to feel that she is odd.

On examination, posture is unexceptional and movements are very full, often without pain. Significantly, the characteristic ache will soon appear if patients are asked to remain in extension, for example. Further, the patient may show a little wriggle, or hesitation (with pain) at about 30°–45° of flexion or extension or both, as she appears to 'ride over a milestone' on the way down or on return. During this arc of pain the patient may grasp the thighs for support. Usually, there are neither distal leg pains, neurological symptoms nor neurological deficit, and straight-leg-raising may be 100° on each side without pain. Blood tests are negative. The patient is very likely to be told she is imagining the pain, or to be regarded by the busy clinician as work-shy, inadequate or a back-slider.[924] Lateral X-ray films at the extremes of flexion and extension may reveal a hypermobile lumbar segment, although often without the 'slip' of degenerative spondylolisthesis, which enlightened palpation during careful passive tests will reveal anyway. The segment is often L4–L5.

Frequently, straight X-rays with the patient in orthodox postures will show nothing. During radiography it is necessary to use positions which will allow the soft tissue insufficiency to declare itself.[1184a]

(c) *The postsurgical patient.* A year or so after surgical fusion of the L4–L5 and L5–S1 segments, a minority of the patients report for follow-up appointments and describe a pain of somewhat different distribution to that of the chronic problem for which treatment was originally sought. The pain is still lumbar but higher up, together with periods of feeling much the same pain as of old. On examination, 'hinging' is plainly visible at the L3–L4 segment, and palpation during a passive test of physiological movement confirms hypermobility at that segment.

There is no sciatica or neurological deficit, and at this stage no thigh pain of femoral nerve distribution.

It may be that the higher backache is sufficient to provoke facilitation of adjacent cord segments, and thus 'lights up' the old and remembered pain of times past (p. 173).

(d) *The 'keep-fit' enthusiast* may be prone to ensure his continuing spinal mobility in a somewhat excessive and obsessive way, and overstress his vertebral connective tissue with vigorous daily exercise. As normal and often clinically silent degenerative changes proceed, the connective tissues binding one particular segment (often L4–L5) are never afforded the chance to undergo the slow and natural adaptive shortening which accompanies degenerative change; the consequence is that of hypermobility of one and sometimes two segments. The site and extent of the excessive intervertebral movement depend to an extent upon the type of 'keep-fit' activity, and the possible incidence of more violent sudden strains as in judo, wrestling and gymnastic mat-work. These recurrent episodes, in the process of disc degeneration with hypermobility, characterise the nature of the syndrome.

Joints which are unduly lax may be injured by minor trauma easily sustained by stable joints during everyday activities, and the facet-joints will share in this segmental overstress. Traumatic synovitis, with serous or haemorrhagic effusions, may lead later to secondary osteoarthrosis.[705] The clinical features are very much the same as in (b) above, but the spinal movements may not be as markedly free as in young women, and the patient may present initially as an 'acute back episode' following some particular stress. An assessment of the temperament of the patient, the nature of his activities and the history of previous episodes, together with the examination findings of palpably excessive movement at one segment, provide a clue to the real background of the patient's problems.

(e) *The young man in his twenties with undetected lumbar osteochondrosis*, stiff middle and upper lumbar segments, and an overstressed, irritable and unstable L5–S1 segment has been mentioned on page 243.

(f) *The mature woman between 40 and 50 with degenerative (group III) spondylolisthesis* (p. 147) will describe being troubled by chronic pain for months, years or decades. It occurs less often in men.

'Long-standing soft-tissue instability causes degenerative changes in the intervertebral joints. Late in life this may result in facet insufficiency and secondary subluxation forward.'[921]

The L4–L5 segment is normally more mobile than other lumbar segments, and is the one most commonly affected.[780]

Pain in the low back, buttock and thigh is almost universal and usually described as a constant, nagging ache. It is rarely severe, but there may have been several past episodes of sharper pain involving first one buttock and thigh or leg, then the opposite haunch and limb in a subsequent episode. Some describe a 'heaviness' and 'weakness', or a 'burning' quality to the pain. The symptoms are frequently bilateral but asymmetrical. Some may present with thigh pain and no current backache, although they may have had backache for years previously; others have bilateral backache but no thigh pain.

Many do not like standing for too long and get relief from sitting, but may need to change this position, too, in favour of moving about lightly or changing the chair. Some patients report difficulties of negotiating kerbs and steps because of their reported limb 'heaviness' or 'awkwardness'. A few may actually limp at times. All of a series of 200 cases[1058] had a smaller lumbosacral angle, i.e. less lordosis, than normal. There may be only minor articular signs apparent on cursory testing, although overpressure at the extremes of a seemingly acceptable range may sharply provoke the back pain, and sustaining the extreme position of a lumbar movement will elicit a steadily increasing ache. *Many can touch their toes with ease.* Besides pain, there may be cramp, tingling and numbness in leg and foot.

Although this is the type of spondylolisthesis most often associated with neurological signs, they are by no means always present, the most constant frank deficit being that of depressed knee- or ankle-jerk.

Muscle weakness of root distribution may need to be carefully looked for since it is often slight, and straight-leg-raising may be normal.

In Rosenberg's[1058] series of 200 patients, the 5th lumbar root was most commonly involved in neurological deficit, and the most frequent sensory change was diminished sensation to pinprick on the lateral aspect of the thigh.

Saddle anaesthesia or paraesthesiae, and sphincter problems, are very uncommon.

On X-ray, the degree of slip is not great, but when L4–L5 is involved the L4 vertebral body is seen to shift forward on flexion and backward on extension. Myelography in severe cases will show an hourglass constriction of the dura at the segment concerned; root entrapment may be due to a diffuse annular bulge and to buckling of the ligamentum flavum, and Macnab (1977)[780] describes it as a form of segmental spinal stenosis.

In a study of 50 patients, 25 with group III spondylolisthesis and 25 without, Gomez et al. (1977)[423] verified the clinical impression that arthrosis of the hands occurs much more frequently in those patients with Group III degenerative spondylolisthesis. As a corollary, there was a higher than expected frequency of degenerative spondylolisthesis in those patients with extensive arthrosis of the hands.

The man 'fearful for his back'

He may be over 40, and in past years suffered a probably minor episode of back trouble. Perhaps because of his temperament, combined at the time with a strongly worded caution from his doctor to take care, the patient has lost all confidence in the health and durability of his vertebral column.

From time to time, further minor episodes serve only to convince him of the dire need to strengthen his defences, and not to 'push his back too far'. He is probably faithfully wearing his fourth or fifth successive lumbar support, from which he is parted with some difficulty, and on being asked to move his back during examination does so with trepidation, needing encouragement to allow his spine to be subjected to a full movement test. Movements are globally limited by stiffness rather than pain, and the dominant features are (a) the patient's caution and (b) the lack of any significant abnormality other than stiffness due to disuse. There are no neurological symptoms or signs, straight-leg-raising is somewhat reduced bilaterally by resistance rather than pain, and on palpation there is no objective evidence of a segment being different from its neighbours, all of them being stiff and eliciting an over-cautious voluntary muscle-guarding response.

Although a degree of degenerative change may be radiologically evident, it is consistent with the patient's age and unexceptional. Provided the patient is sleeping well, has no history of a primary neoplasm or signs of possible ankylosing spondylitis, it is highly likely that he needs to have his confidence restored, and the natural durability of his back demonstrated to him.

'Time-dependent' backache and sciatica (p. 201)

Provocation of pain in backache and sciatica is as a rule 'stress-dependent', i.e. particular movements or postures aggravate the pain, and other movements and postures tend to quieten it down or relieve it; in general these particular movements and postures are known well enough, and are useful in gaining clues as to the likely nature of the patient's problem. For example, the patient who hates standing and walking and prefers to sit, especially with his elbow resting on his knees, is more likely to be suffering from mild degenerative trespass into a congenitally narrow spinal canal than from a frank disc trespass into a roomy neural canal.

There is a singular group of patients whose symptoms and signs appear to be time-dependent, i.e. characteristically their symptoms steadily increase throughout the day, from a comparatively pain-free morning to a regularly pain-racked evening, almost regardless of their occupation and activities during the day, and these have a 'saw-tooth' behaviour.

On rising in the morning, the patient is virtually symptom-free but by the late evening the symptoms have come on with real force and the patient is glad to get to bed. While in the late forenoon or early afternoon standing or walking may give more relief than sitting, neither of these give any relief at all by late evening, and the patient must needs lie down. This regular diurnal waxing and waning of symptoms according to time rather than stress characterises the syndrome, and the important factor appears to be that of increasing gravitational compression, i.e. whether sitting or standing. This is just another form of stress, of course, but the more dominant factor appears to be time, and this remains true whether the complaint is backache alone or backache with sciatica.

For example, a 31-year-old housewife with left low lumbar pain, coccydynia and posterior thigh and calf pain to the heel regularly awoke with minimal pain and stiffness, and just as regularly suffered her worst pain and disability by late evening. Previous bouts of pain every 9 or 12 months appeared to have had their origin from when, aged 18, she had fallen heavily on her back. The pain distribution during the last three episodes was similar to the present episode, which began in the back without identifiable cause and spread to the heel within a few days. The coccydynia waxed and waned with the other pains. The whole leg felt numb and cold, as did the four outer toes, but only the lateral border of the foot had any objective sensory loss. The pain steadily increased throughout the day, and was aggravated by sitting, driving and bending; coughing produced a jab of back pain but no leg pain. Standing and walking were easier than sitting at first, but later in the day walking provoked the same pain as did sitting. Rising from the sitting position was painfully slow and awkward. Posture was unexceptional; lumbar extension provoked the backache only, flexion was limited by back and posterior thigh pain when her fingertips reached mid-shin. Straight-leg-raising was left 75°, limited by left lumbar pain, and right 90° with similar left-sided pain beginning at 75° and increasing to 90°. On palpation, the L5 spinous process was very sore to Grade 1 central pressures, as was the left lamina. On passive physiological-movement testing the L5–S1 segment was patently hypermobile. There were no other palpation signs of note, and the coccyx was only moderately tender.

The chronically overstressed labourer's back

The patient is typically 45–55 years old and a strong, solidly built stocky man,[421] commonly a steel erector, agricultural worker, gravel-pit or building labourer, whose characteristic appearance is that of large muscular shoulders mounted atop a long lordosis. The abdominal wall is strong and the patient's belly is protuberant in a long curve from sternum to groin. The glutei are large and strong, and the patient stands on massive legs with a four-square John Bull stance.

Pain is reported as lying across the middle and low lumbar region, spreading to loin and upper buttock and often into the inguinal region on one side. There are neither sciatica, neurological symptoms nor signs of root involvement.

The pain, which began insidiously some months before, appears to be as solidly implanted as the patient's stance on earth, is not very reactive and is virtually continuous.

The dominant factor is pain behaviour, in that it increases within one hour of work at his usual occupation and it disturbs sleep. The patient cannot work, and is not getting proper rest.

Lumbar movements, which are limited not by pain but spontaneously by natural resistance, provoke the pain only moderately, and the patient has difficulty in describing which movements hurt most, since none of them are especially more painful than others, although each may hurt a little. If anything, side-flexion away from the painful side hurts more than side-flexion towards. Flexion has some slight resemblance to bending forward, in that the whole magnificent edifice of the patient's trunk is ponderously lowered a little in the general direction of his feet, with little apparent change occurring in the curvature of the trunk; the movement does not increase the pain. Straight-leg-raising is never more than 65°–70° bilaterally, and has little effect on the pain. Manual testing of segmental accessory movement is likely to do more damage to the therapist's hands than to the patient and only reveals that there is no irritability. Passive physiological-movements test (PP–MT) reveal a *relative* lack of movement (there is not much anywhere!) at the L2–L3–L4 segments.

The X-ray appearances are characteristic with generalised sclerosis, somewhat rounded upper and lower edges of the lumbar vertebral bodies, and 'bowing' into the spongiosa of the hyaline cartilaginous plate. The bowing is markedly outlined by sclerosis.

Slow-onset backache and sciatica (the 'equinox' syndrome)

In the sense that sudden backache may include pain beginning at once or within three or four hours of a period of physical stress or a traumatic incident, there is a different type of onset characterised by a more delayed response. Typically, the patient has become filled with the 'divine discontent' of spring, or with irritation at the sight of autumn leaves cluttering the flower beds, and in either case spends many hours of unaccustomed physical effort in the garden. Other typical histories are those of moving house, some hours of enthusiastic but amateur bricklaying or laying a concrete path. Alternatively, the patient may have taken a long car-ride to visit aged parents and spent a night or two in a very soft bed. The mild lumbar stiffness and trivial discomfort pass off after a hot bath but by next morning, or sooner or later during that day or the next, backache comes on with real force and is accompanied by severe lumbar stiffness. Either then or within hours or days of the onset of the severe lumbar symptoms, pain may either be felt spreading distally to buttock or posterior thigh, or may be felt simultaneously in the upper calf and buttock of one limb. The pain may distribute itself in a fairly common pattern which more or less accords with a dermatome (Fig. 2.20) but just as frequently remains a patchwork, e.g. of pain in the low back and buttock, upper calf and outer border of the foot. Some patients will declare their worst pain to be at the posterolateral haunch, others will point to the calf as the worst pain. Some will describe 'a long band of toothache' from buttock to toes. There may be some low lumbar pain on the contralateral side.

Passive neck-flexion aggravates the backache and often the sciatica, and a cough but more particularly a sneeze may savagely provoke a jab of pain from buttock to heel. The patient walks with difficulty, but prefers to stand or lie than to sit. A dining chair is more comfortable than an easy chair, and when the patient rises from either the process is a slow and cautious rearrangement of lumbar posture. For a minute or so the patient may not be able to stand fully erect.

While sphincter disturbance is rare, it can occur (p. 150), and appears due to involvement by trespass upon the 4th sacral root.[218]

Much more common is a degree of constipation because sitting and straining at stool is painful and attention to toilet equally so.

The sciatic leg may feel cold, and *be* cold, and there may be paraesthesiae and a sense of numbness of the whole limb or only the posterolateral part of it; sometimes the patient declares the whole foot to be numb, or can be quite precise in that the three outer toes are known to have some loss of sensibility. The extent of objectively diminished sensibility is generally somewhat smaller than that reported, and more often lies distally. Some patients report 'strips of cold' down the outer aspect of the limb, and others complain bitterly of cramp in the calf. Unpleasant 'burning feelings' are less frequently described.

The patient sleeps more comfortably on a firm mattress on the floor, yet still wakes feeling painfully 'locked' for an hour or so in the morning. Depending to an extent upon whether a single root of the sciatic nerve or more than one root is involved, and the extent of the involvement, there may be some difficulty in walking, not only because the whole limb is painful but the foot also feels useless. In severe cases there may be a dropped foot.

Physical tests. The patient stands uncomfortably and prefers to put most weight on the unaffected leg. Extension is limited and may hurt in back and buttock only or in the whole of the painful limb. Side-flexion towards the painful side is more likely to do the same than side-flexion away from it. Flexion is cautiously attempted, because it is usually the most painful and limited movement. The pelvis may tend to rotate to the opposite side. Neck-flexion when supine aggravates the lumbar pain and sometimes the sciatica. The jugular compression test (p. 63) may do the same, more especially when simultaneous pressure is applied to the abdomen. Straight-leg-raising may be reduced by 10°–15° on the painless side, but is frequently less than 35° on the affected side, with provocation of pain from buttock to heel. The test may 'light up' paraesthesiae for some time afterwards.

Neurological deficit (which is not confined to this syndrome only) (see p. 160) tends to follow patterns of root distribution, although not as consistently as is sometimes asserted; ascribing the lesion to this or that segment on the basis of neurological findings is not an exact science.

Muscle weakness does not necessarily accompany every episode; by no means does every patient show 'the full hand of cards' of neurological deficit.[1207] Many patients with disc prolapse have minimal neurological signs.

Thus a patient with lower sacral, coccygeal or perineal pain and with no neurological deficit must not, willy-nilly, be taken for an L5 lesion with idiosyncratic pain reference; the possibilities of a lower sacral root lesion (see below) must always be borne in mind.

The infrequent L3 involvement is declared by weakness of quadriceps and sometimes psoas, and a loss or diminution of the knee-jerk.

Provocation of pain on the 'femoral nerve stretch test' does not always occur, and conversely, this test often provokes back pain arising from lesions at the L4–L5 and lumbosacral segments.

If the L4 vertebral segment is involved, there may be postural deviation (listing) to one or other side, or the patient may be straight when standing but list to one side or other on flexion. Power loss in L4 root lesions occurs most frequently in the foot dorsiflexors, and the knee-jerk may be diminished or absent in some.

Postural deviation may also occur in lesions at the L5–S1 vertebral segment.[833] Lesions of L5 root are manifested by loss of great toe extensor power and weakness of tibialis posterior, with loss of the great toe-jerk.[1207]

S1 root involvement is declared by loss of power in peronei, calf and hamstrings, and a depressed or absent ankle-jerk. On buttock contraction the gluteal mass may feel less hardened than its unaffected neighbour.

S2 root palsies do not involve the peroneal muscles, but the calf, hamstrings and gluteus maximus are weak.

S3 root interference is declared by pain in the upper inner and posterolateral thigh, a lack of deep tendon reflex or muscle power changes, and pain encroaching upon the perineal region.

Pain, numbness and paraesthesiae in the perineal and genital area characterise S4 root involvement, and to lesions of this root are ascribed weakness of bladder and/or rectum.[218] On the other hand, Ross and Jameson (1971)[1062] hold that single nerve root lesions are unlikely to cause bladder dysfunction.

Because the cauda equina is more likely to be trespassed upon by central protrusions, which need not declare themselves as dramatically as in 'Presumed tear of annular laminae' (3) (p. 256), it is prudent to enquire about 'saddle' area sensory changes and the function of sphincters in *all* cases of backache (see p. 150).

A common clinical course is as follows: Severe leg pain usually diminishes with the appearance of neurological signs, but the limb may remain cold, feel numb in a variety of distal distributions, and also feels somewhat weaker than its fellow. The sensory changes largely disappear, not infrequently leaving a small circumscribed patch of objective sensory loss for two or three years or longer.

Unless the neurological involvement is multiradicular (p. 107), normal muscle power is recovered in some 10–30 weeks, depending upon the nature of involvement.[1369] If more than one root is involved, power may still be reduced two years later (see p. 108). Operative treatment gives no better prognosis for rate of muscle power recovery than does conservative treatment.[1295]

WHAT HAS HAPPENED IN THE LUMBAR SPINE?

The attractive black-or-white explanation on the basis of 'disc in' or 'disc out' has much to commend it, since it has the charm of nice, simple revealed truth[514] and this is always popular, even when descriptions include *varieties* of 'disc in' and 'disc out'.

The simplistic view that disc lesions are either cartilaginous or pulpy will no longer do; histological examination[1203] demonstrates that the extruded material is something of a mixture.[780]

A real difficulty is that we cannot always know, but what

we can be sure about is the variety of changes, and combinations of these, which may be underlying the clinical features. Awarness of the types of disc herniation and prolapse (p. 145), formulated on the basis of an incidence of 0.0001 per cent, should be accompanied by awareness of other documented changes, e.g. the seemingly irritant nature of the products of disc degeneration and the presence of arachnoid adhesions and trespass by tissues other than the intervertebral disc (see p. 151).

Since myelographic evidence of disc trespass need not be accompanied by either symptoms or signs[552] the presence of disc herniation or prolapse should not invariably be taken to indicate the single cause of clinical features.[445]

Hirsch, in 1971,[549] suggested that a bulging disc narrowing an intervertebral foramen is not the only cause of pain, and that it was not rational to consider only the intervertebral discs as sites of stress. Having passed through an 'extreme operative phase' in the management of low back pain, he mentions the possibility of actually creating disability by cutting into discs which are not bulging and interfering with nerve roots or perhaps otherwise causing pain.

Certainly, root pain and root signs for which no adequate cause can be found at operation are common enough.[137, 545] Therefore, it might be more compatible with observed fact to adopt the premise that some patients have sciatic pain of root distribution because they have an irritated hyperalgesic nerve root;[750] they may or may not have a 'disc lesion' accompanying it. They do not have to have a 'disc lesion', and even if they do, it need not necessarily have anything to do with *causing the pain*, other than possibly making it worse.[445]

Sciatica without backache

With no period of backache preceding the appearance of unilateral leg pain, it begins insidiously in youngish men and for no apparent reason, starting more often in the posterior thigh but occasionally in the upper calf. The pain then proceeds more or less as in the syndrome just described, except that frank neurological signs do not often accompany the pain, which is seldom very severe. While there is no pain in the back, lumbar movements aggravate the pain, especially flexion but sometimes also side-flexion towards the painful side. Flexion is sometimes very limited and the patient may rotate his pelvis to the opposite side during the attempt to bend forwards; straight-leg-raising may be less than 35°. Sciatica without backache is unusual, and in a series reported by Lansche and Ford[695] the incidence was only 1 per cent. Those handling spinal problems all day and every day will probably note a slightly higher incidence.

Presumed adhesions of lumbar roots and/or sciatic nerve

The patient, more usually a mature young man, back at work after a recent bout of backache and severe sciatica, describes minimal pain in back, buttock and leg, but considerable restriction because he cannot bend lower than to touch his patellae or tibial tubercle, and appears to rotate his pelvis to the opposite side when attempting flexion. Sitting up in a bath, or sitting up having breakfast in bed, are impossible. Both flexion and straight-leg-raising on the affected side, which is reduced to 40° or so, are limited more by strong resistance than by pain, and such pain as there is may be felt in the low back but especially down the posterior thigh to the knee.

A dominant feature is the lack of any other articular sign; some residual weakness of the calf, for example, and absence of the ankle-jerk, are not noticed by the patient, whose main complaint is that of the functional restriction (see p. 461) imposed on dressing and bending to the floor. Long periods of sitting, as in driving a car, may increase the backache and leg 'stiffness' but these are mentioned by the way, and not as the main nuisance-restriction of lack of flexion.

N.B. An underlying causal relationship[466] between chronic cervical degenerative change and changes in superficial connective-tissue attachments of upper limb muscles (e.g. 'tennis elbow') is now more widely considered than in the past, yet the same relationship between low lumbar degenerative change, and changes in the attachment-tissues of lower limb muscles, does not seem to be as well appreciated. For example, many patients with chronic lumbar degenerative changes may report 'sciatic' pain which is worst over the lateral aspect of the knee joint, and may spread down the anterolateral leg almost to the ankle. Careful palpation may not infrequently detect that the most acute provocation of this pain is caused by rubbing a fingertip across the anterior ligaments of the superior tibiofibular joint. While some of this group of patients do, in fact, have a coexisting joint condition for which the superior tibiofibular joint requires mobilising in its own right, many can be relieved of this 'sciatic' pain by transverse friction alone precisely directed to the ligament mentioned.

Sciatic scoliosis

Following the progression of acute backache (p. 256) to sciatic pain, or more commonly the *insidious onset* of backache and then sciatica (p. 262) with neurological signs, a proportion of patients will show newly acquired lateral lumbar deviation on standing, and this will usually be secondary to the joint problem.

The incidence of slight lateral listing is higher than seems generally supposed, because minor degrees of deviation may be undetected or are ignored.

On the basis of surgical findings, the vertebral segmental characteristics may be as follows:

L4–L5—protrusion is often lying in the root 'axilla'
  the listing is towards the side of pain

passive neck flexion in supine lying does not provoke back pain
contralateral straight-leg-raising does hurt.

L5–S1—the listing is usually away from side of pain
passive neck flexion does hurt
contralateral straight-leg raising does not hurt.

The side to which the spine is listed is explained on the basis of nerve-root and disc-protrusion relationships[218, 239, 780] (p. 200). The mechanisms postulated are as follows:

1. When the protrusion is lateral to the nerve root the patient will lean away from it.

2. When the protrusion is medial to the root, i.e. in the root axilla, the list will be towards the side of pain, and during flexion the deviation will often increase. In both of these cases the posture assumed is regarded as that which seeks to relieve the pain of root compression or irritation.

Macnab (1977)[780] believes these observations to be somewhat simplistic, since the sciatic list disappears on recumbency. He mentions that the loss of lateral curvature on recumbency differentiates sciatic scoliosis from structural scoliosis; spinal deviation and sciatic pain are not necessarily interdependent, as we have seen (p. 254).

3. A contralateral list may change to an ipsilateral list while the sciatic pain remains in the same limb, and this can be due to a nerve root stretched over the summit of a protrusion.[794]

4. Alternatively, a particular type of mid-line protrusion may underlie the phenomenon of an alternating list with alternating sciatica, depending upon posture and movements of the lumbar spine.

In (3) and (4), the space-occupying effects of a mobile, pedunculated or sequestrated mass of disc substance can be underlying the changes of spinal posture. Alternating deviation is sometimes regarded as diagnostic of a disc protrusion at the L4 segment.[218]

The criterion that an absence of *vertebral* rotation, in standing, distinguishes (a) the 'sciatic list' secondary to recent joint problems from (b) the compensated postural scoliosis requires, like most rules of thumb, some qualification.

In postural scoliosis due to a short leg the vertebral bodies tend to rotate to the side of the convexity, but rotation need not always occur and when present, is not always to the convex side.

Stoddard (1969)[1180b] reports a study[54] of 545 erect radiographs, which showed that 45 per cent of spines showed a convexity to the short-leg side, 32 per cent showed convexity to the long-leg side, and 23 per cent showed a straight spine. These were not clinical assessments, but observable and reproducible signs; a little more than half of the patients with unequal leg lengths *not* showing a convexity to the short-leg side.

It must therefore be accepted that a fully reliable datum on the basis of vertebral rotation, for comparison between sciatic listing and postural scoliosis, does not exist, at least so far as the factors of lateral curves and vertebral rotation are concerned.

If we make the assumption (which may or may not be justified) that there were no examples of horizontal plane *pelvic rotation* in this series, the criterion holds good for about 75 per cent of cases only, and then only so long as the side of the convexity is ignored.

Should *pelvic rotation* also have occurred in this series, which it does in some cases of leg length inequality, then it might be recalled that a degree of pelvic rotation inducing vertebral rotation is not rare in sciatic scoliosis.

Two of the more reliable factors helping distinction between the two conditions are:

1. A history of 'listing' coinciding with onset of the current joint problem, and having been absent before it (yet patients are sometimes blissfully unaware that they are moderately listed to one side, and may have been so for some time).

2. A plumb line from the external occipital protuberance does not lie in the gluteal cleft but to one side of it.

Sustained and persuasive manual correction procedures are usually unsuccessful in both sciatic scoliosis with neurological deficit and in postural scoliosis which has been compensated. Patients with sacroiliac joint problems may also suffer sciatic scoliosis.

The factors of intrapelvic asymmetry, as well as postural rotation of the whole pelvis, must enter into consideration. It is known[105] that there is in some patients a tendency for the ilium, on the long leg side when there is leg length inequality, to be 'rotated' backwards, and that this induces the sacral ala of that side to shift backwards and downwards, tending to impose a rotation to that side of the 5th lumbar vertebral body, presumably by reason of attachments of the iliolumbar ligament. The opposite ilium tends to 'rotate' forwards. Since the longer leg will often induce a general postural convexity to the *opposite* side, and the lumbar vertebrae will tend to rotate towards the convexity, while the L5 vertebra is induced to rotate towards the side of the concavity, there must be set up opposing mechanical stresses which might be (a) sources of the pain accompanying these postural abnormalities, and (b) a possible explanation of the variety of lumbar postural changes seen on standing X-ray films.

Two of the writer's recent patients exhibited quite weird combinations of pelvic distortion, unilateral lumbar flattening, lumbar and thoracic scoliosis with rotation, accompanied by sciatic pain to the popliteal space but no neurological signs. The marked asymmetry and deviated restricted movements were normalised during a single treatment session in which only localised sacroiliac techniques were employed.

Clinical experience suggests that a simple sacroiliac joint shuffle (for want of a better word) can, at least in youngish women, underlie some cases of so-called sciatic scoliosis.

Further anomalies (p. 24) of the lumbosacral region are common, and among these are a tilted upper surface of sacrum and a trapeziodal-shaped fifth lumbar vertebra (Figs 1.28, 1.29, 1.30).

These considerations can never be left out of assessment of what has transpired to cause the listing in sciatic scoliosis (see also p. 254) and assessment of the sometimes weird postures demonstrated by these patients during lumbar movements.

A transitional L5 vertebra will sometimes produce lateral deviation which very closely simulates sciatic scoliosis, and these patients may present with a history of mild aches but a recent and sudden onset of low back pain, associated with some stress such as reaching into a car. One such patient (Fig. 1.30) had a perfectly level pelvis but her spine was listed to the right side. The X-ray revealed a transitional and trapezoidal L5 vertebral body, and manual prevention of deviation during active flexion aggravated the pain which accompanied normal forward bending. Her pains were completely relieved by moderate posteroanterior pressures on the *left* posterior superior iliac spine; the writer is unable to explain this.

As ever, and like the vagaries of referred pain (see p. 192), the single factor of infinitely variable biological plasticity may serve to produce mechanical postural 'solutions' (of the various opposing stresses) which can be highly individual from patient to patient and which often are not amenable to snap judgements or facile authoritarian pronouncements as to their true nature. Simply, we cannot always know.

Patients with sciatic scoliosis usually list away from the side of pain, and if the deviation is accompanied by lumbar rotation when standing, it *may* not have anything to do with the current sciatic episode (*vide supra*). Some may present with loss of lordosis and deviation to the less painful side, while a few will show a fixed lordosis with deviation to the painful side. When extending, the lumbar spine may deviate further to the affected side, but when flexing, the pelvis may rotate to the unaffected side. Others will initially deviate further on flexion and then straighten out to bend forward with a perfectly straight back, returning via the same lateral deviation to assume a standing posture with its characteristic list. Many will progressively increase the degree of lateral list during their limited range of flexion.

Side-flexion to the side of the list is the most free and least painful movement, but also sometimes provokes the pain to a degree. Surprisingly, some patients are able to moderately side-flex to the opposite side, although there may be a short jab of pain during the restricted movement. In both slow onset backache and sciatica (p. 262) and in

sciatic scoliosis, when surgical exploration has been planned on the basis of myelographic findings of disc trespass, the intensity of the pain seems to have no relationship to the size of the disc protrusion.[91]

The clinical features otherwise resemble those described in the 'equinox' syndrome (p. 262), with the exception that patients with sciatic scoliosis tend to be referred for surgical opinion rather more frequently since a recent and dramatic alteration in the patient's posture usually initiates a more energetic plan of action.

Young people may retain some lateral deviation for a year or more following relief of back and limb pain by conservative measures; among mature adult cases who come to surgery the relief of symptoms is not always accompanied, either immediately or for many months, by straightening of the spine. Some adults appear subsequently to go through life with a more or less permanent slight list to one side, in the presence of an otherwise normal radiographic appearance.

Provided there is no sphincter disturbance and pain is neither intense nor prolonged, immediate surgical attention is not necessarily indicated, although a recent and *disabling degree* of spinal deviation does amount to the need for surgical opinion.

Patients who may be flexed forward and deviated away from the painful side, and walk into the treatment room with a recently acquired lumbar posture which resembles a banana, will almost certainly be suffering from the trespass occasioned by *oedema and effusion*, whatever else may have occurred, and it is a mistake to abandon conservative treatment before fluid congestion at the site of the lesion has had time to settle; a gratifying change to a virtually straight spine in standing, and a considerable lessening of pain within two to three weeks can occur, although the neurological changes will alter little in that time.

The 'listing' which also occurs in juvenile spondylolisthesis resembles that due to lumbar joint derangements; by eliminating the source of irritation the spondylolisthetic scoliosis corrects itself spontaneously.[91]

THE SOFT TISSUES AND LOW BACK PAIN

Movement-techniques used in treatment cannot help but be applied for the most part to the soft tissues, and in a real and important sense one is very often not mobilising or manipulating joints so much as mobilising the soft tissues, with all the potentialities for affecting nerve impulse traffic, skeletal and also smooth muscle tonus, tissue fluid exchange and arteriolar, venular and lymphatic flow. The soft tissues are of primary importance (pp. 110, 196).

As between changes in an articulation as such and changes in the soft tissues related to it, the genesis of many chronic joint problems is not easy to clarify in terms of which are primary and which are secondary effects.

The following factors have been discussed:

1. The probable contribution of secondary muscle spasm to the total pain produced by an *acute* joint problem (p. 197).

2. The factor of *chronic* 'spasm' or muscle shortening, with accompanying changes in relative population of fibre-types, which appear to be the secondary and established sequel to chronic degenerative change in joints (pp. 117, 199).

3. The likely *genesis* of chronic vertebral joint conditions, secondary to established imbalance of muscles because of abnormal occupational or habitual postural use of musculature (p. 113).

Burnell (1974)[143] made an e.m.g. study of patients with back pain who had undergone rhyzolysis procedures (p. 520), and was interested to observe that quite large segments of the sacrospinalis muscle had been denervated. Since it is not possible for rhyzolysis procedures, by cutting, to denervate the apophyseal joint itself, Burnell has suggested the distinct possibility that denervation of muscle may be the factor which is responsible for relief of pain achieved by these procedures.

In passing, a somewhat similar observation was made[1100] after a number of arthrodeses of the sacroiliac joint had been performed for intractable painful conditions which followed low spinal surgery. Patients lost the intractable pain immediately after the operation, and the authors concluded that relief of pain might well be due to neurotomy of fine nerves, performed incidentally during the approach to the joint.

Burnell considers the muscles as being of more significance, in the causation of back pain, than may have been appreciated, and that any techniques which will reduce muscle spasm and pain are well worth trying. An important factor, perhaps, is that patients who undergo rhyzolysis, either as a first treatment or because they have been referred to Pain Clinics specifically for the procedure, have usually had an intractable joint problem for some time, and the factor of *more chronic secondary changes in paravertebral muscles* may be of first importance.

The facts that (i) the pain is very frequently relieved completely, and (ii) functional abilities are quickly restored, (iii) nothing is done to *the joint* itself, indicate that the observations of Burnell and others are of importance in the management of back pain.

In the absence of *recent* violent muscular stress, acutely tender areas along the spinous processes, and maximally over the tips of the transverse processes[143] may be palpated; they appear to resemble a particular type of tennis elbow in which chronic and unremitting strain is an important factor. That vertebral *joint* problems may initially have induced a low-grade collagenosis in these specific regions of muscle-attachment tissues (see p. 188) should not be discounted, but the condition resembles that of lateral epicondylitis, and appears to be related to chronic stress.

The lordotic low back

Among the middle-aged, a common presentation is that of symmetrical low back pain, associated with a lordotic posture but unassociated with limb symptoms or neurological signs and occurring somewhat more frequently in men. Pain is aggravated by standing (patients frequently mention museums and art galleries) and walking, but relieved by sitting. The patient stands with a hollowed low back and a somewhat lax and protuberant abdomen, sometimes giving the impression of 'too much beer, too many babies'. Extension and either side-flexion movement provoke the characteristic pain, while flexion does not, but during painless bending forward (which may be a little restricted but otherwise unexceptional to cursory examination) the low lumbar lordosis does not change and movement occurs largely at the middle and upper lumbar segments; similarly, the soft tissues overlying the lumbosacral region will appear flattened on a tangential view during flexion.

Straight-leg-raising is of normal and virtually painless range for the patient's age-group. Palpation reveals a degree of stringiness and a lack of plump resilience, which normally characterises the feel of healthy relaxed muscle, overlying the low lumbar segments. The fifth lumbar vertebral spine is tender, as are the immediately paravertebral regions on either side. The lumbosacral segment is also stiff on passive physiological-movement tests.

The syndrome is distinguished from spinal stenosis (q.v.) by the *absence* of limb pain, paraesthesiae and neurological signs.

It appears to be a chronic muscle-tightness entity because simple treatment procedures which stretch the lumbosacral soft tissues, and strengthen the abdominal wall, frequently relieve all the signs and symptoms of it (Fig. 6.8).

Common variants are as follows: Middle-aged patients may present with a bilateral chronic lumbar ache, worse on one side than the other, with pain spreading bilaterally into the upper posterolateral haunch area, but additionally into the groin and anterior thigh of one side. The groin and thigh pain is worse at night and commonly the backache is not, although both are painfully stiff on rising in the morning.

Movements are stiff, and all provoke the pain to a degree; extension, and side-flexion to the side of the groin pain, are the more painful. Flexion is characteristic in that the low lumbar area takes little part in the movement, a localised lordosis being maintained in flexion. Straight-leg-raising is commonly almost full for the patient's age but limited on the side of groin and haunch pain; there are no neurological signs. Examination of the hip on the most painful side reveals that it, too, shares in the limited movement. Plainly the patient has combined low lumbar joint problems, chronic lumbar muscle change and an early osteoarthrotic hip joint.

Besides the localised attention required for the early arthrotic hip, there is a lack of complete response to soft-tissue stretching procedures only, for the low lumbar musculature; it appears that both spondylosis and arthrosis of the lumbosacral segment are contributing to the clinical features and need treatment attention in their own right.

Sometimes there appears to be no *joint* problem at any segment other than L3–L4, in which case this is the one which requires localised treatment together with the other procedures, and at other times the lower three lumbar segments will all require attention.

Meralgia paraesthetica, a burning pain on the antero-lateral aspect of the thigh with numbness and tingling, is often attributed to compression or irritation of the lateral femoral cutaneous nerve as it passes through the lateral end of the inguinal ligament, i.e. an entrapment neuropathy. Investigation of changes in nerves at the site of soft-tissue entrapments does not always yield positive evidence of damage (p. 100), and it is perhaps significant that the patients are mostly obese,[222] and very often have a pronounced lordotic posture.

The so-called entrapment features are frequently relieved by eradicating the lordosis by flexion exercises, improving the patient's posture and strengthening the power of the abdominal muscles and it may well be, therefore, that the real cause is foraminal constriction of a root of the femoral nerve, due to an habitually lordotic posture reducing the vertical dimensions of the intervertebral foramen.

Meralgia paraesthetica may also follow surgical fusion of the L4-L5 facet-joints, but the symptoms usually subside within a few weeks of operation.[326]

Internal disc disruption

Crock (1970)[211] has observed that, 'The whole issue of disc lesions is wider and more complicated than can be explained on the simple basis of disc-tissue prolapse alone', and describes the clinical features of a large group of patients with a singular type of disc pathology, which involves:

1. alteration in internal structure of the disc
2. changes in its metabolic function
3. local tissue changes in the immediate environment of the disc but excludes escape of disc material from its normal confines, i.e. physical trespass does not occur.

Depending upon the site of the disc involved, the patient describes a deep-seated dull ache, with pain in an associated limb of an intolerable aching character. The symptoms become more widespread, and a constitutional illness is declared by intractable spinal pain (usually un-influenced by physical measures such as manipulation or traction), nausea, weight loss and severe headache. There may be visual upsets, altered temperature appreciation in

limbs and transient episodes of weakness in the affected limbs, so that there is difficulty in gripping or walking. There is a very low tolerance of physical activity and the patients dislike travelling in bumpy vehicles. There is restricted spinal movement, but rarely any signs of somatic root interference; straight-leg-raising is usually unaffected.

The pathology is not fully understood, but appears to span the fields of biochemistry and the mechanics of disc nutrition.

During interbody fusion procedures, the sympathetic trunk may be found matted to the disc affected, and para-vertebral lymph nodes may be enlarged. Adjacent vertebral bodies show increased vascularity, marked softening and altered density. The disorganised disc tissue is soft, slightly yellow and has altered staining properties. Amorphous tissue, and fibrillation of the annulus, are seen.

The relationship of these changes to disc disruption is uncertain, and disc narrowing is not observed.

The clinical features might be due to irritation of structures adjacent to the disc by leaking of disc metabolites, and/or the production of autoimmune reactions by the same metabolites entering the general circulation.[547]

SPONDYLOLYSIS AND SPONDYLOLISTHESIS: Group I and group II

[Degenerative (Group III) spondylolisthesis is described under Lumbar Instability (p. 258), and Groups IV and V on p. 147.]

Spondylolysis and spondylolisthesis need not *per se* be responsible for symptoms. Severe degrees of slip may fortuitously be discovered in patients who have no backache and whose physical activity is vigorous. The coexistence of (i) neural arch defect, with or without olisthesis, and (ii) back pain, sciatic and/or neurological signs need not mean that the radiological and the clinical features are directly associated.

Juvenile spondylolysis without olisthesis or slip
(see p. 146): Group II

While the pars articularis defect is not a congenital lesion, its familial incidence has been clearly demonstrated,[91] and there is a strong hereditary component in the aetiology of this fatigue fracture.[1326] The incidence of appearance of *the lesion* is greatest between the ages of $5\frac{1}{2}$ and $6\frac{1}{2}$ years, and the reason for this is not known; it is not rare for the pars interarticularis defect to be discovered very much earlier.[1329] There is uncertainty as to whether the pars fracture is due to an extension injury[1250] or a flexion stress.[327]

The average age for appearance of *symptoms* is 14 in girls and 16 in boys, and the clinical manifestations are those of lumbar instability.[922] In a group of 59 patients under 19 years, with spondylolysis,[91] boys outnumbered girls 50 to 9. A little over a third of the 59 patients gave a history of significant trauma at the time of onset of symptoms, most of these traumatic incidents occurring during school athletics. Fifty-five complained of pain in the back; 4 had no pain and the pars defect was incidentally discovered. Of the 9 girls, 8 had back pain, half with trauma and half without trauma. Only 12 had *unilateral* defects of the pars, and in 55 of the group the lesion was at L5. When the lesion is at the lumbosacral level, the average age of the patient is lower and the lesion more likely to be associated with spina bifida occulta; there is often attenuation of the bone.[921]

Some patients with the defect will have symptoms severe enough to warrant surgical fusion, others will not. Of the 59 mentioned above, 24 had minimal symptoms and no neurological signs and on follow-up over 1 to 9 years 18 of them had no significant discomfort. Most of the remainder of the group, while suffering some discomfort which necessitated lumbar supports and some restriction of activity, had neither disabling pain nor neurological deficit and did not require surgery.

Juvenile spondylolisthesis

'The difference between spondylolysis and some types of spondylolisthesis is probably only a matter of degree, dependent upon variations in the age of onset, stability and subsequent stresses and strains.'[922]

Forward slipping is permitted by (i) facet deficiency or subluxation (group I); (ii) loss of pars continuity (group IIa); (iii) attenuation and elongation of the pars (group IIb).

While facet dysplasia is a congenital defect, it is probable that all three deformities can be acquired as a result of soft-tissue failure, excessive lordosis and trauma; the latter two occur frequently in toddlers.[922]

The most severe degrees of slip are seen[1188] in those with group I (dysplasic) spondylolisthesis, where congenital abnormalities of the upper sacrum or the arch of L5 allow the olisthesis to occur.[1329] Girls outnumber boys by two to one.[1188]

Group IIa occurs more commonly in boys than in girls, and is at the lumbosacral level with a defect in the pars interarticularis of the 5th lumbar vertebra. Many have no symptoms and need no treatment.

In group IIb spondylolisthesis, the forward slipping seldom increases after the age of 20 and is more common in adult males.[780]

Bianco (1971)[91] describes 114 patients aged 7–19 years; boys outnumbered girls by 78 to 36. The severity of slip was graded as 1 or 2 (p. 146) in 97 patients, and graded 3 or 4 in 17 patients. In an overwhelming majority of them (110), the spondylolisthetic segment was L5. Spina bifida was present at either L5, S1 or both segments in 27 of the group. Only 17 (14.9 per cent) had associated scoliosis. Significant trauma occurred in only 30 cases.

The onset of backache may be quite sudden and this type of onset is termed by Macnab (1977)[780] 'the listhetic crisis', although when the patient is seen the main complaint may only be that of back pain of long duration. A few complain only of postural deformity, of changes in trunk contour and attitude. The patient presents with a rigid lumbar spine, and in a handful there will be a scoliosis due to spasm, this scoliosis resembling the 'list' of sciatic scoliosis (p. 264). There is flattening of the buttocks, anterior rotation of the pelvis,[91] a flat and prominent sacrum and sometimes severe hamstring spasm inducing the patient to stand and walk with bent knees.[780]

In severe degrees the site of the lumbar slip may be visible, and there is apparent shortening of the trunk, sometimes with bilateral loin creases. On forward flexion, the patient is sometimes unable to reach beyond the patellae.

There are varying degrees of straight-leg-raising limitation, with gross bilateral limitation sometimes.

Of the 114 mentioned above, 15 had varying degrees of hamstring tightness. Less than 20 per cent had neurological signs.

Fifty-three of the 114 patients were treated by surgical fusion, and neither during the operation not at myelography were any disc protrusions observed. Patients with the highest grade of slipping tended to have the least back pain.[91]

Adult spondylolisthesis

It has been suggested[1313] that spondylolysis and minor degrees of spondylolisthesis may be a commoner cause of chronic low back pain than is appreciated.

Group IIa spondylolisthesis is a common *incidental* finding in mature people, but may give rise to clinical features in some (Fig. 1.29c). Group IIb is found mainly in middle-aged men, usually at L4–L5 but at higher levels, too.[1188]

Trespass may give rise to radicular symptoms, with much leg pain from lumbar root involvement added to the back pain. The fibrous tissue thickening, at the spondylotic break in the pars interarticularis, is responsible for most of the trespass upon the 5th lumbar root.

The clinical features of lytic lesions (group IIa) will depend on the level at which they occur. After 20 years, increased slip at the lumbosacral level is rare, probably because of the stout processes and firmer attachments, via the iliolumbar and lumbosacral ligaments. At the L4 and L3 levels, the degree of slip may increase in adult life, more especially if L5 is sacralised.

Increased mobility due to a pars defect at L4 increases the stresses imposed on the 4th lumbar disc, hastening degenerative processes. There is also an increased incidence of trespass upon the cauda equina, and consequent neurological symptoms and signs, since the neural canal is normally slightly stenotic at vertebral segments L2, L3 and L4. In some, a marked deterioration in symptoms occurs with the increased slip.[597]

Spondylolysis predisposes the subjacent disc to early degenerative change; spondylolisthesis does not occur without disc degeneration. 'The local causes of pain in spondylolysis, with or without a slip, are instability, foraminal encroachment on the nerve root, extraforaminal entrapment of the root, and disc degeneration.'[780]

Making the radiological diagnosis of spondylolisthesis does not mean that treatment for 'the slip' is necessarily indicated. In mature adult patients with low back or limb pain, the question to be answered is: 'Does the pain come from the olisthesis or from the associated disc degeneration?'

It may be difficult to separate those patients in whom a discogenic (spondylotic) episode is underlying the presenting symptoms. A lengthy history of periodic episodes, rather than continuous difficulties, favours a discogenic cause.[983] Also, if pain is unilateral and worse on sitting, it is likely to be arising from the degenerative disc changes and not from the slip, but if pain is bilateral and worse on standing, but easier on sitting or flexion, it is likely to be due to the slip itself, since flexion tends to reduce the shearing stress on the segment involved.

The younger the patient the more likely is the pain to be due to the slip itself, and Macnab (1977)[780] suggests that in the combination of spondylolisthesis and back pain, (i) if under 30, the defect is likely to be the cause of symptoms; (ii) if between 30 and 40, the defect might be the cause of symptoms; (iii) after 40, the spondylolisthesis is uncommonly the cause of symptoms.

An exception is that in group III (degenerative) spondylolisthesis, when neurological signs are present they are likely to be arising from the unstable spondylolisthetic joint, and this is frequently the L4–L5 segment. He tabulates the possible causes of pain derived from, or associated with, spondylolisthesis as follows:

Instability at the defect
Foraminal entrapment of a nerve root
Degenerative disc changes above or below the slip
Hyperlordosis
Degenerative changes at the thoracolumbar region
Unrelated pathological lesions in the spine, such as neoplastic disease
Psychogenic low back pain.

The appearance of the back is characteristic, with an unduly long sacral region, possibly a degree of scoliosis and pronounced but asymmetrical loin creases. There may be a visible depression overlying the fifth lumbar vertebra, depending upon the nature of the spondylolisthesis. The three clinical manifestations[922] are:

1. Symptoms due to *instability*, i.e. pain in the back and spreading to both buttocks and thighs; this is of mesodermal origin from connective-tissue structures and muscles with their attachment-tissues.

2. Symptoms due to *root involvement*, which are not uncommon.[780] There may be chronic irritation of spinal roots by the mass of tissue surrounding the defect in the pars interarticularis;[922] decompression by removal of the loose neural and surrounding tissues has provided good results.

While the intervertebral foramen is enlarged by the forward slip of the vertebral body, the free neural arch may be tilted forward,[780] and trespass downwards upon the nerve root. The pedicles of the listhetic vertebral body may also descend upon and thus kink the root on each side, and the corporotransverse ligament may do likewise. Disc prolapse, much more commonly at the level *above* that of the subluxation, has also been found responsible for root involvement.

3. *Cauda equina lesions* may be precipitated by trauma and stress upon the defect producing sensation loss in the buttocks, backs of thighs and calves, and bladder dysfunction.[922]

Spondylolysis in the aged
The accepted incidence of 5–7.5 per cent of spondylolysis[780] in the white population does not appear to hold good for all age-groups. A radiological study of 125 unselected geriatric patients, aged over 65, revealed an incidence of 12 per cent.[899] Very frequently, a prespondylolytic stage was observed, in which it appeared that attenuation and weakening of the pars interarticularis was caused by compression of the bony isthmus by articular processes of the vertebra above and below, probably contributed to by thinning of discs. Thus the acquired nature of the condition, at one end of the age scale, is evident.

Lateral pelvic tilt (Fig. 8.8)
Assessments of body alignment and symmetry can only begin at the pelvis, with its 'abstract ideal' posture accepted as a hypothetical norm and employed as the datum for assessing the presence or absence of changes in (i) the support of the pelvis, i.e. the lower limbs; (ii) symmetry and posture of the pelvis itself; (iii) symmetry of superincumbent structures, i.e. the spinal column.

We must first find abnormality, and then decide whether it is significant and thus a likely factor in producing the symptoms reported; somtimes it is not.

Recognition of the infinite range of biological plasticity, the infinite potential of the body for adaptation of both structre and function, efficiently and painlessly, seems sometimes to be lacking when we determinedly take up the hunt for 'rules of thumb' which will make our clinical preoccupations less onerous.

Clinical impressions are that many patients with back-

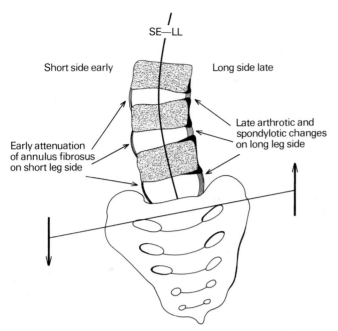

SE—LL

Short side early   Long side late

Early attenuation of annulus fibrosus on short leg side

Late arthrotic and spondylotic changes on long leg side

Fig. 8.8 Scheme of anteroposterior view of tilted pelvis due to leg-length inequality.

ache can be shown to have leg-length differences of more than 1 cm, but, 'There is no detailed information on the effect on the spine of a lateral pelvic tilt due to leg-length discrepancy' (Farfan, 1973).[326]

'Almost every pathological change to which back pain has been attributed has subsequently been demonstrated in the symptom-free population.'[1248] Conversely, Stoddard (1969)[1180b] showed that more than twice the number of patients presenting with backache had a short leg, compared to a control group without backache, although 40 per cent of the group with backache did not have leg-length inequality.

Hult's (1954)[580a] statistics indicated that differences of up to 3.75 cm were not often associated with backache.

Nicholls (1960)[931] observes:

There is no general agreement on the incidence of leg length inequality in otherwise normal subjects, or on how much this difference may be associated with symptoms. The recorded incidence of difference in leg length will depend upon the methods of assessment and the selection of subjects. The smaller the unit of measurement the greater will be the incidence, and the larger the unit of measurement the greater will be the agreement between observers.

Estimation of relative leg lengths is difficult by any clinical test.[105] Accurate clinical assessment of the horizontal alignment of iliac crests is also more difficult than may sometimes appear, not least because spinal column deviation from the mid-line may unwittingly influence visual assessment, e.g. because on sagittal viewing the spine is not straight, it is subconsciously assumed that the pelvis *should* be tilted to one side or other. It is not always easy to avoid finding what one wants to find, or

expects to find, and nowhere is this more true than in clinical assessment of pelvic posture in the frontal plane and in assessment of the presumed changes in intrapelvic relationships.

The presence of congenital anomalies such as a tilted upper surface of sacrum and/or a trapeziodal-shaped body of L5 help to compound the difficulties, by slightly inclining the low lumbar spine to one side or other; these can exist in the presence of a level pelvis (Figs. 1.28, 1.30). Conversely, it is extraordinary how deceptive appearance can be, and that the iliac crests appear level and the spine appears straight is no guarantee that an a-p erect film of the whole pelvis and lumbar spine will not reveal postural and bony anomalies *to which, were they not known, few clinicians would think of ascribing the genesis of low lumbar backache* in the presence of the clinically assessed straight spinal column.

Combined changes in normal orientation of the pelvis can also occur due to leg-length differences, with resulting kyphoscoliosis.

If, for whatever reason, the upper surface of the sacrum is not level, it is reasonable to assume that asymmetrical strains are imposed upon the lumbar, and very probably thoracic, spines, yet it does not invariably follow that *pain* will ensue, or if it does, that pain reported must be due to the abnormal strains.

Other factors given, it seems equally reasonable to assume that a child who grew up with leg-length inequality would simultaneously also develop the joint-and-soft-tissue adaptations which provided developmental compensation for this asymmetry. Evidence is not lacking[220] that this occurs at the other end of the spine where although the forces are lighter, so also are the weight-bearing masses of bone which sustain them.

Developmental asymmetry in the lower half of the body can take a number of forms and can occur in a number of anatomical locations, e.g. leg length, angulation of the femoral neck, form of the ilia, shape of the sacrum and the lumbosacral disc and configuration of the articular facets concerned.[1093]

Solonen (1957)[1157] describes the disposition and area of sacroiliac joint surfaces as not always similar when sides are compared in the same individual.

Farkas (1932)[339] quotes precise measurements to indicate that a physiological scoliosis exists, with a curvature to the left in the cervical, upper thoracic and lumbar region in 80 per cent of people, and a compensatory lower thoracic curvature to the right. In the remaining 20 per cent, the curvatures are reversed, and the factor of stronger thoracic muscles on the right side is mentioned as a cause. Plainly, occupations which involve heavy unilateral use of upper limb muscles during adolescence and early manhood may accentuate this tendency.

When there *is* a lateral pelvic tilt due to inequality of leg length, it would be expected that in some young people compensatory adjustments could occur in the soft tissues, with slight but significant changes in the joint-surface dispositions of the sacroiliac and pubic joints, the lumbosacral segment and succeedingly higher segments of the lumbar and thoracic spines. In many, there occurs a lumbar convexity to the short leg side and a thoracic concavity to the long leg side. In others (see Sciatic scoliosis, p. 264), convexities and concavities are reversed, and in yet others the spine remains straight; Stoddard (1962)[1180a] gives radiographic evidence that in this last group with straight spines, the leg-length discrepancy appears to have been taken up in a proportion of patients by adaptations of the sacroiliac joint disposition, with the result that the erect posture at lumbar and thoracic spines remains undisturbed. Thus, a short leg does not necessarily produce a pelvic tilt, nor a scoliosis,[1180a] nor *need* it produce pain, as we have seen.

Neither, at least in children does compensatory or other torsion of the sacroiliac joints, where these can be assumed to have occurred, disturb the horizontal level of the iliac crests.[736]

Backache does indeed occur due to the strain created by lateral pelvic tilt in some, if only on the basis that provision of a heel lift on the short leg commonly, though not always, eradicates the back pain. Sometimes the back pain is made worse by a heel raise (q.v.) and in 28 per cent of the control group of Stoddard's[1180a] series with a short leg of 0.5 cm or more (8 per cent with 1 cm or more) there was no backache.

In summary, the purpose of these observations is to suggest that things are not always what they seem, and that 'deformity need not make pathology' could be added to our rules of thumb.

Where unequal leg lengths have produced a lateral pelvic tilt, changes seen on the short leg side from behind are:

A flattering of normal curved outlines of both loin and haunch
A wider gap between hanging arm and loin
The iliac crest is lower
A lower posterior superior iliac spine dimple
A lower gluteal mass
The gluteal cleft is tilted to the short leg side
The gluteal fold is at a lower level
Lumbar scoliosis with convexity to the short leg often occurs, but it can be to the opposite side in some[1180a] and in others there is no scoliosis
In flexion, a tangential view shows the pelvis to appear rotated to the long leg side.

If the postural changes completely disappear with the patient sitting on a hard flat surface, leg-length inequality can reasonably be assumed. If the postural changes wholly or partially remain, this can suggest well-established soft-tissue changes and/or that there may be congenital or acquired changes in the pelvis itself.

Persisting soft-tissue changes, e.g. psoas spasm,[736] can disturb the orientation of pelvic joints in children, and it is not always easy to decide when this factor of alteration in soft tissue may be the primary cause, or secondary effect, of postural changes affecting the pelvis in young people.

Further, Schmorl and Junghanns[1093] have suggested, 'These anatomical facts should not blind us to the fact that the psyche has a profound influence on posture.'

Changes of pelvic joint disposition are discussed on page 279. Often there is no history of injury or occupational stress, but some patients will date the onset of joint problems from a particular incident, which is frequently more trivial than the extent and nature of the pain would suggest.

Backache and leg pain secondary to lateral pelvic tilt have a tendency in some to present according to a chronological pattern (Fig. 8.8):

1. Probably because of a degree of elongation and attenuation of the annulus fibrosus on the short leg side, disc prolapse with root involvement and sciatica on that side are likely to be the clinical features when trouble starts during the patient's twenties.

2. When problems arise later in life, and it is surprising how late they can be, the features are those of combined arthrosis and spondylosis of the long leg side, with the earlier emphasis on purely discogenic changes and probable sciatica with neurological signs now tending to be absent. In general, the pains are now more localised and less distal.

Thus, the more mature the patient, the more likely are the radiographic appearances of vertebral joint compression on AP films, whereas in the younger patient with quite severe sciatica, straight X-rays may show nothing other than the postural changes present.

Common clinical features of this category of chronic lumbar joint problems are: the patient is usually over 50 and reports recurring episodes of unilateral backache, with sciatic pain to the back of the knee. During the severe stage, pain may spread across the low back, but settles to the usual side as it becomes subacute.

Walking and standing, and sitting without comfortable support, provoke the pain. There is considerable stiffness after immobility, e.g. on rising in the morning, and after sitting, even with comfortable support, for more than 30 minutes. The patient rises cautiously from the chair, and appears to have to 'readjust' his lumbar posture by standing for a moment or two, before he is able to walk away.

Typically there are no neurological symptoms. (Although this does not mean to say that mature patients may not present with symptoms and signs of neurological deficit. They will very frequently describe long previous trauma of some severity to the low back, such as falling heavily on the buttocks on a concrete floor.)

On examination, there is leg-length inequality of some 1.25–2 cm, the pelvis being tilted upward on the affected side. There is pelvic joint asymmetry, in that the posterior superior iliac spine is 'shuffled' backwards on the affected side. The pattern of movement-restriction falls into two subgroups, i.e. a small proportion whose unilateral lumbar pain is aggravated by side-bending *towards*, and a much larger group whose pain is provoked by side-bending *away* from the painful side. In both, extension is limited by resistance as well as provocation of the unilateral pain, and lumbar flexion in both groups is virtually full and painless, the low back rounding well as a rule; in some, a degree of lumbosacral lordosis may still be apparent in full flexion, albeit the movement is uninhibited and much the freest of all.

The straight-leg-raising is free, unrestricted and normal for the patient's years. Usually there are no neurological signs.

A variant of this particular group is represented by the example of a 43-year-old gamekeeper, who had been discharged from the Army 20 years before with 'a slipped disc'.

Following some stress three weeks before, when he had pulled a loaded trailer behind him for some distance, he presented with a pelvis tilted up 2 cm on the left side and a left low lumbar and buttock ache which spread to the popliteal space on walking, and also changed to a throbbing ache then. He had a constant, moderate but variable ache, with a symptom-free right side. He slept well, and was not especially troubled on rising in the mornings. Sitting aggravated his ache, initially and briefly, and then it subsided. On rising from sitting, however, and on getting out of a car after a moderate journey, his epithet for the severe but temporary aching stiffness was 'bloody murder'. A cough or sneeze hurt him in the back but not in the leg. Lumbar extension and both side-flexions were stiff and limited by resistance, not pain. He could flex only to touch his upper shins, the range being limited by left lumbar pain as well as resistance. The assumption that his normal flexion range was probably more than this was based on the straight-leg-raising range, which proved to be right 80° and painless, but left 55° and limited by left lumbar pain.

While passive neck-flexion in supine slightly provoked his lumbar pain, he had no neurological symptoms or signs.

Gentle repetitive central vertebral pressures to L5 provoked the throbbing ache associated with walking, but also improved his left straight-leg-raising by 20° to 75°. His flexion range remained unaltered. Flexion had increased by 6 cm at his next attendance, and by adding double-knee flexion to the mobilisation treatment, his straight-leg-raising increased to 80° and he flexed to his ankles. Six months later, he remained trouble-free.

Adults in their thirties and forties may have a lateral tilt which is well enough compensated in standing and walking and when sitting in soft chairs, but not after prolonged sitting on a hard chair. If such a person changes to an occupation which involves being seated thus for many hours, unaccustomed backache may begin.

There are other consequences of leg length inequality[261] which are not considered here.

Sagittal pelvic tilt

It is commonly stated[326] that the cervical, thoracic, lumbar and sacral vertebrae form a continuous curve in the foetus and the impression may be gained that the same applies to the newborn child. So far as the lumbosacral angle is concerned this is not so[1287] and in relation to the long 'C' of the rest of the column, this lumbosacral 'reverse' curve is conspicuously present as normal anatomy in the neonate. The plane of the upper surface of S1 vertebral body forms an angle with the horizontal of about 30°. The more the sacrum is tilted forward the greater the angle, and vice versa. The lumbosacral angle is here taken to mean this angle, as a measure of sacral tilt in the sagittal plane; it cannot refer to lordosis of the whole lumbar spine, which is a compound curve although some authorities, e.g. Rosenberg (see pp. 139, 260), use the term to mean the angle between the lumbar spine and dorsum of the sacrum. There is no significant difference between the female and the male lumbar curve.[326]

While the three factors of (i) an abnormally increased lumbosacral angle; (ii) gravitational stress, and (iii) low lumbar degenerative joint disease, appear interrelated to a degree in some, the notion that this is a direct consequence of some failure of natural evolutionary processes, because man has adopted the erect posture, is fallacious.[1338]

Variations of sacral disposition in the lateral view, when the angle may vary from 20° to almost 90°, and of the sacral profile itself, have frequently been considered together with 'abnormalities' of sagittal spinal curvature, and a diathesis to one or more joint conditions of the lumbar spine, pelvic girdle and hip joints has been postulated on the basis of these observations.[445]

In a series of 182 lumbar spines, there were only 3 examples of Schmorl's nodes occurring at the lumbosacral joint, and this might possibly be due to inclination of the segment to the line of gravity.[326]

In a study of static postural effects upon the aetiology of arthrosis of the hip, Guttman (1970)[476] differentiates three pelvic types according to the magnitude of the lumbosacral angle, i.e. the 'steep' pelvis with angle greater than 45°, which is said to overstress the hip joint; the 'neutral' pelvis with an angle between 36° and 44°, and the pelvis with an angle of 35° or less, when the longitudinal axis of the sacrum is nearer to the vertical than to the horizontal.

Investigations on 132 healthy people showed that roughly one-third belong to each category. The significant point may well be '132 healthy people'. Highly competitive athletic activity during adolescence[880] is probably just as important in the genesis of hip arthrosis as that of an aesthetically undesirable and 'abnormal' lumbosacral angle.

Schmorl and Junghanns (1971)[1093] assert: 'The differing degrees of angulation play an important role and influence the statics and dynamics of the spine as well as the birth canal. ... Critical evaluation of all available investigative results makes it difficult to diagnose an abnormal lumbosacral angle and it is even more difficult to consider it as a cause of pain.'

In general terms, an habitual posture of segmental or regional hyperextension of the lumbar spine appears responsible for more joint changes and recurrent backache than the posturally flat lumbar spine,[335, 780] but not all authorities are agreed on when a lumbosacral angle may be regarded as abnormal, and some still advocate the cultivation of a lumbar lordosis during resting positions and occupational activity.

Farfan[326] observes that in spines with large lumbosacral angles, it would appear the discs are better able to withstand compression loads; also, the fifth lumbar joint appears better protected from torsional strains. The latter effect would seem to depend upon the orientation of facet-planes, although Lumsden and Morris[769] found that this factor seemed to be of no consequence in governing the amplitude of rotation at the lumbosacral joint. Whether the 5th lumbar vertebra is seated deeply in relation to the iliac crests, or is carried somewhat higher, is not considered to be of any particular significance.[1326]

The important factor, so far as lumbar joint disease is concerned, seems to be not so much that a subject's normal posture may incline more to a hollow low back or a flat back, *but occupational and recreational activities which habitually and continually induce hyperextension of the lumbar spine*; for example, the persistent wearing of high heels, combined with an occupation which involves standing and reaching up. Forceful approximation of posterior structures in weight-bearing positions is damaging to the lumbar spine, in that undue loading falls on the synovial facet-joints and interosseous connective tissue structures (see pp. 23, 85).

Janda (p. 114) has emphasised the tendency for predominantly phasic muscle to lenthen and predominantly tonic muscle groups to shorten, and this is a not infrequent finding in low back joint problems.

The factor of *prolonged* approximation of the posterior elements is important, and Macnab (1977)[780] regards the most common manifestation of disc degeneration to be that of secondary recurrent backache due to hyperextension strains of a posterior joint, or to persistent posterior joint subluxation. The *habitually lordosed* back is regarded as having no safety factor of absorption of functional extension movements, and thus the undiminished force of extension stress will give rise to painful capsular lesions of the facet articulations and to arthrosis of these joints.

A normal lumbar posture of being slightly more lordotic than the average is probably of no real consequence, so long as the individual's occupation and habits do not involve prolonged hyperextension, but include a proportion of the day in more flexed positions such as sitting or bending. Whether the individual's normal posture is average or lordotic, a degree of *prolonged and habitual hyperextension*, combined with a degree of abdominal muscle weakness and shortening of dorsal soft-tissue structures (see p. 267) will cause pain sooner or later. Sometimes an abnormally increased lumbosacral angle really means an aesthetically undesirable lumbosacral angle and rationalisation will surely follow.

La Rocca and Macnab (1969)[697] studied two groups of 150 people between the ages of 35 and 40 years; the subjects had been engaged in heavy work all their lives. Those of one group were under treatment for low back pain; the other group were pain-free and denied any history of low back pain at any time.

There was no statistical difference in anatomical variants seen on X-ray and measurements for lordosis and lumbosacral angle were evenly distributed in both groups. Likewise, there was no correlation between anatomical variants and the degree of disc degeneration. The only correlation observed was that between disc degeneration and age.

To regard it as an advantage for the horizontal sacrum to allow the lumbosacral facet-joints to bear more weight is a doubtful hypothesis. Conversely, it is not unknown for diagnoses of postural pain due to flat back to be applied to cases of unrecognised Scheuermann's disease of the low thoracic and upper-with-mid-lumbar spine, causing manifest segmental irritability at the L5–S1 level (see p. 243).

Transitional vertebrae and backache

Schmorl and Junghanns[1093] refer to the 'pain-causing transitional vertebra' syndrome (*sacralisation douleureuse*) and mention that the presence of a transitional vertebra in itself does not necessarily cause the pain, but that additional changes will be the initiating factor (Fig. 8.9).

Anomalous fifth lumbar vertebrae give rise to most trouble when the transition is unilateral and incomplete,[509] since the syndesmosis attaching the sacralised half to the sacrum permits some movement, less on the sacralised side than the normal side.

These changes can cause backache and sciatica in some and symptoms develop more often and more severely on the side which is not sacralised. Others may present with 'added' joints on both sides of an incompletely sacralised L5, and one or other of the joints may present with the

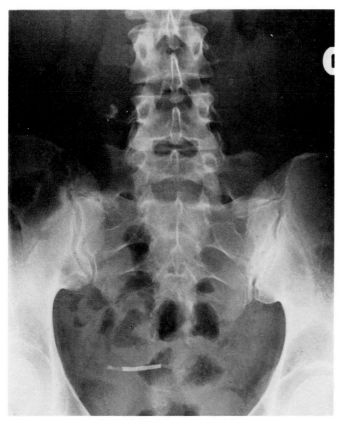

Fig. 8.9 Transitional fifth lumbar vertebra with adventitious joints between sacral ala and 'transverse process' on both sides. Transitional vertebrae *per se* need not be responsible for symptoms. This 30-year-old lady's intractable back pain was successfully treated on the basis of clinical findings, which were those of a sacroiliac rather than a lumbosacral problem. To what degree the anomaly had predisposed her to sacroiliac joint dysfunction is not known, of course.

radiographic evidence of arthrotic change (Figs 1.26, 1.27, 1.28, 1.30).

In lumbarisation or partial lumbarisation of the first sacral segment, injection of irritant saline into the joint (or pseudo-joint) produced pain spreading over the buttock to ischial tuberosity and under the buttock.

For example, this lady of 40 (Fig. 1.27) had deep, persistent bilateral low back pain, spreading to the right haunch and anterior thigh, after an initial bout of right sciatica. The back pain was constant and had the unusual effect of doubling her forwards into a crouched position after 20 minutes of walking and carrying shopping; she could only continue walking after resting against a wall. On examination she had a slightly sway-back posture, and her movements were generally good except that extension and side-flexion aggravated her low back pain. There were no other signs of note. On palpation, the haunch pain could be provoked by lateral pressures on the L1 spinous process but it was difficult to provoke her lumbar pain by palpation. The X-ray showed a transitional and thus partially sacralised L5, with 'added' joints between sacral ala and transverse process on each side; the joint on the patient's right showed degenerative change.

A great deal of orthodox mobilising and traction was ineffective, despite careful assessment and ringing the changes of technique. There was the forlorn hope that transverse mobilising of the degenerating adventitious joint at L5–S1 on the right might help, and by the simple technique of opposing lateral pressures to L5 and the sacrum, she was gratifyingly freed of her distressing functional disablement, although she still had slight thigh symptoms when making a bed, for instance, and a lumbar ache on sustained flexion when washing her hair.

Mooney and Robertson (1976)[867] have experimentally produced buttock and ischial pain by injecting hypertonic saline into the pseudo-joints of transitional vertebrae; the pain was relieved by further injection of 2 to 5 cc of 1 per cent xylocaine.

SPINAL STENOSIS (pp. 28, 104)

Although there are several degenerative spinal diseases, not until 1960 was spondylotic caudal radiculopathy accurately diagnosed and properly treated. For nearly 20 years the syndrome was confused with that of a protruded disc. Medical opinion to the contrary was either disregarded or unpublished. Evidence suggests that compression of the cauda equina in a smaller than normal spine has long existed but the clues leading to its discovery were repeatedly misinterpreted.[1300]

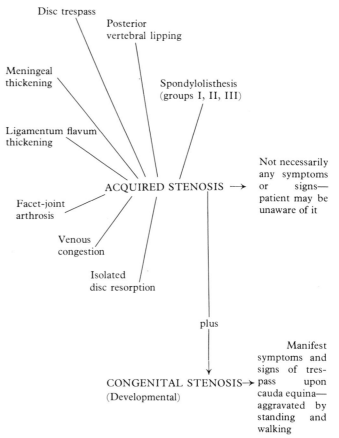

Scheme of relationship between degenerative change and the presence of a developmentally narrow lumbar neural canal

In patients who have an abnormally narrow lumbar spinal canal, the onset of degenerative change may cause a critical decrease in the available space which gives rise to clinical features unlike those of isolated, unilateral disc trespass (Figs 1.32, 1.33).[956]

The mean age of onset is the fourth decade, but the range is 10–60 years. In a comparative study of simple disc herniations and spinal stenosis of varying aetiology, Paine (1976)[963] gives an overall sex distribution ratio among a group of 455 patients (Table 8.4).

Table 8.4

	Male	Female	Ratio
Herniation of nucleus pulposus	86	56	1.5 : 1
Herniation of nucleus pulposus and degenerative stenosis	39	16	2.4 : 1
Herniation of nucleus pulposus and congenital/developmental stenosis	39	13	3 : 1
Herniation of nucleus pulposus with degenerative and developmental stenosis	20	6	3.3 : 1
Degenerative stenosis	69	33	2.1 : 1
Degenerative and developmental stenosis	38	15	2.5 : 1
Congenital/developmental stenosis	8	1	8 : 1
Spondylolisthesis	10	6	1.7 : 1
Total (455)	309	146	2.1 : 1

Where the discogenic changes were associated with developmental stenosis, the average length of symptoms before surgery was three years, but where acquired stenosis was secondary to degenerative change, the average duration of symptoms before surgery was longer, being nine years.

Pain. When the cauda equina is compressed there is usually great pain in the legs; radicular pain is often intense, and bilateral. Pain with a changing pattern of mid- and low lumbar and radicular involvement *according to activity* is a common feature.[315]

In general, the back and leg pains of lumbar spinal stenosis do not occur in the same pattern as do discrete and periodic spondylotic episodes, but tend to be chronic, grumbling, long-continued and progressively worsening.[963] They may be bizarre and vague, and this has led to opinions about psychoneurosis, malingering, or a desire for compensation.[660]

Back pain is usually less acute than in patients with a herniated disc; in more extensive cases of degenerative stenosis the pain may involve higher lumbar regions as well. Many get painful stiffness on inactivity, but pain also progresses through the day with increasing activities, thus showing a degree of time-dependence as well as stress-dependence.

Leg pains are sometimes indistinguishable from those of uniradicular root involvement, but tend more often to be extrasegmental in distribution, i.e. down the back of thigh and calf to heel, but also into the anterior leg and front of foot. Males, particularly, tend to have pain spreading to anterior thigh and medial knee, and perhaps not reaching the ankle.

The male lumbar neural canal is narrowest at the L3–L4–L5 segments, and that in the female at the L5–S1 segment.

The patient with stenosis may be relatively comfortable *at rest in flexed positions* even during the period of having an acute attack. On standing for long, walking or climbing stairs, for example, uni- or bilateral leg pains, with or without muscle weakness and giving way of legs, may come on within 200 yards, to be relieved after some minutes on sitting down and bending forward; the symptoms begin again on renewed standing and walking. It is a mistake to expect that all patients with spinal stenosis should exhibit this claudication on walking. Many will not, and will only describe progressive worsening of pain on prolonged activity.

Where neurogenic claudication is present, it will be different from that of peripheral vascular disease; in the latter case, the 'claudication distance' is fixed, and remains the same on repetition of walking for that distance.[1127] The patient with spinal stenosis will suffer the discomfort at progressively shorter distances, if he attempts to repeat the exercise.

Typically, the claudication pains of peripheral vascular disease disappear if the patient stands still, whereas in neurogenic claudication the pains are more completely relieved by sitting down and flexing forward so as to enlarge the lumbar neural canal. This is substantiated by the observation that a myelographic block can be freed by flexing the lumbar spine.[911] Also, the exercise-provoked pain of neurogenic claudication *does not disappear almost immediately* on sitting down, as would the pain due to peripheral vascular disease.

Often, the patients will also complain of night pains, leg twitching and restlessness in bed, leg 'soreness' and 'burning feeling'. Coughing and sneezing do not necessarily provoke the pain. Since supine lying on a flat surface, e.g. a sitting-room floor, produces a lumbar lordosis, it is understandable that some patients will report provocation of their symptoms when lying this way.

While the phrase 'intermittent claudication of the cauda equina' may express the difference between neural canal trespass and peripheral vascular disease, it is a misnomer, since claudication means 'lameness' or 'limping' and the cauda equina cannot walk.

The reason for symptoms and signs of intermittent claudication is quite probably local vascular changes of the spinal roots. Exercise increases blood flow to the cauda equina and this extra fluid may be enough to provoke or aggravate the root pain. Conversely, the claudication has been attributed to an ischaemic neuritis of the cauda equina, produced by exertion;[1292] the vasodilatation and hyperaemia occasioned by an increase in local blood volume thus aggravates the local compression in the neural canal. It has also been suggested that cerebrospinal fluid dynamics are disturbed, with the creation of a high local pressure secondarily impairing venous drainage and thus causing congestion.

Frank postural deformities are less common in the stenotic patient than in those with unilateral disc trespass[963] and similarly, *spinal movements* may be quite free, especially flexion. The patient may often appear to be normal on examination,[1188] so history-taking is important.

A common pattern is pain provoked by extension, and side-flexions, with flexion full and painless. If extension does not provoke the pain immediately, it will frequently do so if the extended posture is held for some 10–20 seconds. Likewise, straight-leg-raising may be full and painless; if it is limited by back and/or leg pain, the degree of restriction will be the same bilaterally, even if the pains troubling the patient are only unilateral.

Neurological changes. Bilateral neurological deficit is frequent, and besides involving the commonly affected L5 and S1 roots, there may often be signs attributable to trespass upon the L4 and L3 roots, and occasionally L2 root.[963] Absence of ankle-jerk and depression of knee-jerk is frequent; *sphincter disturbance is not, although it occurs.*[315]

More severe cases will report patchy sensory impairment in the legs, and limb weakness on standing and walking.[956]

In some, limitation of straight-leg-raising and depressed ankle-jerks may not show unless the patient is asked to walk around for 10–20 minutes and return for further examination.

Dombrowski[265] in describing chronic nerve root compression secondary to progressive spinal stenosis, mentions that myelography may demonstrate a complete block in the absence of neurological signs; e.m.g. findings often correlate poorly with the degree of block on myelography. Many of his patients had either normal or only slightly abnormal electromyograms but almost complete block on myelography.

The investigation technique of ultrasonography (p. 374) can now demonstrate the oblique sagittal diameter of the neural canal, and thus can be used to assess the clinical significance of the canal dimension in association with lesions of trespass.

When comparing 73 patients and 200 normal subjects, it became evident that the available space in the neural canal is a highly significant factor underlying the clinical features of degenerative or other trespass (Porter *et al.*, 1978).[1001]

Bohl and Steffee (1979)[100] indicate that lumbar spinal stenosis may be a cause of continuing pain and physical restriction after total hip replacement; the authors suggest that the causal factors are probably the preoperative stress which the lumbar spine suffers as a consequence of the

limited hip motion. An increased level of activity following surgery probably unmasks the neurological changes and the intermittent claudication in some.

Isolated disc resorption (see p. 92)

A particular type of lumbar spondylosis may occur, characterised by progressive narrowing of a single disc space over a number of years.[214] A normal disc height of between 15–20 mm is reduced to around 3 mm, and on X-ray there is marked sclerosis of vertebral body margins. It commonly occurs *as an isolated affection in an otherwise normal lumbar spine* and there are repeated attacks of acute but short duration low back pain, which last for three or four days and then disappear completely.

Additional trauma or stress to this type of low back condition, as in falling on the buttocks, initiates severe bilateral buttock and leg pains, which in some cases are aggravated by walking and physical activity. It is unusual for these patients to have associated neurological findings of straight-leg-raising restriction or absent lower limb reflexes. Associated disc prolapse is not seen in the established case since the disc has disappeared by resorption, rather than by transference of some of its mass to trespass upon the neural canal. One of the striking features is that at operation the disc space is virtually empty, and clearly recognisable vertebral end-plate cartilage will be found causing the lumbar nerve root canal stenosis.

Backache in generalised degenerative joint laxity

Mature women in the 55–65 age range, with degenerative changes of mild laxity in multiple joints, may report chronic lumbar pain and troublesome morning stiffness of the low back. They also describe walking with a waddling gait until the morning stiffness is eased by activity, and find their aches aggravated by walking or standing for too long, and climbing stairs. Other than in passing, shoulder girdle problems are not mentioned and polymyalgia rheumatica need not be further considered.

Around all peripheral joints the parenchyma of muscle appears to have lost the battle with fat, and ligamentous tissue appears to be following suit; the periarticular soft tissues are pudgy and thickened.

The patient's valgus feet are decidedly flat, together with bilateral metatarsalgia and calloused skin beneath the metatarsal heads. There is often a degree of bilateral genu valgum, with poor tone in the quadriceps. Hip joints are surprisingly mobile, and painless straight-leg-raising is some 120° or more on both sides. The patient's abdomen is corpulent and weak, and all upper limb joints have the same mild hypermobility and deficient stabilisation which is evident in the lower limbs; Herbeden's nodes may be evident at the interphalangeal joints.

The patient stands with a lordosis. Lumbar movements are characteristic in that extension hurts across the lumbo-sacral region and bilaterally into the buttocks, side-flexions are unexceptional and by excessive hip mobility the patient can reach downward to almost place palms on the floor without pain; the lumbar lordosis remains virtually undisturbed.

Palpation findings are also characteristic, and reveal that the lower three or four lumbar segments are stiff, sore and somewhat irritable, i.e. the existing joint problem is a *regional* rather than a segmental one.

The salient features are: (i) the presence of regional spinal stiffness, and pain because of it, in a patient with manifest laxity of most peripheral joints, and (ii) the lack of any sagittal abnormality of vertebral body relationships on lateral films; there may be a loss of disc space in the low lumbar segments, but there is no alteration in vertebral body alignment.

There are no neurological signs.

The chair-bound backache

The patient, a man in his forties or fifties, has been physically active in the past but has risen professionally to assume responsibilities which entail much administrative work. His weight has increased with the decline in his musculature, and these are most obvious abdominally. Symptoms reported are lumbar stiffness on rising in the morning, a lumbar ache on sitting for more than two hours or standing for more than an hour, and a reduced physical capacity.

On examination, the lumbar movements are a little reduced but do not provoke pain to any degree. Straight-leg-raising is 75°–80° bilaterally depending upon the patient's body-type, and apart from some hamstring restriction are unexceptional. There are no neurological signs and radiographic appearances are normal.

Since it appears that the intervertebral disc 'lives by movement and dies for lack of it' (p. 21), the remedy is plain, so long as clinical examination has excluded contraindications to physical treatment.

'Collapsed back' with kissing spines

The patient is more often a somewhat portly woman in late middle-age and she reports diffuse thoracic and lumbar aches on standing, with a more insistent low lumbar pain which considerably reduces ordinary activities. There are usually other problems such as chronic degenerative change in one shoulder, an arthrotic knee or bilateral hallux valgus, but the patient is manifestly seeking help for the spinal problem alone, which is depressingly painful and severely limiting physical endurance. The pronounced kypholordotic spine appears to have slumped and settled down into itself like an old cottage.

Because of degenerative changes in many segments, sometimes associated with developmentally broad spinous processes, low vertebral bodies or the coexistence of both,[315] there is approximation and eventually bony contact of the upper and lower edges of the lumbar spinous processes. Occasionally, the essential cause is a particularly well-developed lumbar spinous process, but much more commonly the changes are secondary to degeneration and occur simultaneously at a number of segments. The chronic trauma and thus injury to interspinous soft tissues is accompanied by ligamentous changes (p. 85)[1042] and sometimes the virtual disappearance of true ligamentous tissue.

On lateral films, the posterior margins of the vertebral bodies have settled backwards and downwards upon the subjacent body, the retrolisthesis thereby reducing both the AP and vertical dimensions of the intervertebral foramina. The tip of the superior articular process thus projects above the lower border of the vertebral body above.[780] The disc spaces have a 'wedge' silhouette which converges posteriorly, and the bony contact of vertebral bodies is marked by sclerosis, more pronounced posteriorly. The edges of the spinous processes are in contact, with opposed bony edges flattened and in some cases smeared out a little to one side or other, which is evident on the AP view. The area of contact is marked by sclerosis and a pseudo-joint may be formed, sometimes with an adventitious bursa.

The chronic impaction of spinous processes (Baarstrupp's disease)[49] interferes considerably with vertebral mechanics (Fig. 1.29D). Changes sufficiently established to have caused the X-ray appearance described will inevitably have also produced arthrosis of synovial facet-joints, and it is likely that the persistent chronic pain is partly due to this, and probably due also to the chronic impaction of vertebral bodies posteriorly; this is the only region of the intervertebral disc which is innervated by nociceptors.

Of the lumbar movements extension is the most limited and is sharply painful in the low back. Rotation to either side also hurts considerably; while side-flexion and flexion are painfully limited to a degree, the pain is less severe.

In the early stages the patient may describe being most comfortable when sitting at ease in flexed positions, but in the more chronic phases many will mention that sitting only partly eases the pain, and that they are most comfortable in a reclining position with slight lordosis maintained by cushions.

The foraminal encroachment may be evidenced by neurological signs which are bilateral in some, but there seems no direct relationship between the extent, or presence, of neurological deficit and the X-ray evidence of foraminal trespass; many patients have no clinical evidence of root involvement.

The assertion[780] that of itself this entity, of spinous process approximation, is a doubtful cause of back pain may be compared with the report[1180b] of a patient whose low back pain of eight years' standing was relieved by a single injection of local anaesthetic between the spinous processes. Dixon (1976)[262] confirms the analgesic effect of injection between the impacted bony areas of the spinous processes. The changes described may, as a late sequel to surgical fusion, occur at a single segment which is unstable to a degree; on lateral films the X-ray appearances are as described above.[523]

The changes may also occur as a component of group III (degenerative) spondylolisthesis (p. 260).

Paget's disease (osteitis deformans)

The popular image of the bent and bow-legged old man with a large head dies hard and Paget's description in 1877 of a patient in the advanced state with a kyphotic vertebral column, enlarged cranium and bowed femora and tibia is very rarely seen.

The condition affects the vertebral column and particularly the lumbosacral region more often than any other part of the skeleton, and the lumbar vertebrae and sacrum are involved in at least three out of every four cases. Nevertheless, it may occur in any vertebra from the atlas downwards, and frequently both the lumbar and thoracic spines are involved.[315]

In a descending order of frequency, the bones affected are sacrum, spine, cranium, sternum, pelvis and lower limb; the tibiae come ninth in this order. The incidence among 2268 men was 3.5 per cent and among 2353 women was 2.5 per cent and in a large series of patients the incidence of spinal involvement was sacrum (55.8 per cent), individual vertebrae (50.0 per cent) and the entire vertebral column (6.5 per cent).[1093]

Although the bony lesions may be multiple in that more than one vertebra is involved, and perhaps a single focus in the skull may also exist, the greater part of the skeleton shows no abnormal changes; the condition is never a generalised bone disease.[896]

The abnormal appearance of the vertebra, described in considerable detail by Schmorl and Junghanns (1971),[1093] is quite variable, with the changes involving only a small area or the whole vertebra.[315] This does not necessarily mark the early stage, as the solitary focus may represent a late stage of evolution;[896] in many the disease is completely unsuspected. The changes appear to be those of concurrent bone formation and destruction, with an abnormal architecture of the bone being laid down.

Occasionally, Paget's disease of one vertebral body may be seen to extend along bridging osteophytes to adjacent vertebral bodies.[1093]

The patient is almost invariably over 55 years and *there are no distinctive clinical features other than aching pain*, which may be quite severe, in the affected part.[896] The pain does not ease with rest, or spontaneously disappear within forseeable periods as does the pain of spondylosis. It may be provoked simply on movement, on physical exertion such as lifting, or when getting warmed in bed. Posture does not as a rule provoke it much. Lumbosacral and buttock pain is common when the sacrum is affected; this may be due to disturbance of the normal ligamentous

stress because of sacral softening, and when osseous lesions such as Paget's disease involve the periosteum and thus its nociceptor system, pain will be more intense than otherwise.[1362]

The abnormal bone is always soft and may easily be cut with a knife; vertebral fractures may occur from trivial injuries and heal by a characteristic type of callus observed in the disease.[1093]

The bone affected is hyperaemic and if subcutaneous it will feel warm to the touch.

The characteristic hyperaemia is caused by blood-flow through the affected bone which may be 20 times the normal.[983]

Excessive bone formation may produce spinal stenosis (q.v.) and signs of spinal cord compression, but the trespass may be confined to foraminal encroachment with consequent root pressure, although this is not common. The need for surgical relief is occasionally urgent.[315]

Medication for Paget's disease has improved markedly in the last few years, and three groups of drugs—calcitonins, diphosphonates and mithramycin—have wrought impressive effects on the symptoms, biochemistry and histological features of the disease.

PELVIC ARTHROPATHY

The sacroiliac joint

It may be appropriate here to mention the occasional comment: 'sacroiliac strains, apart from those following parturition, are excessively rare though commonly diagnosed. The mere complaint of pain over the sacroiliac joint and the demonstration of local tenderness do not justify the diagnosis of sacroiliac strain.'

Indeed not, yet how many experienced workers do hold that such generalised signs justify this diagnosis?

Macnab (1977)[780] quoted Steindler (1962):[1171] 'It is dangerous to arrogate to oneself the opinion that what one cannot explain does not exist.' It might be added here that it is also unreasonable to mention X-ray evidence as proof of the lesion when it is common knowledge that pain and X-ray appearances are not necessarily related.[791] It is as unrealistic to hold that most sacroiliac area pain arises from the joint itself as it is to solve difficult problems by asserting, 'it all comes from the lumbar spine'.

Humanly, we seek a guru with the short and certain answer to our difficulties of assessment, that we might be relieved of the discomfort of swimming in a sea of relativity, and of making up our own minds on the evidence before us. Yet while seeming to ease the difficulties, dogma dulls the wits, and in assessing the clinical states of this mysterious joint we need all the discernment we can muster.[451]

Certain knowledge of the *nature* of common noninflammatory sacroiliac joint problems is small in proportion to the amount of speculation, controversy and assertion about them, but as to their frequent *incidence* in both sexes there is now much less doubt.[662] An increasing number of skilled and experienced therapists who have established high standards of examination, assessment and treatment, are more frequently detecting and treating common sacroiliac joint conditions. As the relative dearth of certain knowledge of the nature of *vertebral* joint conditions has been no bar to quickly successful treatment[450] based on the signs and symptoms in themselves, so also are sacroiliac problems amenable to successful treatment even though their precise nature may not yet be clarified fully. The difficulty lies in detecting them, and trying to understand why they present as they do. That we cannot always explain them is no reason for trying to deal with our uncertainty by imposing an arbitrary and artificial regularity[862] where, for the time being, none can exist.

The sacroiliac joint is more than a mute transmitter of body-weight to femoral heads.

The vagaries of referred pain, and our difficulties because of this, do not justify the convenient generalisation, 'it all comes from the spine'; nor perhaps relieve us of the obligation to examine comprehensively both regions, as well as the hip joint, since patients can present with problems at two, or all three, of these areas. In assessment of this joint, more than at any other articulation, the therapist needs to bear in mind the infinite range of biological plasticity, and the infinite variety of presentation of common joint problems. For this reason alone some observations on the clinical presentation of pelvic arthropathy may be in order.

The variety of presentation of sacroiliac problems seems matched only by the variety of methods of detection and classification of them, this in itself indicating the basic uncertainty.[59, 163, 209, 219, 258, 369, 376, 451, 590, 791, 862, 1180b]

It is unwise to regard visual and palpable evidence of bony point (ASIS and PSIS) asymmetry as the *sine qua non* of sacroiliac lesions. The sacroiliac sulcus may palpably be deeper on the affected side and, other criteria being satisfied, a so-called posterior innominate be present and responsible for the symptoms reported, when the PSIS is higher, lower or at the same level as its fellow; bony point asymmetry in the horizontal plane is not a prerequisite for sacroiliac joint pain. Further, the factor of structural anomaly must always be in mind.

Sacroiliac joint surface configurations differ considerably between individuals, and may also differ between sides in the same individual, as AP X-ray views of the normal pelvis of a dozen subjects will show. As stressed throughout this text, manual treatment should primarily be based upon the actual clinical response to manual testing procedures, and not largely upon theoretical notions of disturbed biomechanics, which appear to rest on assumptions of bilateral symmetry as the norm.

Since Weisl[1301] has, by cineradiographic studies, clearly demonstrated that the axis of simple sagittal movement of the sacrum is highly variable, by as much as 5 cm, and lies 10 cm below the sacral promontory and in front of the joint, the notion that slight abnormal shifts of relationship occur by movement around five axes (among them an axis of sagittal movement at the S2 segment) is probably more belief than established fact.[862] Neither is it necessary for a shift in joint relationships, however slight, to have occurred before sacroiliac joint pain will occur.

While the precise mechanical nature of a sacroiliac joint problem (in those cases where a shift in relationships *does* exist) may defy analysis, this does not mean that relief may not be obtained by simple manual mobilising techniques, the final choice of which depends more upon continuing assessment of treatment effects than an arbitrary selection based upon theoretical concepts.

History. It is not rare for sciatica to arise from the sacroiliac joint, in the absence of inflammatory disease.[542] The sacroiliac and pubic joints as well as the hip, of course, should be given special attention when:

1. Pain is unilateral, rather than bilateral or central, and is not of typical root pain quality.
2. There are no lumbar articular signs, or symptoms (though not infrequently patients have lesions at both areas) and the lumbar spine is clear on palpation.
3. There is an absence of signs and symptoms in the leg attributable to the lumbar spine (e.g. neurological deficit).
4. There may be asymmetry of posterior superior iliac spine (PSIS) and anterior superior iliac spine (ASIS) levels—often but not invariably found.

Special points
1. Dull buttock, groin or posterior thigh and calf ache (N.B. check hip).
2. Subjective heaviness, deadness, 'dullness', of limb.
3. Turning over in bed, or getting onto plinth, or stepping up with affected side leg, produces twinges of pain.
4. Recent pregnancy, falls, twists, strains, such as pushing a motor-car, or leaping a ditch.
5. Habitual sloppy standing, habitual work stance and stresses, twisted-sitting posture.
6. Nature of sports (e.g. fast bowler) and nature of other activities, e.g. physiotherapist, ballet dancer, footballer, hurdler and high-jumper.

A glance at the arrangement of the sclerotomes and myotomes of the lower extremity will show why deep pain reference from the sacroiliac joint may vary so considerably in distribution.[928] For example, isolated phases of abdominal pain have been found to be ameliorated by injection of local anaesthetic into the sacroiliac joint, despite the fact that myelography demonstrated a disc protrusion.[935]

Similarly, abdominal pain in the region of Baer's point

(q.v.) may be relieved for a time by injection anteriorly at the points of emergence superficially of lower thoracic nerves. While the eradication of a local pain by local injection does not necessarily demonstrate its source, it most certainly demonstrates incorporation of the tissue injected into the sites of referred pain, referred tenderness and sometimes muscle spasm, too. The common rule of thumb, that pain on sitting should immediately raise the suspicion of lumbar discogenic problems, may sometimes hinder a balanced assessment of a patient's low back problem.

Very frequently, pain on standing and walking is experienced by those with acquired spinal stenosis due to discogenic trespass and this pain is *relieved* within some 10–15 minutes by sitting. While it is well known that low lumbar intradiscal pressure is higher in sitting than in standing[890] this does not mean that sitting may not also be uncomfortable (see p. 22) in sacroiliac joint problems.

Similarly, while the pain of sacroiliac joint problems is often exacerbated by bearing body-weight on the affected side, as in the support phase of walking and climbing stairs, it is by no means uncommon for the patient to dislike standing with weight equally supported on both feet.

Signs. A common *but by no means invariable* combination of signs is as follows:

1. The patient tends to bear weight on the unaffected side in standing and sitting, and to step up with the unaffected leg.
2. The painful side posterior superior iliac spine is lower, and the anterior spine higher, than its fellow. There need not necessarily be any change in the horizontal level of iliac crests.
3. The sacral apex may deviate slightly to the painless side, with slight asymmetry of the gluteal cleft.
4. The buttock contour is flatter on the painful side; occasionally it is more prominent. The flattening is probably due to loss of gluteal tone, consequent upon the blocking of the sacroiliac joint on that side (see p. 282). For the same reason, the *supine* patient will lie with the affected-side ASIS at a lower horizontal level than the opposite side, almost regardless of the mechanical nature of the joint problem, while the *prone* patient will often lie with the affected leg more inwardly rotated.
5. Piedallu's sign (q.v.) is positive (this finding is present in some, but less frequently than sometimes suggested).
6. Hip rotation abnormalities are present, in that the normal amplitude of rotation remains, but is shifted to favour inward rotation as a rule, because of the hypotonic external rotators.
7. The affected side adductors are tight, while the tensor fasciae latae of the opposite side is hypertonic.
8. There are tension-differences in the sacrotuberous

ligaments, although the disposition of laxness and tightness will sometimes confound theoretical concepts of unilateral iliac rotation.
9. Straight-leg-raising is limited by 10°–30° on the painful side.
10. Iliac gapping tests will hurt, if there is more than moderate pain.
11. Passive testing reveals less movement on the painful side, sometimes associated with severe irritability.
12. On palpation, the sacroiliac sulcus appears deeper on the affected side. There is localised undue tenderness at the symphysis pubis and unilaterally at the adductor attachments, Baer's point (iliacus spasm), over the anterior acetabulum and just medial to the posterior inferior iliac spine. There are painful soft-tissue indurations along the iliac attachment of the gluteal muscles, and the gluteus maximus feels soft and flaccid. The region of the posterior inferior iliac spine is palpably thickened.

Not all of the signs will be present in the same combination in all patients, and the mere presence of some of them does not necessarily indicate that the patient's complaint is due to a sacroiliac problem.

Occasionally, the painful side is opposite to that of the asymmetry described in (2). Patients may present with signs (1), (4), (7), (9) and (10) only, and sometimes after recent pregnancy with no more than unilateral pain and signs (7) and (12).

Movements. Patterns of movement-limitation and provocation of pain will differ from patient to patient. Surprisingly, a few patients have no provocation of pain on movement other than rotation towards the painful side. Lumbar rotation, tested to its extreme range by overpressure, is an important parameter in the examination of sacroiliac problems, and this becomes more apparent with increasing experience. *It is the attachments of the ilio-lumbar ligament which dictate that this movement should always be carefully assessed.*

Many will have pain on extension only or as much pain on extension as they do on side-flexion towards the painful side. Others will manifestly provoke severe pain on bending away from the painful side and on flexion, and yet others will experience equal provocation of pain on both side-flexions.

Taking the variety of benign sacroiliac joint problems as a whole, there is no one characteristic pattern of pain on movement, although there is usually provocation of pain on at least one movement and there are very frequently inequalities of straight-leg-raising and prone-knee-bending.

Our tendency to seek a set of rules of thumb for a 'therapeutic kit-bag' and then to apply these rules of thumb willy-nilly with less than full discrimination, can act in ways which may not always be to the patient's advantage. Just as soon as we have formulated what appears to be the characteristically abnormal articular pattern, it has to be modified in the light of further experience and increased knowledge. For example, pain referred to the calf from sacroiliac joint problems will frequently inhibit toe-standing on that leg, but this must not be promptly taken to indicate that a neurological deficit of S1 and S2 root conduction exists.

The frequency with which patients report a numb, heavy leg often adds weight to the notion that upper sacral root interference may be present, and since it is well known that a depressed ankle-jerk need not accompany *true* S1 root involvement, such an assessment may seem reasonable enough.

With regard to *hip rotation*, the presence of abnormalities will need to be assessed not only in relation to the possible slight disturbance of pelvic joints, the tethering effects of large muscles in spasm and sometimes the more established adaptive shortening of important soft-tissue structures, but also the limitation which is secondary to possible coexisting early arthrosis of the hip.

Laban *et al.* (1978)[690] analysed 50 patients with lumbosacral and inguinal pain associated with an unstable symphysis pubis. None had previous trauma or surgery.

A shift in excess of 2 mm was shown at the symphysis on alternate leg standing. On the symptomatic side, hip abduction and external rotation were reduced. For associated pubic and sacroiliac joint instability, the authors mentioned intra-articular steroid injection, support and physiotherapy. Careful and attentive examination will reveal that early degenerative change is more often detected by the hip flexion/adduction test revealing unilateral groin discomfort than by seeking arbitrary and stereotyped patterns of movement limitation (Fig. 9.22).

Leg lengths. However difficult it is to find acceptable terminology for what presents as a movement abnormality, from clinical experience it appears that the pelvis can become stuck or blocked at the sacroiliac joint, not necessarily in a position of torsion but sometimes so, in people with *equal leg lengths*. When torsion *is* present, this may give the appearance of unequal leg length, when measured from the anterior superior spines.

Decisions about 'anterior innominates' and 'posterior innominates' are sometimes made on the basis of slight apparent differences of leg length in various postures during clinical examination, and the patient treated for sacroiliac joint problems on a basis which *at times* may owe more to rules of thumb and therapeutic bias than to sober clinical assessment.

With regard to Piedallu's sign (p. 329) (Figs 9.4; 9.5) during the sitting-flexion and standing-flexion tests, the occasionally observed apparent increase of leg length on that side during reaching for the toes in long sitting, the

value of this test appears to rest on several assumptions which could bear inspection, viz.:

1. That the ilium rotates around an axis somewhere near the S2 segment. Weisl[1301] has clearly shown that it does not.
2. That pelvic asymmetry invariably denotes a sacroiliac joint condition.
3. That apparent leg-length differences in long-sitting-flexion are invariably significant, even though they do not appear to give rise to any change of lateral pelvic tilt during flexion in standing, when the feet are perforce symmetrically placed.

While the so-called Yo-Yo test, i.e. one leg becoming relatively longer when changing to the long-sitting position from lying, is sometimes associated with reversible pelvic-joint asymmetry, the sign is not necessarily pathognomic of reversible sacroiliac 'shuffling' lesions (for want of a better name). When an apparently longer leg *does* exist on the same side as a sacroiliac joint problem, and a manual backward rotation of the ipsilateral ilium relieves the pain and articular signs, this relief is not necessarily accompanied by an equalisation of leg lengths, although it sometimes is. Neither is there any guarantee that the relief *is* due to changed sacroiliac joint relationships.

Because a mobilisation or manipulation technique moves the structures in which we are presently interested, we should not overlook the host of other structures also being moved, notably the hip joint and particularly the lumbosacral facet structures.

Pelvic joint dysfunction can present in a variety of ways which far exceeds the most accommodating of stereotyped lists of syndromes, and distinguishing between a painful lumbosacral facet and a sacroiliac joint problem is not always easy. For example, a proportion of patients with unilateral 'sacroiliac' problems who, on the basis of an assumed forward rotation of the ilium, respond well to a backward rotation of that ilium, will be found to respond equally well to flexing *both* knees together onto the chest. This circumstance invites consideration that the lumbosacral facet may have been the culprit—more so when the pelvic joint asymmetry and leg-length inequality are seen to remain undisturbed.

It is of interest to note the effect of sacroiliac blocking on tone of the gluteal muscle mass. This has been demonstrated electromyographically.[474] Many people have slightly unequal leg lengths, which are probably insignificant and would not normally be noticed. Where there is shortening of one-quarter of an inch or more, there is a natural tendency for the pelvis to take up a torsional position which most nearly rights the upper sacral surface.

Stoddard[1180a] observes that: '... a short leg gives rise primarily to sacroiliac strain and secondly to lumbosacral or lower lumbar strain', and '... the first compensation occurs in the sacroiliac joint of the *shorter* side.'

The ilium on the side of the longer leg tends to be shuffled backwards, and the pubis slightly upwards, with the sacral base on that side also moving backwards. *Not all patients with leg inequality may show this, presumably because the necessity for, and the nature and degree of, postural compensation may differ between individuals.* For example, a laterally tilted pelvis does not *invariably* give rise to the so-called posterior innominate on the high side. It is not rare to find a depressed PSIS on the high side, accompanied by ipsilateral haunch pain which is relieved by techniques which induce a backward or posterior 'shuffle' of the ipsilateral ilium. Following this, the degree of lateral tilt is sometimes reduced but not eradicated. Explanations of this phenomenon probably lie more in the field of idiosyncrasies of joint configuration, and particular exciting causes, than in hypothetical biomechanics. An important point is that the body cannot read the book, and joints cannot know what is confidently expected of them by the theorist, the logician or the biomechanic.

Conclusions about pelvic distortion in terms of a 'posterior innominate' are sometimes made on the basis of rotation backward of one ilium; or an 'anterior innominate' when forward rotation of one ilium is believed to have occurred. How these concepts can be reconciled with an articular arrangement of opposed surfaces which manifestly exhibits two planes angulated to each other, and sometimes three, is not elucidated.

Pregnancy. Ligaments may remained softened and lengthened for 6 to 12 weeks after delivery, and sometimes for much longer. Among 10 patients in the latter group, a very important clinical sign was a bilaterally positive Trendelenberg sign, and during this examination three patients experienced a snapping sound in the symphysis while vertical symphyseal movement could be demonstrated by palpation (Hagen, 1974).[481]

Less serious movement abnormalities of the sacroiliac and pubic joints, besides lumbar problems, are a common cause of persistent postpartum pain, and after careful exclusion of problems from the intervertebral joints, simple mobilising techniques localised to the sacroiliac joint structures are very effective. Not all require manual treatment; Lewit (1970)[736] describes results at follow-up examination after delivery and of seven cases of sacroiliac displacement, four had disappeared spontaneously.

Obstetric and gynaecological surgery (p. 153). What is the nature of the lesion in these postoperative cases? Certainly, some patients present with pelvic asymmetry, usually with the lower posterior iliac spine on the painful side; others, on postural examination, have a symmetrical pelvis but local irritability on sacroiliac gapping tests and a painful limitation of hip abduction on the affected side. Other hip movements are normal, but the area over anterior acetabulum is very tender to deep pressure. Whether to call

this block, irritability or strain is a matter of opinion. Perhaps sprain might be acceptable, because it certainly seems to result from stress.

Ankylosis or surgical fusion, and adjacent hypermobility (p. 155). In my experience, patients with chronic low lumbar instability, having undergone fusion of L4–L5 and L5–S1 segments, sometimes begin to report a different pattern of pain localised around the posterior haunch area and on the same side as a more mobile and now irritable sacroiliac joint; previously there was no irritability, and less mobility. In some cases the compensatory mobility occurs at the L3–L4 segment and not the sacroiliac joint. In others, only very minor and temporary postsurgical symptoms arise and they do not seek help at routine follow-up interviews.

The surgical procedure of removal of iliac bone for grafting is sometimes followed by pelvic instability, and one report describes how this was demonstrated radiographically in six patients.[207]

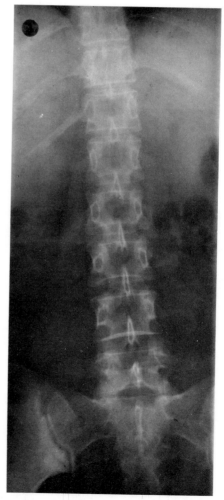

Fig. 8.10 Osteitis condensans ilii, a stress condition which need not have anything to do with pregnancy. Note sclerosis on the iliac side of the patient's right sacroiliac joint.

Trauma and stress. Sacroiliac joint problems giving rise to pain which is sometimes disabling, in childless young women and in young men, are more common than is generally supposed. *One concludes that either the condition goes unrecognised, or because of authoritarian and intimidating pronouncements about its non-existence, the likelihood of the condition is not included among the many factors for assessment, and a careful comprehensive examination of the joint is not conducted.*

Footballers, ballet dancers, high-jumpers, fast bowlers and physiotherapists commonly present with sacroiliac joint problems of this nature, ranging from a painful, irritable and hypermobile sacroiliac and/or pubic joint in a pelvic girdle which may or may not be asymmetrical, to a greater or lesser degree of seemingly irreversible torsion of the pelvis. The consequences of excessive and violent stress in dancing, games and athletics, repetitive unilateral stresses of heavy work and strains imposed upon the pelvis by an arthrodesed hip or an amputation prosthesis will declare themselves by the cardinal signs of: (1) disturbed mobility of pelvic joints and (2) sooner or later, condensation or sclerosis to buttress the bony face sustaining the stress, factors with which we are so familiar in the vertebral column itself as osteophytosis.

The stress condition *osteitis condensans ilii* (Figs 8.10, 8.11) is an example of this. A study of 50 patients with a long history of disease, congenital or acquired deformity or defect of one or both lower limbs, showed that of 45 who had a unilateral disorder of one lower limb, 35 had radiological evidence of bone sclerosis at the opposite sacroiliac joint. This sclerosis is usually more marked on the iliac side of the joint. 'In the light of this small series of cases it is probable that sex and deliveries have no bear-

ing on the aetiology of increased density of iliac bone.' (Solonen, 1957.)[1157]

At this late stage, radiographic evidence of osteitis condensans ilii is still solely regarded by some as supporting evidence of incorrect reposition of the pelvic joints after pregnancy, despite the fact that it has been shown to occur in men!

Newton (1957)[928] mentions that arthrosis of the sacroiliac joint is frequently associated with old trauma in the region of the joint and with contralateral hip disease.

Some of these patients have pain over the joint, but referred from the lumbar spine; others have no pain and are unaware of the condition, and occasionally there may be severe and chronic irritability of one or both sacroiliac joints.

The presence of osteitis condensans ilii, as determined by radiography, does not necessarily imply that coexisting low back and haunch pain is a consequence of the iliac sclerosis, although it may be. Asymptomatic individuals may fortuitously show the changes when X-rayed for other reasons.

Helbing (1978)[531] suggests that while arthrodesis of a hip joint alters the statics and dynamics of functional use, secondary arthrosis of a sacroiliac joint, as a consequence, is apparent more often radiographically than clinically.

Ligamentous lesions. These are sometimes described as present when by bringing the flexed hip and knee of a supine patient into (1) strong adduction, (2) towards the opposite shoulder, and (3) towards the same shoulder, pain is produced in the groin, L5–S1 dermatomes and lower sacral region, respectively (Lewit and Wolff, 1970).[736] Conclusions are that ligaments will be involved in the order (1) iliolumbar ligament, (2) sacroiliac ligament, and (3) sacrotuberous ligament, but since these tests put stress on many structures and also disturb joints and the pain may be being referred into a sclerotome or dermatome distribution, the conclusions seem somewhat arbitrary. Dermatomes are by no means fixed anatomical entities.

Degenerative joint disease. On the basis that radiographic appearances and clinical features are not associated *pari passu*, degenerative changes in the sacroiliac joint are probably not an important factor in assessing the genesis of pains in the buttock, haunch and groin, although they should be borne in mind.

The presence of a mobile painful joint in a man over 50 and a woman over 60 may be something more serious than a musculoskeletal problem, but this should not inhibit normal treatment of the joint when clinical features point to the likelihood of a benign joint condition. The radiograph is important, of course.

Sacroiliitis. The pain of sacroiliitis is usually unrelated to position. Radioactive scanning may reveal acute *osteomye-*

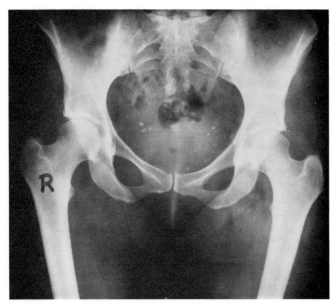

Fig. 8.11 Bilateral osteitis condensans ilii, more marked on the right. This 40-year-old lady frequently landed heavily on her seat when roller-skating and both sacroiliac joints were irritable (see text).

litis of the joint[1232] when it has not been suspected; its involvement appears to have an incidence of some 5–10 per cent in acute haematogenous osteomyelitis.

A hot thermogram over the sacroiliac joint is a reasonably reliable indicator of inflammatory activity in these joints, before this is evident radiographically.[9]

In a group of clinically interrelated disorders, which are termed the seronegative spondylarthritides,[866] i.e. ankylosing spondylitis, psoriatic arthritis, Reiter's disease, the intestinal arthropathies, e.g. regional ileitis (Crohn's disease), ulcerative colitis and Bechet's syndrome, a particularly striking feature was the central position of sacroiliitis as a common denominator to each member of the group.

In *Crohn's disease* the synovitis, in combination with other features like conjunctivitis, appears to be the expression of an immune response to the enteric lesion. In 80 patients there were 3 cases of polyarthritis, 6 of spondylitis and 6 of asymptomatic sacroiliitis.[254]

True bony ankylosis of the sacroiliac joint appears never to occur except as the result of acquired disease (see p. 156).

Newton (1957)[928] reiterates the four cardinal signs of *ankylosing spondylitis*:

1. Spinal stiffness
2. Diminished thoracic expansion
3. Raised ESR
4. Radiological sacroiliac joint changes.

The author describes an extraordinary lack of awareness of the early manifestations of the disease and found during a long-term follow-up study that the average time taken to reach diagnosis was a little more than six years from the age of onset of symptoms. Clinical awareness of the nature of the disease can reduce this period to nine months and much less. Many cases bear no resemblance whatever to classical descriptions of the disease.

Iritis is an important presenting symptom in spondylitis, as is a painful heel, and it has been suggested[226] that all men between the ages of 18 and 30 presenting with calcaneal periostitis and spurs will have spondylitic changes in their sacroiliac joints.

Newton also suggested that, in the presence of other good evidence, a diagnosis of ankylosing spondylitis should not be discarded because the patient is a female and over 35 years old.

Women with ankylosing spondylitis appear to have a lower frequency of radiographic changes in the sacroiliac joint than do men,[171] and its involvement in the changes of ankylosing spondylitis is not invariable.

Resnick *et al.* (1976)[1028] described a clinical and radiological survey in 98 patients, 80 men and 18 women. The disease appears to be 4 to 10 times more frequent in men than in women, although the lower incidence in women may be accentuated by difficulties in recognising mild abnormalities. In general, women differ from men in:

1. An earlier age of onset.
2. Initial and frequent involvement of the lumbar spine.
3. Frequent cervical spine involvement.
4. A milder clinical course with minimal deformity and less systemic manifestations.

The spinal ascent of the disease may become arrested at any stage, although radiographic changes in the sacroiliac joint without vertebral change are unusual. Among the 98 patients, 10 had sacroiliac abnormalities and normal cervical, thoracic and lumbar radiographs; three of this group were women.

Among 116 women, 50 of whom aged 21–71 had backache and 66 with other conditions, 2 of the group of 50 had abnormal X-rays of the sacroiliac joint.[227] Scintillography scanning techniques revealed inflammatory changes in 22, nearly half of the group; the changes were unilateral in 8 and bilateral in 14.

Thus, sacroiliitis is a fairly common cause of backache in women. Scintillography is perhaps the best method of diagnosis. The conditions responded well to anti-inflammatory medication.

A *forme fruste* of ankylosing spondylitis, in which sacroiliitis cannot be radiographically demonstrated, is far more common than has been appreciated.[303]

When radiographic changes are present, the X-ray findings in *renal osteodystrophy* can simulate those of early ankylosing spondylitis, together with associated degenerative changes in the articular cartilage of the joint.[1027]

A study[14] of 143 patients with *primary gout* revealed 24 with radiographic changes of the sacroiliac joint attributable to this disease. All of the 24 had tophi, earlier onset of gout, a longer duration and a more rapid course into chronicity. There may be acute, recurrent gouty attacks, or clinically inactive tophaceous involvement of the sacroiliac joint. Gout of the axial skeleton is more frequent than commonly thought,[801] but involvement is usually found in patients with manifestations of gout over many years.

Tuberculosis of the sacroiliac joint[1153] usually occurs in young adults between the ages of 20 and 40 years. The disease is associated with tuberculosis in other regions of the body, the spine being a favourite skeletal site; the fifth lumbar vertebra was the site most often involved in a series of sacroiliac joint tuberculosis. So far as the latter is concerned, its onset is commonly announced by pain in the posterior iliac or hip region; sciatic radiation is present in about 25 per cent of the patients.

When serious disease has been excluded (so far as this is possible), assessment of pelvic joint problems should take account of several clinical possibilities:

1. Asymmetry in the adult sometimes appears to be long-standing, is frequently irreversible by passive movement and can exist without causing symptoms; patients may

present with sacroiliac area or haunch pain arising from low back and/or hip, the pelvic asymmetry and pelvic joints playing no detectable current part in production of pain.

2. Following stress, trauma, pregnancy, obstetric and gynaecological surgery and the effects of habitual working postures, local and referred pains from the sacroiliac joint can be relieved by specific mobilisation or manipulation. In some, clinically detectable pelvic asymmetry coexists with the painful condition and appears to be associated with it, because of the frequent and characteristic combination of a lower posterior iliac spine and pain on the same side. The asymmetry is not always reversible.

3. Joint irritability, sometimes severe, can be present in the absence of infective or metabolic sacroiliitis, *or any clinically or radiologically detectable postural change.* These clinical states appear to be a subdivision of possibility (2).

4. In a symmetrical pelvis, there may occur a painful movement hindrance of one sacroiliac joint, frequently responsible for buttock, lower abdominal, groin and anteromedial thigh pain—a separate group because the history offers no likely clue to aetiology.

5. The sacroiliac joint, usually but not invariably on the long leg side, can be responsible for symptoms when sustaining stress as part of the natural compensation for unequal leg lengths, although sacroiliac joint pain need not accompany leg asymmetry.

6. A localised very painful and tender area, lying unilaterally between the median sacral crest and posterior superior spine, can sometimes arise in the absence of lumbar articular signs, and appears to be a lesion of superficial connective tissue. (It is difficult to resist thinking of it as 'a tennis elbow in the backside'.)

7. Abnormalities of hip abduction and rotation need not arise primarily in the hip joint, but can be present as part of a sacroiliac joint problem.

8. Disorders of hypermobility in sacroiliac joint and symphysis pubis are interdependent.

9. Painful conditions of this joint in more mature and elderly people should be regarded with a degree of suspicion; bone pathology or serious disease are more likely, although this does not mean to say that benign mechanical problems of the joint may not occur in mature people.

When treating sacroiliac problems by manual techniques, one does not necessarily have to manipulate them. Gaymans (1973)[402] has suggested some useful hold–relax techniques for sacroiliac blocking.

There can be clinical advantage in remembering the subtle effects, on lower limb function, of covert sacroiliac problems. Pains about the ankle and foot, appearing to stem from local changes which themselves seem not to fit into a recognisable clinical entity, are frequently relieved by careful examination and appropriate treatment of the sacroiliac joint on that side.

Bourdillon (1973)[105] has given some examples of this.

It is quite common, for example, to find patients with a lateral pelvic tilt upwards on the side of the painful sacroiliac problem, who also have some restriction of extension of the ipsilateral knee joint. Both will need treatment, and it is wise to also check the tibiofibular and more distal joints.

Not all of this group will conform to this pattern. A 44-year-old woman, who reported left popliteal space pains which were provoked when going upstairs and rising from a chair, had less pain when walking in shoes with a heel and more pain when barefoot or in slippers. The pains had begun after a long walk over uneven ground about a year previously. Her pelvis was tilted up on the right, yet the deeper sacroiliac sulcus and prominent iliac spine were on the left. Although she had no lumbar or lumbosacral pain, she felt a hamstring 'pull' discomfort on lumbar extension, left side-flexion and flexion, which were not limited. The straight-leg-raising test was positive, with left-leg raising restricted to 50 degrees by a 'pull' at the knee; the right leg was normal at 80 degrees. There were no neurological signs.

There was nothing significant on lumbar palpation, but her left posterior superior iliac spine was tender. Extension of the left knee was some three to five degrees limited with a hard 'end-feel', and flexion was limited by pain at 10 degrees.

The knee-joint restriction and straight-leg-raising restriction were cleared up in one treatment of knee mobilisation; the sacroiliac joint was left alone.

Two years later, she reported again with knee pain, this time over the left superior tibiofibular joint, and accompanied again by diminished left straight-leg-raising. The only abnormality at the knee was a slight extension 'block'. It is noteworthy that comprehensive examination then also revealed a degree of atlantoaxial rotatory fixation with a thickened and very tender left craniovertebral region, about which she was unaware until examined. Her lateral pelvic tilt was still present.

While a causal relationship between the described findings was not established, of course, there is reason to believe that the changes may have been interdependent, since painstaking examination very frequently reveals these changes, associated in this distinctive way.

Sacroiliac joint syndromes

Considering the powerful musculature, like psoas major, which crosses the joint, or attaches to the ilium, like the iliacus and gluteal muscles—and ligamentous attachments like the ilio-lumbar ligament, capsule of hip joint and the lumbodorsal fascia—it follows that abnormalities of the joint are highly unlikely to remain without effects, mechanical and/or neuromuscular, upon interdependent structures and functions.

The purely specific, localised, unilateral sacroiliac joint lesion is something of a *rara avis*, other than in pregnancy.

Much more frequently, quite correctly called 'sacroiliac dysfunction' in men and non-pregnant women is reflected by detectable articular signs in the ipsilateral lumbosacral, sacroiliac and hip joints—sometimes involving the contralateral joints, too, and not infrequently accompanied by radiographic evidence of pubic symphysis asymmetry.

The term sacroiliac dysfunction is justified when treatment *localised to that joint* relieves the signs and symptoms.

Because the various clinical presentations involving this singular and mysterious joint are, with some exceptions,[105] not described as often as those of the vertebral joints, some outline case histories are given. Prophylaxis and back-care advice to the patients is not described.

The case histories are grouped as follows:

1. Sacroiliac joint irritability
2. Sacroiliac problems in men
3. Sacroiliac conditions in childless women
4. The sacroiliac joint in pregnancy
5. Combined sacroiliac and craniovertebral joint problem
6. Combined sacroiliac condition with low lumbar lordosis, together with thoraco lumbar kyphosis and C0–C1 joint problem.

1. *Sacroiliac irritability*

Patient D.G., 40 years. From the age of 9 this patient was fond of roller skating and frequently sat heavily on her bottom. As a girl she began having pain across her upper sacral area, worse on the right side; throughout her adult life and the raising of four children she continued to have the pain, which was exacerbated by pregnancies.

Examination: On observation her posture was unexceptional. She was reluctant to step up with her right leg or take weight on it. Extension, right-side-flexion and flexion were reduced, with provocation of right sacroiliac area pain. Baer's point was acutely tender on the right, as was the symphysis pubis and the right sacroiliac sulcus. Testing pressures on the spinous process, and the right paravertebral sulcus, of L5 revealed marked soreness there. Right hip abduction was reduced and painful, as were both hip rotations on that side. She had no neurological signs. Gapping tests of the sacroiliac joint revealed acute irritability, and sacral apex pressure hurt her severely at the right sacroiliac joint. Right straight-leg-raising was reduced slightly by pain, as was the prone-knee-bending test on that side. Figure 8.11 shows osteitis condensans ilii, more marked on the right.

Treatment: This was commenced by gentle rotatory mobilisation, in left-side lying for the right lumbosacral joint. As these were unavailing, treatment was localised to the sacroiliac joint, consisting of very gentle approximation of anterior superior iliac spines with the patient in left-side crook-lying; and similar repetitive pressures on the right posterior superior iliac spine with the patient prone. Ten attendances were required, and ultrasound was used occasionally to settle excessive irritability. At the termination of treatment she was almost, but not completely, relieved of her symptoms, and she was sign-free. Her sacroiliac joints remained somewhat irritable and her bony points unduly tender

to deep pressure. Nine months later, she replied to a postal questionnaire with: 'I am having no trouble with back or hip—no pain, no twinges.'

2. *Sacroiliac problems in men*

(i) *Patient G.B.*, a 24-year-old press tool maker noticed the insidious onset of right posterior, lateral and anterior thigh pain, spreading posterolaterally to the foot, after four years of repetitive lifting strains while standing; these also involved repetitive rotation. The right leg felt heavy and weak, and the limb 'dead'; symptoms were aggravated at times by twisting his pelvis to the left, or turning to the left.

On examination, there were no articular or palpation signs in the lumbar spine, no neurological signs in the limbs and no evidence of hip involvement. On comprehensive examination of the sacroiliac joint, the right was relatively immobile, with the sulcus deeper and the sacrotuberous ligament more easily palpable on that side. A manipulative thrust (Fig. 12.77) to the right PSIS had cleared his leg pain within 10 days, when a second thrust reduced his symptoms to 'slight twinges in the joint area only'. The asymmetry remained virtually unchanged.

(ii) *An insurance agent, B.M.*, with a five-year history of acute episodes of back pain after gardening, coughing while flexed and a blow on the lumbosacral region, complained of bilateral buttock and groin pain, and posterolateral with anterolateral right thigh and upper calf pain. He drove a lot and was active in gardening and house maintenance. Pains were constant, but variable in intensity and distribution. All pains were aggravated by sitting for one hour, standing for 30 minutes, gardening, stretching forward or upward and coitus. Pains were transiently eased by sitting after a period of standing, or moving around lightly after sitting for too long. Although there was no objective loss of sensation, transient feelings of numbness in the ball of both feet followed standing, walking or driving for too long. His posture was unexceptional for a man of his body type, except that the whole posterior surface of right ilium was more prominent than the left.

Extension was reduced to half range by pain over L5 and spreading to the right buttock. Both side-flexions were reduced, in that he could only reach to 8 cm above his knee-crease, and both provoked pain in the right buttock and haunch. Flexion was limited by right thigh pain when his fingers reached the mid-shin level. (It later transpired that this was his normal range of flexion.) There were no neurological signs, and the straight-leg-raising was reduced to 50° on the left by pain in the posterior thigh, and to 60° on the right by pain the lumbosacral region. The prone-knee-bending test was positive, both sides provoking lumbosacral pain. The whole lumbar spine was slightly tender to palpation, with most marked tenderness at L5 centrally and on the right, also over the right sacroiliac sulcus and localised to the right posterior inferior iliac spine. Hip rotations were unexceptional, but combined flexion/adduction of the *left* hip hurt a bit in the haunch of that side. X-rays were unavailable. He had a mildly troublesome hiatus hernia but was otherwise fit and very active.

The *current* problems were assessed as primarily sacroiliac and secondarily lumbosacral; he was not able to attend daily.

A precis of the treatment notes is as follows (for symbols see p. 438):

First treatment 22.10.76

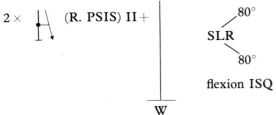

No more treatment was done this day, because examination was prolonged.

27.10.76

'No soreness, but ISQ'

Signs. ISQ with SLR at L. 50°, R. 65°

Treat lumbar spine

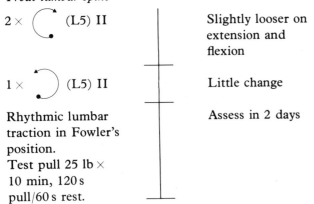

Slightly looser on extension and flexion

Little change

Assess in 2 days

Rhythmic lumbar traction in Fowler's position. Test pull 25 lb × 10 min, 120 s pull/60 s rest.

29.10.76

'Queasy after LT—hiatus hernia—but feels a bit easier' (Stop LT)

Signs. Movements remain slightly freer—not much in it

SLR L. 50°, R. 70°

Treat as S–I Jt problem

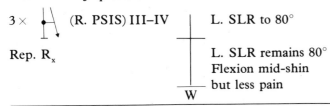

L. SLR to 80°

L. SLR remains 80°
Flexion mid-shin but less pain

1.11.76

'Was OK rising a.m. Saturday—did decorating and wallpapering and now it hurts a bit L. haunch and R. groin.'

Signs. SLR L. 65°, R. 80°

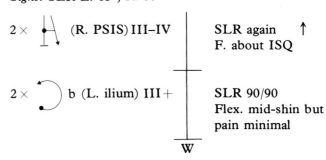

SLR again ↑
F. about ISQ

SLR 90/90
Flex. mid-shin but pain minimal

3.11.76

'Can sit for 2½ hr—residual but minimal R. groin pain'

Signs. SLR L. 90°, R. 90°

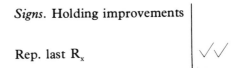

SLR 90/90
Flex. to mid-shin and painless

10.11.76

'Can do more for longer, and suffer less—still some slight R. groin pain'

Signs. Holding improvements

Rep. last R$_x$

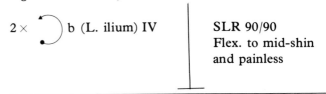

Demo. abdominal isometric flexion exercises and back care

His lumbar spine was not treated after 27.10.76.

When contacted 14 months later, the patient reported a trouble-free interim.

(iii) *Patient R.S.M.*, an active 72-year-old man, subject to back trouble for some 30 years, was on his knees gardening when, in his own words, 'A bolt of lightning struck me in the backside.' He retired to bed with great difficulty, but by 2 a.m. was in such severe localised pain that he contacted his general practitioner, who sedated him and suggested physiotherapy in the morning.

Pain was localised to the left posterior iliac crest and posterior superior and inferior iliac spines; visibly, the patient had been shaken by its intensity. Strangely, there was no limitation of lumbar movement, by neither pain nor resistance, but left hip and knee flexion provoked very intense pain, accurately localised by the patient's index finger to the left posterior inferior iliac spine. The patient had attended for backache some months before, and his range of straight-leg-raising was known to the physiotherapist; it was unaffected by the current episode.

A precis of treatment is as follows:

16.7.77

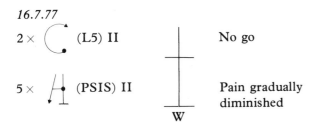

2 × (L5) II — No go

5 × (PSIS) II — Pain gradually diminished

W

18.7.77

'Very much better' Pain still PIIS but plainly less

Signs. Hip flexion still hurts PIIS

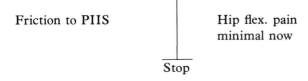

Friction to PIIS — Hip flex. pain minimal now

Stop

The therapist was as astonished as the patient that this simple technique gradually settled the vicious pain.

It is difficult to know what this man had done to himself, and one cannot discount a locked lumbosacral facet-joint as the cause of his pain, nor possibly an acute derangement of an accessory sacroiliac articulation (see p. 29). His response to a localised sacroiliac technique was manifest, and the technique could also have mobilised the left lumbosacral region, of course, but this does not explain the further rapid improvement by localised frictions to the posterior inferior iliac spine. He had remained well when contacted eight months later.

The treatment of low back pain in elderly patients can yield far more encouraging results than is often suggested.

Kirkaldy-Willis (1978)[661b] describes the helpful effects of manipulation and other treatments in the facet-joint syndrome and benign sacroiliac joint problems, for example.

(iv) There is probably no such thing as a purely localised sacroiliac joint problem; the attachments of the iliolumbar ligaments, for example, make such a possibility highly unlikely. Also, there is more in acute or chronic low back pain episodes than can easily be explained by the orthodox theories of discogenic changes.

Ingpen and Burry (1970)[591] describe a large group of patients whose condition is of less well-defined aetiology, variously named low back strain, iliolumbar strain, sacroiliac strain or lumbosacral strain. After careful assessment, the authors conclude that the syn-drome is that of a strain of lumbosacral facet joints and iliolumbar ligaments.

As an example of manual sacroiliac joint techniques fully relieving the signs and symptoms of a low back episode, the following clinical history is not untypical.

Patient H.W.B., a portly little 53-year-old man, felt his low back 'give' as he stooped forward to weld a pipe-section the day before. In constant pain, which radiated from his lumbo-sacral region into both buttocks and upper posterior thighs, he was unable to work, although was fairly comfortable lying on a firm mattress. Getting up to dress was painful, and both neck-flexion in sitting, and coughing, hurt him in the centre low back. He stood with severe bilateral muscle spasm; his pattern of movement was:

Extension—virtually nil because of rising lumbosacral pain.
Left side-flexion—two-thirds, limited by pain at centre and right lumbar.
Right side-flexion—two-thirds, limited by pain at centre and right lumbar.
Flexion—fingers to tibial tubercles, limited by pain across lumbosacral level.
Left rotation (in sitting)—cautious, but full range and pain-free.
Right rotation (in sitting)—reduced a few degrees by lumbo-sacral pain.
Straight-leg-raising was (L) 80° with central lumbosacral pain and (R) 75° with similar pain.

There were no other articular signs of note and he had no neurological symptoms or signs. Apart from acute tenderness over the right transverse process of L5 vertebra and centrally over L4, and slight tenderness centrally over L5, he had no detectable signs at the lumbar or sacroiliac joints.

Treatment. Five repetitions of left rotation (grades II− and then II+) improved his straight-leg-raising to 90°/90°, and his flexion was increased by 5 cm. At his second attendance three days later, his condition had deteriorated and straight-leg-raising was now (L) 60° and (R) 45°, with flexion still considerably reduced and pulling on the right lumbosacral region. Pelvic rotation to the left (grades II to IV−) were of no avail. Three grade III mobilisations of the right posterior superior iliac spine (see Fig. 12.61) relieved all signs immediately, with free straight-leg-raising and free lumbar movement. A few days later, he reported being back at work with no problems.

These events do not necessarily suggest that there might have been some sacroiliac problem, but do suggest that the lumbopelvic articulation was affected in some way, and the joint condition was resolved by minimal movement of the painful-side ilium, with the iliolumbar ligament probably transmitting movement to the L5 vertebral body. Herein may lie a partial solution to the vexed question of what 'sacroiliac strain' may be in some.

(v) The known propensity for sacroiliac and midlumbar joint problems to occur together can produce an odd mixture of symptoms and signs.

A 41-year-old office worker, who was athletically active in his leisure hours, reported a bilaterally symmetrical low lumbar pain, which radiated down the back of his *right* thigh to the knee, and also to the *left* groin much more than to the right, 'when bad'. There was no left thigh pain.

He stood with a slight lateral pelvic tilt upwards on the left—this disappeared when sitting, and in both postures his spine appeared straight. Lumbar articular signs were:

Extension—unexceptional.
Left-side-flexion—fingers to knee crease without pain.
Right-side-flexion—an identical range of movement but now provoking right more than left lumbosacral pain.
Flexion—fingers to toes, painlessly, but retaining a localised lumbosacral lordosis.
Rotations—unexceptional.

Straight-leg-raising was left 85° with *left* lumbar pain, and right 85° but painless. The hip joints were normal, but *left* prone-knee-bending hurt in the left loin and was a little limited by this pain and by resistance; the right was normal.

There were no neurological signs, and on palpation the left sacroiliac sulcus was tender, the left PSIS more prominent posteriorly and the L2–L3 segment was thickened on the left with noticeable tenderness of the L2 and L3 spines and left transverse processes, elicited by moderate pressure.

He was assessed as a combined lesion and treated by left p-a PSIS pressures for the sacroiliac component and right rotations for the L2–L3 problem. His left straight-leg-raising and right-side-flexion pain diminished markedly after the sacroiliac technique, and diminished further after right lumbar rotation.

He was shown a corrective postural lying exercise for the pelvic asymmetry and a bilateral knee flexion exercise for the localised lumbosacral lordosis.

Within an hour or two of treatment, his right sciatic pain reappeared for some hours, then disappeared. A week later, his pattern of articular signs was the same, but the amount of pain on the positive testing movements was considerably less.

A single localised grade V right rotation to the upper lumbar segment cleared the straight-leg-raising restriction, and a single thrust technique to the left ilium cleared the remaining restriction of right-side-flexion.

He has remained sign and symptom free.

Joint problems do not invariably respond to manual treatment:

A 26-year-old builder, with left buttock and posterior thigh pain of insidious onset six weeks before, stood with lateral pelvic tilt upward on the left. He was a bulky and strong man who used his back heavily at work. Walking quickly, bending to work and sneezing all provoked the left buttock pain. When sitting on a flat surface, the pelvis was virtually level. The only traumatic incident in the history was a road traffic accident four years before in which he sustained a fractured right femur; this may have been responsible for shortening of that limb.

On extension he appeared to hinge at the L4–L5 segment, but the gross range was normal and only slight buttock pain was provoked. Side-flexions were unexceptional other than that the movements were of unequal range. Rotations were normal.

On flexion, he deviated well to the right, with a flattened left buttock and slight pain there; fingertips reached mid-shin. He lay supine with the left leg markedly externally rotated. Straight-leg-raising was left 45°, limited by hamstring tightness and less

so by buttock pain, and right 90°. There were no neurological signs, and careful palpation revealed a normal lumbar spine but marked deepening of the left sacroiliac sulcus.

After three treatment sessions, during which every sacroiliac, and subsequently lumbar, technique known to the writer failed to do other than produce only slight improvement (i.e. slightly less pain and improved flexion range), active treatment was stopped and the patient recommended to daily practise an exercise to restore what appeared to be the cause of his pains—a backward-shuffled left ilium.

During the ensuing three months, his symptoms slowly and steadily regressed.

Flexion range had increased but slightly, although the range of left straight-leg-raising had improved to 75° and there was much less pain when hamstring spasm imposed the limitation. He was advised to raise the right heels of all shoes by 1 cm (⅜ in).

3. *Sacroiliac conditions in childless women*

(i) *Dancer: Patient G.D.*, a slim 22-year-old professional dancer complained of persistent sacroiliac area pain after an hour's practice or rehearsal of modern dance routines. X-rays were unremarkable. Her right posterior superior iliac spine was more prominent and lower than its fellow, and the right anterior superior iliac spine higher than that on the left. Her iliac crests were level in standing and sitting.

The most remarkable feature during examination was the unmistakably clear exhibition of Piedallu's sign (q.v.). Other than this, her only articular signs of note were some 10° restriction of full flexion, by resistance and 'tightness' with only moderate pain, and a 15° restriction of right straight-leg-raising by the same factors. Rotations were unexceptional even to strong overpressure. The lumbar spine was clear on palpation, but the posterior inferior iliac spine on the right was markedly tender to localised pressure—the buttock was not. The sacral apex pressure test was negative, and she had no neurological signs.

Her condition defied all treatment methods and combinations of technique, for sacroiliac joint, lumbar spine and hip known to the author; her symptoms and physical signs remained unaltered, and on cessation of treatment she was seriously considering changing her career. Whether she was subsequently relieved by another practitioner and other treatment, or did give up dancing, is not known because she disappeared from follow-up.

(ii) *Patient LD.*, a 23-year-old physiotherapist, gave a three-month history of beginning to feel stiff in the upper right buttock region after the day's work. Two months later, at a period when she was lifting many patients, the pain became sharper, and bed rest for a week was prescribed. At that time the pain spread down the posterior thigh and calf to ankle, with tingling in the 5th toe. The left leg was unaffected.

X-ray showed a Schmorl's node at L4–L5, a slightly reduced L5–S1 disc space and the possibility of a partly transitional S1 vertebra.

When seen at the end of the three-month period, she described upper buttock pain only; this was worsened by sitting for more than a few minutes, by stooping and by lying on the right side. These did not hurt her low back. On observation, her right posterior superior iliac spine was plainly more prominent than the left, but her pelvis was level and there was no detectable postural spasm of back muscles. Right-side-flexion was reduced by 5° and provoked her pain, and on bending forward she could reach just below her knees, with similar provocation of pain. Her straight-leg-raising was L. 90°, and R. 45° limited by pain over the sacro-iliac joint. Apart from a 5° limitation of R. hip abduction she had no other signs of note, and on careful, specific and persistent palpation it was difficult to find anything worth recording at the lower three lumbar segments. Her right posterior inferior iliac spine was a different matter, being acutely tender—there was otherwise only mild diffuse tenderness over the rest of the buttock on that side.

She was assessed and treated as probably a combined lumbo-sacral and sacroiliac problem, with the latter causing most of her current difficulties, i.e.:

22.8.74

$2 \times$ ⊣ (PSIS) II   SLR ↑ 15° Flex. ↑ 3″ (8 cm)

$1 \times$ R(ASIS) thrust   Not much better
in lumbar rotation
loc V.

W

27.8.74

'Was pretty sore, but functionally much more able'

Signs. Flex. gain maintained-SLR 55°

$2 \times$ ↔ (R. leg) II   SLR 90/90
Flex. to mid/lower shin

Stop

It was suggested that her hospital colleagues continue the gentle rhythmic leg traction as indicated and that she report again in a month.

25.9.74

'Doing very well, no problems except cannot sustain stooping for too long'

Signs. Movements √ √

R. SLR resistant over last 10° but goes to 90°
R. PSIS still prominent in standing.

At this time she attended as one of a group of patients being presented during follow-up demonstrations to the candidates of an annual comprehensive Manipulation Course.

In retrospect, the mistake in treatment was the localised grade V technique on 22.8.74; this was unnecessary. Nevertheless it probably contributed to her progress, although it raised the questions of 'environmental manipulation' in that it involved left pelvic rotation for positioning, and this cannot help but rotate the lumbar spine, too. Thus we are left with the plain fact of immediate improvement in straight-leg-raising

and flexion (22.8.74) after a technique which was as carefully localised as is possible; single leg traction is not a localised technique. Since these were the only objective clinical criteria available, assessment of the nature of her problem may be acceptable as a reasonable one.

Eighteen months later the lady sent a brief report of her condition—'All systems are "go", and have been since.'

(iii) *Patient I.G.* had noted the insidious onset of right haunch pain three months previously, on getting up from sitting. The pain settled to a constant dull ache, relieved only by lying on the left side. The only trauma recalled was a heavy fall from a motor-bike on to her right buttock, 20 months previously.

On examination, the pelvis was laterally tilted to the right and the trunk very slightly deviated to the left, the left posterior superior iliac spine was prominent and the left buttock flattened. There were no lumbar articular signs other than a painless and slight deviation to the left on extension, but not on flexion. Other than slight left buttock flattening, with no detectable gluteal weakness, she was neurologically clear. Straight-leg-raising was 90° and painless. Right hip lateral rotation was painlessly reduced, left hip medial rotation likewise.

On her right side, iliac gapping and approximation were positive, the adductors tight with their origins tender, and Baer's point and the anterior acetabular area very tender, with mild tenderness of the third, fourth and fifth lumbar spinous processes. There was severe localised pain on palpation of the right posterior superior iliac spine and sacroiliac sulcus. She was treated by two applications of the technique in Figure 12.20 (grade II and then III), after which her lumbar extension was symmetrical. The next day her pain was '50 per cent better'; the mobilisation was repeated. By the third day her right haunch pain was slightly worse again, but the gapping tests were no longer positive. She was not treated that day; examination on the fourth day revealed no haunch pains, symmetrical hip rotations and adductor tensions, and no tenderness at Baer's point or the acetabular area.

During the following three days her pain had gone and she had enjoyed dancing, although the right sulcus was still tender on palpation. Two days later, because of a return of mild pain, she was manipulated (Fig. 12.78) but this did not effect any immediate further improvement; however, she continued steadily to lose all her symptoms without further treatment.

(iv) *Patient L.M.* This young lady of 20 years reported a lumbosacral ache, worse on the right and 'violent' after 15 minutes of badminton, with daily episodic jabs. Sitting eased her pain sometimes, standing or walking for 30 minutes made her uneasy. Sustained stooping hurt and she returned to the erect with some difficulty, feeling a 'click' as she did so. Her pain was time-dependent to a degree, in that it always built up to the end of the day. She could recall no trauma.

Her pelvis was tilted up on the right. Extension and side-flexions were a little reduced and hurt the right lumbosacral region; she flexed to touch her tibial tubercles with a somewhat flat back but little added pain, only a manifest reluctance to go further. Gentle overpressure to further flexion was resisted because it alarmed her. Straight-leg-raising was left 90°, right 55° with rising buttock pain, and the prone-knee-bending test hurt similarly on the right though it was not limited. She was neurologically normal. Firm unilateral pressures at L5 on the right hurt moderately. The right posterior inferior iliac spine was acutely tender, her buttock was not.

Right straight-leg-raising improved by 20° at the first treatment of localised right PSIS pressures, and straight-leg-raising was 90/90 by the second. Her residual pain and limitation of flexion was cleared by adding left rotational mobilisation for the lumbar spine. She adapted comfortably to a 1 cm (⅜ in) raise on the left heel, and on check-up after 14 days was out of trouble.

4. *The sacroiliac joint in pregnancy*

(i) *Patient S.W.* A 29-year-old mother, following right lumbar and sciatic pain during her first pregnancy three years before, described a recurrence of symptoms during the fourth month of her second pregnancy, which continued thereafter for eight months to the time of admission. She could not stand for long or push the pram without severe pain, and was understandably very depressed. Sudden trunk movement or a jar stirred up the pain for several hours, although there was no cough impulse. On examination, trunk extension was of good range but produced a jab of pain down the limb to the ankle; there were no other articular or neurological signs. Straight-leg-raising was normal; the right posterior superior iliac spine acutely tender.

After three mobilisations (Fig. 12.61) (grade II—) to the right posterior superior iliac spine, extension range was virtually painless. At the second session two days later, extension was normal, but iliac gapping still hurt. The technique was repeated four times up to grade III— and she reported five days later that the pain had considerably reduced and she was able to do more. The technique was progressed to grade IV, together with an added technique (Fig. 12.59) on the right anterior superior iliac spine (grade III) for the pain on iliac gapping. Thereafter she remained trouble-free and sign-free up to her discharge a fortnight later.

(ii) *Patient M.I.* A 29-year-old mother with a child of two years was 22 weeks into her second pregnancy when she developed right sacroiliac area pain, two days previously, on standing up after lying at rest. There was no backache or left leg pain, but posterior thigh pain from right upper buttock to the popliteal space. Each time she subsequently stood from sitting she experienced numbness and pins-and-needles in the sole of the right foot for a few minutes. When seven months pregnant, two years previously, she had experienced a similar episode which had settled of its own accord before her first baby was born.

On examination she was hardly able to walk the few steps from car door to treatment room. All movements were severely limited by pain in the right sacroiliac region, and because of her distress straight-leg-raising was not tested. Careful palpation, progressed to fairly firm pressure, revealed no tenderness or other signs in the lumbar segments.

The right posterior superior iliac spine felt depressed, in relation to its fellow, and the sulcus was acutely tender. Gentle sacral apex pressure hurt severely at the right sulcus, and there was severe tenderness localised to the right posterior inferior iliac spine. Her distress was visibly relieved by gently manoeuvring her into a left-side-lying position with right hip and knee well flexed, and the left hip and knee well extended. She was shown how to dispose her limbs in this way if she had a further attack; she declined a 6-inch crepe bandage cummerbund support, and was able to walk the 400 yards home. Until the birth of her baby, she

experienced the occasional jab of right buttock and thigh pain when walking, but was otherwise trouble-free. When contacted a year later she had remained trouble-free.

(iii) *Patient H.B.* A 26-year-old, eight and a half months pregnant woman had five days previously felt a stab in the right upper buttock on reaching upward to a cupboard. The pain was localised to the right lumbosacral region and below, and spread distally to the right heel when she lay in bed. The continuous upper haunch pain was aggravated by sitting, dressing, bending, and moving about after immobility. She had no lumbar articular signs other than that flexion provoked right haunch pain when her fingers reached to the upper shin. Straight-leg-raising was 90/90 and there were no neurological signs.

Palpation in side-lying revealed no lumbar signs but acutely tender right posterior superior and inferior iliac spines.

She was treated by gentle repetitive pressures on her right anterior superior iliac spines, while in comfortable left-side-lying, after which she was able to flex to the floor and easily put on her shoes. Her pregnancy was uneventful and she remains comfortable.

5. *Combined sacroiliac and craniovertebral problem*

A housewife of 51 years, with constant left lumbosacral and sacroiliac joint area pain, reported the spread of pain to left anterior haunch and groin when presssure was applied to the left posterior superior iliac spine. Later during the treatment sessions she reported an 'inverted saucer' of vertex cranial pain whenever 'her back was bad'.

Her 15-month history of buttock, haunch and groin pain was initiated by a bout of flu, and the 'backache' of her flu then settled in her left haunch area, the groin pain only being provoked as described.

Some 30 years before, she had slipped and landed very heavily on her ischial turberosities, and 15 years after that had 'left sciatica pain' spreading to heel, for which she had been given exercises and a corset. Her back pain was time-dependent as well as stress-dependent, always being bad in the evenings. The 'constant, nagging ache' was slowly increasing, and aggravated by lying on her back, standing on the left leg and pressing her pelvis against the seat of a dining chair. Sitting in any kind of chair produced increasing haunch discomfort after 30 minutes. Walking eased the pain to a degree. She had recently been clinically examined twice, and after each occasion she had noticed transient slight numbness at the posterior left thigh. On observation, she had bilateral sacrospinalis spasm and her trunk was slightly 'windswept' to the right. Her pelvis was level. Her lumbar spine articular pattern was:

Ext.—⅓ with pain in left sacroiliac area
LSF—⅓ with pain in left sacroiliac area
RSF—⅔ with 'pull' pain in left haunch and groin
Flex.—'Kick' of pain left sacroiliac area at 45°/55°, then full painless flexion. 'Kick' coming up, too
LR—⅔ with pain left sacroiliac area
RR—¾ with pain left sacroiliac area.

Because of her manifest soreness, the sacroiliac joint was not tested, and examination of hip and prone-knee-bending were also postponed. Straight-leg-raising was R. 90°, and a slightly limited L. 85° by left sacroiliac area pain. On return of the left leg to horizontal, there was a 'kick' of pain at 45°. Brudzinski's test provoked her sacroiliac pain; she had no neurological signs. Palpation findings were as follows:

○ Tender
● Sore

X Stiff Segment
III Thickened (deep)
≋ Elicited Spasm

ϡϢϡ Hypermobile
         Segment
⊗ Prominent

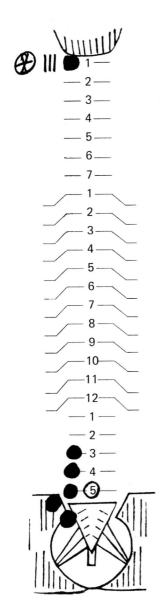

The record of her treatments is as follows:

30.10.74 (day of examination)

$2 \times$ (L5) I   ISQ

W

31.10.74

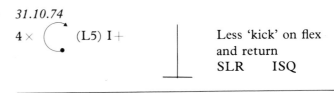

$4 \times$ (L5) I+   Less 'kick' on flex
                          and return
                          SLR   ISQ

5.11.74

'Sting gone from pain, sleeping better and can lie on back now'

Signs. F few°. No 'kick' and pain a little less

$2 \times$ (L5) II   F. easier
                          E. and LSF range ↑

$2 \times$ (L5) III   F. steadily easier
(getting   LSF=RSF now
sore)

6.11.74

'Very sore indeed'

Signs. F. regressed a
little

$3 \times$ (L5) I   Assess 24 hours

7.11.74

'Feeling better but still sore'.
Also reports vertex headache whenever 'back is bad'

Signs. Less tender L5.
F. no 'kick' but otherwise ISQ
Tender and thickened C1 on left. Suboccipital pain on left Ext/side-flex/rot quadrant sustained.

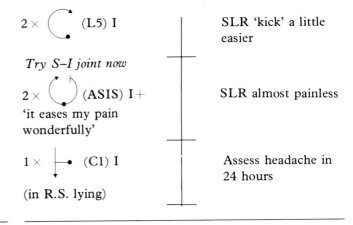

$2 \times$ (L5) I   SLR 'kick' a little
                          easier

Try S–I joint now

$2 \times$ (ASIS) I+   SLR almost painless
'it eases my pain
wonderfully'

$1 \times$ (C1) I   Assess headache in
                          24 hours

(in R.S. lying)

8.11.74

'Going well after 4 hours slight soreness—little headache'

Signs. Lumbar movements ✓✓ except slight pain on extreme of ext.
SLR 90/90 with very slight 'kick'

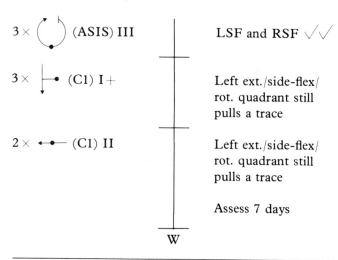

$4\times$ (ASIS) II+   Assess 3 days

$3\times$ (C1) I

12.11.74

'Has been really good. Can stand longer, no headaches, no pain on pressing back in chair'

Signs. Flex. and SLR ✓✓
Slight pain on overpressure to LSF and RSF

$3\times$ (ASIS) III   LSF and RSF ✓✓

$3\times$ (C1) I+   Left ext./side-flex/ rot. quadrant still pulls a trace

$2\times$ (C1) II   Left ext./side-flex/ rot. quadrant still pulls a trace

Assess 7 days

W

18.11.74

'No problems'

Signs. She's right!   Stop.

In retrospect, this patient is a good example of those who do not mention associated problems unless asked. This diffidence is sometimes due to unawareness that apparently disparate pains may indeed be associated, and at other times because the patient has in the past been subjected to ridicule or had her reports brushed aside. The author has very frequently observed respected and able clinicians saying to the patient, 'You cannot possibly be having a pain *there*.' Subsequently, rather than to look or feel a fool, the patient takes care to pull up the drawbridge, and will only mention pains which are 'neat and tidy'. Later, other clinicians handling her succeeding problems are put at a disadvantage, and it is likely that the patient's problem is recorded as a neat little statistic representative of a particular kind of clinical pattern, when in fact the total presentation may not be in the least 'neat and tidy'.

Precisely what the association *is*, between craniovertebral joint problems and low back with sacroiliac problems, is difficult to explain on any basis other than that expressed by, 'no vertebral segment is an island', but as to the *existence* of this association experienced practitioners have no doubt.

6. *Combined sacroiliac condition with low lumbar lordosis, together with thoracolumbar kyphosis and C0–C1 joint problem*

This lady of 31 presented with a history of 'hip and knee' trouble when aged 15–16 years, falling down a flight of stairs at 17, and backache as a teenager. The backache eased during her early twenties. She had an episode of 'right sciatica' in 1975, with pain to the popliteal space, and during that time the dorsum of her right foot had felt cold.

Three months before her attendance, she had a miscarriage at 18 weeks.

Her area of worst pain was the right upper buttock; this was a constant background ache with several episodes of 'shooting across' the lumbosacral region. She had more diffuse ache over the lower thoracic and upper lumbar region, and episodic left occipital and frontal pain. Her back felt 'unstable and likely to go at any minute'. She slept well enough, but always woke uncomfortably bent forward and leaning to her left, not being able to straighten until she had a shower. After more than an hour's sitting, she could get out of a chair carefully but remained bent and deviated to the left for a few minutes. Dressing, standing for more than an hour and bending over a work-top aggravated her buttock pain; she returned from sustained stooping very cautiously. The pain was eased by a hot shower, a hot water bottle or massage to the back. A cough or sneeze hurt the lumbosacral region.

On examination, the thoracolumbar junction region was kyphotic and she had a pronounced but localised lumbosacral lordosis. Her pelvis was laterally tilted upwards on the right, and her right posterior superior iliac spine was more prominent than its fellow.

She stood deviated a little to the left.
Articular signs were:

Ext.—$\frac{1}{2}$, stiff, with pain across lumbosacral level.
LSF—$\frac{2}{3}$, with 'pull' right lumbosacral.
RSF—$\frac{2}{3}$, with pain right lumbosacral.
Flex.—Fing. to lower shin, little pain, keeps lumbosacral lordosis, lower thoracic/upper lumbar kyphosis. Deviates left.
LR—$\frac{3}{4}$ with pain to right lumbosacral.
RR—$\frac{3}{4}$ with pain to right lumbosacral.
Her pelvis levelled up when sitting.

Straight-leg-raising was $55°$ on both sides and limited by lumbosacral pain. Passively testing the right hip combined adduction/ flexion 'quadrant' hurt her badly in the buttock; the left was normal. Prone-knee-bending on the right was reduced by some 10°, the left was normal. There were no neurological signs and Brudzinski's test (q.v.) was negative. There was little to find other than localised lordosis on central palpation of the lower lumbar spine, but L5 was sore to grade II unilateral pressures on the right. The postural kyphosis at upper lumbar and lower thoracic segments was markedly evident on palpation, and segments T10–L2 were manifestly stiff. There was also marked tenderness and elicited spasm on middle-range central pressures over this region. On sacroiliac joint examination, the right Baer's point was very tender as was the right anterior acetabular area. The right sulcus was deeper, and the right posterior inferior iliac spine very sore; the sacral apex pressure test was strongly positive in that it hurt her at the right sacroiliac sulcus.

She was analysed as a possible right sacroiliac joint and lumbosacral joint problem, almost certainly an old Scheuermann's disease of the kyphotic region with compensatory lumbosacral lordosis, and a concurrent left craniovertebral joint condition.

It was decided to approach her problem from below upwards, the treatment plan being:

— R. PSIS and shoe raise L.

—localised stretch of lumbosacral fascia plus isometric abdominal exercise
—mobilise thoracolumbar kyphosis, plus corrective exercises
—mobilise C0–C1 R.

Confining the description to treatment of her pelvic joints:

2× (PSIS) III–IV | SLR 85/85 and painless
Flex. much more confident.

The essential point is that her upper buttock and lumbosacral pain had probably more to do with her sacroiliac condition than her low back, but plainly her needs were much more than just mobilisation techniques.

It is always difficult to ascribe several pains to their proper source, and in the absence of feeling on sure ground one must proceed on the provisional first analysis and a basis of the greatest weight of likelihood; the gathering of positive findings begins with the result of the first mobilisation procedure employed. Either it helps, or it does not. In this case, unravelling 'the tangled ball of wool' (p. 350) had begun on the first day.

The use of a unilateral heel and/or buttock raise is discussed on page 475.

The 'piriformis' syndrome, the 'theatre—cocktail party' syndrome, the 'lumbo-pelvo-hip' syndrome

The 5th lumbar vertebra, the sacrum and the sacroiliac joint are sometimes regarded[59, 60] as comprising a structural and functional unit (the 'sacroiliac unit') which can exhibit a characteristic syndrome.[837] Other writers include hip conditions, and speak of a 'piriformis syndrome', and others a 'lumbo-pelvo-hip complex'; experienced therapists will recognise the syndrome being described.

Barbor (1978)[60] has observed that much pain is referred from spinal and pelvic ligaments, i.e. intervertebral ligaments, the iliolumbar ligament, sacroiliac ligaments, sacrotuberous and sacrospinous ligaments, and holds that these can refer pain according to dermatome distribution; the sacrotuberous ligament, for example, can refer pain to the calf and heel.

The 'numbness' and 'deadness' of the limb (without objective sensory loss) which, in the author's experience, patients sometimes describe, is said to be due to lesions of the sacrotuberous ligament, and if this ligament is injected with local anaesthetic, the calf and heel 'numbness' disappears. Further, it is observed that groin and sacral pain can be referred from lesions of the lumbosacral segment, and the iliolumbar ligament. A reminder of the phenomenon of pain reference according to sclerotome distribution (p. 190)[592b] together with the vagaries of referred pain (p. 192) will indicate the possibilities for difficulty in ascribing pain to a specific soft tissue in the pelvic girdle.

According to Barbor[60] the *symptoms* of 'sacroiliac unit' joint problems of insidious onset are:

1. Sitting causes pain (theatre, car-driving, sedentary jobs).
2. Standing causes pain (e.g. cocktail parties).
3. Walking eases the pain.
4. Worse on waking a.m., but gone in half-an-hour or else hot bath eases it.
5. *Leaning* forward hurts, e.g. washing up, ironing. *Bending* forward may not.
6. Cough or sneeze may hurt in acute sacroiliac strain.
7. Sleep may be disturbed by the pain, which is eased by walking around the room.
8. Slouching in chair, so that weight is taken by sacrum, instead of ischial tuberosities, may ease the pain.
9. Sensation of pins-and-needles in back of thigh and calf, is not uncommon.
10. Daily nagging leg pain for many months or years (too long for root irritation without root palsy developing).
11. A nagging pain at back of thigh, ending behind the knee.
12. Groin pain on standing or sitting (this is said to inculpate the iliolumbar ligament).
13. The symptoms may exist in the presence of a completely negative lumbar spine examination.

The *signs* are:
1. *Lumbar movements* are usually full:
Flexion usually full, but hurts if sacrum is displaced forwards.

Extension frequently hurts if sacrum is displaced backwards unilaterally.

Side-flexion may hurt towards painful side.

In flexion, lumbar spine may deviate from S1 if the sacrum is tilted, the spine deviating to the side of sacral tilt.

2. *Straight-leg-raising*

Can be limited, as hamstrings pull on ischial tuberosity and put a strain on the sacrotuberous ligament.

The limitation of straight-leg-raising is not sudden as in discogenic root pressure; the limb can usually be pushed further after pain begins.

Full straight-leg-raising may hurt the opposite side, when straight-leg-raising on the affected side is pain-free.

3. *Flexion of hip, and then adduction in supine lying*

Is positive uni- or bilaterally, unless only supraspinous ligaments are affected when passive flexion of *both* knees and hips in supine lying hurts when lumbar spine is fully flexed.

The amount of flexion of hip can guide towards which ligaments are affected, i.e. the more hip flexion and less adduction the lower the site of the lesion (see p. 284).

4. When these signs and symptoms occur, even after root palsy due to a disc lesion, sclerosants will often rapidly relieve the remaining ligamentous strain.

5. Tenderness is usually present.

6. Palpation may cause referred pain.

The '*piriformis syndrome*', although not regarded as the primary lesion, is said to manifest itself as a secondary or accompanying clinical feature in many conditions of the lower lumbar spine, sacroiliac joint and hip. Many of the lower limb girdle pains described by patients are believed to have their origin in changes of this muscle.

According to McQueen,[837] the clinical features are, among others: pain radiating into buttock or hip, because of ischaemia of the muscle; pain aggravated by sexual intercourse, and/or by defaecation; tenderness locally over piriformis; pain on external rotation of the hip.

Mennell (1952)[851] also speaks of piriformis syndrome, ascribing this to irritation of part of the sciatic nerve when it passes through the substance of the piriformis muscle. He suggests that the pathognomonic sign is that of sciatic pain provocation, by internal rotation of the straight lower limb, when it is just short of that point at which raising the neutrally rotated limb provokes the characteristic sciatic pain (see p. 317).

The muscle is related to many important structures, i.e. intrapelvically on the left side to the rectum; and by its upper border to the gluteus medius and superior gluteal vessels and nerves, and by its lower border to the coccygeous and gemellus superior. Emerging between the latter muscle and the piriformis are the inferior gluteal and internal pudendal vessels, the sciatic, posterior femoral cutaneous and pudendal nerves. Muscular branches from the sacral plexus also pass between the piriformis and the gemellus superior.

An important point is the action of piriformis.[437] *It laterally rotates the neutrally positioned thigh, but abducts the flexed thigh. Thus combined flexion and adduction of the hip joint (with knee flexed) is the one movement which puts most tension on the piriformis (as well as its immediately neighbouring muscles, of course).* It will have been noted that various slight changes in the *proportions* of adduction and/or flexion during this testing movement are said (p. 284) to inculpate this or that ligament, as the causative lesion underlying the patient's complaint. A moment's consideration indicates that a great many highly differentiated and important soft tissues are disturbed in one or other ways by this single physical test, and will also indicate the real difficulty in confidently ascribing positive signs to changes in this or that tissue. When the *range* of the movement is limited, the pain elicited is in the groin and the operator can detect a *localised* 'block' to further probing *at the same instant* as the patient experiences a momentary twinge of groin pain, some kind of change localised in the hip joint may seem to be a reasonable conclusion, but there is no absolute certainty of it.

Kirkaldy-Willis and Hill (1979)[662] have noted that the clinical history of sacroiliac and piriformis syndromes is broadly the same as that of the posterior facet syndrome (p. 289), in that there is buttock, trochanteric and posterior thigh pain. Since the muscle is closely related to the anterior surface of the joint, spasm of piriformis may lead to strain of joint; alternatively, strain of the joint may result in muscle spasm. In passing, much the same relationship between the iliacus muscle and sacroiliac joint problems in children has been noted by Lewit (p. 152).

Resisted external rotation of the hip provokes pain—as does the passive application of tension to piriformis (among the other tissues which are perforce included in these passive tests).

Taking sacroiliac and the piriformis syndromes as a whole, the authors suggest that when injection of the piriformis muscle (p. 515) dramatically relieves the pain, the diagnosis is confirmed.

Also,

Manipulation specifically directed to restore the small range of movement normally present in the upper or lower part of the joint or to both of these is a most helpful diagnostic aid. When it results in restoration of movement as described above, or in relief of pain, or both, these also confirm the diagnosis.

It is suggested by Pace and Nagle (1976)[961] that a typical history in the piriformis syndrome is that of an incomplete fall, affecting females six times more frequently than males. The pain overlies the groin, hip, buttock or posterior thigh, being provoked by static abduction, and by lateral rotation in sitting; medial rotation is limited. Rectal examination reveals a tender piriformis where it overlies the proximal ischial spine.

It has been noted by Maxwell (1978)[821] that patients with sciatic pain, affecting the side of an apparently longer leg, do not respond to chiropractic therapy (presumably for sciatica) as well as those with sciatic pain on the shorter leg side. Careful analysis revealed a piriformis muscle syndrome on the side of the longer leg.

Because *muscle tenderness* of itself has not engendered elsewhere in the body a host of muscle syndromes like trapezius syndrome, deltoid syndrome, sacrospinalis syndrome, gluteal syndrome, gastrocnemius syndrome and so on, it may appear somewhat indiscriminative to attach such importance to the name of a tender muscle as to propose a clinical entity on the basis of what is almost certainly a secondary consequence.

Sacroiliac joint problems are common on the side of an apparently long leg. Painful joint problems tend to produce tenderness in overlying muscle. The piriformis syndrome tends to disappear after quite moderate mobilisation, guided by assessment, of the sacroiliac joint on the painful side, perhaps also by mobilisation of the ipsilateral hip joint and sometimes a small raise on the heel of the shorter leg.

In summary, while our knowledge of the nature and behaviour of non-inflammatory pelvic arthropathy remains patchy, we are in no position to be completely confident about which pains are coming from where, when a single test disturbs so many structures, and we can only logically treat on the basis of signs and symptoms in themselves, rather than on the doubtful principles of 'selective tension' (see p. 316) and an overreliance on the neat and tidy reference of pain into dermatomes.

Coccydynia

The single fused mass of four coccygeal vertebrae is separated from the sacrum by a fibrous intersection, which permits a small amount of movement.

Abnormalities at the low lumbar segments can produce trespass upon the coccygeal nerves of the cauda equina; also, ventral movement of the coccyx can exert traction on the filum terminale, which attaches to the dorsal coccygeal surface.

Because the incidence of sacrococcygeal transitional vertebra is somewhere around 10 per cent,[1093] conclusions about X-ray appearances of fracture of the coccyx, non-ossification, partial ossification and angulation of the coccyx may be difficult in some cases.

Coccygeal pain, which has been erroneously said to be confined almost exclusively to young women:[983] (i) may be referred from the lumbosacral segment; (ii) may be the sequel of direct trauma, such as sitting heavily, or a blow on the tip of the coccyx; (iii) may follow parturition stress of coccygeal soft-tissue attachments.

Also, congenital axial deviations of the coccyx may cause symptoms after long periods of sitting. Stoddard (1969)[1180b] observes that coccygeal pain is rarely psychogenic, but that preoccupation with rectal and perineal functions may focus attention to the coccyx.

Richards (1954),[1036] who regarded psychogenic factors as secondary rather than primary, reviewed the possible causes of coccydynia after a study of 102 cases, in which less than half gave a history of injury. He believed that in many cases the coccygeal pain was caused by central disc prolapse at a low lumbar segment. Nearly half of the patients with coccydynia had initial low back pain or sciatica, and most of the remainder later developed similar symptoms. Many patients gained relief from coccygeal pain after the application of a plaster jacket for the lumbar spine.

Rose (1954)[see 1036] also reported success in the treatment of coccydynia when employing the same methods; this infers the link which is frequently perceived between lumbosacral joint problems and coccygeal pain.

Lewit (1967)[733] observed often that patients who complained of low back pain, but not coccygeal pain, had tenderness of the coccygeal tip; further, that his score of successes in treating the lumbar pain improved when manipulation of the coccyx was included. In some, treatment of the coccyx alone was sufficient to relieve the 'lumbago'.

Of 112 cases with coccygeal tenderness, 22 had coccygeal pain, 79 had low back pain. A proportion had buttock and hip pain, and 15 of the women reported menstrual pain. He recommends examination of the coccyx as a routine measure during investigation of low back pain, and in his group of 112 patients (28 men and 84 women) the coccygeal findings were:

the most important in	38
one among other significant findings in	45
of secondary importance in	23
not observed for sufficiently long in	6
	112

Clinical features.

1. *Referred coccydynia:* Low lumbar and/or sacroiliac joint problems very frequently coexist, and when the latter is present the coccygeal pain may possibly be partly referred and partly due to connective tissue-tension differences between sides of the pelvis. An intrapelvic cause should be borne in mind when assessing the nature of referred coccydynia in men. Taking a lumbosacral joint problem as an example:

The pain is diffuse, and may include the buttock and gluteal fold.

The coccyx itself, as well as its locality and the lower sacrum, may be tender.

There may be pain during sitting, but there need not be. Some patients describe the pain being provoked only by the lumbar movements of sitting down, and standing from sitting.

Coughing may hurt, and pain can be exacerbated by straight-leg-raising.

The referred pain together with the lumbar pain may be aggravated by straining at stool.

Some women may have menstrual pain.

2. Coccydynia due to localised cause:

The localised pain may be due to an acute traumatic periostitis or to adhesions following direct injury to the sacrococcygeal joint.

The coccyx may be deviated to one or other side by trauma, or may be anteverted, sometimes to a right angle, although asymmetry of appearance on X-ray is not conclusive evidence that trauma has occurred.

Many patients have coccygeal pain on sitting which is lessened by leaning forward in a chair; those with a coccyx well covered by soft tissue may not be too uncomfortable when seated.

Stepping up with either leg may provoke the pain.

The tip of coccyx is acutely tender, and a testing of lateral movement, per rectum, is especially painful.

Movements involving gluteal-attachment traction may hurt, and the patient may notice a click on getting up from sitting.

Myofascial strains following parturition may produce tenderness which is localised to one or both sides of the coccyx; these strains may also occur other than in childbirth.

In about 6 per cent of all pelvic fractures, there is an associated coccygeal fracture.[1093]

The symphysis pubis

The structural and functional interdependence of soft-tissue and bony pelvic components, which form an architectural entity, has been mentioned (p. 155) as has the strength of the interpelvic ligaments (p. 29). The symphysis pubis plays an important role in the stability of the pelvis, and it may be involved in changes occurring because of disturbances between sacrum and the ilia; conversely, primary disturbances of the symphysis pubis will have repercussions involving the sacroiliac joint (Coventry and Taper, 1972;[207] Schmorl and Junghanns, 1971).[1093]

A radiographically evident uneven position of the pelvis (Fig. 6.11) is an important indication of loosening of the pelvic ring (Kamieth and Reinhardt, 1955).[628] These points are neatly demonstrated in an a-p view, depicting the radiographic appearance of an adult female pelvis, in a comprehensive text on anatomy.[437]

The minor distortion may be either current, or the fossilised evidence of events much earlier in the patient's life. Schmorl and Junghanns (1971)[1093] observes that permanent stress of the pelvis as is common, for example, in soccer players, occasionally leads to osteoarthrosis of the symphysis. In the study (Harris and Murray, 1974)[506] (p. 156) of pubic symphysis changes in athletes, clinical features were pain in the pubic area radiating to groin or lower abdomen, and clicking in some, indicating instability. A chronic stress lesion in the iliac component of

a sacroiliac joint was found in 20 out of 37 athletes, and 13 of them had instability at the pubic symphysis.

A further study (Durey and Rodineau, 1976[284] (see p. 156) also demonstrated pubic arthropathy in sportsmen. Pubic or inguinal pains, sometimes bilateral, radiating to lower abdomen and progressively more easily provoked, accompanied sport and eventually walking, climbing stairs and rising from sitting. The authors observed radiological changes from simple sclerosis of pubic margins to changes resembling those of pubic osteitis. Dystrophic changes were observed proceeding through definite stages to stabilisation.

The evolutionary radiographic changes occur in four stages, described by Luschnitz *et al.* (1967):[770]

1. A florid stage, characterised by marginal notches of the opposed symphyseal margins.
2. An intermediate stage of sclerosed fringes of symphyseal margins.
3. A stage of sclerosis.
4. Finally, a stage of exostoses projecting at the margins of the obturator foramen.

Other appearances commonly seen were double contrast images, notching of the superior or inferior angle of the symphysis, a widening of the symphyseal gap and instability of the pubic joint when the subject was supported on one leg.

As the abnormality recedes with rest the 'notches' fill up, there is a lessening of marginal irregularity and a narrowing of the symphyseal gap. After several years the symphysis regains an almost normal radiographic appearance, although sclerosed joint margins may still persist together with osteophytes at superior or inferior angles.

The authors assert that pubic arthropathy in athletes is far from being an infrequent condition, and also that the factors which seem to favour pubic arthropathy are pelvic imbalance caused by inequality of leg length, and concomitant changes in the sacroiliac joints and lower lumbar discs.

Certain factors seem to favour changes in the pubis: the morphology of the player, i.e. hypermuscled lower limbs and general lack of suppleness; the temperament of players, those having the tendency to train a great deal, and to be especially intense physically, appearing to be more prone to the condition.

We have already seen (*vide supra*) that the joints of the pelvic ring are architecturally interdependent.

Harris (1974)[505] reviewed previous reports of pubic arthropathy in women, and described in detail the changes occurring in three women with disabling pain in the pubic region. The radiographic appearances resembled those in athletes but there were certain differences. Instability was common, and manifested by a clicking sensation at the pubis. The clinical and radiological features were considered to be those of infection in the retropubic space resulting in venous stasis and thrombosis, which in turn led to an avascular necrosis of the pubic symphysis. It was surmised that instability caused most of the symptoms, on the basis that successful relief of long-standing symptoms followed a surgical stabilisation procedure in two of the patients. Aetiological factors were thought to include multiple pregnancies, pelvic operations, or both, together with pelvic sepsis.

Other authors (Huskisson and Hart, 1973)[583] have reported the radiographic similarity between pubic arthropathy in athletes and osteitis pubis in women.

With regard to asymmetry of the pubic joint, and the radiographic appearances of osteitis condensans ilii, this is still regarded by some authorities[262] only as evidence of incorrect repositioning of the pelvis postpartum, despite the fact that both conditions are well known to occur in male athletes.

Changes occurring at the pubis during and after pregnancy have been mentioned on page 153. Particularly in multiparous women, the symphysis pubis may occasionally become a truly mobile joint, with pelvic instability as a consequence (Schmorl and Junghanns, 1971).[1093]

Spinal dysraphism

Abnormal splitting of the notochord can involve the central nervous system, the axial skeleton, the skin and the viscera;[1079] the spinal abnormalities resulting from incomplete closure of a split notochord can cover a range from slight widening of the vertebra to a complete anterior and posterior bifida.

At birth, occult forms of spinal dysraphism are not usually evident, and spinal cord function may not be impaired.

In 73 of 100 confirmed cases, however,[605] the external cutaneous changes associated with spina bifida were manifest, i.e. 57 had lumbar hypertrichosis or lipoma; 16 had either a naevus, dimple, sinus or a slightly pigmented and scarred patch of skin.

As growth continues the dysraphic defect begins to prevent the naturally changing relationships of spinal cord segments and vertebral segments. There may be pressure from the growth of abnormal tissue, e.g. a lipoma or dermoid. Possible inversion of laminae may interfere with growth of the spinal cord within a consequently narrowed neural canal. The trespass will interfere with segmental blood supply by producing ischaemia, and neuronal function may also be disturbed by direct compressive effects. Sensation abnormalities and muscle imbalance will follow.

Spina bifida occulta (cleft spinous processes)

The incidence of this condition varies between 10 and 33 per cent, according to the estimate consulted.[605, 315] Sandifer (1967)[1079] regards it as a common and usually symptomless malformation. The vertebral anomaly, in its mildest form, is a lack of fusion of the neural arches of one or several vertebrae. The most frequent location is the fifth lumbar neural arch, and next the first sacral segment; the existence of both lesions is not rare.[315]

Spina bifida, of itself, probably never causes symptoms, except through the associated abnormalities of nervous tissue (see p. 24). It is sometimes associated with myelodysplasia, with symptoms according to the level of the defect.[1079] The neural tube may be open, as in myelocele, or closed.

When present, the neurological symptoms are bilateral and often symmetrical, and there are signs of congenital atrophic paralysis, with wasting of calves and feet; the feet are clubbed and the ankle jerk absent. Sensory loss can be severe distally and will underlie trophic changes; there may be blueness and coldness of the feet.

The sacral region may also be involved in sensory loss, and sphincter function disturbed. The neurological defects are not static, and may increase as growth inflicts further damage, either by the physical trespass of compression, or the effects of increasing traction or progressive gliosis.

The symptoms of spinal dysraphism may be delayed, because the neurological signs vary in severity. They are often diffuse and complex, and difficult to interpret.[509]

The spinal cord or cauda equina may be unable to 'ascend' relative to the vertebral segments during growth, and the tethering lesions may be of various kinds,[1079] including a tight filum terminale.

Young people may complain of back and other spinal problems during the adolescent growth spurt (girls 12–14 years, boys 14–16 years) and the presence of mild bilateral pes cavus, shortening of the tendocalcaneus and a history of enuresis as a child, without a clear history of any neurological disease, should raise the suspicion of dysraphism as the root cause of the patient's difficulties.

Slight swelling of the lumbosacral region (meningocele), and pigmented or hairy skin, may have been missed during cursory examination. There may well be a lesion tethering or compressing the lower end of the cord or the cauda equina;[1079] re-examination commonly reveals a shortening of one leg and foot, though this is not always present.[605]

Drug-induced joint and muscle pains

Huskisson and Hart (1973)[583] observe that, 'aches and pains in joints and muscles may on occasions be caused, or precipitated, by drugs', and they give a detailed description of drug effects. While these effects are likely to be more manifest in peripheral joints, one needs to be aware of the possibility of drug-induced pain. For example:

1. A variety of muscle aches have been reported with the oral contraceptives.

2. Sodium depletion may cause muscle aches and cramps with overenthusiastic diuretic and spironolactone therapy.

3. Crush fractures in osteoporotic vertebrae may cause considerable discomfort, the corticosteroids often being responsible.

4. The barbiturates may rarely cause arthralgia accompanied by contractures.

5. Acute haemoarthrosis may occur with anticoagulant overdosage. The affected joint is swollen, red and very tender, but settles within a few days.

6. Repeated intra-articular steroid injections may cause destructive changes in a limb girdle or a more peripheral joint, although there is more recent evidence to the contrary.

NEOPLASMS

The salient clinical features of vertebral tumours have been tabulated[983] as follows:

Possible symptoms: mild, severe or catastrophic pain
weakness of legs
unsteadiness of gait.

Possible signs: deformity of the spine
painful and restricted movement of the back
swelling of soft parts of the back
paraplegia.

Radiographically: wedging and flattening of *one* vertebral body with normal discs above and below
ballooning of one vertebral body
erosion of the anterior border
change in the lamellar architecture
increased density.

Occasionally, excessive vertebral involvement may be manifest only as an apparent diffuse osteoporosis, and this may be the X-ray appearance of multiple myeloma.[780]

(a) Cervical spine

Intracranial tumours, e.g. meningioma, may present with cervical and occipital pain[417] when symptoms can have been present for a few months or years. Among three such patients, none related a history of nausea or vomiting and the ESR was normal in each, although all had papilloedema and cervical flexion was the most limited movement in all of them. They all described pain as maximal in the posterior neck, spreading upwards to occiput and *unaccompanied by significant neck stiffness*. The incidence is not high, e.g. Frykholm[392] describes how, over a period of 15 years, three patients with migraine transpired to have intracranial tumours, but nevertheless needs to be remembered.

Mid- and lower neck. When cervical pain of some duration is due to malignant deposits or infection of *cervical* structures, the neck may be held virtually rigid,[1370] but the early clinical presentation may simulate cervical spondylosis. A Pancoast tumour in the early stages, for example, may amount to no more than aching over the upper trapezius on that side, and some vague but persistent discomfort on cervical movements away from the affected side (see below).

In a series of 179 cases of confirmed intraspinal cervical neoplasms,[1291] 133 were extramedullary. In 60 per cent of the cases the initial presenting symptom was distinctive pain. Holt and Yates' (1966)[565] description of benign cystic lesions at the junction of posterior cervical roots and posterior-root ganglion includes their belief that in certain cases brachial neuralgia may be caused by them.

(b) Thoracic spine

Peripheral bronchial carcinoma (Pancoast). When a tumour lies in the apex of the lung, and later involves the adjacent vertebrae and ribs, it may present with a peculiar combination of motor, sensory and sympathetic effects.[257] Pain and disturbed movement in the associated upper limb, and atrophy of the small muscles of the hand, are probably caused by disturbances of the limb girdle architecture as well as by involvement of the lower cords of the brachial plexus. Horner's syndrome may be evident, with contracted pupil, ptosis, enophthalmosis and absence of sweating. There may be hoarseness due to paralysis of a vocal cord, but the signs of bronchial obstruction may only develop later and this allows time for the neural features to be declared first.

Neurinomas[175] are especially common in the thoraco-cervical area and may occur as part of generalised neurofibromatosis.

Over 25 per cent of patients with spinal metastases present with neurological dysfunction, and over 80 per cent of the tumours producing neurological deficits occur at *thoracic* cord level.[780]

The prognosis is poorer the more cranially the lesion, the more rapid the onset, the longer the signs have been present and the more manifest is sphincter involvement.

In a series of more than 1000 patients[1130] with surgically proven bone tumours involving the vertebral column, including the thoracic region, 38 were preoperatively diagnosed as protrusion of lumbar intervertebral disc.

All the symptoms associated with disc changes, *not excluding abnormal movement patterns*, may occur in tumours of vertebral bone.

While the pain of discogenic backache is usually intermittent, the pain of intraspinal tumours tends to be constant and intractable.

Epstein *et al.* (1979)[319] report three patients with thoracic spinal cord tumours, who presented with primary signs and symptoms of lumbar spine abnormality. The evidence of spinal cord disease was minimal and could easily have been overlooked. They suggest that total myelography, in cases of suspected lumbar disc disease, is mandatory since myelographic changes in the cervical and thoracic spines can be clinically important, notwithstanding the presence of marked changes in the lumbar region.

(c) Lumbar spine and pelvis

Soft-tissue neoplasms like meningiomas, neurofibromas and schwannomas are likely to present initially with the clinical features of single somatic root compression. Differentiation between vertebral tumours and intraspinal soft-tissue tumours by clinical and radiological means is not always possible;[1140] sometimes the nature of the growth may not be clarified until surgical exploration and inspection decide the issue. Signs and symptoms of back pain and nerve root involvement, with evidence of spinal block, occur in each group and there is often no way of clinically establishing the difference.

(i) *Benign tumours.* Neurinoma and meningioma are most common.[912] The coexistence of severe backache and scoliosis may indicate a benign tumour. Idiopathic scoliosis is rarely painful.[780]

The presence of non-malignant intradural neoplasms may eventually be declared by the signs of extrasegmental involvement, among which in the lumbar spine is frequently an absent knee-jerk.[1188] Their presence is confirmed by myelography.

Benign osteogenic tumours occur more often in patients under 30 and usually involve the vertebral apophyses rather than the vertebral body.[780] They present with pain which is not especially severe, and it may have been present for some time before X-ray reveals the lytic lesion.

A *hemangioma* occurs in some 12 per cent, the incidence increasing with age. It is not necessarily associated with backache.

Osteoid osteoma occurs in children and young adults and is associated with backache and vertebral spasm and with scoliosis which does not show the usual features of idiopathic scoliosis. There may be trespass upon the spinal cord.[1140]

An *osteoblastoma* occurs in the neural arches of lumbar spine and sacrum. Males are affected more than females and 80 per cent of cases are under 30. There may be a neurological deficit.

Aneurysmal bone cysts are the only benign spinal tumours which may extend from one vertebra to another. They occur in older children, adolescents and young adults,[1140] equally among the sexes. Bone destruction is marked.

(ii) *Malignant tumours.* With a malignant tumour in the *limb* bones, pain is the first symptom; later the patient notices a lump. When this sequence is reversed, the tumour is not as a rule malignant.[983]

For obvious reasons, the rule of thumb cannot be so easily applied to the vertebral column; nevertheless, the important point is that pain is commonly the first symptom, and as always it is *the characteristic behaviour of pain related to time, posture and activity* to which the clinical worker must give the fullest attention.

Malignancy occurs most frequently in patients over 30; the older the patient the more frequently they occur and the more likely is the tumour to be malignant. They usually involve the vertebral body rather than the apophyses. Backache is commonly the presenting symptom, and it is wise not to rely on X-ray appearances; in autopsy specimens with neoplastic changes, quite gross disease may not be visible on postmortem radiographs in 85 per cent of the specimens.[780]

The pain is characteristically worse on rest, and particularly at night; early in the history it will awaken the patient from sound sleep, but later the patient is awake for more time than asleep. Discogenic pain may be bad at night, but is more commonly provoked by *movement* in bed, and its intensity is generally less than when the patient is trying to move about during the day[91] and suffering the effects of gravitational compression.

Turning over and changing limb positions often relieves the pain of degenerative joint disease, but gives no relief from the pain of malignancy, and frequently the patient must get up and walk about in an attempt to distract himself.

It should be remembered that *disc space infection* has a different characteristic,[91] in that it may be so severe at night that movement in bed is not even possible, and the patient is *unable* to sit up, or get out of bed.

Once the pain begins, the symptoms steadily become virtually constant, tending to remain so regardless of position or movement.[1180b] This does not mean to say that active movements, asked of the patient during clinical examination, will not provoke pain. Contrary to what seems to be believed, an active movement may provoke a very severe jab of pain; rotation of the thoracic spine, for example, may make a patient gasp with the viciousness of provoked fulgurant pain which disappears as quickly as it arose. The usual analgesics provide no relief.

While continuous and harrowing distress may be the dominant feature of pain from malignancy, the emotionally disturbed patient with psychogenic pain may try to give the same impression, but tends to describe suffering rather than symptoms, and the histrionic extravagance of description may invite the suspicion that while the patient may certainly be in pain, the kind of help they manifestly need is not that indicated for malignant disease.

Changes in blood levels of calcium, phosphorus, alkaline and acid phosphotase, and globulins, may accompany malignant disease, and the ESR is commonly raised.[780]

Where spinal movements are *not* painful, they will certainly be so once a kyphus has developed due to vertebral body collapse, and before this, a gentle flat-handed vertebral springing test (p. 353) will evoke the characteristic sharp reflex guarding of vertebral muscle contraction[1180b]—in this respect the spinal response will represent that of a suitably similar palpation test of 'the acute abdomen'.

Primary tumours

Chordomas. These are more commonly seen in men between 40 and 70, but it is a rare lesion.[1140] The slowly growing tumour infiltrates adjacent structures and tends to recur after excision. It almost invariably causes death by local involvement of the central nervous system.

Myelomas are the most frequent primary malignant tumours of the spine. They are uncommon below the age of 50 years[780] and are seen more often in men. In myelomatosis, the disease may be declared by the sudden onset of severely painful backache because of a pathological fracture, or the condition is revealed by the onset of paraplegia.

Often there is slowly increasing backache, and there may be weakness, weight loss and other constitutional features such as an ESR of 50 mm per hour. There may be anaemia and pyrexia.[1180b]

Metastases

Marked osteolysis is seen in hypernephroma, thyroid tumours and carcinoma of the large bowel, and osteoblastic secondaries may occur when the primary is in the breast, bronchus or prostate.[780]

Secondary carcinoma usually occurs in older women, with a primary in breast or uterus, not always discernible during life.[983]

The lumbar vertebrae are frequently involved and the second lumbar vertebra seems a favourite site. Weakness of hip flexion, when tested by static contractions against resistance, may be significant, as may difficulties in walking. In multiple metastases, bone may be riddled with metastases and yet not cause symptoms.

Other tumours

Slowly expanding lymphomas in the epidural space can for some time mimic the clinical presentation of disc disease. A retroperitoneal malignant tumour, e.g. lipofibromasarcoma, may be the inciting factor in meralgia paraesthetica.[365]

SUMMARY

The recognition of neoplastic disease, earlier rather than later, depends more on awareness, vigilance and suspicion rather than a set of rules. One must *always* be thinking of it, all the time and every time. Whenever it is confirmed, tracking back on the clinical features, or lack of them, may sometimes reveal where history-taking or physical examination might have been more attentive or more comprehensive.

The factors which may provide warning of the possibility of neoplastic disease could be summarised as follows:

1. Occipital pain which is aggravated on neck-flexion but which is not accompanied by vertebral movement-limitation and in which palpable signs of upper vertebral involvement are absent.
2. The 'globally' rigid cervical spine with all movements greatly reduced, in the absence of trauma and other factors significant enough to warrant the clinical articular signs
3. The combination of shoulder girdle pain, neurological signs in the distribution of C8–T1 and Horner's syndrome
4. Severe intractable pain accompanying muscle spasm and vertebral deformity in young people. Sciatic scoliosis is not *invariably* a simple joint problem.
5. Disturbing or more severe and inexorable pain at night, in middle age or later, unrelieved by resting and uninfluenced by changing position of trunk or limbs.
6. Meralgia paraesthetica which is accompanied by intractable pain at night.
7. Backache in a patient with a known history of malignancy during the past two years.
8. Sciatic pain with bizarre extrasegmental sensory symptoms, and neurological deficit, but no backache.
9. Backache with pronounced loss of hip flexor power is always suspect.
10. The spontaneous onset of backache in late middle age, in the absence of a previous history of back pain, is more likely to be due to osteoporosis or malignant disease than to benign joint problems.[1180b]
11. Pain which is severe enough to be uninfluenced by the usual analgesics, and requires morphia for more than 48 hours, is likely to indicate malignancy.
12. Persistent backache which is not quietened or reduced by rest, and not influenced by posture. The older the patient, the more is malignancy suspect.
13. Shock, vomiting and loss of spinal function following a trivial spinal jolt or stress; the cause is likely to be pathological fracture.
14. Back pain with weakness, sphincter disturbance, malaise and pyrexia.
15. Back pain with marked difficulty in walking, in the presence of normal foot, ankle, knee and hip joint function.
16. The coexistence of back pain and ankle clonus, with a normal range of straight-leg-raising.

9. Examination

INTRODUCTION

No diagnostic laboratory test for joint disease is completely specific (Hollander, 1978).[560]

Tests which may be strongly suggestive when positive do not rule out disease when they are negative. Many cases of joint pain can be diagnosed from clinical findings alone, although careful attention to the history, together with a precise physical examination which is planned on the basis of it, is mandatory.

Having established the salient features for which the patient is attending, i.e. pain, restriction, painless loss of function, instability, loss of confidence, attendance following outpatient or inpatient invasive or other procedures, for example, the particular form of examination will differ according to the nature of the salient features of the case.

After analysing the data obtained by two clinicians examining consecutively, during the history-taking of 27 cases of low back pain and the physical tests in 23 cases, Nelson et al. (1979)[913] suggest that if the clinician obtains a large amount of information much of it will be unreliable; if he is prepared to limit the amount of information, its reliability will be increased. In 1053 items in the history, observer disagreement was 33 per cent; on 569 items of testing, 34 per cent.

Redesign of the proforma used resulted in a reduction of observer error during history-taking to 18 per cent, but there remained a 30 per cent disagreement during physical tests.

The importance of careful, precise history-taking, and of standardised meticulous physical tests is thus emphasised. By those teachers responsible for physiotherapy postregistration manipulation courses, and for the better education of student therapists, this need has received careful emphasis for some time.

For example, getting the patient to point with one finger to the precise area of pain (p. 306), rather than relying on verbal descriptions, has been standard practice among clinical therapists for more than a decade.

Therapists who base conservative treatment procedures very closely upon presenting signs and symptoms after comprehensive examination would suggest that reduction of factors for assessment is a retrograde step, and would prefer not that the number of factors for assessment is reduced, but that clinical examinations remain comprehensive, and a detailed, uniformly higher standardisation of physical tests established.

Writing in the same journal, Kirkaldy-Willis and Hill (1979)[662] stress the importance of a carefully planned approach which should include a careful history and physical examination, with repeated clinical assessment of the patient, '. . . other useful tests include facet and nerve injections, the response to manipulation, lateral radiograms in flexion and extension . . .'.

Since the principles of clinical examination are applicable to all clinical disciplines, the following observations about examination of the knee joint are as apt for vertebral joint examination:

In every physical examination there is a theoretical ideal. The examiner tests all anatomic and dynamic aspects of the joint in question (bones, soft tissues, range of motion, muscle strength, vascular and neurological integrity). In a practical examination, however, the key to an accurate diagnosis is often based not on a step by step analysis of all possible factors, but on a specific investigation of the patient's subjective complaint. A thorough, complete examination is always performed, but emphasis is naturally placed on that portion of the examination that has the greatest clinical relevance. This kind of selective examination usually produces the highest yield of information about clinical disease in the shortest time. Frequently, a diagnosis can be made on the basis of the patient's history alone, a judgment that can be supported by a precise, specific physical examination. (Hoppenfeld, 1979)[570]

Planning the most efficient and productive *form* of examination, from patient to patient, becomes easier with clinical experience but first there must be a foundation, and a good beginning is to thoroughly drill oneself in the systematic approach of examining all the separate tissues from which pain and other symptoms *might* be arising.

Knowledgeable trimming and speeding up of the procedures follow naturally in time, as the worker gains clinical experience. Thus basic procedures are described below.

Either at the time of the initial clinical examination, which is essentially a sorting procedure, or at a subsequent examination conducted by the clinical worker who is going to treat the patient, it is necessary to give fullest attention to an 'Indications' examination, which is concerned solely with the *manner* in which the diagnosed joint problem is manifesting itself, and with localising the vertebral segment(s) involved.

Arranged in logical sequence, comprehensive examination by the therapist is the foundation of effective treatment, and it is necessary to acquire an orderly and systematic approach.

Examination should always follow a basic pattern, in strict sequence; this enables the therapist to build up a firmly grasped technique of investigating joint problems and will give increasing confidence in assessment as skill is progressively acquired:

1. 'Listen'   History
2. 'Look'   Observation
3. 'Test'   Test
4. 'Feel'   Palpation
5. Record   Write an account of examination
6. Assess   Sort out priorities of information derived, and therefore of treatment.

Attention should be concentrated on only one aspect at a time.

NB. Sections 1, 2, 3 and 4 are elaborated as needed to elicit full information.

AIMS of this fundamentally important procedure are:

A. *Subjective examination*—to gather all relevant information about the site, nature, behaviour and onset of the *current* symptoms, with their behaviour in the past and details of previous treatment, if any, and to formulate the next step of physical tests accordingly.

B. *Objective examination*—to seek abnormalities of function, using active, passive, neurological and special tests of all tissues likely to be involved, guided by the history.

C. *To apply this information* in planning treatment.

Disturbances of function in the musculoskeletal and nervous system, and their effects, are noted, and the more precise and full is examination the more likely is correct localisation of the joint problem, with a clear appreciation of how movements of the vertebral segment(s) are abnormal.

SUBJECTIVE EXAMINATION—HISTORY

Because the therapist's examination is not a sorting procedure, emphasis on particular aspects, and thus the sequence of examination, are different; it is important to appreciate the reason for this. Assessment and continuing reassessment are the basis from which constructive treatment evolves, and because *pain* and *its behaviour* are the dominant factors: (a) compelling the majority of patients to seek treatment, and (b) guiding the selection and modification of treatment, *a clear grasp of both the distribution and the behaviour of pain are of first significance.*

Since patients depressed by pain tend to describe the onset in a rambling and sometimes emotionally charged fashion, which may thoroughly confuse the therapist with a host of 'red herrings' and prejudice the orderly grasp of essentials, the sequence of history-taking suggested is:

1. Patient's daily activity, at work and play
2. The pain, and other symptoms, *currently* troubling the patient
3. The onset of the attack, and previous attacks, if any
4. Previous treatment, if any, and its effects. (See scheme.)

The patient should be kept to the point, kindly but firmly, and irrelevant elaboration discouraged. The therapist should *listen*, make no assumptions, try to clarify the information being gathered, and help the patient to be as precise as reasonably possible, by:

1. Keeping the questions simple
2. Asking one at a time
3. Getting an answer before proceeding to the next one
4. Avoiding putting words into the patient's mouth
5. Giving equal value to awkward points in the history, though they may be unwelcome in that they may negate favourite theories and bias on the therapist's part.

When writing of the pitfalls of communication, Wright and Hopkins (1978)[1353] point out that in England, some 30 per cent of physiotherapy time is devoted to rheumatic/orthopaedic conditions; the factor of communication with patients is vital.

In assessing the level of tripartite agreement on the meaning of common medical terms between doctors, therapists and patients, the authors compiled a multichoice questionnaire, by which the participants could indicate their understanding of the meaning of about 28 commonly used words and phrases, viz.: 'numbness, weakness of the arm, cramp, sciatica, slipped disc, neuritis, vertebra, spinal cord, morning stiffness, arthritis, deformity, swelling of a joint, anaemia, rheumatism, ligament, locking of a joint, cervical, osteoarthrosis, sacrum, loin, heredity, lumbar, debility, salvage operation on a joint, steroids, spinal cord anatomy (diagram), back (diagram), sciatic nerve (diagram). The three sets of diagrams showed alternative locations of these structures.'

The answer favoured by the majority in each of the groups was clearly indicated by the highest percentage, and the agreement grades were:

More than 70 per cent   good
50–69 per cent   fair
Below 50 per cent   poor

Among doctors agreement was rated as good for the majority of questions but for *weakness of the arm, sciatica* and *sciatic nerve* the agreement was only fair, and for *back* it was poor.

Among patients agreement was generally poor; good agreement was reached only for *rheumatism* and *heredity*. Poorest agreement was for common 'household' words like *arthritis, slipped disc, deformity, ligament, vertebra, spinal cord, lumbar, numbness, sciatica* and *back. Loin* and *groin* were confused by many, and rheumatic sufferers considered *morning stiffness* as a total inability to move.

Some 17 per cent of rheumatic patients took *arthritis* to mean a crippling disease of joints; the authors report a study in which 28 per cent of a group of general practitioners did likewise.

Among both student and trained physiotherapists agreement was good for most of the terms, yet with only fair agreement for *weakness, swelling of a joint, rheumatism, loin, spinal cord anatomy* and *sciatic nerve. Arthritis* and *back* were poorly agreed, and two-thirds of the students got *loin* and *groin* mixed up.

Between doctors, physiotherapists and patients agreement was patchy. On the whole physiotherapists and patients did not appear to share a common language, nor did physiotherapists and doctors appear to have an entirely common language, since agreement was not good for 30 per cent of the terms.

Among the authors' observations are the following:

Patients' answers to questions containing these words and phrases should not be taken at their face value.
Care must be taken in ascertaining what the patient understands by commonly used words.
It should not be surprising that patients do not follow instructions if they do not understand what we are talking about.
The term *arthritis* should be used with caution and with explanation.

Regrettably, the fatuous expression *slipped disc*, which was popularly defined by patients as 'a bone out of place', continues to be perpetuated and probably continues to cause as much real but unnecessary concern as unthinking overuse of the word *arthritis*.

Other than in research projects as here discussed, slipshod expression by clinicians with responsibility has plainly resulted in patients having notions which are yet one further remove from reality.

Important questions: there are some questions which are mandatory, and it is unwise to begin treatment without the required information. (See Contraindications.)

Cervical region   (i) Any dizziness (vertigo), blackouts or 'drop' attacks?
     (ii) History of upper respiratory tract infection? (In juniors.)
     (iii) Any history of rheumatoid arthritis or other inflammatory arthritis? Treated by systemic steroids or anticoagulants?
     (iv) Any neurological symptoms in legs?

Thoracic region   (i) Has the patient been treated recently by systemic steroid drugs? Anticoagulants?
     *(ii) Any neurological symptoms in legs?

Lumbar region   (i) Any perineal or 'saddle area' anaesthesia or paraesthesiae?
     (ii) Any change in micturition habits associated with the back trouble, or sphincter disturbance?
     (iii) Steroids or anticoagulants?

NB. (a) It is desirable that the therapist sees the X-ray, but the more important information is that the patient *has* been recently X-rayed, and the films have been seen by a radiologist.
     (b) General health and possible coexistent disease should be enquired about.
     (c) The significance of inexorable night pain should be borne in mind (see p. 302).

A frivolous mnemonic may help the forgetful (i.e. all of us) to bear these in mind.

XXX Ale dizzily steers 'urting rheumatoid legs to night watering place

XXX Ale   —X-ray and Anticoagulant drugs
Dizzily   —Dizziness
Steers   —Steroids
'Urting   —Upper Respiratory Tract Infection
Rheumatoid   —Rheumatoid Arthritis
Legs   —Leg symptoms
to
Night   —Night pain
Watering place—Micturition disturbance, 'saddle' anaesthesia.

Prolonged heparin sodium medication, e.g. for antepartum iliofemoral thrombophlebitis, can induce spinal osteoporosis. A case of multiple spinal fractures has been reported.[1162a]

---

* These questions are additional to the routine neurological examination of arms with cervical and thoracic regions, and legs with thoracic, lumbar and sacral regions (q.v.).

Pain

The important information is that concerning the *current* distribution of pain and where it is worst; outlined by the patient pointing with one finger if possible (where it is *not* is also important), its nature and characteristics, i.e. its behaviour related to time, posture and activity (p. 276) and the degree of joint and/or root irritability (p. 174).

Distinctions must be made between constant pain, with areas of radiation at times; periodic or episodic pain, and elicited pain, i.e. that which is produced only by certain postures, movements or by later testing examination and/or palpation.

Distribution. Should be interpreted in relation to dermatomes, myotomes and sclerotomes as a likely, but not infallible, help to localisation of cause. For example, the symptom-area outlined by the patient often indicates the need to investigate two or more possible sources, e.g. back pain over the lumbosacral segment, with an ache spreading across anterior thigh from posterolateral buttock to medial knee, should lead to comprehensive examination of hip as well as lumbar spine. *Thus the content of History dictates the scope and planning of subsequent testing.*

Nature. The pain may be:

A dull, persistent ache, lying deep and hard to outline.
Transient, severe pain superimposed on this at times.
A mild catch or twinge, or a severe jab or 'shoot' on movement.
Sickening, severe and disabling 'root' pain.
Inseparably associated as painful paraesthesiae, i.e. prickling, 'burning' or hyperaesthesia.

Irritability. An initial assessment of the degree of joint and/or root irritability (q.v.) should be made.

Characteristics. In seeking the behaviour of pain related to time, posture and activity (see p. 172), a logical sequence of enquiry can assist the patient as well as the therapist, e.g.

How has the pain behaved during the last fortnight—increasing—static—decreasing?
Night pain —how do they lie?
　　　　—sleep disturbed?
　　　　—how? because *pain* wakes the patient without changing position or has patient disturbed joint by changing position?
　　　　—painful paraesthesiae wakes patient in early hours?
　　　　—type of bed base, mattress and pillows?
Rising a.m.—painfully stiff?
　　　　—how long to loosen up?
Day pain —does pain increase steadily as day goes on, or depend upon activity? (i.e. stress dependent/time dependent)

　　　　—which posture or activity aggravates/eases?
Sitting—standing—bending and lifting—arms above head—reaching—housework—coughing and sneezing—deep breath—sustained flexion and returning from—driving—reversing car—sewing—reading—theatre—walking?
Evening —does pain build up regularly in evening?
pain —eases now because can rest?

Understanding the characteristics of pain and the pattern of its aggravation and relief does not necessarily make accurate identification of the tissue responsible any easier, but provides the therapist with the vital criteria which are of fundamental importance in assessment of efficacy of treatment. Painstaking exercise of discernment and a grasp of small detail are infinitely worthwhile, because in time they provide a grasp of joint problem behaviour which no other exercise or education can give.

Downie *et al.* (1978)[274] have noted good correlation between pain 'scores' employing four different rating scales, the correlation holding good when presentation of the scales was separated by physical examination and the series of questions. Since the four scales calibrated well there is good evidence that the same underlying pain variable is being measured. A 0–10 numerical rating (11 points) performs better than a continuous (visual analogue) scale or a 4-point descriptive scale.

Abnormalities of feeling

The *distribution* of dysaesthesia, paraesthesiae and areas of loss of sensation must be noted, together with their characteristics related to time, posture and activity.

Onset (see p. 253).
(i) This may be *insidious*, a mild and sporadic ache demanding attention as it becomes painfully more continuous; the patient may have no recollection of injury or stress, but frequently, long forgotten trauma may be recalled which can reasonably be associated with a current joint condition. This pattern often indicates a problem easier to help than not.

(ii) Onset may be *slow or delayed*, in that symptoms begin some hours or days following stress (see p. 262); this fact can assist in selecting treatment, e.g. lumbar traction.

(iii) *Sudden onset*, in the form of recent severe trauma sufficient to fracture bones, after which the symptoms arising from joints were of secondary importance, can indicate that treatment of the joint condition will progress only slowly.

(iv) *Sudden onsets of a joint locking* are sometimes easier to help than slow onsets over hours or days, but a history of recurrent locking shows the need for treatment-emphasis on preventing recurrence rather than reduction

THE SKELETAL FRAMEWORK OF ORDERLY HISTORY-TAKING

1. Patient's occupation

2. Pain

Where? (and where *not*)
Worst?
Nature?
Behaviour – related to

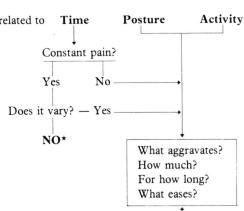

3. Paraesthesiae and concomitant symptoms

(e.g. tingling, 'pins and needles', formication, dizziness, numbness, 'uselessness', 'heaviness', 'coldness', localised 'burning' etc.)

Nature?
Where?
Behaviour?

4. Mandatory questions (see p. 305)

5. Onset

This episode?
Previous episodes?

* Raises suspicion of neoplastic disease, inflammatory arthritis or psychogenic pain.

6. Previous history and treatment and results

of the derangement. Concerning recent stress and injury, it is surprising how often patients will initially disclaim this, to recall by the next treatment session a severe fall three days previously.

Previous history

Degenerative joint conditions, like chronic bronchitis, exist in time as well as space. Knowledge of the past behaviour of joint troubles can help in assessing the nature of the problem and therefore in planning treatment more appropriately. When asked about similar troubles in the past, the answer may include information about, 'only odd attacks of fibrositis and rheumatism' or 'stiffness only'. It is probable that the patient is unwittingly relating information about spondylotic episodes and the significance of this history should be clear to the therapist.

Questions should therefore include:
Similar trouble before?
If 'no'—episodes of stiff neck? Stiff back?
Onset of previous attacks, if any?

Trauma? Site of pain? Radiation?
How long to recover?
Recovered completely?
Treatment given, if any? How effective was treatment?

The answers to these questions indicate the likely pathology and stage of progression, the likely percentage and the rate of improvement, and the possibility of recurrence. The information helps in assessment.

OBJECTIVE EXAMINATION—OBSERVATION

Much information can be gathered by observation, which begins on first sight of the patient and continues throughout the physical tests of the examination.

Initially, way of moving, gait, general posture, manner and willingness to co-operate are noted, and following the 'Subjective' examination the patient undresses sufficiently for the body region to be adequately observed. The patient should be examined in a warm room with a good light; the therapist should be placed to see well, and basic procedures should follow the same sequence every time.

Changes in attitude (deformity), contour (swelling, wasting, muscle spasm), colour (circulation, inflammation), and skin appearance generally are noted, taking into account general build and age.

Neck and thoracic region
Patient sits sideways on treatment couch or on stool, with hands on thighs so that all aspects of head and trunk may be seen.

From the front. Relate head, neck and trunk to an imaginary perpendicular or a purpose-designed grid background. Note horizontal level of eyes, position of chin and neck, contour and symmetry of clavicles, clavicular joints, shoulder joints, subclavicular hollows and the mass of neck, pectoral and arm muscles. Note symmetry of waist contours related to arms. Observe and handle the patient's hands for intrinsic muscle wasting and temperature.

From the side. Relate head and neck posture to trunk posture, and note increased or decreased curvature.

From behind. Check contour of posterior cervical muscle, trapezius, latissimus dorsi and sacrospinalis muscles. Note bulk and symmetry. Check levels and attitude of scapulae, horizontal body curves (ribs) and back muscle contours.

Palpation. Feel sides and back of neck, and trapezius with pectoral muscle for postural spasm.

Lumbar and pelvic region
Patient stands with feet a little apart and the minimum of covering.

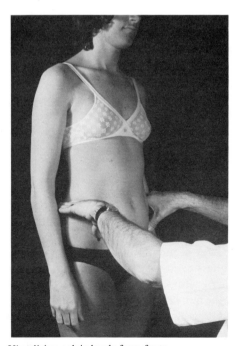

Fig. 9.1   Visualising pelvic levels from front.

From behind. Relate spine and gluteal cleft to imaginary perpendicular, and horizontal level of shoulders and scapulae with pelvic levels. Observe waist contours, symmetry of rib cage and sacrospinalis muscle masses. Check attitude of whole pelvis, level of iliac crests, dimples over posterior superior iliac spines; observe buttock contours, level of gluteal folds, and posterior limb muscles for wasting.

Palpation. Iliac crests and posterior iliac spine levels, muscle mass of sacrospinalis for postural spasm.

From the side. Check if patient stands with pelvis rotated, and with increased/decreased spinal curvature.

From the front. Check symmetry of anterior superior iliac spines, contours of abdomen and muscle mass of thigh, leg and foot.

Palpation. Anterior iliac spines and tubercles of iliac crest.

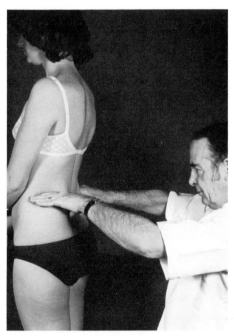

Fig. 9.2   Observation of bony points from behind. It is best to visualise these from about the same level.

Other postures
It is necessary to observe the contours and attitudes of body parts in postures other than sitting or standing, and to compare changes in these two factors when different postures are assumed. These further positions involving movement are described under 'Observation' because it is this aspect of the clinical examination which should be given the most attention during the tests described. The particular arrangement of physical tests will vary from patient to patient; it is essential that examination pro-

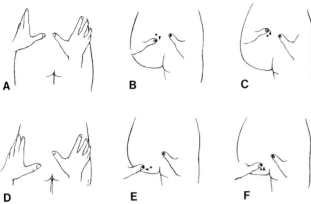

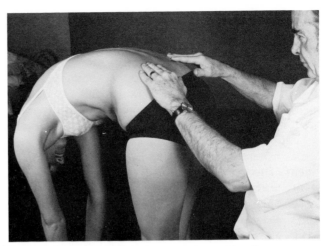

Fig. 9.4 Observing possible changes on forward bending.

Fig. 9.3 Tests for sacroiliac fixation. To test the left side (upper part of joint A to C) (A) Place thumb of right hand over spinous processes S2 and thumb of left hand over the posterior superior spine. (B) and (C) Instruct patient to flex the hip and knee to 90° and observe movement of the thumb. In the normal joint the thumb will move caudally. In the abnormally fixed joint the thumb will move cephalad. (Lower part of joint D to F.) (D) Place right thumb over last sacral spinous process and left thumb over sacral tuberosity. Again instruct the patient to flex the hip and knee to 90°. (E) In the normal joint the left thumb will move laterally. (F) In the abnormally fixed joint the thumb will remain stationary or above cephalad. (Reproduced from Kirkaldy-Willis WH, Hill RJ 1979 A more precise diagnosis for low back pain, Spine 4: 2: 102, by kind permission of the authors and publisher.)

cedures are *planned* on the basis of initial observations and history, and different aspects of the examination may need to be combined if the patient is in much pain. Patients in moderate or more severe pain should not be subjected to prolonged inspection while they endeavour to hold difficult and painful postures, and during the early stages of treatment it is often necessary to make these postural observations *during* the normal tests of movement.

1. *Standing and sitting.* A simple method of determining whether a compensated lateral tilt of the pelvis in young people is probably due to a leg length inequality is to assess the degree of tilt in standing, and then to assess it again with the patient sitting on a hard horizontal surface such as a gymnastic stool (Figs 9.1, 9.2, 9.4, 9.5). When sitting, the patient is supported on ischial tuberosities, and should the tilt be eradicated and the pelvis then assessed as level, a reasonable assumption is that the cause of the tilt lies in unequal leg lengths. The test is less reliable for the more mature patient in whom adaptive shortening may have occurred, and in any event can never be more than a quick and simple test which is less satisfactory than anteroposterior films of the hip joints, whole pelvis and lumbar spine in the standing position. Ideally, whole-spine erect films allow the superimposition of vertical and horizontal plane lines, and the most accurate assessment.

2. *Flexion during standing and sitting.* Besides comparison of vertebral and pelvic posture in the coronal, sagittal and horizontal planes in *standing* and *sitting*, comparisons

may need to be made when the patient bends forward when standing, and bends forward when sitting.

A tangential view, from behind or in front as is most suitable, will not infrequently demonstrate one or more of pelvic rotation, alteration in the horizontal relationship of posterior superior iliac spines (Piedallu's sign, p. 329), flattening of one paravertebral muscle mass, vertebral rotation, visibly disparate amounts of movement occurring in different regions, maintenance of a rigid low lumbar lordosis and lateral deviation to one or the other side. Sometimes a postural lateral deviation in standing will be eradicated in the flexed position, and in other patients a straight spine in standing or sitting will deviate on flexion, either momentarily or progressively throughout the movement (see p. 266).

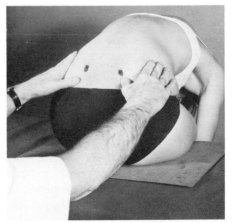

Fig. 9.5 Observing bony points during flexion while sitting.

3. *Contour and attitude in supine lying.* These should be compared to posture when standing and sitting, and the alterations noted. Body contours should be viewed tangentially. The supporting surface should be uniformly even, and care taken that the patient is lying in a neutral

position, so far as this is possible. Many elderly patients will require three or more pillows.

The contours of the neck, the position of the clavicles and the pectoral region together with shoulders, should be observed, and the sides of the thorax compared. Pelvic posture and the horizontal relationship of anterior superior iliac spines should be noted.

With a 'horse-shoe' grasp over the neck of each talus of the supine patient, the examiner places his thumbs immediately beneath each medial malleolus and bends the patient's knees so that the soles of the feet are rested side-by-side on the plinth, with the operator's thumbs in neutral side-by-side contact. The patient is then instructed to gently raise the pelvis off the couch, move it from side to side, and then settle it down again in the most neutral position. The patient's legs are then extended and the relative position of the operator's thumbs, still grasping as above, are compared. Equality or inequality of leg lengths in the supine position should be noted.

Standardised tests should not lead to standardised conclusions, and leg length discrepancy observed by this test has no significance unless incorporated into the overall assessment of posture in the standing and sitting positions; the two ubiquitous factors of (i) lumbosacral/pelvic anomaly and (ii) asymmetrical adaptive shortening of strong connective tissue and muscle, should temporise a ready tendency to ascribe the cause to changes in sacroiliac joints.

Pelvic rotation observed in supine lying which was not present on standing may be due to wasting of the gluteal muscle mass on one side. This is not always easily detectable in standing, and an apparently normal but soft gluteal mass, due to gluteus maximus weakness, is more easily squashed by pelvic weight when lying than its opposite fellow with normal tone.

4. *Prone lying*. With the patient in a neutral prone-lying position, body contours should again be noted by a tangential view.

With a 'horse-shoe' grasp now over the tendocalcaneus, and the examiner's thumb and index finger lying immediately under the medial and lateral malleolus respectively, leg lengths should be compared (a) with the legs in neutral position, and (b) after the grasp has been changed so that the thumbs rest on the middle sole of foot and fingers rest on dorsum of foot, with the knees flexed to 90°. Before assessing a leg-length discrepancy in the position (b), both legs should be moved as one, forward and backward and to the left and right, before being stabilised at 90°. The movements should not be large enough to grossly disturb the resting position of the pelvis. Minor apparent discrepancies in leg length may occur if this preparatory settling down is not completed.

A lateral view of the alignment of tibial tubercles in this position completes the observation of posture in prone lying.

NB. Asymmetry of contour and attitude *need* not be of any significance in the context of symptoms reported by the patient. The sometimes unwitting tendency to assume that 'symmetry is all', and that asymmetry must always be 'normalised' for symptoms to be relieved, is an insufficient basis for planning treatment.

Clinical examination of pelvic posture in standing and sitting, and comparison of leg lengths can be completed quite quickly and should form part of the examination for *all* vertebral regions (see 1. Standing and sitting, p. 309). The reason for stressing the importance of this measure is, of course, the mechanical and neurophysiological *interdependence* of the vertebral column, which declares itself in a variety of ways, some of them subtle; unless borne in mind during examination, the small signs and portents may be missed, and the therapist's grasp of the genesis of clinical features would be incomplete.

Adequate appreciation of this basic premise seems fairly thin on the ground, even among those with some experience of handling vertebral joint problems. The following case-report may clarify the point:

A 27-year-old mother of two reported with right frontal, suboccipital, neck, upper scapular and arm pain of some months' duration, accompanied by paraesthesiae of 'glove' distribution. The symptoms had been waxing and waning for some nine years following a fall on the shoulder from a scooter. The symptoms were aggravated by lying in a bath, neck movements, carrying shopping and any activity involving arm pressure, e.g. cleaning windows, ironing. Sleep was frequently disturbed. The patient did not then complain of backache, although questioned as to other pains. Previous treatments elsewhere included medication, heat, ultrasound, manipulation and a collar.

During examination, a slightly-bulging contour posteriorly over the upper two right ribs was observed. All neck movements were of good range. Extension, right side-flexion, right rotation and flexion provoked the right yoke and upper scapular pain; left rotation and left side-flexion were unexceptional. Sustained hold of neck movements to the right did not provoke a latent exacerbation of the paraesthesiae. Movements of the right shoulder were slightly painful at the extreme of all movements. There were no neurological signs in any limb. X-ray of neck, shoulders and chest were negative.

Palpation findings were as depicted in Figure 9.6.

Treatment. Patient and plodding mobilisation of the craniovertebral, neck, and right upper rib joints, including harness traction during the nine attendances over a period of six weeks, steadily reduced all symptoms to a more tolerable level (i.e. 'some 75 per cent better') but did not completely relieve them. It was then suggested that she should allow time for the problem to settle, i.e. not seek further treatment for a period of three to six months. She later reported chronic, grumbling yoke pain, with occasional headaches and arm pain with paraesthesiae, in the distribution described, but overall had remained improved.

A year later, she again attended with a report of chronic, right upper buttock and haunch pain, provoked by playing squash and

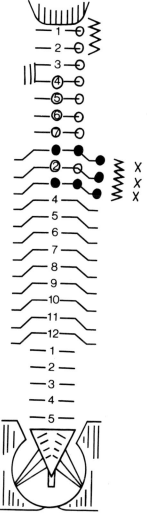

Palpation Findings

○ Tender   X Stiff Segment   ⅏ Hypermobile
● Sore   III Thickened (deep)   Segment
            ≋ Elicited Spasm   ⊗ Prominent

Fig. 9.6 Palpation findings at neck and thorax of a 27-year-old woman with a lateral pelvic tilt, upwards on the right (11.5.77).

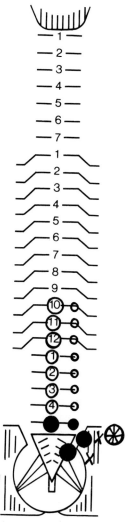

Palpation Findings

○ Tender   X Stiff Segment   ⅏ Hypermobile
● Sore   III Thickened (deep)   Segment
            ≋ Elicited Spasm   ⊗ Prominent

Fig. 9.7 Palpation findings at low thoracic, lumbar and sacroiliac joints of the patient mentioned in Fig. 9.6 (19.6.78).

going to 'keep fit' classes; the unilateral pain had begun at waist level and steadily migrated downwards. She also mentioned that any activity stirred up both the buttock and haunch pains, and also provoked the head, neck and arm pain previously treated. Observation revealed a lateral pelvic tilt, upwards on the right, with a posteriorly prominent right posterior superior iliac spine. The frontal plane asymmetry disappeared on sitting on a flat surface.

Extension was much reduced and exacerbated pain on the right from the thoracolumbar region to the sacrum. Left and right side-flexion were reduced by a third, and very cautiously performed; both hurt savagely as above. Flexion was reduced to reaching the knees only, with pain provoked as above. Rotations were reduced to 60° on either side. Straight-leg-raising was left 75° and right 80°, both limited by right buttock pain. Prone-knee-bending was reduced to 90° on both sides, with similar provocation of pain.

There were no neurological signs.

X-ray, within the year, had revealed no abnormalities.

Palpation findings were as depicted in Figure 9.7.

Treatment. By placing a ⅜ inch lift under her left heel, the painfully limited extension immediately became free and markedly less painful.

The right ilium was very gently mobilised (grade II−), which produced further improvement in extension range and an increased straight-leg-raising. It was suggested she raise the heel of all left shoes, and not attend for further treatment until the effects of the raise became clear. Within a fortnight, all pains (frontal, suboccipital, neck, arm, low back and haunch) with the exception of a localised right yoke pain, had disappeared. The localised right yoke pain remained subject to provocation by working stress, and was completely relieved if stress was avoided.

On retrospective analysis, it is probably correct to assume that the remnant of chronic right yoke pain was, in fact, due to the trauma of falling on that body part some 10 years before, and that this was aggravated together with all other pains, by the depredations of failure to compensate for a laterally tilted pelvis due to unequality of leg length.

The important point is that it is not possible to *know in advance* just how big a factor, in production of symptoms and signs remote from the pelvic levels, the consequences of pelvic asymmetry may be from patient to patient. Stoddard (1962)[1180a] describes three patients with obscure anterior thoracic pains, whose symptoms were relieved by no other treatment than an appropriate heel lift.

While location of the *source* of backache, or a cervical, thoracic or lumbar pain is necessary, there is also the question of the *genesis* of these pains, and the functional interdependence of the spine should always be considered.

In no way does this detract from the importance of accurately localised treatment, but it does clarify the context of that treatment, and might considerably improve an understanding of why vertebral joint problems behave as they do.

OBJECTIVE EXAMINATION—PHYSICAL TESTS

Tests of the tissues mentioned below are related to their function.[217]

1. Joint function is *movement*, and both active and passive tests of voluntary range, and passive tests of accessory range, are necessary.

2. Muscle function, with its tissue of attachment, is first to *develop* and then to *sustain* tension. By resisted isometric contractions, weakness and/or pain on applied tension are noted.

3. Ligaments and capsule *sustain tension, limit and also guide movement and maintain the integrity of joint structures.*

Tension is applied by passive movement, noting whether pain is caused, movement is limited, or the periarticular structures allow undue movement. It should be noted that *localised* tension is much easier to apply to the structures of single peripheral joints than to those of the multijointed vertebral segments.

4. Neurones *conduct impulses*, and the conduction is tested by methods which disclose loss or abnormalities of conduction, e.g., questioning the patient regarding sensation and equilibration changes, observing possible vasomotor disturbance and muscle wasting, observing and palpating for muscle spasm, testing for neurological deficit as muscle weakness and diminution or loss of tendon jerks, and testing skin for sensory diminution or loss.

5. Some special tests, e.g. straight-leg-raising (Fig. 9.17), prone-knee bending and others (see p. 60) are applied to test the freedom of movements of spinal nerve roots and neural canal structures, but are not conduction tests. Special tests may include, for example, (i) trunk rotation with the head stabilised, and (ii) successively tapping the spinous processes with a patella hammer. It should be noted that a single testing procedure, i.e. *resisted isometric contraction of muscle*, may be employed both in (2) to seek abnormalities in the muscle and its attachment-tissues, and in (4) to determine whether motor nerve conduction is normal.

Tests of movement. When symptoms and their behaviour are understood and postural abnormalities noted, the next step is to clarify which vertebral movements, or carefully applied stresses (i) reproduce or aggravate the patient's symptoms; (ii) are in themselves abnormal.

Since arthrosis and spondylosis are largely benign diseases of the joints, consideration of the movement abnormalities resulting is fundamental to devising treatment. They can be manifested in many ways, sometimes obvious during an active test and sometimes remaining undetected until passive tests (q.v.) of both voluntary and accessory movements are completed.

Mobility in multijoint articulations. The physiological range of movement at each vertebral joint, however small in comparison to the larger peripheral joints, is just as important to healthy joint function; when diminished by various causes, limitation at an individual segment is rather more difficult to detect than in peripheral joints in that it cannot readily be seen, although it can easily be palpated with practice.

A typical cervical vertebra takes part in the formation of ten separate joints. One thoracic vertebra takes part in 12 joints (counting each demifacet) and each lumbar vertebra, 6 joints. During degeneration changes and after trauma the natural apportioning of movement to each small component of this kind of complex articulation may be upset, and what appears on cursory examination to be normal movement in gross terms is actually movement achieved by extra strains on those joints adjacent to the stiff segments of the articulation. This abnormality tends to be self-perpetuating, and cannot always be remedied by the patient who has little influence, by way of voluntary effort, upon this defect.[446] Movement may be limited, of full or limited range but distorted, and sometimes excessive in hypermobile joints.

Limitation may be due to:
Pain
Spasm of antagonistic muscle-groups
Other tissue-tension, e.g. as stretch on adhesion formation or other soft-tissue contracture
Tissue-compression, e.g. as squeeze on marginal chondro-osteophytes, periarticular thickening, or intra-articular tissue changes.

During examination of a joint, one *can* only do:

1. Functional test (active movement)
2. Passive test—of functional range (especially the 'end-feel' of the movement)
    —of accessory movement and joint characteristics
    —of surrounding fibrous and other tissues
3. Muscle power test.

Each part contributes information about the state of the joint and its immediate neighbourhood, though the importance of each part varies according to the position and nature of the joint.

While it is not possible to suggest a rigid testing sequence applicable to all joints, a basic *spinal* testing procedure must include the following tests:

Joint movement—active, functional test
    —passive test of active and accessory movement
Joint structures—by local stress—tension, compression, torsion, unilateral approximation
Muscle testing—for muscle and attachments ⎱ by
             localised
    —for neurological deficit ⎰ isometric
             tension
Other neurological tests—tendon jerks, plantar response, ankle clonus, sensation
Special tests, e.g.—Straight-leg-raising (NB. This is not an exclusively neurological test)
    —rotation test for giddiness
    —spinal tapping test, etc.

and these are modified according to the nature and characteristics of the joint under examination.

Testing active movement of vertebral regions

Factors to be noted are:

Willingness to move
Quality of the movement (deviation, asymmetry, adventitious movement)
Limitations of normal range, if any
Amount of limitation
Nature of the limitation —reluctance
        —increasing pain
        —spasm
        —pain and spasm simultaneously
        —inert tissue-tension
        —tissue compression
        —muscle weakness
If painful   —*when?* (e.g. 'arc' of pain, or towards the end of range?)
        —how quickly does pain increase during movement, if at all?

—how much pain is caused, or how easily exacerbated? (Initial assessment of irritability)
—does it limit the movement? (It need not)
—*where* is the pain?
—is it exacerbation of presenting pain only, or spreading further, or a pain not previously reported?
—extent of spread into a limb?
Paraesthesiae and concomi-—elicited or aggravated by
tant symptoms   movement?
        —which movement?

It is important to establish the *factor primarily responsible*[797] (see p. 360) for the abnormal movement, because appropriate treatment procedures (q.v.) should be based on this knowledge; frequently only one of these factors is primarily responsible, although at times this is not so.

Normal movement. To prove that movement is normal, it is necessary to:

1. Repeat quickly
2. Add pressure at extreme of range, which should be tolerable (Fig. 9.8)
3. Give sustained pressure at end of range
4. Sustain pressure on movement towards the side of pain
and it may also be necessary to:
5. Give compression on movement towards the side of pain
6. Test 'corner' or combined movements (Figs 9.9, 9.16, 9.22)

Cursory examination of movement is insufficient, and therefore ranges which appear full and painless should be tested by passive overpressure at the extremes of active range before being accepted as normal.

Overpressure may cause discomfort in normal joints, but this test should not hurt; if it does, the joint is suspect and its degree of involvement requires clarification by further examination.

Again, the orthodox single testing movements, e.g. flexion, extension, rotation, etc., may frequently be insufficient to reproduce or aggravate the patient's symptoms, or to reveal latent joint abnormalities which are underlying the patient's complaint; because of inadequate examination of movement, therefore, joint problems amenable to treatment may remain undetected.

More searching tests of movement include:

a) Combined movements, e.g. extension with side-flexion, or flexion with side-flexion (conveniently termed quadrant testing movements) (Fig. 9.16)

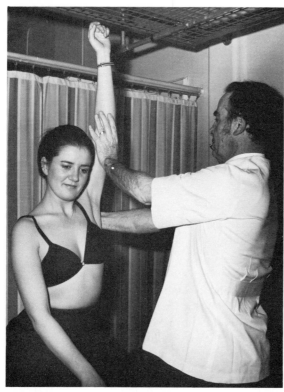

Fig. 9.8 Passive testing of the extremes of shoulder elevation. It is necessary to give overpressure to all apparently painless active-testing movements.

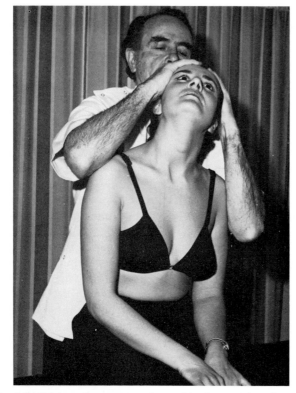

Fig. 9.9 Passive overpressure to the combined movements of extension and left-side flexion.

b) Applying compression or overpressure at the extremes of single or combined movements (Fig. 9.8)
c) Gently holding a vertebral region at the extremes of range of an active movement, single or combined, so that possible delayed or latent effects may be elicited. This test is of value when the presence or absence of 'root' pain (see p. 175) remains undetermined by less searching tests.

A description of combined (or quadrant) movements, and of the method of trying to provoke the effects of physical trespass upon the vertebral artery, are as follows:

Upper cervical spine
Sit or stand at side of patient — —extend at craniovertebral junction
—then rotate towards
—then side-flex towards

Vertebral artery test — —extend head and neck, then rotate each side
—fix head, then patient rotates trunk (Fig. 9.10)

Lower cervical spine
Stand facing patient—one hand on (R) frontal area and other on (L) scapula. (Can do from behind, if facing mirror and can see patient's face) (Fig. 9.9) — —approximate occiput to (L) scapula, then add rotation to the same side

Cervicothoracic
Stand facing patient, place (L) hand on (R) shoulder and (R) hand on (L) low neck, so that palmar aspect of metacarpal heads bears against low cervical transverse process — —press into extension and (R) side flexion, then rotate (R)

Thoracic spine
Stand behind patient (use mirror if possible) — —extend, side flex to (L), then rotate (L)

Lumbar spine
Stand behind patient with hands on shoulders — —extend, side flex to (L), then rotate to (L).

Tests should be repeated to the opposite side.

NB. Do not lose tension or approximation when additional movements are imposed.

Limit of range. This is virtually indefinable in an absolute sense, since the limit of *active* movement varies with the state of the tissues, the time of day, the willingness of the patient, and the speed of the movement performed, and the limit of *passive* movement varies with the tolerance of the patient, the courage or indiscretion of the operator, and the metabolic or vascular state and temperature of the patient's tissues at the material time. Probably a useful working definition is: 'Limit of range is reached when the therapist, the patient, and the joint decide that the movement has proceeded far enough'!

The intensity and duration of increased pain on movement depends upon the degree of joint and/or root irritability

Accurate assessment of this is important, because pain which is easily exacerbated indicates the need for careful handling, both in examination and treatment. The three factors to be considered are the amount of movement required to exacerbate pain; the intensity of the added pain; how long it takes to recede to normal levels.

A small unguarded movement stirring up intense pain for some hours indicates a highly irritable joint. Irritability is also manifest when a quick testing movement elicits spasm earlier in the range than does a more sedate testing movement, and also when both *pain and spasm*, either of which is of sufficient magnitude to limit range, are elicited simultaneously. Pain which is not easily provoked and which settles down very quickly after provocation by a gross movement indicates a much less irritable joint.

Spasm of antagonistic muscle-groups can be elicited, as the primary movement-limiting factor, notwithstanding a degree of pain beginning either before the limitation or being elicited as the point of limitation is reached. The accompanying pain is frequently not sufficient of itself to stop the movement. The variety of ways in which joint irritability can be evidenced is due not only to the state of the joint but also to the variations in central nervous system excitability from patient to patient. In less irritable joints, pain may be limiting the movement at any point on the range. Pain may also begin during a movement and rise only moderately until the movement is fully completed. A painful arc of movement, of greater or lesser amplitude, may be traversed during an otherwise uneventful movement, as may sudden 'jabs' or 'catches' (see p. 259).

If the two factors of inert tissue-tension and tissue-compression are taken together as *resistance*, it is commonly found that arthrotic and spondylotic vertebral segments, giving rise to the complaint of a dull persistent ache, can be limited by this resistance as the primary factor, without eliciting further pain of any consequence. The resistance may be due to changes of long standing or be of more recent origin.

Distortion also occurs during movements, and when asymmetry or deviation from normal paths is noted during active tests, it is important to clarify its significance. If it is the patient's natural way of moving, manual prevention of the deviation during testing will produce discomfort but no pain; when the deviation is an involuntary guarding response against pain during movement, its manual prevention during movement will hurt, and this information helps in selection and accurate assessment of treatment procedures.

Crepitus on movement is more likely to be arising from the synovial joints.

Hypermobility of vertebral segments can either be *acquired*, when pathological instability is underlying it, or be *inherited* as in those patients who are naturally loose-jointed.[705]

Testing muscle function

Static isometric contractions, of vertebral and paravertebral muscle, are more frequently employed as neurological tests, i.e. of motor nerve conduction (q.v.) than as tests of intrinsic changes in muscle and/or its attachment tissues, but where weakness of paravertebral muscle, e.g. the abdominal wall, is believed part of a postural defect, an assessment of muscle-power is necessary, and similarly where it is suspected that forces sustained by joints may have produced tissue-damage to muscles.

Resisted 'static' (isometric) contractions. It is probably wise to accept that while this may be the aim, it is an extremely difficult thing to arrange in practice.

Joint movement always occurs, joint surface compression occurs, and surrounding non-contractile joint structures are almost always disturbed in some way. It is practically impossible *to keep joints quite still* while muscles around them are put into strong static contractions. Thus, when examining the periarticular contractile tissues (of peripheral joints) such as muscle, tendon and tenoperiosteal junction, by applying local tension, the fact that joint compression and joint shearing invariably occurs should be borne in mind. Aggravation of pain by these tests need not necessarily indicate that the lesion lies in these contractile tissues. Meticulous examination will reveal that it is not often a muscle attachment near a joint is abnormal without the joint also being abnormal, and the precise nature of the changes occurring is not as clearcut as is sometimes asserted, especially so in upper limb areas commonly involved in referred pain (and other symptoms) from more proximal vertebral lesions.

When manually testing *the tightness of postural muscles*, a short sustained and uniform pressure should be exerted at a right angle to the direction of muscle elongation—repetitive 'pumping' pressures are likely to elicit facilitation effects and increased tension.

When testing the tightness of hip flexors, for example, the supine patient lies with coccyx at the edge of the plinth, one hip and knee maximally flexed onto the chest and supported there by the therapist.

The iliopsoas and rectus femoris of the freely hanging leg are tested for tightness by:

1. Observing the position of the thigh in relation to the horizontal plane, and exerting a steady perpendicular pressure to the lower anterior thigh.
2. If the rectus femoris is tight a slight extension of the knee will be manifest during this test. Anteroposterior pressure on the shin will result in a degree of hip flexion of the rectus femoris is especially tight.

Testing connective-tissue structures

Local tension (by passive movement or resisted contraction). The term 'selective tension' is not used, since it is extremely difficult to arrange that a single tissue has tension selectively applied to it only. It is usually only possible to dispose the patient in such a way that tension is applied to a whole group of tissues, *including* the tissues one is presently interested in. Active movements apply normal stress and tensions to all soft tissues. When muscles are relaxed the range of passive movement exceeds that which is possible actively, and for this reason the inert capsular, ligamentous and aponeurotic tissues are additionally tested by passively applying further tension; this is regionally localised, so far as possible, by careful hand-placing and grasps.

When assessing the responses to these tests, i.e. in terms of which tissue be giving rise to the pain or spasm thereby elicited, two factors should be borne in mind:

1. Movement of a 'rigid' structure, i.e. a vertebral body, must also move *all* structures attached to it.
2. Pain may be elicited on passive stretching of one aspect of a spinal region, and be re-elicited on following resisted isometric contraction of muscles on the same aspect. This does not necessarily indicate that the lesion must therefore lie in vertebral muscle.

The tests are:

1. The passive overpressure to *apparently normal* gross active movements (described above).
2. Passive questing movements of vertebral regions, to try to ascertain more clearly the nature of factors *limiting* gross active movements, or of other responses, e.g. a test of cervical rotation (see p. 314), or flat-handed pressure on the spine of a prone patient (see p. 353).[1180b]

More localised passive tests are described under 'Palpation'.

Neurological tests

Information that the signs and symptoms of root involvement (see p. 160) are appearing, have become established, or are regressing, is an important factor in assessment, as is the *distribution* of neurological signs. Evidence that more than one root is unilaterally involved, or that there is bilateral evidence of root changes, generally contraindicates many treatments.

Root involvement affecting *muscle strength*, if present, is invariably revealed without testing every muscle and every joint action. Concerning muscle weakness, the absence or presence of neurological deficit is confirmed by testing only one muscle, or joint action, as representative of a given cord segment. In broad terms, the pattern of nerve root supply (see p. 69) will help to indicate the probable level of involvement.

During the therapist's 'Indications' examination, the neurological tests employed are restricted to those providing guides for treatment, and normally the only *tendon reflexes* tested are the biceps, supinator, triceps, knee, ankle and great toe jerks. Plantar responses are also tested and the absence of ankle clonus must be determined. Incipient root involvement may be missed if reflexes are tested once only, and routine 'Indications' examinations should include tapping the tendon *six successive times*, to uncover the fading reflex response which indicates developing root signs.

An additional deep tendon reflex is described by Berlin (1971).[87] With the patient's foot in plantar-flexion and inversion, and the tip of the therapist's finger exerting pressure over the heads of 4th and 5th metatarsals, the dorsum of the examiner's distal phalanx is briskly tapped. In 11 patients tested the reflex was absent in all, while other deep tendon reflexes were variably affected.

When positive, the test is considered an indication of lesions affecting the L5–S1 segment.

While one authority asserts that the state of the tendon reflexes is a valuable localising sign, another may observe that patterns of neurological deficit in lower limbs cannot be relied upon to inculpate a particular root, although it is not always clear whether electrodiagnostic methods have been included in the procedures for establishing the nature of the neurological deficit.

In his series of 26 patients with lumbosacral root compression who underwent a correlated clinical and electrodiagnostic follow-up, Yates (1964)[1369] found that all 23 patients with involvement of the first sacral root showed a depressed or absent ankle-jerk, while those with involvement of fifth lumbar root had normal knee- and ankle-jerks. Subsequent investigation reveals that the two heads of gastrocnemius may be differentially affected by lumbosacral radiculopathy,[1249] the medial head is most commonly affected by L5 root lesions and the lateral head by lesions of the S1 root.

Among 60 consecutive patients with lumbosacral joint problems, 18 had a clinically diminished ankle-jerk, but in only 8 patients were the clinical findings validated by e.m.g. testing, and among these 4 had involvement of the lateral head, 3 had involvement of the medial head and 1 had involvement of both heads. Some had a clinically *enhanced* ankle-jerk on the painful leg side and this was confirmed by e.m.g. tests in one of them.[1249]

When testing for *sensory changes* leading questions should be avoided. Patients should be asked to report, with eyes closed, when tactile sensation is stimulated by simple stroking tests. When areas of complete anaesthesia are reported, or suspected, the testing of skin sensitivity to pinprick is necessary.

NB. When attempting to localise the segmental level of root involvement by distribution of root signs, the overlap of cutaneous supply, and pre- and postfixation of plexuses should be borne in mind, also the discrepancy between vertebrae and roots in the cervical region and the great obliquity of the lumbosacral roots (see p. 24). The precise nature of the lesion affecting the nerve root often remains in doubt in non-surgical cases, and sometimes in surgical cases, also.

SPECIAL TESTS Passive testing movements such as: (1) straight-leg-raising in supine lying (Fig. 9.17);[1314] (2) knee extension in sitting; (3) neck flexion in supine lying and in sitting;[133] (4) knee bending with hip extension in prone lying; either alone or in combination, can exert tension on the spinal nerve roots with their dural sleeves. Thus they provide information on the freedom of movement of those structures, and on the extent of entrapment or restriction imposed by trespass of related structures and/or by intrinsic changes in the tissues themselves. The degree of root irritability is likewise indicated by limitation occurring simultaneously with aggravation of root pain, coexisting with loss-of-conduction signs in that root.

The functional interdependence of spinal structures, particularly the inextensible soft tissues within the neural canal, i.e. the dura and root sleeves, indicate that the following are also highly interdependent factors, which may underlie clinical presentations from 'tight' hamstrings to headache:

1. The position of the head and neck
2. The posture of the thoracic and lumbar spines
3. The position of the hip joint and the knee joint
4. Whether the patient is lying, sitting or standing
5. The presence of lesions producing tethering and thus increased tension and distortion of neural canal structures
6. The dural continuity from the lumbosacral plexus to the intracranial meninges.

Maitland (1978)[799a] has initiated a detailed method of formulating and tabulating normal values for the mean ranges of extensibility of structures in the vertebral canal, and suggests that further investigation is required, so that information might be provided in relation to (i) the use of straight-leg-raising as a treatment technique and (ii) the concept of tight hamstrings.

The field of these *interrelationships* is as yet largely unexplored, although much work has been done on the biomechanics of the spinal cord itself, of course,[121a] and on the basis of their detailed findings on the effects of medial hip rotation, as a qualifying test of the effects of straight-leg-raising, Breig and Troup (1979)[121b] have suggested that in those patients in whom medial hip rotation elicits pain, the piriformis muscle itself may be hyperalgesic.

1. *The Straight-leg-raising test* (Fig. 9.17) places a varying degree of tension on each of the lumbosacral roots, from L4 to S2 inclusive, the most traction being exerted on the first sacral root (see p. 61). Further, a degree of lumbosacral plexus and root traction must occur when the foot is dorsiflexed in addition (Braggard's sign), but it is a mistake to ascribe the increased calf pain, willy-nilly, to the pain of increased root tension.[780]

Exacerbation of 'sciatic' pain, by forcible foot dorsiflexion near the end of a painfully limited straight-leg-raising range,[451] is not always a reliable indication that the extra pain is due to further sciatic nerve stretch; foot dorsiflexion will often produce calf pain at 60°–70° on a normal leg, and simple calf tenderness often accompanies purely sacroiliac conditions, being exacerbated by the dorsiflexion test.

Allowing the knee to flex relieves the pain elicited when the knee is kept straight—while this knee-flexion relieves tension on the sciatic nerve, it also relieves tension on the hamstrings, of course; thus the manœuvre does not provide any more specific information about the *cause* of painfully limited straight-leg-raising.

Similarly, while it is known that internal rotation of the lower limb[121b] exerts tension on the root components of the sciatic nerve (see p. 296), the test is of negligible additional clinical value provided the straight-leg-raising test has been meticulously performed in the first place, i.e. with the knee extended, the foot at 90°, the leg slightly adducted and with neutral rotation. The point at which painful root tension limits further movements (if this *is* the limiting factor) can be adequately determined one way or another, and need not require alternative tests which essentially give the same information. Many people have 5°–10° normal discrepancy between limits of left and right straight-leg-raising, and the normal full range can be anything between an angle of 75°–120°, measured between longitudinal axis of leg and horizontal surface of couch.

Wyke (1976)[1362] asserts that the production or provocation of pain, either by active trunk flexion or passive straight-leg-raising, need not be due to traction on nerve roots, since (i) the spinal cord does not move vertically within the vertebral canal, and (ii) (Brodal, 1969)[130] the nerve roots are firmly anchored to the walls of the intervertebral foramina (see p. 62).

'In both sets of circumstances the intraspinal pressure is increased (and nerve root irritation is thereby increased) because of changes in the transverse diameter of the spinal cord and in the volume of blood in the epidural veins that then occur.'

A positive straight-leg-raising test is not, as had been suggested (Edgar and Park, 1974)[298] a *sine qua non* of root involvement. For example, radiofrequency myotomy of trigger spots in paravertebral musculature can produce an immediate increase in the range of straight-leg-raising, as well as lasting pain relief.[658]

Hirsch *et al.* (1963)[551] have shown that lumbar and posterior thigh pain can be produced by irritant injections into the region of facet-joints, and Mooney and Robertson (1976)[867] have demonstrated (p. 250) that facet-joint changes will painfully reduce straight-leg-raising. Anaesthetic block of the facet-joint restores normal straight-leg-raising within five minutes. The notion that a reduced straight-leg-raising is pathognomonic of lower lumbar disc protrusion[298] could bear some inspection; in 40 per cent of patients who experienced pain relief (with interruption of the pain–muscle spasm cycle by denervation of the facet-joints with a thermistor probe under fluoroscopic control)[658] a marked improvement in the straight-leg-raising test also occurred.

Mooney (1977)[870] also reports patients with a straight-leg-raising reduced to about 45°–60°, and positive e.m.g. readings at the point of limitation. Injection of a single facet-joint is followed by the return of normal range of straight-leg-raising and myoelectrical silence.

Where a limited straight-leg-raising *is* due to root involvement, this need not be due to a 'disc lesion', implying trespass. Fahrni (1966)[334] describes three patients with the classical symptoms and signs of disc protrusion, and consistently positive myelographic findings. *No disc protrusion was found at operation* but the nerve root was densely adherent to the disc. Full and lasting relief was obtained by surgical release of the root, leaving the disc intact (see also p. 264). It is very probable that there need not be any involvement of roots or dura for straight-leg-raising to be limited. The limitation imposed can be due purely to an irritative joint lesion, i.e. involving disc or facet-joint or ligament, or all three, not physically affecting neural tissue yet producing a greater or lesser degree of hamstring spasm.

Where straight-leg-raising is limited by only 10°–20°, the pain is possibly caused by beginning of tension in a root which is abnormally sensitive from causes intrinsic to the root itself, and not inevitably accompanied by any trespass of neighbouring tissues.

Where straight-leg-raising evokes pain with reduction to below 45° or thereabouts, it may probably indicate movement of an already stretched root over a protruded disc, i.e. some of the 'normal slack' has already been taken up by the space-occupying protruded material.

The one important factor to note is *the character of the response* and to use this as a criterion for assessing the efficacy of treatment techniques employed.

The importance of the crossed straight-leg-raising test has been emphasised by Hudgins (1977).[578] In some cases of sciatica, raising the normal side leg exacerbates the sciatic pain in the affected leg.

From cadaver experiments it is known that raising the straight leg not only applies torsion to the ipsilateral roots but also pulls laterally on the dural sac, thus disturbing the contralateral roots. When positive, the sign is regarded by some as almost pathognomonic of disc herniation (although it does not necessarily follow, of course, that the disc herniation is entirely responsible for the pain). Hudgins examined 351 consecutive cases of supposed disc herniation with leg pain, and in 58 of these the sign was positive. The presence of a herniated disc was proven in 56 (97 per cent) of them. Of the 293 patients with painful straight-leg-raising on the affected side only, 188 (64 per cent) had a proven herniation.

Since up to 20 per cent of myelographic examinations may fail to reveal evidence of disc herniation, it is calculated that a patient with a positive crossed straight-leg-raising test and a negative myelogram nevertheless has a post-test risk of herniated disc of some 90 per cent. Hudgins suggests that myelography is unnecessary for diagnosis in these patients, and that it should be disregarded if normal.

Following surgical intervention, pain relief was enough to allow resumption of normal activities in 91 per cent of those patients with the positive crossed straight-leg-raising sign, but only in 70 per cent of those without it, i.e. painfully limited straight-leg-raising on the affected side only. It was therefore suggested that the sign should be sought for every patient with low back and leg pain, since its known implications could reduce delayed referral for surgery and unnecessary investigation procedures.

Perhaps clinical considerations are not as clearcut, since it is a common experience for manual therapists to conservatively treat, with success, many patients with a positive crossed straight-leg-raising test.

Kirkaldy-Willis and Hill (1979)[662] suggest that there should be a high index of suspicion of neuritic rather than referred pain when straight-leg-raising is markedly reduced; more so when the Lasègue test is positive; even more so with the crossed Lasègue sign. The Lasègue test is not quite the same as the straight-leg-raising test, of course.

Frequently, surgeons need to determine whether the cauda equina is the site of significant compression; while disc prolapse is normally accompanied by a positive straight-leg-raising test, a negative straight-leg-raising is *not* a contraindication for surgery in spondylotic stenosis where back pain and/or sciatica are aggravated by lordotic postures and relieved by lumbar flexion.

Disabling spondylotic trespass can exist in the presence of a normal straight-leg-raising.[1300]

2. *If knee-extension in sitting* is passively tested, the mechanics of the cord, meninges and root traction are broadly similar to (1), with exceptions that gravitational compression, adding to intradiscal pressure, now tends to increase the effect of any restriction upon free movement of the

meninges, and this effect will be pronounced if the patient slumps into a generally flexed posture (p. 60).

3. *Neck flexion in lying* (Brudzinski's test). The effect of traction exerted in this way upon the neural canal structures extends caudally as far as the thoracic and lumbar regions and for this reason it is perhaps a more valuable examination procedure for these regions than for the cervical region in that aggravation of low back, pelvic girdle or leg pain by this manœuvre is a useful indication that the source of pain lies wholly or partly in the spine and neural canal rather than in more peripheral tissues.

4. It is sometimes necessary to apply the *combined effects* of (1), (2) and (3) when guides for action in treatment are not clearly afforded by any one of these tests performed alone. Thus it may be necessary to flex the patient's neck while raising the straight leg with foot at 90°, or further, to apply these tensions while the patient sits slumped.

5. *Knee-bending with hip extension*, passively performed with the patient prone and pelvis stabilised, may exacerbate root pain of 3rd, and perhaps the 2nd and 4th, lumbar segment origin, since the femoral nerve lies in front of the hip joint and this test tends to disturb the sensitised root (if there be such) by traction. The range of movement available in the hip after the knee has been flexed is very small, and consequently forward pelvic tilting is difficult to prevent.

NB. It is most important to bear in mind that these manœuvres also put stress on joints, and responses can thus be equivocal when joints also are in an irritable state. For example, the *femoral nerve stretch test* applies compression to the knee and hip joints, torsion to the sacroiliac joint with a forward-tilting effect upon the pelvis and thus also a disturbance of lumbar joints. Similarly, besides its well-appreciated traction effects on the sciatic nerve and lumbosacral roots, the *straight-leg-raising test* also tends to move, because of the lumbar-spine-flexion effect via the pelvis, *joints* which may be irritable, the joints between the vertebral bodies and also the synovial facet-joints. The pelvis is tilted backwards in the sagittal plane, and also upwards in the frontal plane, i.e. a lateral tilt upwards on the tested side. The pelvis is also slightly rotated[445] towards the untested side, all of these effects occurring towards the end of range in the normal person. Hence, while standardised and precisely performed manœuvres are necessary, standardised conclusions are unwise, and the examiner is never relieved of the obligation to *assess*, to weigh the value of what are frequently equivocal responses to standard tests.

Hazlett (1975)[523] observes that in 45 patients with a femoral distribution of symptoms and signs, the femoral nerve stretch test was not particularly useful to diagnose irritative lesions of the upper lumbar nerve roots, because of difficulties in controlling spinal motion on extension of the hip.

6. An additional, *active straight-leg-raising test*, seeking the 'Hoover' sign,[36] may assist in deciding between willingness and unwillingness of the patient to co-operate fully in the objective part of the examination. Normally, when the supine patient is asked to elevate one limb, the heel of the opposite foot is pressed to the couch. With the examiner's palm under the heel, the degree of downward heel pressure should be much the same for either limb in a normal subject. When a weak or painful-side limb is elevated, the opposite and normal-side heel is pressed harder into the examiner's palm than when the normal side limb is raised. Should no downward pressure be exerted by the normal heel, the patient is probably not attempting to raise the supposed painful and/or weak contralateral limb. The test should not be regarded as conclusive in itself, but can at times assist in assessment of clinical features.

7. *Cervical rotation tests.* The effects of head and neck movements on the vertebrobasilar arterial system have been noted (see p. 3), and also the possible mechanisms underlying the distressing symptom of 'cervical vertigo' and 'drop' attacks (see p. 183).

Dizziness is commonly reported by middle-aged and elderly patients, and the cause is frequently not within the province of physical treatment; for example, if it is exacerbated by movement of the head in space, i.e. active neck rotation, but not when the head and neck are kept still

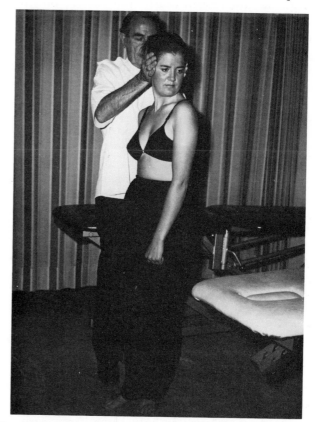

Fig. 9.10 Active cervical rotation, by the model turning her trunk fully to her right, while the therapist stabilises the head. Thus neck rotation occurs without head movement.

while the patient twists the trunk (Fig. 9.10), the exciting factor is likely to be head movement in space and not rotatory cervical stress.

In patients for whom physical treatment is indicated and whose dizziness is aggravated by *both* of the above manœuvres, it is important to avoid rotatory cervical movements in treatment; besides carefully noting the effects of cervical rotation during active tests, it is wise to gently hold the lying patient's head in full rotation to either side for about 30 seconds. Symptoms not aggravated by the active test may appear during sustained passive rotation, and treatment procedures should likewise avoid rotation movements.

8. *Vertebral percussion test.* When it has been established that an ache is most likely to be arising from a thoracic or lumbar joint problem, and examination with careful palpation has failed to localise the vertebral level(s) responsible, gentle percussion of the spine can assist in revealing it. The patient stands with the spine flexed or sits leaning foward with elbows supported on knees, and the therapist gently and successively taps the spinous processes with a patellar hammer, noting at which level(s) the response exceeds that of the mild discomfort of the test.

OBJECTIVE EXAMINATION—PALPATION

It is of interest to observe skilled clinicians carefully percussing the thorax over the lung fields, confident of their ability to gather valuable clinical information by this classical and important method of examination.

For example, the position of the trachea in the suprasternal notch, and the apex beat, are located by palpation. The axillae, supraclavicular fossae and the neck triangles are felt for enlarged glands; and the presence of tactile fremitus over an area of impaired resonance may help in deciding whether the impaired resonance is caused by pleural effusion or not. In other disciplines, palpation of the radial, dorsalis pedis and temporal pulses, of the liver, spleen and cervical glands, or the nature of lower limb oedema does not excite comment, yet failure to include these simple but important tests in the appropriate examination procedures would soon invite observations about negligence and lack of examination method. In discussing the clinical value of palpation in respiratory disease, a standard text (*The Practice of Medicine*[1040]) asserts:

...we must recognise that error is increased by carelessness, haste and indifferent techniques, and may be reduced by a careful routine and the skill born of long practice and experience. Secondly, we must remember that it is in the borderland separating slight abnormality from normality that mistakes are most easily made.

It would be difficult to express more clearly the factors important in *all* examination by palpation, particularly the tactile search for tissue-tension abnormalities in the vertebral structures.

The daily occurrence of orthopaedic surgeons and rheumatologists carefully palpating a synovial sheath at the wrist, or the structures of an ankle, the first carpometacarpal joint, an elbow or a knee, and recording their findings about effusion, synovial thickening or crepitus, exostosis, the presence or absence of ligamentous laxity, patellofemoral crepitus or pain on approximation, and the 'clonks' or 'thuds' of an intra-articular derangement, is regarded not as unusual but proper to the discharge of professional responsibilities.

Further, should a patient report rhythmic twinges of pain over the dorsum of the foot when walking, the clinician does not initially palpate the hip or knee, but the foot itself, the site of the patient's complaint. Plainly, the art of feeling or 'looking with the fingers' has been widely practised by physicians and surgeons for centuries, and much clinical examination would be the poorer for its exclusion from the process of finding out what is wrong. After long practice, clinicians and teachers set great store by their skill and experience in using these methods; they rightly become proud of their expertise and devote time to transmitting their painstakingly acquired proficiency to the medical student.

In this age of diagnosis by computer and other technology, experienced clinicians and teachers, who understand better than anybody the value of a careful clinical search for abnormality, are tireless in reiterating the vital importance of (a) listening to the patient, (b) physically examining the patient, and (c) palpation. Perhaps it is not surprising, therefore, that the manipulatively minded worker (whether surgeon,[105] physician,[1180a] physiotherapist[450] or osteopath[390]) should be at a loss to understand why the similar and logical use of careful segmental palpation, in examination of spinal joint problems, has in the past been regarded with scepticism by some.

For example, when localised and subtle changes of contour and attitude have been observed in relation to the vertebral column, what is more instinctive than proceeding to *feeling* them, examining them by palpation? Often it is only by this means that their relevance or significance can be determined. The existence of manifest abnormality, detected by experienced palpation and with the clinical knowledge of what is normal, does not change because the sceptic cannot, or will not, feel what there is to be felt, or because the means of perceiving its presence by feeling has never been elucidated for him.

Assessing movement-abnormalities (pp. 351, 359) at vertebral segments, or arthrotic knee joints, for example, employs criteria which are common to both, since there are at present no other. The manipulatively minded worker is as earthbound as his colleagues of other disciplines; his clinical ways and means are no more than the ways and means existing, yet by constant attention to what his fingers are telling him, and by practice, he has developed an examination method which employs the criteria in a more localised and specific way, not now to a larger peripheral joint but to a vertebral mobility-segment.

Conclusions about the *nature* of the abnormality palpated, and its significance in relation to symptoms, are a matter for experienced assessment and therefore arguable, but of its *presence* there can be no doubt.[627, 492]

Procedure

A joint, with its immediate periarticular tissues and surrounding muscle tissue, has not been adequately examined unless it has been investigated by localised passive movement and palpation, because these methods obtain information not available by any other means.

Palpation is used to test:

1. The state of the skin, with superficial and deep soft tissues.
2. The state of periarticular tissues (palpation of the *still* joint).
3. The characteristics of segmental vertebral *movement*.

Note that in (3) the range of movement examined may therefore be:

a. That of regional and segmental *accessory* joint movement, which by definition cannot be produced voluntarily, and
b. That of the *voluntary*, or physiological movement between two vertebrae (see below).

Skin, soft tissues and subcutaneous bony points. The temperature, texture and dryness or excessive moisture of skin are noted. Abnormalities such as dysaesthesia (diminished sensibility); hyperaesthesia (unpleasantly increased sensibility); anaesthesia (loss of sensibility) are sought.

Swelling may be palpated, and its nature discerned, e.g. it may be soft and fluctuant, or thickened and indurated. The texture, i.e. pliability and soft resilience, of muscle bellies is noted, as is the presence and distribution of postural spasm. Undue tenderness of superficial bony points, and of superficial tissues including interspinous connective tissue, is sought. Body areas which are normally tender should be borne in mind.

Periarticular palpation (Figs 9.11, 9.12) provides information of possible abnormalities of joint relationship, in the more superficial joints (this refers to a degree of fixation in an asymmetrical position, not subluxation, e.g. as stated by Coutts, 1934,[208] '... a pathological fixation in a position within a normal range of motion'), undue tenderness of deep periarticular tissues, deep thickening and the presence of undue bony prominence. The latter may be anomalies of bone structure (see p. 24) which are of no clinical significance, or degenerative exostosis.

It is wise to note that palpation findings may not be quite the same in the lying position as they were when

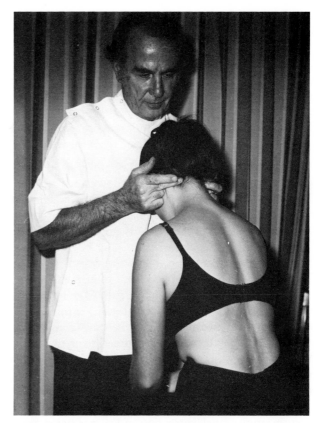

Fig. 9.11 This illustrates important palpation tests, i.e. that of assessment of abnormalities at the craniovertebral junction.

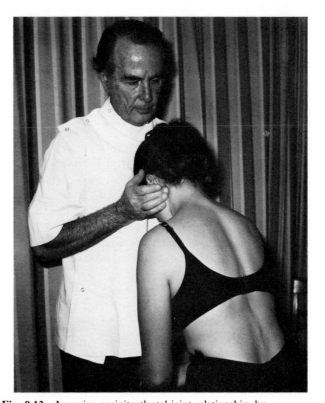

Fig. 9.12 Assessing occipitoatlantal joint relationship, by simultaneous palpation of the mastoid process and lateral mass of atlas. 'Abnormalities' are not necessarily clinically significant.

the patient was sitting or standing. For example, if the occipitoatlantal joint relationships are palpated bilaterally with the sitting patient's forehead resting on the standing therapist's chest, it is not uncommon for a prominent left arch of atlas to change to prominence on the right when the same region is palpated with the patient prone. While we may speculate upon the causes of this phenomenon, it behoves the need to stick to standard testing procedures when assessing, so that reproducibility is assured.

Accessory movement (regional and segmental). (i) Flat-handed pressure, applied vertically downward upon the thoracic and lumbar *regions* of a prone patient, is an important objective test. It elicits much useful information, helpful in the assessment of what is normal from patient to patient, and when abnormality may be present (*see* Assessment in Examination, p. 353).

Passive tests of *segmental* accessory movement are performed by applying thumbtips or pads, singly or more usually together, against vertebral bony prominences. Carefully graded pressures are applied in various directions. Fingers should rest but be spread so as to stabilise the more active thumbs. The lumbar regions in heavy patients may require some of the pressures to be applied via the pisiform of the operator's hand, reinforced and stabilised by the other.

Gentle longitudinal distraction and compression movements may also be manually applied to the cervical region, while the amount of distraction occurring at a mobile segment is palpated. Distraction may also be applied mechanically, via a cervical harness and pulley system.

Thumb pressures used are: postero-anterior central pressures on spinous processes; postero-anterior unilateral pressures over the joints between adjacent articular processes; transverse pressures against the sides of spinous processes; postero-anterior unilateral pressures on the angles of the ribs.[797]

For fullest information, the main direction of testing movements are altered, in that central pressures may be angulated slightly cranially or caudally, transverse pressures may be likewise angulated, and unilateral pressures given a cranial, caudal, medial or lateral bias, sometimes in combination.

During this important stage of examination, most of the criteria (see p. 313) *for testing active movements of vertebral regions are reapplied, because fullest information about the segmental localisation of a joint problem, and the way it is clinically manifesting itself, can only be gained by careful and orderly passive tests and palpation.*

Note: A suggested routine for palpation of accessory movement is included with the tabulated 'Examination Procedures' for vertebral regions.

(ii) Passive tests of the available *functional or physiological* movement between two vertebrae are performed when necessary.

By this examination method the three degrees of freedom—or available range in the sagittal, frontal and horizontal planes—which the spine can traverse by voluntary movement, are passively and rhythmically reproduced by the examiner; adjacent bony points are palpated in turn and their changing relationship is the basis for comparisons, and for assessment of segmental mobility. Translation movement and accessory ranges along the axis of the column, approximation and distraction, are also tested on occasions.

Technique is described on page 336.

REGIONAL EXAMINATION PROCEDURES

A basic drill for the vertebral regions and associated limb girdles is given below, each followed by a suggested palpation routine. These will frequently need elaboration to elicit special information, and should therefore be regarded as minimum essential testing procedure. Since pain is very frequently referred from proximal to distal, and since joints which are situated in areas to which pain of spinal origin is commonly referred often develop secondary dysfunction, which contributes to the total picture of signs and symptoms, all examinations should invariably proceed from the spine to the distal body parts, in an orderly sequence.

CERVICAL REGION—ROUTINE EXAMINATION OF NECK AND FOREQUARTER

1. History ('Listen')
   a. What is patient's usual daily activity (work and play)?
   b. Details of *present* pain
      —site and boundaries—radiation to arm? Hand?
      —headache? Which part of cranium? Face pain?
      —*nature*—deep or surface—shooting?
      —improving or worsening?
      —area of worst pain?
   c. *Behaviour of pain* related to time, posture and activity
      —constant, episodic or occasional?
      —what aggravates?
      —what eases?
      —any functional restrictions, because of pain?
      —night pain?
      —rising a.m.? Day/evening pain?
      —time-dependent or stress-dependent?

d. *Other symptoms*

—paraesthesiae? Where? Which fingers? (Any fullness, puffiness, numbness?) Dizziness? Dysequilibrium? Visual symptoms?

—what aggravates/eases?

—any symptoms in legs?

e. X-rayed? Drugs? Systemic steroids? History of rheumatoid arthritis? Anticoagulants? General health?

f. *Onset* of this, and previous attacks (after *all* details of *present* symptoms understood).

Previous treatment, and result of that treatment?

NB Now *plan* which spinal and peripheral joints need *more* than routine examination (e.g. thoracic joints, shoulder, elbow or wrist, lower limbs—cf. cervical myelopathy).

2. Observation ('Look')

Observe pelvic posture in standing and sitting, with quick check for possible leg length inequality (Figs 9.1, 9.2, 9.4, 9.5).

Patient sitting

Head and neck posture—shoulder levels?

Spasm—asymmetry—any other contour change, especially round deltoid?

Initial palpation. Feel muscle bellies for presence of consistency changes and postural spasm. Palpate eyebrow tissues.

Patient rests forehead on operator's chest. Palpate

—suboccipital region (Figs 9.11, 9.12)

—lateral mass of atlas near mastoid process

—paraspinal region, over neural arches (see p. 321).

3. Function ('Test')   *Patient sitting*

Watch for: Limitations and *reasons* for limitation, i.e. ? pain ? stiffness ? spasm. Always give overpressure to clear, if apparently normal. Repeat if necessary for asymmetrical movement, deviation; watch for level affected—painful/painless when prevented? Employ quadrant movements and compression (localising effect to craniovertebral, midcervical or cervicothoracic as applicable) if need be, to clarify. Seek regions of muscle tightness.

Ext.
LSF
RSF
Flex.
LR
RR

Muscle power —tuck chin in ⎱ C1 and C2 (Figs
(resisted isometric —push chin up ⎰ 9.13, 9.14)
contractions) —press head and neck laterally—C3

Peripheral joints

Temp./mand. joint (Check if face pain)

Clavicular joints —test accessory movement

shoulder girdle —elevation (active) then *resist* (for C3–4)

Shoulder joint —elevation through flexion and through abduction (active)
—passive overpressure to clear

Elbow/forearm —check

Wrist and hand —check

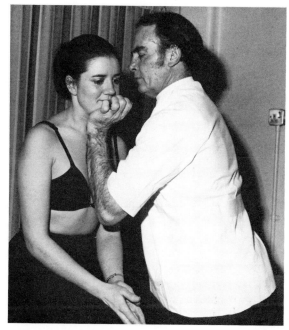

Fig. 9.13 Resisted isometric (static) contraction of muscles supplied by C1 and C2 (a.p.r.). See 'Patterns of somatic nerve root supply' (p. 69).

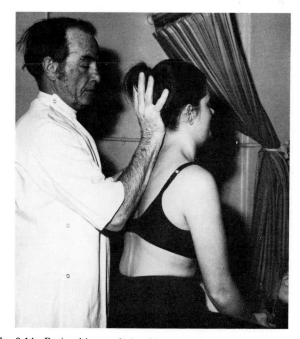

Fig. 9.14 Resisted isometric (static) contraction of muscles supplied by C1 and C2 (p.p.r.). See 'Patterns of somatic nerve root supply' (p. 69).

Patient lying supine

Gently hold head fully rotated for 30 seconds either side, to see if headache aggravated or incipient syncope produced.

Muscle power

Shdr Abd.	Deltoid	(C5)
Elb. Flex.	Biceps	(C6)
Elb. Ext.	Triceps	(C7)
Wrist Ext. or Flex.		(C7)
Thumb Ext.	EPL	(C8)
	EPB	
	APL	
Hand	Intrinsics	(T1)

Reflexes

Jaw jerk	V cranial nerve		
Biceps	C5	C6	test six
Brachioradialis	C6	C5	successive
Triceps	C7		times

Sensation

Stroking test along dermatomes and sensibility to pin-prick if applicable.

4. Palpation ('Feel'). While the patient is supine, palpate the upper three or four ribs, costochondral junctions and intercostal spaces.
   a. Find abnormality (see separate drill)
   b. Decide whether abnormality is significant (sometimes is not)

   NB. Passive physiological movement test (PP–MT) is only included if necessary.

5. Record (Figs 9.40–9.46)
   Write a readable account of findings; asterisk salient signs and symptoms.

6. Assess
   Where to place the first emphasis on treatment.

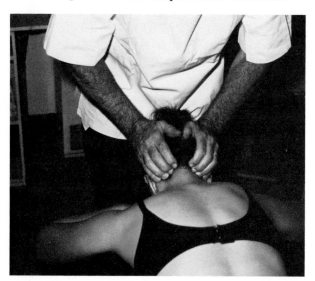

Fig. 9.15 General palpation of the paravertebral sulcus, from the suboccipital region to the upper thorax. The suboccipital region should be palpated when the patient is lying prone as well as sitting upright.

Palpation of cervical spine   Forehead rest, prone lying

General palpation: sweep fingers lightly, paravertebrally, occiput to upper thoracic region.

Seek

—general information of state of soft tissue
—sensitivity of suboccipital tissues to pinching and skin rolling
—tenderness 2 fingers' breadth lateral to suboccipital mid-line
—frank thickening of deep suboccipital tissues

Segmental palpation: feeling:

Allow thumbtips to sink in gently—the harder you press the less you feel. Try to make thumbs more perceptive; visualise the structures you are palpating (Fig. 9.15).

Seek abnormalities: thickening—undue tenderness—undue bony prominences—apparent bony asymmetry.

Moving the joint: by thumb-tip pressure against vertebral prominences, increase movement progressively, grade I–IV; only palpate in depth if indicated

Seek abnormalities: irritability—elicited spasm—diminished or increased accessory movement—provocation of pain and/or paraesthesiae locally and/or distally

Postero-anterior central pressures	—C2–T3
Postero-anterior unilateral pressures	—C1–T3
Postero-anterior unilateral pressures	—Ribs 1–2–3 (plus other levels if indicated earlier in examination)
Transverse pressures	—C2–T3

For fullest information—alter direction of palpation movement:

—cephalad—towards head
—caudad—towards feet
—more medially
—more laterally

If applicable: passive physiological-movement test (PP–MT) of active intervertebral range of each segment.

SHOULDER AND CLAVICULAR JOINTS— ROUTINE EXAMINATION OF SHOULDER

1. History ('Listen')
   a. What is patient's usual daily activity (work and play)?
   b. Pain

   —extent and nature of present pain? Any head, neck, scapular, thoracic or axillary pain?

—radiates to elbow, hand or fingers?

—which aspect of arm? Which fingers?

c. *Behaviour of pain* related to time, posture and activity

—constant, episodic or occasional?

—what aggravates, what eases?

—pain at rest, or only on movement?

—which movements? Of neck? Of shoulders?

—how much pain is caused?

—how long after movement does pain persist?

—pain at night? Can sleep on that side?

—other functional restrictions by pain? (i.e. assess degree of joint irritability)

d. *Other symptoms*

—any paraesthesiae, numbness, vascular changes?

—which fingers?

—any 'deadness'/'heaviness' of arm? What provokes these?

—general health?

e. *Onset* of this attack, and of previous attacks, if any.

NB. Plan examination of more distal joints, e.g. elbow, wrist, hand, if needed.

2. Observation ('Look')   *Patient sitting*

Posture, shoulder levels, abnormalities of contour and attitude (e.g. around head of humerus), postural spasm.

3. Function ('Test')   *Patient sitting*

a. Routine examination of neck and clavicular joints, with active movements of shoulder *girdle*, then detailed examination of:

b. Shoulder   *Note these factors:*

Active (Fig. 9.8) then passive:

—elevation forwards

—willingness to move?

—quality of movement?

—scapulohumeral rhythm?

—elevation sideways (abd.)

—flexion/extension at 90°

—range limited?

—by how much?

—what appears to limit it?

—pain primarily?

—spasm primarily?

—external rotation

—internal rotation

—both?

—inert tissue-resistance primarily?

—muscle weakness?

Pain

—when does it begin?

—how quickly does it increase?

—where is it felt?

—when is it felt ('arc' of pain)?

—is it provocation of presenting pain?

—does it increase without limiting the movement?

—how severe is it?

—how soon does it settle?

Seek: regions of muscle tightness.

Patient lying

c. *Neurological test* of reflexes, sensation and distal muscle (C8–T1)

d. Passive test of 1st rib, clavicular and glenohumeral joints:

1st rib   —accessory gliding

Clavicular   —accessory gliding repeated

Glenohumeral—abduction

—external rotation

—internal rotation

—flexion/extension at 90°

—elevation

} Carefully recheck the factors noted during active movements

e. Resisted contractions with shoulder held still in neutral and elbow bent to 90°

Shoulder: Abductors

Adductors

Ext. rotators

Int. rotators

Flexors

Extensors

Elbow: Flexors

Extensors

Supinators of forearm

Note:

1. Local pain elicited by these tests may indicate that muscle attachments are contributing to the symptoms

2. Do not include these tests if the patient is in a lot of pain, but complete the examination as soon as practicable.

4. Palpation ('Feel')   *Patient lying*

Complete the passive test by examination of accessory glenohumeral joint movement and 'quadrant' test (i.e. combined movement) if applicable (Fig. 9.16)

How does the humeral head move in the glenoid? Is accessory range reduced? Compare with opposite arm

Palpate also for local tenderness, swelling, temperature and palpate the upper three or four ribs anteriorly, the costochondral junctions and intercostal spaces.

5. Record (Figs 9.40–9.46)

Write a readable account of findings. Asterisk salient signs and symptoms.

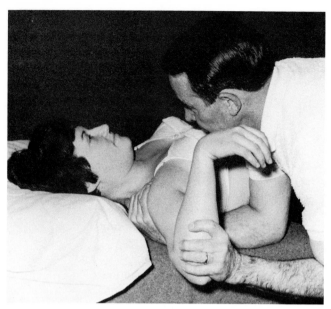

Fig. 9.16 Testing the extremes of the combined ranges of extension/abduction of the glenohumeral joint.

6. Assess

Where to place the first emphasis in treatment, and general treatment approach.

NB. Recall tendency for conditions of heart, liver and diaphragm to refer pain to shoulder and arm.

THORACIC REGION—ROUTINE EXAMINATION OF THORACIC SPINE

1. History ('Listen')

   a. What is patient's usual daily activity (work and play)?

   b. Details of *present* pain

   —site and boundaries?—radiation?—rib areas, breast, sternum, abdomen?—Upper limb?—Neck?

   —*nature*—aching or stabbing?

   —getting better or worse?

   —where worst?

   c. *Behaviour of pain* related to time, posture and activity

   —constant, episodic or occasional?

   —what aggravates?

   —what eases?

   —neck movements?

   —arm movements?

   —trunk movements?

   —coughing and deep breath?

   d. *Other symptoms*

   —paraesthesiae in arms, in legs?

   —any weakness in arms, in legs?

   e. X-rayed? Recently on systemic steroids? Gastrectomy? (Latter two because of possible osteoporosis,

when ribs are especially vulnerable.) Anticoagulants? Rheumatoid arthritis? General health?

   f. *Onset* of this and previous attacks? How treated? Result of treatment?

2. Observation ('Look')

   Observe pelvic posture in standing and sitting, with quick check for possible leg length in equality (Figs 9.1, 9.2, 9.4, 9.5)

   Patient sitting (after checking pelvic levels and leg length in standing)

   Posture: (especially increased a-p curves, e.g. localised or generalised 'dowager's hump')

   Patient crosses forearms in front of body—inspect for rib asymmetry, prominence of trapezius on one side, carriage of scapulae

   Often useful to feel for rib prominence by flat-handed sweep over posterolateral surface of hemithorax.

3. Function ('Test') *Patient sitting*

   Neck: Usual tests (*see* 'Neck examination')

   Try to clarify effects of neck and arm movements on thoracic pain

   Upper limbs: Examine cursorily if no symptoms there

   (NB. Elevation of arms extends thoracic spine)

Thoracic spine:	Slump (sag sit)	Watch for limitation. Give over-pressure to clear if apparently painless and full range. Watch for asymmetrical movement. (Check chest expansion)
(patient places	Ext. (*not from hips*)	
palms on	LSF	
opposite	RSF	
shoulders)	LR	
	RR	

   Deep breath and cough

   Seek regions of muscle tightness.

   Patient lying supine

   Passive neck flexion, then straight-leg-raising, then active neck flexion *with* each straight-leg-raise to clear.

   NB. Neurological test of lower limbs. (Do not leave this out.)

   Sacroiliac joint approximation and gapping of ilia.

4. Palpation ('Feel')

   While patient is supine, palpate costochondral junctions and xiphoid

   Patient prone with arms to side

   a. Find abnormality (see separate drill).

   b. Decide whether abnormality is significant (sometimes is not).

5. Record (Figs 9.40–9.46)

Write a readable account of findings; asterisk salient signs and symptoms.

6. Assess

Where to place the first emphasis in treatment.

Palpation of thoracic spine (Upper thoracic area included in Cervical spine examination)

> *Prone lying—arms to side, head to one side*

General palpation:

> —sweep flat hand, paravertebrally, for state of skin texture and moisture
> —thumbs across sacrospinalis for spasm
> —fingers longitudinally in paravertebral sulcus, for undue prominence and line of spinous processes
> —flat-handed vertical pressure

Segmental palpation: feeling:

Allow thumbtips to sink in gently—the harder you press the less you feel. Try to make thumbs more perceptive; visualise the structures you are palpating.

Seek abnormalities: thickening—undue tenderness—undue bony prominences

Moving the joint: by thumbtip pressure against vertebral prominences, increase movement progressively, grades I–IV; only palpate in depth if indicated

Seek abnormalities: irritability—elicited spasm—diminished or increased accessory movement—provocation of pain and/or paraesthesiae locally and/or distally

Postero-anterior central pressures   —T1–T12
Postero-anterior unilateral pressures—T1–T12
Transverse pressures   —T1–T12

For fullest information—alter direction of palpation movement:

> —cephalad—towards head
> —caudad—towards feet
> —more medially
> —more laterally

If applicable: passive physiological-movement test (PP-MT) of active intervertebral range of each segment.

LUMBAR REGION—ROUTINE EXAMINATION OF BACK AND HINDQUARTERS

1. History ('Listen')

   a. What is patient's usual daily activity (work and play)?

   b. Details of *present* pain

   > —site and boundaries?—radiation to buttock, thigh, leg, foot, toes?

   > —*nature*—deep or surface?
   > —improving or worsening?
   > —area of worst pain?

   c. *Behaviour of pain* related to time, posture and activity

   > —constant, episodic or occasional?
   > —what aggravates?
   > —what eases?
   > —effect of sitting and rising from?
   > —effect of stooping and rising from?
   > —night pain? Rising a.m. (stiffness or pain)?
   > —day pain? Evening pain?
   > —time-dependent or stress-dependent?
   > —other functional restrictions by pain (eg. cough or sneeze)?
   > —standing? Walking?

   d. *Other symptoms*

   > —paraesthesiae? Where?
   > —which toes? 'Saddle' area?
   > —micturition?
   > —weakness in legs?

   e. X-rayed? Drugs? Systemic steroids? Anticoagulants? General health?

   f. *Onset* of this, and of previous attacks (after *all* details of *present* symptoms understood). Previous treatment, and result of that treatment?

   NB. Now *plan* which spinal and peripheral joints need *more* than routine examination (e.g. sacroiliac, hip, knee, ankle).

2. Observation ('Look')

   Pelvic and shoulder levels—spinal posture—iliac crest levels—leg lengths—postural spasm—swelling—other contour changes. (NB. see also Examination of sacroiliac joint.) (Figs 9.1, 9.2, 9.4, 9.5.)

3. Function ('Test')   *Patient standing* (feet a little apart)

Ext.   *Watch* for: limitation and reasons for limitation, i.e. ? pain, ? stiffness, ? spasm
LSF
RSF   Overpressure to clear. Corner extension movements and compression, if need. Asymmetrical movement? (repeat if necessary, and watch for level affected) Deviation? Painful or painless when corrected?
Flex.

Seek regions of muscle tightness.

Muscle power: Toe standing for calf (S1–2). Repeat six times consecutively for each side.

Patient sitting (knees together and arms folded)

(Compare sitting posture to standing posture)

R. Rot.   *Watch* for abnormalities as in standing.
L. Rot.

Patient lying supine

Passive neck flexion—iliac gapping and approximation—hip and knee flexion and rotation—straight-leg-raising—straight-leg-raising with neck flexion.

Test straight-leg raising with hip slightly adducted, and in neutral rotation, and with foot held at 90° (Fig. 9.17).

Functional test: Neck rest crook lying with feet fixed: trunk raise forward.

Muscle power:

Psoas	L1–2
Quad.	L3
T.A.	L4
EHL	L5
Tib. Post.	L5

Reflexes: Knee-jerk (L3) six times, and plantar response

Test for ankle clonus

Sensation: Stroking test, and sensibility to pinprick if applicable.

Patient lying prone

Reflexes: Ankle-jerk (SI). Test tendon-jerk six times

Muscle power:

Ham	S2
Glut.	S1

Femoral nerve stretch test: prone knee bending, with hip extension (stabilise pelvis)

Functional test: feet fixed: head and shoulder raise.

4. Palpation ('Feel')

  a. Find abnormality (see separate drill)

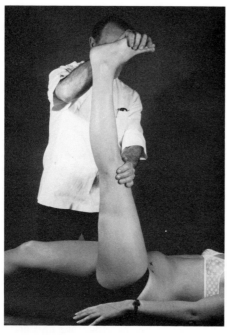

Fig. 9.17 Straight-leg-raising should be tested with the hip slightly adducted, in neutral rotation and with the foot held at 90°. Near the normal limit of SLR, the foot should not be too strongly dorsiflexed as this can produce pain in a *normal* limb.

  b. Decide whether abnormality is significant (sometimes is not)

  NB. Passive physiological-movement test (PP–MT) if necessary, in appropriate positions.

5. Record (Figs 9.40–9.46)

Write a readable account of findings; asterisk salient signs and symptoms.

6. Assess

Where to place the first emphasis in treatment.

Palpation of lumbar spine

Standing—feel for postural spasm

Patient in prone lying (arms to side, head to one side)

General palpation:

  —sweep flat hand, for skin state
  —thumbs across sacrospinalis, for spasm
  —fingers longitudinally in paravertebral sulcus, for undue prominence and line of spinous processes
  —flat-handed vertical pressure.

Segmental palpation: feeling:

Allow thumbtips to sink in gently—the harder you press the less you feel. Try to make thumbs more perceptive; visualise the structures you are palpating.

Seek abnormalities: thickening—undue tenderness—undue bony prominences

Moving the joint: by thumbtip pressure against vertebral prominences, increase movement progressively, grades I–IV; only palpate in depth if indicated.

Seek abnormalities: irritability—elicted spasm—diminished or increased accessory movement—provocation of pain and/or paraesthesiae locally and/or distally

Postero-anterior central pressure   —L1–L5
Postero-anterior unilateral pressure—L1—L5
Transverse pressure   —L1–L5
Whole of sacroiliac sulcus
Tip of coccyx

Use pisiform pressure technique if indicated.

For fullest information—alter direction of palpation movement:

  —cephalad—towards head
  —caudad—towards feet
  —more medially
  —more laterally

If applicable: passive test of physiological intervertebral movement (PP–MT) of each segment.

PELVIC JOINTS—ROUTINE EXAMINATION OF THE SACROILIAC JOINT

The comprehensive examination of this joint should be regarded as an expanded section of the 'Routine examination of back and hindquarters' (q.v.). The sacroiliac joint should not be examined comprehensively until the lumbar spine, hip and lower limb examinations, including neurological tests, have been completed.

This self-discipline is necessary because of our ubiquitous tendency to jump to conclusions about supposed sacroiliac joint conditions as the cause of the patient's low back pain and/or sciatica. A good rule of thumb might be: 'Deformity or asymmetry does not always mean pathology.'

Examination. Because the joint lies in an area to which pain is very frequently referred from the lumbar spine and occasionally from the hip, it is desirable to exclude lumbar lesions, lumbosacral conditions, conditions of one or both hips and serious disease of the sacroiliac joint before admitting the probability of a benign sacroiliac condition as responsible for the symptoms reported and likely to respond to the appropriate manual techniques. This is desirable, but not always possible. Following thorough examination, one must sometimes proceed initially on a basis of greatest likelihood, thereafter depending upon continuing assessment of the results of treatment to provide more guidance.

When lumbar and sacroiliac joint signs are equivocal, which frequently happens, a good rule is to give priority to the lumbar spine, and to proceed thereafter by a process of exclusion based on assessment of treatment effects. If the problem *is* sacroiliac rather than lumbar, it will declare itself soon enough.

The distribution of pain can be important, yet its segmental significance is not always easy to clarify because:

1. Dermatomes are neurophysiological entities, whose boundaries can fluctuate with the levels of facilitation at cord segments
2. Patients vary considerably in their patterns of pain reference or projection from similar, common joint abnormalities
3. Pain may be referred to sclerotome areas, which differ from dermatomes.

Proceeding in a logical sequence of comprehensive tests for the suspected joints, we ask: 'What does it look like?' and 'What is the X-ray appearance?' but most importantly: 'Which applied compressions or tensions and other stresses aggravate or reproduce the symptoms reported by the patient?'

Examination techniques

It is good practice to try to restrict testing procedures on the lying patient to either the lumbar spine or the sacroiliac joint, and not test both together. This is difficult (e.g. the iliolumbar ligament presents problems) but it is worth attempting at all times. The number of tests is legion. Some so-called tests do not merit description while others

induce quite gross movement in the lumbar spine and are much too unspecific; a few are seemingly based on the idea that rotatory movement of the ilium, around an axis at S2 level, is the only important movement occurring at the sacroiliac joint. Yet others are so subjective that description of them is an irrelevance.

Observation

Gutmann (1970)[475] mentions that while the cervical spine and the craniovertebral joints are important in disturbances of vertebral *mobility*, the lumbo-pelvo-hip region is more important in disturbance of *posture*; a careful analysis of pelvic posture is necessary.

Feeling and looking simultaneously can cause confusion; when clinically testing for symmetry, it is wiser to localise thumbs or fingers on bony points without also visualising the area, and then to observe the levels being palpated. Whether the thumbs are settled upwards or downwards onto bony points is unimportant. One should resist the tendency to find what one would like to find (Figs 9.1, 9.2, 9.4, 9.5).

Piedallu's sign. With the patient sitting on a hard flat surface, one posterior superior iliac spine, more frequently on the painful side, is lower than its fellow. On forward flexion, the position is reversed, the previously lower bony point now becomes the higher of the two.

Maigne (1972)[791] explains it as being due to muscular contracture; Piedallu asserts that the blocked joint moves solidly as one, while the sacrum on the painless side is free to move through its small range with the lumbar spine. Whatever the explanation, the sign is that of an unmistakable movement abnormality with a torsional component.

A method of detecting movement abnormalities, in the standing patient, is that of palpating the changing relationship of bony points of the sacrum and posterior ilium when the patient flexes the hip and knee of the unsupported side. This test, included in the teaching on post-registration manipulation courses in the UK since 1970, is well illustrated in Figure 9.3.

The fact that the ischial tuberosity moves laterally during hip flexion, while the PSIS moves downward during the same movement, is a clear indication that normal movement of the ilium, at the sacroiliac joint, is other than simple rotation.

Neurological tests

The presence of lumbosacral nerve root and/or cauda equina involvement, due to the consequences of spondylotic changes and/or other pathology, should be accepted if:

There are manifest neurological signs currently associated with the episode being treated.
Coughing and sneezing produce a smart exacerbation of the pain, more especially in the limb.

Brudzinski's neck flexion sign is positive in that it aggravates haunch and limb pain.

Bilateral jugular vein compression also aggravates the pain within a short interval, often almost immediately.

A sacroiliac condition can of course coexist.

Patients with sacroiliac problems often report paraesthesiae in the absence of neurological signs, which appear to simulate the consequences of lumbosacral root involvement; also a diminished ankle-jerk and some residual muscle weakness may be the tombstone of a past discogenic episode and may have no connection with a current sacroiliac condition.

Straight-leg-raising is not an exclusively neurological test; besides its tendency to disturb lumbar joints in various ways it also applies stress to the sacroiliac joints, and this can at times be used as a differentiation method. If straight-leg-raising on one side is restricted to 70° by a jab of haunch and leg pain, and the contralateral leg can be raised to a painless 90°, then raising both legs together to a painless 90° indicates that reduced range on the affected side is due to unilateral torsional stress on that sacroiliac joint. This test does not preclude a possible coexisting lumbar problem, it only indicates the cause of straight-leg-raising restriction, yet this is clearly helpful when assessing. Exacerbation of sciatic pain, by forcible foot dorsiflexion near the end of a painfully limited straight-leg-raising range (Fig. 9.17) is not always a reliable indication that the extra pain is due to further sciatic nerve stretch; foot dorsiflexion will often produce calf pain at 60° to 70° on a normal leg, and simple calf tenderness often accompanies purely sacroiliac conditions, being exacerbated by the dorsiflexion test.

Iliac gapping and approximation test

The importance of these tests is their usefulness in excluding joint irritability, hypermobility and serious disease. They should never be left out, yet they are frequently negative in the presence of benign sacroiliac problems, which are confirmed by other tests, and which can be relieved by mobilisation or manipulation techniques applied specifically to the joint.

Hip extension

When there is hypomobility in one sacroiliac joint, an additional test may serve to conform it. The therapist stands level with the pelvis and leans over the prone patient to stabilise the sacrum with the palm of one hand, while the other hand passively extends the hip with an above-knee grasp. The leg on the hypomobility side feels heavier and cannot be extended as much as its fellow.

Prone knee-bending hip-extension test

When pelvic asymmetry, in patients with equal leg lengths, accompanies unilateral sacroiliac joint pain, e.g.

on the right, the right pubic ramus and anterior superior iliac spine will often be a little forward and higher, respectively, than the same bony points on the left; similarly, the right posterior superior iliac spine will be a little lower than on the left. The prone knee-bending hip-extension range on the right side is often restricted, sometimes painfully, since the attachments of rectus femoris on that side have been drawn slightly apart. That the range is not invariably restricted or painful is a reminder that backward rotation of one ilium is not the only form in which pelvic asymmetry can present; confident pronouncements about a 'posterior innominate' as the cause of the patient's pain are not always justified, because the painful side is occasionally on the left in the example quoted, and at times there appears to have occurred a slight bodily shift of one ilium, with little 'rotation.'

The clinical states of this mysterious joint have not yet been satisfactorily clarified and are by no means understood. Attempts to clarify problems by dogmatic assertions serve only to cloud the issue and to retard real understanding. For example, the objective evidence, of palpable asymmetry of the posterior margins of the ilium on the side of pain, is not always most manifest at the posterior superior iliac spine, but equally manifest along the whole length of the posterior margin; thus it is apparent that the asymmetry can be more of a slight shift in relationships rather than a pure rotation, which is plainly not possible at such a joint. Whether this asymmetry has anything to do with what the patient reports by way of symptoms is a matter for experienced assessment.

Radiography

Not surprisingly, a patient with unremarkable X-ray appearances may be in considerable pain from a sacroiliac lesion. Continental radiologists have developed the technique of sacroiliac radiography in the craniocaudal axis. The tube is positioned above the patient who leans the trunk forward a little while sitting on the cassette (Fig. 9.18). The view gives better detail of the bony joint surfaces, particularly of the ventral aspect at the level of the pelvic brim; the circumscribed opacities seen in orthodox views can be shown to be intra- or extraosseous.

In osteitis condensans ilii, the thickness of the involved ilium can be shown. Whether it will become possible to radiographically show subtle yet painful changes in joint relationship remains to be seen. Incidentally, Figure 4.59 on page 445 of the 35th edition of *Gray's Anatomy* beautifully depicts a right-sided so-called 'posterior innominate' sacroiliac lesion in a female patient!

Palpation

The joint can be palpated in one locality only, i.e. at its inferior extent in the region of the posterior inferior iliac spine. Acute unilateral tenderness here and thickening is very common in painful sacroiliac conditions, and when

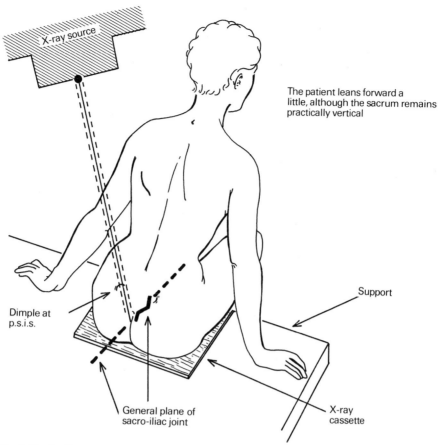

The patient leans forward a little, although the sacrum remains practically vertical

X-ray source

Support

Dimple at p.s.i.s.

General plane of sacro-iliac joint

X-ray cassette

Fig. 9.18 Radiographs in an inclined parasagittal plane so that the main ray is in the general plane of the sacroiliac joint of that side. (After Hayes J, Hayes E February 1979 Brit. Assoc. Man. Med. Newsletter.)

well localised (as opposed to a general referred tenderness of the whole buttock) is a useful confirmatory sign. When palpating for movement abnormalities in the sacroiliac sulcus, it is impossible to feel movement in the joint; what one senses is a rhythmic, shifting relationship of adjacent bony prominences. After a little practice, changes in tension and springiness of the sacrotuberous ligament are surprisingly easy to feel through the gluteal mass, although gluteal tenderness must be taken into account before admitting the value of this test in individual cases and assessing the differences in tension, if any.

A change in joint relationships, which tends to approximate the sacral and tuberous attachments of the ligament, will slightly reduce the tension on one side, and vice versa, provided such a change has occurred. We have already noted that pain from the joint need not be accompanied by asymmetry.

Sacral apex pressure test

This is one of the most valuable tests because it is the most localised and specific, when applied on the prone patient (Fig. 9.19). On a firm surface, the pelvis rests on a tripod of two anterior superior spines and the pubis. Sacral apex pressure tends to shear the sacral joints and the lumbo-

sacral joint on the stabilised ilia. While apex tenderness alone is inconclusive, exacerbation of the unilateral sacral pain complained of is strong supportive evidence of a sacroiliac problem. The fact that lumbosacral shearing may also be referring pain to the sacroiliac joint must be borne in mind—one is never relieved of the obligation to assess.

In many patients the only *signs* will be the slight unilateral deepening of a sacroiliac sulcus, the subtle flattening on one buttock, asymmetrical hip rotations without range discrepancies and the provocation of localised pain by craniocaudal and anteroposterior stressing of the joint surfaces (Fig. 9.20).

Pain provocation, by the various methods of stressing the joint, are really no more than developments of the simple apex pressure test; it is a mistake to rely too heavily upon these developments in examination, and like all other tests the findings by these methods should be incorporated into the clinical assessment as a whole. In this respect, one should bear in mind that sacroiliac movement includes angular and parallel (shuffling) movement, as well as so-called rotations. Stressing first one and then the other ilium and the sacrum in opposite craniocaudal directions may at times reveal a consistent pattern of provoca-

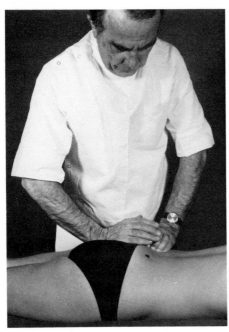

Fig. 9.19   Rocking sacrum by pressure at its apex or caudal end with medial edge of right hand. Left hand palpates changes in left sulcus.

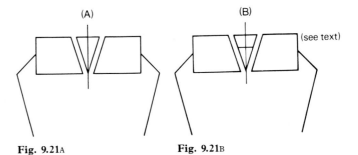

Fig. 9.21A   **Fig. 9.21**B

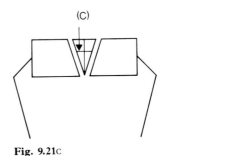

Fig. 9.21C

Fig. 9.21   Scheme of posterior aspect of pelvis

tion or relief of symptoms, with particular combinations of pressure, and these palpation findings may assist in selecting the therapeutic movement.

For the purposes of examination by palpation with the patient prone, the sacrum is functionally divided (Fig. 9.21A and B) (A) into two paramedian halves and (B) an upper and lower half; and by carefully localised provocative pressures, it can be determined which stress is most effective in aggravating the symptoms (Dietzel, 1978).[258]

The affected side is always that on which the greatest palpable soft-tissue changes and the greatest aggravation of pain by provocative pressures can be demonstrated.

With a left-sided joint problem (Fig. 9.21C) provocative pressure on the left half of the sacrum, in a caudal direc-

tion, is the most effective in aggravating the pain (testing pressures are shown as continuous lines).

Thus, in the example (Fig. 9.21D), other combinations of craniocaudal movements which might also *provoke* the pain are as shown. Reading from left to right:

    left ilium cranial
    left lower sacrum caudal
    right lower sacrum cranial
    right ilium caudal
    traction on right leg

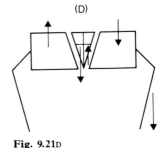

Fig. 9.21D

Similarly in Figure 9.21E, different craniocaudal movements (now as broken lines) which may tend to *diminish* pain are as shown from left to right:

    traction on left leg
    left ilium caudal
    left half of sacrum cranial
    right half of sacrum caudal
    right ilium cranial

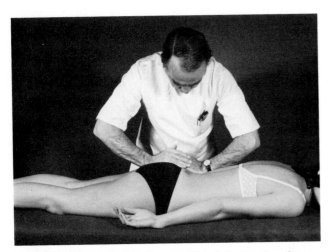

Fig. 9.20   Stressing the joint in a caudal/cephalic direction. Sacrum towards the head with ilium stabilised.

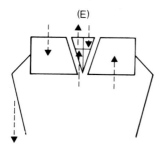

Fig. 9.21E

It will be apparent that in those cases where the most potent provocative pressure is *caudally* on the *right* ilium, the direction and side of the other movements depicted will be reversed.

The clarity of these findings will differ between patients, and clinical presentation does not always fit neatly into these somewhat systemised textbook patterns. Also, pain may be provoked when both ilia are pressed cranially, or both halves of the sacrum are pressed caudally (Fig. 9.21F).

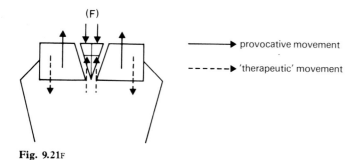

Fig. 9.21F

> ⟶ provocative movement
>
> - - - - ⟶ 'therapeutic' movement

By imagining an upper and lower half of the sacrum (but not placing an imaginary rotatory axis in any particular location, since the movements are highly unlikely to be purely rotatory) we can distinguish which *ventral* pressure, on the upper and lower halves of each side of the sacrum, also tend to provoke or diminish the patient's pain.

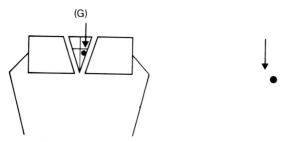

Fig. 9.21G

In this example (Fig. 9.21G), either or both of the pressures (↓ right half of sacrum caudally and ● right lower sacrum ventrally) are the most provocative pressures, while ventral pressure on the remaining three small quarters (i.e. upper right and two left) will tend to be more comfortable for the patient.

As with cranial/caudal pressures, the intensity of provoked pain and the degrees of relief on ventral pressures are variable; once the graphic method is agreed, it is possible to symbolise with economy the two main provocative movements. For example:

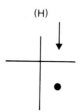

Fig. 9.21H

If the dorsal aspect of the sacrum is represented by a cross (Fig. 9.21H), cranio/caudal pressures are represented by arrows and ventral pressures by dots. The most provocative of the testing procedures are then seen at a glance, and the movements most likely to assist in relieving pain can, after consideration of other factors, be selected for initial trial and assessment of results.

A suggested examination drill may be tabulated as follows:
observation—testing movement—palpation
(*Patient stands with feet a little apart and parallel*)
    Symmetry of general spinal contours?
    Stands with pelvic rotation?
    Buttock contour? Level of gluteal folds? Asymmetry of gluteal cleft?
    Level of iliac crests, and tubercle of crests? (Fig. 9.1)
    Swollen appearance over one or other joint?
    PSIS levels from behind? (Fig. 9.2) ASIS levels in front?
    Lateral pelvic tilt? Real or apparent leg shortening?
    Observe pelvic posture during Trendelenberg's test.

(*Patient bends forward*)
    Skyline view of gluteal mass from in front of patient.
    Reobserve and repalpate PSIS for asymmetry (Piedallu's sign). (Fig. 9.4)

(*Patient sits erect on hard level surface, and then bends forward*)
    Repeat observations and palpation of bony points from behind, in both positions—lateral pelvic tilt still present or previous lateral tilt in standing now eradicated? (Fig. 9.5)
    Many patients have anomalies of bony points; interpret findings conservatively.
    When testing, compare sides and seek unequal movement, loss of movement (Fig. 9.3), tissue contracture, hypermobility, undue tenderness, irritability.
    Before using thigh as a lever, check that there is no hip joint involvement.

(*Patient lies supine*)

Check for leg lengths and 'set' of the pelvis, with patient lying straight (see p. 309).

View horizontal levels of ASIS; observe how the limbs fall into rotation.

Examine hips: Compare tension, by passive stretch of:

Abductors, and iliotibial band

Adductors, i.e. abduction of flexed limb with foot alongside opposite knee (Patrische test)

Iliopsoas, i.e. with opposite hip fully flexed to allow passive extension of affected side

Passive flexion-adduction test (Fig. 9.22). Hurt in groin or buttock? End-feel?

Add pressure down length of femur, with opposite ASIS stabilised in this postion. Hurt?

External and internal rotation. Limited?

Static isometric contractions of hip abductors and adductors. Painful? Where?

Examine sacroiliac joint:

Iliac gapping and approximation tests with flat hard pillow under patient's lumbar spine

Palpate in sacroiliac sulcus of same side while repetitively flexing, and then flex-adducting, hip. Movement abnormalities?

Straight-leg-raising—either leg, then both together

Palpation:

Baer's point (iliacus spasm and tenderness). Compare sides.

Adductor insertion, for undue tenderness.

Anterior acetabular region.

Configuration of symphysis pubis, and undue tenderness there.

(*Patient lies prone, with arms to side*)

Skyline view of gluteal mass, and view degrees of rotation of resting legs.

Check leg lengths in extension and in knee flexion (see p. 310).

Examine hips:

Passively extend each hip while stabilising sacrum with opposite hand. Extension limited and 'heavier' leg on affected side?

Compare tension of rectus femoris, e.g. press heel to buttock with pelvis stabilised, then gently extend hip. Limited? Hurt?

With knees flexed 90°, check hip rotation

Examine sacroiliac joint:

Flex far knee to 90° and medially rotate far hip repetitively; with pelvis stabilised by operator's chest, palpate near sacroiliac sulcus.

Movement abnormalities? (Fig. 12.60)

Rock sacrum by repetitive pressures to its apex (at sacrococcygeal joint), compare movements at sulci.

Does it hurt at sacroiliac joint? (Fig. 9.19)

Stress sacrum upwards and ilium downwards and vice versa. Painful?

What is the pattern of provocation and relief? (Figs 9.20, 9.21)

Palpation:

Relative depth of sulci.

Undue tenderness medial to PIIS.

Symmetry of sacrotuberous and sacrospinous ligaments through gluteal mass (which may itself be tender).

Record (Figs 9.40–9.46)

Write a readable account of findings; asterisk salient signs and symptoms.

Assess

Where to place the first emphasis in treatment.

Discussion

Plainly, indications for treatment will become more marked in an almost direct relationship to the number of factors which are accurately assessed. The more comprehensive the examination, the more likely appropriate treatment will be found, as the weight of emphasis gradually mounts up during examination. Therefore it is of first importance to be thorough and comprehensive, and to place more reliance on observable facts than on an over-imaginative interpretation of them.

Nevertheless, the vagaries of referred pain can cause great difficulty, and it is wise to remember that combined sacroiliac and symphysis pubis conditions tend to refer pain to haunch, groin and anteromedial thigh; also that it is not rare for a sacroiliac problem to be accompanied by abnormalities at the third lumbar segment.

ROUTINE EXAMINATION OF THE HIP

The comprehensive examination of this joint should be regarded as an expanded section of 'Routine examination of back and hindquarters' (q.v.). Some of the tests here are included in that routine. Nevertheless, exclusion of problems at the lumbar spine and sacroiliac joint, and neurological tests of the lower limbs, should accompany the more detailed hip examination set out below.

Pain in the hip region need not arise from the hip joint, and that due to a hip condition is not necessarily felt in that area.

Because the hip joint is the proximal end of a weight-bearing and dynamically stabilised column, examination procedures should reflect this in their emphasis on functional weight-bearing tests.

1. History ('Listen')

a. What is patient's usual activity (work and play)?

b. Details of *present* pain

—extent and nature?

—any back, buttock, trochanter, groin, thigh/leg pain?

—what aspect of limb? Which toes?

c. *Behaviour of pain* related to time, posture and activity (Assess degree of joint irritability)
—continuous, episodic or occasional?
—pain at rest, or only on movement?
—what movement? Of back? Of hip joint?
—how much pain is caused?
—how long after movement does pain persist?
—pain at night? Can sleep on that side?
—other functional restrictions by pain? Standing? walking? stairs? driving? dressing?
—how far can patient walk comfortably?

d. *Other symptoms*
—paraesthesiae? Numbness? Blanching or flushing due to vascular changes? Which toes?
—any 'deadness'/'heaviness' of limb? What provokes this?

e. X-rayed recently? Drugs? Systemic steroids? Anticoagulants? History of rheumatoid arthritis? General health?

f. *Onset* of this, and previous attacks? Previous treatment? Result of treatment, if any?

NB. Now *plan* which more distal joints need *more* than routine examination, e.g. tibiofibular, knee, ankle joint, foot.

2. Observation ('Look')   *Patient standing*
Changes of contour—swelling—wasting?
Changes of attitude—stance?

3. Function ('Test')   *Patient standing*
Observe:
—standing from sitting
—walking
—standing and flexing alternate knee to chest, and extending, abducting and rotating non-weight-bearing leg
—hopping lightly on one leg
—wide stride standing
—stepping up on stool on either leg
—full squat position from standing

Equilibrium test:
—patient stands on one leg, with eyes closed, and is lightly supported by one hand. Check stabilisation efficiency of each hip when vision is denied.

Patient lying supine
Passive test:
of all ranges compared with other limb, with overpressure and assessment of 'end-feel' (i.e. assess nature of limiting factor, if any), especially of combined ranges, e.g. flexion-adduction (Fig. 9.22).
Test compression and distraction
Seek regions of muscle tightness

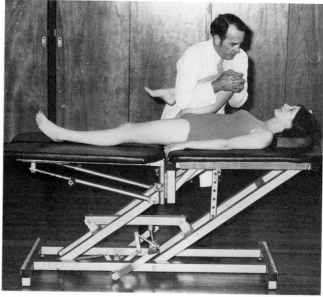

Fig. 9.22 Passive test of the 'end-feel' of combined flexion-adduction range of the right hip joint.

Muscle power: resisted isometric contraction
Flexors
Abductors
Adductors } of hip
Extensors
External rotators
Internal rotators

Palpation:
Baer's point (flexor spasm)
Swelling
Wasting
Tenderness anteriorly and laterally over bursae
Temperature

Patient lying prone
Press heel to buttock with pelvis stabilised—extend hip joint
Muscle power: resisted isometric contraction
Hamstrings, as knee flexors and knee rotators
Palpation:
—ischial tuberosities and posterior trochanter area
—bulk of gluteus maximus when statically contracted

4. Record (Figs 9.40–9.46)
Write a readable account of findings. Asterisk salient signs and symptoms.

5. Assess
Where to place the first emphasis in treatment, and general treatment approach.

PASSIVE PHYSIOLOGICAL-MOVEMENT TESTS (PP–MT)

Because examination of intervertebral movement may employ both *accessory*-movement tests and *physiological*-movement tests, it is necessary to distinguish clearly between them, and for this reason the following procedures are named as above.

Descriptions of examination procedures are best used as companions to practical teaching sessions, because the method cannot be adequately learned from a text; familiarity with the nature and extent of movement at the different segments takes some time to acquire.

There are many ways of perceiving movement, and the techniques described are somewhat basic; they can be developed as the therapist gains skill. Some therapists test each segment in both weight-bearing and non-weight-bearing positions.

The examiner should adopt a procedure which comes most easily to hand and is methodical; apart from modifications to suit a particular patient's physique, it is better to stick to the method chosen—the same tests should be done in the same way every time.

Procedure: Any *apparent* positional abnormalities should be noted first (in this connection, transverse processes are more important than spinous processes), tests for segmental mobility are then applied. No more pressure than is needed to adequately detect the ranges of movement should be used. It is important not to 'waggle' but to produce precise, rhythmic movements of fair amplitude and regular frequency.

C0–C1

Patient lies supine with head on a flat pillow
Therapist stands at head with patient's vertex in contact with his abdomen

Side-flexion:

Support occiput with fingers of left hand while left thumbtip rests between lateral mass of C1 and mastoid process.
Place right hand as required for efficient support of patient's head.
Repetitively side-flex craniovertebral junction to right side as thumb perceives amount of gapping between C1 and mastoid on the left. Isolate movement to upper cervical *only* (Fig. 9.23).
Repeat to opposite side after changing grasp.

Rotation:

Stand a little clear of head and rotate it away from palpating thumb. Repeat to opposite side, with changed grasp (Fig. 9.24).

Flexion:

Rest patient's occiput on small block and place palm (fingers caudally) on patient's fore-

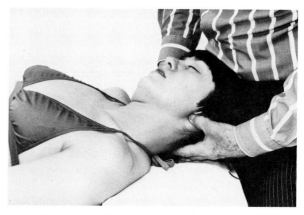

Fig. 9.23 Passive physiological-movement test (PP-MT) of side-flexion of C0–C1 segment. It is important to isolate movement to the craniovertebral junction.

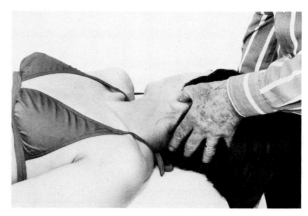

Fig. 9.24 Passive physiological-movement test (PP-MT) of the small degree of rotation between the atlas and occiput. The neck itself should be held in the neutral position so far as sagittal movement is concerned.

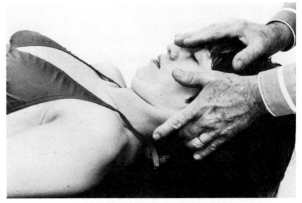

Fig. 9.25 Passive physiological-movement test (PP-MT) of the range of flexion at the craniovertebral junction (C0-C1).

head. Press forehead caudally so that chin is repetitively depressed by movement at craniovertebral junction. Palpate, with finger or thumb, the left and then the right basiocciput at the joint as the head flexes (Fig. 9.25).

Extension:

Remove block, and with patient's vertex in therapist's abdomen, together with each forefinger against the joint on that side, repetitively extend the patient's head at the craniovertebral junction by flexion of therapist's knees (Figs 9.26, 9.27).

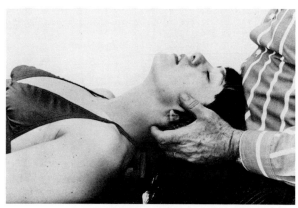

Fig. 9.26 Passive physiological-movement test (PP-MT) of the extension range at the craniovertebral junction (C0–C1). The point of contact between patient's vertex and therapist's abdomen moves through an arc, the axis of which is the craniovertebral joint. This necessitates considerable movement of the therapist's trunk, hips and knees.

C1–C2

Patient lies supine. Therapist stands at head.

Rotation with side-flexion:

Support head with palm of left hand, while the index or middle finger is rested on the tip of C2 spinous process. The right hand rests as convenient on that side of the patient's head, and helps to guide the testing movement. With the left palpating fingertip kept in the mid-line, the patient's head is side-flexed to left and right; the degree of offset of the spinous process of C2 to the opposite side is a measure of both side-flexion and rotation range, since these two degrees of freedom are interdependent. (For alternative method see p. 341) (Figs 9.28, 9.29).

Flexion:

Support head with palm under occiput, and pads of middle fingers resting on the posterolateral aspect of the C1–2 joint; check that it is not C2–3. Flex head repetitively and compare movement.

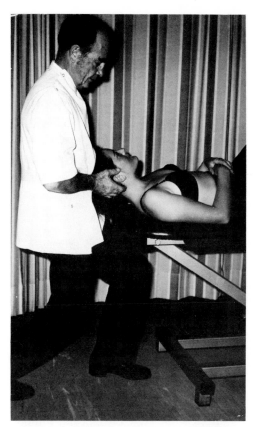

Fig. 9.27 Passive physiological-movement test (PP-MT) of extension at the craniovertebral junction, illustrating the considerable movement of the therapist's trunk, hips and knees.

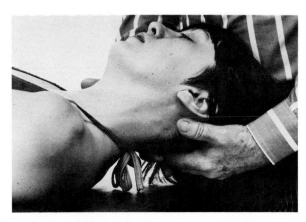

Fig. 9.28 Passive physiological-movement test (PP-MT) of rotation-with-side-flexion of the atlantoacial joint C1–C2.

Extension:

Extend head, keeping movement confined to upper cervical region only.

C2–C6

Patient lies supine on high plinth.

Flexion:

Therapist sits or crouches at patient's head, supports occiput with one palm (fingers towards patient's vertex) and repetitively flexes

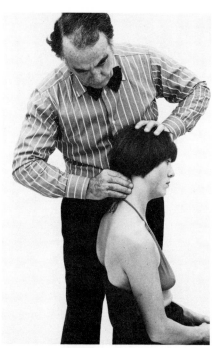

Fig. 9.29 Passive physiological-movement test (PP-MT). Alternative method of examining the physiological range of combined side-flexion and rotation of the atlantoaxial joint (C1–C2).

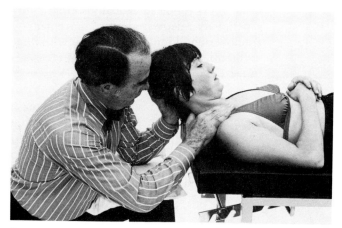

Fig. 9.30 Passive physiological-movement testing (PP-MT) of flexion, between segments C2–C6.

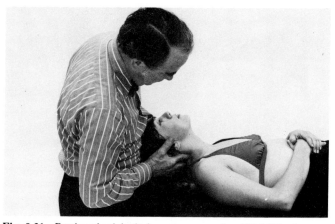

Fig. 9.31 Passive physiological-movement testing (PP-MT) of extension at cervical segments between C2 and C6.

neck while edge of opposite thumb palpates gapping between successive spinous processes from above downwards.

Flexion is gradually increased for the lower segments (Fig. 9.30).

Extension:

The therapist stands at patient's head and supports occiput with the non-palpating hand. With palm of the palpating hand conveniently placed, the therapist places index or middle finger (or one reinforcing the other) over the junction of adjacent vertebral arches, and pushes the neck into extension. The therapist's trunk is somewhat involved in the movement. Repeat on opposite side (Fig. 9.31).

Side-flexion:

The therapist places the right foot a pace out and forward; otherwise the starting position is virtually the same.

Side-flexion is palpated during bending the patient's neck towards the right by some movements of the therapist's body.

Movement is gradually increased for the lower segments.

Change starting position and repeat to opposite side.

Rotation:

The therapist stands facing the side of the patient's head and cups the occiput in the fingers of the cranial hand, with palm near to the patient's ear.

The palm of the caudal hand is placed over the patient's far zygoma and cheek, while the pad of middle finger rests postero-laterally on the far vertebral arches.

Rotation movement is perceived by a reciprocating action of both hands, turning the head towards the therapist.

Repeat to opposite side.

C6–T3

All of the movements of this region are examined with the patient in side-lying and the therapist facing the patient, resting his sternum on the deltoid area of the uppermost folded arm to provide some stabilisation of the patient's trunk.

The therapist's cranial forearm supports the patient's head, with fingers curling round the patient's lower neck—the medial fingers are more active in grasping, while the therapist's cranial forearm and trunk take part in the movements. Avoid stress on the patient's neck.

Flexion, extension, rotation and side-flexion are all tested in this position, while one finger of the caudal hand palpates movement between adjacent spinous processes (Fig. 9.32).

Side-flexion and rotation are repeated to the opposite side.

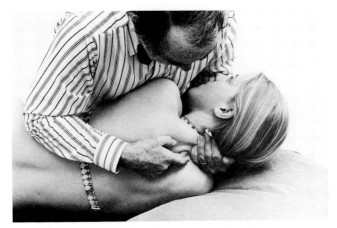

Fig. 9.32 Passive physiological-movement testing (PP-MT) of rotation, between segments C6–T3.

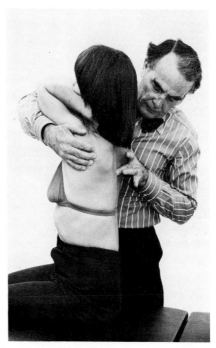

Fig. 9.33 Passive physiological-movement testing (PP-MT) of extension, between segments T3–T10.

T3–T10

Flexion:

Patient sits sideways at end of plinth in 'neck rest' position with elbows together, i.e. adducted.

Therapist stands at side, reaching *over* the patient's forearms to grasp the opposite upper arm and hold the patient's trunk against his own.

Movement is palpated between the spinous processes with the free hand, while the therapist repetitively flexes the patient's trunk by dipping his own in a side-flexion movement.

Extension:

Patient as above, with elbows still adducted but now raised forward.

Therapist as above, but now reaching *under* patient's arms to place hand on lateral aspect of opposite scapula.

Both patient's and therapist's trunk are rhythmically moved to produce extension as the spinous processes are palpated from above downwards (Fig. 9.33).

NB. In the two tests above it is important that the therapist moves his trunk as one with the patient's trunk.

Side-flexion:

Patient in 'neck rest' position as before.

Therapist stands at side, reaching across the patient's upper pectorals and under the opposite axilla to grasp as in extension testing. The patient then rests both arms on the therapist's forearm.

The palm of the therapist's free hand is placed on the near hemithorax, with index or middle finger against the near side of adjoining spinous processes. The patient's trunk is repetitively side-flexed, by a reciprocating movement of both hands. Movement is palpated either as gapping or approximation of the bony points.

Rotation:

Patient is in crook-side-lying with arms folded and adducted. The therapist sits in the 'crook' of the patient (or stands facing the head) and stabilises the pelvis by placing his near axilla on the patient's upper trochanter. The therapist's outer hand is placed over the patient's upper arm, and movement is produced by rhythmically pushing the trunk away from the therapist into rotation. The therapist's free forearm lies parallel with and against the trunk, assisting in stabilisation of its lower part as the middle finger, reinforced by the index, is placed from below upwards on the sides of adjacent spinous processes. The fingerpad fixes the lower spinous process while the tip perceives rotation movement of the upper process (Fig. 9.34).

NB. Passive testing of *combined* physiological movements may also yield important information (Fig. 9.35).

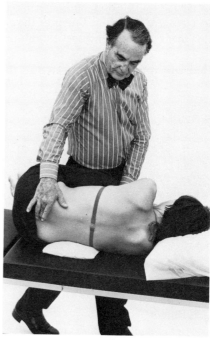

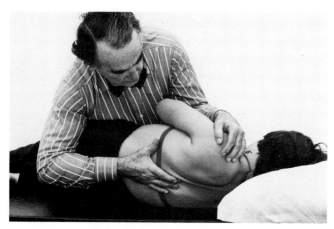

Fig. 9.34 Passive physiological-movement-testing (PP-MT) of rotation, between segments T3–T10.

T10–S1

(A small flat pillow under the patient's loin will keep the lumbar spine in neutral position.)

Flexion:

The patient lies on side with knees and hips bent. The therapist, in walk-standing facing the patient's head, supports the patient's shins across his lower abdomen by clasping the lower bent knee with his outer hand. The index or middle finger of inner hand rests between adjacent spinous processes, and perceives the amount of movement as the patient's knees are rhythmically moved towards his head by

Fig. 9.36 Passive physiological-movement testing (PP-MT) of flexion, between segments T10–S1.

the therapist's pelvis in a forward and backward rocking movement (Fig. 9.36).

Extension:

The operator turns to face the patient, maintaining the shin–lower abdomen contact, and also changes his grasp so that the caudal hand now supports the patient's underneath leg.

The therapist's cranial hand now palpates movement between adjacent spinous processes, as extension is rhythmically produced by movement of the therapist's trunk (Fig. 9.37).

Side-flexion:

The flat pillow is removed and the therapist, facing the patient, applies his caudal arm

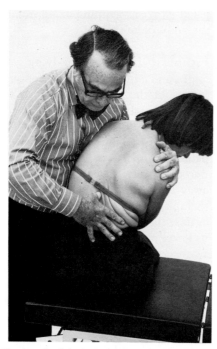

Fig. 9.35 Passive physiological-movement testing (PP-MT) of combined flexion, side-flexion and rotation, of segments T3–T10.

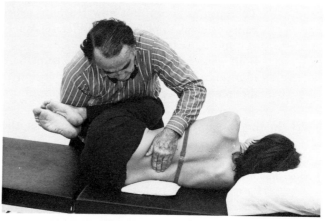

Fig. 9.37 Passive physiological-movement testing (PP-MT) of extension, between segments T10–S1.

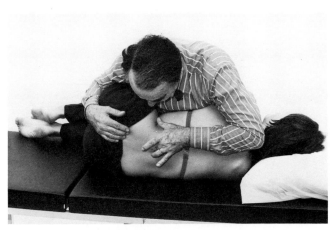

Fig. 9.38 Passive physiological-movement testing (PP-MT) of side flexion, between segments T10–S1.

round the whole of the patient's upper rump. By a rhythmical side-sway of his own trunk towards the patient's head, the therapist produces a side-flexion movement which can be palpated either as gapping or approximation by a finger of the cranial hand. Repeat to opposite side (Fig. 9.38).

Rotation:

The flat pillow is replaced and the therapist places the palm of his caudal hand on the patient's upper trochanter. By leaning his cranial-side axilla on the patient's upper ribs, his forearm lies along the lower thoracic spine and a reinforced finger can rest against adjacent spinous processes.

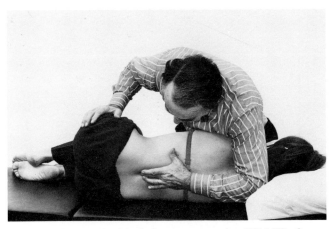

Fig. 9.39 Passive physiological-movement testing (PP-MT) of rotation, between segments T10–S1.

Rotation is perceived as the patient's pelvis is rocked backwards and forwards (Fig. 9.39). It is not always necessary to repeat on the opposite side, but this should be done at first.

C1–C2

An alternative method of testing rotation and rotation-with-side-flexion is as follows:
Patient sits on a low stool or plinth.
Therapist stands at side (Fig. 9.29).

Rotation:

Palpate or grip spinous process of C2 with finger and thumb of one hand, and with the other hand placed on the vertex spin head about 30° from side to side. Perceive degree of head rotation at which C2 begins to move.

Rotation with side-flexion:

Head is side-flexed and degree of side-swing of C2 spinous process to the opposite side is assessed.

Notes

It will be apparent that more than one starting position is employed in testing most of the spinal regions, and when a complete vertebral examination is done, less time is taken up if a sequence of sitting, lying and side-lying is adopted, and findings at the different levels recorded out of numerical order.

RECORDING EXAMINATION

A systematic and accurate record of examination facilitates quick reference during treatment to salient findings, which should be noted especially (see listed Examination Procedures).

Methods of setting out information are varied to suit requirements; shorthand symbols save time and are desirable so long as their meaning is agreed.

A specimen Recording Chart is set out below with one side devoted to subjective examination and the other to objective examination, with remarks on initial assessment and the first choice of treatment. This double-sided vertebral examination recording sheet (Figs 9.40, 9.41) may be adapted for recording information from only the upper half of the spine (Figs 9.42, 9.43) or the lower half (Figs 9.44, 9.45).

Examples are given in Figure 9.46 (A) to (F).

Name _____ No. _____ Age _____ Activity:

Work _____
Play _____
Date _____

SITES OF PAIN   AND PARAESTHESIAE

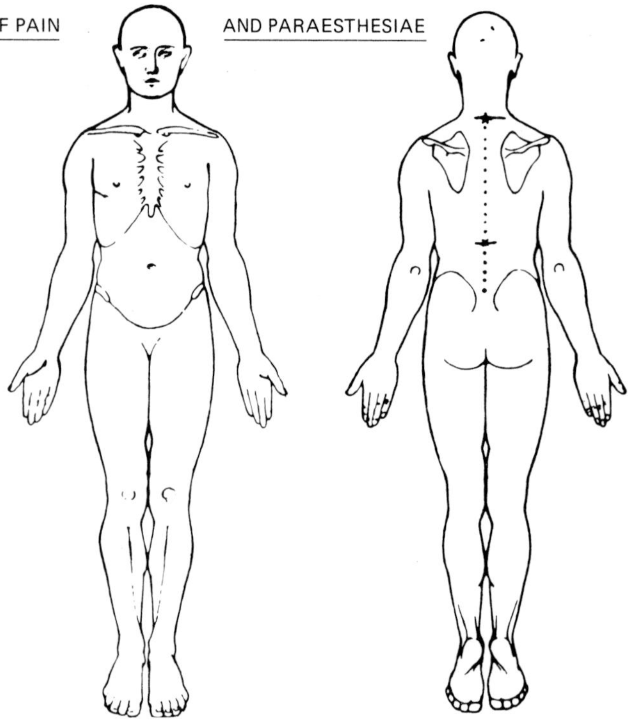

PARAESTHESIAE and Other Symptoms:

Rheumatoid Arthritis

Dizziness

Micturition

Drugs

General Health

PAIN Degree		
Nature		
Constant	Periodic	Occasional
Increasing	Static	Decreasing
Night Pain		
Pillows	Bed	
Rising a.m.		
Aggravates		
Eases		
Sustained Flexion	Rising from	
Sitting	Rising from	
Cough/Sneeze		
Deep Breath		
Day Pain (overall)		
Evening		
IRRITABILITY		

Current History

Previous History, Treatment and Results

Fig. 9.40 Vertebral examination recording chart: subjective examination (symptoms).

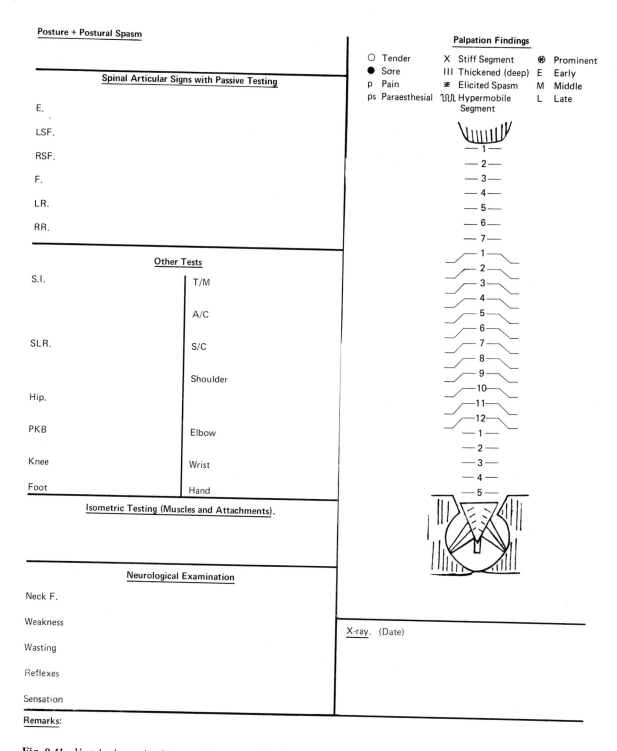

Fig. 9.41 Vertebral examination recording chart: objective examination (signs).

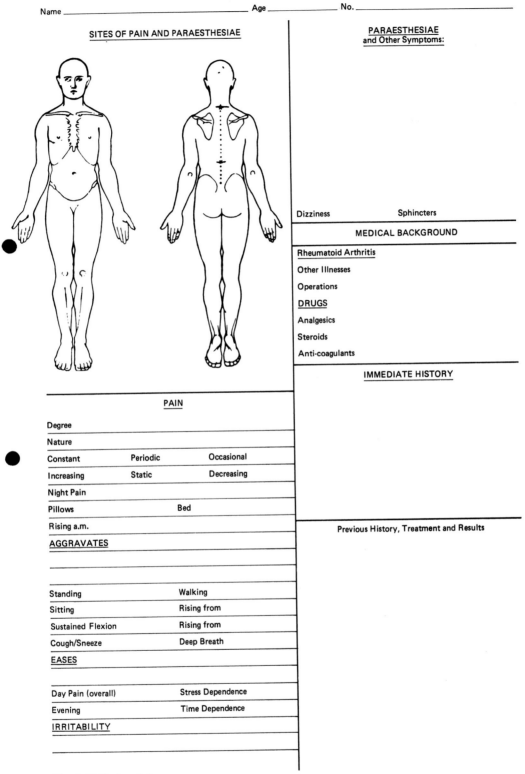

Name _____ Age _____ No. _____

SITES OF PAIN AND PARAESTHESIAE

PARAESTHESIAE
and Other Symptoms:

Dizziness   Sphincters

MEDICAL BACKGROUND

Rheumatoid Arthritis

Other Illnesses

Operations

DRUGS

Analgesics

Steroids

Anti-coagulants

IMMEDIATE HISTORY

Previous History, Treatment and Results

PAIN

Degree		
Nature		
Constant	Periodic	Occasional
Increasing	Static	Decreasing
Night Pain		
Pillows	Bed	
Rising a.m.		

AGGRAVATES

Standing	Walking
Sitting	Rising from
Sustained Flexion	Rising from
Cough/Sneeze	Deep Breath

EASES

Day Pain (overall)	Stress Dependence
Evening	Time Dependence

IRRITABILITY

Fig. 9.42 Neck and thorax.

Posture + Postural Spasm

Spinal Articular Signs with Passive Testing

E.

LSF.

RSF.

F.

LR.

RR.

Other Tests

T/M

A/C

S/C

Shoulder

Elbow

Wrist

Hand

Isometric Testing (Muscles and Attachments).

Neurological Examination

Neck F.

Weakness

Wasting

Reflexes

Sensation

Remarks:

Palpation Findings

○ Tender	X Stiff Segment	⊛ Prominent
● Sore	III Thickened (deep)	E Early
p Pain	⇌ Elicited Spasm	M Middle
ps Paraesthesiae	∿ Hypermobile Segment	L Late

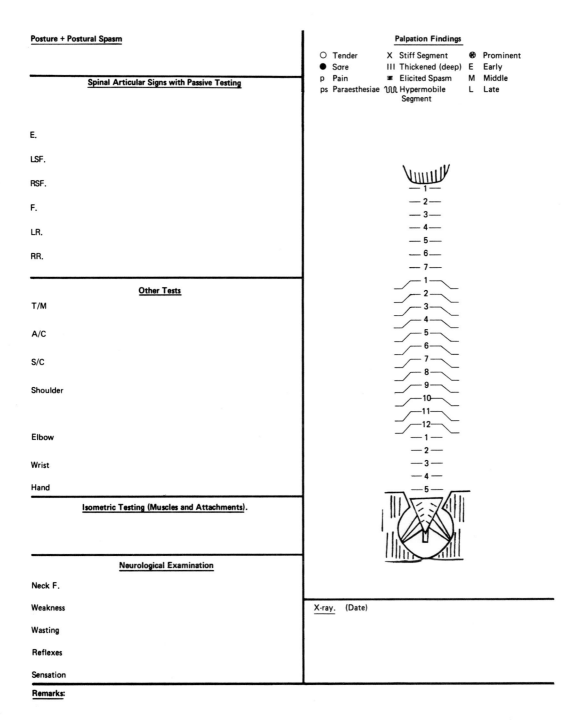

X-ray. (Date)

Fig. 9.43 Neck and thorax.

Name _____ Age _____ No. _____

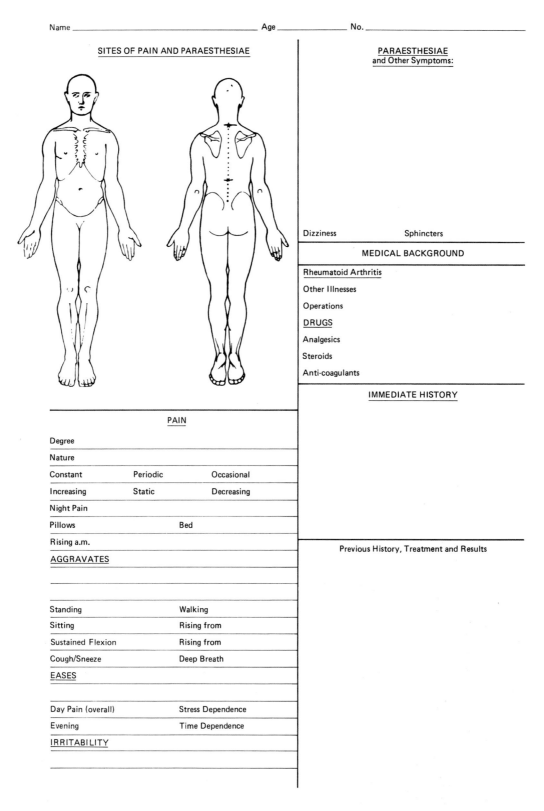

SITES OF PAIN AND PARAESTHESIAE

PARAESTHESIAE
and Other Symptoms:

Dizziness   Sphincters

MEDICAL BACKGROUND

Rheumatoid Arthritis

Other Illnesses

Operations

DRUGS

Analgesics

Steroids

Anti-coagulants

IMMEDIATE HISTORY

PAIN

Degree

Nature

| Constant | Periodic | Occasional |
| Increasing | Static | Decreasing |

Night Pain

Pillows   Bed

Rising a.m.

AGGRAVATES

Standing	Walking
Sitting	Rising from
Sustained Flexion	Rising from
Cough/Sneeze	Deep Breath

EASES

| Day Pain (overall) | Stress Dependence |
| Evening | Time Dependence |

IRRITABILITY

Previous History, Treatment and Results

Fig. 9.44 Low back and pelvis.

Posture + Postural Spasm

Spinal Articular Signs with Passive Testing

E.

LSF.

RSF.

F.

LR.

RR.

Other Tests

S.I.

SLR.

Hip.

PKB

Knee

Foot

Isometric Testing (Muscles and Attachments).

Neurological Examination

Neck F.

Weakness

Wasting

Reflexes

Sensation

Remarks:

Palpation Findings

○ Tender	X Stiff Segment	⊗ Prominent
● Sore	III Thickened (deep)	E Early
p Pain	⩧ Elicited Spasm	M Middle
ps Paraesthesiae	∿ Hypermobile Segment	L Late

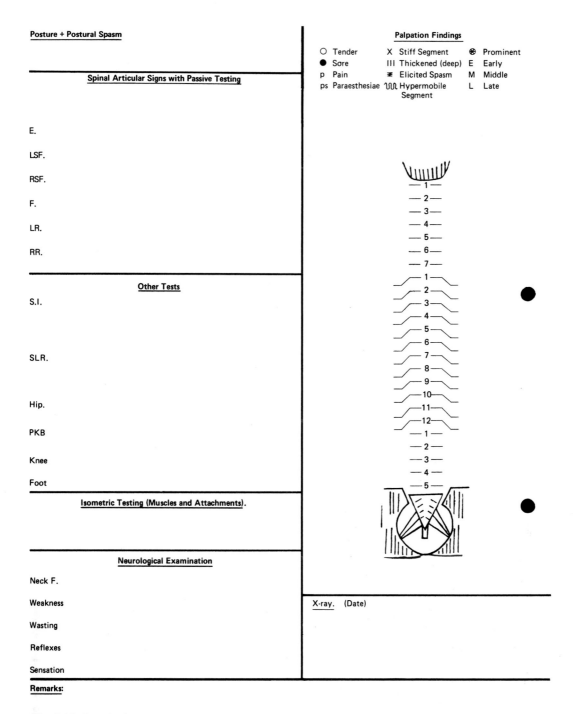

X-ray.   (Date)

Fig. 9.45 Low back and pelvis.

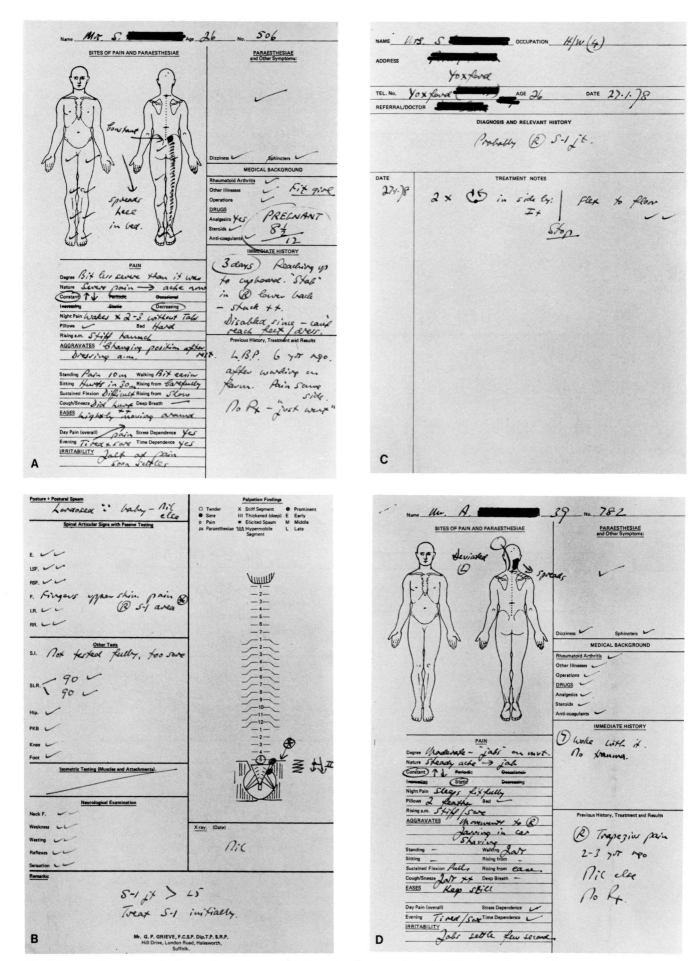

Fig. 9.46 A–F Illustrate simply the use of recording method. Examples of more prolonged treatment are given elsewhere in the text.

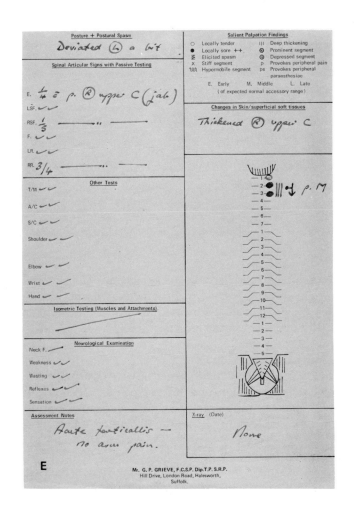

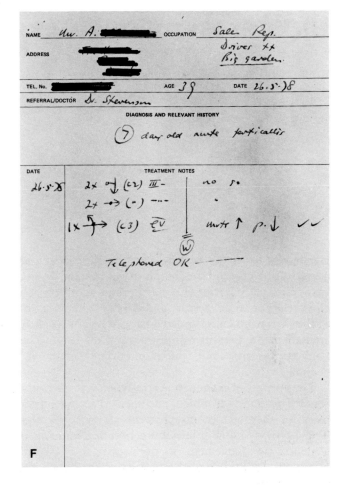

10. Assessment in examination Prognosis

Depending upon the patient's pain, temperament and degree of anxiety, and the complexity of the joint and soft tissue changes, descriptions of symptoms and their behaviour related to time, posture and activity amount at times to the therapist being handed a tangled ball of wool. Examination and assessment must unravel the tangle, clarifying the priorities and relative importance of the signs elicited.

The purpose of examination is to fully and clearly grasp *how* the patient is troubled, and then to seek a physical basis for these symptoms, in terms of objective signs. These provide initial guides for action in treatment, but a degree of judgement is necessary, and therefore *assessment*—of the patient; of the relationship between the symptoms reported and the signs of disturbed function; of priorities, when two or more aspects need attention— is equally important, so that the first choice of treatment method is closely related to the findings.[444, 456, 797]

This may not be easy when patients are treated in groups, or when specific treatment prescriptions must be followed precisely, but an endeavour always to relate treatment and its results to examination findings and assessment is repaid by a better understanding of the behaviour of degenerative joint disease.

Some mention of assessment during examination has already been made in preceding pages.

History
There is considerable variation in the way patients describe their symptoms and functional difficulties; some make less of their troubles than others, and may find difficulty in recalling the important time-sequence of developing symptoms. The therapist must assess how complete, fulsome or sketchy an account is being given.

Pain intensity is not always proportional to objective findings; also a patient's response to pain may appear average, low or high. Accounts of pain intensity will vary with the patient's temperament. It is important to note that the site of a previous and painful limb injury will be disproportionately painful if referred pain of vertebral degenerative disease later invades that limb. The central nervous system appears to retain a memory for previously well-trodden neurone pathways, and pain at the old site is easily rekindled in later years.

Observation
Patients' functional difficulties can be noted when they are undressing, reaching to demonstrate painful areas, reaching for shoes, getting onto the plinth, and moving on it. Sometimes their agility belies the difficulties reported.

Objective tests
Logical treatment depends upon finding signs which are reasonably compatible with symptoms presented by the patient. A thickened and stiff spinal segment may be the 'tombstone' of a past episode, and not directly responsible for the pain currently troubling the patient; also it is unlikely that paraesthesiae of the three middle fingers, with a weak triceps muscle, would arise from a tender and irritable C2–C3 segment.

For example, pain in the upper medial pectoral area can arise from the sternoclavicular joint, pain more laterally may be referred from the cervical region and/or shoulder joint, and lower paramedian pectoral pain can be referred forward from upper thoracic segments.

Objective tests by active and passive movement, and careful palpation of all joints and associated tissues likely to be giving rise to the pain, will help to clarify the cause by a process of exclusion.

Again, the distinction between (a) muscular aches in the region of the vertebral joint problems, due to causes outlined (see p. 172), and (b) the pain *referred* into more distal limb muscles from the vertebral lesion, and (c) pain also referred distally from a coexisting limb girdle joint problem, is not always easy, but is an important part of clinical assessment. For example, during assessment of the priorities of treatment of the ubiquitous neck/shoulder problems, a helpful guide may be:

1. Where (i) the cervical and upper half of the thoracic spine and the clavicular joints show no significant clinical

abnormality, and (ii) the pain of a single resisted shoulder movement is dominant among the clinical features, and (iii) there is clearly no restriction of shoulder mobility on active and passive careful testing (although the movement which stretches the tendon concerned may be painful) attention localised to the rotator cuff tendon appears indicated.

2. If (i) there are clinical abnormalities of the lower cervical and upper thoracic spine, (ii) restricted shoulder movement is more dominant in the clinical features, and (iii) more than one resisted movement is painful, there might be clear indications for giving attention to both vertebral and peripheral joints, with the first priority being the spine.

In general terms, the amount of pain referred distally into a limb from spinal problems is an index of difficulty (the further distal, the more difficult) in applying quickly successful treatment.

PALPATION IN ASSESSMENT

PALPATION

The examiner should always bear in mind that palpable asymmetry of segmental contour, attitude and movements are not necessarily abnormalities[220]—findings must invariably be assessed in terms of their relation to the symptoms reported and signs previously observed.

We may paraphrase our knowledge of the functional interdependence of the spinal column by asserting 'no vertebra is an island', and because (p. 364):

1. Few musculoskeletal testing procedures are unequivocal (pp. 319, 329)
2. Of the vagaries of referred pain, referred tenderness and spasm of muscles in areas to which pain is referred
3. There is so much overlap of dermatomes, and a fluctuation of their boundaries according to the state of facilitation at cord segments
4. Sclerotome boundaries transgress axial lines, and correspond only very roughly with dermatomes
5. The innervation of vertebral structures may be derived from cord segments two, three or more distant
6. Patterns of innervation may vary by prefixation and postfixation of plexuses

the greatest weight of assessment, when endeavouring to localise the segmental level of vertebral joint abnormalities, rests on what is found by palpation, and passive tests of intervertebral movement.

As we have seen (p. 320), palpation includes feeling the state of the skin surface, the superficial and deep soft tissues including muscles and attachments, the configuration of superficial and deep bony prominences, and the deeper periarticular connective tissues—*while the joints remain still*.

For appreciation of the characteristics of vertebral *movement*, methods include passive tests of: regional accessory movement; segmental accessory movement; functional or physiological movement.

1. Palpation with joints at rest

a. *Undue tenderness.* Tenderness can be very misleading, e.g. the first rib, the clavicle and the midthoracic spinous processes in young women are naturally tender, and of no significance when this tenderness is unaccompanied by other signs or symptoms. Tenderness as such does not necessarily indicate abnormality unless, in relation to neighbouring structures of the same region, it is marked—and is accompanied by symptoms and signs reasonably associated with the marked tenderness of that structure.

Tenderness just medial to the posterior inferior iliac spine in suspected sacroiliac joint problems, for example, is of less significance when the whole of the gluteal mass is tender (probably referred tenderness) but decidedly of significance when (i) accurately localised and (ii) this positive finding is buttressed by negative findings elsewhere.

The problems of assessment are compounded by referred tenderness as well as referred pain (see p. 168) and this factor should be borne in mind.

b. *Postural spasm*, i.e. hypertonus of vertebral muscle in the static postures of sitting, standing and lying, is not as a rule localised but tends to be regional. It can be palpated in the sternomastoid and trapezius muscles, axilla-boundary muscles and the sacrospinalis, for example.

When a vertebral region is obviously fixed by postural spasm, which remains largely unchanged whether the patient is standing, sitting or lying, its cause is likely to be a lesion whose degree of irritability is not gravity-dependent. Rarely, this may be gross facet-locking by overriding, or an apophyseal fracture, conditions requiring inpatient attention, but far more often it appears due to a localised soft-tissue derangement, which can be freed by manual mobilisation. The important point is that traction, or distractive techniques, are less likely to help in this case than in lesions whose postural fixation by spasm immediately disappears-with the patient lying down. In these cases, where the degree of irritability and postural spasm is plainly gravity-dependent, distractive techniques are very likely to help, whether applied manually or mechanically, and may be the sole type of mobilisation needed.

It is wise to remember that the muscles of an area to which pain is being referred may be in a degree of postural spasm, and also that 'spasm' may be the natural expression of the patient's anxious temperament, in which case its *distribution* and degree, relative to the musculature as a whole, is the important assessment factor.

In addition to the sensory changes which accompany joint problems, there is the facilitated motor response which has been well demonstrated by Denslow (1944).[252] Stoddard (1969)[1180b] observes that: 'Segmental motor reflex thresholds were determined by measuring in kilograms the amount of pressure applied to the spinous process of each segment which just evokes contraction of the paravertebral muscles at that segmental level. Muscular contractions were detected and evaluated by electromyographic recordings.' Vertebral segments showing movement abnormalities invariably required weaker stimuli than did those with normal movements.

c. *Undue bony prominence.* Complete anatomical symmetry of paired structures probably does not exist; close observation of the body contours, and palpation of the vertebral column, in a large group of healthy young people tends to confirm this impression. Cervical spinous processes are asymmetrically bifid, the lateral masses of most atlases show asymmetry, and thoracic spinous processes are very often deviated from the 'mid-line'. Less so do asymmetry of rib angles and of vertebral body laminae in the thoracic region occur, and asymmetry of the lumbar laminae is not frequent.

For this reason, undue prominence of a single rib angle or vertebral lamina is more often than not of significance; this does not mean to say that malalignment or subluxation is thought to be present; only that there may be a degree of fixation at some point on the normal range of movement, and that in one or more of the joints of that vertebral segment or costovertebral region there are soft-tissue changes hindering free movement. When these findings exist in the absence of other signs, and there are no symptoms, treatment is certainly not merited on account of the asymmetry, unless there is a clear case for regarding the abnormality as part of an interdependent clinical entity incorporating the changes at that segment and causing symptoms in other vertebral regions (see p. 364). Neither is localised treatment likely to be profitable when localised changes of contour and attitude are clearly the result of long-standing adaptive shortening, although it is often of help to the patient if the mobility, and thus tissue-fluid exchange, of soft tissues are improved *adjacent* to the site of fibrotic contracture.

In general, it is wise to conservatively interpret 'undue prominence', or asymmetry of the bony structures of normal anatomy, and to be slow in ascribing vertebrogenic pain to their presence alone. The easily felt exostosis of degenerated cervical facet-joints is another matter, and this may well be significant when assessing the segmental level of joint changes giving rise to pain.

d. *Thickening.* Not surprisingly, thickening is very frequently localised over the site of painful joint problems, even though the joint itself cannot be directly palpated. It is probably indurated oedema, at times combined with a degree of capsular and ligamentous thickening due to fibrosis, although on occasions one may also be palpating the belly of small intersegmental muscles in a degree of postural spasm. Further intensification of the spasm will be produced by palpation which is too aggressive or rough, and these findings are common in the suboccipital region and at the cervicothoracic junction. When not accompanied by symptoms, painless thickening combined with a degree of movement restriction should be left alone, but see (c) above and page 364.

2. Palpation of accessory movement

a. *Diminished/increased accessory movement.* Perception of diminished or increased accessory movement by manual testing requires (i) an appreciation of the wide variations of body type and normal regional range of movement, and (ii) a familiarity with the normal accessory ranges of each segment.

A normal vertebral *region* may feel generally: hard and springy; soft and yielding; soft and springy; tight, tough and unyielding.

Further, comparisons between the normal amplitude of anteroposterior *accessory* movement, e.g. of C2, C6 and C7, in the order of millimetres, can with attention and a little practice be made quite readily, and the differences would be as follows:

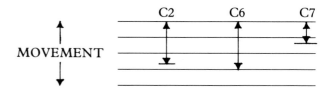

Vertebral segmental accessory movement may be *restricted*, as is often detected in tests of anteroposterior gliding between proximal and distal rows of a carpus, for example, or it may be *increased*, as is frequently detected during anteroposterior gliding tests for cruciate ligament laxity at the knee, and in applying passive abduction/adduction strains of the same joint when testing for instability.

(i) If segmental accessory movement is *limited* the examiner must then ask: What is the amount of limitation? What is the nature of the limitation? Is it pain, primarily, evidenced by voluntary muscle guarding? Is it irritability, evidenced by eliciting involuntary and well-localised spasm very early in the small range of movement? Is it not so much pain, or irritability, but moderately painful restriction (felt as resistance to free movement) imposed by connective tissue thickening? Is it virtually painless and old-established fibrotic contracture? In what way, if any, are these findings related to the symptoms reported by the patient?

(ii) If segmental accessory movement is *increased*, are the testing movements painful, or painless? By how much is the movement increased? Does the increase arouse suspicion of an unstable segment?

When assessing examination findings during this fundamentally important procedure one is doing no more and no less than in exactly similar assessments being carried out by professional colleagues many hundreds of times on the same day during examination of shoulders, hips and knee joints. The findings are, as in all clinical assessments, incorporated into the larger context of the patient, the symptoms, and the unique combination of all factors so that formulation of precise individual needs may be made and treatment planned.

b. *Elicited spasm*, e.g. that provoked in response to testing movements of a reactive irritable joint, is sometimes very localised indeed, and one needs to know on which side, and to which vertebral level, it is most localised, and particularly whether the response is elicited in the early, middle or late part of the available accessory-movement range. A knowledge of what the normal regional and segmental accessory movement should be, from spine to spine, is presupposed, and the point on the range at which spasm is provoked allows an assessment of the grade to employ for the initial mobilising technique, i.e. the degree of irritability is a fundamental factor governing the grade of mobilisation.

c. *Provocation of pain and/or paraesthesiae locally and/or distally:* This provides vital information and is a valuable localising sign. As in testing voluntary movements (p. 312) the therapist seeks to reproduce or aggravate the patient's symptoms, or at least find evidence of abnormality which could be underlying them. For example, the patient's response to a regional flat-handed pressure (p. 302) may vary in that:

(i) if local guarding spasm is immediately elicited, and pressures either side of the locality do not elicit spasm, the presence of a vertebral lesion is generally confirmed, and more detailed segmental tests are indicated

(ii) if a brisk guarding response involving the whole thoracolumbar spine is elicited, pathology of a more serious nature may be present, and further tests of movement should not be made until the suitability of physical treatment has been confirmed

(iii) a slightly delayed response may indicate a wish to impress the examining therapist.

Similarly, if repetitive gentle pressure localised to the 6th thoracic spinous process provokes the submammary pain of the patient's complaint, and pressure on T5 and T7 produces slight local pain only, the joints and associated tissues likely to be responsible are those related to T6. When postero-anterior movement applied to the spinous process of L5 aggravates or provokes pins and needles in the forefoot of a sciatic limb, and the same movement applied to the fourth and third segment does not, (a) it is very likely that there is already a degree of trespass upon the root by related structures, and (b) treatment techniques should be carefully chosen so as not to further provoke the irritable root; likewise if postero-anterior unilateral pressure on the C5–C6 facet-joint provokes paraesthesiae in the forefinger of the same side.

Further, if the same kind of testing movement on C2 inferior articular process reproduces the hemicranial pain of the patient's complaint, while testing other segments on the same and opposite sides does not, it is perhaps reasonable to assume that the lesion responsible is associated with the C2–C3 segment on the side palpated, since this is the segment moved most by that particular pressure, and to treat initially on that basis. The same applies to posterior axillary and upper arm pain on palpating the second or third rib angle on the same side.

Further, if simultaneous transverse vertebral pressure in opposite directions, on the spines of two adjacent vertebrae of the painful region, provoke or aggravate the patient's pain, and no other combination of transverse pressures does this, or to such a degree, it is reasonable to assume that the segment responsible has been localised (Fig. 10.1). Postero-anterior unilateral pressures then assist localisation; further considered on page 355. In contrast to this when, in the absence of neurological signs, the uni- or bilateral upper limb 'glove paraesthesiae' diagnosed as of vertebral joint origin, are provoked by central pressure on T345 segments, this cannot be due to a C5678 somatic root involvement (other than possibly a spread of

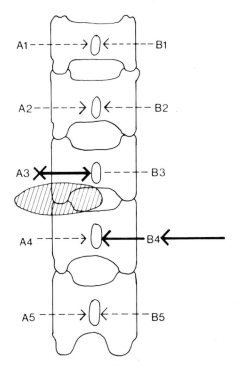

Fig. 10.1 Stabilisation of the middle vertebral spine by pressure A3, with simultaneous movement to the opposite side of the subjacent spine by pressure B4, is the only combination of pressures which provoke or aggravate the patient's pain. Frequently, transverse pressure B4 alone, in the direction indicated, and posteroanterior unilateral pressure between A3 and A4 is enough.

excitation by facilitation to those cord segments) but is more likely to be due to mediation via the autonomic neurones accompanying somatic nerves to the limb. Here, mobilisation of those segments by this same technique is a reasonable procedure to begin with, and it will often relieve the paraesthesiae, whatever the true explanation of the phenomenon may be.

d. *Crepitus.* This is more evident on active movement and often reported in the cervical region, occasionally at the sacroiliac joint, by patients who are anxious that the 'noisy' movement might be ominous evidence of 'the crippling disease of arthritis'. During examination by passive movement, it is sometimes felt during cervical rotation in extension, but more usually the simple act of lying down reduces crepitus-on-movement considerably.

It is probably due to the approximation and rubbing together of roughened facet-joint planes, is more subdued during rotation in flexion, and is seldom encountered in the thoracic and lumbar regions, other than the scapulothoracic crepitus which very frequently accompanies 'the scapulothoracic syndrome' (see p. 236). It is, however, occasionally encountered in the lax sacroiliac joints of young mothers, and indicates the need for external support.

3. Palpation during functional or physiological movement

Functional mobility varies with posture; it may not be the same in standing as it is in sitting, or lying, and may also vary with the time of day, there being less mobility early in the forenoon and in the evening, and rather more in the middle hours, as a rule.

The functional range of a vertebral 'mobility-segment', i.e. movement between two bony points of adjacent vertebrae, is difficult to detect at first, and requires long, constant and attentive practice. Movement of a typical cervical segment is perhaps the hardest to assess. Assessments of segmental mobility must take into account the different general nature of spinal movements from person to person, e.g. lax and loose jointed; tight jointed.

Movement is assessed as:

4—Hypermobile
3—*Normal*
2—Reduced
1—Trace
0—Ankylosed.

These are assessments of mobility, and not diagnoses of the *cause*, for example, of what is assessed as 'ankylosis' at a segment.

Fused vertebrae are not rare in the cervical spine, or transitional vertebrae in the lumbosacral region; further, the degree of postural gap palpated between two spinous processes in any vertebral region is not a reliable indication of the mobility of that segment. The sole criterion is the amount of movement, since assessments of postural bony-point relationship would already have been made prior to these procedures.

Technique is described on page 336.

EXAMINATION AND ASSESSMENT METHOD

Many workers (i) use physiological-movement testing infrequently and place much more reliance on careful segmental examination of *accessory movement*, noting the effects of the variety of testing movements employed and which of these either reproduce or aggravate symptoms reported by the patient, and to what degree. In this way, having previously noted the history of pain behaviour during everyday functional occupations, and its behaviour and changing distribution during the regional spinal movements (single and combined) of active tests, the examiner seeks the fullest grasp of the relationships overall, that the subjective and objective effects of segmental treatment techniques may be wholly observed during subsequent assessments.

Other workers (ii) regard passive testing of voluntary movements (single or in combinations) as standard examination procedure, and therefore the routine mechanical basis for assessment of joint problems. (See p. 366 for further discussion.)

Further to the theme of assessment when palpating accessory and physiological movement

Schmorl and Junghann's[1093] concept of the 'mobility segment' is a great advance in the way we think about the vertebral column and its benign or more serious abnormalities, yet we have suggested that 'no vertebra is an island'; we may usefully add to this 'and no mobility segment'.

It is wise to note the functional interdependence of the spinal regions (see p. 364). We are not dealing with a simple perpendicular arrangement of bony segments bound together by straps of ligament, but a dynamic body axis in which no localised abnormality can exist without sooner or later affecting more distant segments and ultimately the whole spine. Just as one cannot passively move a vertebra without moving all soft tissues attached to it, so no event, anywhere in the spine, remains completely isolated.

The innervation of spinal structures is especially rich and is often derived from spinal cord segments unusually remote from the innervated structure. Filaments of mixed somatic and autonomic nerves, after being formed from paravertebral plexuses outside the intervertebral foramen enter it and wander up and down the neural canal before terminating. This wandering is particularly marked in the cervical and upper thoracic spine, but occurs in other regions, too.

Because of this diversity and richness of innervation,

the nature and volume of the afferent impulse traffic from vertebral receptors is also rich. The upper cervical spine is especially important in this respect (see p. 3). Voluntary movement is only as good as reflexogenic efficiency, and these arthrokinetic reflexes are disturbed by changes in joints which are degenerating, as evidenced by abnormalities of movement.

Therefore, when transverse vertebral pressure to the left, for example, on C2 spinous process provokes the upper left-sided neck pain and suboccipital pain of the patient's complaint, we have provoked it by disturbing at least *two* 'mobility segments', i.e. C1–C2 and C2–C3. We have disturbed, in asymmetrical ways, soft tissues at those two levels on the patient's right and the patient's left. We have also disturbed the attachments of muscle bellies which may span several segments, connective tissue structures spanning neighbouring regions and, in the foramen transversarium, the vertebral artery with its sympathetic plexus destined for distribution to intracranial structures.

The muscles will include scalenus medius, the intertransversarii, semispinalis cervicis, longus colli, rectus capitis posterior, rectus capitis anterior and lateralis, and obliquus capitis inferior.

Connective tissue structures will include joint capsules, the apical ligament, alar ligaments, accessory atlantoaxial ligaments, anterior and posterior longitudinal ligaments and the ligamentum nuchae.

We cannot ignore the structural, functional and neural interdependence of the vertebral column; it is a constant factor underlying clinical presentation (see p. 129), and further, a constant factor to be borne in mind when examining, assessing, choosing techniques and formulating plans of treatment.

After other tests we seek by palpation irritability, elicited spasm, diminished or increased accessory movement, provocation of pain and paraesthesiae—we are trying to reproduce the symptoms reported by the patient, and if we can do that we have usually localised the focus of the abnormality. We have found the segment(s) responsible, although we may not understand precisely *how* they are responsible.

Here are two examples of palpation findings. In Figure 10.2 a patient complaining only of *left* occipital pain is found to have a prominent, thickened and very tender *right* lateral mass of atlas, movement of which aggravates the pain, with much less tenderness at C2 and C3 on the same side, slight tenderness at C1, C2 and C3 on the *opposite, left side*, and at C2 and C3 centrally. Had we palpated down the *left side first*, and accepted without question that the stiff, thickened and slightly tender C2 and C3 segments were responsible for the left-sided occipital pain, even though testing did not provoke this, we might not have discovered that the left-sided headache was provoked or reproduced *only* by unilateral movement of C1

on the *right*. If localised right-sided movement of C1 provokes the left-sided occipital headache, and left-sided movement of C2 and C3 does *not*, then the important segment to initially mobilise is C1 on the right, not C2/3 on the left. The left-sided stiffness at C2/3 is something of a red herring in this particular clinical presentation, and we are likely to get the patient out of pain sooner by attending to the movement *which accurately reproduces the pain*, than by working on the assumption that the C2/3 stiffness *ought* to be responsible for the symptoms. We have listened to what the joints are telling us, and we have assessed which are the treatment priorities.

To complete the full treatment of that patient one should attend to the stiffened C2/3 segment on the left, after the greatest progress in relieving the patient's headache has been achieved, yet the stiffness may be very old and virtually irreversible; consequently vigorous mobilisation or manipulation may only hurt the patient without profit, and the decision must then rest on whether a painless functional range of upper cervical movement has been rendered possible, as evidenced by repalpation and active tests with overpressure. If these show that further improvement in ranges of movement can be achieved by mobilising C2/3 on the left, the treatment is indicated, but when to stop is as important as when to start (see p. 444).

Referring once more to the example given, had we not been able to provoke the left occipital pain by moving C1 on the right, it would have been proper to accept the left-sided stiffness of C2–C3 as the cause and to begin treatment there, subsequently being guided by assessment of effects.

In the second example (Fig. 10.3), the slight tenderness at C123 on the right side is of no great significance, because we find that unilateral movement of the thickened, tender and prominent C2–C3 segments on the left immediately reproduce the left hemicranial pain, whereas right unilateral movement does not. It is clearly indicated to mobilise C2–C3 on the left, in the appropriate grade. Thus, when assessing the segmental locality of the changes underlying clinical features, our first priority is, 'How can we reproduce them?', and if, despite a careful search, we are unable to do this, we should then proceed on the basis of, 'Which segmental changes have we found which are most *likely* to be responsible?', and the search for these may require testing physiological ranges, too.

Mention has been made of slightly altering the direction of vertebral pressure techniques when examining, i.e. a little caudally, cranially, medially or laterally.

When examining the consequence of degenerative joint disease, we come upon the clearest and most potent expression of the abnormality existing by subtle changes in how we apply the localised testing movements; adding a little bias in one direction or another often makes all the difference between a fairly relaxed, inert patient allowing testing movement to continue, and the sharp response of

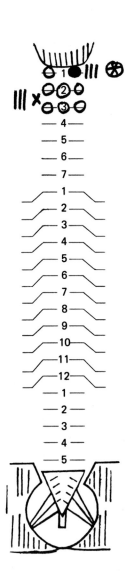

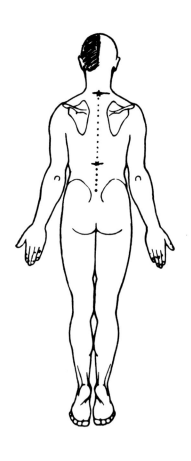

Palpation Findings

O	Tender	X	Stiff Segment	⊛	Prominent
●	Sore	III	Thickened (deep)	E	Early
p	Pain	⇌	Elicited Spasm	M	Middle
ps	Paraesthesiae	∿	Hypermobile Segment	L	Late

Fig. 10.2 Chart of palpation findings in a patient with headache (see text).

involuntary muscle guarding to protect a highly reactive joint, *which is most sensitive to that movement with that bias.*

We may now conceive the view that we do not treat 'mechanical joint problems' so much as *movement abnormalities, highly individualised from patient to patient*—radiological appearances and theories of biomechanics notwithstanding (see p. 359).

The more attentive, searching and subtle is examination, the more comprehensive our grasp of how they are

uniquely presenting. This does not mean we know any more about 'why?', only that we have a better insight into what we are trying to deal with, using treatment methods which themselves are based on movements of one kind, or degree, and another.

When looking for the site of what frequently transpires to be 'reversible diminished movement due to soft tissue changes' (p. 378) expressed as 'limitation', 'restriction' or 'blocking', we must be able to distinguish between hypo-

Palpation Findings

O	Tender	X Stiff Segment	⊗ Prominent
●	Sore	III Thickened (deep)	E Early
p	Pain	⇶ Elicited Spasm	M Middle
ps	Paraesthesiae	ᙡᙡ Hypermobile Segment	L Late

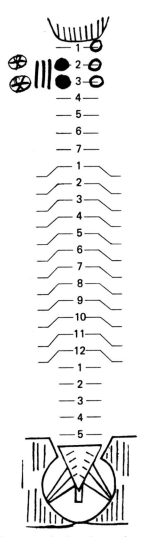

Fig. 10.3 Chart of palpation findings in a patient with headache (see text).

nature of a joint problem, and it is necessary to palpate each segment while passively performing the normal active movements of rotation, side-flexion, flexion and extension (pp. 336–341)—we are not now concerned with accessory movements, and these tests may sometimes be necessary to clarify questions of whether restricted or increased movement of vertebral segments is essentially the change which underlies the clinical features.

Again, in middle-aged men reporting a lumbar ache, there is clearly reason to assume that these symptoms *do* arise from the vertebral joints, yet there seems to be no great tenderness, no elicited spasm, no hypermobility and no undue thickening or prominence, and physiological movement tests are occasionally necessary to clarify the site of diminished movement. These tests are usually more necessary at or near the junctional regions of the spine than the segments between (see p. 365). We should observe that workers of much academic and clinical experience naturally tend to rely on examination methods to which they have become accustomed and by which they work to the best effect.

When testing vertebral segments, different abnormalities can be detected by a sense of tissue-tension, or 'end-feel', and they can be classified as types (see below) familiar to all experienced workers, whatever may be their preferred palpation methods. The differences can be apparent to one worker employing accessory-movement tests only for the majority of patients, because he is experienced in interpreting findings in this particular way. Another will assess the type of 'end-feel' by the routine use of passive physiological-movement tests only, or combinations of them, sometimes reserving the moment of greatest attention to the 'feel' of movement limitation after positioning the segment for a particular technique and just prior to performing the final thrust.

Yet another will place the greatest reliance on the particular pattern and degree of voluntary movement restriction, employing palpation routinely but in a general way and not necessarily deriving precise treatment indications from palpation (see p. 366).

The latter may tend as a rule to employ regional manipulations (see p. 388) as the main therapeutic basis.

Perceiving the nature of factors limiting movement

Distinguishing between *types* of movement limitation is easy when handling normal mobile peripheral joints, e.g. the abrupt stop when testing full extension of elbow or knee is quite different to the squashy feel of soft-tissue approximation when the same joints are flexed to their limit.

As MacConaill[782] has shown, flexed joints are 'loose-packed' and movement is limited by soft-tissue contact, whereas extension movements are limited by 'close-packing', when the female surface is in most complete con-

mobility and hypermobility. Aside from considerations of why it is so, tenderness and pain may arise from both a hypermobile and a hypomobile segment. The latter we try to reverse, the former is certainly not a case for grade V manipulation techniques, although we can significantly reduce pain and irritability by gentle, repetitive mobilisation which is kept well within the normal movement range of adjacent segments.

In a small proportion of cases, the testing of *accessory* movements may be insufficient to fully elucidate the gruence with the male surface, the capsule and ligaments are in maximal tension and it is difficult, although not impossible, to separate the bones by traction.[437] A moment's examination of the close-packed humeroulnar joint in fullest extension reveals that a measure of accessory abduction and adduction range can still be passively produced, without releasing the degree of extension—the limit of extreme movement is always something of a movable feast (see pp. 313–315) and this ability to accurately assess, by observation and by feeling, what is normal and abnormal in peripheral joint movement is served basically by applied anatomical knowledge, the assessment becoming more accurate with clinical experience; this too applies to the vertebral joints.

a. *On giving overpressure at the extremes of voluntary movement of spinal regions.* The 'end-feel' in normal young subjects is mostly that of soft-tissue tension, i.e. the combined resistance in varying degrees of muscle with its attachment-tissues, fascial planes, ligaments, joint capsules and the annulus fibrosus of discs. We know, for example, that the main limiting factors in sagittal lumbar movement is the annulus, although other soft tissues are put on tension; rotation and side-flexion of the three regions, with flexion of the lumbar and thoracic regions, have an elastic resistance to manual attempts to increase range, and the precise end-of-range is difficult to pinpoint; however, comparison between sides allows assessment, and range abnormalities can readily be perceived on overpressure, if not by simple observation beforehand, or both.

That cervical and thoracic extension are limited by bone-to-bone contact (or cartilage-covered bone contact, in the normal) and not especially by soft-tissue tension, cannot fully be perceived manually because all one can feel is a somewhat harder and less elastic stop to the movement, although a degree of elastic resilience remaining is easily detected.

Gently forcing cervical extension produces unpleasant discomfort before a solid limitation, if a normal subject allows this degree of questing. Cervical flexion is limited by approximation of mandible and sternum compressing the soft tissue between, yet movement can be continued for a few degrees as the posterior vertebral tissues are stretched by the 'beer-handle' effect of pressing downwards on the occiput.

Craniovertebral extension is limited by the posterior edge of the atlantal facets engaging the condylar fossae of the occiput; the same movement is limited at the cervicothoracic junction by the inferior articular processes of C7 engaging horizontal grooves below and behind the superior facets of T1. Thoracic extension is limited by contact of inferior articular processes with the laminae below, and by contact of the spinous processes.

At the thoracolumbar junctional region, a 'mortise' effect is produced in full extension by engagement of the articular facets of T11 and T12 (sometimes T12 and L1—see p. 14) and this is one of the few articular mechanisms in the body where a practically solid bony-contact lock occurs at the extreme of movement.[228]

Practically all other so-called bone-to-bone locks, with the exception of dental occlusion and lumbar rotation in neutral or extension, occur to a degree only.

b. *When testing vertebral accessory-movement ranges by rhythmic pressures against the bony prominences available to palpation*, with the patient lying prone in a neutral position, the anatomical and functional criteria governing *voluntary-movement* assessments do not apply on a one-to-one basis at each segment. (See Figs 2.6; 2.7.)

For example, (i) the 35°–45° range of rotation at C1–C2 is not reflected in the degree of movement palpable on postero-anterior pressure on the C2 spinous process—the odontoid prevents this—and to appreciate the limit of available range of rotation it is necessary to turn the patient's head through 90°, and feel how far short of this amplitude the spine of C2 has moved. Nevertheless, should voluntary cervical rotation to one side be limited to 30° or less, by pain arising from changes at the C1–C2 segment of that side, this will be very accurately reflected in the ease with which involuntary spasm and voluntary muscle guarding are provoked on applying unilateral pressures to C1 on the painful side, and transverse pressures to the spine of C2 towards the painful side, with the patient lying in the neutral position.

Again, (ii) in the presence of pain referred forward to the pectoral region and breast which is arising from thoracic joint changes at interscapular levels, cursory examination of voluntary thoracic movement does not invariably reveal positive signs, neither does overpressure at the limit of the customary regional movements always reveal abnormality.

Limitation at individual segments is sometimes concealed from detection during observation of regional movements, only to be revealed on searching tests of combined movements (see p. 314), or more surely on careful and systematic palpation at segments T345.

Further, (iii) stiffness spanning three mobility-segments between L1 and L4 is often detectable by careful observation of the patient's back during active tests, but not invariably so, yet after active tests which may be somewhat inconclusive, a flat-handed downward pressure on the lumbar region declares the probability at once, and segmental palpation confirms it.

Abnormal 'end-feels' on passive testing

A general table of findings of segmental abnormality on passive testing is set out below, with *general* indications. They do not represent diagnoses and they cannot be considered in isolation from assessment of the clinical features as a whole; their presence *per se* does not necessarily amount to an indication for treatment.

The table refers *only* to the differing nature of what can be perceived by *palpation, per se,* and does not include the important factor of *pain,* and other clinical features.

(For more precise relationships between findings and grade of mobilising see 'Range–pain–resistance relationship', p. 360.)

NB. The development and sophistication of radiological methods, e.g. radiculography, stereoradiography, epidurography and image-intensification techniques (see p. 369), together with the highly detailed parameters adopted by German radiologists[37, 38] for clarifying the nature of mechanical changes depicted on plain film, might appear to be overtaking and overshadowing the usefulness of palpation as an examination method. The two are not really in conflict, because while these significant advances add valuable facilities for the better understanding of vertebral abnormalities, our perennial concern as therapists *in the clinical situation* will remain the articular signs and their relation to symptoms.

There appears no effective substitute for passive movement and palpation as methods of seeking, segment by segment, to provoke or reproduce symptoms reported by the patients, by which we assess the need for mobilisation techniques of a particular nature, direction and grade, and further assess their efficacy as treatment proceeds.

Because we enjoy better means, and can apply more detailed criteria, when looking at abnormal joints, general medical and surgical indications are better appreciated; but where manual techniques *are* indicated, the treatment needs of the abnormal joints, and our methods and criteria for assessing these, remain the same.

GROUPING JOINT ABNORMALITIES

To have complete control of the treatment movements we apply, and also to apply them with the most effectiveness, we need to develop two things:

1. A precise *grading* of the mobilising movements and manipulations used in treatment, and
2. A good understanding of the great variety of ways in which abnormal movement may present.

The nature and characteristics of the abnormal movement give us our indications for treatment, both in terms of the grade of movement to use initially, and subsequently the modifications needed as the signs and symptoms change during treatment.[797, 456]

So far as abnormalities of joints, and their effects, are concerned, patients can be placed into one of five main groups:

Group 1 There is plenty of pain from the joint, either at rest and/or on movement; it is very irritable, and

Table 10.1

Type	Comment	General indication
1. Resistance (a)	Elicited spasm	Mobilise (grade I–IV)—degree of irritability governs initial grade
2. Resistance (b)	Negligible spasm; negligible voluntary guarding response. Tissue-tension limits movement before end of range, with elastic resilience detected when stressed. Other movements of the segment feel similar	Mobilise (grade I–IV) May manipulate (localised grade V) later
3. Resistance (c)	'Block'—no elastic resilience when stressed. 'Block' feels firm to attempts at moving it. Only one movement may be involved	Manipulate (localised grade V) if no preclusions (see p. 463)
4. Resistance (d)	Fairly 'hard end-feel' nature of limitation at end of movement, which is reduced. No possibility of much further movement, but may be slight elastic resilience. Other ranges likewise limited. (Chondro-osteophyte contact?)	Persistent mobilisation—and traction, provided adjacent segments are not hypermobile
5. Resistance (e)	'Springy-rubbery rebound' type of resistance to questing movement—feel is similar to that when trying to extend knee joint in fixed-flexion after IDK	Mobilise in positions which gap the joint surfaces—traction alone may be helpful. Only those manipulations (localised grade V) which gap the joint should be considered
6. Resistance (f)	Very little, if any, movement can be detected. Fused vertebrae, or degenerative ankylosis?	Refer to radiographic appearance
7. Hypermobility (a)	Normal physiological 'feel' (i.e. detectable elastic resistance at end of range) but range is greater than normal. May or may not be painful	If not causing symptoms, or provoking those reported, leave alone. If painful, mobilise within normal range for pain only
8. Hypermobility (b)	'Boggy', 'squashy' unphysiological feel; amplitude of movement is greater than expected, and 'end-feel' may not be encountered. May or may not be painful, but usually is. When elicited spasm is provoked, it is widely generalised	Likely to be serious pathology. Stop testing movements and do not treat. Check history again, and leave alone until indications for treatment have been reconfirmed

the pain and irritability limit the movement early in the range

Group 2 Resistance (either as contractile-tissue tension, i.e. spasm; or inert tissue-tension, i.e. adhesions and fibrosis; or tissue-compression) and *pain*, are *both* responsible (in varying combinations) for limiting the movement. This is a very large group

Group 3 *Resistance*, as inert-tissue tension or compression, is manifestly the range-limiting factor. It may hurt *slightly* to test the joint, and there may be a trace of spasm, but these latter two are negligible in the face of resistance as the movement-restriction factor

Group 4 There is a 'catch', or momentary 'twinge' of pain, either *during* a movement which is otherwise of full range and painless, or more often at the end of it. This group often show the twinge or catch of pain at the end of *combinations* of movement, such as combined extension and side-flexion of the neck, or combined abduction with extension of a shoulder

Group 5 comprises those patients in whom an accurate and confident diagnosis of *joint derangement*, often confirmed radiologically, can be made; we need not consider this group any further in this particular context.

Notice how the criteria for categorising these patients are the factors of abnormal movement. It is not the pathology which is of first importance, but the particular phase of the pathology the patient is in. Even then it is still not the pathology we give our main attention to, but how the abnormalities are manifested in terms of movement.

Examination and assessment must be accurate enough to elicit which group the patient falls into, and subsequent reassessment must be accurate enough to detect when the joint is moving from group to group. The joint abnormality may move from group to group in one treatment—it may not move from one group to another in a week of daily treatments.

The essence of good examination and assessment of joint problems lies in extracting, from all the material presented by the patient, a clear mental picture of the interaction between the various factors we can measure, or estimate, i.e.

1. The patient's story gives *some* information regarding the probable degree of joint irritability, the amount of pain at rest, and the functional restrictions
2. The active test of movement gives *more* information regarding the functional range, and its possible limitation, as described above
3. The passive test of functional and accessory ranges gives the *most* information (and often confirmation) regarding:

a. amount of pain, and spasm and other resistance during applied movement
b. their point of onset on the range of movement
c. the relationship between these factors
d. their rate of increase of effect, in bringing the movement to a halt
e. the primary nature of the limit to further movement.

Only this depth of attention, observation and perception during palpation will allow us to assess the 'Range–pain–resistance' relationship which gives us our treatment indications for each joint problem we handle. The nature of the range-limiting factor invariably decides the grade employed in treatment, and frequently also the positioning of the patient's joint, and the particular technique.

Movements of abnormal joints are usually, but not invariably, limited, and since the available excursion of movement is reduced the grades of treatment are proportionately reduced (see p. 421).

ASSESSMENT AND USE OF GRADES IN TREATMENT (see p. 366)

It is not possible to describe the very many varieties of presentation of abnormal joints, with permutations of the 'Range–pain–resistance' relationship, but an outline guide to initial grade selection is useful provided subsequent selection is guided by careful assessment of results; the two factors of: (i) treatment position of the joint, and (ii) technique selection being given.

By combinations (see p. 361) of these five simple steps, the 'Range–pain–resistance' relationship for any one movement can be clearly expressed.

Validity of programmes of research, into the nature and magnitude of movement-limiting factors in degenerative joint disease, would depend upon precise data and meticulous recording, but in clinical work the need is for a quick and clear graphic record of the assessment by which the treatment plan is formulated. Advantages of this method are speed and simplicity because the need for abscissae and ordinates, calibrated for joint range and for magnitude of limiting factors respectively, is avoided. The important clinical findings to record are: (i) the *point of movement-limitation*, as a proportion of normal range; (ii) the nature of the *primary* range-limiting factor; (iii) the nature and magnitude of secondary factors.

These can be clearly expressed and be read at a glance, and although easier to apply to careful manual tests of peripheral joint movement, the method has been found of much value in 'Examination-and-assessment' training programmes during which candidates, after some tuition and practice, are able to express their findings, after vertebral-segment tests, with a degree of interobserver error which is gratifyingly small.

This is probably the best use of 'joint pictures', i.e. as a means of developing perception of the *characteristics* of joint abnormality as they differ from patient to patient.

Joint pictures may be used for each of two or more passive movement tests of single vertebrae or for two or more active tests of a vertebral region, but reach their most sophisticated development when employed for the single accessory vertebral movement which is being given priority as an assessment parameter during treatment.

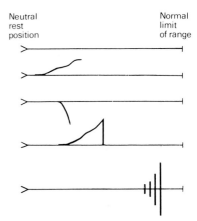

Examples of findings follow, with *a method of graphic description* in which:

the horizontal line represents normal range and movement is from left to right

pain is depicted above it

spasm is depicted below it

movement-limitation is represented by a vertical line from the dominant factor responsible

resistance (other than spasm) is represented by a number of vertical lines which always cross the range line.

Assessment	*Joint picture*	*Initial grade* (see p. 421)
1. Joint irritability is manifest with pain at rest and/or provoked early in the testing movement		I
2. Spasm elicited by the testing movement limits it quite early in the range, with pain less dominant	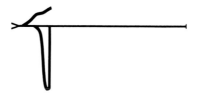	I or I+
3. Elicited spasm and pain inseparably limit the movement early in the range	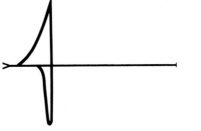	I
4. Spasm limits the movement much earlier with a quick probe than with a slow probe, indicating latent irritability	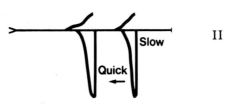	II

Assessment   *Joint picture*   *Initial grade*
(see p. 421)

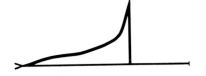

5. In the absence of resistance, slowly rising pain limits the movement after ½ range

II

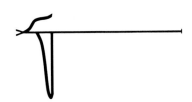

6. Pain and 'resistance' (as either spasm, other tissue tension or tissue compression) are *together* limiting the movement. The grade employed depends upon: a) which is the dominant factor, b) when the limit occurs

I or I+

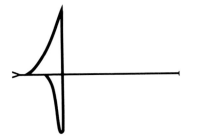

   i) Pain and/or spasm encountered early in the range have been described in (2) and (3).

I

   ii) Limitation by pain and virtually spasm-free resistance in roughly equal proportions

      a) before ½ range

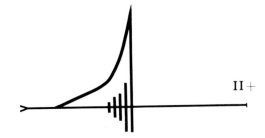

II+

      b) after ½ range

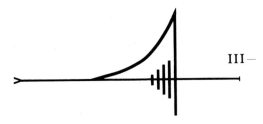

III−

   iii) Spasm limits the movement beyond ½ range with little pain

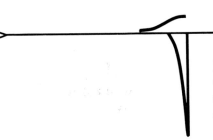

IV (up to point where spasm is about to be elicited)

Joint picture   *Initial grade*
                                    (see p. 421)

iv) Limitation by the resistance, without spasm, of tissue tension, or compression, is encountered at or beyond ½ range; pain rises to its maximum then but is much less dominant than resistance and by itself would not limit the movement

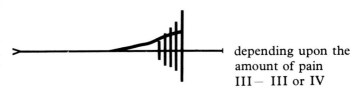

depending upon the amount of pain
III— III or IV

7. In the virtual absence of pain or spasm, resistance limits the movement (a) either before, or (b) after ½ range

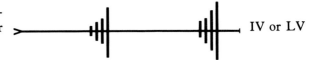

IV or LV

8. Resistance, including spasm, is encountered well beyond ½ range, with minimal pain

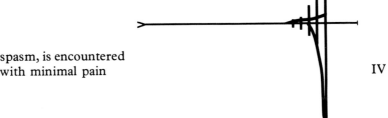

IV

Notes

1. The notion that grades denote progression of treatment in time is incorrect, since the nature of the movement-limiting factor governs initial choice of treatment grade and it has been shown that, from the first, this may be grade IV.

2. Neither do the grades symbolise an ascending scale of aggression in treatment. 'Grade IV' indicates a particular amplitude, and position, on the available excursion of movement, and not *necessarily* the greatest vigour in mobilising.

3. One should make up one's mind whether one is treating primarily *pain*, or *resistance*, because this is fundamentally related to the grade of mobilisation which is chosen. Most of the more serious manipulation accidents,[630, 759, 1096, 1148, 438] a few of them catastrophes, which have been reported in the literature have followed overvigorous or rough treatment, more often to the upper cervical spine. But there is a dilemma here—certainly nothing untoward, but also nothing of any therapeutic value, is going to result from aimless, undisciplined, oscillatory waggling applied to the upper cervical area or any other body part.

Technique should be precise, specific and controlled,

yet mobilisation is by no means always gentle—as it has frequently and erroneously been defined—and in the appropriate circumstances is quite vigorous. If mobilisations grade I to grade IV, and traction, do not produce sufficient improvement, it is time to consider the indications and contraindications for manipulative thrust techniques.

4. An intervertebral segment may present as (1) above while another segment in the same vertebral region will present as in (6 ii a). Treatment of the former should take priority.

5. When employing grade III or IV, possible treatment soreness should be alleviated by using lower grades on alternate days.

6. Indications for grade V techniques are on page 463.

7. *Recording method*
As an exercise for beginners it is useful to symbolise, as treatment proceeds, the changing relationship of pain, resistance and point of limitation of one movement; an example is given on page 364.

Although not all joint problems require more than one treatment; for example if patients present with joint problems in stages (v) and (vi) a single localised grade V technique may be indicated.

Recording Method Example

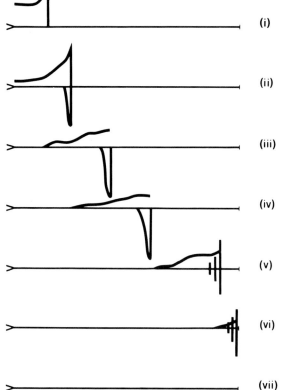

(i)

(ii)

(iii)

(iv)

(v)

(vi)

(vii)

SUMMARY

As one generally handles highly irritable joints and/or nerve roots, with much respect, and less irritable joints with less respect, technique grading is guided in the first instance by *pain:*

1. If pain is constant even at rest and rises quickly on movement into range, *or* it appears early in the range and rises to a level sufficient to stop the movement well before the normal limit, the techniques should be of small amplitude, gentle and confined to the beginning of available range, i.e. grades I, I+ or II−.

2. If there is no pain at rest, and it only begins after more than half range has been traversed, then the mobilising technique can move into the pain a bit, and even up to the limit, with care.

3. A 'block' by spasm, more than pain, can be treated by a grade IV technique up to the point of spasm so long as it occurs beyond half range. If it occurs before that, one should use a lower grade—the earlier the spasm, the lower the grade.

4. A block by inert-tissue tension, or compression, with negligible pain or spasm, should be treated with a grade IV technique, and a grade V technique may be indicated.

During treatment, movement into pain depends not entirely on the pain as such, but also on its characteristics, its quality or its nature: with much pain and irritability, low grades are employed; with dull aches, one can often manipulate immediately, that is, use a single, short-amplitude, high-velocity thrust technique, a grade V, provided all other factors are favourable and there are no contra-indications.

The ability to grade techniques accurately depends upon a working knowledge, from clinical experience and trained perception, of the voluntary and accessory range of all vertebral segments. Yet when palpating we must always remember the patient's age and the natural varieties of individual spines, i.e. hard and springy; soft and springy; soft and yielding; inelastic, tight and tough.

In brief:

1. Examination and assessment must elicit the range–pain–resistance relationship existing.
2. The depth of mobilising must be right for the range–pain–resistance relationship.
3. Subsequent assessment must be precise enough to guide technique and grading in accordance with the changing requirements of the abnormal joints.

Having decided whether one is treating *pain* primarily, or *resistance* primarily, the broad principles for choosing the patient's position, the technique and the grade are as follows:

Pain. Mobilise the range of accessory movements with the joint in a painless position, or use physiological movements in a painless part of the range.

Resistance. Both accessory and physiological ranges are mobilised *at* the available limit of movement.

IMPORTANCE OF JUNCTIONAL REGIONS

With a step-by-step process of exclusion, beginning with the history and proceeding through observation, active-movement tests, regional and then segmental palpation, the essential purpose of examination is to precisely localise the *source* of symptoms reported. Assessment of the *presentation* of the movement abnormality, i.e. how it is manifesting itself, then provides the guide for action, even though we may not be able to know all we would like about its true *nature*.

Self-education in the accurate localisation of spinal joint problems is probably the most important single aspect for the beginner to develop following training courses; one learns the importance of going like a dog after a cat for the *precise level* of vertebral involvement. Sooner or later, however, depending upon the 'mileage' of patients treated, it will become evident that the interdependence of the vertebral column is asserting itself in various ways, e.g.

1. Postero-anterior unilateral movement of T1 or the first rib provoking the unilateral hemicranial pain reported by the patient

2. Cervical rotation and side-flexion restrictions disappearing on mobilisation of T1
3. Lumbar side-flexion improving on mobilisation of the sacroiliac joint of that side
4. The frequency with which patients report with concurrent upper cervical and lumbosacral joint problems.

There are many further examples of this phenomenon, simple explanations of which are always attractive; one could analyse (1) on the basis of scalenus muscle spasm, since the scalenus medius has partial attachment to C2 above and to the first rib below, and analyse (4) on the basis that should the foundation of a structure be disturbed its most superincumbent parts are likely to be affected most. Since the craniovertebral articulation is a prime organ of equilibration, the analogy is a reasonable one, whatever the biomechanical and neurophysiological mechanisms may prove to be when comprehensive analysis ultimately becomes possible.

The analogy does not take into account, of course, whether the craniovertebral abnormality might have developed first, with subsequent effects upon more distant but interdependent segments.

Further to (1) above, Frykholm[392] describes the observation that many patients with brachialgia, due to a cervical rib, have also suffered from cervical migraine, which was relieved by adequate decompression of the brachial plexus.

A clinical and radiological survey[1028] of 98 patients with ankylosing spondylitis was undertaken to evaluate male and female differences in clinical features. Radiographic differences in the 18 female patients included a high incidence of cervical spine abnormalities and a combination of sacroiliac and cervical spine involvement, with normal intervening thoracic and lumbar regions. Spondylitis is not spondylosis, but these findings may help to stress the important factor of perceiving the vertebral column as an interdependent functional structure. Meanwhile, our present knowledge of vertebral column structure, innervation and neurophysiology is more than enough to support the contention (Wyke)[1362, 1363] that we not only mobilise, and thereby affect, joints but by our procedures are affecting complex arthrokinetic systems, disturbing the musculoskeletal neurophysiology of the whole patient.

In this connection, the junctional regions of the spine are frequently found to show movement restrictions when the pain reported can be provoked at segments distant from them. *While the treatment of the segments giving rise to pain remains the priority, a careful check of the junctional regions and subsequent attention to any movement abnormalities found can be worthwhile, since the more comprehensive the examination and the more effective the treatment, the less do the problems seem to recur.*

Bourdillon (1973)[105] observes that: '... errors in exact localisation of the lesion are surprisingly common even to those with experience. They form the main indication for a repetition of the localised part of the examination on every occasion before treatment is undertaken.'

Examination findings allow an assessment of the length of treatment likely to be required. Aches and pains of moderate intensity localised to vertebral and paravertebral regions, with little or no reference to limbs and no neurological involvement, may often be significantly reduced by treatment counted in days rather than in weeks.

'Experience with manipulative treatment shows that it is rarely sufficient to mobilise the affected joint on one occasion only. The number of treatments required varies enormously from patient to patient.' (Bourdillon, 1973.)[105]

The need for periodic medical treatment of diseases with episodic exacerbations, like chronic bronchitis for example, is unquestioned, yet the similar need for periodic attention to a like disease, which also has existence in time as well as space, i.e. vertebral degenerative joint disease, is seemingly not understood as plainly as it should be. For some, it seems that manipulation means getting everything tidied up with one expertly applied manipulative thrust, and anything other than this is not properly manipulative treatment.

Those who wittingly or unwittingly hold this view may have conceptions, but the one thing they do not have is first-hand shop-floor clinical experience of common vertebral joint problems.

Progress is likely to be slow in the following situations:

1. When there is a localised distal area of objective numbness
2. When there is marked muscle wasting, as a consequence of degenerative joint disease
3. When there is severe limb pain, or when the worst pain is more distal than proximal
4. When pain is sufficiently severe to produce facial distortion
5. When neurological deficit indicates involvement of the following nerve roots (in order of difficulty): L3, S1, S2. Patients with neurological signs from L4 and L5 are easier to relieve
6. Where postural spasm is maintaining:
   a. a lumbar spine deviation towards the painful side, or
   b. marked lordosis on attempted flexion, or
   c. a flattening of the lumbar curve, or
   d. a frank lumbar kyphosis.
7. When extension is grossly limited, and either produces or exacerbates arm or leg pain
8. When straight-leg-raising is severely restricted unilaterally and especially bilaterally
9. If palpation at a single vertebral level elicits brisk protective spasm over a much wider area

10. Where symptoms are felt locally *and* referred, from one acutely tender spinous process
11. Long-standing cases
12. Result of recent trauma
13. Moderate or severe whiplash injury during last three to four years
14. Juniors and adolescents.

The nature of pain is a further factor in duration of treatment. A generalised ache or a restrictive nuisance is more quickly relieved than is a throbbing intense pain, or a shooting, stabbing pain.

NB. It is uncommon for spinal joint problems to be single[105] and where multiple problems require careful analysis and appropriate treatment, the process cannot be achieved by the facile production of a single joint 'click', however prevalent may be this conception of what manipulation is about.

Some other common fallacies are:

1. That the obese patient is more prone to discogenic lumbar joint problems, and to recurrences, than is the slimmer person.[326]
2. That postural asymmetry of the pelvic joints must *necessarily* be responsible, sooner or later, for low back pain; it is more than likely, but not inevitable.
3. That in suitable cases a corrective heel raise, for patients well over 40 who have chronic lumbar pain due to a laterally tilted pelvis, cannot quickly relieve intractable symptoms; the prognosis need not be gloomy in these cases, simply because the patient is mature.
4. That joint conditions of sudden onset are invariably easier to relieve than those of insidious onset; this is by no means true.
5. That the longer a joint problem has existed, the more difficult it will be to relieve.
6. That restricted straight-leg-raising indicates discogenic trespass upon a root of the lumbosacral plexus, and that the prognosis is therefore that of neurological involvement.
7. That provocation of the unilateral midlumbar and anterior thigh pain by the 'femoral nerve stretch test' is corroboration of an irritative lesion of a root of the femoral nerve, and justifies a like prognosis.

DISCUSSION—THE USE OF PALPATION IN ASSESSMENT

An outline of how palpation is used in conjunction with treatment methods, which emphasises one aspect or another, is given on page 354, and approaches (i) and (ii) were briefly described.

A short description of some of the differences between these two categories may be helpful to the less experienced.

In (i), the use of persuasive, segmental repetitive mobilising movements (grades I–IV) is the main therapeutic basis, and manipulative thrust techniques comprise less than 20 per cent of the treatment procedures employed.

In (ii), the therapist also employs repetitive, persuasive segmental movements in treatment, as well as manipulative thrust (grade V) techniques, with a tendency to conceive the latter as the lynch-pin of therapeutic method in this field of work.

Having reached consideration of examination methods by palpation, we need to consider the fundamental difference between two common rationales of treatment by manipulation, which may lie at the source of much of the beginner's confusion and which are rooted in the two cardinal factors of palpation and assessment.

Procedures are *primarily* based on either:

(i) *the constant relationship to pain of particular physiological movements in a spinal region,* or
(ii) *which specific segmental movements, i.e. flexion, extension, rotation, of vertebra are most restricted.*

In (i), *clinical assessment* of patients and their pain is the basic skill and fundamentally important, and in (ii), *mechanical assessment of mobility by palpation* is the important factor, although both approaches employ both of these factors in different combinations in their method.

The difference is illustrated by the example of a single vertebral segment which may have two or three of its possible movements restricted, and which is found to be the segment giving rise to the patient's symptoms. We can either mobilise that segment:

(i) *Guided primarily by the distribution and behaviour of pain,* without being unduly concerned with abstract geometrical considerations of the correctness of the particular movement found to be therapeutically effective, and this is the first approach, *or*
(ii) We can use techniques which specifically loosen each of the *restricted segmental movements* assuming thereby that relief of symptoms and signs will follow as a consequence of restoring movement—and this is the second approach.

In the first, (i), distribution of pain and its behaviour (and behaviour of other symptoms) are more important than mechanical considerations, and for this reason the first principle governing application and modification of techniques is not their supposed mechanical suitability for the known configuration of joints being moved, but their suitability and effectiveness as evidenced by continuing assessment, for each patient's unique presentation of pain.

In the second, (ii), mechanical considerations are virtually paramount, and it is a basic tenet that therapeutic passive movements which are not applied either in the plane of the facet-joints (gliding) or at right angles to them (gapping), are 'incorrect'. Very much the same basis governs what is thought 'correct' for peripheral joints, also.

Yet another approach is based on the prime importance of *patterns* of movement limitation, with commonly occurring abnormal 'articular patterns' being integrated into a corpus of teaching which relies to a degree on extrapolation to formulate conceptions of the precise nature of trespass, derangement or other lesions believed to be underlying the signs and symptoms. Thus philosophies of treatments, which govern selection and type of procedures used, arise naturally from conceptions of the nature of the abnormality, or from acceptance of the fact that more often than not we cannot know its true nature.

It should be emphasised that we know very much less, about the true causes of much vertebrogenic pain, than we sometimes care to admit.

Because of the real paucity of necessary facts it comes about, as in other walks of life, that the way people think governs what they do.

We have already noted above that the differences of approach and therefore method tend, in shop-floor clinical practice, to become matters of emphasis only, yet the fundamental dissimilarity remains, and if this is grasped early in the day by the beginner, much that is initially puzzling in manipulation teaching may be easier to understand.

The differences of approach are roughly analogous to the professional preoccupations of mechanical and telecommunications engineers whose fields of activity overlap considerably.

A basic difficulty is that each manipulation philosophy, when first encountered, appears so logical and so reasonable. A further, painful difficulty for the tyro may not even be recognised, let alone resolved, until after two or more years of clinical experience in manipulative work, when more knowledge and familiarity with the behaviour of common joint problems allows retrospective analysis and a sobering comparison between how much is understood from lectures and technique demonstrations and what actually transpires in the clinical situation. For some reason, which may have something to do with a therapeutic method involving physically handling the tissues of another, manipulation, more than any other therapeutic discipline, seems prone to advocacy based almost entirely on the supposed merits of this or that *technique*. Having completed a long and devoted training in many different techniques of *handling*, e.g. massage, maintenance movements for neurological and inflammatory arthritic conditions, proprioceptive neuromuscular facilitation techniques and other manual resistance methods, the beginner tends to see manipulation almost totally as an art, believing some essential potency of effect to reside in the technique itself; thus working and practising incessantly to emulate what appears to be the teacher's practised facility and dexterity of technique. As clinical experience grows, manipulative work is better seen as a slowly growing science, subject to ordinary physical laws like everything else; treatment techniques are then rightly relegated to no more than another instrument to serve a widening understanding of the clinical features of degenerative joint disease, i.e. why, and which, patients suffer it.

Thus the experienced worker actually manipulates only a handful and often none of the daily quota of patients, the essential needs of most being perhaps some modes and undramatic localised mobilising, local segmenta exercises, regional strengthening exercises, harness traction, temporary or more permanent support, simple advice and guidance, very frequently *a restoration of confidence in their spines* or a combination of these allied to the medical and surgical procedures which may be indicated. Throughout a professional career, a few may not develop beyond the point of believing expertise in technique to be paramount; for most it is but a stepping-stone to more effective work with joint problems—*it is palpation and assessment which make the stepping stone.*

Sometimes, arbitrary and perhaps impatient attempts to impose order, reason and logic from without on the irrational behaviour of signs and symptoms in common joint problems may be misguided and counter-productive. The body cannot read the book, and joints cannot know what is confidently expected of them by the theorist, the logician and the biomechanic. In our enthusiasm for this or that therapeutic revelation we sometimes overlook the infinite range of biological plasticity of response, and of individual uniqueness, which makes fools of us all at one time or another. Perhaps it is wiser to 'allow joints to speak for themselves', especially in the matter of palpation findings, and to assess and treat joint problems on the basis of acceptance of what is there to be observed, while views about its genesis must often remain unproven.

In our condition of only limited albeit slowly increasing certainty, careful and clinically responsible empiricism, and moderation in the use of vigour during treatment, seem to be prudent things.

These matters are most pertinent to fundamental questions of how palpation is used, its value as an examination method, how closely clinical presentation may be related to palpation findings and how justifiable is the heavy reliance on palpation in clinical assessment.

Undeniably, if the examiner can keep an approach which is flexible and receptive, and try always to relate palpable vertebral abnormality, which presents itself in such a variety of ways, to the features of degenerative joint disease, a valuable method of clinical self-education comes literally to hand, and the question of manipulation philosophies assumes less importance. The joint is thus allowed to speak for itself, and real learning begins to take place because one is now listening—by feeling.

It is during this time that we vitally need the ability to live with a little confusion and doubt, because it is absolutely certain that if we do examine patients well, progressively improve our palpation skill, and do not sweep awkward and unwelcome facts under the carpet, we will feel more and more the need to rearrange concepts and ideas about the passive movement of joints which have perhaps served well enough in tne past. The time is now—and yesterday has gone.[444]

11. Investigation procedures

Measuring spinal mobility

Several clinical methods of measuring spinal mobility have been reviewed and compared by Reynolds (1975)[1032]. They are:

1. The Dunham spondylometer, described by Dunham (1949)[283]
2. A skin distraction method, described by Schober (1937)[1124] and elaborated by Moll and Wright (1971)[865]
3. An inclinometer or pendulum goniometer using the principle described by Loebl (1967)[760]

Reynolds observes that the main clinical application of this type of measurement lies in the follow-up examination for cases of ankylosing spondylitis.

While clinical examination remains the best diagnostic procedure, a number of sophisticated developments in radiographic method, and an increasing variety of other investigation procedures are providing more specific data. Information about these highly specialised techniques should be sought in appropriate texts, but some brief comments are included in the following list, which is not comprehensive.

Radiography

X-rays make good policemen but poor counsellors, in that while the straight radiograph may exclude serious bone disease and significant mechanical defect, it does not often provide much guidance about how to treat the patient. Even when frank mechanical defect is revealed, it may have little or no clinical significance. In 151 people whose occupations involved strenuous manual labour or vigorous physical activity, but who gave no history of back pain, the radiographs revealed: 8 with spondylolisthesis, including one complete forward dislocation; 5 with pseudospondylolisthesis (group III); 30 with transitional vertebrae, including 10 with accessory or adventitious joints and 5 with scoliosis.[97]

Radiologists tried to discover some correlation between lumbar spinal bony joint configuration before and after manipulation.[1047] Nothing significant came of their careful measurements (using the methods of Begg and Falconer, 1949,[79] Froning and Frohman, 1968,[388] and Pennal et al., 1972).[980] Radiographs of the lumbar spine and radiographic assessments of spinal motion were of no value in predicting or assessing the response of patients to manipulation; they contributed little to the management of such patients except to exclude serious spinal pathology before any form of physical treatment was commenced.

Carstairs (1959)[159] makes the point that in most patients with musculoskeletal conditions, the problem is not to make a completely accurate diagnosis but to make sure that treatment, although probably empirical, will be safe. For this reason alone, radiography is necessary to exclude infective and neoplastic disease before manipulation or traction.

A grading of the radiographic appearances of diseased joints[644] is as follows:

Apophyseal joints of cervical spine

Changes of disc degeneration are not included and should be disregarded in grading.

Grade I: Doubtful osteophytes on margins of articular facets of apophyseal joints
Grade II: Definite osteophytes and subchondral sclerosis in apophyseal joints
Grade III: Moderate osteophytes, sclerosis and some irregularity of articular facets
Grade IV: Many large osteophytes and severe sclerosis and irregularity of articular facets.

In lateral films narrowing of apophyseal joints cannot be assessed accurately.

Cervical disc degeneration

Changes in the apophyseal joints are not included and should be disregarded in grading. The most severely affected disc space determines the grading.

Grade I: Minimal anterior osteophytosis
Grade II: Definite anterior osteophytosis with possible

narrowing of disc space and some sclerosis of vertebral plates

Grade III: Moderate narrowing of disc space with definite sclerosis of vertebral plates and osteophytosis

Grade IV: Severe narrowing of disc space with sclerosis of vertebral plates and multiple large osteophytes.

Thoracic disc degeneration

Grade I: Possible sclerosis and osteophytosis at anterior margins of disc space

Grade II: Definite but slight osteophytosis and sclerosis of vertebral plates

Grade III: Moderate narrowing of disc space with sclerosis of vertebral plates and osteophytosis

Grade IV: Severe narrowing of disc space, marked sclerosis of vertebral plates and large osteophytes.

Lumbar disc degeneration

Grade I: Minimal osteophytosis only

Grade II: Definite osteophytosis with some sclerosis of anterior part of vertebral plates

Grade III: Marked osteophytosis and sclerosis of vertebral plates and marked narrowing of disc space

Grade IV: Large osteophytes, marked sclerosis of vertebral plates with marked narrowing of disc space.

Back pain in disc degeneration need not be the result of the degeneration as such nor need its severity have any relationship to the severity of the X-ray changes, but may be due to other factors including fracture of the hyaline cartilaginous plate or the growth of granulation tissue into the disc after annular rupture. By analogy with degenerative arthrosis in other joints, the symptoms probably arise from changes in the surrounding soft tissue rather than from the structures of a deranged joint. *Further, they very frequently arise from tissues remote from the site of the most severe radiographic evidence of joint 'disease'.*

NB. X-ray appearances associated with clinical conditions are mentioned briefly with their description (see 'Clinical Presentation') (p. 205).

X-rays with a much higher degree of resolution, some ten times better than with standard apparatus currently in use, have recently been used to analyse bone defects with a precision impossible for conventional methods.[304]

Discography

The technique of injecting radio-opaque material into the nucleus pulposus of intervertebral discs is not new. Lindblom[see 315] experimented in 1941 by injecting red lead. The accuracy of interpretation of lumbar discograms depends upon the assessment of three main findings: (i) the amount of contrast material which can be injected; (ii) the reproduction of the symptoms, and (iii) following injection, the radiological appearances of the disc system.

The normal disc has a limited ability to accept injected fluid, and 0.5 ml may be adequate to exclude abnormality. Degenerative fissuring of the annulus may allow dispersal of the fluid, and relatively large amounts may be injected; thus the acceptance of around 3 ml may demonstrate abnormality of the disc system,[970] e.g. small tears in the annulus, without disc rupture, may permit extravasation of the dye in patients over 30 years of age.[780]

Cloward (1959)[184] advocated cervical discography as being superior to myelography. Some authors[315] have noted no real correlation between the amount of material used and the intensity of symptoms provoked and do not use either cervical or lumbar discography as routine procedures.[664, 564, 293]

The recent advantages of image-intensification and direct television viewing, and contrast media of low toxicity, have allowed easier technique and reduced pain for the patient.

Macnab (1977)[780] describes the most effective use of lumbar discography as in those instances when the myelogram is negative, venography findings are difficult to assess, the root infiltration test is technically impossible and electromyography gives equivocal findings. He also regards discography as of inestimable value in determining the extent of surgical fusion required in spondylolisthesis, i.e. if discography shows the disc above the level of an L5–S1 slip to be normal, a localised L5–S1 fusion is all that is required.

Other authors[1328] strongly believe that even a severely degenerated disc, as evidenced by discography, has little to do with symptoms.

Schaeffer (1976)[1087] has mentioned that all a discogram will show is a degenerate disc, but what it will not show is whether the degenerate disc is a cause of the symptoms.

Brodsky and Binder (1979)[132] reviewed 199 patients who had undergone lumbar discography, and found that management decisions were influenced by the discogram findings in 155 cases (78 per cent). One hundred and six patients (53 per cent) had negative or equivocal myelograms but positive discograms.

Myelography

Introduction of negative or positive contrast material into the subarachnoid space allows the identification of lesions of trespass. Gas myelography,[528] using either air or oxygen, renders the subarachnoid space more transparent than adjacent tissues, and thus the spinal cord shadow has enhanced density.

With air myelography,[315] the spinal cord in the thoracic and cervical canal can be demonstrated with considerable accuracy; conventional radiography can be used, particularly when investigating the cervical canal. Positive contrast material, originally the non-absorbable and oil-based materials like Lipiodol, and more recently water-based and absorbable Dimer-X, can be used to opacify the spinal canal.[875, 1004, 1159, 1143, 678, 595] The introduction of foreign material into the subarachnoid space may be followed by a sterile, irritative meningitis, the cellular response and increased protein generally being transitory.[594]

The changes may be more permanent when oily contrast media (e.g. Lipiodol, Pantopaque, Myodil) are used, and an adhesive arachnoiditis may occur.[1308] There is marked thickening of the leptomeninges, and infiltration by chronic inflammatory cells. A vasculitis may also ensue, with the possibility of occlusion of pial blood vessels.

Radiographs of the spine a year or two after myelography with these media usually show globules of contrast material, i.e. a form of internal pollution. In the theca, it is slowly absorbed at about 1 ml a year.[1348]

Myelography is of value in demonstrating central disc prolapse or large eccentric trespass impinging on the dura,[970] but the viscosity of iodised oil does not allow clear delineation of lumbosacral root sheaths.

Diagnostic difficulties with myelograms are sometimes due to:

1. Poor filling of the nerve root pockets
2. Ectatic dilated veins
3. An abundance of fat
4. False localisation of the lesion, which happens occasionally when transitional vertebrae are present
5. A clinical syndrome suggesting disc prolapse, but with a normal myelogram.[10]

Radiculography (Myelography with water-soluble contrast material)

Radiculography allows better visualisation of the lumbosacral nerve roots, and more accurate assessment of lateral disc trespass.[1143, 970] The technique differs from conventional myelography.

Epidurography

This is an investigation method in which water-soluble contrast medium is injected into the extradural space, and which is not in general use;[970] synonyms are peridurography, epidural myelography and canalography. Thus it is distinguished from injections into the subarachnoid space. The contrast material, when introduced into the lumbar epidural space via the sacral hiatus, outlines the sacral canal, the cauda equina and the lumbar spinal canal.

Mathews (1976)[820] discusses the relative merits of myelography and epidurography.

Tomography

This method of radiography was introduced by Ziedses de Plante in 1933[1380] and focuses an organ or successive planes of the body structures eliminating the confusing shadows of plain radiography. Used in conjunction with myelography employing a water-soluble medium, myelotomography can be of considerable help[10] in clarification of preoperative cases with negative routine myelograms.

Transverse axial tomography

This is a radiological technique[601] showing an undistorted cross-section of the spine. An X-ray tube and film cassette are placed at opposite ends of an eccentric C-arm, which rotates around the supine patient in a 220° arc—the axis of rotation is the spinal axis of the patient. Axial tomography allows the preoperative detection of lumbar stenosis, and may also be used to evaluate the patient with new or recurrent symptoms after surgical fusion, for example.[602]

Computerised transverse axial tomography (Scintography)[685]

This is a radiological scanning technique showing an undistorted cross-section of the spine or other body part; hence the term EMI Scanner.

By a combination of X-rays and computer technology this precise method of producing pictures of the inside of the body (sometimes called a scintogram) is probably the most significant advance in investigation procedures since Röentgen's discovery of X-rays in 1895.

A fan beam of X-rays, rotated through 180°, is scanned across the supine patient; on the other side of the patient, and diametrically opposite the source of X-rays, an array of highly sensitive scintillation detectors count all the X-ray photons transmitted through the patient's tissues.

A picture of tissue density measurements is built up following calculations by a computer.

In a total of 180° one-degree intervals, some 29 000 readings are recorded from a single tomographic slice, enabling the computer to ascertain the density of a volume of tissue of 1.3 cm³. Each reading can be represented as a square in a matrix containing 25 600 squares. What is produced is a tone (or shade) picture, which has 16 values between black and white.

The representation is not the same as a conventional X-ray tomogram, but the pictorial record of a computerised analysis; thus visual X-ray interpretation does not arise.[947]

The whole-body CT Scanner[864] offers advantages when investigating orthopaedic conditions. The bony framework of the neural canal, including the pedicles and facet-joints, can be clearly visualised, as can the presence of bony spinal stenosis, and soft-tissue masses can be delineated. Computed tomography has been employed to confirm a diagnosis of diastematomyelia.[1299]

The technique has also been employed to diagnose rotatory fixation of the atlantoaxial joint (p. 212),[355] spondyloschisis (cleft of the vertebral arch) of the atlas,[755] fractures of the atlas[636] and a lumbar vertebra,[943] and a Ewing's sarcoma.

Body scanners expose patients to about the same amount of hazardous X-rays as the conventional techniques, yet if the tissues are scanned more slowly to improve the level of definition by reception of more X-ray photons, the exposure increases to levels approaching those of the most hazardous conventional X-ray procedure (Wall et al., 1979).[306] The authors recommend that the need for an improved quality of image must be balanced against the increased risk of bodily injury or cancer.

As applied to scanning of the lumbar spine,[144b] computerised tomography is a remarkably short-term advance in the technology of investigation and a marked improvement on many of the invasive diagnostic tests such as myelography.

Recent research indicates the important potential of high-resolution zoom scan modifications, dose reduction technique, various forms of three-dimensional display, oblique plane capability and better coronal and sagittal displays.

There is more precise knowledge of the degree of physical trespass by disc disease, deformities of the articular processes and joint spaces, and thus of central and lateral stenosis; CT scanning techniques give a much better picture of the sequelae of discectomy, hemi-laminectomy and dorso-lateral fusion procedures. For example, identification of the degree of trespass by over-growth after fusion indicates the need for re-evaluation of some surgical techniques, and in the whole field of radical treatment for lumbar spinal problems these new visualisation methods will ensure that surgery is undertaken only after more accurate and comprehensive analysis—also, that surgery is less likely to usher in a further series of undesirable changes.

The Mayo Clinic has recently developed the Dynamic Spatial Reconstructor by which cone-shaped X-ray beams circle the patient continuously and cover a broader area of the body. A single scan takes in a cylindrical volume 20 cm long and up to 40 cm in diameter. The DSR can 'look inside' the body from any angle, and could find a small lung tumour behind a rib which by conventional X-rays might otherwise be undetectable.

Xerography

This is a new radiographic technique with an increasing range of application.[864] The X-ray technique is standard, with the exception that an electronically charged selenium plate replaces the standard film in a cassette. Radiation impinging upon the plate causes the charge to 'leak' in proportion to the quantity of radiation. A dusting of toning powder will then adhere to the plate in proportion to the residual charge; by a further process the resulting pattern is fused by heat to present a permanent xerographic record, either in the negative or positive forms. Areas of low contrast, like soft tissues, are better demonstrated than in standard radiography.

Radiographic stereoplotting[603]

This is a method enabling three-dimensional measurements to be taken from a pair of X-ray films; the paired radiographs can be obtained with any conventional X-ray unit. Between exposures the X-ray tube is shifted a known distance along an appropriate axis of the structure being examined.

This technique allows detailed examination of radiographs in a manner not readily available by conventional means. Binocular stereovision enables examination of the apophyseal joints and observation of degenerative changes with a clarity that is not apparent when viewing either of the two radiographs in a conventional way.

A better visualisation of facet-joints, by stereoscopic radiography, has allowed an analysis of the changes in these joints in rheumatoid disease. Stereoscopic views showed erosions of facet structures which resembled the rheumatoid erosions observed in other joints.[1135] It was observed that these changes may be due, among other causes discussed, to analgesic or steroid therapy.

Interosseous spinal venography (Epidural phlebography)

The introduction of contrast material into the vertebral venous system via injections into a lumbar spinous process, for example,[22] allows identification of lesions and trespass upon neural cord structures.[1272] The rich plexus of intervertebral veins is outlined by contrast, and in lumbar disc herniations the protuberant disc trespass can be recognised on lateral films by the backward displacement of epidural veins from the posterior surface of the intervertebral spaces. Other space-occupying lesions can also be detected. Epidural veins may also be outlined by percutaneous catheterisation of the femoral vein, with advancement into the external vertebral vein under X-ray control.[778]

The radiological change of venous occlusion by trespass is readily observed.[948]

Vertebral artery angiography

The vertebral arteries are particularly subject to compression by spondylotic and arthrotic changes, and the segmental level of impingement can be anywhere between C1 and C6 segments.[285]

The vertebral arteries can be visualised by retrograde pressure injection of the brachial arteries[315] and a right brachial angiogram will opacify the right vertebral artery from its point of origin to, and including, the basilar artery.

The vascular condition of 'subclavian steal' may produce symptoms which closely resemble vertebrobasilar insufficiency, and vertebral artery angiography, via a midstream injection into the ascending aorta, is of value in elucidating the cause of symptoms.

Cineradiography and fluoroscopy

These two methods of dynamic visualisation[348, 349, 1331] are ideal to study normal and abnormal movement of the cervical spine[981] but do not allow precise measurement of ranges of movement. Enlargement of individual frames of cine-film is of limited value, since the loss of fine detail compares poorly with a standard radiograph. Further, the patient may 'run off' the screen during dynamic studies of movement.

Some authors suggest that a combination of radiographic methods may be necessary to clarify the causes of neck pain, for example, and advocate the use of odontoid views, oblique films, lateral films at extremes of movement, pillar views, tomograms and cineradiography, in the patient with obscure neck problems.[1332]

Among the large number of non-radiographic investigation techniques, some are:

Thermography

A healthy body shows a symmetrical temperature distribution, with a surface temperature range of about 12°C. Limb temperature falls off distally by about 2–3°C towards fingers and toes. A thermographic or heat camera measures the body's infrared 'glow', which is proportional to temperature, and transduces it to electrical impulses which can then be recorded as a multichromatic photograph. Surface body temperature is very closely linked to blood flow, and abnormalities due to drug effects, disease or injury may cause the abnormal tissues to become hotter or colder than the normal surrounding tissue.[609]

While the technique has considerable application in detecting the degree of vascularity of the extremities, it can also be an aid in assessing the *extent* of some types of neoplasm. It is also capable of detecting inflammatory processes in joints, and a 'hot' thermogram may uncover sacroiliitis before the characteristic radiographic changes become manifest (p. 285).[1074]

A thermogram of the asymptomatic individual's back reveals a symmetrical tadpole-shaped area—the 'paravertebral warm area'. In patients with back pain, thermography frequently revealed a paravertebral area which was asymmetrical, lacked continuity and was accompanied by 'cold patches' over the gluteal region in some. In pain-free subjects, the gluteal 'cold patches' were absent.[1215]

Nerve root infiltration

The infiltration with local anaesthetic of an involved nerve root at its point of emergence will eradicate the sciatic pain and thus demonstrate the site of the lesion.[780] Placement of the needle requires different approaches for the fifth lumbar and first sacral roots.

After localisation of the needle a contrast material is injected, and if placement is correct the root sleeve is outlined on radiography as a tubular shape. Local anaesthetic is then injected.

Electrodiagnosis

Electromyography is valuable in that while it may not provide the specific clinical diagnosis[175] it is able to localise specific root involvement, and the presence of multiradicular involvement; evidence that more than one root is involved can be of prime importance in assessing the indications for conservative or surgical management of the patient (see p. 107).[569, 613] Electrodiagnosis also offers a means of distinguishing between a neurapraxia and more severe nerve injury, and thus prognosis.[1038] The e.m.g. is valuable in assessment of hysterical paralysis.

The major e.m.g. changes associated with nerve root compression are fibrillation potentials and positive sharp waves at rest; there is also a decrease in the number of active potentials on voluntary contraction. Macnab (1977)[780] observes that myelography and electromyography should be used to supplement each other.

Magora *et al.* (1974)[785] examined 57 patients with headache syndromes and found e.m.g. evidence of neuropathic or spinal lesions in the seminspinalis muscles in a high proportion of them.

The second remarkable observation was the high incidence of neuropathic lesions disclosed by e.m.g., even though a careful neurological examination did not reveal any pathological signs.

Troup (1975)[1247] demonstrated by e.m.g. that the two heads of gastrocnemius are differentially affected by lumbosacral radiculopathy; the medial head most commonly by L5 root lesions and the lateral head by lesions of S1 root.

Electroencephalography

The use of e.c.g. has demonstrated that acceleration and deceleration trauma (whiplash injuries) to the neck and head can cause a similar clinical picture, and similar e.c.g. abnormalities, to those resulting from a direct blow to the head.[1231]

Electronystagmography and cupulometry

The basis for e.n.g. recording is the corneoretinal potential. The cornea is positively charged with respect to the retina, effectively transferring the eye into a rotating dipole.[679, 1341]

Four e.n.g. electrodes are placed around the eye to record vertical and horizontal nystagmus, the fifth electrode acting as a ground. Vestibular dysfunction demonstrated by this, and other, tests still remains for several years after whiplash trauma, and may later be responsible for recurring symptoms under conditions of physiological or pathological stress.

Intervertebral disc manometry

The *in vivo* intradiscal pressures are measured by a specially constructed needle with a pressure-sensitive membrane at its tip.[883] The pressures are recorded on an electromanometer to which the needle is connected. The needle is introduced into the nucleus pulposus, a discogram serving as a guide that the needle is correctly located in the nucleus pulposus.

In the last decade intradiscal pressures have been recorded in a variety of postures and during a variety of voluntary activities, and have contributed significantly to knowledge of forces sustained by the lumbar intervertebral disc.[890]

Cystometry

Occult bladder dysfunction appears to be a major manifestation of lumbar nerve root compression.[1059] In 100 patients with the provisional diagnosis of lumbar root involvement, routine bladder evaluation by cystometrogram showed that the characteristics of bladder dysfunction were present in 83 per cent. Residual urine was found in 20 per cent of the group.

The authors suggest that it may now be clear why some patients require catheterisation postoperatively, despite what may have been a relatively atraumatic surgical procedure; this proportion of patients probably had occult hypotonic bladders preoperatively, and the problem became overt postoperatively (see p. 150).

Radioactive isotope studies

Radioisotopes emit radiation while retaining their ordinary chemical properties, and thus by the rate of their breakdown demonstrate activity rather than structure.

A compound such as technetium polyphosphate, for example, will be concentrated at a bone tumour or an abscess, and will thus produce a 'hot spot' when recorded on a scanner. Radioisotope examination is the method of choice for demonstrating multiple lesions such as neoplastic deposits in bone.[864]

Radioactive scanning techniques of the sacroiliac joint, for example, can reveal early cases of sacroiliitis some six months or more before radiographic examination shows abnormality. The radioisotope strontium (^{85}Sr) can be employed, and patients are given an intravenous injection of 50 microcuries; the uptake of strontium in the sacroiliac joints is measured 8 to 9 days afterwards.

While radiography gives an index of the difference between the integrals of the rates of bone formation and resorption, radioactive scanning techniques provide an index of the rate of bone formation. An increased uptake of strontium (^{85}Sr) indicates an active process.

Radioactive scanning of the uptake of fluorine-18 has detected acute osteomyelitis of the sacroiliac joint, when initial radiographs were interpreted as normal.[768]

Ultrasonography

This is a non-invasive investigation method in which a pulsed beam of ultrasound is passed through a body part; the beam is reflected from surfaces perpendicular to it and is recorded by oscilloscope. The type of scan may be linear or three-dimensional. Use of the method in bone is hampered by difficulties such as echoes from normal bone.[864]

Nevertheless, by inclining a transducer at 15° to the sagittal plane of lumbar spines, Porter *et al.* (1978)[1000] directed a 2 cm diameter beam of ultrasound through the thin bone of a lamina, and thus obtained three major echoes: (i) from the posterior surface of the lamina, (ii) from its anterior surface and (iii) from the posterior surface of the vertebral body.

A sagittal, or more lateral, movement of the transducer causes high absorption of sound by the spinous processes and the facet-joint structure, respectively.

The mean oblique sagittal diameter of the spinal canal can be measured with a high degree of accuracy by the inclined transducer beam. This non-invasive technique can thus demonstrate the degree, and cephalocaudal extent, of spinal stenosis (see p. 275); it may reveal bony encroachment which is not detectable by myelography, and measurement at each lumbar level will help planning of the surgical decompression.

Psychometry and personality studies

There is clear recognition[1309] that when personality factors are unfavourable, a poor prognosis of the effectiveness of surgery for lumbar pain is virtually certain, no matter how accurate the anatomical diagnosis or how skilled the surgeon.

Studies have demonstrated that some patients with certain personality traits, which can be evinced by tests, are less likely to respond to treatment than are those not exhibiting these traits.[891]

Since an individual's response to pain is very much a psychological phenomenon,[407] the development of a reliable formula for prediction of how a given patient is likely to respond to surgery has considerable advantage. Psychological tests such as the Minnesota Multiphasic Personality Inventory (MMPI) and the Cornell Medical Index (CMI) have been found to be of value. Combined with the surgeon's preoperative evaluation of the degree to which symptoms might be of psychogenic origin, the preoperative use of the MMPI, CMI and Quick tests on a group of 130 patients having chymopapain injections allowed the derivation of an easily applied prediction formula.[1328]

Patients with low scores on the MMPI hysteria and hypochondriasis scales were 90 per cent certain of having a good or excellent symptomatic improvement, while only 10 per cent of patients with high scores showed this amount of improvement.

Nuclear magnetic resonance

Herman (1979)[536] has described how the measurement of nuclear magnetic resonance, an analytical method well established in chemistry since the 1940s, can be adapted to analyse small body regions; the analysis can be expressed as a black and white density image, i.e. a photograph.

The method is based on a physical phenomenon in which radio waves stimulate transitions between the spin states of nuclei in a magnetic field.

The atomic nuclei of hydrogen atoms, which are present in tissue in enormous numbers, act like tiny magnets. Each nucleus precesses (like a spinning top) thereby becoming a receiver or emitter of short-wave radio-frequency radiation. If a radio-frequency magnetic field is applied to the atom it absorbs energy and tips over. If the radio-frequency field is then removed the atom loses energy and eventually returns to its initial state of equilibrium. The rate of return is an exponential one with a time constant which depends upon the atom's environment. In viscous surroundings the return will be slow; in a more fluid one it will be faster. The wavelengths of the absorbed radiation, and the duration during which the nucleus returns to its original state, can reveal much about the chemistry of the environment of the nucleus.

Researchers are experimenting with methods of enhancing the signal strength by injecting tiny 'permanent magnets' (paramagnetic ions) into the blood stream; the method is roughly analogous to the injection of contrast media to show up the radiotranslucent areas in X-rays.

The images produced so far by physicists, chemists and computer experts have been maps of the density of mobile protons; in other words, the water content, yet by taking the NMR spectra of a number of different atoms (protons, phosphorus, sodium and possibly carbon and nitrogen) a complete chemical analysis may be possible.

Since the tissues of a 70 kg person contain some 42 kg of water, this investigation method plainly has promise.

There is some evidence that the environment in a tumour differs from that in the normal tissue, and a map of relaxation time in principle would indicate the location of a tumour. Thus the technique holds special promise for the detection of tumours in soft tissue.

The method may be able to give clear information about areas of oedema and it may well, eventually, be a useful tool for monitoring blood flow and the movement of other body fluids and for imaging inaccessible anatomical regions such as the spinal cord and brain stem.

This possible method of non-invasive diagnosis appears to have no risks attached, so far as is known at present. NMR has similar applications to computerised tomography but also has important advantages. It does not use potentially dangerous forms of radiation. It does not *necessarily* require contrast media to be injected to make some tissues show up. It can take pictures directly of sections at any angle through the body. And by adjusting a few settings, the NMR equipment can produce pictures in which different tissues show up differently. Images of high quality have recently been produced, one clearly confirming a suspected cerebral neoplasm in a 22-year-old woman, and another demonstrating healthy intervertebral discs. The technique allows soft tissue discrimination.

12. Principles of treatment

Although largely benign and eventually self-limiting, degenerative joint disease of the spine resembles chronic respiratory disease, in that its slow progression over many decades is marked by exacerbations which are frequently related to functional, environmental and other stresses; as in the management of chronic bronchitis, for example, treatment aims must be realistically assessed against the known natural history of the disease.

The pace and degree of degenerative changes in joints and their associated tissues differ widely from person to person, and in general terms the morphological changes of degeneration have little direct relationship to the amount of pain or functional disablement suffered by an individual at any particular time.

In clinical practice, the classical division between conservative and radical treatment becomes less important as the combined skills of the medical, surgical and paramedical team are applied to help the patient. Consequently, treatment methods are discussed under the headings of general principles, one of which may be the guide for medical, physiotherapy, and surgical procedures. For example, in the management of three patients, *relief of pain* is the dominant reason for the three treatments of:

—medical prescription of analgesic drugs
—carefully graded manual mobilisation to the vertebral segment
—surgical removal of prolapsed disc material or overgrowth of bone for relief of severe root pain by decompression.

Again, the principle of *stabilisation* of a vertebral segment may underlie:

—provision of a supportive collar for the neck
—exercises to strengthen the abdominal wall muscles in low back pain
—segmental strengthening of intrinsic muscle like rotatores and multifidus
—surgical fusion (arthrodesis) of an unstable segment.

Further, one method of treatment may meet different requirements; for instance, while support in the form of a stiff cervical collar may temporarily or semipermanently *stabilise* a painless but dangerously unstable segment, for which surgical fusion may not be feasible, for another patient the purpose of a soft collar is to *ease the pain of an irritable spinal segment by resting it* for a short period.

Spondylosis and arthrosis
When symptoms and signs indicate a predominantly *spondylotic* pattern, the emphasis of treatment is placed on:

1. Rotatory manual mobilisation.
2. Traction—sustained or rhythmic, but always sustained if there is nerve root involvement with root irritability.
3. Stabilisation—by mechanical support if necessary, and by surgical fusion if indicated, but often by correction of muscle imbalance with strengthening exercises.
4. Surgical decompression for intractable symptoms.

The latter, for example, may take the form of a cervical hemifacetectomy, for relief of root pressure, or removal of protruded lumbar disc material for the same reason.

When the clinical features are predominantly those of *arthrosis*, the main treatment emphasis is on:

1. Localised movement, whether produced by manual mobilisation, manipulation, rhythmic traction (in the absence of irritability) or specific exercise.
2. Supports, which are less indicated in degenerative conditions of synovial joints, but may be required for a limited period to ease pain by allowing irritability to settle.

Therefore, while not all of the treatments tabulated under 'Principles' are applied in all cases, and the management of the patient may include perhaps analgesics and heat, with postural correction and prophylactic advice, the emphasis of *active treatment*, if indicated, will be on traction for spondylosis and movement for arthrosis, *when the clinical features are clear enough for the distinction to be made* (p. 378).

AIMS OF TREATMENT

The primary treatment aim is restoration of normal painless joint range by:

1. Relief of pain and reduction of muscle spasm
2. Restoration of normal tissue-fluid exchange, soft-tissue pliability and extensibility, and normal joint mobility
3. Correction of muscle weakness or imbalance
4. The stabilisation of unstable segments
5. The restoration of adequate control of movement
6. Relief from chronic postural or occupational stress
7. Functional reablement of the patient
8. Prevention of recurrence.

The aims will assume differing orders of importance between individuals.

The following tabulated list, which is not exhaustive, is arranged as examples of method to indicate the variety of ways in which the principles of treatment may be applied.

Relief of pain

Injection of
—local anaesthetic
—hydrocortisone
Oral analgesic and/or anti-inflammatory drugs
Heat—SWD
    —MWD
Ice
Ultrasound
Rest
Support
Massage, e.g. inhibitory pressures
Mobilisation
Stretching
Manipulation
Traction
Acupuncture
Operant conditioning
Electro-analgesia
Counter-irritation

Surgical
Epidural injection
Chymopapain injection
Rhyzolysis:
 (i) by stab injection
(ii) by radio-frequency
Disc fenestration
Disc enucleation
Decompression
Fusion by arthrodesis

Movement

Active mobility exercises
—regional
—segmental
Hydrotherapy
Massage
Mobilisation
Manipulation
Traction

Surgical
Joint manipulation under anaesthesia
Nerve root stretch under epidural and/or general anaesthesia

Stabilisation

Support
Muscle-strengthening exercises
—regional
—segmental
Correction of muscle imbalance

Surgical
Fusion
Sclerosant injection

Postural correction

Passive stretching of contracted soft tissue
Active exercises to stretch contracted tissues
Re-education by postural exercises
Correction of sleeping posture
Unilateral heel raise, for example

Functional reablement

Restoration of confidence
Job analysis
Ergonomic correction of
—work posture
—driving posture
—lifting and handling
Prophylactic advice

Surgical
Postoperative rehabilitation

They cannot always be clearly differentiated. Consequently, so far as physical treatment is concerned, a *working hypothesis* may be stated as a set of principles:

1. There is relatively little relationship between radiologically evident degenerative change and the symptoms reported by the patient.
2. There is a very close relationship between *loss of function, or abnormal function*, and signs and symptoms.
3. Loss of function is very frequently found at sites other than those of degenerative change as such.
4. Chronic degenerative changes will remain when normal function consistent with age is restored, and symptoms are partially or completely relieved.
5. Loss of function is, for the most part, manifested in terms of abnormalities of movement.
6. Treatment is directed, in the main, to *states of reversible diminished movement due to soft-tissue changes*, with their consequences; but also at times to mild degrees of hypermobility.
7. Methods are essentially regional and localised movement (including traction) begun and graded according to examination findings.
8. Syndromes of instability are treated by measures to stabilise vertebral segments.

Because the common vertebral (and peripheral) joint problems are, in the main, abnormalities of movement for one reason or another, it follows that treatments involving the application of movement would form the lynchpin of therapeutic methods, together with one or more associated treatments; it is for this reason that treatment by movement forms the bulk of the methods described in this text.

Common vertebral joint problems, and more especially low back pain, comprise by far the most costly ailment of modern society.[869, 1339]

While there is a gratifying increase in recognition of the value of manipulative procedures, *a much more important development is recognition of the potential of informed and experienced manipulative therapists working ethically as part of the medical team.*

Mooney and Cairns (1978)[869] emphasise this aspect:

We believe that there is a role for passive assisted joint mobilisation (manipulation?) by the therapist. There is every reason to expect that a joint unable to proceed through its full anatomic range is abnormal. If mobilisation by manual therapy can increase this range, the joint should benefit. If this is the only therapeutic manœuvre it is a short-sighted one, but when incorporated into a progressive exercise program focused on improving function and enhancing strength and endurance, it has a useful role. Physical therapists functioning in a responsible medical environment offer the greatest potential for this manœuvre to be pursued in an ethical setting wherein comparison of results with other methods can be challenged.

DEFINITIONS

For commonly used procedures, descriptive terms and phrases may vary between groups of workers and from country to country, e.g. the word 'manipulation' may for one group refer specifically to localised thrust techniques of short amplitude and high velocity, while for another national group the word may be used mainly as a general term covering *any* manual or mechanically applied movement of body parts. Again, the one word may correctly be employed in either the general or the specific sense.

Definitions are given below for terms used in this text:

Passive movement is any movement mechanically or manually applied to a body part; there should be no voluntary muscular activity by the patient. Such treatment therefore includes:

1. Massage
2. Maintenance movement
3. Mobilisation
4. Manipulation
5. Stretching (A) (See also Stretching (B) in 'Massage')
6. Traction.

1. *Massage:* Passive movement of soft tissues, usually manually but sometimes mechanically applied.

2. *Maintenance movement:* Passive movement to preserve existing joint mobility, soft tissue extensibility, and kinaesthesis, where voluntary movement is not possible or is temporarily undesirable.

3. *Mobilisation:* The attempted restoration of full painless joint function by rhythmic, repetitive passive movements to the patient's tolerance, in voluntary and/or accessory range *and graded according to examination findings.* The patient is at all times able to stop the movement if so wished. This may affect a whole vertebral region or be localised so far as is possible to a single segment.

4. *Manipulation:* An accurately localised, single, quick and decisive movement of small amplitude, following careful positioning of the patient. It is not necessarily energetic, and is completed before the patient can stop it. The manipulation may have a regional or a more localised effect, depending upon the technique of positioning the patient.

5. *Stretching (A):* Sustained or rhythmically intermittent force applied manually or mechanically to one aspect of a body part, to distract the attachments of shortened soft tissue. Both of the therapist's hands are in firm contact with body points providing attachments for the shortened tissue.

6. *Traction:* Sustained or rhythmically intermittent force, manually or mechanically applied in the longitudinal axis of a body part, and thus to all aspects of it.

In 1–6, there should be no voluntary muscular activity by the patient, although involuntary spasm is often present and may be the reason for treatment.

Massage: mobilisation of soft tissues

In the final analysis, all movement techniques whether mobilisation, stretching, manipulation or traction, are movements of the soft tissues, and the justification for a separate classification is to draw attention to the prime importance (see p. 113) of including techniques which have the specific purpose of improving the vascularity and extensibility of the soft tissues.

Because:

(i) Normal muscle function is dependent upon normal joint movement
(ii) Impaired muscle function perpetuates and may cause deterioration in abnormal joints (p. 115)
(iii) Muscles cannot be restored to normal if the joints which they habitually move are not free to move

the treatment of joint disturbances should include measures which relax *muscle* and restore its normal vascularity and extensibility, while restoration of *normal painless joint range* remains the primary treatment aim. The classical use of massage, as a method of relieving pain, promoting relaxation and the reduction of muscle spasm, reducing swelling and improving circulation must be as old as pain itself, and is well described in many texts.[850, 1180a]

Similarly, the importance of deep transverse frictions and the technique of their application are described by their innovator, Dr James Cyriax.

The following description of treatment methods for soft tissue is restricted to those which are commonly employed in the management of vertebral joint problems:

a. Stroking
b. Stretching (B)
c. Inhibitory pressure
d. Kneading
e. Vibration
f. Frictions

a. *Stroking, or effleurage*, may be firmly and deeply applied with the greatest possible area of hand contact, to relieve fluid congestion of a body part, but is more usually employed as a method of inducing relaxation in a tense, anxious patient. A minute or two spent in slow, rhythmic stroking over a region of muscle spasm is often worthwhile, since it not only allows time for the patient to begin settling down but also gives the therapist an opportunity to become more familiar with the state and texture of the soft tissues.

b. *Stretching (B)* is applied either along the length of a muscle or transversely across its belly, and while the technique is called muscle stretching it will be plain that all musculoskeletal soft tissues are influenced by it in varying degrees. Distinguished from Stretching (A) because the therapist's hands, fingers and thumbs remain in contact with soft tissue only.

In longitudinal stretching techniques, the slow, deep finger, thumbpad or heel-of-hand traction movements are rhythmically applied with the body part disposed so that elongation of muscle and connective tissue is possible; when giving transverse stretching movements across muscle bellies, the same disposition of the patient is necessary.

c. *Inhibitory pressure.* With the patient comfortably disposed and the attachments of the hypertonic muscle(s) approximated, pressure is applied over the belly of the muscle by finger or thumbpad, thenar or hypothenar eminence. Pressure is slowly increased and as slowly relaxed, after a minute or so of sustained contact. Pressure may be repeated at the same locality or on an adjacent section of the muscle, and is continued until the palpable contraction is felt to relax, or it becomes plain that the hypertonicity will not respond to this particular technique.

d. *Kneading and petrissage* are not dissimilar in that both techniques are directed to improving the tissue-fluid exchange, vascularity and normal texture of subcutaneous and deep soft tissue. The various manipulations all have the quality of alternate traction, picking-up or squeezing and relaxing movements of a localised mass of tissue held between fingers and thumbs, or between hypothenar eminences; a muscle mass is treated by handling small sections of it at a time until the whole region has been treated. The method may be combined with stretching (which is only a regional variant of kneading) or with inhibitory pressures, and an important effect is that of assisting muscular and general relaxation.

e. *Vibrations* may be applied by fingertips, but effective technique is difficult to acquire and requires long practice; further, the method is less suitable for the large muscle masses of the trunk and limb girdles, and since a powered vibrator is much easier to use as well as being effective, it seems sensible to employ one.

The tonic vibratory reflex (de Domenico, 1979),[236] a reflex increase of tone in response to a vibratory stimulus of low amplitude (>3 mm) with a frequency of around 100 Hz, is useful in the re-education of weakened phasic muscles, where these are the antagonists of tight postural musculature (see p. 114).

The slow tonic contraction lasts for some 20 seconds, and repeated applications of the vibrator produce an augmented response.

Notwithstanding its use to facilitate a weak voluntary contraction, or to initiate one, in neurological conditions, clinical impressions are that vibratory treatment of paravertebral regions of referred pain, and of the secondary muscular aches segmentally associated with spinal joint problems, is also a valuable adjunct in improving vascular exchange within the muscle. The paradox that such a *stimulus* may often induce a following *after-relaxation* remains unexplained, although it has been suggested that frequencies of 20–50 Hz tend to produce inhibition[567] and also an effect upon the autonomic nervous system.[345]

Mastny (1974) stresses the value of vibratory treatment in the management of traumatic and degenerative joint conditions.[814]

f. *Frictions* may be applied transversely to the localised attachment points of muscle, tendon, aponeurosis and ligament, or in a firm circular fashion with thumbpad or heel of hand along an extensive bony attachment such as the iliac crest.[217]

Connective tissue massage

Superficial soft tissue manipulation, by rhythmic and carefully applied fingertip traction strokes, can achieve physiological and therapeutic effects which are difficult to explain,[290, 377] other than on the basis of somatic and visceral structures sharing a common segmental neurone pool in the spinal cord.

In this connection, it is important not to overlook the rich and varied innervation of the one structure which lies between us and our environment, i.e. the skin with its superficial connective tissues, together with its equally rich central nervous system connections.

Careful palpation of superficial structures reveals areas of tightness and hyperaesthesia which are often unknown to the patient, and which when appropriately treated by the stroking techniques can improve the blood supply of extremities and assist in the treatment of back pain.

The zones for treatment are based to a degree upon the topography of Head's Zones (p. 178).

NB: The benefits of improved vascularity, tissue-fluid exchange and restoration of normal extensibility may well be an important factor in the therapeutic effects of treatments like regional mobilisation, specific mobilisation or rhythmic traction, although there is no absolute certainty that this is so.

Maintenance movements

As previously defined, these movements sometimes have a place in re-education of postural abnormalities of the vertebral column, but for the most part find their best use in the management of inflammatory arthritis and neurological conditions.

Mobilisation and manipulation

In the general sense, *any* movement technique applied to musculoskeletal tissues mobilises them by manipulation, which may be manual or mechanical and, further, may be localised or regional.

These passive movements may be categorised as follows:

Techniques under the control of the patient
Soft tissue techniques (massage)
Regional mobilisation
Specific or localised mobilisation
Stretching (sustained or rhythmic)
Traction (sustained or rhythmic)

Apart from sustained stretching and sustained traction, all of these techniques have the quality of rhythmic repetition, and are under the control of the patient in that the patient can stop the movement at any time if so wished. Mobilisation as defined (p. 378) is a graded movement (see p. 421).

Techniques not under the control of the patient
Regional *manipulation* (including distraction techniques)
Specific or localised *manipulation* (including distraction techniques)

After careful and precise positioning of the patient, these techniques are single, high-velocity movements of short amplitude, and are not under the control of the patient, since the movement is completed before the patient can stop it. They are distinguished by the speed of movement, and are categorised as grade V techniques when vertebral *regions* are manipulated, and Localised grade V techniques when every effort is made to localise the movement to a particular *segment*. There is probably no such thing as a completely segmentally localised vertebral manipulation; true isolation of effect to a single segment is virtually impossible.

MANIPULATION IN GENERAL TERMS

The history, development and various types of treatment by orthopaedic surgeons, orthopaedic physicians, physiotherapists, osteopaths, chiropractors, naturopaths and bonesetters have been described in very many texts.

Manipulation belongs to no man, nor to any professional group; indeed, it has the happy knack of being all things to all men. Some professional groups seem to claim it for their own, while for the timid and overconservatively minded it can conveniently be cast in the role of an Aunt Sally, or scapegoat.

Occasionally, there is justification for this, e.g. when patients unfortunately have been subjected to imprudent treatment by the euphoric rogue-elephant manipulator.

It is an equally convenient platform for the clinical worker who, at heart, is no more than a rule-of-thumb bonesetter, with a reach-me-down set of concepts about things being 'out' and requiring to be 'put back' or 'sucked back'.

Historical descriptions which attempt to clarify the various schools of manipulative treatment, and then somewhat rigidly categorise them, are of limited use because while an individual who is well experienced in a particular method may have a working acquaintance with other methods, no one person can really know enough of each to pronounce with full knowledge and impartiality on all of them. Hence it becomes a matter of opinion and of inclination. Further, human frailty and curiosity being what they are, what is vehemently preached from any particular pulpit is never quite the same as what goes on between the pews, because congregations are people; all of us have our supposed falls from grace, we incorporate something from all treatment philosophies in what we do, and rightly so. It is also human to do what one wants or likes to do, and then to rationalise afterwards, or to make a virtue of expediency.

Jacob Bronowski (*The Ascent of Man*, 1973)[134] reminds us, '... there is no absolute knowledge. Those who claim it, whether they are scientists or dogmatists, open the door to tragedy. All information is imperfect. We have to treat it with humility. That is the human condition.'

When rationalisation becomes threadbare and contrived, and reveals only an overriding wish to impose arbitrary order by *diktat* upon things which nobody really understands very well anyway, Bronowski's homily has especial meaning for us.

a. PROCEDURES AND RATIONALE

Briefly, *orthopaedic surgeons* tend to employ manipulations with the patient under general anaesthesia; the movements are more frequently gentle and prudent, and comprise a passive traverse of normal voluntary joint range, so far as the underlying condition allows. The spinal techniques amount to regional, rather than segmental, manipulation.

Orthopaedic physicians dislike manipulating a generally anaesthetised patient and commonly employ regional mobilisation or manipulation techniques (what we might term 'environmental manipulation') whose effect can be reported by the conscious patient; thus the manipulator is guided by the changing patterns of signs and symptoms. Where possible, the manual manipulative procedures include traction; where not, they do not, and thus the declared virtues of applied traction during manipulation are only partially applicable.

Physiotherapists tend to rely on repetitive persuasive and accurately localised techniques which are carefully modulated according to the highly variable nature of the single or combined movement-limiting factor, and particularly according to the joint's, and the patient's, tolerance. Specific or regional single grade V thrust techniques are occasionally used. Traction techniques, either manually or mechanically applied, are used in their own right and are not routinely combined with other techniques. Segmental and regional vertebral exercises are an important part of treatment procedures.

The chiropractic method favours direct manual intervention methods applied to the bony prominences of the vertebrae, with a speed and vigour which takes reflex defences by surprise.

The osteopath (a meaningless word, but no more so than many terms in current use; for example, spondylosis merely means 'an excess or fullness of the spine', and arthrosis merely means 'an excess or fullness of the joint'). The osteopath tends to employ soft tissue techniques and regional or specific 'articulation', i.e. mobilisation, as a preparatory treatment before using specific thrust techniques. These are localised by using shorter or longer levers[1180a] and/or by skilfully fixing and protecting the chain of vertebral joints by what are termed 'locking' positioning techniques (see p. 425); these are not always without strain on uninvolved segments. Frequently, the preparatory treatment is enough, and thrust techniques transpire to be unnecessary. Gutmann (1968)[474] observes, '*The intervention of the two latter methods is carried out on the basis of a local diagnosis, and appears to take no account of factors other than movement-dysfunction of the joint in question.*' [My italics.]

Bonesetters have been referred to above.

There is no essential difference between the principles of manipulation for vertebral and peripheral joints,[450] so the principles can be expounded in relation to the vertebrae alone, bearing in mind the additional complications of the spinal cord and nerve roots, autonomic nerve trunks, important vessels and the ubiquitous intervertebral discs.

Defined by the *Oxford English Dictionary* as, 'to handle, deal skilfully with, manage craftily', manipulation, in the professional sense, can be held to cover any manual procedure applied passively to a relaxed body part, often for the restoration of joint range and functional relationship. The idea that force and flamboyance must necessarily accompany a manipulation is quite wrong. A specific joint movement of short amplitude and high velocity is occasionally indicated, yet by far the majority of effective manipulative work requires only the use of simpler, much more gentle and less dramatic mobilising procedures.[443]

Because of the most tenacious and traditional association of manipulation (in its general sense) with concepts of 'putting joints back',[1095] 'reducing subluxations', 'adjustment',[1180a] 'repositioning', 'correction' and so on, proffering a different approach to the manual treatment of common joint problems requires considerable persistence. The difficulty is compounded by the well-known therapeutic results of 'reducing' an intra-articular derangement of, for example, the knee, by manipulation. Yet to approach the passive-movement treatment of vertebral, sacroiliac and peripheral joint problems with only this somewhat simplistic doctrine in mind is considerably to reduce the possibilities of improving an understanding of the infinite variety of presentation of joint problems, gradually improving the number of successful treatments, and gaining the professional respect of peers and colleagues.[451]

Bearing in mind what has been said previously on asymmetry and anomalies (p. 280), the standpoint that 'symmetry is all' and asymmetry and distortion must always be 'normalised' becomes less tenable.

However, when a bony prominence of a vertebra appears to remain blocked or fixed in a position normally adopted during a natural asymmetrical movement, while the rest of the vertebral column (i.e. its adjacent or neighbouring segments) are in a neutral and resting relationship, it is always worth while considering the adaptation of techniques to influence these clinically detectable shifts of normal relationship *when assessed as of recent origin and associated with production of the symptoms reported. The important point is that 'reduction' is not always necessary for symptoms to be lastingly relieved.*

Those without special experience in this field often conceive manipulative treatment to be that of restoring range to a stuck joint, most often dramatically, by a single manual procedure. The restoration of movement and the relief of pain are conceived ideally to be instantaneous and accompanied of course by the obligatory click. The click has a certain value because patients are sometimes impressed by it and clinical workers are naturally interested in it, but apart from this it is of no especial importance.[1258]

Lewit (1978)[743] has suggested that manipulation is effective if: (a) there is some passive movement restriction, and (b) we achieve normalisation of mobility. He further suggests that if pain and exaggerated mobility coexist, manipulation is futile and may even be harmful.

Maitland (1977)[797] has carefully described the appropriate use of passive movement techniques when successfully treating pain associated with hypermobility, and thus the matter under discussion hinges around what is meant by manipulation.

Lewit[743] mentions the click, a typical articular phenomenon, as the sign of a successful manipulation. Not all workers would agree with this; while some successfully manipulated joints 'click' synchronously with the executive thrust, others do not. Often, the production of a 'click', perceived at the segment treated, is not accompanied by manipulative success, and the patient is no better.

A most superficial survey of the daily case-load of accident and emergency, orthopaedic, rheumatology, rehabilitation and sports injury clinics, and the multifarious needs of these patients with vertebral and peripheral joint pain in terms of passive movement techniques of one kind or another, suggests that to see manipulation proper as *only* the production of a click by facet-joint (or any other joint) gapping, is greatly to restrict its considerable and rightful place in physical medicine.

Edwards (1969)[307] has noted the successful application of passive-movement techniques in treatment of low-back pain, among the normal case-load of a general hospital. Patients treated with those techniques (Maitland, 1977)[797] were got better in about half the time taken for those treated by more traditional physiotherapy techniques.

It is also believed by many that manipulation necessarily means forceful treatment, and that this force is likely to damage joints and other structures.[443] Treatment by manipulation is the prerogative of no one professional group, and it does not follow that because orthopaedic surgeons, orthopaedic physicians, osteopaths, chiropractors, bonesetters and naturopaths use particular techniques, that only these techniques will relieve the signs and symptoms of a particular joint lesion (see p. 367), nor is it true that sudden, dramatic manipulations necessarily make the patient suddenly, dramatically better.

The release of fixation or blocking of a joint is a common everyday experience—most people have shaken about an elbow or knee, and on doing this have experienced a release of a temporary block to free movement. The author has a patient whose intractable headache was completely relieved when she stumbled down some steps and jolted her neck! (Her iatrogenic relief was unaccompanied by a click.) The experience may be likened to overcoming the immobility of a stuck drawer in a chest of drawers by rattling it about.

In relation to atlantoaxial dysfunction, Coutts (1934)[208] has defined what may be called a blocking, as 'fixation in a position possible to a normal neck', and this excellent working definition is a useful starting point for discussion of the purpose of treatment by passive movement.

What is the fundamental nature of the functional block to free movement? The plain truth is that we do not know, yet it is very likely that the phenomenon described occurs only in the synovial vertebral joints.

Research findings[313, 677, 743, 789, 1230, 1382] begin to indicate the possibility that locking may involve some derangement of the synovial meniscoid villus or fringe which projects into the joint cavity at nearly all spinal synovial joints; also, at times, the painful, fixed engagement of roughened, arthrotic facet-joint planes. It is no accident that the prime aim of many manipulative thrust techniques (some of which, it is important to recognise, were evolved mainly by the osteopathic school, at a time when the 'osteopathic lesion' was considered the essential mechanical vertebral abnormality) is to produce gapping of articular surfaces, thereby freeing the joint. Nor is it accidental that traction techniques figure so largely in passive movement for vertebral joint problems, albeit the notion of 'sucking back the disc' has been a factor in the past.

Were the concept of facet-joint blocking to be our only clinical preoccupation life would be simple, but the occasions when a vertebral joint fixation, because of a locked or blocked joint, is freed by a single manipulative thrust technique comprise only a very minor proportion of manipulative work. The one-shot dramatic manipulative treatment which *completely* relieves signs and symptoms is much more of a rarity than we are sometimes led to believe, or more importantly, would like to believe. Much more commonly necessary is the attentive, plodding analysis of joint problems, often occupying more than one treatment session, by orderly and logical method, and the progressive familiarisation of oneself with the salient clinical features which guide treatment procedures, and which differ so much from patient to patient.

The degenerative changes of spondylosis, osteophytic trespass, fibrosis, acquired stenosis, spinal root irritation, secondary contracture of soft tissue, segmental instability and segmental stiffness (for one reason or another) provide the major bulk of what we might term a family of 'abnormalities of movement', and since only 1 in 10 000 subjects progresses to the stage of myelography and major surgical procedures, i.e. 0.0001 per cent,[723] conservative treatment is of the utmost importance.

Lewit (1972)[739] observes that when *manipulative treatment relieves pain, it has succeeded in doing so purely through the normalising of disturbed function.*

There are many ways of normalising the disturbed function of structures which comprise the moving parts of the body, and even the most superficial acquaintance with the many schools of manipulation makes it plain that while they all have their successes the basic premise, rationale and treatment procedures adopted by each seem to differ considerably.

Greenman (1978)[440] observes that:

There is a wide and varying range of techniques that now fall under the term manipulation, or spinal manipulotherapy, and if one picks up various textbooks on the subject, one notes whole different systems. They vary from mild mobilisation or from very slight movements to various forms of massage, to gross nonspecific movement using femurs and shoulders and so on, to minute specific kinds of adjusting techniques which put a specific contact on either a transverse or a spinous process and give a very short, sharp thrust. So there is great variation in techniques by people who claim to be spinal manipulators, and a generalisation can never be made from a single qualified practitioner to the entire field of manipulation. Nevertheless, *all* of manipulative therapy is often dismissed on the basis of one technique.

Haldeman (1978)[787] has tabulated some hypotheses, from times past to the present, of the nature of therapeutic effects of manipulative therapy:

Theory	*Author*
1. Restore vertebrae to normal position	Galen (1958)[395]
2. Straighten the spine	Pare (1958)[969]
3. Relieve interference with blood flow	Still (1899)[1176]
4. Relieve nerve compression	Palmer (1910)[966]
5. Relieve irritation of sympathetic chain	Kunert (1965)[686]
6. Mobilise fixated vertebral units	Gillet (1968)[408]
7. Shift a fragment of intervertebral disc	Cyriax (1975)[218]
8. Mobilise posterior joints	Mennell (1960)[852]
9. Remove interference with cerebrospinal fluid circulation	De Jarnette (1967)[237]
10. Stretch contracted muscles, causing relaxation	Perl (1975)[986]
11. Correct abnormal somatovisceral reflexes	Homewood (1963)[566]
12. Remove irritable spinal lesions	Korr (1976)[675]
13. Stretching or tearing of adhesions around the nerve root	Chrisman *et al.* (1964)[174]
14. Reduce distortion of the annulus	Farfan (1973)[326]

It is plain that differing principles of approach, the considerable varieties of methods and the many hypotheses about effects leave us with little that is common to all of them.

If the technique and effects of simple massage are put to one side, then on further acquaintance, there appear to be only two factors which are common to all manipulative disciplines, namely: (i) skilful and confident handling; (ii) joint movement.

We might consider these factors as follows:

(i) Skilful and confident handling
Although adult patients are likely to stoutly reject the idea, most experienced practitioners might agree that those who present with varying degrees of painful damage to their locomotor apparatus, or who are temporarily disabled for their normal work and activity by pain, are actually in a state of mourning for their partial loss of physical function; many are also needlessly frightened of what the future may hold, in terms of an expected and fearful restriction of their locomotor freedom.

Perhaps in a part of their psychic, emotional world they have unconsciously become children again, and instinctively long for the omnipotent mother to take hold of the injured part, to handle it with loving care, skill and sympathetic interest; and to make them better—one way or another. Emotional maturity, social aspiration and intellect notwithstanding, it is very common indeed for people with restricting aches and pains from joints instinctively to seek out the therapeutic 'handler', whether orthopaedist, physiotherapist, osteopath, chiropractor, masseur, bonesetter or football team trainer.[138b]

Confident, gentle and skilful *handling* by whatever technique is a very powerful therapeutic weapon, and therapists who handle their patients with insight and understanding, and examine them attentively with care for detail,[629] have already won half the battle; willy-nilly, they have already been psychologically cast by the patient in the role of 'the sympathetic handler who will make me better', and the confident and skilful therapist fulfils the role, satisfying a deep and unconscious psychological need. Only so far as this powerful psychological need is concerned, the actual clinical method of handling pales into insignificance; so much so that, even should the therapist not make the patient sign- and symptom-free, the burden of pain may be considerably relieved, and the patient calmed and reassured.[138b]

Physical contact through the touch or palpating hands of doctors or physiotherapists is felt by patients as a particular expression of care and concern for them. Many acknowledge an almost electric sensation about their neck and back, in the area of the superficial trapezius muscle, or over their arms or hands, at the very prospect of physical contact, of massage, of attention. While physicians now largely express their concern and care by deep thought and the contemplation of the outcome of tests, physiotherapists still represent the most direct and natural expression of the impulse to help. The amount of physical contact with patients—particularly the lonely, the frigtened and the elderly—should never be reduced.[301]

So long as the human animal suffers benign but painful restriction of free bodily movement, so long will there be a need for those skilled in therapeutic handling. All the more desirable that the handling should be informed, prudent and of the highest academic standard.

(ii) Joint movement

The manual treatment of limbs and the spinal column has always maintained its place in official medical practice ... with the hand we are mechanically able to influence certain conditions of the tissues; above all the mobility of joints as well as the relationship between joint partners. However, *we also set in motion reflex effects* [my italics] and thereby the human hand may influence the regulation and control mechanisms of postural and movement systems. In a narrower sense, we mechanically try by manual therapy to restore *disturbed joint function* [my italics] to normal, so far as is possible.[474]

There is ample evidence that nociceptor activity giving rise to pain also generates extensive reflex effects; there is similar evidence (*vide infra*) that the simple passive movement of joints likewise generates reflex effects.

It is untrue that treatment by mobilisation and manipulation can be adequately discussed only on a mechanical cause-and-effect relationship; while we continue to regard musculoskeletal joint problems as simple mechanical ones, while we conceptualise only like mechanical engineers, our potential for better results will remain restricted.

Millions of asymptomatic individuals are walking about with mechanical joint problems.

Because of the work of B. D. Wyke[1354, 1357, 1361, 1363] and P. Polacek[998] we have every reason for progressing to the point where we begin to think like telecommunication engineers—since the most basic acquaintance with spinal joint neurophysiology and recent research findings indicate that the phenomenon of joint pain and its relief by mechanical techniques involve effects which transcend simple mechanical ones, e.g. widespread reflex changes in the degree of facilitation in spinal motor neurone pools, voluntary and smooth muscle tone, vasomotor and sudomotor tone and alterations in pulse rate, cardiac output and blood pressure.

If we add to this the effects of treating chronic changes at the junctional vertebral regions (p. 364), and that of modulating the chronic changes in texture and extensibility of the soft tissues (p. 113), simple therapeutic concepts of 'putting back' things which are 'out', or hoping to routinely deal with joint pain by manœuvres restricted to a single segment, begin to be seen as inadequate.[397]

There are many alternatives to high-velocity thrust techniques. For example, Jones (1964)[616] described the technique of spontaneous release by positioning, in which the patient is passively disposed in the position of greatest comfort and held there for some 90 seconds. After that interval, the patient is very slowly returned to the neutral position. Muscular hypertonus is released and voluntary guarding becomes unnecessary. The technique is applicable to both spinal[763] and peripheral joints, and is particularly useful in treatment of the painful shoulder.

Although treatment of a single segment is often sufficient in the very early stages of dysfunction of that segment, where none existed before, the greater majority of joint problems present as a complex of chronic changes.

There is no magic in the manipulator's hand, there is no mystique of manipulation. But there is a central mystery, and *it lies in the variety of responses of the abnormal joint to the different things we do in the way of treatment by passive movement of one kind and another.*

Joints cannot read books, or understand theories about technique; what suits one joint problem will not suit another. We must learn to be humble in the face of this mystery, we must learn to listen to what the abnormal joint is trying to tell us—in short, we must learn to *assess*.

b. NEUROPHYSIOLOGICAL EFFECTS

In the business of getting the patient better, the technically desirable movement, the movement which is logically based on biomechanical concepts, on the orientation and configuration of facet-joint planes, for example, is by no means always *the successfully curative movement;* we can only learn which is the therapeutic movement from the initial *responses* of the joint, and it is the author's belief that the ultimate understanding of this central mystery can be served, among the study of other factors, by improving our appreciation of the neurophysiological aspect of our work.

One essential point is that when applying the principles of mechanics to the prevention and management of back pain, the other biological factors which are relevant must be taken into account; in particular, the epidemiological, neurophysiological and psychophysical aspects.... Pain implies neurophysiological dysfunction, and its relationship to the pathomechanics of lumbar spinal disorders dominates the interpretation of signs and symptoms ... (Troup, 1979).[1250b]

Korr (1978)[676] has made some pertinent observations in this respect:

Manipulative procedures, even in the hands of the same practitioner, vary according to the findings and their changes in each visit; they vary from practitioner to practitioner, from patient to patient, and, for the same patient, from visit to visit. Manipulative therapy is no more a uniform therapeutic entity than is surgery, psychiatry or pharmacotherapeutics. Clinical effects are thought to be achieved through improvement in musculoskeletal biomechanics, in dynamics of the body fluids (including blood circulation and lymphatic drainage) and in nervous function.... It has been clear for many decades that the nervous system is a major mediator of the clinical effects of manipulative therapy, yet the precise mechanisms are still, for the most part, obscure.... According to our hypotheses, both the changes in afferent input and the transinduced changes in excitation and conduction of neural elements produce, in turn, changes in the central nervous system and in the periphery, reflected in aberrant sensory, motor and autonomic functions.

In an orthopaedic environment, there is much emphasis on: the protective role of the vertebral column; its function of giving attachment to muscle, and its biomechanical characteristics, for example, but it also has a much neglected *neurophysiological* function, i.e. of serving a neuromuscular reflex system which drives the perceptual and reflex basis of posture, movement and respiration;[1361, 96] of being a prime organ of equilibration.

Joints move only when muscles induce them to do so or allow gravity to do so. Muscles only do what nerves tell them to do, after the muscles have informed the nerve centres of their states of tension. The forces acting on joints and connective tissues of the vertebral column itself tell the nerves what to tell the muscles to do. Vertebral joints are extensively 'wired up', to the muscles which move them, by a very complex feedback or servo system; not only to the muscles which move them but to all other musculoskeletal systems including that of respiration, and also to vascular and visceral systems governed by autonomic nerves.

The afferent discharge from type I and type II corpuscular mechanoreceptors in the facet-joint capsules of the neck (p. 11), for example, produces reciprocally co-ordinated reflex effects on vertebral and limb musculature;[1363] thus disorders of posture and movement of the head, spine and limbs may result from traumatic, inflammatory and degenerative changes in the cervical joints. Unnecessarily vigorous manipulation and traction techniques may produce disturbances of this powerful cervical arthrokinetic system[1358] which can exert effects upon mandibular and external ocular musculature[1363] as well as that of spine and limbs. Conversely, repetitive and persuasive passive movements, within the tolerance of the patient, may be used to enhance mechanoreceptor afferent activity and thereby reduce awareness of pain.

All articular reflexogenic systems are polysynaptic—the afferent impulses from type I and type II mechanoreceptors operate through the fusimotor neurone-muscle spindle loop system, while those from type III mechanoreceptors (absent from spinal joints) and type IV nociceptors operate through the alpha motoneurones only.

Stimulation, whether mechanical or chemical, of *the nociceptor systems* in the connective tissues of the vertebral column also produces polysynaptic reflex contraction of the related portions of the paravertebral musculature (see p. 196)[979] and *examples of effects mediated via the nervous system in vertebral and peripheral joints* are as follows:

(i) Brief mechanical *stimulation of nociceptors*, in the facet-joint capsule of a spinal cat, will simultaneously evoke a large number of reflex alterations in the body, e.g. reflex spasm of the segmentally related musculature, as well as alterations in cardiovascular, respiratory and endocrinal function.[1356]

'It is the combination of all these spontaneously-occurring physiological changes, ... in the presence of pathological irritation of nociceptors, which makes up the totality of the patient's experience of pain.'

(ii) 'associated with the *active and passive movements* of joints in various parts of the body, and with the application of *limb and spinal traction*... afferent discharges from joint receptors exert potent reflex influences on the activity of the limb, paravertebral and respiratory musculature at spinal and brain-stem levels.'[1357]

Dee (1969)[244] presented the simultaneous electromyographic record of bilaterally co-ordinated arthrokinetic reflexes, as widespread changes in muscle tone in the ipsilateral and contralateral hip musculature of a lightly anaesthetised cat, during *passive abduction and adduction* of one isolated hip joint.

(iii) Electromyograms of articular reflexes in the intrinsic muscles of the cat's larynx (Fig. 12.1) recorded from pairs of needles inserted directly into the muscle, demonstrate the changes reflexly produced during movement of the *cricothyroid joint*.[1354]

(iv) Electromyograms of arthrokinetic reflex responses in the leg muscles of a cat, after a cuff of skin was removed from around the joint region and all tendons operating over the joint were divided, demonstrate rapidly and slowly adapting motor unit responses (Fig. 12.2) accompanying *passive movement* of the ipsilateral ankle joint.[1354]

(v) An electromyographic record of responses to *passive movement* of an ankle joint, before and after electrocoagulation of the joint capsule, demonstrates the absence of motor unit responses following electrocoagulation (Fig. 12.3).[1354]

Mechanoreceptor and nociceptor reflex effects upon the cervical musculature (Figs 12.4 and 12.5), and the reflex effects of cervical traction (rapidly applied to the apophyseal joints of a single cervical segment) upon the muscles of all four limbs (Fig. 12.6), leave no doubt about the widespread neurological effects of passive movement of the vertebral column.

While the research findings briefly referred to above provide an insight into the complexity and extent of neuromuscular changes which accompany joint abnormalities, our clinical grasp of the totality of these and other changes *occurring in the joint problems of individual patients* remains patchy. We do not just mobilise and manipulate joints, we mobilise complex arthrokinetic systems, which are functionally and neurophysiologically interdependent.

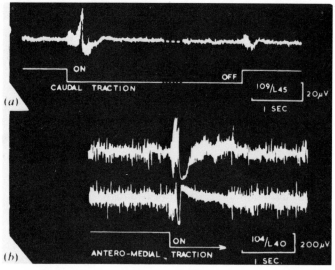

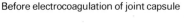

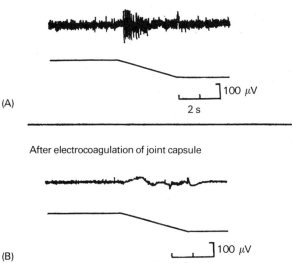

(A)

Before electrocoagulation of joint capsule

100 μV
2 s

After electrocoagulation of joint capsule

(B)

100 μV
2 s

Fig. 12.1 Electromyograms of articular reflexes in the intrinsic muscles of the cat's larynx, recorded from pairs of needle electrodes inserted directly into the muscles.

(A) Rapidly adapting motor unit discharges provoked in the detached left cricothyroid muscle at the onset and cessation of passive caudal displacement of the isolated ipsilateral cricothyroid joint. The interrupted line indicates a period of 60 seconds during which constant joint displacement was maintained. (From Kirchner and Wyke, 1965.)

(B) Reciprocally co-ordinated, rapidly adapting articular reflex responses in the thyroarytenoid muscle (above) and posterior cricoarytenoid muscle (below), displayed in simultaneous recordings during anteromedial displacement of the isolated ipsilateral cricothyroid joint. Note that, immediately following the joint movement, brief facilitation of motor unit activity in the (adductor) thyroartenoid muscle is accompanied by transient inhibition of activity in the (abductor) posterior cricoarytenoid muscle. Note also that slowly adapting changes in motor unit activity are absent in each of the tracings in (A) and (B).

(From Wyke 1967 The neurology of joints. Annals of the Royal College of Surgeons of England 41:25. Reproduced by kind permission of the author and the Editor.)

Fig. 12.3 Abolition of articular reflex responses in the leg muscles to passive movement of the ankle joint by electrocoagulation of the joint capsule. Both electromyograms were recorded from the same muscle (tibialis anterior). (A) Motor unit responses evoked in the tenotomised tibialis anterior muscle by passive plantarflexion of the isolated foot. (B) Following capsular electrocoagulation, the motor unit responses are absent. The myotatic reflex (not illustrated) was still elicitable in the muscle. (From Wyke BD 1967 The neurology of joints. Annals of the Royal College of Surgeons of England 41:25. Reproduced by kind permission of Dr B. D. Wyke and the Editor, Annals of the Royal College of Surgeons of England.)

Fig. 12.2 Electromyograms of articular reflex responses in the leg muscles of the cat to passive movements of the ipsilateral ankle joint. Prior to the recordings a cuff of skin was removed from around the joint region, and all tendons operating over the joint were divided and freed.

(A) Rapidly and slowly adapting motor unit responses in the tenotomised tibialis anterior muscle to plantarflexion of the foot.

(B) Rapidly and slowly adapting motor unit responses in the tenotomised gastocnemius muscle to dorsiflexion of the foot.

(From Wyke 1967 The neurology of joints. Annals of the Royal College of Surgeons of England 41:25. Reproduced by kind permission of the author and the Editor.)

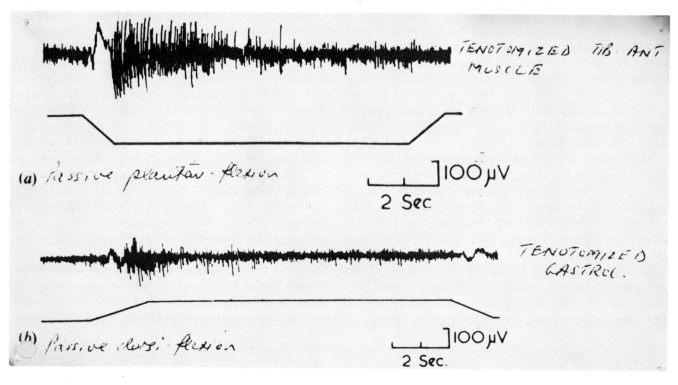

(a) Passive plantar-flexion

TENOTOMIZED TIB. ANT. MUSCLE

100 μV
2 Sec

(b) Passive dorsi-flexion

TENOTOMIZED GASTROC.

100 μV
2 Sec.

CERVICAL REFLEXES

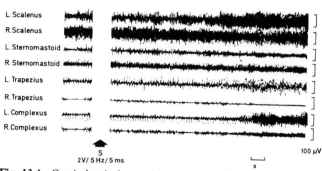

Fig. 12.4 Cervical articular mechanoreceptor reflex effects on neck muscles. At the arrow (S), a single cervical articular nerve supplying the left C3–C4 cervical apophyseal joint (isolated by microdissection in an anaesthetised cat) was repetitively stimulated electrically for 3 sec with stimulus parameters (indicated below signal) that selectively excite the mechanoreceptor afferent fibres in the nerve. The tracings are simultaneous electromyograms from homologous pairs of neck muscles, displaying the co-ordinated, long-duration reflexogenic effects; of articular mechanoreceptor afferent activation.
(Figs 12.4–12.6 reproduced from Wyke BD 1979 Neurology of the cervical spinal joints. Physiotherapy 65:72, by kind permission of Dr B. D. Wyke and the Editor.)

CERVICAL REFLEXES

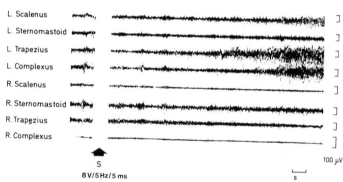

Fig. 12.5 Cervical articular nociceptive reflex effects on neck muscles. At the arrow (S), the same cervical articular nerve as in Figure 12.4 was repetitively stimulated electrically for 3 sec with stimulus parameters (indicated below signal) that excite the nociceptive (as well as the mechanoreceptor) afferent fibres in the nerve. The simultaneous electromyograms (from the same neck muscles as in Figure 12.4) display the altered patterns of reflex activity evoked by the additional activity of nociceptive afferents coming from the C3–C4 joint.

A pertinent observation is that the sinuvertebral nerve, which re-enters the intervertebral foramen from the paravertebral plexus (q.v.) and contains mixed somatic and autonomic fibres, is not a single filament but may consist of up to six filaments, which have a known propensity to wander up and down for several segments before their termination as end-organs.[299]

By our localised, and regional, procedures we may modify the whole musculoskeletal neurophysiology of the patient, and as yet we do not know nearly enough about their effects.

CERVICAL REFLEXES

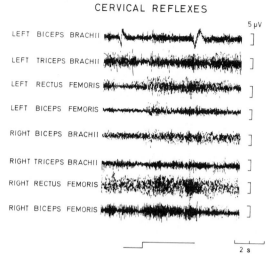

Fig. 12.6 Reflex effects of cervical articular manipulation. At the event signal, vertical traction was applied rapidly across the apophyseal joints between the C3 and C4 vertebrae (isolated by surgical microdissection from all tissues other than their nerve and blood supply in an anaesthetised cat). The simultaneous electromyograms from homologous pairs of upper and lower limb muscles display the articular mechanoreceptor reflex effects of such cervical manipulation (the accompanying reflex effects on the neck muscles are not illustrated here).

Seduction is more satisfying, and more effective, than assault, and for this reason alone, the method of localised persuasion is preferred, at least until the clinical terrain is understood; as in other walks of life, it is often less damaging to the object of our attentions and very frequently more productive.

c. MANIPULATION TRIALS

While some of the reported manipulation trials[270, 413] and other reports[253] suggest that manipulation is no better than any other treatment, this may well have come about because the right questions were not being asked in the right way.

Taking as his criteria: (i) full subjective and objective relief; (ii) detectable changes in spinal mobility Rasmussen (1979)[1014] studied a small group of 24 male patients with non-radicular low back pain of less than three weeks. The randomised treatment was either shortwave diathermy three times a week for 14 days, or manipulative treatment for the same period. Of the manipulative group, 92 per cent were free of symptoms in 14 days, and in all of them the mobility had improved. Of the shortwave diathermy group, 25 per cent were free of symptoms in 14 days and 50 per cent showed objective improvement of mobility.

The value of manual therapy in a very common benign joint condition, i.e. cervicobrachialgia, has been clearly presented by Kogstad et al. (1977).[669] One-third of the patients, referred in 1972 to a physical medicine department, had cervicobrachialgia. From 350 patients initially examined, 50 of them (38 men and 12 women, aged 23–65) satisfied the criteria of:

1. Age: under 65.
2. Pain of more than three weeks radiating from neck to shoulder/arm, with or without paraesthesiae.
3. Pain reproduction by testing neck movements (most frequently by a combination of extension, side-flexion and rotation to the painful side, i.e. reducing the size of the intervertebral foramina).
4. Hypomobility of the lower cervical region measured by 'the hemispheric test' (a recording of movement in degrees using the projections of a fixed indicator on the head in standard position on a hemispheric scale) and 'Myrin's vigoromotor test' (using the recordings from a compass in standard position on the head); and in addition osteopathic segmental mobility tests.

Excluded from the trial were psychoneurotics and patients with psychosomatic symptoms related to the neck, shoulder or arm; those with functional disorders in the neck/shoulder/arm region (e.g. tendinitis and tenovaginitis) and those with general pain or stiffness in muscles or tendons of the upper extremity.

The patients were randomly divided into three groups:

(i) *Manual therapy*—40 minutes twice a week for 4 weeks. Each session included heat, soft tissue treatment, specialist specific manipulation and instruction on posture, etc.

(ii) *Conventional therapy*—60 minutes three times a week for 4 weeks. Each session included heat, soft tissue treatment, isometric exercises, 15 minutes intermittent traction, and instruction.

(iii) *Placebo*—one placebo tablet three times a day for 4 weeks. These patients were informed about the disease, given simple ergonomic advice and asked to contact the hospital if they got worse.

The results of the treatment are shown in Table 12.1.

Table 12.1 Results of treatment

	5 weeks			18 months		
	No.	Worse/ no change	Symptom- free Much better	No.	Worse/ no change	Symptom- free Much better
Manual therapy	13	8%	92%	13	15%	85%
Conventional therapy	21	19%	81%	20	23%	77%
Placebo	16	50%	50%	15	50%	50%

Northupp (1978)[938] suggests that we should keep in mind that the musculoskeletal spinal lesion is not a *thing*—it is a complex process, a lesion of *motion*, and not something which can be sectioned or biopsied or seen on the autopsy table.

Sometimes the type of procedure will vary considerably, but the end point ... is always the same, and that is restoration of physiological motion within the normal constraints of that joint. To restore it to its maximum efficiency of range of motion. There are various ways of doing that.... And this is precisely the problem with clinical trials that purport to evaluate the efficacy of manipulative therapy and which use a standardised manipulative procedure on all of the patients. That is totally unrealistic. If you are going to evaluate manipulative therapy, then you ought to test it as practised. Every patient that I see—even the patients with the common complaint of back pain—I treat differently. Each patient is different, with a different kind of musculoskeletal problem, requiring an appropriate manipulative approach. I would never use the same treatment on a series of patients, because my experience tells me that it would be at least as frequently inappropriate as appropriate. (Greenman, 1978.)[440]

It is precisely for this reason that Maitland (1977)[797] has advocated basing the selection of procedures on *the unique way in which each individual joint problem presents*, and why assessment is so important. Unless trials of manipulation are imaginatively formulated with this in mind, they will continue to be a waste of valuable time, money and effort, and will only add to the general confusion.

d. GROUPING OF TECHNIQUES

The following *representative* examples of techniques, with observations about their use, are grouped according to the author's personal view (p. 381). A few examples of techniques for the limb girdle joints are included, since the treatment of vertebral joint conditions frequently requires some mobilisation of proximal peripheral joints.

For complete descriptions and illustrations of the great variety of manipulative methods (in the general sense), appropriate texts should be consulted.[390, 627, 797, 798, 1180a, 850, 851, 852, 217]

While some of Maitland's techniques (among others) are briefly described (p. 413), readers are referred to his textbooks.[797, 798] For applied movement which is *not* under control of the patient see page 422.

Because every joint movement also affects the soft tissues; almost every soft tissue technique disturbs joints to a greater or lesser degree; the grouping of treatment methods is often governed by treatment rationale rather than by the actual nature of the movement, there is no universally acceptable arrangement of the various categories.

Where the techniques, or adaptations of them, described by Maitland (1977)[798] are illustrated, the grade of movement is given.

Some of the symbols used by the author are in general use; some are not.

A. Soft tissue techniques
B. Regional mobilisation
C. Mechanical harness traction and manual traction
D. Localised mobilisation
E. Regional manipulation
F. Localised manipulation
G. Limb girdle joint techniques.

A. SOFT TISSUE TECHNIQUES

The object is mobilisation, and frequently a degree of stretching, of connective and muscle tissue. Relaxation is assisted and tissue-fluid exchange is stimulated; joint movement almost invariably occurs.

The restoration of normal painless joint range is the primary treatment aim. When the function of a joint is abnormal, there will follow sooner or later as a consequence, abnormalities of the muscles which cross it, e.g. spasm, weakness, wasting, tightness and ultimately a degree of fibrosis. These clinical features must be treated, but the primary attention must be given to the testing and treatment of the *joint*, even though the use of massage, for example, may occasionally be necessary to induce relaxation so that the joint can be treated.

While the *soft tissue techniques* of Stretching (A) are intended to affect specific muscles or groups of muscles, they are essentially regional techniques by reason of their field of effect.

1. As a first step, chronically shortened tissues should be stretched (i) passively and steadily; (ii) after maximal contraction, and by this stretching the inhibitory effect on weakened antagonistic muscle will be lessened.

2. Other factors (age, chronicity, etc.) given, if a satisfactory balance between the opposed muscles and other soft tissue is not achieved after three to five treatments of the shortened postural muscles, a specific training programme for the phasic muscle group must begin.

The ligamentum nuchae and other posterior soft structures in the suboccipital region sustain a localised stretch when upward and forward pressure applied to the occiput (Fig. 12.7A) is accompanied by a reciprocal downward and backward pressure, applied via the lower jaw.

A more generalised tension is applied to posterior cervical structures when the whole neck is flexed (Fig. 12.7B), while the upper thoracic region is stabilised by downward pressure on the upper sternal region. A degree of localisation may be obtained by shifting the occipital hand so that its heel applies the pressure lower down the neck (Fig. 12.7C). It is imperative to be gentle, and to apply the tension for two or three short periods, with a rest in between.

Transverse frictions are sometimes applied to aponeurotic muscle attachments at the nuchal line of occiput (Fig. 12.8).

Unilateral tension may be applied to the soft structures linking head, neck and shoulder by combining side-flexion and rotation away from the shortened side, and adding a degree of unilateral traction (Fig. 12.9). While the heel of the stabilising hand rests on the outer pectoral area (and not painfully on the point of the shoulder), the palmar surface of the therapist's right index finger can apply a degree of localisation, depending upon its positioning, by bearing

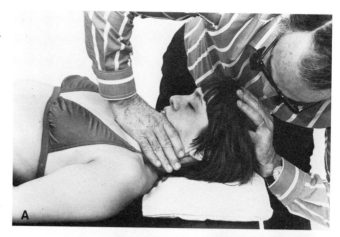

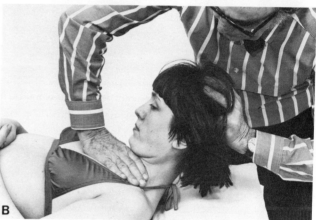

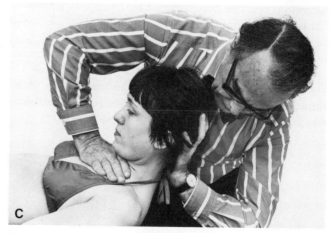

Fig. 12.7 Soft-tissue stretch of posterior cervical structures. (A) Suboccipital; (B) whole neck; (C) more localised to lower neck.

against a transverse process. While the therapist's stabilising hand remains unmoved, the patient's head and neck are returned to the neutral position by fairly large and rhythmic excursions of the therapist's body.

The scapular soft tissue attachments often need mobilising, and it is convenient to have the patient in side-lying, with the hips and knees flexed to 90°; this helps to stabilise the trunk. The patient's upper hand should lie under the chin.

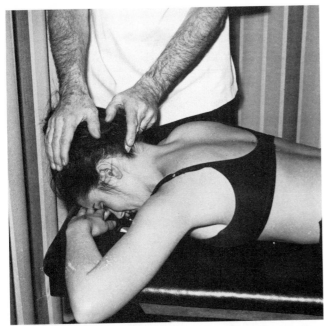

Fig. 12.8 Transverse friction to aponeurotic attachments of muscle to nuchal line of occiput.

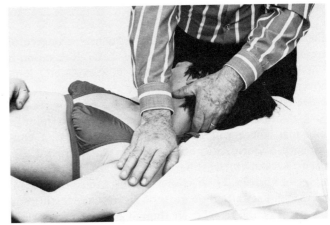

Fig. 12.9 Rhythmic unilateral soft-tissue stretching of structures common to the neck and shoulder girdle.

Finger grasp of the medial border of scapula, and sternal pressure on the patient's deltoid area, remain unmodified throughout the movements of scapular lifting (Fig. 12.10A), protraction (Fig. 12.10B), retraction, cranial and caudal mobilising. Thus these fairly large scapular excursions must be accompanied by equally large movements of the therapist's body.

The sacrospinalis muscle group, and associated connective tissues, may need unilateral stretching and mobilisation. This may be achieved in part by orthodox massage techniques, or by using methods which also have a considerable effect upon the more intrinsic joint structures.

In Figure 12.11, the patient is positioned as in Figure 12.10 and the therapist stands astride facing the patient

with his forearms resting on the patient's posterior axillary and gluteal regions. These regions are distracted by flexion of the therapist's hips and by simultaneous lateral movement of his forearms, while his fingertips lift the upper side muscle mass away from the spinous processes as he repetitively leans upon the patient. By extending the hips and allowing the forearms to approximate, distraction is released; the movement is rhythmically repeated. The effect is enhanced by a small hard pillow under the patient's loin, and further enhanced by exerting the finger pressure to 'lift' the spinous processes, as shown.

The lumbosacral region may require a unilateral distraction technique (Fig. 12.12A) with the patient in a side-lying position, over a hard pillow under the loin, and close to the plinth edge so that the degree of hip extension is minimal.

The patient's under hip and knee are comfortably flexed, and the upper limb lowered over the side of the support. By gentle pressure over the lower lateral femur with the caudal hand, and a stabilising pressure on the patient's gluteal region with the cephalic hand, a sustained

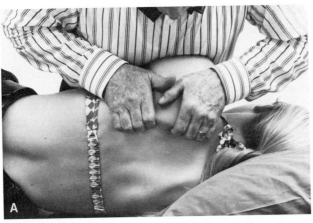

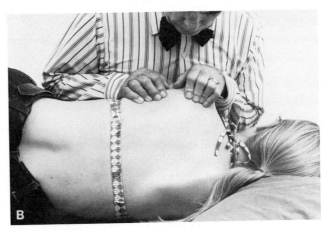

Fig. 12.10 (A) and (B) Mobilisation of the scapulothoracic articulation, by stretching techniques for soft-tissue attachments.

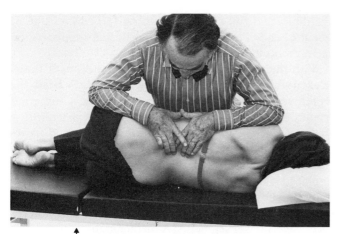

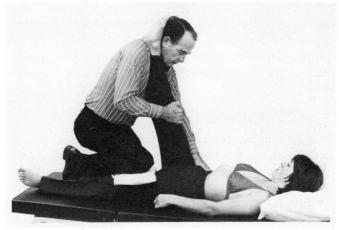

Fig. 12.11 ↑   Soft-tissue mobilisation of the paravertebral mass of the sacrospinalis muscle.

Fig. 12.13 ↖•   Unilateral mobilisation of restricted range of straight-leg-raising when root or joint irritability is absent and *restriction*, rather than *pain*, is being treated.

or rhythmic unilateral distraction of the lower lumbar region is achieved.

The technique may be adapted for vertebral listing or deviation (Fig. 12.12B, C).

Straight-leg-raising may be unilaterally restricted, and accompanied by chronic and stable root symptoms and/or unilateral hamstring tightness; these will require stretching.

With the patient supine on a low plinth, the therapist stabilises the pelvis and opposite limb by (i) palm pressure on the ipsilateral iliac spine and (ii) knee pressure on the lower contralateral thigh, which is protected by a flat pillow (Fig. 12.13).

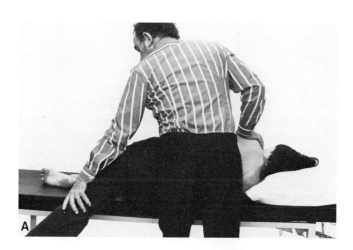

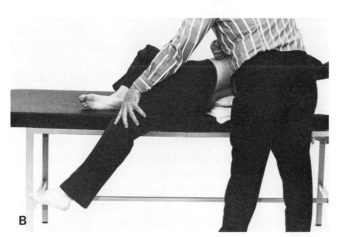

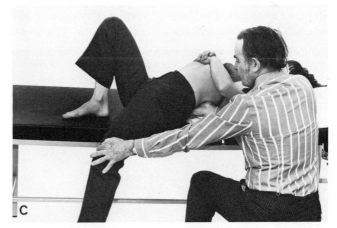

Fig. 12.12 (A) (B) (C) ⤝   (A) Unilateral stretch of lumbar and lumbosacral soft tissues of the patient's left side (or right side). When there is evidence of ipsilateral sciatic nerve root involvement, the technique is unsuitable since a further increment of root tension would be applied.[121b] The technique may also be adapted (B), to aid in the slow correction of listing, or listing with flexion, directly associated with a recent lumbar joint derangement but not complicated by established lateral pelvic tilt or neurological involvement. The patient should initially lie on the side deviated towards, with a loin raise of small hard pillows. The uppermost limb, at first resting on the plinth, is gently lowered to the floor. After some minutes the patient will become accustomed to the position and the therapist's supporting hand can be removed. The slow step-by-step rotation to the supine position may take up to thirty minutes. If pain is provoked at stage (B), and does not diminish with a few minutes' rest, it is wise to stop and slowly return the patient to the starting position. Following either the completed manœuvre, or its attempted completion, the patient intersperses floor resting, in a neutral position, with self-correction exercises before a mirror. The disposition of the lower limbs, e.g. degree of flexion of the under hip and knee, the height of the loin raise and time spent in getting the patient supine are variables which must suit the patient.

The therapist's other foot rests on the floor, while the free hand stabilises the patient's limb, with knee extended, against the shoulder of that side.

The stretch is imparted by a forward and upward movement of the therapist's trunk, by extension of hip and knee.

B. REGIONAL MOBILISATION

This description correctly applies to a wide variety of techniques, when defined as repetitive, rhythmic passive movement applied to vertebral *regions*, or at least to more than two segments.

Rhythmic manual or mechanical traction (p. 396) is perforce also regional mobilisation in this sense, although by careful positioning of the patient every effort may be made to produce the majority of the mobilisation or traction effect at a particular segment.

The osteopathic term 'articulation' refers to the same type of movement, with the important qualification that the effects are often carefully localised to a single segment, and commonly employed to improve the diminished range of a single movement of that segment.

Thus the word articulation,[1180a] when applied to techniques used in this way, might be equated with localised mobilisation, and these localised techniques are described later (p. 413). As will be seen, they are more often distinguished by the use of direct contact, through the soft tissues, with the bony apophyses of a single vertebral body.[798]

Cervical rotation. The patient lies supine with head and neck supported, beyond the edge of the plinth, by the therapist who stands at the patient's head. For left rotation, the therapist's left hand comfortably grasps the patient's chin, with full contact of palm and fingers on

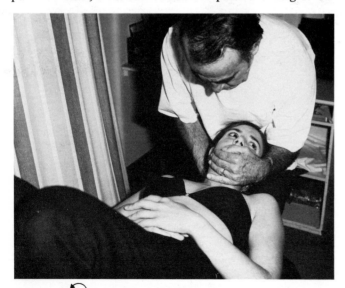

Fig. 12.14   Cervical rotation to the left, within a grade I amplitude, for a C2–C3 joint problem. For lower cervical segments, the neck would be more flexed.

mandible, and full contact of ventral forearm on side of face and head. The therapist's opposite hand supports the patient's occiput.

With the therapist's trunk held still, and upper limbs relaxed while positively supporting the patient's head, the repetitive, rhythmic left rotation movement is imparted around an imaginary longitudinal axis; *the movement is oscillatory because the hands move reciprocally and all excursions have equal value* (Fig. 12.14).

Localisation, in the sense that a particular segment may be placed in its most favourable disposition for movement, is achieved by maintaining the neck in a neutral position for craniovertebral movement, with increasing flexion for successively lower segments. A further method of restricting the effect is to transfer the palmar surface of the index finger of the 'occipital' hand so that it unilaterally bears against the transverse process of C4, for example; the head and all segments to C4 are then rotated as a unit, with a localised effect on the C4–C5 segment.

Below C6, the small but important *Cervicothoracic region* movement very often becomes restricted.

(i) Flexion (Fig. 12.15A) limitation is conveniently treated with the patient in an elbow-lean prone lying position. While the forearm of the therapist's stabilising hand lies along the thoracic spine, the finger and thumb grasp a spinous process; the therapist's opposite thenar eminence applies rhythmic distracting pressure to the next spinous process above, by contact just distal to the therapist's carpal scaphoid. The forearm must be kept vertical.

This technique *looks* specific, but a regional mobilisation effect is difficult to prevent.

For (ii) extension of the same region (Fig. 12.15B), the patient clasps her fingers behind her neck allowing the therapist, who stands at her side, to gather both elbows in a grasp from underneath.

The therapist stabilises one spinous process by thumb pressure, so that a careful and moderate extension movement can be applied by lifting with the opposite forearm. While a degree of localisation is achieved by the thumb pressure, the attachment of latissimus dorsi and pectoralis major will dictate a regional effect. This is diminished as much as possible by firm pressure of the stabilising thumb, and by not allowing the extension movement to involve the whole thorax. The potentially powerful leverage should be used with caution.

Thoracic extension (Fig. 12.16) is more often limited than flexion, and a suitable position for the patient is neck-rest-sitting on a stool, with the fingers clasped. The therapist stands behind the patient with one foot forward, and applies the lateral haunch of that side to the patient's back. By reaching over the patient's arms and grasping them close to the axillae, a gentle and rhythmic extension movement of the thoracic spine can be applied by leaning back-

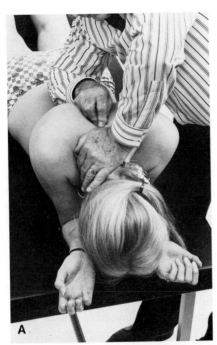

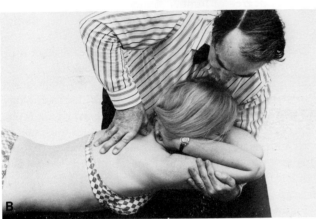

Fig. 12.15 Flexion (A) and extension (B) of the cervicothoracic region (see text).

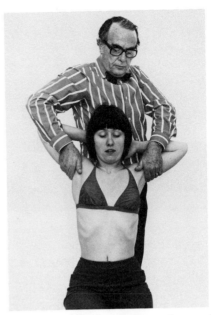

Fig. 12.16 Soft-tissue mobilisation of contracted pectoral and anterior thoracic structures. The potentially powerful leverage must be used gently and cautiously.

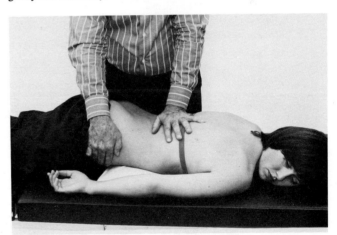

Fig. 12.17 ↻ A moderate range of lumbar rotation, which is more useful for encouraging relaxation (preparatory for other techniques) than for much else, can rhythmically be performed with the patient lying prone.

ward. The excursion of movement should be moderate, since it is not easy for the patient to quickly prevent overenthusiastic stretching.

Lumbar rotation (Fig. 12.17), albeit with a degree of extension combined, may be employed for its relaxing effect as well as its mobilising effect, when muscle spasm prevents other techniques, or the patient is temporarily unable to lie on either side.

The prone patient lies over a small flat pillow under the abdomen; the therapist stands at the side and reaches over to gently grasp the far anterior superior iliac spine, resting the other hand on the low thoracic region. By gently raising and lowering one side of the pelvis, a rhythmic rocking lumbar rotation of small amplitude is produced. A degree of localisation will obviously occur when the therapist's thumbpad engages the near side of a lumbar spinous process.

Lumbar rotation in side-lying[798] can be precisely graded. Figure 12.18A shows a grade II left rotation of the pelvis (and thus the lumbar spine) with the patient's lower limbs arranged so that the L3–L4 segment is most favourably disposed to benefit from it, i.e. with hips and knees flexed a little less than 90°. (The disposition of the patient may need to be modified slightly, following assessment of the effect of the first attempt.)

With forearms aligned with the patient's thighs, the therapist stands behind, level with the patient's low back, and places a palm on the iliac crest and the greater trochanter. The patient's upper wrist lies on her loin, so that the slightly retracted shoulder girdle adds to the mild inertia of her trunk, as the pelvis is repetitively rotated to

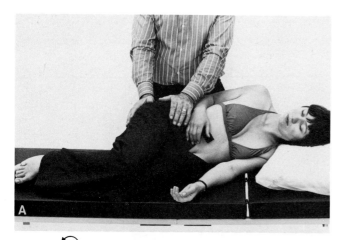

Fig. 12.18 (A) Rhythmic lumbar rotation, to the patient's left side.

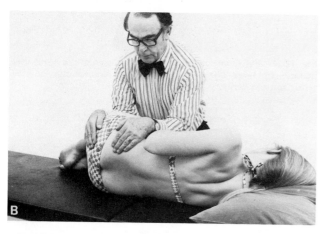

(B) Lumbar rotation (in grade II) by a slightly built therapist for a heavy patient.

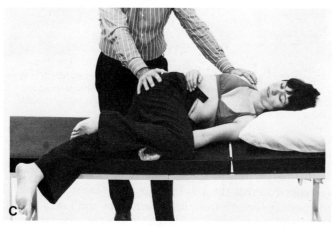

(C) A grade III lumbar rotation.

the patient's left through the middle amplitude of the available range of movement.

When handling a heavily built or very tall patient, the therapist modifies the technique (Fig. 12.18B) by standing in front of the patient and crouching a little, so that both of the patient's knees may be stabilised in the therapist's lap.

Hand pressure on a tender buttock region should be avoided, while the repetitive lumbar movement is applied as above, with the difference that stress upon a slightly built operator is considerably lessened.

For a grade III lumbar rotation which is repetitively taken to the limit of available range, the patient's position is modified, in that the under shoulder girdle is shifted forward to add more thoracic rotation (Fig. 12.18C). The under limb is extended at the knee and rotated externally, which also extends that hip a little; the upper knee is flexed, with the foot conveniently hooked behind the opposite knee. Because friction between the patient's upper knee and the plinth surface often prevents free movement, it is useful to interpose the patient's under forearm, which must be kept relaxed.

The therapist's stance should be such that the patient's upper shoulder can be lightly steadied but not completely stabilised, and the lumbar spine can be observed while rotatory movement is being imparted.

As the degree of lumbar flexion or extension is modified, so the therapist's stance must also be slightly changed.

Double hip and knee flexion is a most useful technique, partly because a proportion of lumbar backache appears to arise mainly from chronic approximation of posterior joint structures, in the absence of frank disc pathology, and also because chronic tightness of the overlying fascial planes (i.e. lumbodorsal fascia) and vertebral musculature must be released before postural correction is feasible. Further, the technique may be modified to produce thoracic flexion, with the main effect directed to a particular segment.

Figure 12.19A depicts a grade II— movement, in the early stage of the available range. It is important for the therapist to stand widely astride, imparting the movement by small excursions of his trunk and not by flexing the forearm which supports the patient's thighs.

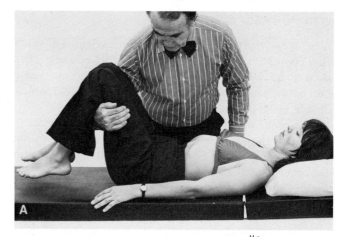

Fig. 12.19 Passive lumbar flexion (see text). (A)

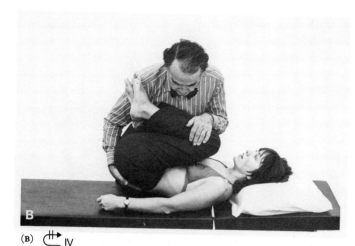

(B) ⟳ IV

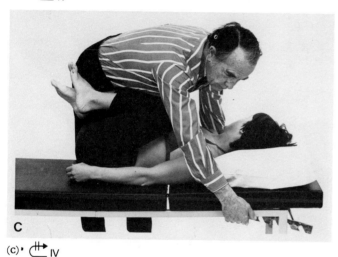

(C)' ⟳ IV

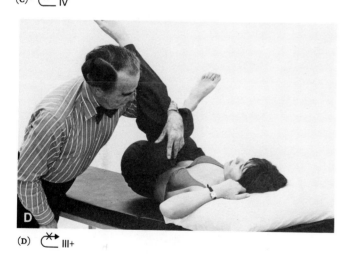

(D) ⟳ III+

As potentially powerful forces are applied whenever the therapist's body-weight is employed in a downward direction, these techniques must never be imprudently used.

If the therapist, standing at the side, crosses the patient's near knee over the far one and grasps the near knee after passing a forearm under the far knee, large amplitude flexion and side-flexion regional movements can now be applied to the lumbar area. By adopting a wide stride standing position, and using equally large amplitude movements of his own trunk, the therapist can approximate the patient's knee to her head, and thus produce flexion as far caudally as the upper thoracic spine. By stabilising one thoracic spinous process with his cranial hand, the therapist can increase the effect upon the mobile segment of which that vertebra forms the upper part, but this hardly justifies grouping the method among localised techniques.

When the lumbar and thoracic flexion movement is imparted by approximating the patient's knees to the near axilla (Fig. 12.19D) an additional side-flexion stretch is also imparted to the near-side lumbar structures.

Sacroiliac joint problems often respond to quite gentle procedures; techniques need not be flamboyant and dramatic.

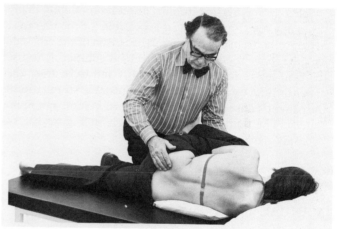

Fig. 12.20 ⟳ A modest and undramatic sacroiliac mobilising technique, when the painful side is that of a relatively depressed posterior superior iliac spine, and the lumbar spine is not involved.

Figure 12.20 depicts the patient in side-lying over a small flat pillow which maintains the spine in a neutral position. With the underneath limb extended slightly at the hip, and stabilised there by the outer aspect of the operator's leg which is placed on the plinth, the sole of the patient's upper foot is placed against the operator's anterolateral loin. While supporting the patient's upper knee with one hand, and palpating in the upper-side sacroiliac sulcus with the other, the operator can produce mild shearing effects upon the upper sacroiliac joint by repetitively moving his pelvis forwards. Since the operator stands on one leg, although also supported by the leg on the

In Figure 12.19B the therapist applies a grade IV movement by leaning his cranial forearm on the patient's upper shins, adding to the stretch of dorsal lumbar soft tissues by lifting the patient's sacrum with the caudal hand.

A degree of localisation to the low lumbar area can be achieved if the therapist also leans on the patient's shins and applies additional pressure in a downward and caudal direction (Fig. 12.19C).

plinth, it is as well not to have an arthrotic or unstable left knee!

While a degree of localisation is achieved, this cannot be called a localised technique—as may be determined by a third person palpating the L3–L4 segment, for example.

By reason of the a–p distance (some 7–8 cm) between the sacroiliac joint and the acetabulum, *longitudinal distraction of one lower limb* will tend to induce a combined downward and forward movement of the ilium on that side.

The lower leg of the prone patient is fixed between the operator's crossed thighs, while he leans forward with straight arms to stabilise the sacrum, by placing one palm on its dorsal aspect, further stabilised by the other palm on the dorsum of his hand.

The technique (Fig. 12.21A) is performed entirely by repetitive distraction movements of the therapist's lower limbs.

The effects of this useful technique may be further enhanced by also distracting the ipsilateral anterior superior iliac spine with one hand (Fig. 12.21B) or by increasing the tension in rectus femoris by bending the patient's knee and applying the distraction via the uppermost region of the calf (Fig. 12.21C). This latter technique needs some practice before it can easily be performed.

When using this longitudinal distraction method many times in a day (Fig. 12.21A) it is possible for the therapist to painfully strain one knee joint, by reason of the crossed-leg grip above the patient's malleoli. A solution is to use the bent leg technique (Fig. 12.21C) and to distract the patient's limb by looping a broad adjustable strap around the patient's upper calf and the therapist's trunk (not illustrated). The limb is then distracted as in Figure 12.21A by trunk movements.

C. MECHANICAL HARNESS TRACTION AND MANUAL TRACTION

Introduction. Because guides for various therapeutic procedures are basically notions about the nature and purpose of these procedures, rationale is fundamentally important. Also important is the wisdom of revising concepts as knowledge increases.

Traction is widely used in various ways in orthopaedic practice, but in association with manipulative treatment of spinal joint problems its use in the past has been restricted to attempts to restore presumed shifts of disc material to its 'proper' place, most often by way of a sustained pull repeated daily.

So long as the nature of common pathological changes underlying neck pain and brachial neuralgia, and backache and sciatica, is basically envisaged as 'a slipped disc' and the sole basis for using traction is the notion of mechanically 'putting it back', or 'shifting it off the nerve

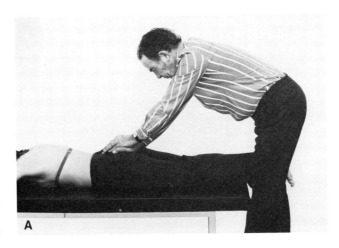

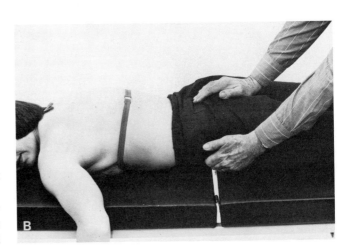

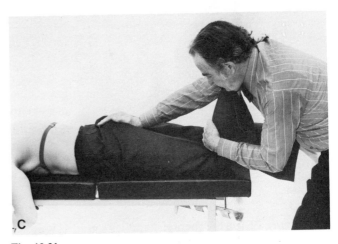

Fig. 12.21

(A) Distraction of the left lower limb and ilium while the sacrum is stabilised.
(B) Enhancement of effect by simultaneous distraction applied at the same side a.s.i.s.
(C) Further enhancement by flexing the knee and applying distraction at the popliteal space. The height of the support is a critical factor when using this modification, which requires much practice.

root', the therapist is denied a much wider range of application of this useful treatment method.

Alternatively, if traction is conceived as a flexible and freely adaptable method of mechanical mobilisation, its field of usefulness is considerably broadened.

Experimental evidence and clinical experience support the view that many abnormalities may combine to produce the syndromes treated (see Pathological Changes, p. 125), and among the factors are:

1. Spinal stenosis, congenital and acquired
2. The blood supply of the spinal cord, cauda equina and brain stem
3. The great variability of arterial distribution
4. The tendency to partial ischaemia of spinal cord cells lying in so-called 'watershed areas' of end-artery supply, and the particular pattern of arterial distribution in individual cases
5. The vertebral venous plexuses, and their tendency to engorgement in benign as well as malignant space-occupying lesions
6. Buckling of the ligamentum flavum, as a part of degenerative change, with trespass anteriorly into the neural canal
7. Degenerative change of facet-joints, and consequent trespass by exostosis and thickened, indurated soft tissue
8. Disc degeneration, herniation and prolapse
9. Root irritation and compression by physical trespass of related tissues
10. The seemingly irritant nature of the products of disc degeneration, and their possible role in nerve root inflammation
11. The complex neurophysiological interdependence of supply to the vertebral structures
12. The importance of afferent impulse traffic from the mechanoreceptors of facet-joints, particularly in relation to equilibration
13. The tendency for joints, ligaments and dura to be supplied by filaments derived sometimes from segments five or six distant—this applies particularly to innervation of structures within the neural canal
14. Reactive fibrosis of the nerve root sleeve
15. Segmental instability or hypermobility, and segmental stiffness or hypomobility; often existing side by side
16. The phenomena of referred pain, and 'remembered' pain, and the difficulties sometimes in accurately localising the segment(s) responsible for signs and symptoms, and localising the treatment.

Similarly, in a discussion of traction technique, taking cervical traction as an example and bearing in mind: (a) the condition/diagnosis, i.e. the whole nature or family of pathological changes likely to have occurred; (b) its unique presentation in any one patient; (c) the effects it is hoped to produce, and (d) coexisting conditions which may complicate techniques, there are about a dozen factors to be considered:

1. Type of apparatus and suspension points available
2. The position of the patient
3. The physique and weight of the patient
4. The head/neck angle (i.e. the relative lengths of occipital and mandibular straps)
5. The neck/trunk angle (i.e. the rope angle, decided by position of the fixation point)
6. The force or poundage
7. The weight of the apparatus, between neck and attachment point
8. The duration of the traction
9. Whether sustained, or rhythmically varied and the periodicity of pull and release phases
10. The frequency of traction sessions
11. The presence of difficulties, such as: an overtender suboccipital area; a painful arthrotic temperomandibular joint; badly fitting dentures, and so on
12. Finally, the question: 'What are we doing it for?'

The principles of treatment of the lumbar spine require much the same consideration, while for thoracic traction there are one or two additional factors requiring attention.

Some effects of traction. Undoubtedly, traction is capable of producing (a) measurable separation of vertebral bodies, and (b) centripetal forces exerted by the tension applied to surrounding soft tissues.[817] These effects are valuable and important in the treatment of signs and symptoms considered due to particular stages in the process of disc herniation and prolapse; yet myelographically demonstrated disc trespass into the lumbar neural canal frequently coexists with the complete absence of symptoms or signs, this having been shown to be so in 37 per cent of 300 normal subjects.[552]

Traction has other and equally important effects, some of which are likely to be most valuable when it is employed rhythmically, or modified so as to produce oscillatory longitudinal movement rather than a frank distractive effect.

Among these may be:

1. The simple mobilisation of joints with reversible stiffness
2. Modification of the abnormal patterns of afferent impulse traffic from joint mechanoreceptors
3. Relief of pain by inhibitory effects upon afferent neurone traffic subserving pain
4. The reduction of muscle spasm
5. The stretching of muscle, and connective tissues
6. The improvement of tissue-fluid exchange in muscle and connective tissue
7. The likely improvement of arterial, venous and lymphatic flow

8. The physiological benefit to the patient of rhythmic movement, and of the lessening of compressive effects.

Use of technique. Since only about 1 in 10 000 of the population with backache and sciatica, for example, come to myelography and operation,[723] conservative treatment is of prime importance, yet by this very circumstance we are denied a view at open operation of the lesion as it exists in each patient, and by the nature of these lesions their mortality rate is practically nil; significant opportunities for comparing clinical findings and post-mortem appearances are few indeed. There are X-rays, there is extrapolation, there is intelligent guesswork, but at best only a sketchy correlation between, on the one hand, the known serial tissue-changes in an ageing joint or in one insulted by trauma, and on the other hand the signs and symptoms presented by any one patient. In benign joint problems of the spine, confident and precise diagnosis is difficult.

Further, since we do not know fully and precisely what mobilisation, manipulation or traction does to a joint and its associated tissues, we can only use the treatment logically, i.e. select and modify it, on the basis of signs and symptoms and how these change as treatment proceeds; it is not wise to base selection of procedures on diagnostic concepts only, or to regard traction treatment solely as a means of creating possible suction effects, measurable separation of vertebral bodies, and ligamentous stretching. The immense amount of information now available about the intervertebral disc and the great variety of biochemical and physical changes which can occur in it and its closely related structures, should caution us not to conceive it simply as a sort of badly packed suitcase. Clinical experience teaches that a relatively small poundage, sufficient to equal the natural apposition tendencies maintaining the integrity of resting joints, is often enough to relieve pain and limitation.

Joint apposition forces are small,[64, 65] being due to: (a) the slight elastic tension of muscle, tendons and aponeuroses, the joint capsule, ligaments, periarticular connective tissue, deep and superficial fascia and skin; (b) the slight negative pressure within joints, some 5–10 mmHg below that of atmosphere.[1354]

In passing, the presence of elastic fibres has been demonstrated in the annulus fibrosus of intervertebral discs.[139]

To summarise this point, it is often useful to regard traction as (a) a moderate (sustained or rhythmic) amplification of the effect of negating gravitational compression by simply lying down, and (b) another form of passive mobilising technique. To do this, it is not necessary to employ cumbersome apparatus which may resemble the weight and construction of a battleship, or harness resembling the trappings of a brewer's dray.

It has to be admitted that the mechanism of pain production in common joint problems is not yet completely understood, nor enough known in every case about why the procedures relieve the symptoms and signs. Neither is it possible to explain the puzzling fact that 5 to 15 minutes of daily traction can have potent therapeutic effects on a joint which is otherwise subject to some 12 or more hours daily of gravitational compression amount-

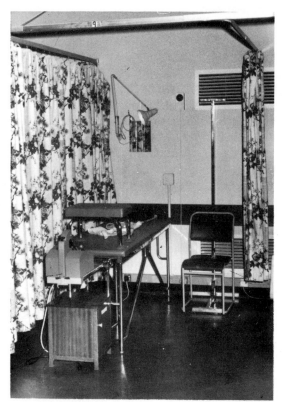

Fig. 12.23 shows the Tru-Trac table, machine and 'Fowler position' stool, with the chrome stand and an ordinary chair for sitting traction in the near-neutral position.

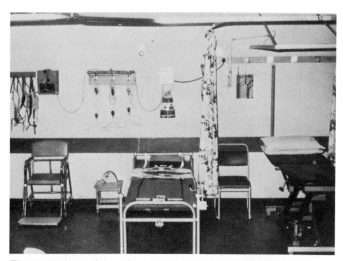

Fig. 12.22 shows, from left to right, a selection of cervical harnesses, Tru-Trac machine, with tilting-type chair, three Maitland-type double-pulley systems, a modified 'Scott' traction frame with 'Scott' harnesses and an 'Oldchurch' manipulation plinth. The 'Scott' frame has been boarded over and covered with vinyl to reduce friction and thus dissipate force factors.

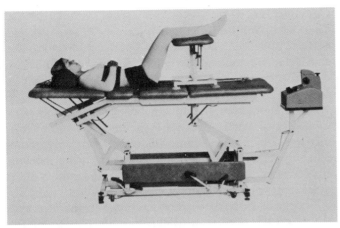

Fig. 12.24 The more recent Tru-Trac ('Tru-Eze') incorporates a number of improvements, particularly that of variable height. For example, lumbar traction in flexion may be achieved either by using the leg support, or by lowering the table relative to the traction machine, or by a combination of both methods.

ing to many times more than the poundage employed in treatment. In the face of this embarrassing ignorance, it is surely sensible to place the most reliance on what is much more clearly known, i.e. the relationship between common and uncommon sets of signs and symptoms, and the varying grades and types of treatment procedures. Here, the ground becomes more sure in direct relationship to the completeness of our grasp of: (a) the signs and symptoms in themselves, and (b) the full potential of the treatment methods.

Plainly, the therapist's prime concern must be: (a) careful and comprehensive examination, and (b) continuous development of treatment methods, neither of which relieve us, of course, of the obligation to improve our imperfect understanding of the nature of the lesions we treat.

Technique. The response of the signs and symptoms to the initial procedure selected should be the dominant factor, e.g. in the case of testing the response to one of the manual techniques, or to the initial trial of traction.

Since a frequent objective of treatment is to produce movement, and most movement will occur when a joint is positioned in the midposition of all the other ranges of

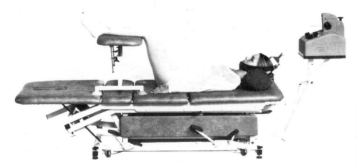

Fig. 12.25 Cervical traction may be arranged with a 45° angle between the line of pull and the horizontal, although this does not mean, of course, that the angle of neck with trunk will also be 45°. Again, the angle of pull can be varied by modifying the height of the table.

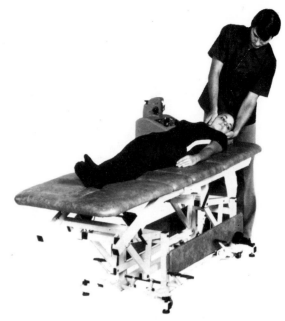

Fig. 12.26 The facilities of a breathing hole for the prone patient, provision for swinging aside the traction machine, and depressing the head end, allow the plinth to be adapted for both manual mobilisation and other treatment such as postural drainage.

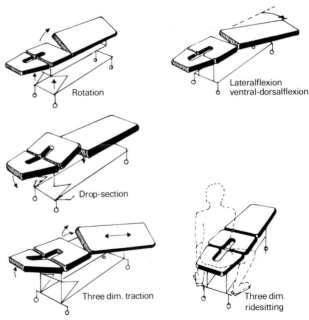

Adjustment of table segments.

Fig. 12.27 A scheme of a three-dimensional treatment table devised by F. Kaltenborn. Adjustment of the adaptable sections allow a variety of dispositions of the patient's trunk and limbs. NB For those not well experienced in particular methods of treatment, it is wise to bear in mind that excellent and effective work is perfectly possible using a simple horizontal support and a variety of hard and soft pillows, together with a traction harness and pulleys. Sophisticated apparatus does not add therapeutic effectiveness as a matter of course in direct relation to its complexity, although it may be labour-saving.

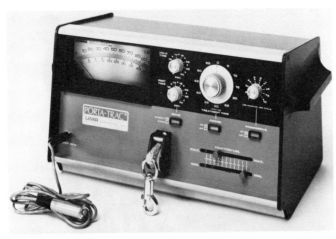

Fig. 12.28 The Porta-trac Unit allows traction to be progressively applied in increments of 1 to 10 lb (0.5 to 4.5 kg), and in cycles from 2 to 30 seconds, to a maximum of 100 lb (45 kg) or 200 lb (90 kg) with the poundage doubler.

which it is capable, the lordotic areas of the spine (cervical and lumbar) should be positioned more in neutral or slight extension when treating the upper parts, i.e. C1–C2, L1–L2, and in increasing flexion as the lower areas are treated, i.e. C6–C7, L4–L5, L5–S1. This applies especially when treatments with a generalised or regional effect, i.e. traction, are being used, but less so when specific vertebral contact techniques are employed.

Apparatus is of many kinds (Figs 12.22, 12.23, 12.24, 12.25, 12.26, 12.27, 12.28, 12.29) and provided funds allow there is advantage in having choices of method, and of harness.

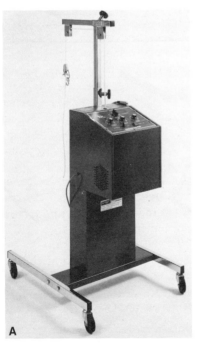

Cervical traction

Signs and symptoms due to involvement of articular and periarticular tissues at the neck and upper/middle thoracic spine respond well to passive movement techniques, of which cervical harness traction (sustained or rhythmic) is only one.

Cervical traction should not be regarded solely as a treatment in itself; patients sometimes benefit from a mixture of techniques. Some will improve on harness traction only, though manual mobilising can be more specifically localised to vertebral segments affected, and is often quicker in appropriate cases.

Flexion of the neck, without traction, separates the vertebrae posteriorly—it also increases the tension in the dura, meningeal ligaments and nerve roots;[130] this tension is increased if there is already a degree of *congenital* or developmental stenosis, and further increased if there is *acquired* stenosis due to: disc pathology; osseous bars and bosses; ligamentum buckling; facet-joint changes.[120]

Flexion also aggravates the tension of meningeal adhesions.

With the patient half-lying or lying, the resultant of the forces acting on the neck is that of: (a) the weight of the head; (b) the weight of the harness, spreader and rope; (c) the angle of rope; (d) the poundage (Fig. 12.30), and without accurate knowledge of all four components it is impossible to know just how much stress, in which particular direction, is being applied to the cervical spine and soft tissues. For this reason alone it seems wise to start fairly cautiously with low levels of stress and increase if need, on the basis of careful assessment of each treatment.

Some conclusions derived from research[191, 192, 193, 1260, 1261] findings are:

1. Most experimenters, with poundage above 20 (9 kg), some of them very high, separated the vertebrae by about 1–1.5 mm per space, measured at posterior vertebral levels.

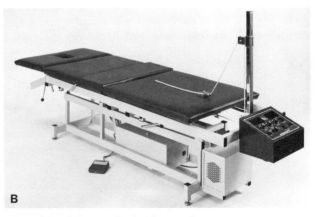

Fig. 12.29 (A) and (B) The TX Traction Unit, which can be adapted for sitting traction by the use of an adjustable-angle chair, also incorporates a fully adjustable treatment table which can be used alone for mobilisation and manipulation treatments. The tension range is 0–200 lb (0–90 kg) with hold and rest periods of 0–60 seconds each. Types of traction provided for are static, intermittent, progressive static or progressive intermittent.

RESULTANT

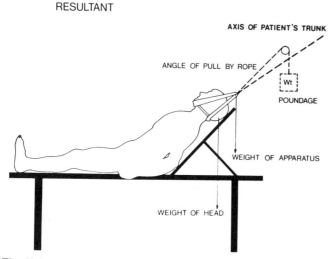

Fig. 12.30 Some factors which must be known before the effects on the neck of distraction forces can accurately be predicted.

2. By far the greatest separation occurs posteriorly, and is greatest with increasing flexion.

3. The normal cervical lordosis is eradicated at pulls of about 20–25 lb (9–11.5 kg).

4. A traction force of 30 lb (13.5 kg) for only 7 seconds will separate the vertebrae posteriorly, the amount increasing with greater flexion.

5. At a constant angle, a traction force of 50 lb (22.5 kg) produces greater separation than 30 lb (13.5 kg), but the *amount* of separation is not significantly different at 7, 30 or 60 seconds.

6. When separation of vertebral bodies *is* desired, high tractive forces for short periods will achieve it.

7. Upper cervical segments do not separate as easily as lower cervical segments.

8. Rhythmic traction produces twice as much separation as sustained traction.

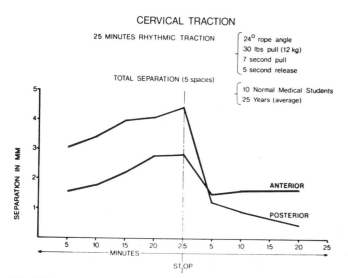

Fig. 12.31 Following cervical traction, the posterior structures will return to normal more quickly than anterior structures.

9. When traction forces are removed, restoration to normal dimensions is four to five times quicker in posterior structures. Restoration anteriorly is much slower (Fig. 12.31).

10. As would be expected, less separation occurs in 50-year-old patients than in normal 20-year-olds.

11. In one comprehensive trial, patients with frontal headaches and vertigo-like symptoms etc. did not do well on traction given in slight or greater flexion.

With regard to traction for neurological symptoms and signs:

... cervical spondylosis can only be regarded as a predisposing factor for the development of nerve root symptoms ... it is quite amazing to what extent a nerve root can become squeezed and deformed by a slowly growing osteophytic protrusion, without any clinical evidence of irritation or dysfunction. Reactive fibrosis may also involve the root-sheaths and periarticular tissues, obliterating the root pouches—yet the root remains functionally intact. Such changes, however, always make the root extremely vulnerable to all kinds of stress and pain.[392]

When a nerve root is stretched or otherwise injured by trauma, in a mature patient, and begins to hurt (i.e. after months or years of being steadily squashed and distorted by slow, painless degenerative trespass[282, 1194]), are we giving traction to try and reverse the serial tissue-changes which have given rise to the current syndrome of root pain and root signs, or do we better devote our time to gently trying to reduce the current inflammatory response?

'There appears no evidence to suggest ... that actual disc protrusion can be reduced by this means.'[105]

Since heads and necks are dissimilar in shape and size, a supply of different harnesses is useful. A desirable harness is adjustable in all three dimensions—occiput to spreader, chin to spreader, and chin to occiput—this allows comfortable adjustment of the head/neck relationship without necessarily affecting the degree of neck flexion which may be required by the treatment. Single pulleys and weights are often used but a double pulley with a small spring balance (or better still, a tensiometer or statimeter) in series allows a more graduated application and removal of traction.

Localisation of effect: The main traction effect should be directed to the vertebral segment involved and the patient so positioned that the segment is at midpoint of its available sagittal movement.

It follows that: (a) interpretation of the segmental significance (if any) of the distribution of signs and symptoms, (b) palpation for extra spinal tenderness, local guarding spasm, thickening around joints and diminished accessory movement, and (c) a passive test of physiological movement to find the mid-range of affected segment(s) are necessary parts of examination.

It also follows that: (a) the patient's position (e.g. sitting, lying, half-lying), (b) the angle of the neck with head, and neck with trunk, (c) the adjustment of harness straps to individual requirements have a bearing on the effects produced and are therefore important.

Generally, since the most movement is achieved when a joint is positioned at the midpoint of all its available ranges, the occiput–C1 and C1–C2 joint should be treated in the neutral or slightly extended head/neck relationship, with increasing flexion of the neck for lower cervical and upper thoracic levels, but the best position for each patient is entirely governed by the requirement to produce the movement (traction effect) at the vertebral level intended, and by the response to the initial treatment. Hence, assessment of effects produced is also important.

The duration of treatment and amount of force applied to the vertebral column in all of these techniques need not be as great as is commonly employed; good results are often achieved with minimum poundage. Occasionally up to an hour's traction with heavy poundage (30–40) (13.5–18 kg) is required; in these cases a few minutes' rest halfway is wise.

A more or less standard force/duration 'recipe' for all patients does not amount to planned treatment, neither does a steady progression of one or both factors as a routine procedure.

No passive movement technique should be continued beyond that necessary to relieve signs and symptoms.

NB: Behaviour of symptoms *during* traction is of no special significance (relief of signs or symptoms during traction by no means indicates that they will remain relieved *between* tractions, which is the aim of the treatment) and it is not an infallible guide to modifications of technique, *except*, if very severe pain is dramatically relieved during the first gentle traction treatment, carefully take the harness down at once and reapply with reduced poundage and duration on next attendance. These patients suffer a prolonged and severe exacerbation afterwards if care is not taken.

It is the assessment immediately preceding the treatments which should dictate modifications (if necessary) of angle and pull, force applied, and duration of traction, but, *for the first treatment*, apply the minimum amount of traction necessary to improve the signs and symptoms when assessed immediately following.

Sustained traction with patients lying or half-lying: single pulley and weight; double pulley and spring balance; Tru-Trac apparatus.

(i) *Initial treatment:* Explain procedure to patient.

Lay patient down, with head supported on pillow(s) while harness is applied. It is often more comfortable for patients to have knees flexed. If using adjustable harness, secure straps so that pull is comfortably and evenly applied to occiput and mandible, and the head/neck relationship in sagittal plane is consistent with the need

to produce the main effect at specific intervertebral levels.

Fix spreader and pulleys, etc., and arrange attachment of upper traction hook and the height of pillow(s) so that the intended angle of *neck flexion on trunk* is produced (this may need to be adjusted after assessment). The line of the rope is usually at a slight angle to the longitudinal axis of the neck. For this reason, traction in flexion is best done in lying or half-lying, and traction in neutral in sitting, although traction in slight flexion while sitting can be done.

By gently applying and releasing moderate traction force (8–10 lb) (3.5–4.5 kg) in a rhythmic way, and by palpation between spinous processes, ensure that the movement produced is occurring mainly at the vertebral level intended. Adjust angles of pull until this is achieved, and note the minimum poundage required to do so. Increase the latter if intervertebral movement cannot be detected.

Then give a short two to five minutes pull at this poundage.

Remove traction and reassess salient signs and symptoms.

Guides for action are:

a. If adequate subjective improvement (i.e. symptoms) and adequate objective improvement (i.e. signs) are evident, repeat treatment at subsequent attendances with same position/poundage/duration, as long as adequate improvement continues.

b. If worse, do no more at first session, but modify apparatus for head/neck angle, and fixation point for rope angle, at the subsequent attendance.

c. If no change, add 3–5 lb (1.5–2 kg) and repeat traction with same duration; if still no change, repeat increased poundage with duration increased by five minutes.

(ii) *Subsequently* (if patient is having traction treatment only): Assess changes in signs and symptoms before each treatment, and if the patient continues to improve adequately there is no need to alter angle, poundage or duration. Cervical traction is not necessarily like a 'progressive weight resistance' exercise regime.

Patients having traction and manual mobilising during the same sessions should be assessed after each application of technique.

NB: Try to achieve results with minimum duration and poundage.

As a rule of thumb, patients of average physique should have treatment progressed, when indicated, by increments of 3 minutes and/or 3 lb (1.5 kg), with a maximum of 20 for both; higher amounts are necessary for some patients. Traction is unlikely to help if significant improvement has not occurred in three attempts.

A guide follows (Fig. 12.32):

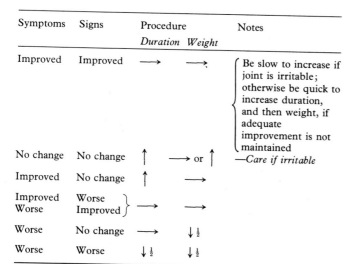

Symptoms	Signs	Procedure Duration	Weight	Notes
Improved	Improved	→	→	Be slow to increase if joint is irritable; otherwise be quick to increase duration, and then weight, if adequate improvement is not maintained —*Care if irritable*
No change	No change	↑	→ or ↑	
Improved	No change	↑	→	
Improved / Worse	Worse / Improved }	→	→	
Worse	No change	→	↓½	
Worse	Worse	↓½	↓½	

Fig. 12.32 A guide to modification of duration and/or tension, when necessary, after the initial treatment by traction

Rhythmic traction (or variable traction): Tru-Trac apparatus; chrome stand and Tru-Trac table; tilting chair; ordinary plinth (Figs 12.22 and 12.23).

Technique is not very different, except that the apparatus requires the inertia of the patient's weight for its operation and many patients try to 'go with the rope' when the pull is applied. They need to be reminded to remain still and relaxed, and allow their body weight to act.

Set the poundage, duration and periodicity required and proceed then as for sustained traction except that: with severe symptoms—relatively long periods of 'hold' and 'rest' should be employed (i.e. less movement); as symptoms become less severe—shorter 'hold' and 'rest' periods are more effective (i.e. more movement).

NB. Since the upper cord attachment may be stationary, the degree of neck flexion can be modified by raising or lowering the head of the plinth, or the whole plinth if this is not possible, if the patient is lying or half-lying. When the extended headboard of the older Tru-Trac table is being employed to treat a supine patient, the greatest possible flexion is only 24°. Traction in neutral can be done with the patient sitting under the apparatus. A tilting dentist-type chair is then useful for altering the neck/trunk angle, for traction in flexion.

Thoracic traction

The not infrequent clinical finding, that cervical traction is capable of provoking pain from a latent and undeclared middle/lower thoracic, and sometimes lumbar, problem is a useful reminder of the mechanical interdependence of the vertebral column, and of how far into the thoracic area cervical traction is felt. In general, the principles governing thoracic traction are the same as for other regions, with the exception that the application of tension is not as direct. Cervical and lumbar harnesses can be designed to utilise convenient bony configurations, e.g. occiput and mandible, contours of upper loin area, lower loin and iliac crests, but because there are no conveniently shaped body areas which allow an upper attachment for traction to be applied specifically to the thoracic spine, the treatment requires adaptation of:

a. the cervical traction method, for the upper three-quarters of the thoracic spine (T1–T9), and
b. the lumbar traction method, for the lower quarter of the region (T9–T12).

Segments T1–T9. When applying experimental cervical traction with a horizontal pull to a supine subject of average physique, a pull of around 60 lb (27 kg) is required before the traction is sufficient to overcome body weight and friction, and begins to move the patient bodily along the plinth towards the attachment point. (The pull required will vary somewhat with the patient's physique and clothing, and the nature of the plinth surface.) For this reason, when giving thoracic traction via a cervical harness, the weight of an inert and relaxed patient is often sufficient to provide counter-traction with pulls below 50 lb (22.5 kg); poundage of this order and sometimes above may be required when attempting to influence thoracic joint problems below the T6 segment. With higher poundages counter-traction by the lumbar traction pelvic harness may be necessary. Down to the T6 level, lighter poundages are quite effective, and and for the T1 to T3 segments, pulls in the middle and upper ranges of cervical traction poundages are usually sufficient.

It goes without saying that any degree of *cervical* pain, and irritability, will preclude this method of harness traction for the thoracic spine problem, and manual mobilisation (including manual thoracic traction) must be the treatment of choice.

Technique. By a passive test of thoracic flexion and extension in sitting, assess when the segment to be treated is in the mid-position between extremes of these sagittal movements and try to reproduce the general thoracic posture which accords with this requirement when the patient lies down.

Existing postural curvature differs widely between patients, of course. Raising the end of the plinth and placing two or three pillows under the patient's head and upper thorax may be necessary.

The cervical harness is applied and the fixation point arranged so that the neck/trunk angle is around 45°; this may need modification following a pretreatment manual test of whether the traction is affecting the segment intended. This is palpated by the therapist as test pulls of the selected treatment poundage are rhythmically applied with the therapist's other hand. A double-pulley system reduces manual effort.

Before proceeding, assess joint irritability, intensity of pain and nature of the pain; providing no exacerbation has occurred following the test pull, and the traction is clearly reaching the affected segment, apply the traction for four minutes, then reduce the tension slowly and considerately. The signs and symptoms are then assessed as for cervical traction with the exception that when poundages around 50–60 (22.5–27 kg) are being employed for the middle/lower thoracic segments, and there is no change after the initial session, repeat the four-minute pull but with the same poundage. If there is still no change, do no more at that session—the guide for subsequent sessions is as for the cervical spine (Fig. 12.32)—bearing in mind that proportional increases in poundages, as for cervical traction, are not always desirable when the middle/lower thoracic segments are being treated.

The effect of friction between patient and plinth, and thus the amount of applied pull which is dissipated because of it, is not easy to assess—many factors (termed 'dissipated force factors' by B. D. Judovich)[620, 621, 622] contribute to the proportion of applied poundage required to overcome resistance, e.g. (i) the weight of the patient; (ii) the surface area of contact; (iii) the nature and shape of the contacting surfaces. Added to this, the weight of the patient's head and neck, acting downward at an angle of approximately 135° to the line of the rope, when the latter is at 45° or so, contributes to the fraction of the poundage which is neutralised so far as clinical usefulness is concerned.

For example, during horizontal lumbar traction on a fixed plinth surface, a force equal to some 25 per cent of the patient's body weight must be subtracted from the poundage selected, the remainder representing the force actually being applied to the lumbar joint structures; and while dissipated forces of this order would not apply to the T1–T9 thoracic traction method described, it remains a factor to be eliminated, or reduced as much as possible.

The poundage dissipated is very much lessened by a non-friction, rolling half-section of the plinth, but not quite so completely as in horizontal lumbar traction because of the large angle between the lines of pull and the direction of the rolling section movement, at least when the patient is propped up by two or three pillows and the fixation point is somewhere overhead.

When a rolling plinth-section is not available, simple methods which help to reduce the proportion of dissipated force are: (i) placing a small nylon sheet, doubled, between patient's upper trunk and pillow; (ii) carefully lifting the patient's trunk, after poundage has been applied, and then lowering it back on the pillow. The lower the segment being treated the more important are these considerations. Forces applied can be measured in various ways, e.g. by a statimeter or a tensiometer in series with the rope, by a single spring balance reading up to 56 lb (25.5 kg), or by a bank of two light spring balances, reading up to 25 lb (11.2 kg) each, and arranged in parallel by common attachment points at either end of the bank. With this method, which is somewhat cumbersome, each balance shows a half of the tension applied.

Segments T9–T12. The lumbar traction plinth and harnesses are employed with the thoracic belt applied higher than when treating lumbar segments; if the Scott harness is used, the lower of the three straps should be more firmly applied. Small folded towels may be needed in the axillae to prevent discomfort. The pelvic harness is applied as usual.

Vertebral mobility in the sagittal plane is *least* at the T9–T10 segment, amounting to 2°–4° only, and the mid-position of this range is more difficult to assess. So long as the supine lying posture is comfortable, and the patient is relaxed, the mid-position is achieved in many patients. Nevertheless, it is always worth ensuring that this is so because, depending upon the patient's posture type, pillows considerably placed beneath the knees 'for comfort' may well put the low thoracic segments into an undesirable amount of flexion. The amplitudes of movement are small, and therefore critical.

The aim of *localising* the pull to the segment concerned is more likely to be achieved by placing the segment immediately over the division between fixed and rolling sections of a friction-free plinth.

Technique. The initial test treatment, and immediately following assessment, are conducted virtually as for lumbar traction, bearing in mind that treatment on a non-sliding section plinth requires incorporation of the dissipated force factors into assessment of the tensions needed. There is also the factor of the fraction of pull which is effectively neutralised by the springy thorax, and the slightly extensible vertebral segments lying in series between the low thoracic spine and the sacrum.

Lumbar traction

Some reports[746, 756, 815] in the recent literature indicate that clinicians are investigating lumbar traction in new ways, and attempting to provide added information on its application and usefulness. Yet in a majority of papers the writers appear to remain preoccupied with the factors of:

1. Increasing the height of the intervertebral space
2. Altering the profile of the annulus fibrosus
3. Reducing the intradiscal pressure and thus creating a suction effect
4. Exerting centripetal pressure by increasing the tension of circumferential soft tissues.[817, 819, 568, 648, 973, 831]

Probably because there have been clear demonstrations that conditions favouring these effects are readily produced by traction, questions of its efficacy continue to be largely discussed only in relation to disc trespass, sciatica and neurological deficit;[1294, 708, 710] yet it has been estimated that motor weakness occurs in less than 15 per cent of hospital cases of sciatica.[1369] For example, brief reports of four trials, all of which admitted patients with sciatic pain, many of whom also had neurological signs, are of interest. Some reported good results, others indifferent results:

1. Thirty-seven patients with sciatica, neurological deficit and positive myelographic signs were treated by rhythmic traction of one-third body weight on a friction-free table. A control group of 35 with similar clinical findings were treated by simulated traction with trivial poundages for the same period. There was no significant difference in treatment results, in these 72 patients with clear evidence of root involvement.[1294]

2. Forty patients, most of them with neurological signs, were treated by 55–70 lb (25.32 kg) rhythmic traction on a friction-free table for 20 minutes daily, producing 'excellent' results in 6 cases, 'good' in 15 and 'poor' in 19.[568]

3. A double-blind controlled trial of sustained traction excluded patients with recently acquired neurological deficit, although one criteria for admittance was the presence of sciatica, defined as severe and well-delineated pain in the limb. The 'control' group (14 patients) received simulated traction with trivial poundage. Improvement in the treated group (13 patients) did not achieve statistical significance, albeit the groups were small.[819]

4. Sixty-two patients with low back pain, and sciatic pain of more than a month's duration, were assigned to one of three groups comprising: (a) heat, massage and exercises, (b) hot packs and rest only, and (c) 20 minutes rhythmic traction in the Fowler position with pulls of one-third body weight plus 30–40 lb (13.5–18 kg), combined with abdominal and hip extensor muscle strengthening. Briefly, the patients in group (c) showed a significantly greater improvement than groups (b) and (a).[746]

Some other conclusions derived from research findings are:

1. With high poundages, the L4–L5 space is increased by 1.5 mm and the L3–L4 space by 2 mm, i.e. narrowed disc spaces are returned to something like their normal width, but the spaces return to their pretraction level after release of tension and on standing up.[241a]

2. *Vide* other reports, high poundages are apparently not necessary; in general, pulls of half, or a little more, of a normal subject's body weight will increase the lumbar vertebral space by about 1.5 mm, if this be the aim of treatment, and reduce the intradiscal pressure by about 25 per cent.[888]

When some of these reports prompt unfavourable opinions in medical journals of international standing, wholly questioning the value of traction and suggesting that it should be abandoned as a routine treatment,[708, 710] there is justification for reiterating the value of traction used in other ways and for other reasons.

When selecting manual and mechanical passive movement techniques in the treatment of lumbar and lumbo-sacral joint problems, there may well be an advantage in setting aside the classical and almost automatic tendency to associate (a) sciatica with or without neurological signs, and (b) sustained traction.

Perhaps a greater flexibility of approach, based primarily on the signs and symptoms *per se* and the degree of joint and root irritability, rather than on classical concepts of mechanical changes as the necessary causes of these clinical states, may lead to wider appreciation of the infinite variety of their presentation, and the formulation of a wider and more appropriate field of indications for using traction.

Lumbar traction should certainly not be regarded as a treatment apart from other mobilising techniques. It is a passive technique which can be interspersed or changed with others as indicated.

Perhaps we are optimistic to expect that prolapsed disc material can be restored to its former position by traction. Many patients who benefit from this treatment may not have sustained this particular type of joint derangement, and if we believe that some have, it is not necessarily the sole cause of all the symptoms. Consequently, it is not easy to know precisely why traction is beneficial, especially when applied with low or moderate poundage.

The object of treatment is to relieve signs and symptoms *between* treatments and relief of pain *during* traction does not always indicate that this object will be achieved, although the initial trial of traction can be employed to note its subsequent effect.

Movement on and off the treatment table. Patients who are unable to modify their functional movements to lessen pain should lie down and get up from the plinth with the lumbar spine held in the neutral position.

Lying down.
1. Sit on plinth with back straight and a right angle at hips, knees and ankles
2. Keep knees and ankles together all the time and lower the trunk sideways to a side-lying position with the back held still. As the trunk is lowered the legs are raised sideways, the body moving as one piece
3. Roll on to back
4. Stretch out legs.

Getting up. This is an exact reverse of this procedure. Do *not* allow the patient to get up by initially raising the head and shoulders forward. Legs must flex first, then roll on the side, then sit up.

Stretcher patients should roll, or slide with knees bent, on to the treatment table from trolley placed alongside.

Technique A (Sustained traction on a flat support). The following sequence applies to the Scott harness, used on a *non-sliding platform*.

Initial procedure is broadly the same as for cervical traction (q.v.).

Know the patient's salient signs and symptoms before applying traction, and assess them after the initial trial; subsequently, assess before each treatment session.

Shoes, belts, corsets and restrictive clothing should be removed. Shirt or petticoat may be kept on but should be loosened upwards before straps applied.

On a flat treatment table, low lumbar lesions are better treated supine with hips and knees flexed, and mid/upper lumbar with less flexion, though the optimum position for each patient must be found by assessment.

Arrange thoracic and pelvic bands on the table before the patient lies down and test the salient sign chosen as the assessment marker (often straight-leg-raising). Estimate the angle at which limitation, if any, occurs, noting its characteristics, e.g. if painful, where the pain is being provoked, and record it on the patient's card.

1. Padding: Some harnesses need to be padded; the Scott harness is often better without padding.

2. Thoracic band: Patient puts arms through the thoracic harness and the straps are secured. The band should be placed immediately below the greatest diameter of the thorax (i.e. its upper edge at the ziphoid level) so that it cannot slip upwards, and securely fastened. Respiration is bound to be somewhat restricted; try to achieve a good pull with the minimum discomfort to the patient.

3. Pelvic band: The band is secured resting on the iliac crests (or sacrum, if prone)—some patients prefer it resting on the greater trochanters, and if it can be comfortably secured in this position there is no objection to this; it makes no difference to the ultimate effect but compression of gluteal vessels may produce transient paraesthesiae. Secure the thoracic straps to the head of the apparatus, taking up all slack by hand. Steadily pull the straps of the pelvic harness, and take up all slack by hand before securing them to apparatus. The patient should wriggle a little to settle harness comfortably, and do this again during the application of the traction. The pelvic band should be settled round the patient's pelvis *at right angles to the horizontal* and tilted anteriorly, or posteriorly, if assessment of early treatment shows the subsequent need for this.

First application. Wind patient out slowly and progressively to about an indicated 40lb (18 kg), and check straps; friction effects will reduce *the applied tension* on the lumbar spine to about 20–30lb. The patient's reaction to a short and gentle initial pull of ten minutes or less provides valuable information for future procedures, and his confidence is gained if he is introduced to an unusual experience gradually. He is told to report the slightest discomfort.

NB: If severe pain is dramatically relieved with the first gentle pull, lessen it carefully at once, otherwise a very severe pain reaction will occur.

Assess results immediately afterwards, as described for cervical traction, employing duration increments of five minutes and poundage increments of 10–15lb (4.5–7 kg).

Subsequent treatments. Pull in an indicated range of 40–100lb (18–45 kg) (very occasionally up to 150lb (67.5 kg), depending upon the physique of the patient) and for up to 20 minutes *daily*, although 15 minutes often suffices, using the 'guide' (Fig. 12.32) given for cervical traction but with the increments mentioned above. Around 25 per cent of the force of the traction is 'mopped up' by the springy thorax and soft tissue generally, and by friction between patient and plinth (which is lessened considerably with a sliding friction-free platform). The spring balance will show a decrease in pull, but the decrease during treatment will be negligible if slack is taken up efficiently beforehand. If the straps are slipping they must be reapplied more effectively after slowly winding the patient in.

Notes: a. Explain what the treatment involves and what reactions may be expected.
b. Instruct the patient not to have a heavy meal before treatment.
c. Warn the patient to try to avoid sneezing or coughing while on full traction.
d. Patients should expect a possibly irregular improvement, with some stiffness immediately following each treatment.

End of treatment. Wind in slowly and smoothly until all straps are slack. Release all buckles carefully and slowly—a sudden release of a tight thoracic band can be severely painful. Warn patient not to inhale deeply immediately as this can also be painful. After treatment, the patient should lie for a minute or two to collect himself. Assist him up by the method described. The main assessment is carried out the day *after* treatment, i.e. prior to the next one.

A basic treatment has been described but there are many variations. Patients may be treated prone or supine, one or both bands may be used upside-down. (Patients treated supine on the unmodified Scott frame are bound to be in flexion due to the canvas sagging a little; this does not suit all patients.)

It is usual to start with most patients supine on a firm surface and thereafter to modify the technique individually according to findings—we cannot know exactly how the lesion is affecting the joint and we can only find the most effective procedure by trial and error with each patient. The consistent factors are (a) a steady pull repeated daily at first, and (b) assessment of suitable poundage by behaviour of signs and symptoms, and the patient's physique.

Spinal traction is effective but often undramatic; it involves the patient in some discomfort, and so the length of treatment should be kept as short as possible by giving an adequate session at each attendance.

Traction should be abandoned when (a) there is no improvement after three sessions, or (b) there is deterioration in terms of increased pain and/or further movement restriction during the first two days, despite variations in the application of pull. Patients having sustained traction for severe root pain should be carefully checked for the appearance of neurological signs at each visit, because a lessening of pain may actually be the change which often accompanies increasing root compression and this may indicate the need for a short trial of increased poundage and duration; watchful assessment of effects is important at this stage. As the pain becomes less severe and less variable, rhythmic traction can be substituted with advantage.

Technique B (On friction-free Tru-Trac table—rhythmic or static).

Setting up. 1. See that the sliding lumbar section of the table is locked in its fixed position, by pushing the black knob on the left-hand side of foot end of table.

2. Release the cream formica sliding platform by pulling out the chrome spring on its right side, and sliding the platform out a few notches. Leave the platform in the horizontal position.

3. Clamp the machine, dials upward, on the end of the formica platform and screw the black knob tight.

4. After assessment of salient signs, fit the thoracic and pelvic harnesses over minimal clothing to the patient while standing; some recent changes allow harness to be applied with patient lying. Make sure the harness is comfortable but firmly applied.

5. The patient lies supine with feet towards the machine and with hips and knees flexed so that calves rest on small stool and pillow. The intervertebral segment being treated should be level initially with division of table.

6. Attach thoracic harness to clips at head of table. With 'Poundage' knob positioned at 'Cord Release' position, pull out the cord, pass it under the stool and clip it to the lumbar harness rings.

7. Adjust (a) length of thoracic straps, (b) position of formica platform until the set-up has minimal slack and will allow the sliding lumbar section to move horizontally as the traction comes on.

There is an extra length of adjustable cord with the equipment.

Treatment. 1. Instruct the patient about using the 'Help needed' bell and the method of switching off the treatment, should this be necessary.

2. With sliding platform locked in position, set the poundage to two-thirds of total available (lower if dealing with an irritable joint), and apply a short 1–2 second pull to settle the harness firmly, while patient wriggles pelvis to assist the process. Friction due to the locked platform will reduce tension actually applied to the joint.

3. Release the sliding platform lock by pulling out the black knob on left side. Set switches for 'Static' or 'Inter-

mittent', set 'Hold' and 'Release' periods if applicable, set poundage required, and start the treatment by turning timing dial to the right for the required period.

4. The timer mechanism switches off the machine and releases the traction at the end of the set period.

After treatment. 1. Carefully assist the patient to lift buttocks a little, so that sliding platform can be gently closed up and locked.

2. Release the harness and remove the stool. Lock the sliding platform before the patient gets off the table. Instruct the patient to get off the table after a short rest by rolling onto side with knees and hips bent, and lowering legs as trunk is brought to the vertical.

3. When indicated, modify duration and poundage according to the Guide (p. 403) given for sustained traction.

Notes: a. Since the traction is virtually 'friction-free', poundage indicated on the dial is probably that being applied to the joint.
b. As the table is relatively high, some patients may need to be helped down.
c. Patients may also be treated in the prone position, with standard or reversed application of harness.

Oudenhoven (1978)[959] describes *gravitational lumbar traction* as a method of treating pain considered secondary to nerve root or sinuvertebral nerve inflammation.

By employing the thoracic harness only, and tilting the support in progressive increments, distraction is applied to the lower half of the torso, gravity beginning to produce a traction effect at about 35° of tilt. Hence frictional resistance is progressively negated.

Inpatient treatment sessions are 30–60 minutes, six to eight times daily, depending upon tolerance. The angle of traction is progressively and regularly increased, and when pain is relieved, treatment sessions are continued at this angle of tilt for similar durations for a further three days, after which the patient is discharged to continue a home traction programme as indicated.

The treatment was considered unsuitable for referred pain from the lumbar musculature or apophyseal joints, and to this end the differential was established by the response to local anaesthesia of the posterior primary rami at L3, L4 and L5 bilaterally—the injections were under fluoroscopic control.

Those patients whose pain was relieved for the duration of the anaesthesia were considered unsuitable for gravitational traction.

The study was not intended to assess forms of conservative treatment other than gravitational traction, although the patients in this review had failed to benefit by other conservative measures.

The 121 patients were divided into:

Category I: those who had had no previous operation—87 (72 per cent)

Category II: those who had undergone one or more surgical procedures—24 (28 per cent).

In Category I, 69 (87 per cent) of the 81 patients without a true disc herniation were no longer occupationally disabled, and in Category II, 13 (45 per cent) of the 29 patients who had not had a spinal fusion continued to have good pain relief.

It was postulated that the treatment failures in Category II may have been due to postoperative fibrosis, and Oudenhoven suggests that the technique of gravitational lumbar traction warrants careful consideration in the management of chronic back and leg pain.

Intermittent or repetitive rhythmic lumbar traction with sliding plinth sections. The physical behaviour of the clothed lower half of the torso, lying on a sliding-section platform and being subject to intermittent longitudinally applied tension, is not the same as that of a simple helical spring; it is likely that a degree of residual or resting elongation remains, even when the pulling cord is slack during the rest phase of rhythmic pulling cycles.

It is important to bear in mind that once an initial distraction to the set maximum has been applied, a sliding-section platform will rarely go back to rest in the previous fully closed-up starting position after the pull phase has been completed, unless a system of springs or some such is provided to draw it back.

A moment's experiment will demonstrate this, and so long as there is no provision for both the sliding-section platform and the patient's lower half to be incorporated into a single mass which is distracted *as a whole*, notions of what happens to body tissues between pull phases may be fallacious.

This is a factor which must be included in any consideration of the use of this or that traction method, and what is believed to be happening during its application.

Much the same considerations probably also apply to cervical traction in supine, but less so in the half-lying position and probably not at all to traction from a suspension point directly overhead, when the patient is seated.

Similarly, the physical behaviour of a torso, under rhythmic or sustained traction, is not the same when prone as when supine; the differences can be reduced if the harness is always arranged so as to be in contact with the sliding-section, but this may not always suit the aims of the treatment method and the differences will remain. An experiment will verify that the nether end sliding-section will be distracted more (for a given tension) when the patient is supine, and the harness straps under the patient, than when the patient is prone and the harness is arranged to pull on the dorsal aspect of the trunk. With the latter arrangement, excursion of the moveable part of the table is lessened and the benefits of a sliding-section table are considerably reduced.

Multipurpose table

The Akron traction table, which can double for both traction and manipulation treatment, allows a variety of applications covering most clinical requirements for rhythmic or sustained traction and may also be used, with the longitudinal plug removed, for progressive resistance exercises with weights (or springs, with a floor attachment) in the rehabilitation of amputees and the treatment of weak hip musculature.

The couch is divided into a friction-free roll-top pulling half, which can be raised for half-lying positions, and a fixed but longitudinally divided half with removable central plug when a prone breathing facility is required. It is a stable support and being slightly lower than standard plinth height allows easier mounting for short patients and those disabled by backache. The mechanism operates on the principle of a weight sliding on a bar as in weighing machines, and provides for a scale of tensions from 5–10 lb (2.2–4.5 kg) to 115 lb (52 kg). The degree of tension is selected by sliding a weight so that its central marker is opposite the calibration on the scale, which is marked in pounds or kilograms. A timer-switch, with 'pull-duration' and 'rest-duration' controls for any combination of rhythmic traction from a few seconds to over three minutes, together with the sustained-traction switch, are mounted on a small portable hand-box which has a hook to attach to the horizontal part of the framework.

Fixation points are adaptable for use with types of traction harness in common use; but a cloth harness for pelvis and thorax, and a cervical harness with adjustable occipital and mandibular straps probably allows the greatest range of adaptability for the different requirements of patients. Via a cord attaching the mechanism to the moving end of the plinth, an electric motor takes up the slack until the weight is in balance. As the harness settles on the patient, the motor maintains in equilibrium the inert resistance of the patient and the poundage set by the operator. If sustained traction is selected, the motor is reactivated immediately tension falls off (due to slight tissue and harness stretch) and equilibrium to set poundage is restored.

The manufacturers state that the mechanism is accurate with tension above 10 lb (4.5 kg), provided instructions are followed. When requiring accurate tensions between 5 and 10 lb (2.2–4.5 kg), in the early stages of treating very irritable cervical joints, manual pulley systems incorporating a spring balance would probably be preferred.

When employing rhythmic traction, a duration of 15–20 seconds should be allowed for the selected tension to be reached, and also fully released.

NB: The back-rest should never be raised without securing the rolling top by means of the hand wheel provided.

Techniques. With the machine connected to the mains supply with mains switch 'on' there remain two switches to operate, *viz.* the 'on-off' switch with green light indicator at the side of the machine, and the red treatment selector key on the remote control box. When commencing treatment it is advisable to always operate these switches in the sequence of green light on, then red treatment selector key from rest position to 'rhythmic' or 'hold' (sustained traction), and in the reverse order when finishing the treatment. It is especially important, after switching the treatment selector key back to 'rest', to wait until the mechanism is *fully* released before operating the green light switch, since the mechanism retains the previous instructions and should it be operated again without having previously been allowed to return to 'full release', it will complete this phase before obeying the new instructions. This will be confusing to the operator following, whose instructions are apparently being ignored by the mechanism, at least initially. The use of switches in the sequence recommended will prevent this confusion.

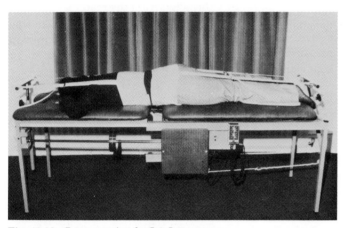

Fig. 12.33 Prone traction for L4–L5 segment.

Lumbar traction (prone position) (Fig. 12.33). With all switches, other than the main, at 'off' position remove the transverse plug and slide the rolling section firmly against the fixed section; secure the rolling section with the hand wheel to keep it stable while preparing the patient. The longitudinal plug is also removed. Before the patient lies down, the harness is firmly and securely applied, with the straps centred symmetrically over the dorsal thorax and buttocks. As with the Scott harness, the less padding the better; so long as there is one layer of clothing between patient and harness and no skin contact by the Velcro material, the harness will be quite comfortable. The remarks on page 406 apply also to the Akron harness.

The patient lies prone with face between the fixed-section padding and feet towards the pulling end, and with the lumbar segment to be treated lying directly over the division of the table. For accurate tensions, the horizontal T-bars should be 11 inches (27 cm) above the centre of the pulling-bar fulcrum (a small mark is filed on the vertical of the T-bar to indicate this height when level with the top of the outer tube).

All slack in the system is taken up by hand; in the case of the pulling section the T-bar should be drawn up against the metal frame, thus extending the spring which covers the pulling cord.

See that:

1. The patient is comfortable
2. The harness is symmetrically placed
3. All slack has been manually taken up and the T-bars are secure
4. Both switches are to 'off'
5. The poundage selected is correctly indicated by position of the central marker on the sliding weight
6. The hand wheel securing the rolling section is now unscrewed to release the rolling mechanism.

For rhythmic traction. The knobs on the control box are set to 'hold' and 'rest' positions desired, and switches then operated in the sequence described; the red key to 'rhythmic'. Remember the 15–20 second allowance referred to above.

For sustained traction. The 'hold' and 'rest' knobs are ignored, and the red key is switched right across to the 'hold' position.

At the end of the treatment period, switch off in the recommended sequence, waiting for the tension to be fully released and *then* turn off the green light switch. Before releasing the patient, gently slide the rolling section against the fixed section, and secure the rolling section with the hand wheel before the patient gets off the plinth.

NB: Older versions of the table can be secured by placing the transverse plug across the gap at the pulling end.

The general considerations, precautions, indications and contraindications of lumbar traction apply (q.v.).

Alteration of poundage during treatment. This facility is unlikely to be required, but tension may be altered during traction with the exception that during sustained traction, the poundage should not be *reduced* without returning the red key switch to rest for a few seconds.

Lumbar traction (supine position) (Fig. 12.34). Preparation of the table is the same, with the exception that the harness is placed on it before the patient lies down. Preparation of the patient is similar, and pillows or the leg-rest flexion stool, available with the apparatus, can be used if a degree of flexion is required.

Treatment procedure is as described in 'Lumbar traction—prone position'.

Thoracic traction (half-lying position—segments T1–T9) (Fig. 12.35). The greatest degree of neck flexion possible, with the cervical traction mast in place and fully extended, is around 30°, and depending upon the patient this may be insufficient to affect thoracic segments below the T6 level, as mentioned previously. Also, with the patient in a modified half-lying position on the horizontal treatment

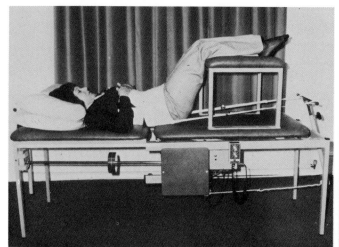

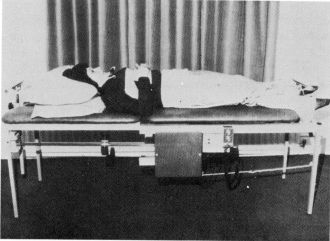

Fig. 12.34 Supine traction in Fowler's position for L5-S1 segment. Whether a patient be treated in this degree of hip flexion would depend upon the purpose of the traction. In the example illustrated, the purpose is to stretch the dorsal lumbosacral soft tissues, and it is for this reason that hip flexion is considerable. (NB The postures depicted are examples only—the position for each patient is a matter for assessment, and there is no 'standard' position.)

Fig. 12.36 Supine traction to affect T12–L1 segment.

table, supported by pillows arranged under upper thorax and head, it is not possible to use the traction mast. A convenient adaptation is to dispense with the cervical traction mast and pass a longer cord through a separate pulley, attached overhead to a weld-mesh support. The cord is attached to the cervical harness, and by its other end to the grip-cleat which is hooked to the T-bar. The patient may then be treated with the back-rest placed a little raised for comfort.

The procedure is otherwise as described previously. A spring balance is necessary to ensure that tension being applied to the patient is that selected, since varying positions of the overhead pulley, height of T-bar, angles of pull, and friction, will be responsible for discrepancies. A small and neat 56 lb (25 kg) spring balance is obtainable

from a well-known maker; the weight of harness and spreader should be subtracted from the reading obtained.

Some therapists prefer to replace the single cord with a neat double-pulley system, although the factor of measuring tensions *applied to the patient* remains to be considered.

When applying traction to the *mid- and upper thoracic segments*, a half-lying position with the back-rest raised and the cervical traction mast extended to its limit is recommended, although the optimum set-up for individual treatment must be found by assessment.

Thoracic traction (supine or half-lying—segments T9–T12) (Fig. 12.36). This may be done in two ways: (i) with the patient supine on a flat table as in supine lumbar traction (described above), or (ii) with the patient in a degree of half-lying on a raised back-rest, employing the cervical traction mast and strong cervical spreader for attachment of the thoracic strap (Fig. 12.37).

In both cases, the thoracic harness must be attached cranially and not caudally to the segment to be treated,

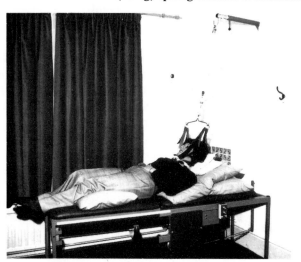

Fig. 12.35 Midthoracic traction, via cervical spine flexed to 45°, to affect T7–T8 segment.

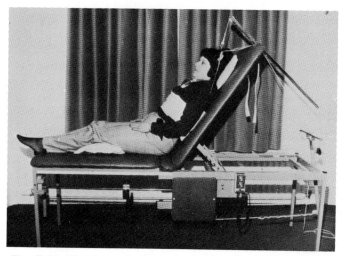

Fig. 12.37 Traction to the thoracolumbar junction, in ½ lying position.

and the axillae suitably protected. For women patients, padding to protect the bosom should take account of individual needs.

In technique (i), the degree of flexion of hips would be the important factor deciding the mid-position of the segment to be treated, which should, of course, be placed directly over the division of the table. Because of this requirement, most patients must lie with legs apart to allow movement of the T-bar at the foot end.

In technique (ii), flexion of the knees (and thus further flexion at the hips) also puts a low thoracic segment into a flexed position—this can be ascertained by palpating the segment and raising/flexing the knees with the other hand.

Cervical traction (supine lying). It is probably better to avoid trying to give 'neutral' traction with the patient lying, and pulling with the rope parallel to the horizontal plinth, because there is always a tendency for the mandibular strap to apply the lion's share of the tension; also, the amount of friction between head and pillow precludes the best estimate of the amount of pull actually being applied to the upper cervical structures.

To produce a pull the resultant of which is virtually in the longitudinal axis of the upper neck, it should be arranged that the rope angle is some 10°–15° above the horizontal, counteracting the effect of gravity on the head; this arrangement ensures a pull in the neutral position (Fig. 12.30). Yet there is still the factor of friction to be considered, and for this reason neutral cervical traction is probably best applied in sitting (Fig. 12.40), with a double-pulley and spring balance set-up, because the tension then being recorded is that being applied to the patient (less the weight of the harness and spreader, which are between spring balance and the patient) and it may be necessary in the early stages to pull with low tension,

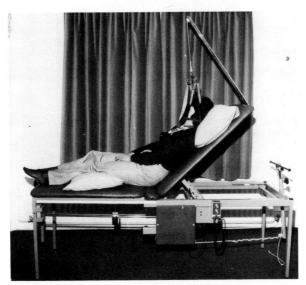

Fig. 12.38 Cervical traction in neutral position of craniovertebral segment.

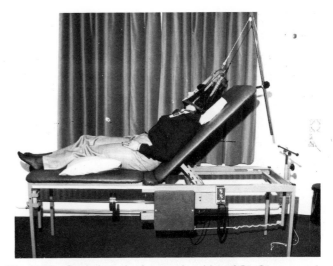

Fig. 12.39 Cervical traction in neutral position of C5–C6 segment, i.e. flexed to about 25°.

i.e. just sufficient to allow the beginning of movement to be perceived by a palpating finger.

When neutral cervical traction in the supine or virtually supine position is the treatment chosen, the principles governing the first and subsequent treatments are as given above and procedure with the Akron table is as follows:

The extensible cervical mast is not used, but after application of the cervical harness, the cord is attached to the spreader, and the grip-cleat adjusted to take up the slack. The grip-cleat hook is attached to the T-bar, which should be raised high enough to allow a 10°–15° rope angle.

Operation of the mechanism is as described previously except that with the T-bar raised to a height of 22 inches (56 cm) from the pulling-bar fulcrum, the manufacturers state that tension being applied to the patient is only half of that indicated by the sliding weight.

Cervical traction (half-lying) (Figs 12.38 and 12.39). With the back raised to the third or fourth notch, a much more flexible arrangement of angles of pull becomes possible, and traction in flexion or in neutral is then easier to arrange. With a pillow under the patient's knees, and a pillow supporting the head, the support for the cervical traction mast is slotted into place. The height of the mast is adjusted by sliding it in the friction-grip, which on tightening the black knob stabilises it at the required height. A few turns of the cord around the knob will hold it there while the harness and spreader are being applied to the patient and then attached to the cord. The grip-cleat is hooked to the middle of the T-bar (at a height of 11 in—27 cm—from the pulling-bar fulcrum) and then adjusted so that the T-bar is pulled forward against the frame of the apparatus. The operation of the table and the principles of treatment are as previously described.

To ensure that the tension selected is that being applied to the patient, a spring balance (25 or 56 lb) (11 or 25 kg)

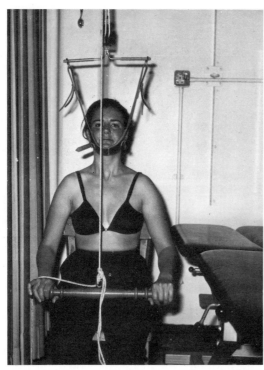

Fig. 12.40 Autotraction to the upper cervical region. The patient sits beneath a double-pulley system attached overhead, and grasps either end of a spreader lying across the upper thighs.

should be incorporated between spreader and pulley, and the weight of the harness and spreader subtracted from the 'balance' reading.

The lack of sophisticated equipment need not preclude the use of rhythmic cervical traction. The patient sits beneath a double-pulley system attached overhead, and grasps either end of a spreader lying across the upper thighs. When the therapist has attached the harness and applied the *maximum* degree of tension required (best measured by a small spring balance in series), the cord is firmly secured to the spreader where it is held by the patient, thus maintaining the tension. By lifting the spreader gently from the thighs, the patient eases the tension applied, and by pressing the spreader down to the thighs again, reapplies the tension. The degree of cervical flexion, the poundage, and the 'hold' and 'rest' periods are variable according to the aim of treatment, and the muscle-work of repetitively pressing the spreader to the thighs does not increase the tension of the cervical musculature. An advantage is that the patient's thighs prevent application of a tension greater than that set by the therapist (Fig. 12.40).

Manual traction. Failing the provision of any equipment at all, rhythmic traction can be applied to the upper cervical spine, lower cervical spine, cervicothoracic region, midthoracic area, thoracolumbar region and low lumbar area, by manual techniques. They can be tiring if not performed correctly and with a good stance, yet are surprisingly easy

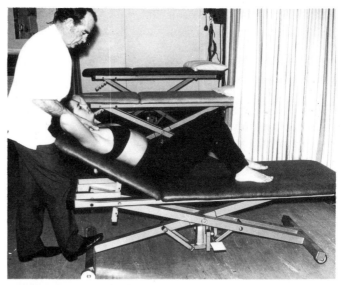

Fig 12.41 Gentle rhythmic manual traction to the cervicothoracic segments.

when the techniques have been mastered (Figs 12.41 and 12.42).

Autotraction (lumbar). A method of autotraction[748] which is achieving good results has been developed at the Rode Kors Syke Huset, Oslo, Norway, by the physiotherapist Oddbjørn Bihaug.[95] The supine patient is stabilised in the Fowler position on a split table by a pelvic band, and applies the tension by pulling with one or both arms, thereby distracting the sliding section of the plinth. The system allows variations in application of tension, and adaptation to individual requirements.

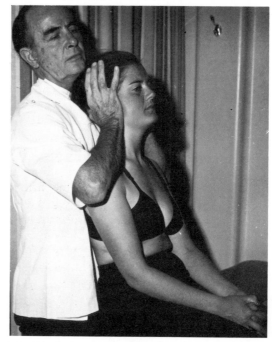

Fig. 12.42 Rhythmic manual traction for the upper cervical region. NB This is not 'oscillatory longitudinal movement'.)

D. LOCALISED MOBILISATION TECHNIQUES

Localised mobilisation techniques are those in which every effort is made to restrict the effect of movement to a single segment. This is easier in some anatomical locations than in others.

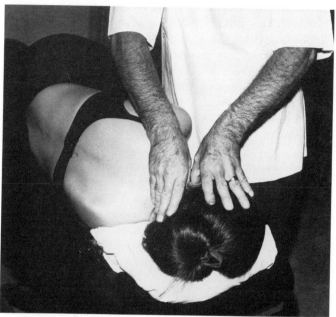

Fig. 12.43 →•→ Transverse vertebral movement of the atlas towards the painful side.

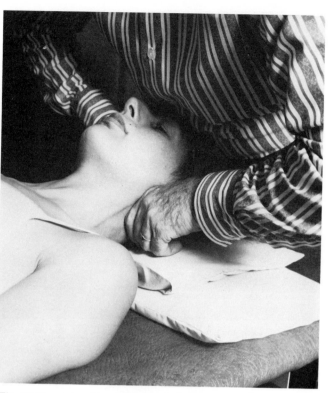

Fig. 12.44 →•→ Transverse vertebral pressures, to the patient's right, of the atlas. Alternative technique.

The occipitoatlantal joint very frequently requires a passive movement and Figure 12.43 shows a method for transverse movement which is easy for both patient and therapist. The patient lies with the painful side on a flat, firm pillow. The therapist stands facing her and contacts the tip of the lateral mass of atlas with one thumbtip; the opposite thumb is placed alongside and helps to stabilise the thumb primarily imparting the small-amplitude, grade I oscillatory movement in a downward direction. Contact must not be lost; the atlas and both thumbs should move as a unit.

Because of a coexistent shoulder or upper rib-joint condition, the patient may not be able to lie on one side; the technique is adapted (Fig. 12.44) so that with the patient supine, the operator's palm replaces the firm pillow against the painful side, and the lateral aspect of the operator's second metacarpal head replaces the thumbtip contact with the lateral mass of atlas on the painless side. It is important to keep the forearms aligned with the gentle movements being imparted via the contact with the lateral tip of atlas.

Extension at the craniovertebral joint can be mobilised by standing at the head of the supine patient (Fig. 12.45) and stabilising the posterolateral apsects of the atlas by a finger-and-thumb grasp from underneath. By gentle,

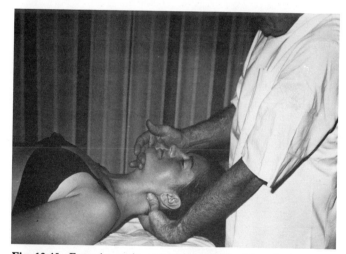

Fig. 12.45 Extension at the occipitoatlantal joint. The atlas is relatively fixed and the occipital condyles are moved by repetitive mandibular pressures.

repetitive grade II cranial movements applied by finger-pressure to the inferior aspect of the mandible with the other hand, the craniovertebral joint is rhythmically extended.

Unilateral postero-anterior gliding of the atlas (Fig. 12.46) is easily achieved with the patient again in side-lying and with her head on a small, firm pillow. The therapist stands facing her shoulders and gently stabilises the head with the far-side palm; the thumbtip or pad of the near-side

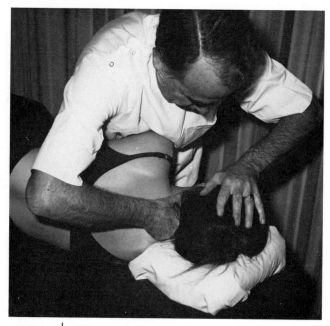

Fig. 12.46 (C1)   Unilateral posteroanterior pressures to the left lateral mass of atlas, with the patient lying on the right side.

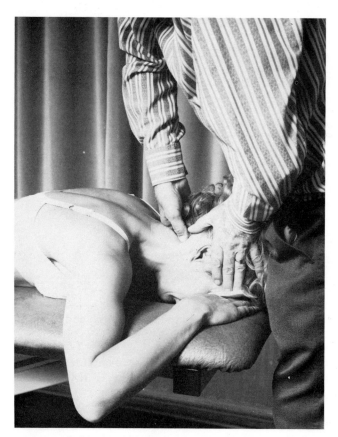

Fig. 12.47 (C1)   Posteroanterior unilateral vertebral pressures to the right lateral mass of C1, synchronously with small-amplitude gapping of the joint by side-flexing the head to the patient's left.

hand bears against the upper posterolateral mass of the painful-side atlas, with the therapist's forearm aligned in the direction of the gentle grade II repetitive postero-anterior movement. Again, atlas and thumb must move in the small amplitude as one.

An alternative method (Fig. 12.47) is with the patient prone and her forehead resting on an Evazote pad on the dorsum of her fingers. Standing at her head, the therapist applies the palm of his hand to the temporal region of the painful side, gently inducing side-flexion away from it in rhythm with the downward, inward and cranial pressures applied by his opposite thumbtip. The thumbtip contact must be precise, delicate and evenly maintained through-out the movement, which may be a grade I, II or III movement.

Restriction near the extreme of rotation at the atlanto-axial joint (C1–C2) may be freed by turning the prone patient's head to the side of limited rotation (Fig. 12.48) and apply-ing unilateral, repetitive postero-anterior pressures to the back of the transverse process of axis with both thumbtips. Movement is imparted to the straight thumbs by excur-sions of arms and elbows, and not by the intrinsic muscu-lature of the hands.

Since much of the available range of C1–C2 rotation movement is taken up by the positioning, the movement is graded as II+, III− or IV, unless the available range of movement (p. 421) be taken as that available with the patient in this particular position.

Side-lying techniques are valuable when treating local-ised problems of irritability and/or adjacent stiffness and hypermobility. Localisation can be very precise, by stabil-

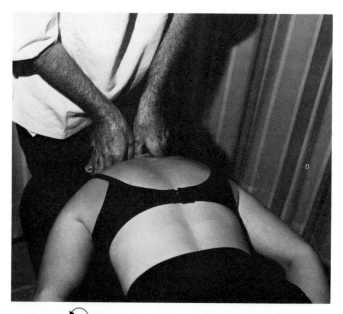

Fig. 12.48   Mobilisation of left rotation at the atlantoaxial (C1-C2) segment, near the extreme of rotation range.

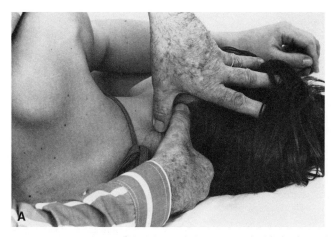
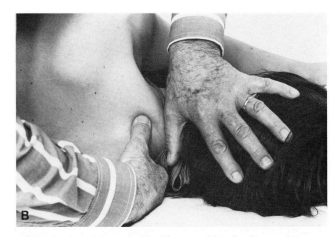

Fig. 12.49 (A) and (B) Side-lying techniques are valuable in the early stages of treating irritable cervical problems, and localisation can be very precise. The thumb positions illustrated are self-explanatory.

isation of segments which need to be kept virtually still (Fig. 12.49).

Established stiffening at the cervicothoracic junction often requires firm and persistent mobilisation, and where firmly applied techniques are used in the presence of flexion limitation, it is helpful to place the patient resting on her approximated elbows, with the head and neck drooping downwards in the space thus provided (Fig. 12.50).

The therapist stands at the side level with her shoulders, and applies one thumbpad reinforced by the other against the side of a spinous process. The repetitive transverse

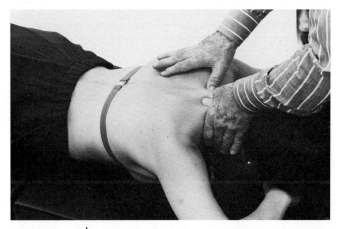

Fig. 12.51 ➙⊣↓ Simultaneous transverse pressures to the patient's right on the spinous process of T1, and posteroanterior pressures on the right transverse process of the same vertebra.

pressure is directed to the painful, or most painful, side; this is one of the few instances when intrinsic thumb muscles are brought into play, so that the patient is not bodily rocked about by the firm pressures being applied.

When limitation of flexion is not such a dominant feature, an alternative method (Fig. 12.51) is for the therapist to stand at the head of the patient, who rests her forehead on the backs of her fingers with an Evazote pad interposed. While the therapist's left thumbpad applies unilateral, postero-anterior pressures to the right lamina of T1 vertebra, for example, the right thumb and forearm are more horizontally disposed to apply reciprocating transverse pressure to the left side of the spinous process of that vertebra.

The costovertebral and costotransverse joints of the first rib may be mobilised by direct rib pressures. There are many techniques; the one illustrated (Fig. 12.52) employs the standard prone position previously described.

The therapist stands facing the patient's opposite hip and applies one thumbpad, reinforced by the other, to the costal arch of the first rib beneath the bulk of the trapezius

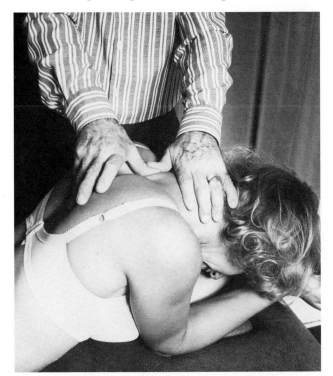

Fig. 12.50 ➙⊷ (C7) Firm transverse vertebral pressures of the C7 spinous process to the patient's right. Used when there is established stiffness with some flexion limitation.

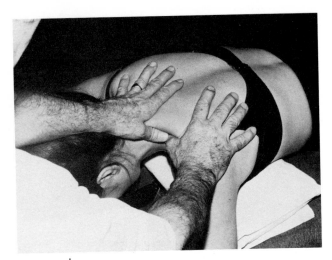

Fig. 12.52 ↓──● (1st Rib)   Mobilisation of the first rib by repetitive pressures, applied anteriorly to the upper trapezius and against the upper rib surface, and directed to the opposite hip.

muscle. Repetitive mobilising pressures towards the patient's opposite hip are applied by movements of the therapist's shoulders and elbow joints via the point of thumbpad contact; the intrinsic hand muscles take no part in producing movement, which is graded according to examination findings.

Anteroposterior mobilisation of the second rib can be of value in the 'second rib syndrome' (p. 235).

With the supine patient's elbow supported against her anterolateral upper abdomen by the therapist's loin, the therapist's near-side thenar eminence engages the left second rib. With the thenar eminence of his other hand engaging the medial aspect of the coracoid process, an anteroposterior and outward movement is imparted to the rib—this is aided by the rhythmic elongation being applied to the pectoralis minor muscle (Fig. 12.53).

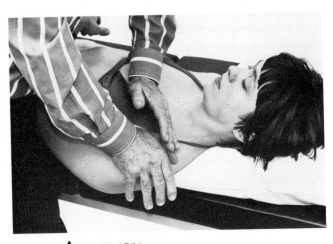

Fig. 12.53 ↑──● (2nd Rib)   Anteroposterior and outward movement imparted to the second rib, aided by rhythmic elongation of the pectoralis minor muscle.

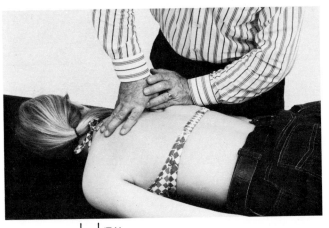

Fig. 12.54 ●↓──↓ (T4)   Simultaneous posteroanterior unilateral pressures on T4 transverse process and posteroanterior unilateral pressures on the angle of the fourth right rib.

The joints of the 4th thoracic vertebra and its associated 4th rib can be mobilised by a combined pressure technique (Fig. 12.54).

With the patient prone, her arms by the side and her head rotated to the treatment side, the therapist stands facing her and places the cranial thumbpad unilaterally over the 4th thoracic lamina and the pisiform bone of the caudal hand on the angle of the 4th rib. The fingers of this hand engage the other, thus ensuring synchronous pressure by both thumb and pisiform.

An alternative to pressures on acutely tender thoracic

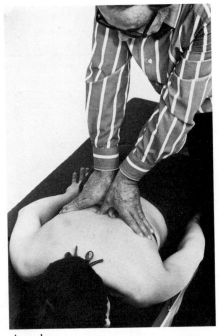

Fig. 12.55 ↓──●──↓   Placing the pads of crossed thumbs over the transverse processes of a single thoracic vertebra provides an alternative to posteroanterior central vertebral pressures. The movement imparted is not quite the same as in posteroanterior central vertebral pressures and should not be regarded as its equivalent for assessment purposes.

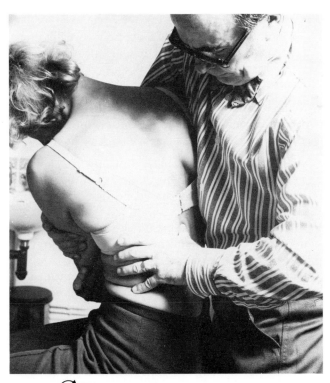

Fig. 12.56 ↻ (T8)   A degree of localisation of right rotation, at the T8–T9 segment, is achieved by stabilising T9 spinous process by left-side pressure and 'tightening' all thoracic segments above T8 by the combined positioning of the trunk.

spinous processes is that of bilateral pressure on transverse processes (Fig. 12.55).

Rotation in the lower thoracic region may be mobilised by positioning the patient so that a majority of effect occurs at a single segment (Fig. 12.56) and this method employs the principle of endeavouring to stabilise a chain of vertebral joints by combinations of movements in positioning (see p. 425).

The patient sits and clasps her elbows. Standing behind, the therapist passes his right arm over the patient's right shoulder and in front of her torso to grasp the left upper arm. Placing his left fingers in her left loin and his left thumbtip or pad against the left side of T9 spinous process, for example, the therapist flexes and then left-side-flexes the patient's trunk. While not allowing any release of these combined positioning movements, right trunk rotation is added; it is important to concentrate on the feeling of increasing soft tissue tension detected by the thumbtip, as the range of available movement is increasingly taken up, from above downwards, by the positioning technique.

Right rotation (in this case at the T8–T9 segment) can be gently or more firmly increased, either by repetitively rotating the patient's trunk against the stabilising pressure of the thumb, or by taking up the combined movements to the existing limit of range and then sharply increasing

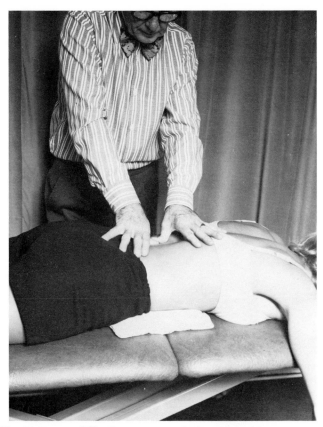

Fig. 12.57 ↦ (L2)   Transverse vertebral pressures to a mid-lumbar spinous process, towards the painful side.

rotation by a single short amplitude movement of the therapist's right hand.

Because a neck-rest position of the patient's hands puts maximum tension on the latissimus dorsi muscle and lumbodorsal fascia of the side to which the trunk is rotated and from which it is side-flexed, this adds unnecessary restriction and the elbow-clasp position is probably more suitable.

While the rotatory effect is probably maximal at the T8–T9 segment, the combined movements produce considerable regional stress, and the effects of these cannot be ignored because one is primarily interested in T8–T9.

Transverse vertebral pressure is a useful technique for *unilateral midlumbar joint problems* (Fig. 12.57).

The patient lies prone over a small hard pillow, with the arms hanging down or at the side. The therapist stands on the painless side and applies one thumbpad to the near side of the spinous process, the other thumbpad reinforcing the first. The oscillatory pressures towards the painful side are imparted by movements of the therapist's shoulders and elbows and not by the intrinsic thumb muscles.

Chronic degenerative stiffness of the lumbosacral segment sometimes requires persistent localised movement (Fig.

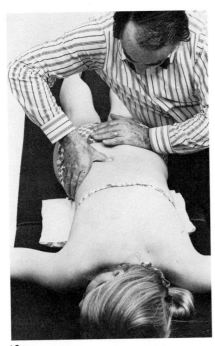

Fig. 12.58 ◄•►| Transverse vertebral pressure, on the patient's right, to the spinous process of L5, while the sacrum is stabilised by the heel of opposite hand.

12.58). The technique is also useful in the presence of the type of adventitious joints which are sometimes associated with transitional vertebrae, and which seem especially subject to degenerative changes (see p. 276).

With the patient prone over a small hard pillow at the lower abdomen and her arms hanging down, the therapist sits on the edge of the plinth and applies the heel of his outer hand to the lateral aspect of the sacrum. By leaning over the patient, the thumbtip of the other hand is applied to the spinous process of L5, so that firm, repetitive pressures may be applied towards the therapist while the sacrum is being stabilised. The technique should be used in either direction, between assessment of effects, so that the more effective direction may be confirmed.

Mobilisation techniques for the sacroiliac joint should be as localised as is possible, because this materially aids assessment of joint problems in a region notoriously liable to confuse the therapist by the equivocal nature of symptoms and signs. The attachments of the iliolumbar ligament will ensure that the fifth lumbar vertebra takes some part in most of the so-called specific sacroiliac techniques, and it may well be that there is no such animal as a purely musculoskeletal sacroiliac condition.

Since the step-by-step palpation methods (p. 331) are essentially similar to the examination method developed by Maitland (1977)[797] and Maigne (1972),[789] the experienced therapist will recognise several choices in the direction of the therapeutic mobilising movement. This can be:

(i) according to the principles of gently repeating the most painful movement in the appropriate grade, or

(ii) according to the principle of Maigne (1965)[787] in which the most painless movement (usually directly opposite to the painful one) is that selected for treatment technique, or

(iii) according to the asymmetry when present.

While it is not always easy to know beforehand which particular movement will be the most helpful, *a basis for selection* of the initial movement might be as follows:

a. where pelvic joint asymmetry is plainly detectable, and assessed as underlying the clinical features, the initial mobilising movement should be that which is most likely to correct it;

b. where step-by-step palpation and provocative pressures have clearly established a pattern of aggravation and relief, and asymmetry is present but barely detectable, the choice of therapeutic movement is that directly opposite to the provocative movement;

c. where pain is manifest but symmetry appears undisturbed, and the results of testing by provocative pressures are equivocal, the prime need is to reduce joint irritability, and thus the initial procedures should either (i) gently gap the joint structures, or (ii) gently and rhythmically repeat the most painful movement, *to the patient's tolerance.*

Whether (a), (b) or (c) are continued with depends upon assessment of results, which is always the final arbiter.

The classic maxim: 'Find it, fix it and leave it alone' does not apply quite so much to sacroiliac joint problems, in the sense of a single and correctly arranged manipulative thrust relieving the joint condition. Several sessions may be needed before satisfactory relief is given to the patient, particularly in chronic and unrecognised cases, where adaptive soft tissue changes have begun to occur as a consequence of the subtle but persisting change in joint relationship. In many patients with an apparent prominence of one posterior superior iliac spine, the range of combined hip adduction/flexion on that side will feel 'tight' and sore, especially in the posterolateral haunch. There will be a mild reduction in the ranges of hip abduction and extension, and there may well be unequal rotation ranges when compared to the unaffected side.

In some, detectable 'tightness' may simulate the earliest soft tissue changes which normally raise the question of an 'early arthrotic hip' and concomitant with manual techniques for the sacroiliac joint itself, the tight tissues will need attention, in their own right, by selective and moderate stretching techniques.

So far as vertebral segments are concerned, our prime aim is to see that they are *moving* as much as they should, and no more than they should. On the other hand, when dealing with mechanical sacroiliac joint problems, the normal mobility is so slight, and the consequences of a

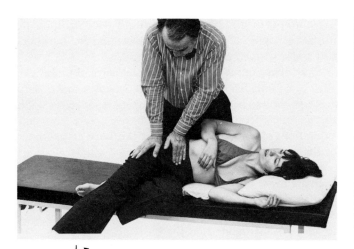

Fig. 12.59 Repetitive gapping of right sacroiliac joint, with mild shearing effect due to the disposition of the uppermost lower limb.

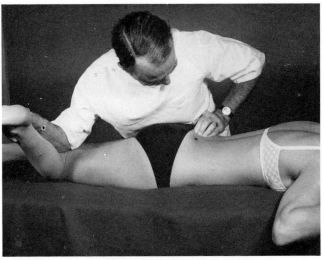

Fig. 12.60 This examination technique, for palpating the degree of sacroiliac joint mobility, can be adapted for its mobilisation effects when treating mild fixation of the joint nearest the therapist.

slight but persisting change in joint relationships can cause such chronic discomfort, that here the emphasis shifts to getting the relationship right, and keeping it right.

When frank sacroiliac joint *hypermobility* is underlying the patient's discomfort, stabilisation is rather easier than in the vertebral column, since a 'binder' (of one form or another) is not difficult to arrange.

Figure 12.59 shows a forward-shearing technique which is indicated in mild degrees of sacroiliac joint irritability associated with a slightly posterior position of the right posterior superior iliac spine (see p. 281).

The patient lies on her side over a small hard pillow under the loin; this ensures a neutral position of the lumbar spine. The under hip and knee are flexed to provide a cradle for the upper leg; this is extended at the knee, and slightly flexed and internally rotated at the hip. The therapist stands behind, level with the pelvis, with his cranial palm on the anterior superior iliac spine and his caudal palm over the greater trochanter. While both hands repetitively induce a shearing influence on the ilium, in the direction of the patient's upper thigh, the therapist's cranial hand adds a measure of sacroiliac gapping by downward pressure on the anterior iliac crest.

In manipulative practice, testing procedures are frequently used as subsequent treatment procedures and Figure 12.60 illustrates such a one. In stabilising the patient's near ilium by the pressure of his lower chest, the therapist has left both hands free; repetitive internal rotation of the patient's far hip joint, by caudal forearm pressure against the medial calf of the patient's flexed leg, allows palpation in the near-side sacroiliac sulcus of the movement occurring. Thus the gentle repetitive movements can be very precisely graded, and this is especially important when joint irritability is present.

Provided the buttock is not unduly tender, the technique is useful in treatment of the 'posterior innominate' of osteopathic terminology.

Mobilisation procedures of more firmness may be required, and in Figure 12.61 the sacrum of the prone-lying patient has been stabilised by palm pressure of the therapist's caudal hand. The heel of the cranial palm has engaged the medial aspect of the posterior superior iliac spine on the far side, which is repetitively mobilised in a downward, outward and caudal direction, by pressures directed in the line of the therapist's forearm.

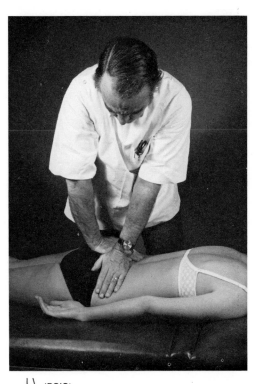

Fig. 12.61 (PSIS) Downward, outward and caudal mobilisation of the patient's right ilium, while the sacrum is stabilised with the opposite hand. From the painless side, the therapist leans over the patient.

Mobilising method

Whatever may be the chosen *method of treatment* by persuasive passive movement to the patient's tolerance, there has been ample demonstration that it does not need to be applied in the plane of the facets, or at right angles to these planes, to be therapeutically effective. This does not mean to say that such movements should not be an integral part of any repertoire of mobilisation techniques; but only that they are certainly not the only effective way to treat patients.[797, 307, 296] For example, one commonly used technique of postero-anterior vertebral pressures ↓ applied by thumbpads or heel of hand to the spinous process of a cervical, thoracic or lumbar vertebra (Fig. 12.62) will plainly produce accessory movement of a dissimilar nature at each region because: the morphology of the vertebrae differs considerably; the orientation of facet-planes is different; the nature of connective-tissue attachments is not the same in each region.

Notions of the vertebrae 'just going up and down' in response to these repetitive pressures plainly will not do, since a moment's consideration of vertebral anatomy indicates that the small movements are likely to be complex, and also to vary considerably between individuals.

As a little bias is added to the movement (see p. 355) by way of a caudal, cephalic, medial or lateral inclination of the direction of pressures, a full and precise biomechanical analysis of the small movement becomes difficult. When transverse vertebral pressures —•→ are applied to spinous processes, equally complex movements are produced.

Whether either, or neither, of these techniques is ultimately employed in the successful relief of signs and symptoms would not depend upon something approaching a *diktat* in a textbook, but would depend upon the initial responses of the abnormal joint and its associated soft tissues, since each patient is unique.

Since these modest and economical ways of mobilising vertebral joints have been shown to occupy a most useful place in the range of available techniques, it follows that therapeutic effectiveness does not derive solely from considerations of what is thought to be the 'correct' geometry of the direction of movement.

Expressed otherwise, the responses of each abnormal joint are more important than 'logical' and arbitrary rules of manipulative method.

A treatment method[797] which would seem appropriate to adopt is formulated on the basis of:

(i) Examination procedures in which the therapist *assumes nothing* but provides opportunities for the nature of the joint abnormality to fully declare itself, in terms of the 'range–pain–resistance' relationship (p. 360)

(ii) Giving the greatest weight to the unique individual combination, and degree, of the abnormal signs and symptoms, rather than to generalised diagnosis

(iii) Grading the degree of applied movement in accordance with detailed examination findings, and

(iv) Changing the technique and/or the grade of applied movement according to the changing nature of the joint abnormality during treatment

(v) Employing the least vigour which will achieve the desired effect.

This treatment approach is by no means the prerogative of any one school of manipulation,[1180a, 627, 217] yet in the author's opinion Maitland (1977)[797] has developed it to the highest degree, and so far as applied movement under

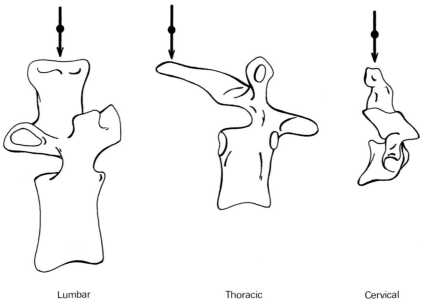

Lumbar   Thoracic   Cervical

Fig. 12.62 Posteroanterior central vertebral pressures on spinous processes will produce different segmental movements according to regional characteristics.

the control of the patient is concerned, the following observations on *grading* concern this particular method.

Grades of manual mobilisation treatment

Each grade (I–IV) has: (a) a constant *position* on the available excursion of movement, and (b) *amplitude*, which is a constant proportion of it.

Grades I and IV are small amplitude movements at the beginning and end, respectively, of available range, while II and III are larger amplitude movements occupying mostly the middle parts of available movement.

Grades are applicable to whatever treatment movement is chosen, be it the available excursion of the active range of a single joint or complex of joints, or that of an involuntary accessory movement.

For normal joints, grades can be depicted in various ways (Fig. 12.63A–E):

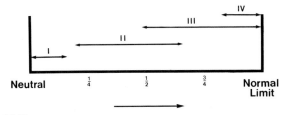

Fig. 12.63A

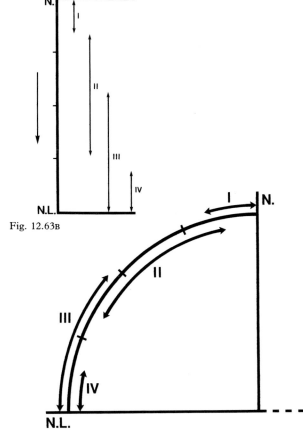

Fig. 12.63B

Fig. 12.63C

Movements of *abnormal* joints are usually, but not invariably, limited, and since the *available* excursion of movement is reduced, the grades of treatment are proportionately reduced, i.e. (Fig. 12.64):

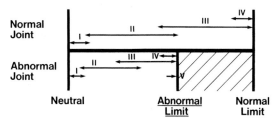

Fig. 12.64 Grades adapted to the reduced available range of movement of an abnormal joint.

Thus, when the 'treatment grade' is expressed or recorded, it refers to grades on the *available* excursion and not the normal range, unless the range of movement is

POSTERO-ANTERIOR VERTEBRAL GLIDING

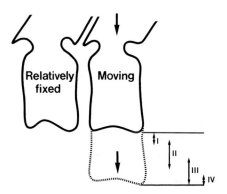

Fig. 12.63D

CARPAL OR TARSAL JOINT GLIDING

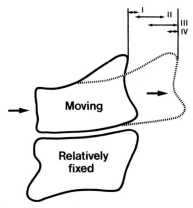

Fig. 12.63E

Fig. 12.63
(Range of accessory movement has been exaggerated for clarity)

not limited, e.g. the abnormality is manifest by painful movement only.

The nature of the range-limiting factor, together with the degree of limitation invariably decide the grade employed in treatment, and frequently also the positioning of the patient's joint and the particular technique; thus when recording palpation and passive movement findings it is necessary to record not only the point of encounter on the expected normal range but also the nature of the limiting factor (see Palpation in Assessment, p. 351).

During examination, it is probably easiest to note the former as being in the 'early', 'middle' or 'late' part of the expected normal range.

In summary:

(i) Palpation findings during *examination and initial assessment* are expressed as factors encountered during the 'E', 'M' or 'L' part of the expected normal range, these being conveniently recorded on a spinal chart alongside the segment concerned

(ii) The *treatment* grade employed refers to the *available* range.

E. REGIONAL MANIPULATION

It is sometimes necessary to employ grade V manipulative thrust techniques, near the limit of available range, when improvement in signs and symptoms achieved by progressive and adequate mobilisation (grades I–IV) has reached stalemate, and assessment of the condition indicates that further improvement is possible.

While the aim of manipulative procedures is more often that of influencing a particular vertebral segment, the term 'regional manipulation' is here taken to include the single, quick distraction techniques with a regional effect, as well as the rotational manipulations for the cervical, thoracic and lumbar regions when manual contact with a bony apophysis of a vertebra for the purpose of localisation does not form part of the method.

This somewhat restricted definition includes, nevertheless, some of the oldest and most useful techniques known to therapists.

The technique of regional lumbar rotation is a prime example of manipulation being all things to all men; it is as old as the hills, and to the best of the author's knowledge there is no school of manipulation in the teaching of which it does not form part of the technique repertoire, in one guise or another.

There are many slight variations of technique, of hand placing and method of contact with the patient; the effects are variously described as 'restoring the normal configuration of the disc',[1371] 'shifting the nerve root off the disc', or 'correcting' unilateral sacroiliac joint asymmetry.[376] Our difficulties arise because the techniques may indeed do just this, but the correlation between what has actually

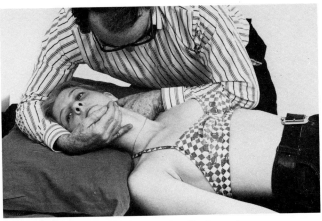

Fig. 12.65 ←•⊣ (C0—C1) loc V A localised gapping manipulative thrust to the left occipitoatlantal joint; this nevertheless has a regional effect and is not a truly localised manipulation.

happened in the large family of soft tissue and joint structures influenced by the manipulation and what we may *believe*, or *hope*, has happened, is manifestly sketchy.

Regional cervical and lumbar rotational manipulations are excellently described in many currently available texts[797, 217] although the aims underlying their use may not include that of regional effect, and Maitland (1977)[797] describes a manipulative distraction technique for the thoracic spine.

An example of distractive manipulation, with a degree of localisation, is that commonly employed for the occipitoatlantal joint (Fig. 12.65). The patient lies supine with her head on a flat firm pillow and the therapist stands on the side to be treated; provided the pillow is firm and so long as the patient's chin, cheek area and vertex are adequately cradled and stabilised by the therapist's cranial palm, forearm and arm, respectively, there is no real need for the therapist to actually support the patient's head from underneath.

Having carefully contacted the patient's occiput, closely adjacent to the occipitoatlantal joint, with the anterolateral surface of the proximal phalanx of his index finger, near the metacarpal head, the therapist slightly side-flexes the patient's craniovertebral region towards himself, and then adds slight extension and rotation to the opposite side.

Three points are then carefully aligned as closely as possible to the paramedian plane, *viz.*: (i) the patients's vertex; (ii) the point of occipital contact, and (iii) the operator's near-side elbow.

This ensures alignment of the forearm to apply a unilateral distraction to the craniovertebral region. While firmly stabilising the patient's head, the available longitudinal movement is taken up by cranial movement of the therapist's forearm, and the manipulative thrust then delivered by a very short amplitude and high-velocity movement with the minimum of energy.

Minor degrees of atlantoaxial joint limitation may be

mobilised by what is in fact a regional manipulation technique (Fig. 12.66) with a localised effect which is dependent upon careful positioning.

The patient lies supine with her head supported, in minimal flexion, beyond the edge of the plinth by the therapist's fingers under the occiput and his thumbs in front of her ears.

Without flexing the patient's neck or inclining the whole neck to one side, her head is gently side-flexed away from the side of restricted movement. The chain of typical cervical joints has thus been 'locked' (in osteopathic terminology) in that the concave-side facet-planes have been closely approximated, and the convex-side facet-planes have been distracted to produce ligamentous and capsular tension. The former are said to be 'facet-locked' and the latter 'ligamentous-locked' (see Discussion, p. 425). Thus as a result of careful positioning, the amount of further movement in the typical cervical segments is minimal.

Because rotation range at the *occipitoatlantal joint* is small, and occurs near the extremes of rotation, movement in these joints will also be minimal, more especially if the extremes of cervical rotation are not approached during the technique.

At the atypical *atlantoaxial joint*, however, the rotation range is much freer, and thus this is the only segment which is left exposed to further rotation movement of any degree.

By gentle, small questing movements the therapist carefully tests the precise point of restriction; when this has been established and the rotation is sensed to be at the point of restriction, the manipulative thrust is delivered by a small 3°–5° amplitude of increased rotatory movement, of high velocity and minimal force, by synchronous movement of both the therapist's hands. Full, regional cervical rotation is not approached.

So much for the theory—the small rotatory thrust is often accompanied by an impressive cacophony of clicks,

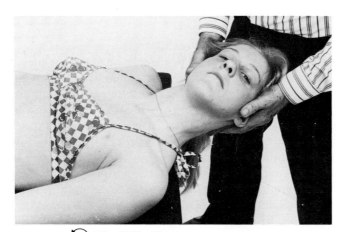

Fig. 12.66 ↻ (C1—C2) loc V   Attempt to localise left rotation to the atlantoaxial joint, based upon positioning by combined movement, according to facet-plane geometry.

and by no stretch of the imagination can this be called a localised technique. It is a regional technique with localised emphasis, like so many other manipulations. The technique has a single indication only—mild unilateral restriction of rotatory atlantoaxial movement in the presence of an otherwise normal neck, and there are much easier and less dramatic ways of treating the patient (see p. 414).

Many descriptions and illustrations of localised or specific techniques plainly show that the positioning for, or execution of, them applies stress to many vertebral segments. This regional stress should not be ignored, and sometimes may well be a factor underlying the indifferent results of manipulative methods which, during the hot pursuit of localisation, overlook the regional stress imposed by positioning.

Care and delicacy of technique will minimise stress to uninvolved segments.

F. LOCALISED MANIPULATION

The basis for preparatory locking of vertebral regions prior to localised manipulation, by methods of positioning which employ combined movements, rests upon the differing nature of vertebral movement from region to region.

Generalised descriptions of spinal movement and of limiting factors need not occupy us here.[437, 631, 994] A detailed knowledge of the morphology of facet-joints is indispensable when devising manipulative techniques with the intention of localising the effect, since the paired facet-joint planes are an important factor influencing the direction, the nature and sometimes the extent of movement in a vertebral district. There are, however, other factors which should not be overlooked, e.g.

1. The spine as a whole is not only an 'empilement' of individual vertebral bones of particular shapes, but also a flexible rod exhibiting three distinct curves in one plane. Its tendency to rotation, when bent in the plane at right angles to these sagittal curves, is no more than can be demonstrated by performing the same experiment with a green and flexible twig; thus an explanation of the physical behaviour of this living flexible rod does not depend *entirely* on the presence or arrangement of vertebral apophyses or facet-joints, except that by reason of their presence its natural physical characteristics are somewhat modified.

2. As we have seen (p. 47), there is some variety in the characteristics of combined vertebral movement between individuals.

3. The effects of anomalies of bone structure and of facet-plane orientation, and of anomalies in the presence of adventitious fibrous bands with unilateral tethering effects which are present in many patients should not be forgotten.

Characteristic movement combinations

Sagittal movement is not 'pure' and cannot occur alone. *Rotation* and *side-bending* are combined, and after the first degree or two of movement one produces a proportion of the other and these physiological combinations of movement cannot be separated. It *is* possible to bend the neck sideways and keep one's nose pointing straight to the front, but vertebral rotation to the same side will occur to a degree anyway, and this voluntary resistance of the natural tendencies of cervical movement will be accompanied by a feeling of strain.

It is these natural, or physiological, combined-movement tendencies which require further examination.

Flexion reduces side-bending and rotation range; it eradicates the cervical and lumbar curves, sometimes slightly reversing the former, often mainly at the C4–C5 segment.

Extension also reduces the range of side-bending and rotation.

Side-bending restricts flexion and extension. Side-bending in the neutral or extended position of the thoracic and lumbar spine makes rotation easier to the convexity than to the concavity; in the typical cervical, and the uppermost thoracic, regions rotation is easier to the concavity. The same applies to the remaining thoracic and the lumbar spine when flexed, as rotation is then easier to the concavity.

Rotation restricts flexion and extension, and is almost invariably accompanied by a degree of side-bending as described above.

These regional combinations of movement are the normal physiological tendencies when the vertebral column is side-flexed or rotated from the flexed, extended or neutral position.

The characteristics of *upper cervical region movement* have been discussed in Vertebral Movement (p. 43), and the only other point to mention is that *flexion* of the cervical region produces a degree of movement restriction, by ligamentous tension at the typical segments, and thus the range of head-rotation on a flexed neck is likely to represent, for the most part, atlantoaxial range.[545]

The physiological tendencies in other regions may be summarised as follows:

Typical cervical region (C2–C6) side-bending is invariably accompanied by rotation to the same side, and vice versa, from all positions of sagittal movement, i.e. whether the neck be flexed, neutral or extended.

Cervicothoracic region (C6–T3). Although movement rapidly diminishes from above downwards, side-flexion is accompanied by rotation to the same side, and vice versa.

Thoracic and lumbar regions. Side-binding is accompanied by rotation to the same side (and vice versa) only in flexion. In the neutral or extended position, side-binding is naturally accompanied by rotation to the opposite side, and vice versa.

Sacroiliac joint. This has been described on page 52.

For those who may be unfamiliar with these movement combinations, it is important not to accept the statements at their face value, but to meticulously work their own spines through the various positions and verify for themselves the tendencies described.

When using specific or localised techniques, the declared *aim* is that of moving one vertebral joint only,[1180a] but since a single typical certival vertebra, for example, takes part in the formation of 10 joints: 4 facet-joints, 2 intervertebral body joints, 4 neurocentral (or uncovertebral) joints, besides giving attachments to very many soft tissue structures which span more than one segment, the view that it is possible to move one joint only becomes untenable.

Similar considerations will apply to *all* other vertebral articulations. This is not to say that, by careful technique and a well-developed sense of tissue-tension, the skilled therapist cannot arrange the patient's position so that the manipulative effect is mainly exerted at a particular segment in a particular way, but only that notions of affecting 'a single joint' should not go unexamined.

Techniques of positioning for localised manipulative thrust techniques (grade V)

The aim is to stabilise adjacent vertebral joints in such a way that the single, quick, short-amplitude thrust is maximally exerted at a single segment in a particular direction; it may be to neatly distract the two planes of a facet-joint, i.e. movement at right angles to these planes, or to translate or glide one upon the other in the existing plane. A further aim is protective, in that careful techniques of controlled fixation of neighbouring articulations where possible will prevent them from being subjected to needless movement; this is also the consideration underlying economy of vigour when applying the manipulative thrust. These are thus the aims.

Let us now examine these considerations, as applied to the cervical spine. In Figure 12.67A, a scheme of the left lateral aspect of the cervical facet-joint planes shows that the planes would roughly converge somewhere in front of the eye. During side-bending to the patient's left, i.e. towards the viewer, the weight of the superimposed head will soon, but not immediately, cause each inferior articular facet to move *downwards*, and then *posteriorly*, upon the upward-and-backward-facing superior articular facet of the subjacent vertebra. On the opposite right side, each inferior articular facet-plane tends to move *upward* and *forward* on the one below. Thus rotation towards the direction of side-bending is imposed by the facet orientation (see Figs 12.67B and C).

If, while holding the neck side-flexed to the left, we

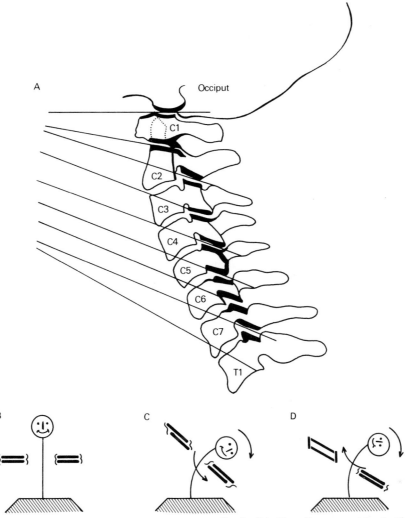

Fig. 12.67 (A) The cervical facet-joint planes are oriented so as to roughly converge at a point somewhere in the region of the eye. (B) Neutral position. (C) Physiological tendency is rotation to the same side on side-bending. (D) Opposite (right) rotation imposed. Facet apposition on (L) and facet gapping on (R).

On the (L) side, a 'facet-apposition-lock' or 'compression-lock' has been achieved by rotating the head and neck in an *opposite* direction to the physiological tendency.
On the (R) side, a 'ligamentous-tension-lock' has been achieved; the facet-planes are maximally distracted and the capsule of the joint is tautened.

impose an opposite (right) rotation, the left facet-planes are markedly approximated, and those on the right strongly distracted. In osteopathic terminology, the left row of typical facets are regarded as being 'facet-opposition-locked', and the right-side row as being 'ligamentous-tension-locked' (Figs 12.67B, C, D).[1180a]

Thus, in the position described above, the facet-lock occurs on the side rotated away from, and the ligamentous lock on the side rotated towards, when the rotation imposed is *opposite* to the physiological tendency of that particular vertebral district.

These positioning techniques which tend to stabilise the vertebral segments of a region by locking do not *ensure* that a small-amplitude thrust will mainly move only the vertebrae to which it is applied, but with careful technique will make it more of a certainty than not.

Bearing in mind what has been said about the regional characteristics of vertebral movement, it will be plain that positioning techniques will vary from region to region, and that the techniques will need careful study and much patient practice before confident precision and economy of vigour gradually replace the hopeful shove.

It should be evident that a sound knowledge of the planes and angulation of the facet-joints, of the characteristics of spinal movement, of the importance of anomalies and individual variations together with a well-developed sense of tissue-tension, are important factors in positioning the patient immediately prior to the manipulative thrust. The German *Fingerspitzengefühl* (literally, 'the sense of perception by fingertip') expresses the importance of this sensitivity.

There is now a further consideration, i.e. while the movement combinations of a typical *cervical* vertebra appear to be fairly well elucidated on the basis of facet-plane orientation, it is not so easy to adequately explain vertebral movement in the same way at all other regions.

As an instance, the behaviour of the segments T6–T3 is much the same as those of the typical cervical region, despite a rapidly diminishing range of movement and the added attachments of the shortest and strongest ribs. To explain this curious phenomenon on the basis that the facet-planes are much like those of the mid- and lower-cervical region is to raise more questions than answers, more so when it is plain that the facet-planes of the T5 segment, for example, are much more like those of T3 than those of T3 are like C7. Yet the typical movement combinations of T5 are directly opposite to those of T3. We can only observe what the characteristic combinations are,[1180a, 489] and employ them for our purpose, while analysis of the biomechanical influences remains to be satisfactorily elucidated. The way in which the patient is positioned to achieve localisation, and the degree of emphasis upon either the positioning itself, or the amount of manual fixation pressure required, will depend upon the observed characteristics of each vertebral region.

For example, at the lower thoracic segments, there is a position of *slight* flexion when rotation to the same side is not automatically combined, and to improve the rotation range of a segment in this particular neighbourhood by a manipulative thrust technique, it is necessary to employ rather more finger and thumb localisation than would be required in other regions.

In general terms, to localise or restrict the main effects of a grade V manipulative technique, the patient is positioned in rotation *opposite* to the physiological tendency. When this is done, the facet-compression lock usually occurs on the side rotated away from, and ligamentous lock occurs on the side rotated towards.

When the objective of manipulation is to free an assumed facet-joint 'fixation', by using thrust techniques to induce movement *in the plane of that joint*, the segment is positioned just short of complete tightness, and this must be sensed by careful and attentive palpation. It is then the manipulative thrust in the plane of the facets which is 'executive', taking the joint to its normal limit, together with a degree of accessory movement, by a short, quick and decisive movement. Here, facet-approximation-locking is emphasised, employing a high-speed manipulative thrust.

When the objective is to emphasise the *gapping* of facet-joints, at right angles to their planes, the emphasis is on ligamentous-tension-locking, and the 'executive' is a slightly slower movement which actually comprises the final synchronous application of the side-flexion and rotation movements which were employed to carefully position the segment.

NB: The term 'locking' is unfortunate, since it conveys a finality of effect. Whether a true lock is ever achieved, excepting perhaps at the thoracolumbar mortice joint (p.

14) on full extension, is debatable. The facet-joint capsules are thin and loose, and even when full capsular tension is applied a rotatory slip or glide is still easily imposed, because the interposed discs (at least in the cervical spine) have the special quality of lateral distortion, which is the physiological basis of sagittal movement in the neck (see p. 46).

For analogy, the fact that the handles of a concertina have been distracted to their fullest limit does not mean that movement of the handles, at right angles to the line of distraction, is not easily applied. Nevertheless the arrangement of facets, and their effect on movement, are important, e.g. although the annular attachments of the strong lumbar disc would, on their own account, preclude a free range of lumbar rotation, the arrangement of the lumbar facets soon prevents this, anyway, by their being firmly approximated unilaterally like the flanges on a railway train wheel engaging the track.

Techniques

NB: It cannot be too strongly emphasised that manipulative thrust techniques, for the vertebral column but also for the peripheral joints, should not be used without instruction which includes a sufficiently long period of adequately supervised practical and clinical work. Manipulative thrust techniques cannot be learned from a text. There is no safe substitute for practical instruction by an experienced teacher, and close supervision in the early stages of clinical work. It is *possible*, of course, to learn from a textbook how to fly a light aeroplane, but only very rarely indeed would the process be without incident.

There are many ways of manipulating vertebral segments; the following selection is *representative of methods* employed to achieve a more localised effect (see also p. 424).

Occipitoatlantal joint (C0–C1). Limitation of side-bending at this joint may be treated by a technique which moves both occipital condyles on a *relatively* fixed atlas, and the direction of the treatment movement is in that of the limitation (Fig. 12.68).

The patient is supine on a low plinth while the therapist stands behind holding the patient's head with whole hand and palmar grasps at the region of the anterior ears.

By flexing the neck, a degree of posterior ligamentous tension is applied to the cervical structures; this leaves the C1–C2 segment still capable of considerable rotation. By side-flexing the neck to the right and rotating it to the left while maintaining the flexion, the right row of typical facet-joints has been approximated (a facet-apposition-lock), and the left row markedly distracted (a ligamentous-tension-lock). Atlantoaxial rotation is also taken up, the atlas having rotated with the occipital condyles. The treatment movement is applied in the normal frontal plane of the occipitoatlantal segment, albeit this has been

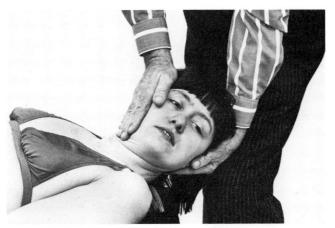

Fig. 12.68 ↘●↗(C0—C1) loc V A gapping/distraction manipulation for the left occipitoatlantal joint. It is vital for the therapist's left hand to remain stabilised against his anterior left thigh.

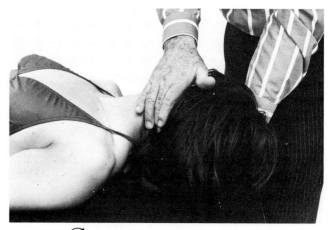

Fig. 12.69 ↺(C2) loc V A manipulative technique for releasing an axis which is blocked or fixed in slight left rotation or left side-flexion. The therapist's under hand does not move.

oriented through some 80°–90° towards the patient's left side.

The increasing tightness of soft structures must be carefully perceived and the very short manipulative thrust delivered without further gross movement of the neck. To this end, by slightly bending his knees, the therapist stabilises the back of his left hand against his lower anterior thigh. With both arms straight, the upper hand delivers a small-amplitude downward thrust as the under hand is synchronously moved upward and outward for the same excursion of movement; the whole cranium is actually moved through the small arc of a curve. Thus right side-bending restriction at C0–C1 is mobilised, and this is an example of localisation achieved without manual contact with a vertebral apophysis. The technique should not be used in the presence of joint irritability at a cervical segment.

The atlantoaxial joint (C1–C2). When the axis (C2) is fixed or blocked in a position of slight left rotation (or left side-flexion, which is the same thing) a pulling technique may replace a thrust technique, albeit the effect is the same.

As shown in Figure 12.69, the patient lies supine and the therapist stands on her right side at the corner of the plinth.

With the patient's head and neck in the neutral position, the head is rotated to the right and supported on the therapist's cranial hand. The therapist's distal phalanx of the index or middle finger of the caudal hand is carefully placed against the left posterolateral aspect of the axis (C2); the patient's head is extended around the fulcrum of the therapist's finger. The rest of the neck is not extended. When the extension and rotation positioning have been taken to the point of tissue-tightness, the manipulative traction movement is a short amplitude pull on the transverse process of C2, along a line joining the tip of the patient's nose and the lobe of the ear. The cranial

hand must be consciously stabilised and still at the instant of the executive movement.

A thrust technique which may be used to free atlantoaxial (C1–C2) rotation restriction is that depicted in Figure 12.70.

With patient supine and the therapist standing at her head, the patient's neck is kept in the neutral position during rotation *to* the restricted side. The therapist's right hand lightly but firmly supports the patient's right cranium, while the left palm engages the patient's left occiput, so that the anterolateral aspect of the proximal phalanx of the index finger engages the left posterior arch

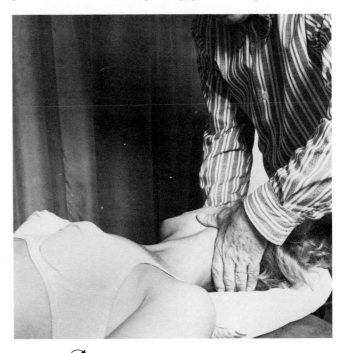

Fig. 12.70 ↺(C1—C2) loc V A manipulative thrust technique (through an arc of some 3° only) to free a right rotation restriction at the atlantoaxial joint.

No cervical technique involving a degree of rotation, or rotation with extension, should be employed without first holding the neck in full rotation with extension for 30 seconds, on either side, to observe its effects.

of atlas. When it is sensed that the point of rotation restriction has been encountered, the manipulative thrust by the left hand is a very quick and delicate increase of rotation which aims at some 3° of movement only. It is important for the ventral surface of the therapist's right lower forearm to limit the excursion of right rotation movement, and the arm should be stabilised as close to the patient's forehead as is necessary to do this.

The latter technique may be modified to mainly affect the C2–C3 segment by shifting the executive hand so that it engages the left posterolateral aspect of C2, in which case *the head, C1 and C2 are rotated as a unit.* In this case, and in other rotatory manipulations for segments below C2, the movement should be in the *opposite* direction to the painful restriction, i.e. a restricted left rotation of C2–C3 or C3–C4 is best treated by a right rotation movement in the first instance.

NB: Rotation rechniques should not be employed before the effects of a test rotation have been noted during the initial clinical examination.

C2–C6. A standard technique (Fig. 12.71) for this vertebral district involves facet-opposition and ligamentous tension locking, and allows modification of emphasis to achieve particular effects. The general effects of applying the combined positioning movements have been described on page 425.

The therapist stands to the right of the supine patient's head, and grasps the chin with his left hand so that the patient's left ear and vertex will be resting against his forearm and biceps muscle, respectively, when the neck is rotated to the left. The anterolateral aspect of the proximal phalanx of the therapist's index finger engages the articular process of the upper vertebra of the cervical mobility segment being treated. Without *inclining* the whole neck to the right, the therapist side-flexes the neck from above downwards, around the stable fulcrum provided by his index finger, by gently pushing to the patient's left side.

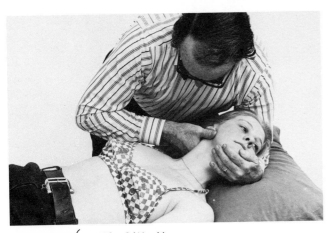

Fig. 12.71 ← (C3—C4) loc V   A unilateral facet-joint gapping technique, in this case for the left C3-C4 segment.

When it is sensed that side-flexion range has been taken up, the side-flexed position is held while rotation to the left is carefully added, until the rotation movement begins to disturb the vertebra in contact with the therapist's index finger. The therapist then adds very slight extension, and confirms that his index finger contact is correct. His forearm is aligned along a line joining his right elbow, right index finger and the patient's left eye, which will ensure that the direction of the thrust is in the plane of the facet-joints.

There are two ways of employing this technique:

1. For right side-flexion limitation at the mobility segment concerned, the therapist takes the combined movements to the point when the restriction is encountered, and then delivers a short-amplitude, decisive thrust in the plane of the facets; the right hand is the executive one and the left hand merely stabilises the combined position. This emphasises the facet-approximation of the preparatory positioning.

2. A modification of the method is to use the ligamentous-tension component for side-flexion (or any other) restriction of the *left* side apophyseal joint. The patient is positioned as before, but the combined movements are not taken completely to the point of restriction; the slower manipulative thrust is applied by a small amplitude, decisive increase of both rotation and side-flexion with the *left* hand, thus producing a gapping effect on the left side of the involved segment. Hence the left hand is now the executive one and the therapist's right index finger remains still as the fulcrum of the movement, or may synchronously add a mild degree of thrust as a secondary accentuation of the movement.

Cervicothoracic region (C6–T3). Acute and chronic conditions of the upper three costotransverse and costovertebral joints are very common, and when manipulation of a single rib is indicated the methods of localisation are similar to those for the typical cervical region.

It is convenient for the patient to lie prone, with the operator standing at her head and slightly to the opposite side of the affected joint. By a combination of rather more left side-flexion and right rotation, together with increased extension, than would be employed for a cervical manipulation, the patient's cervicothoracic region is placed with the left-side facets approximated and the right-side facets distracted. It is important to probe the positioning until the rising tissue-tension can be sensed; since this involves the fixation of a chain of joints which is rather long, it is probably wise to add further stabilisation more locally.

Figure 12.72A shows preparation for a manipulative thrust, which is to be applied to the angle of the patient's first right rib by the distal aspect of the therapist's right pisiform bone. Following positioning, the therapist's left palm and fingers stabilise the patient's neck and occiput, while his left thumb engages the left transverse process

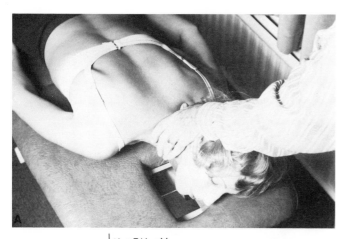

Fig. 12.72 ●——↓(1st R) loc V   (A) Preparation for a manipulative thrust to the right first rib. The patient's head and neck have been side-flexed left and rotated right; the left transverse process of T1 has been stabilised by the therapist's left thumb.

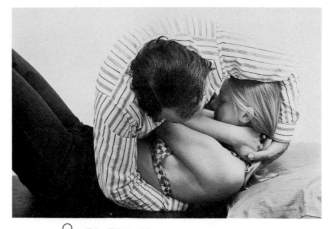

Fig. 12.73 ↓—(T4—T5) loc V   (A) A manipulative thrust technique which may be adapted to free a flexion or extension restriction, at segments between T3 and T10.

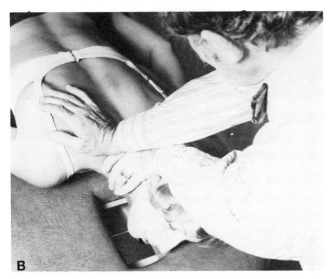

(B) The manipulative thrust is delivered through pisiform contact of the therapist's right hand with the angle of the first rib.

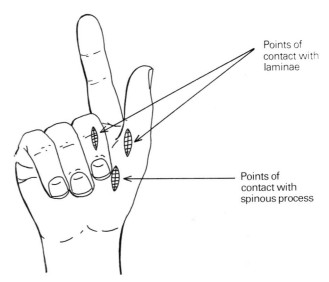

Points of contact with laminae

Points of contact with spinous process

(B) To show the two points of contact, i.e. middle phalanx of middle finger and anterolateral aspect of first metacarpophalangeal joint, which engage the laminae and transverse processes of a thoracic vertebra; a small cottonwool ball may be grasped in the hand to make the points of contact more stable. The spinous process of the vertebra rests alongside the middle fingernail.

of the first thoracic vertebra. Before the downward, outward and caudal thrust is delivered (Fig. 12.72B), some little time should be devoted to ensuring that the pisiform-rib angle contact is precise and firm. The line of the short-amplitude movement is along that joining the therapist's straight arm with his shoulder and the pisiform contact.

Thoracic area (T3–T10). Many techniques for the thoracic region are based upon the effects of ligamentous tension, which is locally emphasised by a degree of manual fixation.

Figure 12.73A shows the patient lying near the therapist's side of the plinth with her knees bent and hands clasped behind her neck. The therapist rolls the patient's upper torso towards himself and engages his right hand (see Fig. 12.73B) firmly against the soft tissues overlying

the laminae and transverse processes of the lower vertebra of the joint to be manipulated. His left palm lies on the back of the patient's hands and his left biceps muscle is against the patient's vertex. By rolling the patient back onto his right hand, and leaning well over so that the patient's upper forearm bears against his lower sternum, the therapist is able to flex the neck and thorax until mounting ligamentous tension is perceived by his right hand. The sharp but short-amplitude thrust is applied by a decisive downward movement of the therapist's trunk while his left arm stabilises the patient's position.

1. *To free a* flexion *restriction*, the thrust is a small but firm increase of flexion, which will be maximal at the segment of which the manually fixed vertebra forms the lower part.

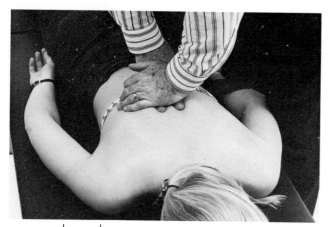

Fig. 12.74 ↓——•——↓ (T7) loc V   A downward thrust simultaneously applied over the transverse processes of a single thoracic vertebra. It is important to position the shoulders vertically over the joint to be manipulated.

2. *To free an* extension *restriction*, the patient's flexed thorax is first locally extended at the involved segment by lowering the patient's shoulders towards the plinth, without releasing the ligamentous tension of the cranial side segments; the executive thrust is then delivered in a downward but cranial direction, i.e. more in line with the patient's upper arms.

The positioning comprises less a 'lock' than a mixture of ligamentous tension with extra localisation by manual fixation.

Extension restriction may be treated by a technique which has elements of the chiropractic method, in that without localisation dependent upon positioning, a direct thrust is applied to vertebral apophyses (Fig. 12.74).

Standing at the side of the prone patient, the therapist applies the palmar-surface of the distal phalanges of his index and middle fingers over the laminae of the lower vertebra of the restricted segment. Leaning well over the patient, the hypothenar eminence of his other hand presses on the dorsal aspect of the two distal phalanges. Instructing the patient to breathe in and then out fully, the therapist closely follows the downward movement of the thorax during expiration and continues to firmly take up the remaining thoracic resilience by a downward movement of his trunk. At the point of encountering the restriction of further movement, a firm but short-amplitude vertical thrust is applied by a movement of the therapist's trunk, and with both hands moving as one.

Techniques of this nature depend almost entirely upon the speed and decisiveness of the thrust, which are much more important than excessive vigour.

Restriction of rotation at a lower thoracic segment may be freed by a manual contact thrust technique following the use of combined movements to assist localisation (Fig. 12.75).

For a right rotation restriction, the patient is seated across the plinth and the therapist stands behind; the patient's

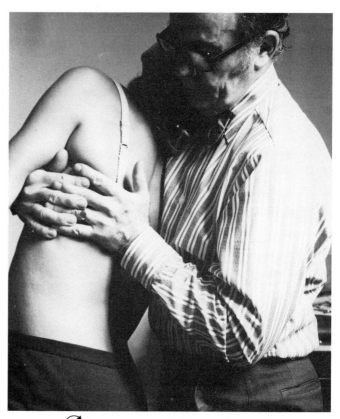

Fig. 12.75 ↺ (T9) loc V   Manipulation to free right rotation restriction at a low thoracic segment. The thrust is upward, towards the patient's shoulder.

arms may be folded but need not be, and many relax better if the arms are ignored. Passing his right arm over the patient so as to engage her right shoulder with his right axilla and her left hemithorax with his right hand, the therapist engages the left transverse process of the upper of the two vertebrae forming the restricted segment, with the pisiform bone of his left hand. The contact must be firm, and with a slight caudal bias, so the upward or cranial direction of the treatment movement is decisively applied. It is convenient to link the fingers.

By gently hugging the patient, she is side-flexed to the right, and then *slightly* extended as the therapist shuffles round to add right rotation, until a sense of increasing tissue-tension indicates that the point of restriction has been encountered. The manipulative thrust with the left hand is a short, sharp upward-lifting motion rather than a rotatory action, and is timed to coincide precisely with the moment that the patient complies with the therapist's quiet instruction that she drop her head onto his right shoulder. A small degree of trunk rotation accompanies the manipulative movement.

It is important (i) to visualise the plane of the lower thoracic facet-joints, and to apply the movement in that plane, and (ii) not to apply more than mild thoracic extension.

Lumbar spine (L3–L4) (Fig. 12.76). When unilateral restriction of movement at a lumbar segment requires manipulative release, the patient lies on the unaffected side in a neutral position. Standing before her, the therapist palpates between the spinous processes of the restricted segment with his cranial hand, and with his caudal hand gently flexes her uppermost leg through a small range until movement begins to be perceived between L3 and L4 spinous processes. At this point the patient's foot can conveniently be hooked behind the knee of the under leg (which need not be straight) or the leg may be allowed to add its weight to the rotatory effect by hanging over the side of the plinth. This may add a degree of undesirable stretch if there is limb pain.

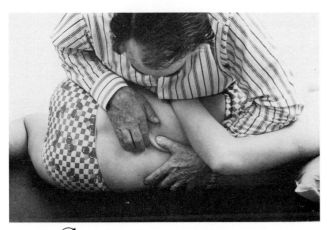

Fig. 12.76 ↻ (L3—L4) loc V Rotational manipulation to gap the L3-L4 facet-joint on the patient's left side. (See text for comments on hypermobility.)

With the spine still in a neutral flexion-extension position, the therapist now palpates the L3–L4 segment with his caudal hand, while rotating the patient's thorax away from himself by pulling upwards on the patient's under arm with his cranial hand. Should the L3–L4 lumbar joint restriction be adjacent to an L4–L5 joint hypermobility, the thoracic and upper lumbar rotation should not be increased beyond the point where the rotation, imposed from above downward, just begins to affect L3–L4. If there is no lumbar hypermobility, a further degree of rotation may be added.

A standard technique is then to arrange the patient's upper palm on her abdomen so that her forearm lies on her loin. The therapist's abdomen bears against the dorsum of the patient's hand. By threading his cranial arm between the patient's arm and trunk, applying his cranial forearm to the patient's outer pectoral area and his caudal forearm to the patient's upper haunch, the therapist has both hands free to localise the emphasis of the rotatory manipulation.

The left trunk rotation is locally emphasised by contact of the therapist's cranial thumb against the left aspect of L3 spinous process, while the right pelvic rotation is emphasised by the therapist's index or middle fingertip engaging the right aspect of the L4 spinous process; the therapist's forearms accentuate the general rotation by contact with the patient's haunch and pectoral regions.

By rolling the patient back and forward, further increments of rotation are successively added, until the point of restriction is encountered. The firm and decisive manipulative thrust is a sharp accentuation of the rotatory movement, by the four points of contact, i.e. cranial forearm and thumb, opposed by caudal forearm and index finger.

When more cautious rotatory manipulations are used to free joint restriction in the presence of adjacent hypermobility, the standard technique is modified, in that if the hypermobility is at L2–L3, for example, the region L3-and-above is held still while the therapist's caudal hand and forearm apply the final rotatory thrust. If L4–L5 is the hypermobile segment, the region L4-and-below is stabilised while the rotatory thrust is delivered from above downwards to L3.

The manipulative thrust is an accentuation of gapping of the left L3–L4 facet-joint. Since the patient is in a neutral position, but somewhat side-flexed to the left by reason of the right-side-lying position, the physiological tendency is for the trunk to rotate to the right (p. 424). By positioning the patient in *left* trunk rotation, the right row of lumbar facet-joints is approximated and the left row distracted.

The basic principles of rotatory manipulation apply to the region T10 to L5–S1, but at the upper part of the region they are considerably modified to accord with its movement, by the four points of contact, i.e. cranial fore-important consideration is the orientation of the lumbo-sacral facet-planes.[1180a]

The sacroiliac joint. It is important to try and localise manipulative techniques, by hand placings which reduce regional effects to the minimum. This is because accurate assessment of sacroiliac joint problems, and the effects of treatment procedures, can at times be uncommonly difficult. The more diffuse the treatment effects, the more uncertain is likely to be assessment of results.

There are many methods; the examples illustrated have been chosen for the reasons outlined. On occasions when assessments can be made with more confidence because of the unequivocal nature of symptoms and signs, the choice of technique becomes wider.

NB: Indications for localised grade V manipulation of the sacroiliac joint occur much less frequently than might be supposed, since the great majority of patients respond to persuasive joint movement by mobilisation, rather than an abrupt insistence on movement by manipulation.

If a posteriorly prominent or rotated ilium is considered to underlie the symptoms reported, their relief by adequate mobilisation has reached a limit and further improvement

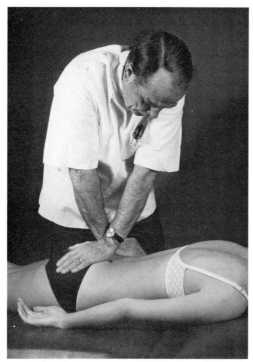

Fig. 12.77 ⊢• (PSIS) loc V A downward and outward thrust to a prominent posterior iliac spine. The therapist's left hand stabilises the sacrum.

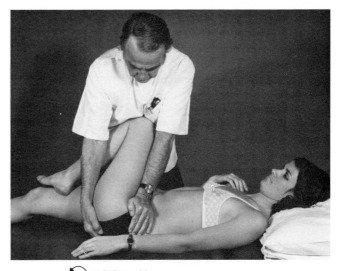

Fig. 12.78 b• ⤸ (ASIS) loc V A gapping with backward 'rotation' manipulative technique for pain associated with a forward ilium on the same side.

is reasonably to be expected, a postero-anterior thrust technique (Fig. 12.77) may be employed.

The therapist stands on the affected side of the prone patient, level with her pelvis. While the cranial arm is held straight and the heel and palm of that hand stabilises the sacrum, the heel of the caudal hand engages the whole surface of the posterior superior iliac spine. The therapist leans a moderate amount of body weight through the caudal arm, which is aligned in a downward, outward and forward direction, for a few seconds before a short amplitude thrust is applied to the ilium in that direction.

On the less frequent occasions when a forward position of the ilium is assessed as underlying the unilateral symptoms, a localised combination of gapping, anteroposterior movement and rotation can be effective (Fig. 12.78). Standing at pelvic level on the unaffected side of the supine patient, and with the affected side hip slightly adducted and flexed to rather more than 90°, the therapist supports the knee against his upper abdomen and leans over the patient, to cup the ischial tuberosity with his caudal palm; his cranial palm rests comfortably on the anterior superior iliac spine.

By slightly flexing his trunk the therapist further adducts the affected-side hip, while not allowing the pelvis to rise from the plinth, and during this slight movement the hand placings are stabilised. The quick but short-amplitude manipulative thrust is a synchronous application of: upward and downward pressures by caudal and

cranial hands, respectively, and by a controlled, short movement of the therapist's trunk, a slight accentuation of the hip adduction and pressure down the length of the femur. It is important to carefully control the degree of applied movement because of leverage on the hip joint.

G. LIMB GIRDLE JOINTS

Vertebral pain syndromes are very frequently accompanied by associated painful conditions of the limb girdle joints (p. 187). Their treatment by manual techniques is a comprehensive subject in its own right,[798] and the few examples which follow may serve as an indication of the importance of gentle distraction techniques, and of improving the range of accessory movements which underlie normal active movements.

Acromioclavicular joint (Fig. 12.79)
The therapist stands on the painless side of the supine patient level with her shoulders. Her upper arm rests on

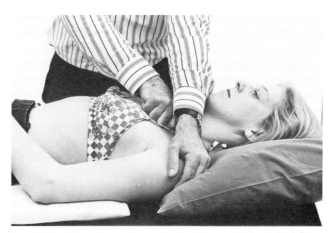

Fig. 12.79 Distraction of the patient's left acromioclavicular joint.

a flat pillow. Stabilising the medial end of the clavicle by a finger and thumb grasp with his caudal hand, the therapist reaches across the patient to place the heel of his cranial hand on the coracoid process and his palm against the head of humerus. The scapular distraction is imparted by protraction movements of the therapist's cranial shoulder girdle, and not by elbow extension and flexion.

Internal rotation of the arm. This is an important functional movement, and a fundamental aid improving voluntary range is to mobilise the accessory gliding and rolling range, in a postero-anterior direction, of the head of humerus in the glenoid foramen.

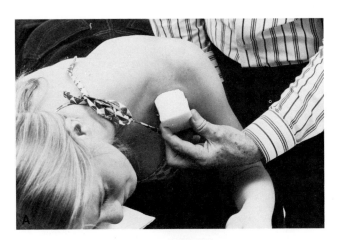

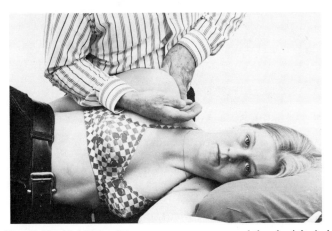

Fig. 12.80 Mobilising the accessory component, and the physiological movement if need be, of the internal rotation range of the shoulder. It is a technique requiring some practice, since there are four things to think about.

Figure 12.80 shows the patient in the side-lying position with her upper limb internally rotated to the point when pain precludes further movement. The limb is safely stabilised at this point by pressure of the therapist's loin, since he is standing behind so that the coracoid process of scapula may be engaged by his hypothenar eminence. The head of the humerus is repetitively mobilised in a forward direction by pressure of the therapist's thumbpad; as the range of internal rotation increases, positioning of the patient's limb is modified so that the gentle mobilisation movements are applied at the point of limitation.

Where resistance is more dominant than pain (see p. 364), forward movements of the humeral head are accompanied synchronously by backward movements of the therapist's forearm, and in later steps of the treatment by downwards (medial) movements of his elbow. Thus the combined movements involve four separate components of the technique, one of which is the unchanging stabilisation of the coracoid process.

Distraction techniques. These form a useful part of mobilisation for shoulder and hip joint conditions.

Figure 12.81A shows the preparation for glenohumeral distraction. A two-inch brick of firm Plastazote is placed

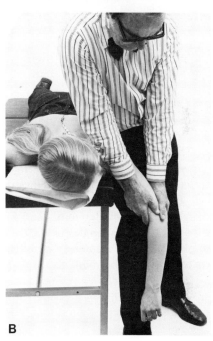

Fig. 12.81 (A) and (B) A distraction technique for the glenohumeral joint, with scapula stabilised by pressure to coracoid process and lateral scapular border.

against the coracoid process, before the patient lies prone and hangs her arm over the edge of the plinth. By standing at the same side and firmly leaning his lateral haunch against the lateral border of the scapula, the therapist further stabilises it; laying the patient's arm over his nearside anterior thigh and slightly flexing the knee of that limb, the therapist grasps the lower end of the humerus with his arms straight (Fig. 12.81B). By this method, even the most slightly built therapist can exert considerable distraction effects upon the glenohumeral joint, by employing bodyweight exerted through straight arms.

Glenohumeral elevation range. This is frequently limited to a slight but painful degree, when tested with the arm close to the head or in full elevation with some abduction from the mid-line.

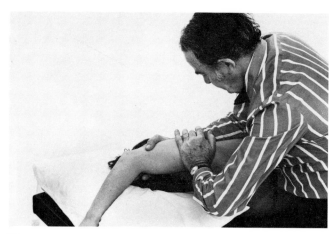

Fig. 12.82 Gaining the last few degrees of elevation at the glenohumeral joint, by small accessory movement anteriorly of the humeral head, with the scapula stabilised.

Restriction of anterior accessory movement of the humeral head in the glenoid cavity often underlies this slight limitation of full elevation.

The patient lies on the painless side with hips and knees flexed to 90°; the therapist stands behind the patient and elevates the arm, to the point of restriction, by grasping its medial aspect just above the elbow (Fig. 12.82). This brings the flexor aspect of his near-side arm against the lateral border of the scapula, which becomes the method of stabilising it. By applying his other palm to the humeral head, just distal to the shoulder joint, and keeping his other forearm aligned at right angles to the patient's arm, the small-amplitude postero-anterior mobilising movements can be localised to the joint.

Distraction of the hip-joint (Fig. 12.83). This is conveniently applied in the line of the neck of femur.[447] The

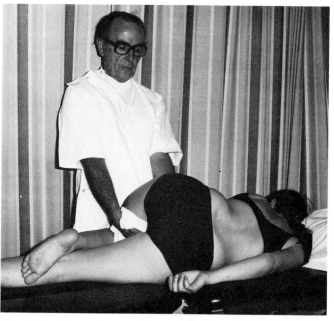

Fig. 12.83 Distraction of the femoral head in the line of the neck of femur. The fulcrum of the movement comprises the patient's knee against the therapist's lower abdomen.

patient lies in a three-quarter prone position with the affected hip uppermost, and flexes this to something less than 90°, hooking her foot behind the under knee.

Standing facing the patient, the therapist stabilises her upper knee in his groin, and with a thick pad of towelling interposed grasps the upper adductor mass with clasped fingers, keeping his arms straight; the positioning thus employs the principle of the third order of levers. By leaning backwards repetitively, the femur is distracted in the line of the femoral neck. Alternatively, a soft canvas sling may be employed to apply the femoral distraction.

13. Recording treatment with clinical method

Because of the prime importance of recording the nature and results of modern investigation procedures, which almost daily become more technical and comprehensive, the volume of accumulated medical information about one individual receiving hospital treatment is likely to be considerable. This will be added to by the more traditional and already comprehensive information recorded about the clinical examination, straight radiography, blood counts, liver, lung or cardiac function tests, etc. and for inpatients a detailed account of temperature, pulse, respiration and other bodily functions, details of monitoring systems, drugs administered, and so on.

There may be a tendency for the importance of this great amount of technical information to obscure its ultimate objective, and to diminish the importance of an equally valid necessity, i.e. an accurate and full notation of the therapeutic *results* of all this attention. This becomes a vital necessity when assessment of the effects of treatment procedures is made for the most part immediately after the procedures; the most effective use of mobilisation, manipulation and traction techniques depends upon precise observation of their immediate effects, and assessment of the meaning and importance of these effects.

Throughout treatment, the therapist must remain in full control of the proceedings and be awake to the significance of *changes* in the signs and symptoms as they occur, whether treatment occupies one or many sessions. Besides the prime consideration of the patient's welfare, there is the importance of learning by experience, and this is facilitated if retrospective analysis is made possible by the orderly habit of precise recording of each step in treatment, and of its effect.

Accurate recording is therefore an unavoidable necessity; all treatment procedures should be fully and precisely recorded, and a common system of expression and notation is desirable.

At present, when the use of manipulative methods by physiotherapists is burgeoning, discrimination between the traditional schools of manipulative method becomes somewhat passé; this is especially so since physiotherapists themselves have made significant contributions in the field.[797, 833, 627, 1053]

The currently available repertoire or vocabulary of techniques is something of a melting-pot, with several new and traditional systems mixed together. Thus there is a difficulty in that the number of manual and mechanical passive movement techniques runs into many hundreds at least; in the absence of an internationally agreed system of notation it is important that therapists use recording methods which are agreed, or at least readily understood, among those of their colleagues who may treat the same patient.

Notation methods arise naturally from what therapists do; where the variety of techniques is considerable, the notation system must be comprehensive and flexible.

Notes would come under several headings:

Examination
Mobilisation
Manipulation
Traction

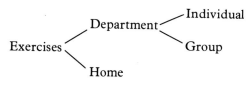

Exercises — Department — Individual / Group — Home

Associated treatments
Prophylaxis and ergonomic guidance
Support.

EXAMINATION

Findings should be written on a Vertebral Examination Recording Sheet, ending with comments on initial assessment and treatment approach selected (see p. 360). Comprehensive examination of peripheral joints can be recorded on a separate sheet.

The author has formulated a layout for recording the

initial vertebral examination findings (see p. 342) which is being adopted, with minor changes, both at home and abroad; there is need for similar method of recording examination of peripheral joints, and head pain. It is probable that separate forms would be required for head pain (including the temperomandibular joint), upper limb and lower limb. It may well be that therapists of the future will employ an electronic method of recording examination, in which the totality of single and combined examination movements, and their effects, are electronically systemised, and thus incorporated into something resembling the modern pocket calculator which could display the salient factors. Certainly, the detailed written account of a comprehensive vertebral and associated peripheral joint examination requires considerable organisation of method.

MOBILISATION TREATMENT (grades I–IV)[797]

Record at each attendance:

On left-hand side	*On right-hand side*
Technique used	Patient's subjective
Grade	assessment of symptoms
Vertebral level(s) treated	(inverted commas)
Number of times	Therapist's objective
Effects *during* application	assessment of signs

and ending with *comments as a reminder for next attendance*

For example:

$\updownarrow$ 11 (C4) ×3   'feels looser'
                         Ext. inc. by ¼ with less
                         pain

If remains improved tomorrow, stop and check after 1/52. Wean from collar.

Thus, a complete but short account of treatment and immediate results is written at each attendance. Shorthand symbols for the techniques employed can save time, and are desirable so long as their meaning is agreed.

MANIPULATION TREATMENT (grade V)

There are many systems of annotating treatment procedures, yet they can be recorded exactly as above; where no symbol is used, or exists, it is wise to write a short description of the technique employed. Whatever recording method is used, it should include these factors:

1. The segment treated
2. The type of manipulation
3. The direction
4. Whether a regional or localised effect was intended
5. Effects (unless it is planned that assessment be after a short period—this must be noted on the record).

Where a technique has been localised, the symbol 'localised V' or 'LV' should be used.

TRACTION (as an outpatient sessional procedure)

Recording should note:

a. whether manual or mechanical
b. apparatus employed
c. position of the patient
d. angle of pull or the suspension (attachment) point
e. the segment(s) for which traction is given
f. force of traction
g. duration of traction
h. whether sustained, intermittent or rhythmic; or manipulative (grade V)
i. periodicity of pull and rest phases, if not sustained
j. effects—if to be assessed immediately. If not, this must be noted.

The difficulty with traction is that there are innumerable ways of applying treatment, and therapists who employ many methods will need a fairly comprehensive recording system, which is flexible enough to meet most requirements.

To distinguish between continuous or sustained traction in bed, and traction treatment on an outpatient basis, the word 'sessional' is probably better than 'intermittent' alone, since the latter could apply to once daily outpatient treatment, or to two applications of sustained traction with a rest between, at a single outpatient attendance.

Manual traction can be specified by the letter 'M'; if this is omitted, the traction can be taken, by agreement of colleagues, to indicate mechanical traction.

If the gross position of the patient is indicated by arrows, e.g.

$\uparrow$ sitting or standing, $\llcorner\nearrow$ half-lying, and $\llcorner\!\!\longrightarrow$ (supine) lying or $\llcorner\!\!\longrightarrow$ (prone) lying,

'SRCT $\downarrow$ (C2–C3)' would denote, 'Sessional rhythmic mechanical cervical traction in sitting for the C2–C3 segment', since it is unlikely that mechanical cervical traction as a sessional treatment would be applied with the patient standing.

'SMRLT $\uparrow$ (L3)' would denote, 'Sessional manual rhythmic lumbar traction to L3', in either sitting or standing, which should be specified.

Where traction is employed as a grade V manipulative technique, the term 'grade V' is added after the segment to be treated.

For example, 'SMMT $\uparrow$ (T5) V sitt.' would denote,

'Sessional manual manipulative traction (T5) grade V in sitting.'

Similarly, 'SSCT ↗ (C5–C6)' denotes, 'Sessional sustained cervical traction in half-lying for the C5–C6 segment.'

Whether the neck is slightly flexed to position the C2–C3 segment at the midpoint of its saggital movement, or further flexed in the half-lying position to do the same for the C5–C6 segment (see p. 402), depends upon careful palpation, and arrangement of the harness and suspension point during preparation for the treatment; therefore the precise positioning adopted is not capable of description unless the suspension point is a standard one, the harness is standard and the patient's position is standard, when degrees of flexion, or a neutral position, may then be recorded.

Nevertheless when cervical traction, for example, is applied in the lying or half-lying position, it is convenient to record details of the number and type of pillows used to support the neck, and these details will naturally follow symbols denoting the patient's position. When normal-sized pillows and small ones are used, the details can be expressed as follows:

'SSCT ↗ 1½ pillows'

'SRCT ↗ 2 pillows'

'SSCT → 1 pillow'

'SSCT ↗ no pillow'.

Thus it is suggested that arrows are used to describe the *gross posture of the patient*, and not the *segmental posture of the joint* to be treated. By specification of the segment treated and the number of pillows used, another therapist subsequently treating the patient would know that the named segment must be so positioned in the sagittal plane that the traction is sustained with this joint in mid-position.

When giving *cervical* traction with standard apparatus providing standard suspension points and using a uniform position of the patient (i.e. degree of neck-flexion on the trunk), there is a method of writing a formula for arrangement of the head/neck angle. Using the Maitland harness[797] the number of strap-holes showing *beyond* the buckle can be expressed in the sequence, for example:

Manidibular strap—3 holes showing
Occipital strap—4 holes showing
Horizontal strap—4 holes showing

Thus, the head/neck angle for a particular individual is written as '3/4/4'.

Slight flexion of the patient's hips and knees by the use of pillows for relaxation and comfort should also be recorded, and this may be noted by the symbol ⌐1 pillow or ⌐2 pillows; this is also of particular importance when treating the thoracic and lumbar segments.

1. Hence, provided the same apparatus is used each time, the recording of a sessional rhythmic cervical traction treatment in half-lying, for C4–C5, with a pull phase of 60 seconds and a rest phase of 30 seconds, could be as follows: 'SRCT ↗ 1 pillow (C4–C5) 3/4/4 8 kg 60/30 × 20 min ⌐ 2 pillows.'

2. Two sustained traction treatments at one session, with a rest between, can be written: 'SSCT ↗ 2 pillows (C7–T1) 2/4/4 20 kg × 20 min × 2 (rest 5 min) ⌐ 2 pillows.'

3. Autotraction (see p. 412) in the sitting position can be recorded as: 'SRCT auto ⊥ sitt. (C1–C2) 2/3/3 5 kg 30/20 × 10 min.'

4. For sustained traction to a low thoracic segment in half-lying, on the Akron table (see p. 410), the recording could be: SSTT ↗ ½ pillow (T10–T11) 24 kg × 15 min ⌐ 1 pillow', indicating that a small flat pillow was used to support the head, and a normal-sized pillow supported the patient's knees in some flexion.

5. Rhythmic lumbar traction in the prone position, for example, would be written: 'SRLT → (prone) (L4–L5) 20 kg 120/30 × 15 min.'

6. Sustained traction to L5–S1 in supine, with some flexion, would be written: 'SSLT → (supine) (L5–S1) 30 kg × 15 min ⌐ low stool.'

SYMBOLS

The major difficulty, in symbolising methods of passive or active movement, is that of trying to represent three-dimensional movement on a two-dimensional surface.

The following are examples of symbols used by the author and some are a modification of those developed by Maitland.[797]

Pending an internationally agreed system (a formidable undertaking), they constitute no more than a contribution for perhaps further modification or development by others. The inclusion of a lateral or medial bias to left or right, or a cranial or caudal bias, should be noted, i.e.: postero-anterior unilateral pressures on the left side, with a slight medial bias, would not be written thus ↓• but thus ↘•; a lateral bias would be written ↙•.

A cephalic or caudal bias could be written, '⊣ ceph', or '⊢ caud', and combinations of caudal and lateral bias can be expressed by '↘ caud', for example.

Symbols which are carried to the reader's right of the centre spot indicate the *patient's* right side, whether standing, sitting, side-lying, prone or supine.

Where a symbol indicates a unilateral technique to the patient's right, the symbol is reversed when it represents a *left* unilateral technique.

Notation method

Vertebral mobilisation and stretching techniques

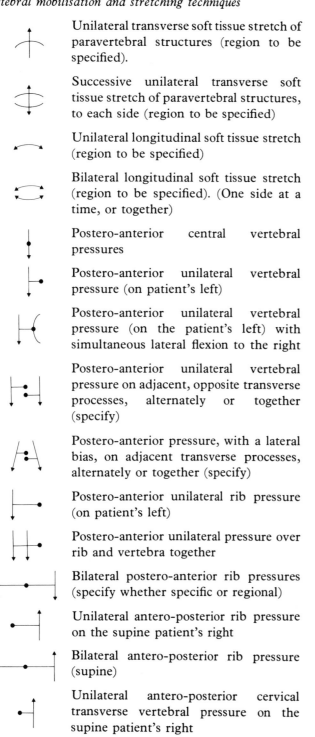

Unilateral transverse soft tissue stretch of paravertebral structures (region to be specified).

Successive unilateral transverse soft tissue stretch of paravertebral structures, to each side (region to be specified)

Unilateral longitudinal soft tissue stretch (region to be specified)

Bilateral longitudinal soft tissue stretch (region to be specified). (One side at a time, or together)

Postero-anterior central vertebral pressures

Postero-anterior unilateral vertebral pressure (on patient's left)

Postero-anterior unilateral vertebral pressure (on the patient's left) with simultaneous lateral flexion to the right

Postero-anterior unilateral vertebral pressure on adjacent, opposite transverse processes, alternately or together (specify)

Postero-anterior pressure, with a lateral bias, on adjacent transverse processes, alternately or together (specify)

Postero-anterior unilateral rib pressure (on patient's left)

Postero-anterior unilateral pressure over rib and vertebra together

Bilateral postero-anterior rib pressures (specify whether specific or regional)

Unilateral antero-posterior rib pressure on the supine patient's right

Bilateral antero-posterior rib pressure (supine)

Unilateral antero-posterior cervical transverse vertebral pressure on the supine patient's right

Bilateral antero-posterior cervical transverse vertebral pressure (supine)

Transverse vertebral pressure (specified whether spinous or transverse process) towards patient's right

Transverse vertebral pressure, to the prone patient's left side, with an anterior bias

Transverse vertebral pressures, in opposite directions, successively or simultaneously on two adjacent spinous processes, which should be named.
NB: When applied first to the left and then to the right at a single segment, the segment should be named

Transverse vertebral pressure to the left, with the subjacent spinous process (or sacrum) stabilised

Combined transverse vertebral pressure to the patient's left and postero-anterior pressure on the left

Transverse vertebral pressure, to the patient's left, with postero-anterior stabilising pressure on the right subjacent transverse process

Oscillatory longitudinal movement (patient lying supine)—cervical spine, cervicothoracic region or one lower limb (specify)

Oscillatory longitudinal movement grasping both legs (neutral)

Oscillatory longitudinal movement, one lower limb in flexion

Oscillatory longitudinal movement, two lower limbs in flexion

Oscillatory longitudinal movement in sitting or standing

Manual or mechanical harness traction in sitting or standing (record whether rhythmic or sustained)

Manual or mechanical harness traction in half-lying

Manual or mechanical harness traction in supine or prone lying

Rotation, of head, thorax or pelvis, to patient's right (add 'Sust.' if sustained)

Cervical, thoracic or lumbar lateral flexion, to patient's right

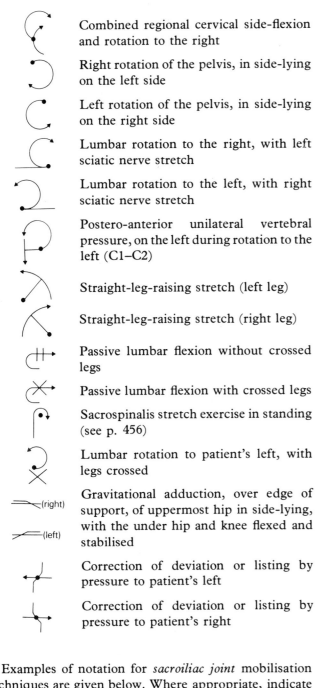

Combined regional cervical side-flexion and rotation to the right

Right rotation of the pelvis, in side-lying on the left side

Left rotation of the pelvis, in side-lying on the right side

Lumbar rotation to the right, with left sciatic nerve stretch

Lumbar rotation to the left, with right sciatic nerve stretch

Postero-anterior unilateral vertebral pressure, on the left during rotation to the left (C1–C2)

Straight-leg-raising stretch (left leg)

Straight-leg-raising stretch (right leg)

Passive lumbar flexion without crossed legs

Passive lumbar flexion with crossed legs

Sacrospinalis stretch exercise in standing (see p. 456)

Lumbar rotation to patient's left, with legs crossed

Gravitational adduction, over edge of support, of uppermost hip in side-lying, with the under hip and knee flexed and stabilised

Correction of deviation or listing by pressure to patient's left

Correction of deviation or listing by pressure to patient's right

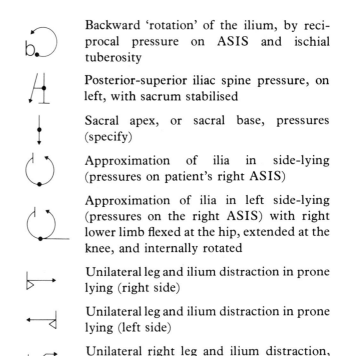

Backward 'rotation' of the ilium, by reciprocal pressure on ASIS and ischial tuberosity

Posterior-superior iliac spine pressure, on left, with sacrum stabilised

Sacral apex, or sacral base, pressures (specify)

Approximation of ilia in side-lying (pressures on patient's right ASIS)

Approximation of ilia in left side-lying (pressures on the right ASIS) with right lower limb flexed at the hip, extended at the knee, and internally rotated

Unilateral leg and ilium distraction in prone lying (right side)

Unilateral leg and ilium distraction in prone lying (left side)

Unilateral right leg and ilium distraction, with bent knee, in prone lying

Examples of notation for *sacroiliac joint* mobilisation techniques are given below. Where appropriate, indicate the side treated.

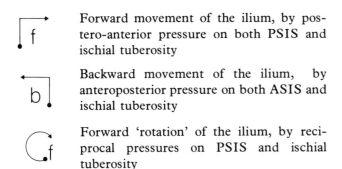

Forward movement of the ilium, by postero-anterior pressure on both PSIS and ischial tuberosity

Backward movement of the ilium, by anteroposterior pressure on both ASIS and ischial tuberosity

Forward 'rotation' of the ilium, by reciprocal pressures on PSIS and ischial tuberosity

Manipulation (grade V)

Note: Add 'LV' (localised grade V) to the symbol if a localised technique and also specify the intervertebral level treated.

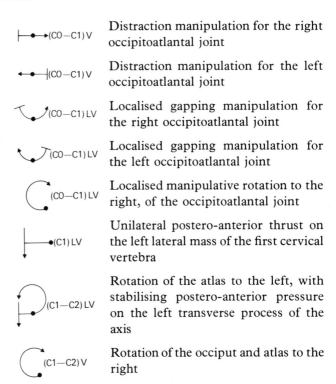

Distraction manipulation for the right occipitoatlantal joint

Distraction manipulation for the left occipitoatlantal joint

Localised gapping manipulation for the right occipitoatlantal joint

Localised gapping manipulation for the left occipitoatlantal joint

Localised manipulative rotation to the right, of the occipitoatlantal joint

Unilateral postero-anterior thrust on the left lateral mass of the first cervical vertebra

Rotation of the atlas to the left, with stabilising postero-anterior pressure on the left transverse process of the axis

Rotation of the occiput and atlas to the right

Gapping manipulation to patient's left (specify whether in supine or prone)

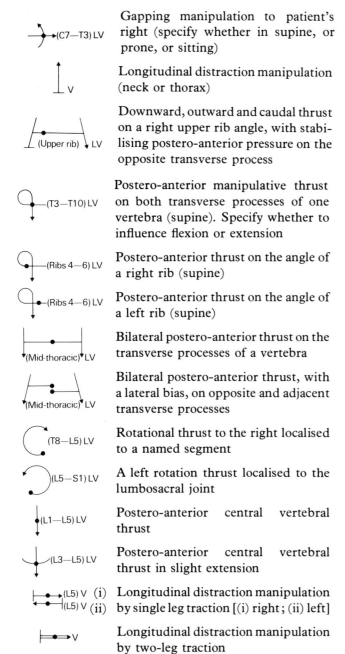

Gapping manipulation to patient's right (specify whether in supine, or prone, or sitting)

Longitudinal distraction manipulation (neck or thorax)

Downward, outward and caudal thrust on a right upper rib angle, with stabilising postero-anterior pressure on the opposite transverse process

Postero-anterior manipulative thrust on both transverse processes of one vertebra (supine). Specify whether to influence flexion or extension

Postero-anterior thrust on the angle of a right rib (supine)

Postero-anterior thrust on the angle of a left rib (supine)

Bilateral postero-anterior thrust on the transverse processes of a vertebra

Bilateral postero-anterior thrust, with a lateral bias, on opposite and adjacent transverse processes

Rotational thrust to the right localised to a named segment

A left rotation thrust localised to the lumbosacral joint

Postero-anterior central vertebral thrust

Postero-anterior central vertebral thrust in slight extension

Longitudinal distraction manipulation by single leg traction [(i) right; (ii) left]

Longitudinal distraction manipulation by two-leg traction

Sacroiliac joint

Forward 'rotation' of the ilium (specify side)

Backward 'rotation' of the ilium (specify side)

Like all good and ultimately productive habits, precise recording is onerous and can be a bore. Yet the need is inescapable, and the benefits make it infinitely worthwhile. Precise assessment of the effects of treatment is not possible without precise recording, and real learning of the craft of therapeutics happens in only one place—the clinical shopfloor. A note of what happens there provides the skeletal framework of self-education.

Paradoxically, we learn more from our therapeutic failures than from our easy successes, and we will make this timeless agent of real learning work much more effectively for us when full and precise recording allows a retrospective analysis.

CLINICAL METHOD

Much has been said about applied anatomy, congenital anomalies, pathological change with or without root involvement, clinical syndromes, examination method, assessment in examination and techniques of mobilisation, manipulation and traction. It will have become apparent that our certain knowledge of the changes underlying common joint problems amounts to an island of knowing in an embarrasingly large sea of ignorance. Similarly, following examination and initial assessment, the times when a therapist is confidently able to forecast precisely *which* technique, or treatment approach, will get the patient better, are not as frequent as we would like.

The previous reminder (p. 420) to 'assume *nothing*' merely states the same truth in a different guise. As one's clinical mileage of patients treated steadily mounts, the knack of more successfully choosing the first technique comes more easily to hand, but acquiring it is a slow process; the tyro who aspires to this state of informed flexibility by short cut is either irresponsible, or has been irresponsibly taught, or both.

Alike in the early and advanced stages in manipulative work, there is no substitute for clinical self-education by step-by-step analysis, expressed by the mnemonic SOAP:

S   Subjective examination
O   Objective examination
A   Assessment
P   Plan of treatment.

The *only* difference between the novice and the advanced worker, in terms of cerebral activity, is that the latter has experience to call upon and progressively works more quickly. At no time does the clinical routine of segmental analysis become redundant.

Assessment continues during treatment (p. 444) and the response to what is done initially, and subsequently, provides guidance for the next step in treatment. Thus it comes about that, by a logical and orderly method of examination, followed by treatment which is planned solely on the basis of the signs and symptoms in themselves, patients are frequently relieved of painful disablements without the therapist ever really knowing the precise nature of the changes underlying these conditions. At times it is possible to be reasonably sure, but more often than not there is insufficient basis for complete confidence that the diagnosis is correct, or has other than a supposed relationship to the changes causing the patient's attendance.

The need to reach a diagnosis is important, but this need is not met by facile, snap decisions which often appear to be made on a patently inadequate basis.

As manipulation, in the general sense, remains largely an empirical form of treatment, so diagnosis, in its precise and clinical sense, often retains some empiricism when applied to common musculoskeletal conditions. For this reason, it is not wise to base the selection and use of passive movement techniques on diagnostic concepts only, although there are certain important clinical features which must be respected for what they infer. For example:

—backache in a patient with a history of neoplastic disease
—joint problems in a patient with advanced diabetes
—mid- and low-lumbar pain in the presence of radiologically-evident osteoporosis
—low backache in a patient with advanced Scheuermann's disease
—thoracic pain in spinal gout.

Nevertheless, the vital principle is that of formulating treatment on the *unique* way in which signs and symptoms present in each patient, while coexistent disease or factors indicating caution are borne in mind. Further, since we do not know exactly what mobilisation or manipulation actually does to a joint and to its associated tissues, we can only use the treatment intelligently, i.e. select and modify it, on the basis of signs and symptoms and how these change as the treatment proceeds. The response of the joint, to the initial procedures selected, is the dominant guiding factor, e.g. in the case of testing the response to one of the pressure techniques or a trial of traction.

Thus *clinical method* is considered under the three headings:

1. Use of technique in general terms
2. Selection of technique
3. Assessment during treatment.

1. USE OF TECHNIQUE IN GENERAL TERMS[456]

Other factors given, the *aim* is to make the joint 'clear', i.e. able to sustain grade IV mobilisation without pain, but it is not always possible, nor advisable, to aim for full restoration of movement, and if symptoms have been relieved it is often better not to attempt to influence joint limitations which are clearly the result of adaptive shortening.

Since the object of treatment is to produce movement, and most movement will occur when a joint is positioned in the mid-position of all the other ranges of which it is capable, the lordotic areas of the spine (cervical and lumbar) should be positioned more in neutral or slight extension when treating the upper parts, i.e. C1–C2, L1–L2, and in increasing flexion as the lower areas are treated, i.e. C6–C7, L4–L5. *This applies especially* when using regional techniques to affect single segments, e.g. rotation.

Two good uses of a technique, in the appropriate grade, at one session, are enough to assess its value in a particular case at a particular time.

In cases likely to progress slowly, four or five *treatment sessions* are sometimes required, before the value of techniques can be assessed.

Unless progress is obviously going to be slow, the therapist should move through the techniques fairly quickly to find the value of each, but this should be well controlled throughout, with techniques adequately performed and with reassessment of signs and symptoms guiding selection at all times. This is quite different from a haphazard and willy-nilly use of whichever technique happens to spring to mind—it is important always to keep the treatment firmly in hand, with a clear grasp of how the signs and symptoms are responding to applied procedures.

Slightly altering the angle when using pressure techniques, or the joint's position in rotation techniques, is often necessary to extract the most benefit. The technique itself need not always be changed.

A technique which produced no change, yet no deterioration either, should be repeated with a higher grade, i.e. more firmly. If the condition continues to remain unaffected, the technique must be changed.

If a procedure helps, it should be continued with. If not, it must be discarded for something that does. There is no gain in persisting with pointless techniques, simply because they may be the therapist's favourites.

Techniques which do not help in the initial stages of a treatment are often found to be successful in the later stages—the therapist should change his ground as the signs and symptoms change theirs, which they will do as the localisation of stress changes during treatment, but he should not discard a particular treatment method until it ceases to help.

When a patient has two or more areas of pain from separate lesions, or a large area of pain appears to have more than one lesion (e.g. a cervical segment and a high thoracic segment) contributing to its existence, it is better to clearly know the effects of treatment procedure on one of these, before a second technique is added in during the same session.

When treatment soreness is such as to make assessment difficult, treatment should be stopped for a day or two to allow the soreness to settle.

When improvement by manual mobilisation has reached a limit, traction should be added or substituted for a little while, after which manual techniques may be taken up again.

It is not always necessary to pursue signs and symptoms with treatment to the bitter end. Often, treatment can be stopped before they are completely cleared, although the patient *must* always be assessed at the end of a few days, when it is frequently found that the joint problem has continued clearing without further treatment.

Gross cervical and lumbar rotational manipulations (grade V) can be repeated two or more times in a single session with benefit (other factors being equal) if the improvement in signs indicates this.

Localised specific manipulations (grade loc V), when indicated, should be done as a rule only once to each side (but see p. 463), and should not be repeated until soreness has settled down in a few days, and then only if signs indicate that a repetition should be useful.

Summary of rules of procedure

1. Bear in mind contraindications, and the conditions requiring extra care and gentleness. DO NO HARM.
2. Examine thoroughly, and carefully assess patient's signs and symptoms for indications of initial technique and likely progress.
3. Always try to localise the problem(s) and work in a specific way, i.e. localise the treatment, too.
4. Begin feeling your way forward by exploratory mobilisation, or traction, and *keep the treatment under control* by frequent reassessment and precise recording.
5. Each step should be reasoned, and governed by the response to the previous steps in treatment.
6. Use manipulative procedures only if necessary; for the most part only when adequately applied mobilisation is not achieving the degree of improvement reasonably expected.
7. If a technique is being effective, do not substitute another until it ceases to produce adequate improvement. Discard or modify techniques which are unproductive.
8. Remember to warn patients about treatment soreness and temporary after-effects; this relieves their unnecessary anxiety between treatments.
9. Do not overtreat; when signs and symptoms are cleared, STOP.
10. NEVER push through spasm when it is protecting the joint you are treating; treat joint irritability with respect.

2. SELECTION OF TECHNIQUE

Tabulated suggestions of what to try first have a tendency to become permanent rules of thumb, albeit qualified; they should be nothing of the sort, since their intention is only that of providing the novice with an initial basis for guidance. As experience is gained, the now more confident therapist will have perceived why the suggested sequence was arranged in this particular way, and will have acquired the clinical basis to know more surely when to transgress the sequence.

For those who have received their initial training in a particular manipulative school, the matter is relatively simple, because their selection of treatment procedures has been inculcated from the first. Those with some experience of many schools may find tabulated schemes irksome, since it is highly likely that they have evolved their own favoured sequence, anyway.

The question uppermost in the tyro's mind is: 'When to do what to which, and how gently or forcefully to do it', i.e. the selection and use of technique. Therefore in the teaching of manipulation, the frequent question: 'I have done a good examination, and found such and such, now what do I do?' must be answered by:

1. Giving the 'Summary of Rules of Procedure'.
2. Providing demonstration of the approach of various schools of manipulation to a given set of signs and symptoms, to show that there are many ways of starting and none of them are 'wrong', necessarily.
3. Teaching contraindications, which help to show when procedures may be unsafe.
4. Producing basic guides for selection of first and subsequent mobilisation and manipulation technique (see below), and stressing the importance of continuous assessment.
5. Assurance that all manipulators have this trouble and that it becomes less troublesome with experience, although all profit from the experience of those who have gone before.
6. Arranging opportunities for course members to be in pairs, ideally, and to work for many weeks on the clinical shopfloor with an experienced teacher.

The following seemingly modest selection of techniques[797] has a very wide range of clinical application; increasing experience of their potential for resolving the signs and symptoms of degenerative joint disease (when their use is correctly applied to the 'range–pain–limitation' relationship, p. 360), is a salutary exercise, and will rightly cast doubt on the proposition that technique must always be based on facet-joint plane geometry. A thorough knowledge of the clinical application of these modest and undramatic procedures is the very best basis for more advanced work.

Selection of technique by distribution of pain

(i) *Central pain, or bilateral symmetrical pain*

CT TT LT (or do unilateral technique to both sides)

(ii) *Bilateral asymmetrical pain*
Usually a good plan to treat as two separate unilateral pains unless they can be shown to be associated, or both pains arising from a segment or adjacent segments, when the pains can be treated as bilateral symmetry.

(iii) *Unilateral pain* (e.g. left side)

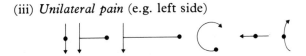

Initially, rotate *away* from the side of pain, and be cautious about rotating *towards* or into the pain, in the cervical region; this guide is modified with experience.

If the initial *lumbar* rotation away from the side of pain is not successful, the opposite rotation is then used without fear of untoward effects because of the direction of rotation itself, other factors given.

Selection of technique in order of efficacy for spinal regions

Traction is mobilising technique, and should be employed as such (p. 398). It is just as correct to change from a manual mobilising technique to harness traction, or vice versa, as it is to change from one manual technique to another. The factor that harness traction may need some three or four *sessions*, before assessment can reasonably be made, does not negate the proposition that it is correctly used in this way, i.e. as a mobilising technique.

Maitland (1977)[797] provides a detailed tabulation of effects of the individual mobilising procedures.

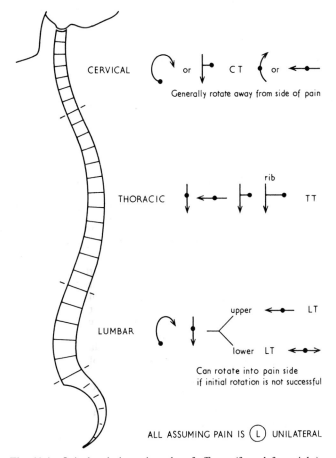

Fig. 13.1 Spinal techniques in order of efficacy (from left to right)

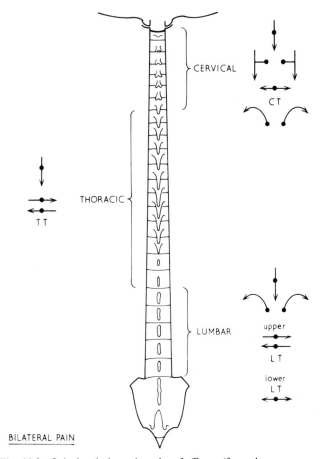

Fig. 13.2 Spinal techniques in order of efficacy (from above downwards)

For more experienced therapists, who have mastered the techniques of careful regional and segmental examination, and understand the prime importance of accurately localised treatment procedures, a precis of clinical method (with some reiteration) might be arranged as follows:

1. During the 'observation' part of the examination for *all* vertebral regions, check leg-lengths, and pelvic symmetry, in sitting as well as standing.
2. Always check the lower limbs neurologically when dealing with neck problems in mature patients.
3. Always check the sacroiliac joints in any case of thoracic or lumbar pain.
4. Note the regions of soft tissue tightness.
5. During palpation, be awake to segmental hypermobility, as well as stiffness and irritability.
6. While primarily seeking the segmental locality of a joint problem, bear in mind the important junctional regions (p. 364) and the covert effects of degenerative change there.
7. Treat specifically at all times, but within the context of regional changes which may also need treatment.
8. Never forget the functional and the neurophysiological interdependence of the vertebral column.

9. Proceed on the basis of:
   a. Specific or segmental joint mobilisation (or manipulation if indicated) by appropriate method
   b. Regional soft tissue techniques, to release tightness
   c. Regional mobilisation, when indicated
   d. Segmental exercises to maintain mobility
   e. Segmental and regional exercises to improve stability, if indicated
   f. Ergonomic advice and guidance
   g. Always aiming to instil the patient's *confidence* in the durability of their vertebral column. Nothing lasts forever, not even joint pain.

   NB: (i) The treatment factors are added in the sequence suggested, as clinical features declare the need, but the set routine may not be necessary, e.g. the gentle release of a recent vertebral joint derangement at C2–C3 may be all that is required.

   (ii) Vertebral segmental exercises are given for the same reasons as exercises for individual peripheral joints.[145]

10. Never lose sight of the whole, while pursuing one's self-education in the many approaches to the treatment of vertebral pain syndromes.

An additional suggested sequence, in broad terms, of localised and regional manual and mechanical techniques, for those with more experience, is given below. Each technique can and should be transposed according to clinical findings, with selections guided by assessment of effects.

Many experienced therapists are competent in the use of techniques derived from various manipulation schools and because this text is not solely devoted to teaching any particular manipulative method, not all of the suggested recording symbols are included in the sequences.

Some standard techniques will be recognised, but it should be borne in mind that in mobilisation of a first rib, for example, the patient may be in the supine or prone position; this variation applies to many procedures, by individual preference.

This tabulation can be no more than a personal recommendation, since a single technique often achieves different effects in different hands.

There are many other procedures for successfully treating the segments and regions concerned, and none should be considered in isolation from the need to restore extensibility and pliability of soft tissue where necessary; some soft tissue techniques have been included.

The formal inclusion of localised and regional grade V techniques is not necessarily a recommendation that these should be employed if preceding techniques under the patient's control have been unsuccessful; some patients may benefit from the use of repetitive mobilising techniques while positioned as for grade V techniques.

Without exception, the use of manipulative thrusts must be carefully guided by the indications (p. 463) and those not adequately experienced in either clinical assessment or manipulation should not attempt unfamiliar manipulative procedures without guidance.

The fact that more than one manipulation is suggested does not mean that more than one at a session should be employed. Again, clinical findings and assessment are the guides for action; techniques should be as localised as possible.

3. ASSESSMENT DURING TREATMENT

In close accordance with the detailed findings during examination and treatment, each session has a beginning, a continuation and an end. The guides for starting, continuing and finishing are solely provided by assessment—there are no criteria other than those wittingly or unwittingly presented by *the patient*. Perceiving when to stop is as important as knowing how to start and recognising how to continue. The better the assessment, the fewer the treatment sessions. Practice makes perfect—there are no short cuts.

Taking as our enemy the changes causing the patient's distress, and regarding the clinical shopfloor as a front line, we are more likely to win battles if we see to our military intelligence, endeavour to objectively understand the nature of the enemy, resist intimidating propaganda about him, do a thorough reconnaissance of the terrain and of his present positions in relation to it, and make an appraisal of the possible moves open to him during the battle and of his present and future intentions. We are also likely to be more successful if we fully understand the nature and potential of our own weapons, economically use our firepower to the best effect and do not deploy our heavy artillery when good marksmanship with a rifle may suffice. Thus we do our best to avoid desecration of the countryside not presently occupied by the enemy.[455]

These observations transpose themselves into the importance of:

a. Developing a comprehensive examination procedure, which allows the joint to speak for itself, and then listening to what it is saying. We will not hear successfully with the deaf ears of preconception.

There are many examples of wide differences in the behaviour of body systems, and a diversity of clinical features which follow tissue damage or abnormal stresses. Three have already been given, *viz.* the vagaries of referred pain (p. 196), the idiosyncrasies of combined movements of the spinal column (p. 47) and the variety of lumbar spinal posture accompanying lateral pelvic tilt.

While there must be reasons for this biological plasticity of behaviour in what appear to be similar changes and we may have elucidated some of the reasons, our certain knowledge remains limited; until it is more complete, attempts by instructors to impose an overall regularity and

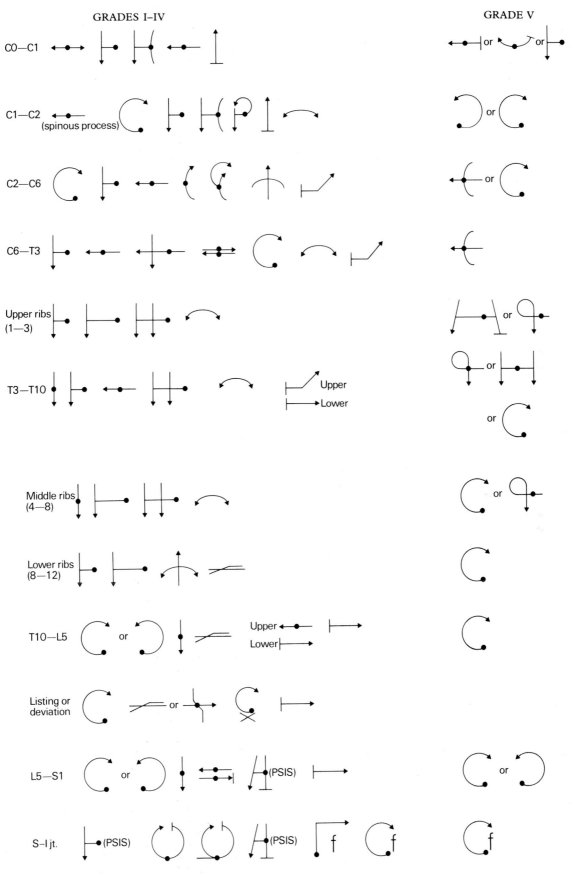

Fig. 13.3   Unilateral, i.e. (L) sided pain

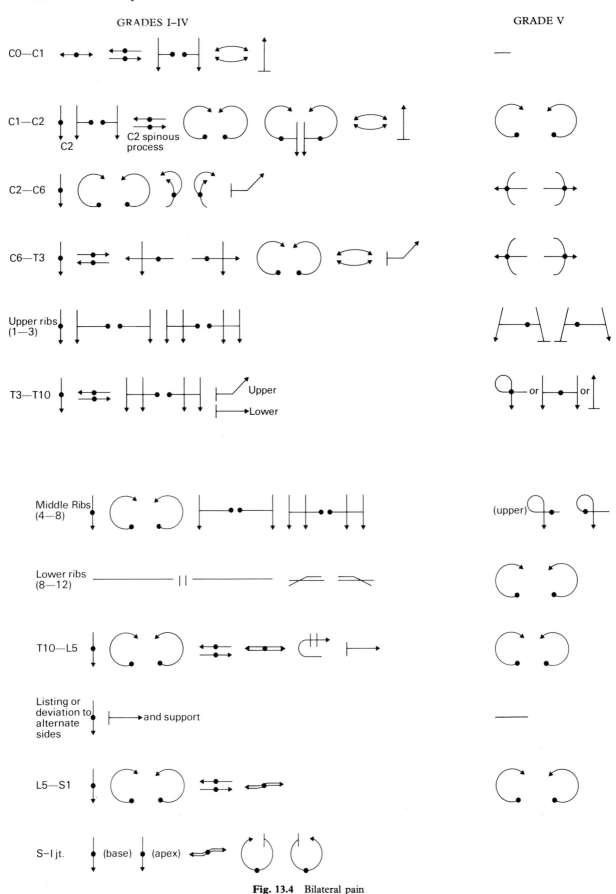

Fig. 13.4 Bilateral pain

seemingly reasoned and logical order, where none can yet exist, are highly misleading for beginners.

No explanation at all is better than authoritarian nonsense.

b. Recognising the biomechanical, neural, vascular, and thus functional interdependence of vertebral structures. This interdependence is a constant factor underlying clinical presentation and further, a constant factor to be borne in mind when examining, assessing, choosing techniques and formulating plans of treatment.

So far as treatment of the joint itself is concerned, the effects of precisely localised and graded passive movements in treatment are better noted if the patient attends daily at first. Once the responses of the joint condition during treatment are understood, attendance can be less frequent.

Not only does assessment give guidance during the continuation of treatment, it also provides the basis for knowing with assurance when treatment can be safely discontinued. Depending upon the nature of the joint condition, and its consequences, attendance will vary between one session and frequent sessions for two or three weeks.

It is important for the therapist to decide (p. 448), 'Can I expect a quick result or is progress going to be slow?' and also to decide (p. 363), 'Am I primarily treating pain or resistance (in its various forms)?'

Assessment of the presenting and then the changing relationships during treatment of pain with movement is a fundamental skill which can be learned, as can the assessment of whether a joint is normal or not. 'Any joint which is not causing symptoms should be able to accept a certain amount of stretch at the limit of its ranges, without pain.'[796] Similarly, Mooney and Cairns (1978)[869] have observed that there is every reason to expect that a joint unable to proceed through its full anatomical range is abnormal.

Assessments of the changes produced by treatment will be inaccurate unless *all* the factors of a movement abnormality are precisely known. Maitland (1972)[796] has well exemplified this:

The behaviour of pain with movement is very important, as is borne out in the following examples of equally restricted lumbar flexion, each with a different pain pattern. The differences are important because they guide the treatment and because, if they are not appreciated, the patient may be made worse by treatment without the physiotherapist realising. In all of the examples which follow, the patient has an ache in his lower back which extends down his leg into his calf. On forward flexion, he first feels a change in his pain when his fingertips reach his knees. With further movement he can reach halfway down his shin with the following differences in the behaviour of his pain:

(i) There is no alteration to the pain, 'half-shin' being the normal limit of his range.
(ii) His back pain increases in intensity until the increase in this pain prevents him from flexing further than halfway down

his shin. His thigh and calf symptoms are not affected by the flexion.
(iii) As movement increases the pain spreads into his buttock but it is stiffness which prevents him from flexing further than halfway down his shin.
(iv) As movement increases so the pain spreads down his leg to his calf.
(v) As movement increases the pain in his back disappears but his calf becomes increasingly painful as the movement reaches the limit of his range.

When pain behaves as indicated in (v) the patient must be treated with much more care than when it behaves in a manner similar to (i). The first indicates a nerve root pain which may be harmed by too zealous treatment. If we are treating a patient such as in (i) and do not take note of the behaviour of pain throughout movement then his pain may change to that of (v) without our appreciating it.

Accurate assessment of the nature of abnormal 'end-feels' on passive testing (see p. 358) will also indicate when further mobilisation (grades I–IV) is pointless, and a grade V thrust technique is indicated. In some cases, this will be indicated from the first, in which case the joint *is* manipulated, provided there are no preclusions (see p. 464). Confidence in safely recognising the indications is based mainly upon methodical assessment of the nature of the range-limiting factor (see p. 360).

Assessments are made: (a) after each use of a technique, during one treatment session; (b) prior to the next treatment.

A selection of two important 'markers for assessment' enables a quick estimate of progress to be made without repeatedly going through the whole examination procedure. The changes in *one symptom*, e.g. the length of time a patient can sit, and *one sign*, e.g. the intensity and precise distribution of pain and/or paraesthesiae during a particular movement, are adopted as parameters; thus assessment of the value of each technique during the treatment session usually hinges on the sign, and the effects of the treatment between attendances upon the symptom, with other information spontaneously proffered by the patient.

Criteria will vary considerably between patients, e.g. an improvement of 2 in (5 cm) in the range of flexion may be significant in one patient, but in another may be judged inadequate improvement to justify continuing with a particular technique.

Choice of the best parameters for assessment is a matter of experience, but patients usually present the dominant symptoms first in their history and this helps selection for *subjective* assessments.

For *objective* assessments, selection is easy if only one movement is painful and/or limited, but it may be necessary to choose the movement which produced the greatest spread of pain, e.g. if both flexion and extension of the lumbar spine aggravate or produce calf pain, it is extension which should be chosen because limb pain on spinal extension movement is a more sensitive index than flexion. This usually also applies to the upper limb.

Although changes in a salient sign and a salient symptom are chosen as the immediate markers of treatment effects, assessment as a whole can be likened to an intensive care unit, in that many factors are continually monitored. Examples are, of course, ranges of movement (both active and accessory), intensity and distribution of pain and of paraesthesiae, neurological signs, degree of tenderness, range of straight-leg-raising and its effects, decrease or increase in asymmetry of movement, changes in the degree of postural deviation, changes in postural spasm and elicited spasm, and so on.

While the routine procedure has been outlined, it is important to make the right interpretation of what patients report. A laconic, 'Not so bad' from a patient who is known to be somewhat monosyllabic, should perhaps be given about the same assessment value as the effusive, 'It's been absolutely marvellous' from a patient who appears unable to make the simplest statement without fulsome embroidery.

If distal pain has become more proximal during the interim, even if the more proximal pain is increased in intensity, this generally indicates improvement. 'The longer the pain the slower the gain', and the progressive centralisation of pain is an important assessment marker which indicates progress. If a patient reports that pain has remained in the same distribution, has come on at the same time of day, and at the same intensity, but its *duration* is 75 per cent less, this is progress. Similarly, if the straight-leg-raising test provokes a grimace at 45°, when it did so at 35° the day before, this is progress, however dramatic the grimace.

Hence the therapist's grasp of the patient's symptoms, and their behaviour according to time, posture and movement, must be complete; patients must be helped to be as precise as they are able. A handful appear incapable of doing other than producing confusion (see apophthegm, Fig. 13.5), and a bit of courteous firmness may be a good idea, i.e. 'You're either better, worse or no different—which is it?'

Improvements are not always due to treatment: in

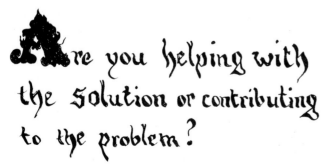

Fig. 13.5 Apophthegm.

mature/elderly patients, whose resilience and powers of recovery are somewhat diminished, it is often more profitable to find ways of reducing joint stress rather than repeating specific treatment which does not hold its improvement. An elderly patient whose pain is always bad on Thursdays, when she carefully negotiates her shopping trolley over pavements by rotating the head to the right to look behind, can be relieved of her regular Thursday pains by learning to pull her shopping trolley with the opposite hand, especially if the regular exacerbation of her right C2–C3 chronic joint problem, by right cervical rotation when pulling the trolley, is undoing the improvement of specific treatment.

Mobilising techniques are grouped as:

a. Localised mobilisation by vertebral pressures
b. Rotation
c. Longitudinal movement and traction.

Examples of treatment guided by assessment follow:

1. Where a quick response to treatment is expected
If, in these cases two uses of the first choice in group (a) do not result in adequate improvement, it is better to proceed next to group (b) than to immediately try all other pressure techniques. If rotation does not produce satisfactory progress, a short traction treatment may be tried, but the next most profitable step is to work through pressure techniques again to find the most effective. The ultimately successful combination of procedures should be achieved solely with the guidance of assessment; wishful thinking and therapeutic favourites are no substitute for objective evaluation of results.

While the patient's report, of changes in symptoms immediately following a technique, are important, some discrimination must temper their face value. For example, if a pain is reported during treatment and it is other than worsening of the particular symptom taken as the marker for subjective assessment, this is not necessarily a negative thing, especially if the signs are unchanged or slightly improved. Transient pain and other symptoms during treatment sessions can be an artefact of treatment, and need not ring alarm bells, unless they infer: incipient or increasing root pressure; vertebrobasilar ischaemia; a deterioration in joint function. For example, during lumbar rotation techniques, the patient may report what appears to be a 'rib-stretch' pain in the uppermost hemithorax. Slight modification of the patient's position will relieve it, and it is of no consequence.

When treating distally referred pain from the lumbar spine, it may transpire that a low-grade rotation technique has moderately worsened the symptoms; the same technique applied in small amplitudes at the limit of available range will frequently produce improvement. The guides for action are (i) that the initial attempt did not worsen the signs, (ii) it was not vigorous enough to have affected the underlying changes, and (iii) it did not produce an exacerbation *during* its application.

2. When it is obvious that treatment will span weeks rather than days

Small improvements or deteriorations in how the patient is troubled are important, and thus the initial examination must be full and precise enough to allow these significant straws in the wind to be recognised. Improvement in symptoms may not keep step with improvement in signs, and vice versa. For example, a patient may report being able to sit for longer, or be able to bend the head over reading or sewing for longer, for some days before any significant change in articular signs occurs. Again, signs may steadily improve for some days before the patient ceases to report 'no change' in symptoms.

In both above cases, the improvements would justify continuing the treatment which produced these results.

If the passive-neck-flexion test (in supine lying) provokes the existing sciatic pain from low back to heel, and after the chosen procedure the test provokes low back pain only, this is improvement.

The patient who, after sitting for 30 minutes, cannot rise directly from the chair and walk away, but has to cautiously 'unwind' and stand awkwardly for some 10–30 seconds before moving, requires patient and persuasive mobilising techniques which can be monotonous to perform, but which are shown to have been the correct approach when the patient returns and reports being able to more quickly stand from sitting.

When limitation of lumbar flexion in standing is accompanied by buttock and posterior thigh pain being provoked at the point of limitation, and mobilisation of a stiff lumbar joint allows an immediate increase of flexion, yet with precisely the same amount of pain, it is very likely that while *movement limitation* was due to the stiff joint, *pain* must be due to some trespass upon the pain-sensitive structures within the neural canal. Hence treatment must be modified to aim at these, and the addition of lumbar traction for example, should be considered. *The point being emphasised here is that pain and movement limitation are not necessarily related.*

If an otherwise fit and strong patient is steadily but slowly improving on mobilisation techniques, and there is no after-treatment soreness or increased irritability, completion of treatment aims should be speeded up.

Articular signs on active tests need not be the only assessment parameter; a reduction of segmental tenderness on palpation, less provocation of pain on segmental accessory movement or provocation of the same pain requiring further excursion into accessory range, are all indications of improvement.

A report that 'my head feels too heavy, I feel I can hardly hold it up' does not necessarily imply cervical segmental instability. Many patients with neck problems

appear to have a type of 'pain inhibition' or a mechanical disturbance of joint function which interferes with postural control of the head, and which very frequently clears up satisfactorily by localised mobilisation of the abnormal segments.

The frequent combination of neck and arm pain need not imply a single cause; many patients will have neck and arm symptoms from a C5–C6 joint problem, together with scapular and arm pain from the T3 segment. It is necessary to be precise about the changing distribution of pain as treatment progresses, and to be aware of combinations of effect.

In contrast, the patient may stoutly say that his or her symptoms are improving while steady deterioration in joint function is objectively plain; the treatment techniques manifestly need modifying in this case.

Examples of signs and symptoms indicating deterioration, and the need for modification or cessation of treatment, are:

The patient's report that a particular symptom is more easily and more quickly provoked.

Periodic symptoms occurring more frequently, with more intensity and for longer duration.

An increase of distal pain, or a proximal pain beginning to spread distally.

Symptoms invoking a suspicion of increasing vertebrobasilar ischaemia (q.v.).

Symptoms changing from an ache to a sharper and more delineated pain, in the same or more distal distribution.

Increasing limitation of movement.

Spinal deformity, or deviation during a movement, becoming apparent.

Symptoms of incipient root involvement, e.g. the advent of paraesthesiae, or sensibility loss.

The emergence, or increase, of neurological signs.

The advent of sphincter disturbance, indicating increasing trespass upon the pudendal nerve.

Neurological involvement. Where the possibility, or probability, of nerve root involvement is suspected, by reason of the patient's description of the *type and distribution* of pain (p. 175), it is wise to carefully monitor the clinical features from session to session, and to include neurological tests, for root tension and of reflexes, as the assessment markers.

When considering *neurological symptoms*, for example, if on cervical side-flexion to the painful side, there is a 12-second latent period for provocation of paraesthesiae in the fingers, and at the next treatment session the latent period is now 3 seconds, this indicates increasing root irritability and the need to modify treatment. Conversely, if the 12-second period has increased to 20 seconds, this gives an assurance that, for the time being at least, the treatment is succeeding.

So far as *neurological signs* are concerned, it is important to distinguish their import in relation to the condition;

for example, the patient with spinal stenosis (q.v.) who has been sitting in a waiting room for 30 minutes before being assessed prior to treatment, may present without neurological deficit, yet if the same patient be asked to walk around the block or stand for 30 minutes immediately prior to examination, a transient neurological deficit may well be present.

If spinal articular signs are in part diminishing, i.e. greater range of some movements before being limited by pain, but the straight-leg-raising test indicates possible pressure on the nerve root because this passive movement is more reduced and painful, the patient's condition has obviously deteriorated.

An increase, or the advent of, a neurologic deficit, and more particularly a report of sphincter disturbance indicate, respectively, the need for a modification of treatment and an urgent surgical opinion.

3. Assessment on symptoms only

Treatment may be necessary for intermittent symptoms which occur during some particular activity during evening hours. There may be very little in the way of joint signs to provide for an objective assessment *during* the patient's attendance, and in order that procedures and their effects may be clearly related on assessment prior to treatment at the next attendance, it is necessary to keep the variety of techniques employed at one session to a minimum, otherwise ascribing good or bad effects to any one of them becomes difficult, and the necessary guides for action are not clear. It is useful to remember that in general, changes in barometric pressure and weather will affect symptoms more than signs.

Relief, or improvement, directly related to treatment procedures will show that treatment was correct, though does not necessarily show that the diagnosis was also correct, since we cannot always know.

If both were *incorrect*, it is better not to have made the patient worse, or the condition more serious; for this reason alone, a fundamental principle is economy in the use of vigour.

In our increasingly technological milieu, the value of subjective and objective clinical assessment should not be discounted or diminished. The predictive value of several highly sensitive and specific serological tests, including the latex fixation test for rheumatoid factor, were subject to investigation.* There were appreciable differences in sensitivity and reproducibility, and some widely used measurements appeared to have little if any real value. Where patients had kept a detailed daily record of morning stiffness and other symptoms, these reports proved to be as useful a measurement as any, and appeared to greatly reduce the variability of assessments by more technical methods. In short, the best measurement of all appeared to be that of asking the patient: 'How are you?'

In summary. Treatment is flexibly adapted according to presenting signs and symptoms; as these change, so should treatment. The guides for action depend upon assessment. This requires concentrated attention at all times; it may be demanding, but it is infinitely more exciting and rewarding than the pedestrian performance of generalised textbook procedures.

* Leading article 1977 Reliability of tests for rheumatism. *British Journal of Clinical Practice* 31:173.

14. Exercises

Voluntary exercises, in many forms, are often necessary to complement passive movement techniques, and at times exercises may comprise the main form of treatment.

Many orthopaedists and therapists appear to hold that the patient has not had a 'proper' treatment unless the therapist has demonstrated and supervised exercises; treatments without exercises being traditionally regarded as incomplete. The suggestion that this or that particular patient does not *need* exercises, because they are not indicated, tends to evince pained astonishment in some.

Common assumptions underlying the general view that 'exercise is a good thing' could probably bear some examination. In a comprehensive analysis of the behaviour of low back pain,[85] it was clear that, 'Patients who regularly participated in physical exercise did not show any dissimilarity in the course of back pain compared to patients who only occasionally or never took exercise.'

In active people and juniors, for example, and also in many mature patients, exercise for the sake of exercise has little point when there are no indications for prescribing exercise with a clear purpose.

The author recalls having to carry out exercises prescribed for strengthening the shoulder girdle elevator muscles of an amateur weightlifter with paraesthesiae of glove distribution in both hands. The patient's musculature was so powerful that he could easily raise the therapist's whole body weight off the floor by elevating his shoulder girdle on one side.

Often, a change of job is much more important than exercise. The load-carrier driver on building sites, who is bounced about on a pitching bucket seat, and the middle-aged telephonist who sits and reaches for heavy directories for hours each day, would reduce stress on low lumbar discs by changing to occupations with more standing, where feasible.

Alternatively, the administrator's chair-bound-backache problem tends to disappear with more physical activity, a better set of abdominal muscles and less weight, the last being rather an indicator of general physical fitness than having much to do with reducing stress on lumbar discs, as is often supposed.[326]

Patients can lose confidence in the capacity of their backs to stand up to the stresses of life. Reassurance and a positive approach during treatment are in some cases more important than the treatment itself, because *a fixed idea of spinal inadequacy is profoundly disabling, and not always justified.*

There is considerable interest in new methods of treating *chronic* pain disability, by a goal-oriented programme aiming to reduce medication intake, to reduce avoidance of activities because of pain, to increase ambulation and selected exercise tolerance and to increase general social and work involvement.

Fordyce *et al.* (1973)[366] refers to 'operant conditioning' as the principles by which the rate, strength and frequency of occurrence of operants may be increased or decreased. Graded exercise programmes form an important part of behaviour-modification techniques, and actively involve the patient in the improvement process.

Mooney and Cairns (1978)[869] refer to the value of the therapist in the training and monitoring of progression through the strengthening exercises.

Group exercises can be a useful method of strengthening vertebral musculature, of improving physical endurance and general locomotor condition and of training in lifting and handling techniques. There is some variation in the organisation of group exercise programmes, since the approach to vertebral joint problems may differ considerably between departments of orthopaedics and rheumatology.[649]

Unless some care is devoted to the clinical examination of each individual whose treatment is solely that of exercises in a particular group, there is a tendency for the person conducting the group treatment to learn very much more about giving exercises to groups than about the precise characteristics of joint problems in the patients being treated.

Individual exercises have many aims. For example:

1. The need to stabilise hypermobile joints by strengthening the environmental musculature, both regionally and segmentally.
2. Mobility exercises for joints liable to become stiff; these may also be regional and/or segmental exercises.
3. Those formulated to assist in stretching contracted soft tissues on one aspect of a vertebral joint.
4. Postural retraining exercises, to diminish the effects of gravitational stress upon particular spinal regions or segments, e.g. where operation is not indicated or is delayed, as in spondylolisthesis or spinal stenosis.
5. Progressive exercise programmes to generally improve muscular strength and physical endurance, and confidence in ability of the spine to stand up to stress.
6. Individual handling instruction, with practice of performance (see p. 509).
7. Preventive or prophylactic exercise.

The aims are often combined.

1. a. STRENGTHENING THE ENVIRONMENTAL MUSCULATURE IN TREATMENT OF A HYPER-MOBILE LOW LUMBAR JOINT

While passive mobilisation techniques are used to reduce the *pain* arising from a segment which may be hypermobile (p. 258), it is necessary that *stability* of the segment be improved.

If the spinal extensor muscles are considered to be weak, or to require extra strengthening, exercises to strengthen them should avoid inner range hyperextension movements, and the starting position arranged so that the resisted movement occurs in middle range and the excursion ceases when normal postural length of the muscle is reached.

Exercises need to be selected with care, since those which stress the joint structures in extreme positions of flexion, extension or rotation are liable to exacerbate the condition. A potent cause of aggravation of low back pain, due to hypermobility, is that of active forced extension in the starting position of prone-lying. It is a very familiar clinical experience to meet the patient who has been religiously performing 'back extension' exercises of this type, and has just as regularly been suffering recurrence of the pains for which these vigorous exercises were prescribed. *They are mentioned only to be condemned as a potent source of continuing back trouble in a particular group of patients.*

During manipulative treatment, with or without anaesthesia, and any other treatment for that matter, including exercises, one of the most common errors is failure to recognise the hypermobile lumbar segment.[279]

Recurrent aggravating backache[780] is one of the most common manifestations of degenerative changes associated with segmental hyperextension, and most of these patients are suffering from recurrent hyperextension strains of posterior joints, or chronic approximation of neural arch structures. Again, the exercise of lying supine and slowly raising the straight legs together, 'to strengthen the abdominal and psoas muscles', is one of the ways in which the symptoms of hypermobile lumbar segments are recurrently aggravated. In the initial few degrees of the movement, the posterior neural arch structures are painfully approximated by the powerful muscle action, as the lumbar spine is drawn into excessive lordosis by the muscles acting with reversed origin and insertion.[151] Similarly, some of the more exotic yoga hyperextension exercises may painfully approximate facet-joint structures, and in the author's recent experience these have more than once initiated an acute and very painful back problem in overenthusiastic patients.

'In the neutral position, moderate extension strains are not painful,'[780] but a segment held in hyperextension has no safety-margin, so that painful capsular lesions result—and keep on resulting as a consequence of repetitive strains.

When progressively stronger isometric 'hold' positions are maintained against the resistance of gravity, with the joint in fairly neutral positions, muscle power may be improved without further joint strain. So far as disc pressure is concerned, isometrically performed exercises are less likely to provoke further pain and disability since it has been demonstrated that they load the lumbar spine less than isotonic exercises.[888] When isometric exercises comprise the only treatment, or they are used together with traction, the results are an improvement upon ordinary flexion and extension routines.[746, 649]

Isometric exercises to improve the power of abdominal muscles are also of value in the treatment of low back pain (*vide infra*)[891] although postural re-education in the importance of reducing the lumbar lordosis by isotonic exercises can be very helpful and Cailliet (1977)[151] provides a few simple and good examples.

There are many types of isometric exercise, and gravitational resistance is not always a necessary component. The following exercises, of which there can be many variations, are suggested as a basis for progression:

Abdominal wall

Starting position: The patient lies supine (Fig. 14.1A) with hips and knees flexed and the feet flat on the support

Exercise: The knees are extended (Fig. 14.1B), that is all; the position is held for increasing lengths of time. The patient must breathe freely throughout.

Progression: With hands on opposite shoulders the patient raises the upper trunk, trying to touch knees with elbows; the degree of hip flexion must not be altered (Fig.

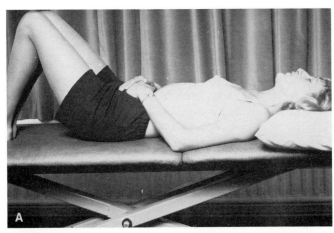

Fig. 14.1 (A) Starting position for abdominal muscle strengthening exercise.

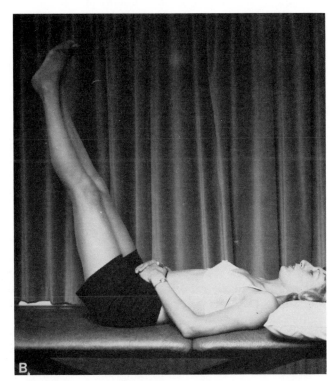

(B) The knees are extended, and the position held for progressively longer durations, without holding the breath.

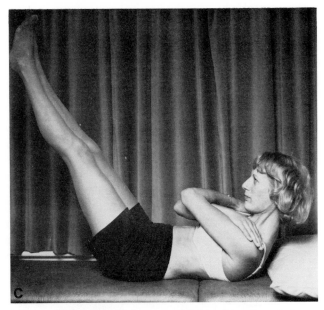

(C) The starting position had been modified by the patient placing palms on opposite shoulders. As the knees are extended, the upper trunk is also raised, without modifying the arm position.

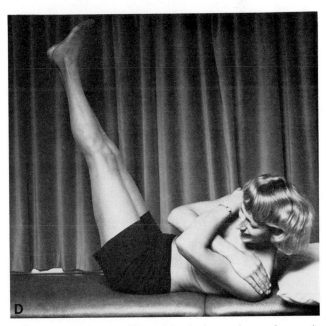

(D) For strengthening the oblique abdominal musculature, the exercise depicted in (C) is progressed by the patient attempting to position one elbow outside the opposite knee. As before, the position is held for increasingly longer periods.

14.1c). Again, breathing must be free, and the position is held for increasing lengths of time, i.e. 3 seconds, 5 seconds, 8 seconds, and so on. When the degree of muscular effort is about to wane, the patient bends the knees, lowering the feet and upper trunk to the starting position, and takes a short rest. The crossed forearms are meant to prevent excessive neck flexion.

Oblique abdominal muscles

Starting position and exercise are similar to above, but now the patient tries to place one elbow outside the opposite knee without releasing the position of hands and shoulders (Fig. 14.1D). Again, the position is held for increasing lengths of time without holding the breath.

NB: It is unwise for these exercises to be performed with the hands clasped behind the neck; the enthusiastic patient often pulls the neck forward vigorously and painfully strains it.

Dorsal extensor muscles

Starting position: (not illustrated) The patient lies prone with trunk on a flat surface such as a kitchen table, the edge of which is covered by a folded towel and approximates to the groin. The hips are flexed so that the toes may rest on the floor, with knees straight. By grasping the sides of the table, the trunk is stabilised; the legs are raised to the horizontal and held there, the isometric hold being maintained for increasing durations (Fig. 14.2). As before, breathing should be free.

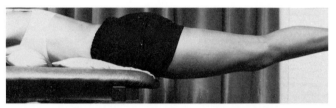

Fig. 14.2 Isometric muscle-work for regional spinal extensor groups. (See text for progressions.)

Progression: This is made by adding weight to the heels, e.g. a light cushion and then a heavier one; the method of performing the exercise does not change. It provides for powerful work by the erector spinae group, with the lumbar joints in what is virtually a neutral position.

1. b. STRENGTHENING THE SEGMENTAL MUSCULATURE IN TREATMENT OF A HYPERMOBILE LUMBAR JOINT

The principle is that of stimulating small but important local muscle groups to work isometrically in maintaining the orientation in space of a single vertebra. This localised strengthening is of fundamental importance, because of clear evidence[619] that lumbar degenerative joint conditions are accompanied by changes in the relative populations of 'fast' and 'slow' fibres in the segmental musculature, e.g. multifidus.

Lateral technique

Starting position: The patient lies prone on the support; the therapist stands at the side and applies his thumbpads to that side of the spinous process of the upper vertebra of the segment concerned. The position is the same as for transverse vertebral pressure (Fig. 12.57).

Moderate but sustained pressure is applied to the bony point, the patient being instructed not to allow the vertebra to be 'displaced'. Initially, a considerable mass of paravertebral muscle is called into play to resist the displacing pressure, but with encouragement and practice the patient begins to localise the muscular effort to a surprising degree. Similarly, there is a need to consciously *relax* muscle groups which need not be called into play and to breathe in a quiet and relaxed way.

Isometric contractions are repeated to the opposite side, and progression is made by increasing the pressures being sustained, and the duration of the 'holds'. The exercise is repeated on the spinous process next below; where two hypermobile segments lie in one vertebral region, both components of each segment must be treated.

Sagittal technique

The patient sits across a plinth, with the buttocks at the rear edge. The therapist stands, crouches or kneels behind the patient, and applies both thumbpads to one spinous process. Moderate but sustained pressure is now applied in a postero-anterior direction, and the patient instructed to not allow the segment to be moved forwards. At first, this elicits a total response of all trunk musculature, but by encouragement to 'think and contract locally' the muscular effort does become much more localised. As before the patient should breathe freely and quietly, and learn to gently wriggle arms, hands, legs and feet to make the point about relaxation of all uninvolved muscle.

Progressions: are made as described above.

The L4–L5 and lumbosacral segments may also be treated with the patient in a prone position; the hips are flexed to 90° (Fig. 14.3) with the patient's feet resting on the floor and the knees some three inches (7 cm) or more above it. The therapist stands at the side, level with the patient's pelvis, and places his cranial palm on the lumbar region immediately above the segments concerned. Moderate, but increasing and sustained pressure is applied to the patient's sacrum by the therapist's caudal hand. The patient must be discouraged from using hip and knee extensor muscles to resist the pressure; the legs should be wriggled about now and then to ensure they are relaxed and taking no part in the movement.

Home exercises: At one attendance, a relative can be taught to give the resistance; the postero-anterior pressures can be self-administered by the patient (Fig. 14.4) and many become highly adept at the exercise.

Thoracic joint problems appear generally to need simple maintenance exercises for mobility than resisted exercises for stability, but where joint pain is arising from a hypermobile segment, resisted exercises should form part of the treatment. They are less easy to administer than at the lumbar spine, but the principles are the same.

Paravertebral muscle of the *neck* may become weakened as a consequence of chronic degenerative joint changes. There are many methods of strengthening the muscu-

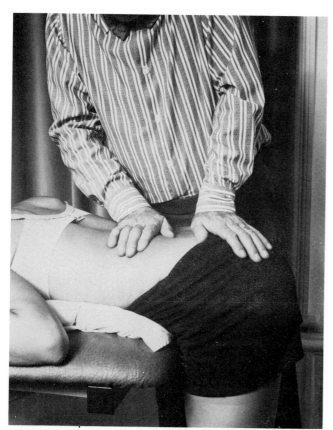

Fig. 14.3 Resisted isometric contractions of lower lumbar musculature, in the treatment of instability. The technique may also be modified, of course, as a hold-relax technique to assist stretching of shortened soft tissues.

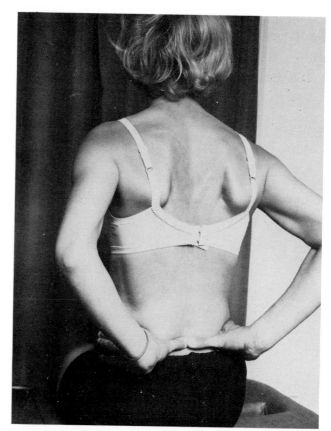

Fig. 14.4 Autoresisted isometric contractions of lower lumbar musculature. The patient can be trained to localise the muscular effort.

lature, varying from (i) somewhat heroic procedures involving the patient lying extended over a kitchen table with a looped towel suspending in space a brick, which is lifted up and down by neck extension, and (ii) proprioceptive facilitation techniques, to (iii) simple self-administered resistance by hand pressure. The latter method is quite efficient, quite effective and does not involve a search for building materials.

Strengthening exercises are by no means always indicated; if localised manual mobilisation, traction and/or a cervical collar have produced relief of pain and freedom of movement, this will allow better muscle function, and thus simple postural-correction exercises and prophylactic advice are more appropriate than strengthening exercises for their own sake.

2. a. REGIONAL MOBILITY EXERCISES

These are well known to all therapists, and all that one needs to mention is the importance of ensuring that the type of exercise given does indeed affect the intended vertebral region. For example, the favourite group of prone-kneeling exercises, to mobilise the lower spine, have much more effect upon the thoracolumbar region than the lumbosacral segments.

Hydrotherapy provides the benefits of relaxing warmth, support and buoyancy, allowing easier voluntary effort and regional mobilisation of stiff spinal joints.

2. b. SEGMENTAL MOBILITY EXERCISES

These previously rather specialised techniques have, in the last few years, become more widely used, and a handy pocket-book text[145] describes some of them. For example, if the right hand is passed across the chest and around the left side of the neck, so that the palmar aspect of the right middle fingertip is placed against the *right* side of the C6 spinous process to stabilise it, active left neck rotation will mobilise the C5–C6 segment. Again, if the patient sits in a high-backed chair, so that the spinous process of T3 bears precisely against the upper edge of the chairback, extension of the head, neck and upper thorax, with a degree of 'chin-pulling-in', will exercise the small extension range of the T2–T3 segment much more than will a generalised thoracic extension movement.

A difficulty with segmental exercises is that many of the manual self-stabilisation techniques are not possible for the mature or elderly patient, by reason of shoulder joint restriction, for example. Sometimes, and in some patients, those who most need them are least able to do them.

Nevertheless, they are an important advance in the treatment of common vertebral joint problems.

3. STRETCHING CONTRACTED SOFT TISSUES

Passive stretching techniques should be accompanied by active movements to maintain the progress achieved. For example, contracture or shortening of the lumbar sacro-spinalis muscle and associated connective tissue may be present and will require stretching; starting positions for exercise should be arranged so that reciprocal relaxation of these antagonists of the abdominal wall may assist in the elongation process.

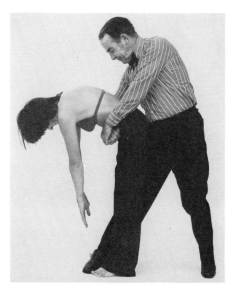

Fig. 14.5 Lumbar flexion resisted by placing a forearm across the patient's lower abdomen. Thus the usually gravity-assisted movement of flexion now requires a strong abdominal contraction, with consequent reciprocal relaxation of dorsal musculature.

The method depicted in Figure 14.5 can be adapted as a 'hold-relax' technique for stretching a tight lumbodorsal fascia overlying the L5–S1 segment. By employing the principle of reciprocal innervation the patient's vigorous flexion efforts can help considerably to stretch contracted low lumbar musculature. With one foot well forward between the patient's feet, and placing his trochanter of the same side against the patient's buttocks, the therapist engages the patient's lower abdomen with the forearm of that side, and leans backward as the patient is encouraged to repetitively reach for the toes. The object is to prevent as much hip flexion as possible, and to ensure that vigorous abdominal muscle contraction will induce a reciprocal relaxation of dorsal muscle.

In *the cervical region*, rounded shoulders and a poking chin are frequently accompanied by established contracture of the posterior cervical soft tissues. Manual stretching techniques (Fig. 12.7) should be complemented by exercises to re-establish a better posture.

Besides 'chin-pulling-in' and 'stretching-up', autore-sisted exercises for the lengthened and weakened anterior neck muscles are needed; these are simply taught to the patient, who is shown how to elicit an isometric neck muscle contraction by manual resistance to the forehead, this being met and held so by static work for the anterior muscles. This is progressed as previously described.

4. POSTURAL RETRAINING EXERCISES

Low backache frequently coexists with excessive lordosis and a lax abdominal wall. Stabilisation of the lumbar spine in a less extended position, by isometric abdominal strengthening exercises while holding a corrected pelvic tilt, is effective in helping to relieve this type of backache.

Spondylolisthesis at a lumbar segment need not cause symptoms, but when the condition does give rise to pain and surgical treatment is not immediately considered, inner range abdominal exercises combined with pelvic tilting will diminish the shearing stress and help to stabilise the faulty segment by reducing lordosis.

5. EXERCISE PROGRAMMES TO IMPROVE STRENGTH AND ENDURANCE, AND TO RESTORE CONFIDENCE, do not require description here

6. INDIVIDUAL ERGONOMIC INSTRUCTION

See page 500.

7. PROPHYLACTIC EXERCISE IN GENERAL TERMS

Other factors given, individuals without vertebral joint problems are more likely to avoid them while they retain the natural resilience, extensibility and vascularity of their soft tissues, strong muscles which are well co-ordinated in isotonic or isometric contraction and reciprocal relaxation, and joints which are freely mobile.

While these are given to the young, the inheritance is often soon to be abused, by competitive trials of strength and endurance which begin the process of unequal muscular development, unequal tightness of connective tissue and certain restrictions of the 'global' mobility of joints.

Plain freedom from pain is not necessarily synonymous with the most efficient functioning of the physical machinery (p. 508) and in particular, the *way* in which we use our bodies is perhaps more a matter of enlightened physical education in human kinetics (p. 500) than pursuing the ideal of excelling in strength and endurance, and little else.

Preventive exercises for the vertebral regions are considered on pages 497, 511.

HOME EXERCISES IN THE TREATMENT OF ACUTE LUMBAR PAIN

The suggestion that a patient may abort, or considerably modify the distress of, an acute attack of low back pain (in the absence of neurological signs) by lying supine or on one side and gently flexing the knees onto the chest, requires some qualification. Unless the manœuvre is first cautiously attempted by the therapist, and its effects observed, it is not infrequent for a severe exacerbation of pain to occur if the advice is given and followed, willy-nilly, by *every* patient with low back pain. Some do better on a different regime (b. below), and a proportion should be at complete rest.

Likewise, the notion that 'environmental' rotatory manipulation of the lumbar spine, or localised thrust techniques to specific segments, will promptly get the patient out of pain.

They are not fail-safe procedures; when they work they do so gratifyingly, but they do not always work.

For example, acute pain arising from falling heavily on the buttocks, or because of an upward jolt when sitting on the hard seat of a truck which has just been driven over a pothole, is often savagely provoked by these procedures. Again, the patient who has probably torn, attenuated or strained the annulus fibrosus of a lumbar disc by a sudden heave in a flexed and rotated position is likely to have the pain severely provoked by a rotatory manipulative technique which repeats the rotatory direction of the exciting trauma.

a. Cautious lumbar flexion, moderately increased as the initial attempts prove to be innocuous and helpful, is of value when posterior structures may have been painfully approximated and, likewise, localised facet-joint gapping manipulations are useful when the arthrotic facet-joint locking in the mature patient, following a weight-free flexion reach, can be established as the cause of pain.

In the greater majority of cases, gentle exploratory oscillatory rotations of small amplitude, or a considerately performed manual traction technique, employing the inertia of the patient's body weight,[1182] are less likely to exacerbate an acute condition, the nature of which is not always easy to assess when the patient is in considerable distress.

If an attack of low backache is regarded solely as 'a severely sprained joint' which indeed *some* of them appear to be, treatment in the initial stages is rest, as in a severely sprained ankle.[780] Since the latter injury would not be subjected to considerable ranges of movement for a day or two, and yet lumbar flexion may help to relieve the gross lumbar muscle spasm in extension, it will be just as effective for the patient to *rest* in a flexed position, either on the back (Fig. 14.6) or on the side with the knees comfortably drawn up. The important point is 'comfortable'; dogged attempts to draw the knees up can be counterproductive in some.

The patient remains at rest, with increasing degree of hip flexion and thus lumbar flexion, as this is found to be comfortable and the pain continues to decrease.

Flexion exercise-manipulations, where the supine patient raises the bent legs above the head for a prescribed number of times each day, are useful when the signs have begun to lessen in severity after the first cautious attempts

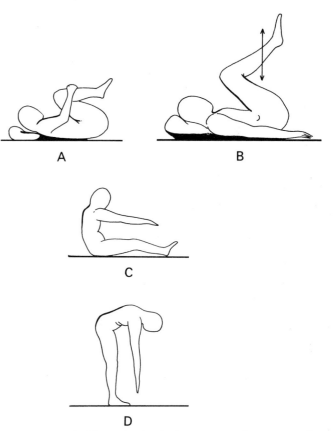

Fig. 14.7 (A)–(D) Home exercises in the treatment of some types of acute back pain (see text). As pain diminishes and confidence improves, the exercise is changed to that of long-sitting and reaching for the toes, and then standing flexion.

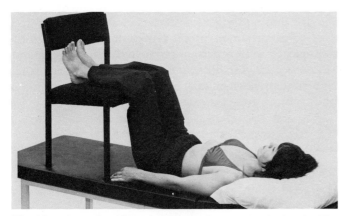

Fig. 14.6 A comfortable resting posture for acute low back pain. The extent of hip flexion and the nature of the calf support are matters of individual preference—there is no arbitrary position.

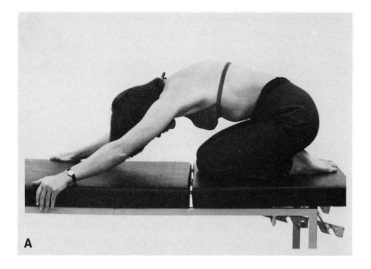

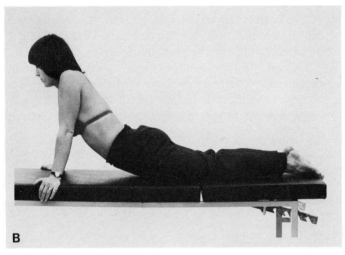

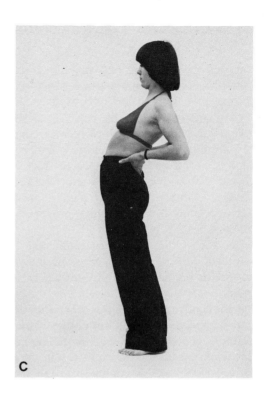

Fig. 14.8 (A), (B), (C) Home exercises in the treatment of localised acute back pain with some loss of normal lumbar lordosis. (See text for cautious progression.) The exercise is initially not suitable for those patients whose neural arches have been painfully approximated by trauma or stress. Allowing the pelvis to sag forward (C) means much less muscle work for the patient (and thus less pain) than bending the trunk backward. The subtle difference is important.

at flexion mobilising; if initial attempts provoke the pain, the exercise should not be employed.

The effect is more easily accomplished if the supine patient merely adds a further movement to that of pulling the flexed knees onto the chest, i.e. from the 'knee–chest' position, the feet are pushed toward the ceiling until the back pain begins to be provoked, and then lowered again. The movement is repeated a dozen times and as pain recedes the knees and hips are further extended, to approach the receding point of provocation. The patient repeats the group of a dozen or so movements at a frequency varying between two and ten or so a day, the number depending upon how the patient feels rather than the magic number of three (Fig. 14.7).

b. For the patient whose painful episode is accompanied by some loss of the normal lumbar lordosis, a scheme of progressive extension may be suitable, following initial assessment.

From the prone kneeling position (Fig. 14.8A, B), with the hands placed forward of the shoulders, the hips and knees are gently extended by carrying the trunk slightly forward over the hands—the position is held for a few

moments before the hips and knees are flexed again by backward movement of the trunk.

From a cautious beginning, by a dozen excursions every hour or so, the exercise is progressed by holding the forward position for longer and by increasing the amount of lumbar extension. The exercise is progressed to lumbar extension in standing (Fig. 14.8c).

NB: Full and vigorous flexion in standing, and full passive extension in prone lying, should be carefully approached until a passive physiological-movement test (PP–MT) has established that there is no segmental hypermobility, which may be aggravated by uninhibited and vigorous free movement.

RECORDING

The orderly nominating of each *type* or *aim* of exercise is a good habit, and its aids assessment. Headings are therefore:

Stability (Power)—Mobility—Stretch—Posture/ Balance/Control—Endurance—Handling.

A record should be kept of the nature of *group exercises*, whether for general strengthening of trunk and cervical musculature, physical endurance or training in lifting and handling techniques.

If we take the example of chronic lumbar pain in a young woman, due to a hypermobile L4–L5 segment, the manual mobilisation treatment (in this case solely for the relief of pain) would be recorded as previously suggested (p. 435). If static isometric contractions are chosen as home exercises for the *regional* improvement of muscle power, it is probable that the therapist has a tried and trusted handful of exercises with the required specific effect, but these should nevertheless be recorded; the aims, type, frequency and duration of exercises must be clear and reproducible for both therapist and patient.

For example, the prescription for an interim week of home exercises may be:

'*Stab*: —abdo. iso. ex. 10 sec hold × 8   ⟋   12 × 4
daily

—neut. ext. iso. exs. 10 sec hold   ⟋   12 × 4
× 8 daily'

and this indicates:

'*Stability*: abdominal isometric exercise with 8, progressing to 12, 10-second holds, 4 times a day
neutral lumbar extension holds for the same periods' (see p. 452).

Progression of the exercise programme for the succeeding weeks should also be recorded. For any progressive scheme of exercises, patients should be encouraged, and shown how, to keep a simple graph of their progress, and to bring it with them on the next attendance.

There is no better reminder of the value of dogged persistence than a manifest indication of steadily increasing muscle power.

For improving the power and functional efficiency of *segmental* musculature, static isometric contractions, against resistance applied to vertebral apophyses, will need to be precisely recorded, and a simple method is to use the mobilisation symbols, differentiated by being enclosed in a circle, i.e.

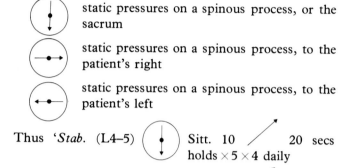

would indicate, 'Segmental stability exercises for L4–L5, as isometric "holds" of 10, progressing to 20 seconds, against resistance applied centrally and transversely to the fourth and fifth lumbar spinous processes. Five holds at each of four sessions daily.'

The fact that the patient can self-administer the central posteroanterior static pressures, but may need an assistant to give the transverse pressures, does not invalidate the method of recording the programme of home exercises.

15. Indications for passive movement techniques and voluntary exercises

Contraindications for passive movement techniques

The following INDICATIONS are given on the assumption that the patient has been through a diagnostic sorting procedure, that treatment by movement is appropriate and, so far as is possible, serious disease and significant mechanical defect have been excluded by X-rays.

The 'Rules of procedure' (p. 442) should be observed without exception.

A. General indications
B. Soft-tissue techniques
C. Localised mobilisation (grades I–IV)
D. Regional mobilisation (grades I–IV)
E. Stretching (A)
F. Mechanical harness traction
G. Localised manipulation (grade loc V) (see also 'Abnormal end-feels on passive testing', p. 358)
H. Regional manipulation (grade V)
I. Exercises.

A. GENERAL INDICATIONS

In general terms, a joint problem is suitable for this treatment if the symptoms are aggravated by activity, some particular movements of the joint and certain postures, and relieved by rest and other ('antalgic') postures—these differ from patient to patient.

Sometimes patients have no immediately apparent articular signs (that is, pain on movement or limitation of gross movement), only an ache, and after passive mobility testing has localised the tight intervertebral segment(s) at a spinal level reasonably compatible with the distribution and nature of their symptoms, they will be found to respond well to passive movement techniques.

It must always be remembered that some types of serious visceral and other pathology, for which these treatments are either contraindicated or pointless, have a tendency to simulate vertebrogenic problems and to refer pain to the neck and back; this pain is not as a rule aggravated by spinal movement but on occasion may be, e.g. in disease of thoracic viscera.

The indications for gentle, moderate or more vigorous treatment become more certain in an almost direct relationship to the number of factors which are accurately assessed. The more comprehensive the examination, the more likely is the appropriate treatment approach to become clarified, as the weight of emphasis one way or another gradually mounts up during the 'indications' examination. Therefore, it is of first importance to be thorough, but also to be quick and not to waste time; for this reason, it is good sense to become skilled in examination procedures as a vital first requirement.

B. SOFT-TISSUE TECHNIQUES

Detailed indications for massage, in its various forms, has been excellently described in many texts[1180a, 850, 1216, 791, 217,] and general indications only are given.

Stroking and light effleurage is used as a preparatory regional treatment when excessive muscle spasm is present in an overanxious patient.

Stretching (B), kneading and petrissage are frequently necessary for the regional soft tissues overlying chronic joint problems; both longitudinal and transverse mobilisation of muscle are needed to soften them, improve their tissue-fluid exchange and local extensibility.

Inhibitory pressures are used for the relaxation or 'decontraction' of muscle spasm.

Vibrations are best applied mechanically.

Fine vibrations are used to reduce the chronic muscular ache resulting from a sustained tension, and are usefully applied to a muscle group *after* a stretching (A) technique.

Coarse vibration stimulates muscle groups which are antagonistic to those requiring stretching; also, some patients may need a vibratory treatment in preparation for instruction in self-applied isometric segmental exercise.

Transverse frictions may sometimes be necessary at the aponeurotic attachments on the nuchal lines of the occiput and at the medial border of the scapula. Their use for connective-tissue changes at the limb girdles, and more distally, has been well described.

Circular frictions are occasionally indicated when

acutely tender and discrete 'nodules' or fasciculi are accurately localised by the patient as a source of discomfort; these accessory treatments should never be used without primary elucidation and treatment of coexisting vertebral joint problems.

C. LOCALISED MOBILISATION (grades I–IV)[456]

Indications for gentle treatment

(i) In the history (elicit by observation and specific questions):
—much joint irritability
—most or all movements hurt severely
—particular postures hurt severely
—much limb pain
—not sleeping well
—cough/sneeze reproduce distal pain
—pain has been severe for some time
—postural spasm protecting the joint area

(ii) During testing (elicit by careful movement tests, noting degree of pain on movement, neurological test, careful palpation):

—pain sufficient to produce facial distortion
—spinal movement produces distal limb pain
—pain and/or paraesthesiae increase some seconds *after* the testing movement has been completed
—elicited spasm
—pain much increased after minimal examination
—pressure on bony points provokes distal pain/ paraesthesiae
—the presence of neurological deficit, unless this is established to be of previous origin

(iii) Result of initial treatment:

—response to first moderate treatment is much increased pain.

Indications for more vigorous treatment, or increased grades (elicited as above)

(i) History:

—moderate pain has been static for some time, and is generally unvarying in intensity
—no joint movement stirs it up much
—when stirred up, soon settles
—sleeping well
—little limb pain, or distal pain
—cough, sneeze or jar does not hurt
—no exacerbation in any particular posture
—no postural spasm

(ii) Testing:

—joint irritability obviously minimal, with no muscle guarding (elicited spasm) on movement

—spinal testing movements may be limited, but do not stir up pain especially
—limitation of movement is more by tissue-tension or by tissue-compression than by pain
—no neurological deficit, or deficit of previous origin only
—spinal pressure does not hurt much, or provoke paraesthesiae, distally or locally

(iii) Treatment:

The initial moderate treatment does not produce any aggravation of signs or symptoms.

Neurological signs. A neurological deficit, manifested by reflex changes, muscle weakness and sensory changes in the distribution of the involved root, need not of itself preclude the use of this treatment to the associated joint(s) so long as: (a) no more than *one cervical root*, on that side, is involved in the upper limb; (b) no more than *one* of the *lumbar roots* is affected, on one side. If the neurological signs span two lumbar segments on one side this is still acceptable provided they are adjacent.

Restricted joint range, and pain at rest or on movement, can still be treated in the presence of the type of neurological deficit outlined above, provided the 'Rules of Procedure' (p. 442) are followed and so long as (a) and (b) are borne in mind.

The *degree of joint and root irritability*, rather than the presence of neurological signs in themselves, which may be old, is the main factor for assessment when planning treatment, and when irritability is marked, or signs are currently developing, the patient must be treated gently, and with caution, respectively.

NB: *Cervical and thoracic joint problems producing neurological symptoms and signs in one or both lower limbs are an ABSOLUTE contraindication.*

Indications for more vigorous treatment (or building up to vigorous treatment) in patients with distal pain and signs of neurological deficit
In the history:

a. When the state of affairs in the preceding week or fortnight has been static. If improving, there would be no need for vigorous treatment.
b. When their answer to, 'What makes the pain worse/ better?' is that nothing does either, i.e. symptoms are generally unvarying in nature.

If the symptoms are easily exacerbated, one should be careful. During examination:

a. Though movements may be restricted, and may reproduce pain distally, or proximally only, it is not *great* pain, even with overpressure. The harder it is to reproduce the pain, the more vigorous treatment can be.

b. Straight-leg-raising is a useful test here. Even if SLR is restricted by 40° or more, and there is only a block with little pain, treatment can be more vigorous. A combination of limited SLR and limited flexion, with other factors pointing as outlined in (a), is a good indication for vigorous treatment.

In treatment:

a. If the initial gentle technique does not produce distal pain, or an increase of it, or a 'latent-period' exacerbation of pain *during* that session, then one can go ahead and build up to more vigorous treatment during the next attendance.
b. By the third session, one should be moving through the techniques fairly quickly, i.e. rotations, pressures, traction, etc. to find the most effective.

D. REGIONAL MOBILISATION (grades I–IV)

Indications are:

a. Localised symptoms arising from degenerative changes and stiffening in several adjacent segments.
b. Thickening, tightness and soft-tissue induration in several adjacent segments, not necessarily degenerative.
c. As a prelude to more specific treatment when the patient finds it difficult to relax (excluding marked irritability).

Massage techniques are often combined with the joint movement techniques; active mobilising and postural exercises are frequently required – some specific conditions are:

a. Ankylosing spondylitis in quiescent periods and preferably early in the course of the disease.
   Quite firm regional and specific manual mobilisation techniques assist the patient to offset stiffness and fixation by regular active exercises, among which respiratory exercises are important, as are movements for upper and lower limb girdles.[1180b, 1275]
b. Postural kyphosis of the thoracic spine, secondary to tightness of anterior structures.
c. Lumbar region stiffness, as a sequel of arthrosis of the hip.
d. Regional cervical stiffening in the subacute and chronic stages of recovery from acceleration and deceleration trauma (whiplash). Localised conditions should be given specific treatment.

E. INDICATIONS FOR STRETCHING (A)

This will be necessary for tightened soft tissue overlying, or associated with, chronic joint problems, e.g.

—the ligamentum nuchae and other posterior cervical structures

—the upper fibres of trapezius
—the scaleni
—pectoralis major and minor
—the concave side of lateral curves due to pelvic tilt in the frontal plane
—the psoas major, which is often unilaterally tight
—the lumbodorsal fascia and posterior lumbosacral structures.

Stretching (A) and regional mobilisation are frequently combined, since the indications are similar.

F. MECHANICAL HARNESS TRACTION[456]

Rhythmic traction

Notes: (for all regions):

With more severe symptoms:	relatively long periods of 'hold' and 'rest' should be employed (i.e. less movement)
As symptoms become less severe:	shorter 'hold' and 'rest' periods are more effective (i.e. more movement)

Progressive traction techniques, in which a set maximum tension is applied gradually by small increments, and similarly released, find their best use in:

a. The very gentle application of low, and later moderate, tension when treating root irritability by sustained traction.
b. Accustoming a nervous patient, or one who has experienced indifferently applied treatment in the past, to traction.
c. The watchful application of traction to the patient with asthma, or other forms of respiratory distress.

Cervical traction
Traction can be used for any musculoskeletal conditions of the cervical spine, either alone or combined with manual techniques.

a. *Sustained*:
   1. Where joint and/or root irritability is high
   2. Recent or developing neurological signs, associated with irritability
   3. Severe arm pain much reducing neck movements towards the painful side.

b. *Rhythmic*:
   4. Acute joint derangements (but see 1. above)
   5. As a mobilising technique
   6. Upper cervical problems not responding quickly to mobilisation (but see 1. above)

7. Much degenerative stiffness coexisting with evidence of gross changes
8. The elderly osteoporotic and degenerative neck (probably more comfortably treated by gentle rhythmic traction than by contact techniques)
9. Established neurological signs *without* irritability.

Thoracic traction

In comparison with the cervical and lumbar regions the sphere of thoracic traction is restricted, while remaining a useful treatment method.

a. *Sustained*:
1. Where joint irritability is high

b. *Rhythmic*:
2. Widely distributed thoracic pain associated with advanced degenerative changes (but check irritability)
3. Thoracic joint problems producing symptoms not aggravated by active movement
4. When manual mobilisation has not produced the fullest improvement considered possible
5. As a mobilising technique.

Lumbar traction

Traction can be considered for most musculoskeletal conditions of the lumbar region, either alone or combined with manual techniques.

a. *Sustained*:
1. Any symptom, of gradual onset without trauma, which is localised to the lumbar spine or referred distally, and accompanied by pain rather than an ache
2. Low back and bilateral, symmetrical leg pain (change to rhythmic traction as symptoms settle)
3. Where joint and/or root irritability is high and root pain is severe

b. *Rhythmic*:
4. Where joint and/or root irritability is low
5. Localised pain from the lumbar spine, not limiting active movement
6. A lumbar *ache*, often accompanying degenerative bony change, or postural deformities, or after old trauma
7. Localised lumbosacral pain, sharply aggravated by extension and side-flexion, but not flexion
8. Lumbar pain with a diurnal rhythm of slowly increasing throughout the day, after a pain-free early morning
9. As a simple longitudinal mobilising technique
10. Where, in the absence of backache initially, the onset of pain is in the haunch or more distally, and is

accompanied by dural tension signs (i.e. neck flexion and/or straight-leg-raising markedly limited by limb pain); traction in prone-lying may be more successful, in some, than in supine lying.

NB: Repetitive, rhythmic traction techniques applied *manually*, other than oscillatory longitudinal movements, are more suitably categorised under 'D. Indications for regional mobilisation'.

G. LOCALISED MANIPULATION (grade loc V)

NB: Grade V techniques should never be used in the presence of spasm which is protecting the segment being treated.

Indications
1. As a progression from adequate mobilisations which have reached grade IV, where the latter have not achieved the fullest improvement in signs and symptoms considered possible.

2. In those joint problems where there are no articular signs, only an ache, and the tight vertebral segment has been localised by passive mobility testing. These cases should not be treated by manipulation if the limited movement at a segment is due to old pathology.

3. Where pain is minimal and does not appear until near the end of the range.

4. Localised symptoms of sudden onset (but see b, c and e below). Localised manipulation must always be preceded by a passive test of functional mobility at each vertebral segment, to localise the level of movement restriction. As a working rule, apply the emphasis of the movement to the lower vertebra of the tight segment (e.g. at C7–T1, it is T1 which should be moved). Techniques are normally done to both sides.

When manipulative thrust techniques are employed for segmental stiffness, they should be done to both sides, although this does not apply to techniques with a bilateral effect, for example that depicted in Figure 12.74. When they are used for asymmetrical restriction of movement, in cases where the opposite movement is free, the techniques are employed to free the restricted movement only, for example Figures 12.75, 12.76.

If we take a further example, i.e. of restricted neck movement, in the absence of any factor precluding grade V techniques, the direction of the manipulative thrust depends, as always, on the direction and nature of restriction.

a. If cervical left-side-flexion feels blocked on the left side, and right-side-flexion feels free and unrestricted, i.e. movement which tends to *gap* the side of restriction is not affected, then a technique which encourages facet-*gliding* on the left side is indicated. Thus the technique employed would be ⟶ taking care while positioning that left-side approximation is not too firmly applied, and applying the emphasis to the thrusting hand rather than the other. If both left- and right-side-flexion were limited, by a left block and a left pull respectively, the technique to use would be ⭰ .

b. If cervical left-side-flexion feels free and un-encumbered, but right-side-flexion is restricted by tethering on the left side, the technique to use is ⭰ , provided that adequate localised mobil-isation had not been fully effective.

Precautions

Besides Contraindications (see p. 465), there are certain clinical factors which preclude the use of manipulation, and these are:

a. Hypermobility of the segment involved.
b. When joint irritability and painful movement are manifest.
c. The presence of spasm, protecting the joint being treated.
d. When segments *adjacent* to the main joint problems are either irritable, or hypermobile, and stresses applied by the positioning for manipulation would aggravate them.
e. Inability of the patient to relax.
f. When the operator senses that the joint will not give— this is felt as a rubbery resistance to the final movement, and must in all circumstances be respected.

Since so much effective work is possible by the best use of *mobilisation and traction techniques which are under control of the patient*, perhaps grade V manipulative thrust tech-niques should be used in much the same way as rheumato-logists use systemic steroid drugs—after extra deliberation and then with watchfulness and care.

As lengthening clinical experience is accompanied by more confidence in recognising indications for grade V manipulations, the therapist uses them more surely, safely and effectively, and with the minimum of vigour. This is no field for the sporting amateur, whose concept of what manipulators do is very frequently the euphoric notion that they spend all their clinical time producing dramatic clicks by exotic techniques.

H. INDICATIONS FOR REGIONAL MANIPULATION (grade V)

Although manipulative techniques *with a localised effect* may involve some movement of a whole vertebral region, this is not the same thing as routinely dealing with lumbar pain by 'environmental' manipulation of the lumbar spine, or routinely treating cervical pain by gross cervical spine manipulations, for example.

They are infrequently indicated; the author's practice is mainly to employ regional lumbar manipulation for those patients who have no detectable clinical signs of any impor-tance, other than stiffness, but who have plainly lost con-fidence in the health and durability of their spines, and need to have its underlying functional soundness demon-strated to them. Even in these cases, vigour is unnecessary, although a purposeful flamboyance may impress the gul-lible.

I. EXERCISES

When the nature and the site of a vertebral movement-abnormality has been established, exercises are indicated as follows:

Segmental instability:
   regional, and segmental, strengthening exercises to assist in stabilising the hypermobile joint, e.g. iso-metric abdominal, back extensor and segmental exercises for lumbar instability.
Postural/mechanical insufficiency:
   postural retraining and strengthening exercises, to diminish the effects of gravitational stress upon a par-ticular spinal segment, e.g. spondylolisthesis.
Segmental stiffness:
   segmental mobility exercises, to maintain the range of movement at a particular segment following local-ised passive mobililisation.
Asymmetrical tissue-tightness:
   exercises to assist in maintaining the extensibility of contracted soft tissues on one aspect of a vertebral segment or vertebral region, e.g. unilateral tissue-tightness as a sequel to lateral pelvic tilt.
Symmetrical tissue-tightness:
   as above, where chronic bilateral contracture has occurred, e.g. (i) the lordosis syndrome, with chronic tightness of lumbosacral fascia and associated soft tissues, and (ii) tight pectoral structures.
Generalised or regional poor posture/balance/control:
   postural correction exercises.
Regional stiffness and muscular inco-ordination in the mature/elderly:
   training in light, rhythmic, co-ordinated regional movements to offset the tendency for facet-joint lock-ing as a consequence of unco-ordinated or impulsive movement.
Recently acquired lateral deviation of the lumbar spine:
   self-administered corrective exercises to restore and maintain normal posture.
Backache due to generalised muscular insufficiency:
   progressive regional mobility and strengthening exercises to restore muscle power and physical endurance.

Spinal stenosis:

    postural retraining in backward pelvic tilt, and strengthening of abdominal muscles, for the standing and walking pain of spinal stenosis, when surgery for decompression is delayed or inadvisable.

Lumbosacral root adhesions:

    flexion exercises to assist in stretching an adhesed root, following the period of acute sciatic pain.

Pelvic joint asymmetry:

    postural positioning exercises to assist correction.

NB: Re-education of regional vertebral movement

In a multijointed articulation like the vertebral column, the restoration of better movement, after months and years of stiffness, may depend on something more than the simple mobilisation of joints. Frequently, patients seem to have a lost or diminished proprioceptive sense of what the normally complex movement *feels* like, and in addition to segmental and regional manual or mechanical techniques they may need to have some simple re-education of movement. A little treatment time spent in this way often pays handsome dividends.

For example, the patient who bends the head back by just tilting the chin upwards with little lower cervical or cervicothoracic movement, may persist in doing this even when the stiff lower segments have been mobilised. Unjustifiably, the therapist may experience a sense of failure to realise aims of treatment, when in fact all that is now required is to restore the lost motor pattern, by exercises which emphasise neck rather than head movement.

CONTRAINDICATIONS TO PASSIVE MOVEMENT TECHNIQUES

Because this heading refers usually to conditions or syndromes for which the treatment under consideration is unsuitable, more for reasons of the dangers involved than because of therapeutic pointlessness, the nature of the treatment should also be discussed.

When physical treatment can be modified to range from the most gentle to quite vigorous, the conditions which might be contraindications can be divided into two groups, i.e. (1) absolute contraindications; (2) those conditions requiring extra care in selection and application of treatment.

NB: One overriding consideration is that any treatment which involves the production of movement or applied stress, either to body regions and tissues or in the form of increased pressures in vessels and vascular sinuses, is *contraindicated* in the absence of a thorough clinical and radiological examination to exclude organic disease.

MANIPULATION

Absolute contraindications (often because of coexisting disease) are:

1. Frank spinal deformity due to old pathology (e.g. scoliosis, or kyphosis due to adolescent osteochondrosis)
2. Most craniovertebral, and some lumbosacral, anomalies (e.g. lack of a stable lumbosacral articulation)
3. Neoplastic disease of skeletal or soft tissue of the spine
4. Bone disease (e.g. osteomyelitis, tuberculosis, Paget's disease, osteoporosis, e.g. due to senility, prolonged steroid therapy, certain hormonal drugs, gastrectomy, or endocrine and other disorders).

   In the presence of calcification in thoracic intervertebral discs, it is probably wise to use manual techniques prudently, especially at the middle and lower thoracic segments.
5. Inflammatory arthritis (e.g. rheumatoid arthritis, ankylosing spondylitis, septic arthritis).

   Manipulative thrust techniques should not be used in the presence of gout.
6. Physical involvement of the central nervous system (e.g. cord pressure *signs* in limbs, cauda equina lesions, neurological diseases such as transverse myelitis).

   An example is a positive Lhermitte's sign, i.e. shooting paraesthesiae in the limb on sudden flexion of the neck. It is seen in disease of the cervical spinal cord, disseminated sclerosis and other demyelinating conditions.
7. Cervical and thoracic joint conditions producing neurological *symptoms* in one or both lower limbs
8. Evidence of involvement of more than one spinal nerve root on one side, or more than two adjacent roots in one lower limb only
9. Advanced diabetes, when tissue vitality may be low
10. Vascular abnormalities (vertebral artery involvement, visceral arterial disease)
11. Congenital generalised hypermobility (Ehlers–Danlos syndrome)
12. Advanced degenerative changes
13. Severe root pain
14. Undiagnosed pain
15. Painful vertebral joint conditions, psychologically reinforced, where manual treatment or manipulation runs the risk of producing an obsessional neurosis of vertebral displacement
16. Warfarin sodium anticoagulant medication.

Further, there are certain clinical factors, confirmation of which is often elicited during examination by palpation, which *preclude manipulation* and these are:

1. Acquired hypermobility or instability at the segment involved

2. When joint irritability and painful movement are manifest
3. The presence of spasm which is protecting the segment being treated
4. When segments *adjacent* to the main joint problem are either irritable, or hypermobile, and stresses applied by the positioning for manipulation would aggravate them
5. Inability of the patient to relax
6. When the operator senses that the joint will not give— this is felt as a rubbery resistance to the final movement, and must in all circumstances be respected.

Pregnancy: A considerately performed manipulation to the cervical or upper thoracic spine may be indicated and necessary, but after the fourth month vigorous rotatory stress should not be applied to the thoracolumbar spine; manipulation should not be employed at *any* time if there is known possibility of miscarriage. Techniques of compression are probably best avoided in the later stages of pregnancy.

MOBILISATION

A consideration of contraindications to mobilisation must include a review of the *purpose* of treatment.

For example, it is known that repetitive small-amplitude movements, applied rhythmically to joints, have an inhibitory effect on afferent impulse traffic from articular receptors subserving pain, and thus the purpose of treatment can be *to relieve pain*, e.g. the pain arising from a hypermobile segment, by the use of gentle mobilisation techniques. In this example there can be no intention to stretch tight tissues, break adhesions, restore displaced material or increase the range of movement.

Similarly, careful mobilisation guided by assessment can be of value for the pain associated with frank neurological signs in the territory of one root on one side. There can be no intention to try to reverse the serial tissue changes culminating in the neurological deficit, only to *relieve the symptoms of it*, and thereby minimise the degree of functional disablement.

Absolute contraindications to mobilisation are:

1. Malignancy involving the vertebral column
2. Cauda equina lesions producing disturbance of bladder and/or bowel function
3. Signs and symptoms of:
   a. spinal cord involvement
   b. involvement of more than one spinal nerve root on one side, or two adjacent roots in one lower limb only
4. Rheumatoid collagen necrosis of vertebral ligaments; the cervical spine is especially vulnerable
5. Active inflammatory and infective arthritis
6. Bone disease of the spine (if no more than a simple osteoporosis of ageing, see below).

The *rules of procedure* should be followed at all times:

a. Careful examination, including the mandatory questions
b. Economy of vigour in technique
c. Treatment guided by assessment and reassessment throughout
d. Discontinuing treatment which begins to produce deterioration in the signs and symptoms.

CARE is necessary in the following situations:

1. *The presence of neurological signs.* While following the rules of procedure, it is important to avoid treatment procedures which reduce the dimensions of intervertebral foramina on the side of the painful limb.

2. *Rheumatoid arthritis.* When prescribed, gentle mobilisation treatment can help the patient, provided:

a. there is no acute inflammation
b. the cervical spine is avoided and the dangers of ligamentous changes and the depletion of bone structure (especially the ribs) are borne in mind.

3. *Osteoporosis.* The condition may be due to one or more of several causes. A loss of approximately 40 per cent of bone salts must occur before osteoporosis becomes radiologically evident, and the ribs are especially vulnerable. Pressure techniques must be used with care.

4. *Spondylolisthesis.* This condition is often symptomless and unknown to the patient. If pain is arising from the affected segment, gentle mobilising can be helpful in reducing pain, but pressure techniques with a degree of energy are contraindicated. The pain may be caused by soft-tissue changes of *adjacent* segments, and in these cases any technique found to be effective in helping symptoms may be carefully used, while mindful of the possibly unstable segment.

5. *Hypermobility* has been discussed above.

6. *Pregnancy.* It is difficult to generalise, but the considerate and moderate use of pressure techniques is possible up to the sixth month and rotations of small amplitude up to the eighth month.

7. *Dizziness* which is produced or aggravated by neck rotation contraindicates the free use of rotation techniques in treatment, but does not preclude careful pressure techniques and traction.

8. *Previous malignant disease* in other than spinal tissues need not contraindicate mobilisation for spinal joint problems so long as the possibility of metastases can reasonably be excluded and treatment is prudent.

TRACTION

Contraindications to cervical traction

NB: Care should be exercised in treating patients who obtain dramatic relief from severe pain with the first application of traction.

1. Those with marked irritability of the temperomandibular joint(s); uncomfortable pressure may be avoided by using a frontal/occipital harness[791] in place of the more usual mandibular/occipital harness. The edentulous patient is often more comfortable with a gauze pad between dentures, or with a thicker pad replacing the denture.
2. Marked ligamentous insufficiency, and segmental instability.
3. Patients who are dizzy, nauseated and sick after the first careful attempt(s).
4. Patients who are unable to relax.

Conditions like neoplasms, active inflammatory arthritis, *rheumatoid erosions and instability*, etc. are not discussed, because the question of traction should not arise.

NB: Without confirmation of rationale with the prescribing physician, spondylotic *cervical myelopathy* is a contraindication.

Contraindications to thoracic traction

Coexisting conditions may rule out:

1. The patient's position, and
2. The pressure of a snugly applied harness, with further pressure as tension is applied. Similarly, pregnancy may rule out harness pressure.

Effective traction may be difficult in:

1. Orthopnoea for any reason
2. Asthma and other forms of respiratory distress
3. Hiatus hernia

4. Recent thoracic and abdominal surgery
5. Old thoracoplasty.

Segmental hypermobility or instability generally contraindicate traction, unless the therapist is able to restrict longitudinal movement to less than the normal of this accessory range. This careful technique is occasionally used for the relief of pain, but is much better done manually.

Thoracic joint problems producing *neurological symptoms and signs in one or both lower limbs are an absolute contraindication*.

Contraindications to lumbar traction

Effective traction may be ruled out by coexisting conditions, e.g. pregnancy. Traction is used effectively for acute conditions of sudden onset in the cervical spine, applied in the line of painful deviation until a normal attitude is possible, but it is unwise to use traction for pain of sudden onset in the lumbar spine (acute lumbago) without a very cautious and short initial trial to test the patient's reactions. The patient whose severe back pain is dramatically relieved with the first gentle pull should have the tension smoothly lessened without delay, otherwise a very severe pain reaction will occur.

1. Recent onset of severe lumbar pain
2. Hypermobility or instability of lumbar segments
3. Undiagnosed pain.

Generally, hypermobility or instability of a segment contraindicate traction, but it may be prescribed, together with abdominal strengthening exercises, for spondylolisthesis, for example.

16. Supports and appliances and adjunct physiotherapy treatments

SUPPORTS AND APPLIANCES

In the treatment of common spinal joint conditions, the most frequently employed supports or appliances are probably cervical collars, lumbosacral corsets, sacral belts and unilateral heel lifts. Thoracic supports are less frequently needed.

CERVICAL COLLARS

At times, these can tend to be a substitute for treatment, in the sense that a minority of workers appear to hold, albeit unwittingly, that cervical spondylosis means pain within half-a-mile of the neck and that the treatment is a collar.

The therapeutic possibilities which might be revealed by comprehensive clinical examination, with consequent procedures precisely based on the findings, are sadly not investigated on every occasion. This regrettable situation is not often engendered by sloth, but more frequently by lack of time and the pressing flood of patients needing attention. The therapist might well echo the death-bed words of Cecil Rhodes: 'So little done, so much to do.'[996]

A perfectly fit but somewhat biddable patient, recently encountered by the author, had been continuously wearing a collar for a period of well over four years. She had been treated for various periods in that time, but was still suffering chronic neck and upper limb pains, worse on the right. The collar had from time to time been renewed, and this itself had convinced her of her dire need for it. A combination of localised mobilisation, cervical traction and isometric strengthening exercises relieved her of all of her symptoms, and dispensed with the need for support.

The important lesson here is that a fixed idea of spinal inadequacy or insufficiency is profoundly disabling, and very seldom justified; one would not lightly take on the responsibility for inducing such a state of mind in a fit individual.

Four sound working rules may be suggested at once:

1. Never supply a cervical support without a plan to eliminate it
2. Never supply *any* cervical support which has not been individually tailored for the person who is to wear it
3. Use easily disposable materials; preferably homogeneous and with a natural resilience
4. If a collar is not completely comfortable and does not soon provide a measure of relief, there is something wrong with it.

Rule 4 needs a little qualification in that a collar, of itself, does not always provide significant and *speedy* relief of severe cervical root pain, for example, but the rule none the less expresses an important principle.

Support, and thus rest, in a neutral position of comfort is usually the rationale for giving a collar, and unless the patient has a dangerously unstable neck because of rheumatoid collagen necrosis of ligaments, is in danger of serious vertebrobasilar ischaemia on movement, or for some other reason needs a semipermanent support, there is not often the necessity to keep the head virtually rigid on the neck or the neck in a virtually fixed relationship with the trunk. When this kind of stabilisation *is* indicated, hospital appliance departments and commercial appliance makers manufacture excellent supports from appropriately rigid materials, but this type of semipermanent appliance is not being considered here.

Although a somewhat firm collar is sometimes essential to stabilise temporarily unstable segments, cervical pain is frequently aggravated and unnecessarily prolonged by unyielding and badly fitting plastic collars, particularly of the type commonly available in outpatient departments. These appliances, often dispensed off-the-peg to an approximate fit by ancillary staff, purport to be adaptable by reason of anterior velcro surfaces which allow modification of the depth of the collar. The upper and lower edges are cut to an arbitrary pattern which is completely comfortable for very few, and the provision of a soft turned edge does little to diminish the unsympathetic pressure of the hard plastic material. More importantly, the notion of 'support in neutral' appears to be equated with the military posture of attention, and an unnecessarily high proportion of the collars given in this fashion push the neck into a degree of extension which becomes steadily more wearisome and painful as the hours pass. A salutory experience is to have one of these appliances fitted to one's self in a position of slight extension and to keep it on for three to six hours.

The cumulative effects of prolonged extension have been recognised, in that the use of bifocal spectacles can easily provoke a cervical radiculopathy where none existed.[614]

Again, the continuous pressure of a semirigid edge against the painfully sensitive suboccipital structures is hard for patients to bear, and when any support calls forth the need for a stiff upper lip to bear the pain of its presence, treatment has tended to degenerate into little other than an exercise in improving the patient's character.

Another approach to the matter of cervical support appears to rest on the hypothesis: 'Since the pain is at the back of the neck, that's where the support should be'; consequently the collar is formed with its greatest depth at the back. A very frequent unsolicited observation by patients is: 'My head feels so heavy, it seems so tiring to hold up', and the insistent posterior pressure of resilient material is not likely to be welcomed.

While it is feasible to satisfactorily fit most patients with a temporary elasticised lumbosacral support by making available a suitably wide variety of sizes (which are paired by incorporating the slightly differing structural needs of the sexes), attempts to supply cervical collars on the basis of a range of sizes are probably a mistake, unless they are constructed of some homogeneous material which combines flexibility with resilience and some resistance to buckling on vertical compression. While the single desirable factor which is thus common to both cervical and lumbosacral supports is *flexibility with resilience, and some resistance to vertical compression* (perhaps rather clumsily described as 'an artificially living substance'), the function of the two appliances (for common vertebral joint problems and in the normal postures of living) are basically

different: (1) the purpose of a cervical support is to gently but firmly *resist upwards* around its whole circumference; (2) the purpose of a lumbosacral support is to *squeeze centripetally* inwards.

There remain the vital factors of individual configuration of the mandible, length of the mandible, shape and length of the neck and weight of the head; the variety and permutations of these is probably not far short of the variety of fingerprints. Hence the importance of rule 2 (above).

Materials: While such materials as folded newspapers (the *Financial Times* is said to be more effective than the *Daily Telegraph*), orthopaedic felt strengthened by plastic struts and hard plastic sheeting may give support, it is not possible to give truly *comfortable* support combined with a degree of resilience, in this way. The desirable qualities of material have been mentioned and these might be met by double layers of one-quarter inch Evazote, or one-half to three-quarters inch sponge rubber. These materials can quickly be cut and shaped, and thus rapidly adapted to their proper purpose, that of comfortably fitting the patient for whom they are intended.

(i) *Evazote*. The inner layer should be one inch proud of the outer layer, and darted so that after heating in the oven provided, it may be folded down (and up) over the inner layer to provide a soft rounded edge *which conforms to the patient's structural idiosyncrasies, since it has been moulded to them*

(ii) *Latex sponge rubber*. Sheets of this material are available, and as the preliminary, a slightly larger outline than would fit the patient is cut to this outline (Fig. 16.1).

By trimming length, width and degree of curvature, the shape is successively modified until it satisfies the main criteria, i.e. gives support, fits comfortably, will not painfully press on sensitive suboccipital tissues, allows a modicum of movement.

While the collar is experimentally held in position by the therapist's cupped hands, the patient moves the head and neck slightly in all directions, reporting any obtrusive edges or lack of support in any part of the collar's circumference.

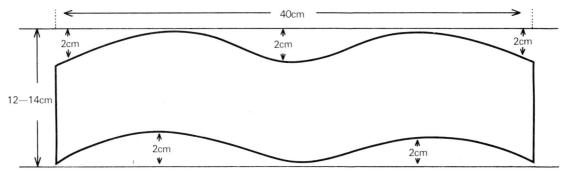

Fig. 16.1   An overlarge pattern for cervical collars. The material (see text) should be trimmed so that it is individually tailored for the person who is to wear it.

The one-quarter inch Evazote and more particularly the one-half to three-quarter inch latex sponge rubber will require binding with a light tubular bandage, and while the Evazote will have sufficient resistance to buckling to need only a method of securing it, the latex sponge rubber requires an additional stiffener in the form of a variable number of turns of tubular bandage around its circumference.

An important factor is the *degree* of stiffening—the soft night collar for reducing sleeping stress is insufficient for absorbing the stress of daily activities, and ideally the patient needs a range of supports which are suitable for some *three* demands: sleeping; working (head down a bit); social activities (head up a bit). One could provide three collars, but this is a somewhat grandiose solution to the problem. The attraction of the sponge-rubber-and-tubular-bandage system is that fewer turns of bandage reduce the degree of resilient resistance and more turns of bandage increase it. The patient chooses and modifies according to changing need, and the only disadvantage is that of uncomfortable warmth in summer. This can be an inducement to use it only when needed, but if a continuous support *is* necessary and uncomfortable warmth is a problem it is probably better to make a thicker Plastazote collar with anterolateral 'windows' for ventilation. Ladies sometimes need reminding of how *interesting* a temporary collar, cleverly concealed by the right piece of silk scarf, can be!

The *indications* for a cervical support, of the kind being described, are:

1. To reduce provocation, by movement, of pain from an irritable cervical nerve root.
2. To settle severely sore, localised cervical joint problems which are being aggravated by mechanical stress.
3. To help support the weight of the head during occupations which necessitate bending the neck for long periods.
4. To prevent jarring of a susceptible cervical or upper thoracic segment when driving continuously in town traffic.
5. To prevent sleeping stress when this is a factor in regularly provoking cervical migraine.
6. In cases of pain from a chronic poking-chin deformity, to hold up the head until pain, muscle imbalance/weakness and soft-tissue contracture have been overcome.

Root pain in the upper limb may be severe enough to warrant a light arm sling, as well as a cervical collar, when the patient is upright.

Cervical joint irritability requires a light and slightly resilient support, which may be needed day and night for some days, or only at night. As in low back problems, measures to improve sleeping posture and avoid stress on joints can be helpful, allowing better rest and reducing the amount of pain and stiffness felt on first rising in the morning. Painful stiffness in the morning may also be reduced by applying a rolled handtowel lightly around the neck, and/or making a butterfly- or bow-tie-pillow to provide neck support and prevent extreme neck positions during sleep. Down-filled pillows are more suitable than those filled with rubber-foam material, the latter tending to resist comfortable indentation by body contours.

Patients wearing collars all day should be warned to be careful when driving a car, moving about a darkened room,[715] using intricate machinery requiring manual dexterity.[1364]

Relative immobility of the upper three cervical segments, together with a lessening of normal compression by the weight of the head, disturbs the pattern of afferent volleys of impulses from mechanoreceptors of these joints; the patient is usually unaware of the transient defects of postural control and upper-limb co-ordination, and for a few days extra care is wise, until a degree of accommodation to the novel situation occurs.

Lee and Lishman (1975)[715] have observed that *vision* is very important in the control of equilibration, and that visual reference (to the verticals and horizontals of one's daily environment) acquired early in life help to train the fine and efficient adjustments of proprioceptive mechanisms for the maintenance of difficult postures and the smooth performances of movement. Later in life, proprioceptive *defects*, which are a sequel to degeneration of joints and the disturbance of mechanoreceptor afferent impulse traffic, can be compensated for, and masked, by vision. If both vision and proprioception are denied by the circumstance of wearing a cervical support and being in the dark, the patient can be in a parlous state.

Wyke (1965)[1364] has unequivocally demonstrated the importance of cervical mechanoreceptors in governing the degree of dexterity in performing intricate manual operations. Co-ordination and equilibratory impulses to all limb muscles are disturbed for a day or two until the patient gets used to the collar.

It would be most interesting to record the changes in muscular activity when driving a car (or, for that matter, piloting a light aeroplane or a mechanical digger). The proprioceptive circumstance is quite singular, with body supported on the backside, the thoracic and lumbar spine curved forward and the neck flexed but the head relatively extended. Since the feet are pushing and releasing pedals, the most constant proprioceptive influence, apart from the behind, is probably from the joints of the hands, gripping a steering wheel or control column. Added to this the whole body is, together with the vehicle, being jogged up and down and from side to side, and fore and aft—it is small wonder that prolonged driving provokes cervical joint problems. The situation is akin to the stress applied to the visual and equilibratory apparatus in trying to read a newspaper while sitting sideways in one of the old London tramcars.[635]

Thoracic pain due to advanced degenerative changes may justify a light general trunk support, but these require much careful fitting and modifying before acceptance by patients, and they may be a short-sighted measure if there is only mild osteoporosis since the condition is further aggravated by reducing normal physiological stress on bone. Shoulder straps are not a good thing—it is better to make a whole polythene jacket—high up to the sternum and over the bust in front, with the back cut well down below the scapulae.

LUMBOSACRAL SUPPORTS

The variety of lumbosacral supports, which range from a light and flexible 'cummerbund' to formidable constructions of steel-braced canvas with many straps, seems matched only by the variety of views of the indications and rationale for their use, and conversely, arguments against their use.

In a survey of the use of external support in the treatment of low back pain, Perry (1970)[987] found that the literature described more than 30 different designs, and by now the number existing must surely exceed this.

If we immediately recognise the factor of a powerful placebo ('that which pleases') effect upon some, of something being given by an omnipotent healer-physician, as an 'encloser', 'supporter', 'warmer', 'protector' and 'identifier' of the injured part, in precisely the same way as a child may regard the bandage (the badge) applied to a cut finger, then having nodded to this factor it may be put to one side; yet not before we also recognise an equally powerful one, i.e. the marked distaste with which many regard *anything* which might draw attention to their functional difficulties. Perhaps we should also recognise that these two standpoints, including the notion that supports weaken the muscles underlie much of the sometimes thinly rationalised argument for and against supports.

When the physician, surgeon, physiotherapist, osteopath or chiropractor flatly asserts: 'It is against my principles to use corsets for back problems because ... (and here follows this or that contention)', one recognises yet again how a philosophy of therapeutics has imperceptibly hardened to the stage of becoming more important than what therapy is *about*, i.e. the infinitely variable needs of patients.

'The prescription of corsets for all and sundry backaches, without proper indications and proper diagnosis, is retrograde and slipshod. It leads to unnecessary expense, unnecessary discomfort, and unnecessary invalidism in many cases. On the other hand, extremists in the reverse direction who condemn all corsets to the waste-paper basket are also making a mistake' (Stoddard, 1969).[1180b]

The widespread and sensible use of many varieties of protective clothing and appliances in industry, the building trades and in sport seems not to engender fears that the part which is supported may be weakened. It is quite extraordinary to observe athletic men, who will be almost obsessive about wearing a supportive wriststrap for an important tennis match, a supportive jockstrap and a protective gumshield for a professional fight, a protective 'box' when defending their wickets against fast bowlers, a scrumcap for rugger and shinpads when playing football and cricket, yet who will show a marked distaste and great reluctance when a lumbosacral support, as a protection against lumbar stress, might be indicated as a transient necessity in the treatment of their painful low back problem.

The enthusiastic amateur footballer who also looks after a demanding garden, and may drive many hundreds of miles weekly in the course of his occupation as an agricultural representative, is not at all keen on the suggestion that a temporary corset, for use only when gardening and driving, may considerably aid the speedy resolution of his back problem.

At times, one cannot help detecting an undercurrent of unexpressed and sometimes unrecognised anxiety—'it might do me a serious mischief—interfere with my muscles (my virility), make me weak (impotent), make me reliant upon it (weaken my natural defences)', and really these are not altogether unreasonable responses. Plainly, suggestions that the region adjacent to the pelvis may need a 'crutch' for a little while, and for part of the day, arouse much greater anxiety in some than similar advice regarding a body part far removed from it, i.e. the neck. That the lumbosacral region differs functionally and structurally from the cervical spine does not invalidate this proposition.

Recent research findings provide the information that wearing a lumbar support, for periods of up to five years, does not 'weaken the muscles'.[887]

The effects of lumbar supports on trunk musculature are that there is no effect during standing and slow walking, but during fast walking the support actually *increased* muscle activity.[1290]

Overall, activity of the sacrospinalis muscle, recorded by e.m.g., is affected very little by the wearing of a corset or brace, although activity of the abdominal musculature is decreased during the time the appliance is worn. Yet over five years the muscles are not weakened. A tight and embracing lumbar support reduces the intradiscal pressure by about 30 per cent[883] and it has been demonstrated how a raised intrathoracic and intra-abdominal pressure decreases the load on lumbar discs.

Reduction by intradiscal pressure is accompanied by reduction or modification of gravitational and functional stress on all *other* lumbar structures, of course; while the pressure in vertebral venous plexuses is possibly raised to a degree.

Thus, the effects of corsets and supports appear due

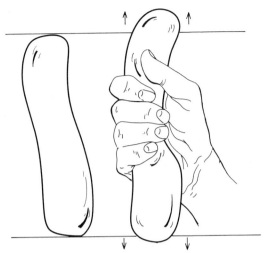

Fig. 16.2 A tubular balloon will increase its length as the middle is constricted.

largely to compression of the abdomen, with a consequent decrease of load upon the vertebral column itself (see Fig. 16.2). These findings corroborate the value of *abdominal strengthening exercises* in the treatment of low back pain. Lumbar supports do not 'immobilise' the lumbar spine; to do this completely, a double-hip plaster-of-Paris spica, extending from just above the knees to the upper thoracic vertebrae, or a plaster bed would be necessary.

Van Leuven and Troup (1969)[1265] unequivocally demonstrated that the range of sagittal movement was virtually the same whether the healthy symptom-free subject was wearing an 'Instant' corset, a tailored lumbar corset or no support at all! While the fearsome strap-and-buckle, canvas and metal-framed type of support may make some movements *uncomfortable*, it does little to *prevent* them.

By the insertion of Kirschner wires into the lumbar spinous processes of normal subjects, Norton and Brown (1957)[939] observed that commonly used low back braces, and plaster-of-Paris jackets, failed to limit lumbar movement. The brace actually appeared to *increase* lumbosacral movement by restricting motion in the rest of the spine. Lumsden and Morris (1968)[769] found that lumbosacral rotation was only slightly restricted by corsets and braces.

There is now the question: What are the stays for? The provision of these ranges from a pair of light, flexible paravertebral inserts posteriorly, to a virtually rigid, rectangular metal framework at the back and a pair of equally formidable anterior steels ('to stop the patient bending forward') together with at least three and often more straps and buckles to bind the assorted ironmongery and the patient into an uncomfortable whole.

Cailliet (1977)[151] makes the surprising observation that the stays must never be bent to conform to the back, but that the back should conform to the stays. Further, that the appliance should have a small curve caudally to conform to the buttock, because 'this ensures comfort and in general a more desirable posture and appearance'.

The notion that lumbar supports restrict motion of the spine is plainly fallacious, and it may be that *the sole function of the corset is to raise the intra-abdominal pressure and thereby reduce, by something approaching one-third, the load sustained by the lumbar discs.* If at the same time it acts as a placebo, keeps the patient warm, acts as a reminder, improves the patient's silhouette and confers other fringe benefits, this is all to the good, but they remain fringe benefits. The real function of the stays, which function just as effectively if made of the lightest metal or plastic strips, is to prevent buckling and folding of the elasticised material doing the main job, which is that of raising the intra-abdominal pressure. The 'navvy' of times past did not wear a leather belt just to keep his trousers up, since this function was usually performed by braces. 'The most important component of a spinal brace is the abdominal binder',[780] and the rigid steel supports, especially anterior or anterolateral ones, are a waste of mineral resources and an unnecessary addition, doing little more than producing discomfort and alienating many patients who would otherwise cheerfully accept the temporary need for an efficient and light 'cummerbund'.

Constructional details

Thompson (1969)[1214] describes in three short paragraphs a simple temporary lumbosacral support which is within the reach of the smallest physiotherapy department, and consists only of Tubigrip and adhesive Moleform; it can successfully be washed.

If a support has been made by an appliance department it must be fitted, and thus the posterior steels (if there be such) need to be shaped to the patient *by the prescriber* after the appliance makers have completed it. *Detachable steels are desirable* for bending to fit—the corset should be wrapped around the patient in standing, and the top of the corset marked on the skin. The steels should be removed and bent to the patient's shape. They should not be pushed too far into a great lordosis in standing, for when the patient sits the lordosis disappears and the corset is pushed backwards. STEELS SHOULD BE BENT TO FIT THE PATIENT'S WORKING POSTURE.

The corset must have sufficient 'waisting' (flare) top and bottom to suit the patient with regard to sex differences, i.e.:

Men —'V' torso, small hips, big gluteii
—corset does not tend to move up as women's do. Straps between legs are not necessary if it fits well

Women—'Parallel' torso, bulging hips, small gluteii
—corset does tend to move up. Needs a longer 'skirt' for them to sit on and keep it down; suspenders for stockings are not enough.

Alternatively, the 'Instant' type of elasticated support with a single Velcro fastening may be worn with the single encircling belt in the lower of the two loops provided, thus gripping the patient below the iliac crests rather than above them.

Perry's review[987] (*vide supra*) mentions the following clinical situations in which one or other variety of support was indicated:

—postoperative fusion
—spondylolisthesis
—pseudoarthrosis
—preoperative trial
—disc syndrome
—chronic pain
—obesity and pain
—acute strain.

Plainly, it is the prerogative of the orthopaedic surgeon to decide whether a support is indicated in conjunction with surgical procedures, and to prescribe the type of support to be supplied; again, the indications for stabilisation, in a proportion of the cases not considered for surgery, may require the prescription of supports of a particular type. Yet this number is very greatly exceeded by those who need support for a limited period, and who benefit most from its provision without delay.

So far as the *provision* of lumbosacral supports is concerned, the interval between recognition of need and meeting the need has now become unacceptably long. With the unabating flood of patients referred for conservative treatment to hospital physiotherapy departments from many sources in a region, it follows that experienced therapists, in those departments which have a section specialising in handling musculoskeletal problems, would have the wit to know when the immediate provision of a simple and temporary support is indicated. Thus an ample supply of a range of supports for both sexes would have a markedly higher cost-effectiveness than the provision of two new short-wave diathermy machines.

Like justice itself, the wheels of appliance-supply, in too many hospitals, grind exceeding slow, and too many therapists have too often experienced a wistful confrontation with the facts of life, i.e. 'this patient doesn't need a corset in six to eight weeks—it is needed *now*'. Bearing in mind the important rule, 'never supply a support without a plan to eliminate it',[987] *the indications for support are* segmental hypermobility, or insufficiency, of which there can be many forms,[1093] e.g.

a. Insufficiency may be due to advanced regional degenerative change in mature patients, where severe chronic spondylosis and arthrosis have markedly increased vulnerability to stress
b. Hypermobility may be due to a single lifting stress in a young nurse, or to grade III spondylolisthesis at L4–L5 in a mature woman
c. Recurrent attacks of lumbar articular derangement, where exacerbations are related to trivial occupational stresses
d. That type of time-dependent lumbar pain which regularly and steadily worsens during the day after a pain-free morning
e. Temporary social and occupational demands, e.g. where a patient *has* to attend a wedding, or other unavoidable engagement; the harvest will not wait for the farmer's acute back pain to subside.

It follows that improving the strength of the trunk musculature (p. 452) and ergonomic guidance (p. 500) are the methods of dispensing with the need for support and that its provision can only be a part of treatment, usually a secondary part.

As cervical collars and some types of cervical traction harness may painfully press on very tender soft tissues, so may a lumbar corset press upon a tender haunch and be difficult for the patient to bear. When support is imperative, this tenderness can be overcome by a vapocoolant spray over the tender region and/or by the interposition of plastic foam sheeting.

Plaster-of-Paris jackets

Like lumbar traction and other treatments beginning to acquire some antiquity, an assessment of the purpose and value of plaster jackets should include a appraisal of why they came into vogue in the first place. This is because old treatments are often adapted to be used more successfully in different ways for different reasons; while they are less often used nowadays, the rationale for applying a plaster jacket in the treatment of acute back pain seems not to have changed much in the last three to four decades, i.e.

—literally to hold the patient up, if such is the patient's need
—to provide local rest by 'immobilisation'
—to allow acute lumbar joint irritability, and acute pain, to settle down
—to attempt the straightening of lateral spinal deviation of recent onset.

In some cases these aims were achieved; in many they were not, the net result of some four to six weeks in a jacket amounting to little more than having been decidedly uncomfortable for that time, having carted around a few extra kilograms and having had one's choice of wardrobe somewhat restricted.

If the patient is not undoubtedly improved, i.e. definitely less restricted by pain within five to eight days, there is no point in subjection to the further inconvenience of wearing it; the simple passage of time has probably conferred a better likelihood of success with alternative treatments of mobilisation, manual deviation-correction and traction. If the patient *is* improved, the jacket can be removed anyway, and an elasticised lumbosacral support and/or other treatment substituted.

Application: The plaster jacket must be a good, close fit, and should be quickly applied by an experienced technician who is adept at protecting bony points and avoiding a thick rim of plaster under the axillae. This type of plaster cast should never be applied by the enthusiastic amateur.

Because of the need to avoid fixing the lumbar spine in a lordosed position, the patient should stand with the hips and knees a little flexed, and the pelvis tilted a little backward; by slight hip and knee flexion most patients quickly get the idea of a backward pelvic tilt and can hold the position for long enough, even when in pain. It is for this reason that all the materials required, including measurement and preparation of the front and back 15 or 20 cm wide 'slabs', should be made ready and close to hand, so that no time is lost.

The arms must not be above the head and there is no point in applying the jacket 'under slight traction', i.e. with the patient grasping a bar above the head. This throws the lumbar spine into lordosis, and in any case, it is doubtful whether any degree of spinal elongation remains when the arms are lowered.

After an inner lining vest of stockinette is applied, the patient's hands may be clasped lightly behind the neck, with the elbows allowed to fall together anteriorly; if this position is hard for the mature patient to maintain, the arms may be supported in some abduction by canvas slings suspended from a ceiling hook or light suspension bar.

Anteriorly, the plaster should extend from upper pubic region to the manubrium, by rounded tongues which are graduated laterally, and posteriorly from the midsacral level to just below the inferior angles of the scapulae (Fig. 16.3). A degree of abdominal compression is important; the jacket must leave no room anteriorly.

Front and back strengthening 'slabs' are incorporated between the encircling turns; some use diagonal slabs also. Before the patient is allowed to go his freedom to sit without uncomfortable groin pressure is confirmed; if this is not possible the plaster must be modified.

It is kinder to patients, and better for the jacket, to give a light dusting of talcum powder over the whole exterior surface, so that it becomes incorporated with the drying plaster and leaves a smoother external coat. Patients should be warned not to scratch itches by poking pencils, etc., between plaster and skin, since they easily become irretrievable and may necessitate removal of the jacket.

SACROILIAC SUPPORTS

A mild degree of hypermobility of one sacroiliac joint, in the absence of severe trauma to the pelvis, can cause nagging, wearisome and intractable symptoms, and is much commoner than seems supposed.

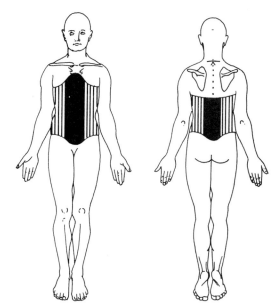

Fig. 16.3 Plaster of Paris jacket. The patient must be able to sit comfortably.

The presence of painful clicking or crepitus when standing on one leg, or radiographic evidence of a vertical pubic shift on changing from one leg to the other, allow easy recognition of gross hypermobility, but it is not until careful palpation tests are made that mild hypermobility, also, can be recognised for what it is, and appropriate treatment given. To require, among other signs, the evidence of a Trendelenburg 'lurch' when walking, before reaching a diagnosis of sacroiliac strain, is to place the requirement much too high.

After repetitive athletic or other stress to the pelvic joints, and after recent pregnancy, a painful and mildly lax joint may need external support; there seems a preoccupation with strap-and-buckle appliances when the degree of support need not always resemble the securing of a cabin trunk. As some cervical collars do need to provide firm support, but most need not be quite so restrictive, so the measure of support for the pelvic joint is a matter of degree, and this requires assessment. A low 'cummerbund' of 15 cm crepe or rayon elastic bandage, or an old girdle or roll-on folded into three and sewn inside a new roll-on, or even a firm roll-on itself, are often quite sufficient to give the degree of temporary support needed, and for sacroiliac joint irritability to settle. Some may prefer a rayon elastic bandage kept in place by a light girdle; this may suit the plump patient.

Not a few patients with sacroiliac joint hypermobility *also* have a lumbar joint problem; there should be no difficulty in accepting the simple proposition that repetitive occupational stress, a vigorous athletic effort or a losing of one's footing when pushing a car, may affect both lumbar spine *and* one or other of the pelvic joints, particularly when torsion figures largely in the stress; thus a patient may need some temporary support for both low back and pelvis, and in these cases the 'Instant' type of corset, with the light belt threaded through the lower of the two loops, is a useful measure.

Recurrent irritability of the sacroiliac joint, as a consequence of hypermobility, may need treatment by injection of a sclerosant solution.[58] Gross hypermobility will necessitate a tailor-made support of considerable firmness, and if this measure does not succeed surgical arthrodesis may be necessary.

CORRECTION OF LATERAL PELVIC TILT

While considerations of deformity and its consequences must take into account many factors, a congenitally short leg, producing lateral pelvic tilt, can be the cause of backache and sciatica (p. 264 and 270); clinical experience indicates that thoracic and cervical joint problems, in some, can also be an indirect consequence of lateral pelvic tilt.

Bearing in mind that a short leg[1180a] or pelvic joint asymmetry *need* not disturb the horizontal alignment of the iliac crests, or cause a scoliosis,[736] and also that lateral deviation of the spine can be due to an uneven upper sacral surface and/or a trapezoidal-shaped 5th lumbar vertebral body (see Figs 1.28–1.30), it is wise to closely consider the factor of lateral pelvic tilt whenever dealing with common vertebral joint conditions (p. 310). This does not mean to say that correction of a tilt by a heel-lift is a 'hole-in-one' therapeutic measure, only that if this factor is not considered among very many others, the items for assessment are incomplete.

Reach-me-down concepts of the causes of backache, and similar approaches to conservative treatment, are no longer enough. The gambit of assessing pelvic levels in standing, and then in sitting erect on a hard level surface, often tells the experienced practitioner much more than 'scientific' mensuration with a tape-measure, which so often employs bony points which are topographical 'districts' rather than distinct eminences. It is a matter of assessment, and erect X-ray films are an advantage, since they can reveal disconcerting bony anomalies, and also scolioses and rotations which sometimes defy analysis.

In general terms, segmental abnormalities of *position* are much less important than abnormalities of *movement*, but the marked exception to this rule is that of the pelvis, where the order of precedence is reversed.[1180a] Leg length discrepancies of one-quarter inch are common, and much greater differences in leg length can be present without apparently causing symptoms, because adaptation by the soft tissues during the adolescent growth spurt has probably been sufficient to compensate for the discrepancy. The cost of this compensation, in many, appears to be a reduced ability to withstand the stresses of ordinary activities; backaches of insidious onset in adults, without apparent cause and without much movement-limitation (although some movements may be painful), are very fre-

quently the clinical features of this failure of compensation.

A very experienced clinician (Stoddard, 1969)[1180b] has observed:

The cumulative effect of one-quarter inch of leg shortening over many years is considerable, and this is a proven aetiological factor in backache of ligamentous origin as well as in pathological conditions of the disc. ... Nature appears to make more effort to compensate for gross structural faults than for minor ones ... many patients with over one inch of shortening are thoroughly compensated and symptom free, yet with one quarter inch of shortening other patients suffer from backache which can only be relieved by using a quarter-inch heel cushion.

The provision of a heel lift must depend upon accurate assessment, as should its effects. A reduction of pain on back movements, when retesting them with small raises underfoot on the short leg side, clarifies the nature of the problem, but assessment is not complete in under two to three weeks.

Side-flexion is usually freer to the side of the short leg, and the patient may deviate to that side on flexion. It is not wise to raise the height of a shoe if side-flexion of the trunk to that side is painful *early* in the range of movement.

As an example, let us consider two patients, one a young woman with left-sided backache and posterior thigh pain, and the other a mature man with right-sided low backache.

In both (see p. 272), the pelvis is laterally tilted upwards on the right because of a short left leg:

a. In the younger patient, with symptoms attributable to low lumbar discogenic changes on the side of the short leg, the unilateral pain is often provoked early in the range of left-side-flexion movement, and a heel lift is less likely to help; it should nevertheless be tried.

b. In the more mature patient, left-side-flexion (although the freer-range movement) is more likely to provoke the right-sided pain than is right-side-flexion, and paradoxically, a heel lift on the left shoe is much more likely to be of value, immediately reducing pain on movement and indicating that the raise should form part of the treatment; this may often need to include stretching techniques for tightened dorsal lumbosacral soft tissues, and strengthening exercises for the abdominal muscles.

If the backache is minor, and there are no signs of chronic changes or marked irritability, a *permanent* heel raise may be all that is required. The raise may be added to one heel, or removed from the heel of the longer side; a heel pad inside one shoe may be sufficient; but the use of soft or resilient material for a pad in the heel is not of much use, the repetitive pounding of multiples of some 100–150 lb (45–70 kg) of body weight soon reduces its height and effectiveness.

Women should have both heel and sole thickened if they wear high heels. In young people, the amount of raise should be a little less than the discrepancy, e.g. an assessed half-inch discrepancy should have one-quarter to three-eighths of an inch lift. In more mature patients, the amount of raise which can be tolerated may be less, yet it is surprising how effective can be a heel raise in patients over 50. Often, mobilisation of the low lumbar joints, followed by a degree of raise as a trial, is required. Patients with a well-compensated leg length discrepancy may have little pain when standing, but a lumbar ache when sitting for long, since the ischii are then bearing weight and a level pelvis is, for them, a strained position. A small flat pillow as a unilateral buttock raise will help.

It should not be overlooked that leg length inequality can produce sacroiliac joint problems as well as lumbar problems (see p. 282), and thus treatment priorities must reflect the detailed findings on examination and assessment.

There is no point in relying entirely on a heel raise in those patients, with pain of fairly recent origin, who maintain a similar degree of lateral pelvic tilt in both the standing and sitting positions; plainly a comprehensive examination of the pelvic joints is the first step.

At times, the effects of a heel raise may defy analysis, in that they can be directly opposite to what is reasonably expected.

For example, a 55-year-old engineer, whose hobby was racing motor-bikes, was push-starting a machine and leapt side-saddle onto the seat of the moving bike, landing on his right buttock. His immediate acute right buttock and right groin pain necessitated a week of complete bed-rest, during which any other than cautious and minimal movement provoked severe jabs of buttock pain. He was seen 14 days after the incident—the pelvis was tilted upwards on the right by some 2 cm and the right posterior superior spine was more prominent than the left, with a deeper sulcus on the right. The pelvic asymmetry appeared well established, and may have been secondary to a left ankle injury (see below).

The lumbar spine was flat, with bilateral lumbar muscle spasm. Cautious lumbar movements were considerably limited by right buttock pain as well as apprehension; flexion was the most free movement, although restricted and with the spine flattened; extension was the most limited and careful. Straight-leg-raising was left 75° and right 45°, both limited by right buttock pain. By reason of a long-past severe ankle injury, the left calf was weak and wasted and the left ankle-jerk absent but there were no other signs of neurological involvement.

All lumbar segments shared in the generalised stiffness which was apparent when testing accessory movement, with marked tenderness and thickening at the right lumbosacral level. The right sacroiliac sulcus and PSIS were also tender to palpation. Mobility testing revealed no detectable difference in sacroiliac movement between sides.

He was initially assessed as more likely to be suffering from an acute right unilateral lumbosacral segment compression insult, than a sacroiliac 'shuffling' lesion, but in the event was much improved by successive techniques, individually localised as far as is possible to both the L5–S1 segment and the right sacroiliac joint, each adding an increment of improvement.

At his second attendance, he had reached the stage of being virtually sign-and-symptom-free with the exception of a slight jab of pain over the right sacroiliac sulcus at about two-thirds of his lumbar extension range. His lateral pelvic tilt remained, and since the sacroiliac techniques had made no apparent impression on the pelvic asymmetry, the effects of a left heel raise were tried. A half-centimetre and then a one-centimetre left heel lift reduced his extension range and increased the sharpness of his jab of pain by successively greater increments, while the same two lifts under his right heel, the side of the upward pelvic tilt, did precisely the opposite.

At his third attendance, after a four days interim during which he had returned to work and had also been carrying out a simple home regime of flexion and extension exercises, his extension had improved considerably but flexion had regressed a bit in that the range was a little limited and his lumbar spine remained somewhat flat. Crossing his right leg over the left when sitting also provoked a jab over his right sacroiliac joint. For the latter reason, the technique adopted was that depicted in Figure 12.61; after three applications, he moved normally without pain and his leg crossing restriction was freed. In retrospect, he was probably more a right sacroiliac than a low back problem, and it would probably have been unhelpful to pursue the question of a heel raise.

Like the temporary provision of lumbosacral supports, the temporary use of a unilateral buttock raise when sitting is sometimes indicated.

A 36-year-old mother of children aged 10 and 12 years stoutly maintained that she had had no back problems with her two pregnancies, but had noticed over 10 years that her right hip periodically 'went out' on walking—by this she meant her prominent right haunch. She recalled no trauma of any consequence to her back.

For the last year, her right hip had not 'gone out' but over the last six months a right buttock ache had developed to a level which she was beginning to find intolerable. The ache spread outwards and downwards over the trochanter, around to the ASIS and halfway down the front of the thigh. It was 'very sore—really bad at times' and was provoked after sitting for 5–10 minutes, on crouching when gardening and when dressing in the mornings.

Standing, and lying flat with legs elevated, eased her pain. She stood with a lateral pelvic tilt upward on the right, a prominent right posterior superior iliac spine, a markedly prominent right buttock and trochanter, and her lumbar spine listed to the left. When she sat on a level surface, the pelvic tilt remained.

Her lumbar articular signs were:

—extension   √√
—left-side-flexion only half with a jab of pain right haunch
—right-side-flexion   √√
—flexion to toes but deviated to the right with a noticeable curve, and with moderate pain right buttock
—left rotation   √√
—right rotation full range but with a jab of right lumbosacral pain at extreme of range

The positive sacroiliac tests were:

—iliac approximation hurt sharply over the right sulcus
—Baer's point (q.v.) was tender on the right
—Patrische's test (q.v.) was positive on the right
—sacral apex pressure hurt at the right sulcus

Testing flexion/adduction of the right hip produced right groin pain.

Straight-leg-raising was 90°/90° and painless, and there was no neurological deficit. Apart from some thickening over the right lumbosacral joint, the lumbar spine was clear on palpation; the right sacroiliac sulcus was markedly tender.

On the first day, techniques individually localised (Figs 12.18, 12.61) to both the sacroiliac and lumbosacral joints considerably eased her pain on movement, especially left-side-flexion and rotation. The likelihood of her need for a temporary left buttock raise when sitting was manifest for three reasons; (i) marked provocation of pain on sitting but not on standing; (ii) maintenance of her lateral tilt when seated; (iii) deviation to the *right* on flexion.

These factors suggested the presence of lumbar soft-tissue contracture on the right, and at her second attendance, when she remarked, 'much better, but sitting still hurts', and her left-side-flexion, flexion and rotation pain remained improved, the techniques were repeated and she was instructed to lift her left buttock by a 1 cm raise when sitting. She was also shown a postural correction exercise for the pelvis and a sustained stretching exercise for the right lumbar soft tissues.

After 18 days, she reported that her pains had virtually gone, she had dispensed with the buttock raise within a week and had been able, without discomfort, to assist with the laying of paving slabs and to go for a 200-mile car drive. Her pelvic contour and attitude were much less marked, although still detectable.

When giving rise to pain requiring treatment, lateral pelvic tilt can be expected to be marked by asymmetrical signs, but it can give rise to perfectly symmetrical symptoms: when the tilt is slight, this circumstance can mislead the examiner.

The possibility of well-established soft-tissue changes should be borne in mind, since the pelvic tilt may be manifest in standing, sitting and lying.

A 26-year-old office worker suffered severe bilateral and equally distributed lumbar and groin pain after a hard game of squash, five weeks before being assessed on 21.2.79. He stood with an upward pelvic tilt on the left side and his lumbar spine plainly tilted to the right—he was unaware of both abnormalities (Fig. 16.4A). Notably, his pelvic tilt remained when sitting on a hard horizontal surface, and the X-ray (Fig. 16.4B) revealed its presence when the patient was lying supine. Careful comparison of the two a-p views of the patient in standing erect (Fig. 16.4C) and lying supine (Fig. 16.4D) shows that in both views, the perpendicular distance between the left acetabulum and the highest point on the left iliac crest remains greater than on the right side. This probably reflects the somewhat fixed and slightly abnormal relationship of the pelvic joints, but may also indicate anomalous development of the ilium itself.

The obturator foramen shadows are slightly more symmetrical when standing than when lying, indicating a slight ilium 'shift' when weight-bearing.

Further, while the upward tilt on the left side remains in both the supine (Fig. 16.4B) and the standing erect position (Fig. 16.4A) the lumbar spine is concave to the right in lying and concave to the left when standing erect.

The lumbar articular signs were:

—extension limited by one-third with pain equally across the lumbosacral level
—right-side-flexion was greater than left-side-flexion; both were painless
—flexion, during marked deviation to the right, was limited by pain equally across the lumbar spine when the patient's extended fingers reached mid-shin
—rotations were unexceptional

Straight-leg-raising was left 65° and right 55°, both limited by symmetrical lumbar pain.

There were no neurological sings, and on the basis of a deep left sacroiliac sulcus (see p. 281) together with lumbar pain, the patient was treated on the basis of a combined lumbar and left sacroiliac problem secondary to lateral pelvic tilt.

Localised mobilisation to the lumbar spine, and then the left sacroiliac joint, produced moderate improvement in straight-leg-raising ranges and in flexion, but plainly not enough.

Over a period of three weeks without treatment a 1 cm heel raise reduced his pain to the point where he could play squash without discomfort.

Both straight-leg-raising and flexion ranges had improved considerably. He still had pain on sitting for more than 30 minutes.

A 1 cm right buttock raise when sitting had relieved this residual discomfort 14 days later; whether this relief of

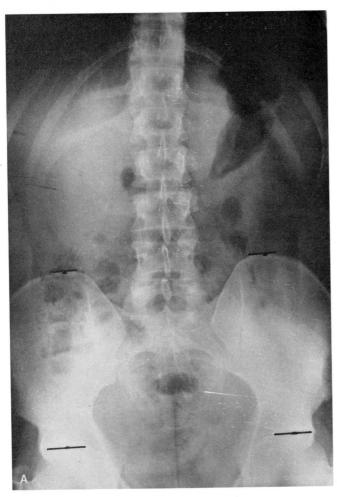

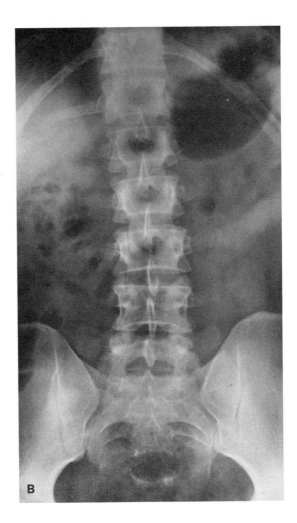

Fig. 16.4 Patient R.M. (See text for comments.)
(A) Standing erect film (22.2.79).

(B) Supine film (22.2.79).

the sitting pain was due to the slowly cumulative effects of the heel raise, or was ascribable only to the added measure of a buttock raise, remains uncertain, although he has now dispensed with the buttock raise. He has since played several games of squash without incident.

A further standing-erect a-p film of lumbar spine and pelvis on 9.4.79 while wearing his 1 cm right heel raise (Fig. 16.4E) revealed that while his pains were satisfactorily diminished, the appearance of pelvic asymmetry had hardly altered at all, although comparison with the standing-erect a-p film of 22.2.79 (Fig. 16.4A) shows the left lumbar concavity to have been slightly reversed; this is probably due to the heel raise but there is no absolute certainty of it.

Several debatable points arise:

a. Was the relief over three weeks due to the delayed effects of mobilisation, or to the heel raise?

b. While a 1 cm heel raise appears not to have modified the pelvic asymmetry, the lumbar spine posture has clearly been modified.

c. Might transient fluctuations, in the tone of paravertebral musculature, modify the posture of a somewhat labile lumbar spine from day to day, and at different times on the same day?

d. Do there exist unknown or ill-understood factors which might account for the variable findings reported by Bailey and Beckwith (1937)[54] (p. 265)?

e. Does leg-length inequality invariably underlie the appearance of lateral pelvic tilt? In many a-p views of the pelvis, there appear grounds for believing that an anomalous difference in the actual height of the ilia may also be the factor responsible—compare Figures 16.4C and 16.4D.

f. Since Epstein (1969)[315] (p. 31) has drawn attention to the importance of torsional soft-tissue strains in producing pain, do we necessarily have to completely 'correct' pelvic asymmetry before pain can be relieved? Is it necessary, as a matter of course, to *manipulate* for manifest pelvic asymmetry, when assessed as the cause of clinical features?

g. Clinical experience indicates that the consequences of a laterally tilted pelvis can be unimportant, moderate, or extensive, from patient to patient. At times the effects of a corrective heel raise will be trivial, partially beneficial or the sole measure required in relieving a host of

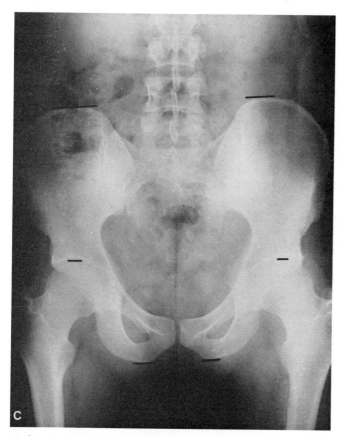

(C) Standing erect: lower lumbar spine and pelvis (22.2.79).

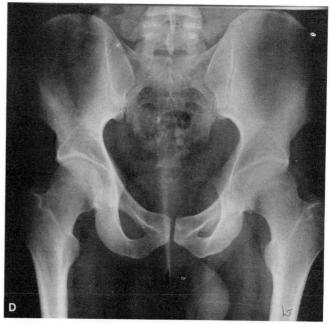

(D) Supine: lower lumbar spine and pelvis (22.2.79).

apparently unrelated joint problems from occiput to low back (see p. 308).

In the field of benign vertebral-joint pain, a prime indication for treatment by a heel raise is as follows:

—unilateral back, buttock and posterior thigh ache
—unilateral scapular region and arm ache
—unilateral neck pain and episodic migrainous headaches

in a young woman of 20 to 25 years of age or so with a lateral pelvic tilt upwards on the affected side (see p. 311).

Sometimes this is the only therapeutic measure required, although a proportion of patients also need localised manual techniques, of course.

An unlevel sacral base is one of the most common findings in patients with low back pain. (Greenman (1979)[440a].)

Use of scales

When pelvic asymmetry and/or leg length inequality are considered present, it is useful to stand the patient on a side-by-side pair of scales. Load differences between sides are noted, and lifts of varying thicknesses placed under the foot of the shorter leg. By this simple measure, the differences can sometimes be eradicated, but whether a simple heel-lift will then be the sole treatment is a matter for assessment.

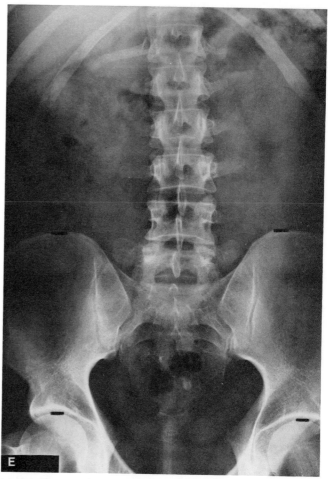

(E) Standing erect film (9.4.79) wearing a 1 cm heel raise on the right shoe.

Later assessment

It is wise to review the effects of a heel raise after some 6 to 12 months, by taking a history of clinical features during the interim and by re-examining pelvic levels, spinal movement and straight-leg-raising. In a small handful of patients, mild thoracolumbar problems may have been initiated.

Clinical impressions suggest that heel raises of something less than 1 cm can have subtle but cumulative effects upon the line of thrust during weight-bearing; in some patients these effects may present as obscure ipsilateral knee pains, for example. Or, after a few months of pregnancy, the 'lateral pelvic tilt' of a year or so before may be observed to be now reversed. Hence *assessment*, a year or so after applying the heel raise, is wise.

ADJUNCT PHYSICAL TREATMENTS

By this phrase is meant those commonly used surface applications to that part of the body from which pains of vertebral origin are believed to arise.

Among these might be included radiant heat, moist heat, hot water bottles, short-wave diathermy, microwave diathermy, ice (or cryotherapy), vapocoolant spray, interferential therapy, ultrasound, localised counter-irradiation by ultraviolet radiation and roller faradism. Electrical muscle stimulation may be used to initiate voluntary strengthening exercises; an alternative use of electrical stimulation (electroanalgesia) has been considered on page 487).

The traditional use of analgesic application to the body surface, for those pains which are now increasingly recognised as arising in the vertebral musculoskeletal and associated tissues, must be as old as pain itself, and it is not surprising that there remains among therapists of all persuasions a powerful instinct to favour this or that application. This is not unreasonable, because the common clinical experience is that they do help, and while the lynchpin of treatment of the moving parts of the body, i.e. the joints and associated tissues, is primarily the variety of forms of therapeutic movement, or modification of movement by temporary support, this does not diminish the value of complementary or associated treatments.

The essential point is that body-surface applications, or such treatments directed to deeper tissues via the body surface, should perhaps not be employed until such time as a comprehensive attempt has been made to elucidate the *nature* of the disturbed function being treated.

Since the nature of common vertebral joint problems is frequently that of a movement abnormality of one kind or another, it must surely be appropriate as a first step to try and elucidate the particular characteristics of the movement abnormality. This does not necessarily mean *diagnosis*, since diagnosis in its proper and classical sense is very frequently not possible; but it does mean that by the application of heat, cold, high-frequency radiations or other applications *without appropriate clinical examination and assessment of the abnormal movements* a basic principle has been ignored, and without constant reference to first principles no progress of any kind is possible.

Thus there is no reason why physical treatment applied in this way need not eventually degenerate into something like coin-operated laundries and dry cleaners, in which those with a painful yoke, interscapular area or low back may deposit a coin in the slot and buy 10 minutes or so of this or that application by holding the affected part a prescribed distance away from, or against, the fixed applicator. In the case of radiant heat, ultraviolet irradiation and faradism this, or something very like it, has virtually happened, of course, and the increasing technology of everyday domestic appliances is an augury that the process may by no means be completed.

The situation becomes completely different when these useful treatment methods are selectively employed to enhance or complement treatment by movement (be it passive or active), muscle strengthening, postural re-education and ergonomic instruction, which itself has been carefully selected on the basis of proper examination and assessment, and whose effects are subjected to continuing assessment.

In the treatment of common vertebral joint problems, adjunct physical methods should probably remain secondary treatments, or to put it another way should not, by the very nature of the lesion under consideration, assume the importance of primary treatment although they may very frequently be the appropriate form of *initial* treatment, as in the field of traumatology, for example.

Mooney and Cairns (1978)[869] have described interesting and effective treatment regimes in the management of patients with *chronic* low back pain, and briefly declare: 'We have not found a role for the various modalities such as ultrasound, diathermy, intermittent traction and transcutaneous nerve stimulation. All seem to avoid the primary goals of the treatment programme, i.e. improving soft tissue control of the degenerated segment and placing responsibility on the patient.'

While chronic low back pain or the 'multiple-operation back' are not the same thing as acute injury and many other painful states, one perceives here a more proper relationship between treatment and its aims than is the case when body surface applications become the primary and single procedure in treating painful vertebral conditions without full assessment. The indications for, and rationale of, their use have been discussed in very many texts.[105, 286, 287, 288, 410, 516, 666, 717, 853, 1023, 1098, 1218, 1234]

Perhaps for ease of application, but also on the basis of clinical experience, the author's use of adjunct treatments is restricted to three methods, i.e. small and flexible electrical heating pads, a mechanical vibrator and an ultrasonic generator with provision for variable frequencies for insonation.

Flexible heating pads serve no other purpose than that of providing comfort by gentle warmth. They are simple and adaptable, and by reason of their flexibility lend themselves to sometimes being incorporated with cervical, thoracic or lumbar traction treatments, with the pad placed against the painful part after the harness has been applied. If there does exist acceptable scientific evidence that they have any therapeutic effect, the author has long since forgotten about or never knew it—perhaps flexible heat pads serve a compassionate streak which is exercised when one changes a nervous and exhausted patient in acute pain into a warm, relaxed and comfortable objective person who is also much more able to give uncoloured information. These considerations may not apply in other than temperate climates, yet simple and hackneyed measures are no less effective for being such. Warmth can also assist the aims of traction, of course.

Electrical safety depends on watchful maintenance of the pads.

Mechanical vibrators have been referred to on page 379.

Ultrasound. If one had to be restricted to but a single method of adjunct treatment, which is most happily allied to techniques of passive and active movement, it would probably be ultrasound.[179]

Therapeutic use of this form of energy is not new; the report of a 1950 international congress on the subject in Rome listed 678 articles, and Curwen (1952)[216] observed that the softening of fibrous tissue by increased permeability was probably the most important effect, this being borne out by clinical experience. In the treatment of 200 cases, the best results were achieved in conditions of superficial scarring, fibrosis and induration. Also, effusions and oedema were more rapidly absorbed under its influence, and inflammatory reactions accelerated.

Curwen considered that calling the mechanical effect 'micro-massage' was an inadequate term for the intense shaking to which tissues are subjected! He regarded the process to be that of increasing the rapidity of fluid exchange within the tissues, under the normal osmotic and hydrostatic pressure mechanisms, due to the shaking of all semipermeable membranes: '... in the way stones in a sieve will pass through the mesh more rapidly if it is shaken than if it is held still'. From that time, when several rheumatology departments commonly gave ultrasound treatments to suitable conditions, its use suffered a decline, to be followed by a steadily increasing interest in its production, technique of application and effects.

As ever, this is reflected in the spate of articles on the subject, and it is of interest to observe that the various clinical states of connective tissue, particularly fibrosis, still comprise the largest single group of conditions for which the treatment is advocated. For example, Dyson and Suckling (1978)[288] provide a table of conditions in which it is nowadays common to use this adjunct therapy, i.e. strained and torn ligaments, inflamed tendons and tendon sheaths, lacerations and other soft-tissue damage, scar tissue sensitivity and tension, varicose ulcers, amputation neuromata, strained and torn muscles, inflamed and damaged joint capsules, fasciitis, treatment soreness after mobilisation techniques.

Ultrasound has been shown to have clinical value in stimulating tissue repair.

An almost routine use of insonation to 'relieve the soreness of mobilisation techniques' may satisfy a compassionate streak, but tends to diminish the possibilities of accurate assessment of the effects of manual mobilisation.

Other than heat pads as a *pretreatment* measure to aid relaxation and assist examination, it is the author's practice never to use any adjunct treatment for movement abnormalities until such time as the nature of the abnormality, and its response to initial procedures, have been assessed. Perhaps it is a matter of inclination and priorities.

Method: Pulsed ultrasound is said to be most effective in recent soft-tissue lesions, and in particular to injuries of the back.[974]

It is very common, but fallacious, to suppose willy-nilly that the earlier *all* back injuries, for example, receive some kind of active therapeutic intervention, the easier they are to resolve. A proportion of acute and painful low back injuries are preferably left entirely alone in the initial stages, an example being those patients with severe bilateral lumbar and buttock pain, in whom movements are 'globally' limited by increasing pain, after a fall onto the buttocks or other application of upward force to the ischial tuberosities. Yet many cases of back injury are considerably assisted by the early use of ultrasound; for example what appear to be minor low back muscle strains and also in the initial treatment of more severe injuries which may include stress fractures of transverse processes.[974] In this connection, the certain identification of minor paravertebral muscle strains by palpation is not as easy as might appear, since the phenomenon of referred tenderness can bedevil the most careful examination; as always, it is a matter of assessment and reasonable likelihood rather than certainty (see p. 258) and the precise nature of the exciting trauma is a vital factor in deciding the treatment approach.

Clinical impressions are that in the great variety of painful joint conditions primarily due to degenerative disease—itself hastened by repetitive stress, or trauma in times past—continuous beam ultrasound at low intensities is effective in assisting to reduce pain. The merits of applying a given quantity of energy emission either intermittently or continuously are plainly arguable, and are not considered here.[794, 944, 182]

Therapists will not need reminders of the necessity for careful recording of any adjunct procedure; with regard to insonation, Oakley (1978)[944] has provided an admirable example of precise recording of treatment.

Vapocoolant spray. Relaxation of muscle in spasm can be achieved by a spray of vapocoolant. The muscle or muscle group is placed on the stretch while the spray is applied to the overlying skin.[1237]

17. Medication and alternative methods of pain relief

MEDICATION

In 1972 a current *MIMS* monthly index listed some 100 items under analgesics and antipyretics and, under anti-inflammatory drugs another 60.[513]

Huskisson (1974)[584] has remarked: 'The clinician choosing a drug for his rheumatic patient is presented with a bewildering array of analgesics, anti-inflammatory, immunosuppressive and other medicines; the same drug also appears under different names in different dosages, combinations and formulations', e.g. the many forms and combinations of salicylates.

Drugs in the anti-inflammatory group which have proved their worth in the rheumatoid disorders have also proved to be gastrointestinal irritants.

The number of available medicines continues to increase, and the following is a simple classification:

1. *Simple analgesics.* Panadol (Paracetamol), Codis (aspirin and codeine), Distalgesic (paracetamol and dextropropoxyphene), DF 118 (dihydrocodeine tartrate), Dolobid and aspirin in small doses.

2. *Analgesics with minor anti-inflammatory properties.* There are a series of proprionic acid derivatives; the group includes the fenamates. They may be prescribed for minor musculoskeletal disorders in which powerful anti-inflammatory effects are not required. An example is ibruprofen, and the analgesic potency is similar to that of aspirin.

3. *Analgesics with major anti-inflammatory properties* are phenylbutazone (Butazolidin), indomethacin (often prescribed for relief of pain at night and morning stiffness) and aspirin in large doses.

4. *Purely anti-inflammatory drugs* are the corticosteroids and corticotrophin, which tend to suppress or affect normal endocrine function. For this reason, no doubt, Mooney and Cairns (1978)[869] observe that steroids have no role in the treatment of chronic degenerative processes.

5. *Drugs employed in rheumatoid arthritis* are gold, penicillamine, immunosuppressive and the antimalarial drugs.

6. *Drugs with a specific action in gout* are colchicine and allopurinol.

Briefly, the use of drugs[513] is as follows:

a. Analgesics

Paracetamol is a mild analgesic with antipyretic properties.

Codeine phosphate is a weak analgesic which may be used in a linctus to control non-productive coughing; the stress of coughing may frequently exacerbate lumbar and thoracic pain, for example.

Phenacetin was present in very many drug formulations, but was rarely given alone. It has a reputation as a nephrotoxic agent and is now seldom used.

Carisprodol has mild analgesic properties and is a 'muscle relaxant' (see below).

Pentazocine (Fortral) is an effective analgesic, with no anti-inflammatory or antipyretic properties.

b. Anti-inflammatory agents

If a drug has an anti-inflammatory effect it will almost certainly have a potential ulcerogenic effect as well.

Aspirin (acetylsalicylic acid) is widely used in its soluble form. The action of aspirin is rapid but short-lived; all preparations, buffered or unbuffered, may cause dyspepsia and/or gastrointestinal bleeding. Forms of the drug are: Paynocil (glycinated aspirin); Bufferin; aloxiprin (Palaprin); enteric-coated aspirin (Nuseals), all of which reduce gastrointestinal side effects. Also, benorylate (Benoral), a combination of paracetamol and aspirin; Safapryn, a similar combination; Levius, which is said to have a more prolonged effect, may be used for the relief of night pain.

Phenylbutazone and oxyphenbutazone are pyrazoles; they are effective anti-inflammatory drugs with an even, prolonged action.

Flufenamic acid and mefanemic acid (Ponstan) are analgesic, anti-inflammatory and antipyretic, and these anthranilates are an alternative if drugs such as aspirin are not tolerated well or are ineffective.

Ibruprofen (Brufen) is a mild analgesic, with anti-inflammatory properties.

Indomethacin begins its anti-inflammatory action within one or two hours of taking. It can produce headache and a variety of cerebral sensations reported as muzziness and giddiness, together with gastrointestinal symptoms.

When degenerative and non-inflammatory conditions are causing sporadic pain only, analgesics with a rapid action may be prescribed. For severe and more constant pain, anti-inflammatory analgesics such as indomethacin or phenylbutazone are more likely to be chosen.

Prednisolone may be given for the early morning stiffness of polymyalgia rheumatica, and *Indomethacin*, *Butazolodin* and *Naprosyn* for night pains and morning stiffness in ankylosing spondylitis.

More recent drugs,[584] with analgesic and anti-inflammatory effects and reduced side effects are:

Alclofenac (an acetic acid derivative)	Prinalgin
Fenoprofen (a proprionic acid derivative)	Fenopron — Proprietary name
Ketoprophen (a proprionic acid derivative)	Orudis
Naproxen (a proprionic acid derivative)	Naprosyn

Other new drugs in the same group are Clinoril, Meturazone, flurbiprofen (Froben) and Tolectin.

Voltarol (diclofenac sodium), a new antirheumatic drug which is said to be well tolerated, also has analgesic and antipyretic properties.

c. Muscle relaxants
In this connection, the views of Mooney and Cairns (1978)[869] are of interest:

Many of the drugs advocated for chronic back pain care are said to treat 'muscle spasm'. It should be noted that myoelectric activity related to chronic pain in the back (when the individual is at rest in a supported position) has never been described. It is hard to understand what spasm is being treated. Our own studies[579] of patients lying in traction in bed complaining of severe back pain and 'spasm', using very thin wire electrodes in the low back musculature, have failed to demonstrate electrical activity.

d. Relief of gout
Three drugs most useful in the rapid relief of acute gout are *indomethacin*, *phenylbutazone* and *colchicine*. Serum uric acid levels may be lowered by reducing urate synthesis, or by promoting the excretion of urate by the kidneys, and uricosuric drugs in common use are *probenecid*, *ethebenecid* and *sulphinpyrazone*; the drug *allopurinol* reduces urate synthesis and is now the most widely used in this group.

ALTERNATIVE METHODS OF PAIN RELIEF

Having mentioned (p. 480) adjunct physiotherapy methods which involve the various applications of heat, cold and some forms of electrical energy, there remains a somewhat disparate group of procedures which are not yet widely incorporated into orthodox physical therapy and which cannot be grouped under those invasive procedures which are themselves intended to exert the therapeutic effect (see p. 514), rather than the implanting of a long-acting device, for example.

A list of these might include:

A. Acupuncture
B. Transcutaneous electroanalgesia
C. Implanted stimulators
D. Operant conditioning, or behaviour modification
E. Relaxation
F. Employment of the biofeedback principle
G. The back 'school'.

A. ACUPUNCTURE

Traditional Chinese medicine[1144] can claim to have been the world's first organised body of medical knowledge. The earliest Chinese medical treatise (*The Yellow Emperor's Classic of Internal Medicine*) was written several centuries before the birth of Christ, and is said to date from 2698 BC and 2598 BC.

Low (1974)[767] mentions that treatment by acupuncture for low back pain is not new.

In America, Bache (1826)[50] described the merits of acupuncture in managing pain in the low back.

In 1825 the French physician *Sarlandiers* used electrical stimulation via needles inserted into acupuncture points to treat back pain, and in 1915 an English acupuncturist, Davis, described the therapeutic value of galvanic acupuncture. A later report (Goulden, 1921),[429] in the *British Medical Journal*, described acupuncture and electrical stimulation in several hundred cases of sciatica.

Smith (1974)[1144] observes:

The theoretical background of traditional medicine is unique, being concerned with the achievement of balance between the two opposing life forces, yin and yang. Illness is thought to be due to imbalance in these natural forces. Practitioners claim that they can identify specific skin areas which become hypersensitive when the function of an organ is impaired—and that the points concerned with a particular organ can be linked to form a line or meridian. The network of these lines and points forms the theoretical basis of the technique of acupuncture.

The Traditional Medical College in Kwangchow teaches that there are 361 acupuncture points; other Chinese authorities have quoted twice as many. It is held that both diagnosis and treatment is facilitated by detailed knowledge of the distribution of these points, and that malfunction of organs is (i) recognised by sensitivity of the point, and (ii) relieved by stimulation of the points.

Thus, acupuncture in Chinese medicine is used both in diagnosis and in treatment.

There are several methods of acupuncture:[462]

Needle acupuncture, or needle insertion in specific acupuncture points. (The points selected may be near the site of the disease or remote from the site, according to traditional meridians.)

Injection acupuncture, the injection of sterile water, saline, local anaesthetic, vitamins or other medication into acupuncture points.

Thread acupuncture, the insertion of thread into one acupuncture point and out through another and the thread left *in situ* for a period of time to produce persistent stimulation.

Pressure acupuncture, the application of digital pressure over appropriate points, and

Moxibustion, which involves the application of heat in the combustion of a piece of artemisia vulgaris.

Auricular acupuncture, which is the stimulation of acupuncture points situated in the ear.

A more recent method of stimulation is the use of electrical current transmitted via needles or surface electrodes (see p. 487).

The use of acupuncture in anaesthesia is very recent, and was not attempted before 1956.

Wall (1974)[1283] believes that social and psychological mechanisms play a dominant part in the effectiveness of acupuncture, but also mentions that while surgical operations are certainly completed under acupuncture, the number of such cases is decreasing. For example, he visited the most active Chinese hospital using acupuncture, and among 5200 major surgical procedures during 1973, only 6 per cent (324) were under acupuncture; the rest were performed under the conventional chemical anaesthesia. In preceding years, the numbers were 845 (1970), 395 (1971) and 350 (1972). He remarks that what *is* new is that the Chinese have developed a combination of three classical techniques for the control of pain: (a) relief of anxiety; (b) suggestion; (c) distraction, and suggests that the undoubted success of acupuncture analgesia involves a number of factors such as the national culture, the personality of patient and doctor, the operation itself and the acupuncture stimulus. Nevertheless, these are assisted where necessary by sedation, narcotics and local anesthesia.

Levine *et al* (1976)[724] observed the effects of needle acupuncture in a small group of 37 patients, 10 of whom had pain associated with nerve damage, the remainder having either acute or chronic pain (the latter defined as pain for longer than 6 months).

In chronic painful conditions, the treatment was effective in producing at least transient analgesia, a high score on psychometric indicators of anxiety and depression being a significant predictor of success in these chronic cases.

Needle acupuncture was observed to produce permanent relief of acute (self-limited) pain, but was not helpful in pain resulting from nerve damage.

Fox and Melzack (1976)[370] treated 12 patients suffering chronic low back pain with both acupuncture and transcutaneous electrical stimulation. The intensity and quality of pain were measured with the McGill Pain Questionnaire. *Acupuncture* was by insertion of a needle into three places on the bladder meridian (points commonly used for the treatment of backache) with a strong manual rotation for one minute at each point. *Transcutaneous electrical stimulation* (see later) was applied, with an e.e.g. disc electrode, for ten minutes at each of the same points in succession. The generator, having a variable output of up to 35 volts, produced 60 Hz sine-wave trains at a rate of three per second, and the voltage was raised to a bearable but painful level. Based on measurement of pain intensity overall, relief was greater than one-third in 75 per cent of patients given acupuncture and in 66 per cent treated by electrical stimulation, the mean duration of relief being 40 hours and 23 hours, respectively. Statistical analyses of the data revealed no significant difference between the two treatments, and both methods appeared to be equally effective.

Gunn *et al* (1976)[464] have remarked on the confusion which appears to exist in China as well as in Western countries (*vide supra*) caused by the inability of workers in acupuncture to demonstrate the exact nature of acupuncture loci, or to identify them in neuroanatomical terms. The authors reviewed 70 commonly used acupuncture points, and found that the loci could be classified into at least three types, *viz*:

I—corresponding to a known anatomical entity, i.e. the motor point of a muscle;

II—corresponding to the focal meeting of superficial nerves in the sagittal plane, and

III—lying over superficial nerves or plexuses.

They append a detailed tabulation of the 70 points, and suggest that as a first step towards the use of acupuncture by the medical profession, a new system of locus nomenclature be introduced, based on relating them to known neural anatomy.

Trigger points associated with myofascial and visceral pains (see Head's zones, p. 178) often lie within areas of referred pain, yet many are located some distance from these areas. Brief, intensive stimulation at trigger points often produces prolonged relief of pain.

For example, the injection of short-acting local anaesthetic at trigger points, or brief stimulation of them by dry needling, intense cold, injection of normal saline or transcutaneous electrical stimulation may diminish or abolish some forms of myofascial and visceral pain for days, weeks or permanently.

Following Travell and Rinzler's paper (1952)[1238] on myofascial pain syndromes, and the phenomenon of pain relief by injection of trigger points, Melzack *et al.* (1977)[848] attempted to determine the correlation between trigger points and acupuncture loci, having observed that the relief of pain by injecting trigger points resembled the relief of pain by needling acupuncture loci. A high degree of correspondence (71 per cent) was noted; the authors suggested that trigger points for pain and acupuncture loci, though discovered independently and according to different treatment philosophies, 'represent the same phenomenon and can be explained in terms of the same underlying neural mechanism'. The authors reproduce clinical syndromes, pain patterns and associated trigger areas described by Travell and Rinzler, and then tabulate the associated acupuncture points with the clinical syndromes.

Shealy (1977)[1119] regards the effects of acupuncture as neither a psychosomatic nor a placebo response, but as due to modulation of nerve function, doing this via the autonomic nervous system. He asserts that many of those in pain are suffering because of overactivity of the sympathetic portion of the autonomic nervous system.

Needle grasp (or the tech'i phenomenon) and trigger point pressure. Needling at acupuncture points and pressure at trigger points (or vice versa), produces a deep aching feeling. While orthodox medicine assumes this to be due to stimulation of an underlying focal pathological change, in acupuncture it is named 'tech'i',[467] and there is evidence that it may be due in part to a local muscle reflex which produces gripping of the acupuncture needle on penetration of subjacent muscle at acupuncture points.

There are two types of needle-grasp—superficial and deep.

Superficial. This occurs when the needle has penetrated the skin for a millimetre or so. When the needle is rotated, the skin around the needle will pucker and be lifted a little as traction is applied to the needle.

Deep. This occurs most obviously at type 1 (motor point) acupuncture loci, a local muscle spasm occurring at the point of stimulation. The needle is observed to be grasped, and this change may occasionally be so intense as to require considerable traction for needle extraction; sometimes the needle is found to be bent.

The phenomenon is most manifest when the needle enters partially denervated or neuropathic muscle, and when the motor point stimulated is already tender.

Gunn and Millbrandt (1977)[467] suggest that the subjective feelings of deep soreness, numbness, heaviness, pressure and aching are probably due to the stimulation of nociceptors and proprioceptors.

An unexplained fact is that the aching feeling is felt at some muscle sites but not others; also unexplained is the nature of the underlying focal pathological change.

Myofascial trigger points are sometimes associated with definite nodules of fibrous tissue. Kennard and Haugen (1955)[650] have observed that trigger points of the pectoral area and back are rare in infants and common in adults, and Korr (1955)[673] has suggested that trigger points develop during the course of growth as a result of musculoskeletal stresses, especially those of the back.

There is evidence that, long after total healing and pain relief, the sites of injured or 'insulted' tissues may be particularly susceptible to the formation of trigger (or acupuncture?) points. It is tempting to equate this phenomenon with the known phenomenon of 'remembered' pain (p. 173).

While the genesis of trigger points in the adult remains to be fully elucidated, it is evident that most of them are relatively invariable from patient to patient and conform to a pattern, while a small percentage, as sequelae of earlier injuries, would naturally conform not to the general pattern but to the type, locality and nature of the injury.

Mann *et al.* (1973)[804] have described the treatment of intractable pain by acupuncture, and Mann (1966, 1967)[802, 803] has provided both an atlas of acupuncture and described the treatment of disease by this method.

Gunn and Millbrandt[465, 466, 467, 468, 469, 470, 471] have noted the phenomenon of tenderness at motor points, and hypothesise that trigger points, acupuncture points and motor points may represent a common underlying basis for understanding much that is as yet unelucidated about musculoskeletal pain.

Weinstein (1974)[1298] has discussed the application of acupuncture in physical therapy, and makes proposals for its possible use.

The techniques of therapeutic local anaesthesia by injection were reviewed by Lewit (1979)[744] and it appeared that the common denominator was needle puncture and not the anaesthetic substance. In 241 patients exhibiting chronic myofascial pain, 312 pain-sites were treated by dry needling, with immediate analgesia without hypoaesthesia in 86 per cent of the cases, when the most painful spot was touched by needle.

Permanent relief of tenderness was achieved in 92 of the needled structures, relief lasting several months in 58, for several weeks in 63 and several days in 32 of 288 pain-sites, on follow-up.

Treatment effectiveness is related to the intensity of pain provoked on needling the trigger zone, and to the precision with which the site of tenderness is localised by needle.

The author observed one feature which is common to the use of local anaesthetic and to manipulation (described as segmental reflex therapy),[741] i.e. after immediate relief pain was reactivated after some hours or next day, the reactivation lasting a day or so before the full therapeutic effect was established.

Comparisons of the undermentioned tabulated pain spots and trigger zones with those of Travell and Rinzler[1238] and Hansen and Schliak,[498] and the periosteal points of Vogler and Krauss,[1273] revealed that there are many such localities and some may have been chosen arbitrarily.

Lewit's localities, and rationale for needling them, are summarised:

Posterior arch of atlas may be the most important single trigger zone in headaches of cervical origin.

Pelvic ligaments. The importance of these ligaments has been stressed by others; pain can be elicited by stretching the ligaments and needling their insertions.

Interdigital fold. An important trigger zone in radicular syndromes. Infiltration is frequently effective if there is a zone of hyperalgesia. Lewit mentions a disappearance or reduction of Lasègue's sign as evidence of success after needling a painful skin fold between the toes.

Head of fibula. Painful spots in this locality may be related to painful leg cramps, a complaint in patients recovering from acute radicular syndromes.

Periosteum of ribs. A frequent source of pain, particularly near the costal angle, in the axillary line, the mammillary line and at the sternocostal junction.

Spinous processes, especially that of C2, probably because of upper cervical muscle insertion.

Upper border of scapula. Insertion of levator scapulae muscle.

Ischial tuberosity. An important muscle insertion point and a frequent site of pain.

In the present climate of interest in acupuncture, much is sometimes made of what is termed 'acupuncture massage', in which circular frictions, transverse frictions or steady digital pressure are applied to muscles at acupuncture loci; in low back pain, for example, the bladder and gall-bladder loci are employed. When the essentials of the technique are considered, they seem to amount to little more than the known method of inhibitory pressures (p. 379).

Duffin (1978)[280] has provided a very good geographical survey of the current interest in and development of acupuncture techniques, yet to suggest that the success of acupuncture in the treatment of pain is explained by what is essentially an hypothesis (the pain-gate theory, p. 168) itself not yet elucidated, is to raise more questions than answers.

Investigation of the effects of acupuncture indicate the possibility that it may stimulate release of endogenous substances with morphine-like biological properties which have an analgesic effect. Brain and serum extracts of acupunctured rabbits injected into untreated animals produced a marked analgesic effect, as evidenced by a great increase in their tolerance of pain.[716]

B. TRANSCUTANEOUS ELECTRICAL ANALGESIA

The initial reference (p. 169) to electrical stimulation, for pain relief, requires further consideration.

In reviewing the results of treating 100 cases of low-back-sprain by surface electrode stimulation at acupuncture points, Gunn and Millbrandt (1975)[462] give the neurophysiological basis for acupuncture as:

1. The development of analgesia depends upon the stimulation of specific acupuncture points, which correspond to certain types of muscle receptor.
2. The transmission of a painful stimulus can be blocked by other afferent inputs at spinal and thalamic levels.
3. There are descending inhibitory influences from the raphe nuclei which are activated by muscle afferents.
4. There also appears to be involved a humoral agent, which has not yet been identified (see above)

The 100 patients with low back pain, 94 of whom completed the treatment and were included in the follow-up study at three months after discharge, were grouped as follows:

Group	No. of patients	
I	29	Non-specific soft-tissue injury
II	7	Disc degeneration (i.e. radiographic disc narrowing)
III	5	Disc generation with only subjective radicular symptoms
IV	13	As group III but with objective signs such as reduced SLR, etc.
V	18	Generalised degenerative changes (some patients had had surgery in the past)
VI	2	Spondylolysis without slip
VII	1	Spondylolisthesis
VIII	11	Recent postoperative cases (original injury not defined)
IX	1	Functional overlay
X	7	a. Lumbar instability—old laminectomy, subsequently required fusion (1)
		b. Compression fracture (2)
		c. Transverse process fracture (1)
		d. Right ilium fracture (1)
		e. Arachnoiditis (1)
		f. Backache superimposed on Marie-Strumpell's disease (1)

Surface electrode acupuncture obviates many of the complications of methods such as needle insertion, e.g. sepsis, transmitted infection and breakage of needles, and also burns from moxibustion.

The technique employs a current with biphasic square wave pulses, with an optimum frequency (found by trial and error) in the neighbourhood of 70–100 Hz and a pulse duration of 0.1 milliseconds. The measured output was from 2 to 6 milliamperes at 2 to 6 volts; this was gradually increased during each session of stimulation, as the patient developed tolerance, working up to 10 mA at 10–40 V.

The stimulation sessions occupied 20 minutes daily, and as improvement occurred the sessions were reduced to thrice weekly. Patients were gradually weaned from stimulation and progressed to moderate or advanced remedial exercise groups, or were discharged.

Placement of electrodes

Whether the symptoms were unilateral or bilateral, electrodes were placed bilaterally, in accordance with traditional acupuncture practice. The anodes were placed on the back, at the segmental levels of spinal nerves, and the cathodes were placed on the limbs according to the distribution of the anterior primary rami. (Root values are those given by the authors.) The points were chosen according to the level of root involvement, and subjective tenderness to digital pressure. In this respect, it is worth recalling (p. 192) that the distribution of symptoms and signs in the lower limb is not a reliable indication of the level of segmental changes responsible for them.

Anodal electrodes were placed as follows:

Acupuncture point	Anatomical locality
Bladder 22	Sacrospinalis L2
Bladder 23	Sacrospinalis L3
Bladder 24	Sacrospinalis L4
Bladder 25	Sacrospinalis L5
Bladder 26	Cutaneous nerve ppr T11
Bladder 47	Cutaneous nerve ppr T12

The *cathodal* electrodes were placed as follows:

a) Posterior aspect of limb:

Acupuncture point	Anatomical locality
Bladder 48	Upper motor point gluteus max (L5–S2)
Bladder 49	Lower motor point gluteus max (L5–S2)
Bladder 50	Sciatic nerve at gluteal fold (L4–S3)
Bladder 51	Sciatic nerve at mid-post thigh (L4–S3)
Bladder 54	Popliteal nerve (L4–S2)
Bladder 55	Sural nerve (L4–5)
Bladder 56	Sural nerve (L4–5)
Bladder 58	Motor point lateral soleus (L5–S2)
Kidney 9	Motor point medial soleus (L5–S2)
Gall-bladder 34	Common peroneal nerve (L4–S2)
Other points	Motor point—gluteus medius (L5–S2)
	Motor point—med. head of gastrocnemius S1–2)
	Motor point—lat. head of gastrocnemius (S1–2)

b) Anterior aspect of limb:

Acupuncture point	Anatomical locality
Gall-bladder 34	Lateral cutaneous nerve of leg (L5–S2)
Spleen 9	Saphenous nerve (L3–4)
Spleen 8	Saphenous nerve (L3–4)
Liver 6	Saphenous nerve (L3–4)
Spleen 36	Motor point tib. ant. (L4–5)

One centimetre diameter stainless steel electrodes were employed.

Results were classified as: (i) Good: relief of signs and symptoms—patient returned to previous employment. (ii) Satisfactory: relief of signs and symptoms, and patient advanced to remedial occupational therapy or referred to lighter employment. (iii) Poor or temporary: no change, or relief only during stimulation.

Group	No. of cases	Good	Satisfactory	Temporary or Poor
I	29	25	3	1
II	7	5	1	1
III	5	4	1	—
IV	13	7	4	2
V	18	8	5	5
VI	2	—	1	1
VII	1	—	—	1
VIII	11	4	3	4
IX	1	—	—	1
X a)	1	—	—	1
b)	2	1	1	—
c)	1	—	1	—
d)	1	—	—	1
e)	1	1	—	—
f)	1	—	—	1

No contraindications had appeared to date, but patients with a cardiac history or with metal in the tissues, such as a plated fracture, were excluded from the series.

The authors compared treatment by surface electrode stimulation with a similar series of patients treated by the standard orthodox regime, and conclude that the former is an acceptable form of treatment comparable to standard orthodox measures, and well worth a trial in those cases resistant to standard regimes.

Gunn (1976)[463] observes that muscle stimulation is maximal at a fairly narrow transverse band, the zone of innervation, near the neurovascular hilus of the muscle and approximating to the motor point on the skin.

Many classical acupuncture points are now seen to coincide with motor points (*vide supra*). Of the many methods of stimulation by acupuncture, the two most employed are transcutaneous neural stimulation using surface electrodes, and needle acupuncture with or without electrical stimulation. The greatest relief of pain is reported to occur following the patient's subjective appreciation of the 'tech'i' phenomenon.

The author discusses the importance of large diameter mechanoreceptors of muscle in relieving pain, and concludes that it would seem logical that stimulation is best applied at the motor point.

Callaghan, Sternbach et al. (1978)[154] examined sensory perception, in those patients with chronic pain in one limb, before and after pain reduction by transcutaneous neural stimulation.

The contralateral limb, and normal subjects, served as controls. Compared to the controls, painful limbs showed considerable impairment of sensory sensitivity; following transcutaneous neurostimulation, however, sensitivity was improved towards normal levels.

Conversely, electrical stimulation slightly impaired sensitivity in normal limbs.

Among the conflicting hypotheses about the mechanism of electrical analgesia, there is slight support for the concept of peripheral small-fibre blockade or fatigue. Findings suggest that, at most, only some small fibres could have been blocked, and this is consistent with the observation that stimulation did not completely abolish the pain but only reduced its severity.

The hypothesis of central inhibition was not entirely supported, either. The results of this research suggest that both peripheral small-fibre blockade and large-fibre stimulation are involved in electroanalgesia; the former is predominant when pain reduction occurs in a painful limb and the later is more noticeable in normal limbs.

Transcutaneous nerve stimulation is ineffective if attempted on the basis of treatment for 30–60 minutes a day, for example. For the majority of patients in whom it may be indicated, the stimulus needs to be applied almost continuously during their waking day, at least initially.[1119] The routines of stimulation must be individually worked out for each patient, with a variety of stimulators and electrodes applied in turn to some 40 different surface points, before the optimum effectiveness is achieved.

For those who will need transcutaneous stimulation on a permanent or semi-permanent basis the treatment plan should aim at transferring responsibility for the use and maintenance of the equipment to the patient; a variety of neat and portable stimulators is now available. The patient will need to attend for a period of familiarisation with equipment, rationale and aims of treatment, the location of motor points and formal dermatome areas, and the need for persistence.

Some may obtain relief fairly quickly, others may need up to four weeks of patient testing with the electrodes in different positions. A combination of using trigger points (p. 118) and formal dermatome areas (Figs 2.18, 2.19, 2.20) is used by some therapists, on a basis of initially placing electrodes proximally to the site of pain and over the spinal nerve root or peripheral nerve trunk serving the painful region.

(i) For central pain which spreads distally, the electrodes are at first placed proximally

(ii) For localised distal pain, and for specific joint pain, electrodes initially are placed in the vicinity concerned

(iii) The use of an interferential technique for localised areas, i.e. four electrodes, may be more successful where two-electrode stimulation has not been successful

(iv) Where there is deep pain, it may be an advantage to initially stimulate with electrodes placed a few segments more cranially.

Some patients will experience pain relief during the stimulation periods only; others will experience relief or diminution for as much as three or four times longer.

It is suggested that stimulation is contraindicated in the presence of cardiac pace-makers, and where pain relief is likely to conceal the symptoms of progressive pathology. TENS (Transcutaneous Electrical Nerve Stimulation)

is particularly suited for use by physiotherapists, and of a recent survey among 196 of them[975a] some 65 per cent employed the technique to relieve chronic pain from a variety of disorders.

Short-term use, and the most common use of the method was in treating low back pain and cervical pain.

C. IMPLANTED STIMULATORS

Wall and Noordenbos (1977)[1284] have demonstrated, following examination of three patients with spinal cord dorsal column lesions, that the subjects did not lose one or more of the classical primary modalities of sensation, but lost the ability to simultaneously analyse the spatial and temporal characteristics of a stimulus. Two of the patients had suffered single stab wounds which cut completely across both dorsal columns and extended into the ventral white matter. Their findings raise questions about the validity of classical teaching, particularly about the nature and physiological significance of afferent impulse traffic in the posterior columns.

Rather more than 10 years ago, following experimental work, the use of electrical stimulation of the central or peripheral nervous system, to inhibit pain, became the subject of much investigation.

Relief of pain by electrical stimulation of peripheral nerves was reported by Wall and Sweet in 1967.[1280]

Since activation of the large A-beta fibres was observed to inhibit nociceptive impulse traffic, stimulation of the dorsal columns of the spinal cord might reasonably offer a method of subduing chronic pain. Experimentally, dorsal column electroanalgesia was found to totally abolish prolonged small-fibre after-discharge (PSAD), as recorded in the upper cervical cord, tegmentum and parts of the cerebellum.

Further experiments, in which electrical impulses of 0.5–1.0 mA were applied to the dorsal columns of cats, demonstrated that noxious stimuli failed to evoke normal responses to pain.

Shealey, Mortimer and Hagfors (1970)[1117] implanted 5 mm square platinum plates into the thoracic spines of six patients, placing the electrodes some four to eight segments above the levels of pain input. The plates were attached to silicone-impregnated Dacron which was sutured to the dura; the pulsed signals were delivered to the implanted radio-receiver, transcutaneously, by a battery-powered radio-transmitter. Biphasic square wave pulse durations of 0.3 ms, repeated 50–275 per second at variable voltages, were controlled by the patients, who seemed to prefer a frequency of 100–200 per second.

Some relief of pain was felt by all the patients. For patients with constant pain, stimulation was constantly required, and there was no lasting after-benefit from stimulation, as is seen in stimulation of peripheral nerves. There was no interference with normal neurological function.

Long (1977)[762] reviews electrical stimulation for the control of pain, remarking that implantable stimulators have been used for stimulation of peripheral nerves, anterior and posterior surfaces of the spinal cord, and the brain; he suggests that peripheral nerve stimulators are the most efficacious of the implantable devices, used specifically for the pain of peripheral nerve injury.

The long-term results of dorsal column stimulation, via the surgical implanting of electrodes close to the dorsal columns during laminectomy, have been reported by Urban and Nashold (1978)[1259] as disappointing, with a failure rate which may be as high as 70 per cent. They itemise the problems as failure to gain effective stimulation referable to the painful region, to derive adequate pain relief from an acceptable level of stimulation and to continue pain relief after initial success.

They describe a percutaneous method of implantation into the epidural space, with electrodes connected subcutaneously to the receiver placed in a subcutaneous pocket in the left loin. Each patient was instructed in the auto-stimulation technique, with variations of frequency and intensity.

The generally poor results of controlling pain by spinal cord stimulation were confirmed, although 7 out of 20 patients were started on 'chronic' autostimulation and only 1 failed to experience continued pain relief.

The advantage of the method is that on failure to respond with satisfactory relief of pain, the system is easily removed.

D. OPERANT CONDITIONING, OR BEHAVIOUR MODIFICATION

Acute, or more especially chronic low back pain, for example, frequently has a number of factors in its pathogenesis.[459]

Disturbances of the skeletal, articular, muscular, cerebrospinal and autonomic nervous systems, and of the viscera, posture and psyche, all need to be taken into account.

It is well known that the intensity or amount of pain (if such can be quantified for analysis other than by common social awareness and subjective evaluation) does not have a one-to-one relationship to the amount of tissue damage presumed to be responsible for it.[846] Beecher (1960)[78] has observed:

Many investigators seem grimly determined to establish—indeed, too often there does not seem to have been any question in their minds—that for a given stimulus there must be a given response; i.e. for so much stimulation of nerve endings, so much pain will be experienced... This fundamental error has led to enormous waste ... there is no simple relationship between stimulus and subjective response ... the reason for this is the inter-

position of *conditioning*, of the *processing component*, of the *psychic reaction*. [my italics.]

In some individuals, pain (or rather more aptly 'pain behaviour') appears to continue for an inordinately long period after presumed tissue damage may be expected to have resolved.

There is something singular and unusual when pain appears to be lasting forever, despite the best efforts of experienced doctors, surgeons and therapists. A proportion of patients appear to have become habituated to pain after chronic disability, and notwithstanding our lack of certain information about the true nature of joint pain, there is reason to believe that pain behaviour may be reinforced, and be continued for disproportionately long periods after the stimulus which gave rise to it has disappeared, if advantage of one kind or another is gained thereby.

'The differences between pain as a sensory system and as a chronic condition are critically important.' (Fordyce, 1973.)[366] Chronic pain allows time for attitudes and types of behaviour to be learned. The set of actions, by which a person in pain will wittingly or unwittingly signal this to others, are called *operants*, e.g. the descriptions of pain, facial distortion, way of sitting down or rising from a chair, reaching out for support, limping, seeking medication or rest and avoiding various fundamental activities or duties. Almost all examples of pain behaviour are operants.

Much behaviour is determined by its consequences.[754] The importance of operants is that they can be influenced, i.e. either steadily reinforced or extinguished, by the consequences which follow them. If a particular behaviour (operant) is repetitively and immediately followed by favourable consequences, it tends to become positively reinforced, and tends to occur again in response to a similar stimulus. Should pain behaviour not be systematically followed by favourable reinforcers, of one kind or another, usually the operant will tend to occur less frequently and ultimately be extinguished. Pain habituation becomes learned when pain behaviour is positively reinforced and well behaviour is poorly reinforced.

Fordyce[367] gives a common example:

A heavy labourer with chronic back pain illustrates positive reinforcement. When he works, his pain increases. When he rests, his pain decreases. If he receives his rest contingent on hurting (engaging in pain behaviour), rest becomes a positive reinforcer. Thus, he must hurt to gain rest. This situation can lead to learning a pain habit—that is, to developing pain behaviour controlled by environmental consequences rather than a pathogenic factor. Although the pain does not start in this way, the arrangement described may serve to maintain or increase the pain even after the stimulus is no longer present.

The description 'psychogenic' is not appropriate, since it assumes the existence of a personality disorder, which is not invariably present. Further, psychotherapy has a low rate of success in treating chronic pain.

Pain behaviour is automatically learned, whether or not the patient has a personality disorder.

Other examples of positive reinforcement for pain behaviour, or secondary gain, are:

(i) The man or woman whose chronic backache, or lower abdominal or coccygeal pain, serves to postpone sexual intercourse, about which there is some aversion because of difficulty, real or imagined.
(ii) Continuing pain eliciting a continuation of extra attention and helpfulness, when 'well' behaviour does not.
(iii) Attention and expressions of sympathy upon pain behaviour are potent reinforcers.
(iv) 'Well' behaviour leading to resumption of unpleasant duties or grappling with painful difficulties.
(v) Hospital inpatients, after a period of chronic pain, may be reluctant to face the sea of troubles which laps the hospital gates.
(vi) Sometimes, a prescription of medication for pain, and rest for pain, may act as reinforcers in some patients, if relief of pain follows.

In each case of long-continued chronic pain, where the changes initially producing pain can reasonably be assumed to have resolved, evidence of a relationship between pain behaviour and positive reinforcers should be sought. For example, there may be a strongly ingrained pattern of using pain as a tool in social relationships.[152]

Operant conditioning refers to methods by which the strength, or frequency of occurrence, of operants may be increased or decreased, and depends upon recognition that pain behaviours are subject to learning or conditioning.

To modify pain behaviour by operant conditioning, the physician and/or therapist must:

a. Establish the behaviour to be produced, increased, maintained, diminished or eliminated.
b. Determine which type of reinforcer (encouragement, withdrawal of attention, praise, disapproval, etc.) are likely to be effective in each individual.
c. Gain sufficient control over the patient's environment to regulate consequences of the behaviour to be influenced.

Mooney *et al.* (1976)[868] described five methods of personality assessment for the psychological treatment of patients with chronic back pain:

(i) Patient pain drawings
(ii) Pentothal pain studies
(iii) Stress score index
(iv) Testing by the Minnesota Multiphasic Personality Inventory (MMPI)
(v) Response to treatment challenge.

In most patients, operants to be diminished or eliminated are medication, and response to pain by non-productive behaviour. Since persons in daily contact with the patient should be trained to become socially unresponsive to pain complaints, and to lavish attention when socially acceptable activities are steadily increased, both professional staff and the patient's family must be appraised of the aims and methods of treatment.

Treatment without altering family reactions to pain and well behaviour is less likely to succeed, or be permanent. This does not mean that medical staff and members of the patient's family are issued with a licence to punish the patient for undesirable actions,[367] and some imagination and compassion should temper the particular type of reinforcers chosen.

Commonly, the aims of treatment are:

(i) Reduction of analgesics
(ii) Extinction of antisocial behaviour
(iii) Diminish avoidance of activities because of pain
(iv) Steadily improve exercise tolerance
(v) Increase walking distance
(vi) Increase work and social activities.

Cairns *et al.* (1976),[152] in describing a method of inpatient management, have found that:

Many patients have viewed surgery as the best, if not the only, method of treatment. Therapeutic blocks are usually seen as second best. Exercises and activity analogous to 'learning to live with it' are viewed as a poor substitute for passive forms of treatment. Our experience indicates that shifting the patient from a passive role to becoming an active participant in his own rehabilitation must receive careful attention. Thus, every effort is made to avoid terminology placing exercises and activities in a tertiary category. Statements to the patient such as 'there is nothing more we can do for you other than exercises' are never made.

Behaviour modification techniques are now being used in the rehabilitation of patients with head injury.[754]

When all is said and done, much of behaviour modification technique is not dissimilar to the timeless process of bringing up children, of helping them to grow up by encouragement and by stressing the positive aspects of steady achievement, self-reliance and socially acceptable attitudes.

Nevertheless, the development and application of this particular method of rehabilitating adult patients is new, and achieving success.[978]

E. RELAXATION

The word 'relaxation' is used in many contexts to describe the single aim of a great variety of techniques—for generally relieving mental and physical tension or achieving 'stillness' of mind and musculature, reducing unnecessary voluntary contraction of skeletal muscle, involuntary skeletal muscle spasm and the tightness of contracted tissues.

Massage, and the exercise technique of 'hold-relax', are methods of inducing relaxation of specific muscle-groups, of course, and there is currently much interest in learning the techniques of meditation and of Yoga, for example.

The physiotherapy methods under consideration are those such as:

(i) Total suspension in slings[473]
(ii) Relaxation exercises for sciatica[1216]
(iii) Deep breathing
(iv) Induction of relaxation by (a) placing the patient in a soothing environment, (b) encouraging restfulness by talking quietly to the patient of pleasant and restful situations[784]
(v) Treatment of migraine, for example, by explanations about stress and fatigue, by shaking and swinging exercises, and tensing then relaxing the muscles of specific body parts, region by region, until all skeletal musculature is in a relaxed state.

Treating painful benign vertebral (and peripheral) joint problems *by using everyday physical means to induce the patient to relax*, is less common than it was. This may be so partly because a much greater variety of treatment methods is now available, partly because the technique never seemed to be quite as effective as was hoped (at least when it comprised the *sole* form of treatment) and partly because slowly improving understanding of the nature of particular joint abnormalities has led to more specific and appropriate treatment.

This is not to say that local and/or general relaxation may not form a valuable part of the aims of many types of current and effective treatment methods, e.g. the rest and relaxation afforded by a well-fitting and individually tailored cervical collar, for irritable neck joints and aching muscles, the timeless value of rest in a position of comfort for an acute attack of lumbago and the methods of biofeedback (p. 493), or that a relaxed frame of mind is not a highly desirable commodity in its own right; only that attempts to induce relaxation, as an umbrella or 'shot-gun' technique for headache, neckache or backache, without first making a comprehensive attempt to understand the genesis of the pain in terms of the proper function of structures believed to be concerned, leaves something to be desired.

As an instance, we know that there are very many causes of headache, some of them pathological changes of serious consequence; it is also known that many causes of 'migraine' (see p. 218) are due to benign upper cervical joint problems which are fairly easily and quickly remedied by specific treatment to the joint abnormality itself. Further, it has been the author's more than occasional experience to encounter patients whose chronic cervical joint condition has never been comprehensively examined, whose description of bizarre symptoms have never been given proper attention and whose indifferent handling by a succession of clinicians and therapists has led to deeply frustrated anger in some, while others have been slowly brought to the threshold of real neuroticism. Cause enough for headache.[295, 296]

While pain, fear, anxiety (often for very sound reasons), overwork, demanding situations and frustrated anger (because of chronic pain) give rise to a general increase in muscle tension, and a reduction of tension is desirable, these factors may more often be provoking or aggravating a covert or overt joint problem than being the sole agent of its genesis.

The factors of listening attentively to what the patient has to say, of handling the patient's tissues considerately and with confident skill and simply getting the patient better, are more potent methods of achieving relaxation than the rather cumbersome and awkward procedure of total suspension in slings, or just talking quietly to the patient in the hope, rather than the belief, that the arthrogenic hypertonus would be induced to just go away.

The methods tabulated above were very time-consuming, and in appropriate cases are not as effective as skilfully applied relaxed passive movement, whether applied to the joints themselves or to the soft tissues or both.

F. THE BIOFEEDBACK PRINCIPLE

Feedback, or knowledge of results, is a powerful factor in the learning process, and amounts to no more or less than the principle of modification procedures being guided by the monitoring of errors.

The same servo-system is the basis for operation of a great variety of control mechanisms in modern technology.

That familar example of feedback, a thermostat, corrects its errors by a series of oscillations of decreasing amplitude as overswing to hotter or colder becomes less and less wide of the mark and the set temperature is reached—the whole cycle starts again as the changes in the environmental temperature make further corrections necessary.

The principle is not new—this was how World War II torpedoes progressively corrected directional errors and finally homed onto and hit the target ship. In biological terms, the shift of glance from near to far or from one thing to another, 'aiming' a hand to grasp an object, and riding a bicycle are all examples of rapid, fine oscillatory corrections which characterise all voluntary activity,[1289] particularly that of homing onto a visual point or neatly grasping a door handle.

Likewise, the 'Donnan equilibrium potential', across the membrane of resting nerve, oscillates very slightly above and below the given average value for resting nerve.

Biofeedback is the technique of using feedback of a normally automatic bodily response to a stimulus, in order to acquire voluntary control of the response, *and in consideration of it we need to discuss posture.*

Roaf (1978)[1045] describes the difficulty of formulating a definition of posture, and it may be that these difficulties will arise whenever we try to charge single, simple and universal words—like 'posture', 'relaxation', 'pain' or 'love'—with scientifically satisfactory meanings. It must always be something of a self-defeating exercise, until such time as science has hived off and then categorised the whole rich variety of emotional, hormonal, mechanical, neurophysiological and social factors to which, by unspoken acceptance, we nod whenever we use these words in ordinary conversation.

This time is not yet, so the words retain their proper expressive value—for example, it is correct to refer to 'sleeping posture' as simple mechanical dispositions of body parts, while accepting the objection to most postural standards, i.e. that they are fixed.

For scientific purposes we have to resort to something of a makeshift, and, as a definition of posture, Roaf proposes: 'the position the body assumes in preparation for the next movement', observing that mere static uprightness is not true posture, since this involves balance, muscular control, co-ordination and adaptation.

Head (1920)[526] had in mind this objection to fixed postural standards when he suggested 'by means of perpetual alteration in position, we are always building up a postural model of ourselves which constantly changes'.

A system of psychosomatic self-regulation, termed autogenic training, was developed in Germany around 1900 and was used to assist in gaining a degree of control over some autonomic functions.[332]

The use of a verbal stimulus for postural re-education, as a type of conditioned reflex, was employed for the correction of tensional imbalance by Alexander (1932)[17, 793] and in the conditioning of pupillary contractions by Hudgins (1933).[577]

In the re-education of improved postural reactions, Barlow (1952)[63] suggested the term 'postural homeostasis' to denote the state of steady motion which underlies all voluntary movements, i.e. 'postural homeostasis in the intact organism is effected by feedback from the eyes, the muscles and the labyrinth, and the information which is fed back is assessed against the postural model'.

This is similar to the property of physiological homeostasis, by which is maintained the constancy of the internal environment (the 'milieu intérieur' of Claud Bernard).

It is the individual's postural model, or body image, which, with his or her co-operation, is made subject to modification by the re-education process.

The principle of biofeedback is always the same: information is made available to subjects about the state of one or other of their physiological systems, in a way that is understandable to them and which allows them to gain control over the function of that system,[517] and thus modify its performance.

If one *associates* a given degree of muscle tension, and its associated *feeling*, with external stimulus, this given tensional balance is, in time, produced by the external stimulus alone, and Barlow's (1952)[63] subjects were taught to project a series of verbal directions which were linked up for them with an improved postural reaction. The exteroceptive stimulus was thus a vocalised word of command, the stimulus gradually and eventually becoming a subvocalised command given by the subjects themselves. In a relatively short period the subjects were able to evoke at will the improved manner of using their bodies.

Barlow found postural defects very common; he considered them present in between 70 to 80 per cent of adolescents and increasing with age. Manual therapists will find interesting his view that postural homeostasis (an improved ability to maintain a correct body image when reacting and adapting oneself to outside stimuli and stresses) is *primarily dependent upon correct equilibration of the head/neck relationship*. His results, in treatment of a group of 50 voice and drama college students, provided powerful evidence of (i) the multifactorial nature of back pain and (ii) the interdependence of the vertebral column.

For example, a voice student, with marked asymmetry of standing posture, had failed an audition because of constant low back pain, and extreme unpredictability of performance. Her body image was inadequate in that she was quite unaware of her postural mistakes and could not correct them; when corrected she felt 'crooked'. Following treatment, her low back pain disappeared, her voice improved and at another audition she was accepted. Other subjects experienced relief from migrainous headaches, and improvement of scoliosis.

Barlow stresses that the re-education was not done by physical exercises but by means of a conditioning procedure which modifies a poor body image and thus improves the capacity for postural homeostasis: 'Various patients with psychosomatic and psychiatric disorders have been treated in this way with success. Remedial exercises or manipulative therapy are inadequate without re-education of the postural homeostasis.'

On the basis that the first function of biofeedback is to make an individual *aware* of what is happening in body systems of which he was previously unaware, with the aim of gaining control over the system, there is evidence that quite considerable degrees of neuromuscular control can be learned.

Clarke and Kardachi (1977)[180] have used more elaborate methods of employing the biofeedback principle in the treatment of facial pain consequent to bruxism, or teeth-grinding at night.

Another method of feedback places the patient in an electronic circuit, which produces an auditory signal related directly to the degree of muscle spasm. Used as a rehabilitation technique, the patient's relaxation and normal muscle activity are aided and guided by auditory evidence of successful reduction of spasm.

Biofeedback procedures have been used in research on the nature of learning and behavioural plasticity, investigating brain/behaviour relationships, and in attempting to quantify the experience of consciousness.[1097]

While modern e.m.g. biofeedback instruments are likely to be used for conditions of muscle overactivity like torticollis, the spasticity of neurological disease, peripheral nerve injuries, rehabilitation of some stroke patients and the correction of gait irregularities, Alexander's successful method (*vide supra*) of using a verbal stimulus as the conditioned reflex clearly demonstrates that electronic circuitry is not essential for clinical exercise of the basic principle, when treating postural defects.

While the evidence of the effects of biofeedback training are interesting, it is presently of a mixed quality and few definite conclusions can be drawn at this stage.[1017] Nevertheless, therapeutic possibilities and the benefits of applying the principles have been energetically pursued and expanded,[73a] with detailed descriptions of biofeedback electronics, selection of patients, a proposed basis for neurophysiological effects, and descriptions of the method in treating psychosomatic disorders and controlling gastrointestinal motility, among many other applications.

Jones and Wolf (1980)[618a] describe the use of e.m.g. biofeedback training during movement, as a method of treating chronic low back pain.

In an excellent review, Hurrell (1980)[581a] suggests that because EMG feedback involves impressive technology, both therapist and patient may be particularly susceptible to the effects of optimistic expectations. Further,

It is important to emphasise that despite the proliferation of publications on the use of EMG feedback, few studies have been conducted with the rigour normally expected in clinical trials of new therapeutic agents or techniques.

G. THE BACK 'SCHOOL'

Nachemson (1975)[889a] remarks that recent studies have shown that both biochemical and mechanical factors are probably of importance in the genesis of back pain, that for the present we cannot successfully treat the chemical component, and should concentrate on the mechanical component. In passing, we might also concentrate on the *neurophysiological* component (p. 384) and the factor of *functional interdependence* of the spine (p. 38).

Knowledge gained from intravital disc-pressure manometry provides the basis for his advocacy of a generalised treatment programme of four instructional group-sessions, in which six patients are led by a physiotherapist. During the first lesson, basic anatomy and function of the spine, and simple information on low back pain, are taught with an emphasis on self-help.

The importance of resting in the 'psoas-release' position (p. 457), isometric abdominal exercises, ergonomic instruction in the techniques of lifting, and the nature of increased disc pressure during functional activities are also taught.

At the end of each instructional session the group practises the exercises and then rests in the 'psoas position' for discussion with the therapist. The treatment programme, for acute back pain rather than the chronic joint problem, is based on rational and well-proven principles:

1. Understanding the nature of the problem makes it much easier to cope with
2. Meeting others 'in the same boat' is always helpful
3. Learning how to rest, and use the body machinery more effectively
4. Strengthening the abdominal muscles by isometric exercise.

The 'group dynamic' is a powerful factor in human psychology; Harding (1977)[500] has emphasised how man's strength lies in the group, the clan, the tribe, and 'for psychological development [he] requires both an outer and an inner environment'. The comforting outer environment, of like sufferers, nourishes and reassures the inner environment.

Again, the knowledge that an examination will be set at the end of the course of treatment is a powerful stimulus to pay attention to the teaching; the writer recalls the notable increase in alertness when a spirit of competition was first introduced to the annual CSP Manipulation Courses in 1968, in the form of theoretical, practical and later, clinical examinations.

Bergquist-Ullman and Larsson (1977)[85] who present a prospective study of acute low back pain in industry and its treatment by group methods, also present an equally convincing exposition of how little is really known about low back pain.

Thus, for a condition not awfully well understood, group treatment is advocated, and the nature of the joint problem is explained to the patient! The observations of Greenman, and of Northupp (pp. 384, 388) are relevant here.

The authors suggest that because several patients are treated at a time, relatively small resources are needed to achieve the same effect as other forms of physiotherapy including manipulative treatment.

A notable feature of the treatment approach was the therapist's visit to the patients' work-site, for about 1 hour at first, and for about 30 minutes a fortnight later, to assess the effects of ergonomic instruction. The arrangement probably works well in large industrial complexes, when the industrial physiotherapist can quickly reach various parts of the workshops or administrative section, but the travelling time and sheer logistics of a therapist making two visits in a fortnight, to the work-place of 70 patients (i.e. the number participating in the trial reported) scattered about a city, rather alters the time and staffing economics of the method.

A logical extension of the principles of group treatment is the development of a thorax 'school', a hip 'school' and neck, shoulder, knee and foot 'schools', which, so far as remedial exercises in groups is concerned, was developed in the early post-war years.[197] This came about because very large numbers of injured men had received treatment consisting of soothing warmth, massage and passive movements. Although in those days limb and spinal fractures, amputations and serious ligamentous injuries comprised the bulk of the conditions which overwhelmingly necessitated a new emphasis on active, energetic and progressive exercises in groups, the classic ingredient of pressure on physiotherapy departments has not changed.

For hospitals and large industrial organisations the central dilemma is that of a flood of patients with musculoskeletal pain, faced by a clinical workforce which is too small and in some cases not specialised enough. Where individual treatment of musculoskeletal pain is not sufficiently precise, effective and speedy, sheer economics will dictate an emphasis on group treatment.

There remains an element of 'umbrella' treatment in the method; for the writer, the inherent defect of any group method of treatment, whether it be the back school, group exercises in lifting and handling or generalised back exercise groups such as were common a decade or two ago, is that of a tendency for the therapist concerned to learn very much more about group treatment than about the infinite variety of ways in which back pain can present, about the comprehensive and multifactorial nature of low back pain and about individually appropriate treatment.

The well-informed modern therapist, who has become accustomed to conducting a thorough and meticulous 'indications' examination and assessment procedure for musculoskeletal problems, is not likely to enjoy giving 'shot-gun-like' treatments (however well founded in general terms) without first making a comprehensive attempt to understand the clinical pattern of presentation so that a treatment plan may be formulated accordingly.

As the advent of virtually routine, successful hip replacement surgery has tended to blunt the purposefulness of research into degenerative arthrosis of the hip, there may be a tendency for group treatment methods for back pain to engender a blunting of physiotherapists' drive to fully comprehend what back pain *is*. When the incentive to learn is removed, we do not learn.

Perhaps the time-honoured and largely unquestioned association of physiotherapy and group exercises may progressively have a ball-and-chain effect upon the development, by physiotherapists, of their fuller potential as highly skilled members of the clinical team.

With respect, one does not need to be especially skilled to give group remedial exercises; in times past the writer was very efficiently taught, among other physical skills, in under six months to do this with confidence and expertise. While we remain tethered and therefore grounded by the classical association of a part of physiotherapy with group exercises, like 'horse and carriage', so long shall we have unnecessary difficulty in overdue metamorphosis into more sophisticated clinical occupations. It may well be that physiotherapy helpers, and not physiotherapists, should be occupied in giving group exercises, and the real talents of physiotherapists developed to the point where appropriate and quickly effective treatment, together with such explanation as fits the case, is given according to the needs of the individual.

18. Prophylaxis

Some people are well aware of which positions suit them, and which postures tend to increase or provoke their particular joint pain, although they seldom have a clear idea how great are the forces developed by usual activities such as sweeping leaves, raking lawns, stooping at a spin-dryer and bending to wash hair at a basin.

Most need help in *analysing the relationship* between what they do, how they do it and why they suffer musculoskeletal pain.

The basic principle is that of avoiding extreme positions or extreme stress for long periods, and the writer's view is that patients should be advised and encouraged to discover by experiment what suits them, following a brief exposition of the effects of sustained stress on soft tissues, so far as it applies to the features of their particular joint problems. (Supports are discussed on p. 468).

An interminable list of instructions can be counterproductive, and frequently focuses an undesirable amount of attention on presumed defects and weaknesses.

The more we encounter the consequences of what has been said to patients in the past, the more plain it is that much anxiety and overconcern about disease and arthritis can be prevented, by never using either word unless it is justified (p. 305). It very seldom is. Degenerative change as such is not 'disease' in the sense that patients conceive it to be.

In the use of prophylactic exercise a distinction should be made between

a. Those which are designed for one patient to complement, and continue the effect of, localised manual treatment to single segments, and
b. Those which are given for home use because they have a generally beneficial effect upon soft-tissue extensibility, ranges of movement and muscle power.

Those given below are for the most part in the second category.

CERVICAL SPINE

(i) Resting postures

Prolonged extension, or the posture of looking upward for even a few seconds, may be sufficient to produce mild syncope. Extension combined with rotation can reduce the lumen of the vertebral artery, with the consequences of vertebrobasilar ischaemia.

Cervical extension tends also to increase root tension at the cervicothoracic junction, where the roots may have undergone two successive angulations before emerging from the foramen (p. 102).

Conversely, prolonged flexion exerts traction on cervical nerve roots and their dural sleeves,[130, 121a] with flattening and broadening of the spinal cord against the osseocartilaginous spurs of spondylotic change,[117] and consequent localised ischaemia (see p. 56).

Side-flexion is usually difficult for the mature or elderly patient, anyway, and since prolonged side-flexion is a posture of strain, it is evident that a *neutral* position is probably the best resting posture for the neck.

This does not mean the military posture of 'attention'—which is a posture of strain (see p. 469)—but that as a general rule the patient should always try to keep the neck as 'long' as possible.

It is sensible to use the support of one hand beneath the chin when reading or writing for long. If the neck feels tired in the evening, a 'bow-tie' or 'butterfly' pillow, with the contents shaken out to the ends and the constricted centre placed in the nape of the neck, gives comfortable support when sitting in an armchair.

Allowing the head to droop forward and to one side, when dozing in trains and armchairs, is a potent cause of painful neck problems. This is quite different from the exercise described below (p. 497).

When sleeping, a good quality down pillow, which accommodates the weight of head and neck and then inertly remains in that configuration, is better than a sorbo-rubber filling which offers an active resistance by its resilience, and is thus less adaptable to the individual's shape.

Again, a 'bow-tie' pillow will support the neck on three aspects. Whether one or two or three pillows are used depends upon the patient's physique and the pillows' thickness; the important factor is support in a neutral position.

Patients who regularly retire at night without a headache and frequently wake up with one, need to give special attention to preventive measures, and may also need a soft night collar for a while. These measures are often more important than treatment, unless frank cervical joint problems are present.

(ii) Activity

Extreme positions or postural stresses for long periods (i.e. driving, reading, sewing, preparing food, looking round, looking up as in decorating, working beneath a motor-car) for more than one hour should be avoided.

Typists who continually look down and to one side should try to modify their work-habits. Fruit pickers who persistently reach overhead, and farmers who look behind to keep an eye on the furrow when ploughing, are also at risk.

Carrying suitcases or shopping in one hand imposes severe stress on the cervical soft tissues and joints. Where possible, the weight should be divided between sides; where not, frequent rest periods are necessary. As soon as the patient *begins* to be aware of strain, the strain should be relieved by doing the opposite for a little while, and moving the neck around a bit. After decorating a ceiling, for example, it is wise to kneel on all fours and allow the head to hang down for a little while; this will relieve chronically approximated neural arch structures by reason of the flexion and the mild traction effect.

Driving is a posture of strain for the neck (see p. 470)—much episodic neck pain is related to driving stress. Thus it may be important for some patients to temporarily wear a malleable collar when driving, so that cervical rotation is possible when needed, yet the head is prevented from sinking further and further forward as the mileage builds up. As important is the need to stop, get out and walk around for a bit—every hour or so, whether the patient has neck problems or not. The back supports of car seats should be high enough, and the head-rest arranged so that the driver's neck may be in a comfortable neutral position. It is not unreasonable to expect that before long, the upholstery configuration of a car driver's seat will be a matter for individual tailoring, by the use of medium-density foam (e.g. Dunloprene D12), and that the shape of the upper thoracic back rest will receive as much attention as the lumbar support.

Neck extension frequently provokes cervical pain. Farhni (1976)[336] has very sensibly referred to the spasmodic neck extension which occurs at the climax of sexual intercourse. Those with cervical joint problems should be advised to try keeping the chin tucked down, and to continue trying until the manœuvre succeeds and its prophylactic effect is demonstrated.

(iii) Preventive exercises

Besides isometric exercises (p. 464) to help overcome symmetrical or asymmetrical tightness, or for other specific purposes, it is wise for healthy people to make two or three full-range excursions of the neck each day. Anterior cervical muscles frequently become elongated and weakened, and this is much easier to prevent than to reverse.

a. A mild traction effect, and prophylactic extension of the ligamentum nuchae, is produced when lying supine with the head on two pillows and the knees and hips bent; the head is smoothly raised and the chin depressed to the chest as closely as possible. After lowering smoothly to the pillow, the exercise is repeated 10–20 times.

b. A more positive exercise is that of sitting in a chair with the arms abducted and the palms, with fingers interlaced, resting on the forehead. While strictly maintaining a neutral neck position, the forehead is pressed against the hands to produce isometric contraction of the anterior neck muscles. The force of the contraction should be built up slowly and smoothly, and over one to three minutes daily.

Although the generalised full-range movement (*vide supra*) are valuable for the neck as a whole, the occipito-atlantal joint may need localised home exercises, and while there exist localised exercise techniques which involve somewhat exotic hand placings for fixation purposes, many patients are just not able to do them.[145]

c. While sitting with the hands lightly grasping the sides of the chair-seat, a simple lateral glide of the head and neck from side to side (like a Balinese dancer), exercises the craniovertebral junction more than the lower segments. If this is *then* followed by simple nodding exercises and full rotation from side to side in the same sitting position, the C0–C1 segment has been given an adequate 'home exercise' treatment in its important ranges. Five excursions in every direction are enough.

CERVICOTHORACIC REGION

(i) Resting postures

The two requirements are that (a) the part should be *relaxed*, and the cervicothoracic region cannot be relaxed unless the cervical, thoracic and lumbar spines are also relaxed by being supported. Thus the support must be from seat to occiput, and (b) the shoulder girdle must be relieved of the weight of the arms, which should lie on arm-rests or pillows. It will be plain that these requirements are seldom fully satisfied for long, even when individuals are supposedly relaxing at home and watching television, for example.

During waking hours, the cervicothoracic region is more or less constantly 'on call', and is probably the hardest-working of all vertebral regions.

(ii) Activities

Patients should be made aware that all activities with the head bent forward, and involving pulling, pushing or pressing movements with the arms (hanging washing, hanging curtains, polishing the car, cleaning windows, pushing recalcitrant motor-cars, prolonged ironing, pull-starters of lawnmowers, outboard engines, etc.) place heavy stress on the 'yoke' area architecture of the spine and shoulder girdles, and these activities must not be prolonged.

It seems almost the rule that the upper thoracic region becomes virtually 'fossilised', so far as joint movement is concerned, in late middle age; this may be because the greater amount, by far, of functional use of the arms involves work in front of the body.

The cervicothoracic region slowly becomes less of an 'empilement' of mobility segments, and more of a region providing a stable attachment for the powerful isotonic and isometric actions of the neck and shoulder-girdle musculature. It follows that connective-tissue becomes progressively thickened, and movement steadily diminishes, as the functional role described above is gradually imposed upon the upper thoracic segments, and structure adapts to function.

This does not necessarily affect the upper two costal joints quite so much—upper rib joint movement abnormalities occur in late maturity, although they are more frequent in younger people.

(iii) Preventive exercises

Paradoxically, the key to relieving, as well as preventing, 'yoke' area pains which are clearly associated with thickened and tender upper thoracic vertebral joints, is that of attending to *shortened and tight pectoral muscles* as well as the joint problem. In general terms, manual segmental mobilisation techniques for hypomobility which are not complemented by exercises to maintain or improve mobility, are not enough; the cervicothoracic region is a prime example of this principle.

Simple exercises are:

a. Stand in a doorway with the arms abducted to 135° and the palms placed against the door jambs. Keep the elbows straight and push the chest (*not* the abdomen, which may painfully hyperextend the low back) through the doorway (Figs 18.1, 18.2).

This exercise is intended for tight pectoral structures, and is not suitable for a painful condition of the glenohumeral joint, unless there is no irritability and treatment has reached the stage of encouraging the last few degrees of elevation in 30° or so of abduction.

b. With the knees bent and feet resting on the support, place one palm behind the occiput and lie supine with the upper thorax over the edge of a stout table (a folded towel relieves painful pressure on the upper thoracic spinous processes). It will be found that resting one ankle just above the opposite bent knee relieves a tendency to lumbar lordosis.[145] Allow the weight of head, neck and arm to

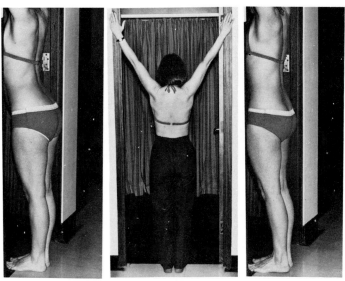

Fig. 18.1 A home exercise for stretching the pectoral muscles (centre). The chest is pressed forward, with the arms stabilised by the door jamb. Producing a lumbar lordosis by pushing the abdomen forward is incorrect (left); the normal posture of the spine should be maintained (right) and it is worthwhile spending a little time ensuring that the patient well understands the procedure.

gently extend the upper thoracic region. The weight of the head should *not* be allowed to hyperextend the neck, by removing occipital support.

c. While sitting, reach the right arm round the left side, beneath the chin, to place the pad of the middle fingers on the *right* side of the C7 spinous process. Repetitively rotate the head and neck to the *left* side. By stabilising C7 (or C6 or T1) in this way, rotation mobility is exercised. Repeat to opposite side. Some patients are just not able to do this exercise.[145]

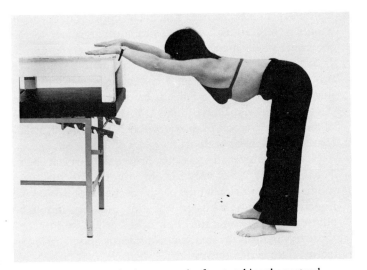

Fig. 18.2 An alternative home exercise for stretching the pectoral muscles. The patient stands with feet astride and, with the elbows kept extended, places the palms on a flat support at about chest height. By repetitively leaning backwards from the ankles, the chest is depressed to the floor, and the pectoral soft tissues repetitively stretched.

THORACIC SPINE

(i) Resting postures

By reason of the continuity and overlapping attachments of the vertebral soft tissues, and thus the physical *interdependence* of the spine, the thoracic region cannot be completely relaxed unless the head, neck and lumbar spine are relaxed by being supported. Hence, supine lying on the floor with the knees bent, the head on a small pillow and the hands lying loosely on the abdomen, is one position in which the thoracic cage *is* relaxed, and its postural tendency to kyphosis counteracted.

(ii) Activity

During heavy work involving grasping, carrying, pushing, pulling and levering objects sideways, the magnitude of forces acting upon the thoracic spine and rib joints is great, and commonly patients have little idea of the magnitude of these forces.[230, 231, 232]

The muscles of neck, shoulder and scapulae, and the erector spinae, abdominal muscles, diaphragm and quadratus lumborum exert great stress upon the thoracic architecture during powerful use of the arms and trunk. Similarly, coughing, sneezing and vomiting considerably stress the thoracic joints.

Activities which stress the cervicothoracic junction (p. 498) also stress the thoracic joints, and should not be prolonged without break.

When pushing an unresponsive motor-car, short steps are better than long strides, since the addition of pelvic rotational stress may be significant in exceeding tolerable levels of stress on thoracic joints. Although the glottis is usually closed at the moment of a lifting heave, it is better to keep the airway open during heavy use of the arms and trunk in pulling and pushing operations. When coughing or sneezing is felt to be imminent, it is wise to bend the knees and hold the lumbar and thoracic spines in a neutral position.

The driving position is important, and a well-raked backrest of the driving seat (as in some low-slung cars with little headroom) makes more work for thoracic muscles. Rosemeyer (1971)[1057] found increased myoelectrical activity in thoracic muscle when the backrest angle was around 140°. The least e.m.g. activity in spinal musculature occurs when the angle is around 120°.[30, 31, 32]

It is difficult to understand why patients are sometimes advised to sit as close to the steering wheel as possible.[780] The height of the backrest should be sufficient to wholly support the thorax, and the configuration should include *lateral* support to improve trunk stabilisation—when the trunk is not sufficiently stabilised there is extra stress on the arms and consequently upon the trunk musculature.[31]

The action of leaning forward when sitting and reaching over a desk to lift a weight of around 2–3 lb (1–2 kg) produces a high magnitude of both intravital disc pressure and myoelectrical back muscle activity. Patients should be warned about this, and advised to stand up, and get support from one hand placed on the desk, before they reach for a weight at the far edge of a desk or table.

(iii) Preventive exercises

The position of relaxed leaning backwards in sitting, against the low back support of a standard office chair, is that in which the intravital disc pressures are lowest[30, 31] and office workers should take up this position from time to time during the working day—many of them instinctively do.

a. A deep inspiration, while raising the arms to full elevation and leaning backwards in the chair, is also a method of reversing the effects of prolonged sitting in a hunched position. Relief from thoracic strain is also gained by lying supine on the floor, with the knees bent and the arms abducted to 135°.

The exercise for maintaining extensibility of the pectoral muscle group (p. 498) is also useful in this respect.

b. Extension mobility of the thorax, and the power of dorsal musculature, is maintained by the exercise of sitting in one's heels on the floor and bending forward to rest the forehead on the floor in front of the knees. The forearms are pronated so that the dorsum of the hands rest alongside the legs. Without altering the flexed posture of the lumbar spine, the thoracic spine is extended, the arms externally rotated and the scapulae approximated, as the head (maintained in a neutral relationship) and shoulders are raised to flatten the thoracic spine. The position is held for an increasing number of seconds as the patient becomes familiar with the purpose and technique of the exercise, which may be fairly strongly progressed by abducting the arms to 90°. Five to ten daily repetitions are enough (Fig. 18.3).

c. Side-flexion and rotation mobility, and mobility of the rib-cage, may be exercised by sitting on a stool or chair with the knees apart. While keeping the pelvis stabilised, one hand firmly reaches for the floor as the opposite arm is elevated to some 150° behind the plane of the trunk, and is looked at by turning head and trunk to that side. The exercise should be done smoothly and easily to full range without jerking. Repeat to opposite side, with 5 to 10 daily repetitions.

Nursing mothers are more prone to thoracic strain than may be recognised, and the exercises described are a useful preventive measure.

The benefits of swimming, badminton and squash are plain, yet patients often need reminding of what they know, i.e. the simple value of free activity. While Yoga exercises have a tendency to produce joint problems in the overenthusiastic, the cult is an excellent way of maintaining thoracic mobility, so long as the fervour to progress too rapidly in ability is kept in reasonable check by a good teacher.

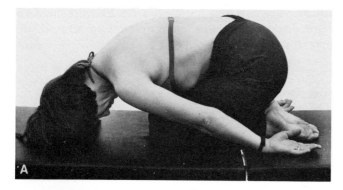

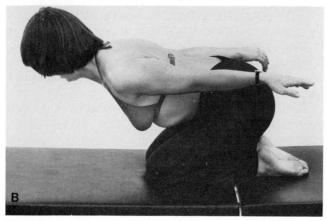

Fig. 18.3 Exercise to maintain thoracic extension mobility and power of dorsal musculature.
(A) Starting position.
(B) Static (isometric) hold in the extended position. The exercise may be progressed by external rotation of the arms, while held closely to the sides.

THE LOW BACK

Introduction
There is not necessarily a direct relationship between the volume of literature on a particular subject and the orderly accumulation of facts about it; the prophylaxis of low back pain is one such example. The mountain of literature on the multifarious aspects of pathology of common spinal articular changes, particularly disc changes, is massive enough to have become all things to all men—it is now so great that each can find in it what they might wish to find, while a great deal is yet unsolved.

Emphasis, in the prevention of low back pain, tends to become polarised around two factors: (a) What is the pathology? and (b) What can we do about it? Yet there are other factors of great importance; for example, questions of human kinetics and good movement appear to figure in prophylaxis much less than they should.[28, 29]

Concepts of the most efficient way to manually handle and lift are too often concentrated on *simple mechanical factors*, at the expense of something which is harder to teach but is of prime importance—training in use of the body so that extensibility and vascularity of all soft tissues

is equally maintained according to their function, and so that the tissues on one aspect of a limb, or the trunk, are not steadily changed to become permanently tighter, shortened, relatively ischaemic and more prone to injury when stressed (see also p. 509).

Anderson (1971)[29] observes:

The difference between good and bad movement is frequently subtle and the distinction often cannot be made without knowing (a) the purpose of the action involved; (b) how the movement was initiated ... there is ample evidence that structural deterioration of the body tissues results from excessive tension in different parts of the body ... mechanisation in industry has reduced the amount of hard labour but it has increased the tendency to *cumulative strain* ... it is unfortunate that, like so many other functional aspects of the human body, the subtle progression of cumulative strain is most difficult to demonstrate by means of laboratory experiments, otherwise many existing conceptions of physical activities would probably have been altered many years ago ... [yet the] immediate reaction to excessive muscular tension and its relation to cumulative strain can be demonstrated by a practical experiment. For example, when the fist is clenched as firmly as possible, with forearm flexed, for about 30 seconds and the fingers are then allowed to relax slowly, it will usually be found that they remain more flexed than normal. Some of the tension remains as a 'hangover', and if this type of action is repeated constantly from day to day, without ever stretching the tissues, normal extension of the fingers will become more and more restricted. Connective tissue as well as muscle fibres will become shortened and it is then reasonable to expect that some capillary occlusion will occur in the tissues concerned. It is, in the experience of the writer, deterioration of this kind occurring in neck, shoulders, and lower back that accounts for the frequency of disabilities and restricted movement in those areas.

Nachemson (1976)[889b] observes that the true cause of back pain remains obscure: '... we do not know where the pain comes from, or at what level we are treating the patient, e.g. at the level of the motion segment, at the level of the dorsal horn neurons in the cord or at higher levels in the brain.'

In much writing, the two factors of bias and advocacy are sometimes more prominent than data. Thus: (a) enthusiastic extrapolation, based upon the considered importance of this or that description of pathological change, and (b) the search for conveniently generalised, standard 'hand-outs' of prophylactic advice for patients have prompted a variety of recommendations for preventing the onset, or the recurrence, of painful joint problems.

Many of the recommendations appear based only on simplified mechanical concepts as they relate to the intervertebral disc, and appear to take little account of the multifactorial nature and behaviour of vertebral pain,[486] or the probability that the true genesis of injury might include steady and selective deterioration of soft tissues over a prolonged period beforehand.

Farfan (1973)[326] has drawn attention to the relatively minor developmental differences which may render an individual susceptible to back pain in later life. These anomalies are common, and many occur in the neural arches or their processes, although low back pain which is considered due to facet-joint arthrosis occurs often enough in the absence of detectable anomaly.

Weinstein *et al.* (1977)[1300] provide a well-referenced description of the many abnormalities found in the posterior (neural arch) structures in lumbar spondylosis.

... two elderly male patients' legs became numb and weak after walking or even standing for just 10 to 15 minutes. Neither of these patients had pulse diminutions in the legs but they developed absence of tendon reflexes in the legs as well as anaesthesias at the height of their walking- or standing-induced attacks. Both of these patients exhibited prompt disappearance of the symptoms povoked by the erect posture shortly after they sat down. One of the two patients, who could ride a bicycle bent over the handlebars and played tennis from a crouch but could not kneel erect without the prompt appearance of numbness and paresis, supports the belief that lordotic posture rather than exercise-induced leg muscle ischaemia was the critical factor. This patient was comfortable lying supine in a hammock but developed his trouble immediately upon turning over to the prone position. Upon exploration of this patient, the yellow ligament between L3 and L4 was found to be pathologically thick; following laminectomy and removal of this ligament, he could walk for hours.[1300]

It is well known that discal injury may occur during excessive loading stress in unsuitable postures, yet back injury involves structures other than discs and although *stooping* is harmful (particularly under load), simple *flexion* is not necessarily so. While the lumbar neural arch structures play only a minor role in pure axial loading (which almost never occurs in normal activity), there is a large strain on these structures during off-centre compression and during posterior compression (extension). Lin *et al* (1978)[747] have shown that the posterior elements transmit considerable force during quasistatic complex loading, and especially so in extension and frontal shear. Other investigators[484] have also indicated the magnitude of forces acting upon facet-joint structures; the damage produced by these forces was demonstrated by Harris and Macnab (1954)[508] more than 25 years ago.

Jayson (1980)[608a] described modern bioengineering techniques to study the strain distribution in cadaveric lumbar spines and observed that:

Under central compressive loads, the compressive strains were greatest in the posterior elements of the spine and tensile strains were greatest at the vertebral rims above and below the intervertebral discs. Disc bulge and strain were greater posteriorly and postero-laterally than anteriorly. When the compressive load was anteriorly offset to simulate forward flexion, the compressive strains on the vertebrae increased anteriorly but the tangential strain increased posteriorly. When the spine was extended, compressive strains decreased anteriorly and increased to *very high*

levels posteriorly (my italics) and particularly in the laminae and apophyseal processes. Disc bulge increased posteriorly but tangential strain increased anteriorly.

Notwithstanding a persistent belief that 'the lower intervertebral disc most likely causes the pain'[889b] there is now ample evidence that changes in the neural arch structures[867] are equally capable of producing the clinical features of back pain with reduced straight-leg-raising which have been regarded as the signs of 'a slipped disc.' The truth is that we do not *know*; this being so, we might get our best guidance from the thing we *do* know about, i.e. *the unique clinical presentation from patient to patient.* For example, Maigne[789] observes that a proportion of 'lumbago' arises not from the low lumbar joints but from the thoracolumbar junction segments, being referred to the lumbar region. This pain is relieved by localised treatment of low thoracic and upper lumbar segments.

Severe aggravation of the clinical feature of spinal stenosis, by lordotic postures, is well documented by Weinstein *et al.* (1977)[1300] yet despite a considerable increase in awareness of the pathomechanics of spinal stenosis, patients with back pain and sciatica continue to be advised of the importance of maintaining, and even increasing, the 'natural' lumbar lordosis, sometimes without reference to that most dominant feature, *the particular nature and pattern of clinical features.*

Improvement in the range of lumbar movements, in the sagittal and in other planes, is a prime aim of treatment for backache, and in general terms a logical basis for prophylaxis.

Hypotheses about changes in the configuration of lumbar intervertebral discs, in particular postures, may have little relationship to what actually occurs (Fig. 18.4), since there is a relative dearth of experiments which might clarify our difficulties.

In the prevention of low back pain, some authorities[335, 336, 151] strongly recommend the flexed posture and eradication of lordosis, while other workers[218, 834] stress the value of maintaining a lumbar lordosis and remind the patient that they are at risk of a recurrence if they lose the hollow in the low back for any length of time.

It is sometimes suggested that African natives do not get backache, because of their tendency to stand with a somewhat exaggerated lordosis, yet from the experience of living in that country for many years the writer knows this to be untrue. Backache is a serious concern to industrial medical officers in continents like Africa.[1340]

Some booklets seem to give patients the impression that the single painful episode which prompted treatment, and prophylactic advice, is unlikely to occur again so long as this or that recommendation is faithfully followed.

For example, the following sentences, by a physician, occur within the compass of a few pages: '... most back pain need never occur if people take sensible precautions

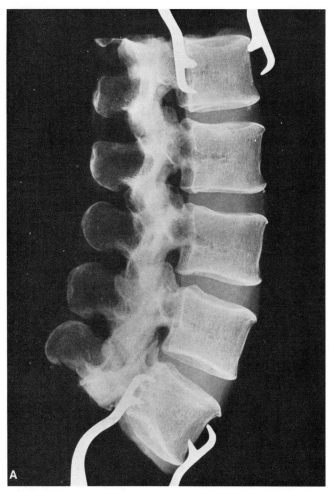

Fig. 18.4 The series (A) to (H) are radiographs of a young girl's lumbar spine, some 12 hours postmortem, being extended and flexed by bone-forceps attached to L5 below and L1 above. The two men conducting the experiment, each to a pair of forceps, exerted all their power to move the specimen to its full limit of sagittal movement. (Reproduced by courtesy of GTF Braddock FRCS. Personal communication, 1979.)

(A) *Extension* and (B) *flexion* with neural arches intact. In extension, the anterior longitudinal ligament is taut; in flexion, the posterior longitudinal ligament is now taut and the discs are bulging anteriorly. There is no posterior bulge of the disc.

against it.' '. . . intelligent planning could prevent you getting backache in the first place.' '. . . we know remarkably little about the causes and cure of back pain.'

It is sometimes overlooked that vertebral degenerative joint change has existence in time as well as space (like chronic bronchitis); that prophylactic measures can only *reduce* the likelihood of painful recurrences is sometimes not made clear to patients.

The unavoidable demands of life, e.g. suddenly reaching to protect a child at risk, having to change the wheel of a car, nursing a sick relative, a night in an unaccustomedly soft hotel bed, will occur sooner or later to induce a painful episode—prophylaxis can only reduce their frequency.

We have no therapy which can compete with the infinite capacity of patients to reinjure themselves.

Prophylactic regimes which include the few well-recognised basic principles of manual handling, together with

sections which owe more to bias and advocacy than to certain knowledge, are probably as likely to succeed in as many cases as those which contain the few basic principles only; we do not yet know why. When very experienced surgeons, physicians and therapists advocate the prophylactic value of lumbar flexion, and other equally experienced physicians and therapists advocate an extension regime, plainly there is room for more certainty.

Reducing the likelihood of musculoskeletal spinal pain, and preventing recurrence of painful episodes, is a field of endeavour in which our sketchy knowledge is evident. To paraphrase Oscar Wilde:[977] 'Truth is seldom simple, and is far from plain.' For example, instruction in manual handling and lifting is almost universally believed to have prophylactic value, although there is no scientific evidence that this has been effective in reducing the severity or frequency of back pain;[412b] while Charlesworth, *et al.* (1978)[168] have no doubt, on practical or theoretical

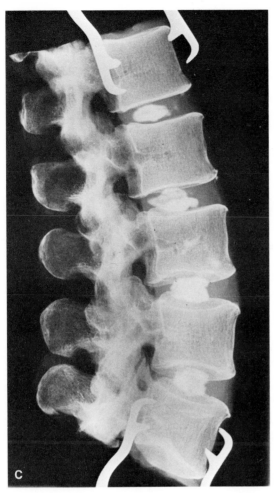

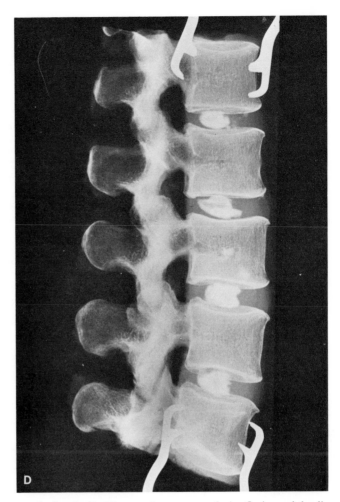

(c) *Extension* and (D) *flexion*. The nuclei have been injected with radio-opaque material. It is plain that the posterior part of the nucleus pulposus of the L2–L3 segment has migrated a little anteriorly, as the posterior longitudinal ligament becomes taut during flexion and the disc bulges anteriorly.

grounds, that such training contributes significantly to the prevention of back trouble.

Neither do we know why there was a 22 per cent increase in back pain episodes, and a 30 per cent increase in their duration, between 1961 and 1967,[1338] long after programmes of lifting training had been instituted in many spheres of industry, in the nursing profession and in physiotherapy, for example, when the writer was active in this field of prophylaxis.

'There is little evidence based on prospective epidemiological studies to prove the value of training but there is no doubt that a well-prepared programme can have satisfactory results, even if one of the mechanisms is a Hawthorne effect, i.e. the initial improvement in performance which tends to follow any change of management.' (Troup, 1979.)[1250b]

Where a high morbidity rate, due to repetitive industrial handling of a specific kind, has provided experience for the formulation of *detailed on-the-job handling techniques*, there appears to be definite benefit from organised training of this kind,[233] but at a meeting of European and American workers in the field of low back pain prophylaxis, it was agreed that there appers to be no evidence of benefit from *general* education in lifting and handling techniques.

While there is some recent and slight evidence[1250b] that the determined application of lifting and handling techniques may result in somewhat less backache, a besetting difficulty is that the techniques appear to their modest best only in those work environments which can be rigorously controlled, and monitored, in a manner approaching the average laboratory research project.

The overwhelming majority of occupational stress occurs during the unforeseeable hurly-burly of daily living—in the care of small children, in household, garden, space-restricted storerooms and loading bays, garages, do-it-yourself jobs, the sports field, multifarious agricultural work, dressing in a hurry, moving house, horseplay with children, walking over difficult terrain and strange hotel beds—any degree of control or monitoring of these chance stresses is unrealistic, though possibly the time is not too far off when training in dynamic body postures will be

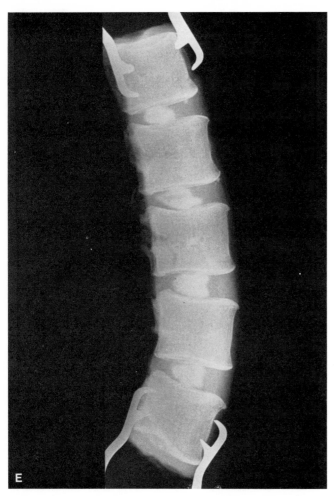

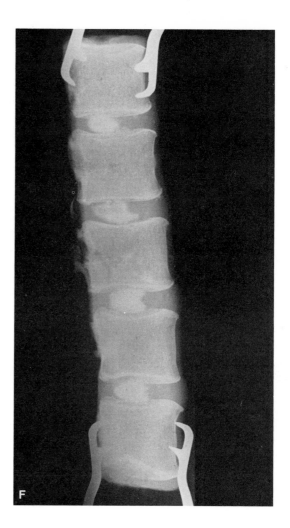

(E) *Extension* and (F) *flexion*. With the neural arches removed, the ranges of movement are virtually identical, suggesting the role of the annulus fibrosus in governing the amplitude of sagittal movement.

as much a feature of education in schools as the ubiquitous calculator.

The abundance of little booklets[168, 248, 335, 527, 671, 1068, 1252, 1321] and advice sheets providing basic information on joint problems, and conflicting advice for lay people, is an uneasy reminder that the few certainties lie buried beneath the weight of vocal advocacy for this or that approach to the problem. One recommends sitting down whenever possible,[780] and another warns against sitting for long.[834] Sit with the back rounded, sit with it hollow, and so on. A likelihood for the patient who reads all of them, in the search for enlightenment and guidance, is that they will become a little confused.

Hutton and Adams (1980)[584a] investigated the forces acting on the neural arch and carried out experiments with a hydraulic servo-controlled testing machine which gave outputs of applied force against joint deformation. They concluded that the lordotic standing and fully flexed postures *both* seem important in the aetiology of low back pain and degenerative changes in the apophyseal joints.

Adams and Hutton (1980)[3a] have also reported a cadaver experiment which strongly suggests that lumbar interbody joints can resist the greatest compressive force when flexed between 4° and 8°. When flexed to greater degrees, the compressive force of back muscle contraction is likely to first damage the supraspinous and interspinous ligaments, and then the intervertebral disc.

Among the many writers of advice booklets for back sufferers, a recent one[722] suggests several options for resting positions and instructs readers to choose the one giving most relief. The important factor of *self-assessment* is a welcome feature.

As might be expected, observations on back pain and prophylaxis, by those who have spent many decades physically handling low back problems on the clinical shopfloor (Stoddard, 1979)[1183b] will be of more practical value than the more generalised observations of others without this hard-won experience.

Some 20 years ago, following a 5-day course of practical shopfloor experience in handling drums, gas cylinders, girders and other heavy industrial weights the writer, who was an active member of the CSP Committee on Posture and Lifting, became convinced of the need to keep the back straight, in a position approaching active extension, dur-

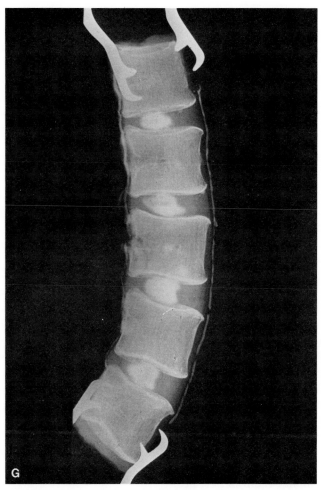

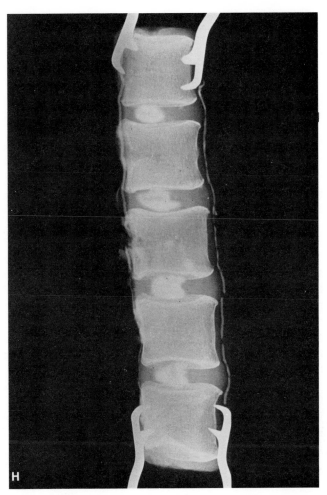

(G) *Extension* and (H) *flexion*. Longitudinal ligaments have been outlined with barium paste. Disc bulging posteriorly during extension at the L4–L5 segment, with anterior bulging at all segments during flexion, is plain.

ing manual handling and lifting (Grieve, 1958).[442] Now sadder and wiser since those days, and more familiar with the infinite variety of forms in which cervical, thoracic and lumbar joint problems may present, it seems plain that advice on prophylaxis, and lifting and handling, after an analysis of household and industrial working difficulties, *should not be too rigid.*

Although they may not be able to articulate their knowledge as clearly as we would like, patients are as a rule much more familiar than the therapist with (i) the *behaviour* of their pain and (ii) with the special ergonomic difficulties of their daily activities, unless a fairly comprehensive analysis during a workplace visit is made, yet very many of them need help to analyse the relationship between the behaviour of their painful episodes and the way they have had to work or the way in which they rest.

The flexible application of principles which are clearly understood is probably better than highly detailed and 'military' instructions gloomily based on the dire need to keep the back straight at all times, or the back bent like a banana at all times.

'There is no "natural" way of lifting which is universal and thus biologically significant.' (Troup, 1979.)[1250b]

It is difficult to equate the advocacy of lordosis with the well-recognised need[326, 746, 780, 331, 151, 891] for improving the power of the abdominal wall musculature. For a proportion of patients with low back pain, sitting in a soft chair provokes the pain, and sitting erect with slight lordosis on a hard chair relieves or diminishes the pain. Conversely, for those whose low back pain is sharply provoked on standing for 15–30 minutes, and whose pain is spread bilaterally to buttocks and thighs on bending backwards for more than a few seconds, sitting (or squatting) is their method of gaining relief, and they may prefer a soft chair.

Quite apart from the clinical features of spinal stenosis, there is this group of patients whose symmetrical low back pain is unaccompanied by sciatica, reduced straight-leg-raising or neurological signs. The only movement which does *not* hurt is flexion (see p. 267). To advise this group to lie prone or supine with the legs straight, which are lordotic postures, and to passively hyperextend the spine as a regular exercise, even when these procedures are *seen* to provoke pain, may indicate that philosophies of treatment can become more important than what the treatment is all *about*, *viz*, the infinitely variable needs of patients (see p. 205).

While the experiment depicted in Figure 18.4A–H may not have completely simulated conditions *in vivo*, it nevertheless provides a valuable clue about the effects on lumbar intervertebral body joints of sagittal movement.

McKenzie (1977)[834] has demonstrated that the application of the few basic principles of prophylaxis in low back pain, including admonitions not to lose the lumbar lordosis, together with a passive extension exercise regime, tended to reduce the frequency of recurrence in a group of patients whose pain was considered due to 'flexion derangement', i.e. worse after prolonged sitting or bending. Patients whose pain could be abolished by flexion, and those with provocation of distal pain on extension, were not advised to follow the regime. It is apparently to this latter group of patients that the two similar 'flexion' regimes are addressed.[336, 780] So far as prophylactic exercise is concerned, clinical experience indicates that a considerable proportion of patients can diminish painful lumbar stiffness in the early morning by gently pulling the knees onto the chest, while lying supine.

Similarly, a flexion-exercise regime, designed to mobilise chronically tightened dorsal lumbosacral soft tissues, is the treatment of choice in some. Again, it is a natural reaction after sitting or driving for a long time, to stand with the feet apart, hands on hips, and to lean backward for a bit, whether one has backache or not.

In others, avoidance of flexion is important, yet this does not necessarily mean that they need to *hyperextend* their spines as a regular routine. The choice of prophylactic measures should be dictated entirely by the occupation and needs of the patient, as deduced from the clinical presentation, and not by the dictates of this or that approach to the problem of low back pain.

(i) Resting postures

Advice about resting postures should be modified to suit individuals' needs. A simplified black-and-white division into two common types of low back pain presentation is perhaps justified in order to make the point, but it has its dangers, since the two simplified groups certainly represent less than 50 per cent of all patterns of low back pain presentation.

Reference to the various clinical patterns described (pp. 250–300) will make this plain. For example, leg length inequality and lateral pelvic tilt are not described, although, in passing, the writer's clinical experience is that a flexion-type regime suits them much better than that of maintaining lordosis.

As an illustration we can describe a simplified '*A*' group who stand with a pronounced lordosis and have a somewhat weak abdominal wall. Their pattern of recurrence is that of:

a. Pain across the low back, initially with some spreading to both buttocks
b. Aggravation of pain by standing, walking, and lying prone or supine
c. All lumbar movements, other than flexion, provoke the pain
d. Flexion is painless, and free so far as tight lumbodorsal soft tissues will allow, with a localised low lumbar lordosis unchanged at the extreme of flexion
e. There are no neurological signs. Straight-leg-raising is fairly free, of equal range and not limited by pain.

That the posterior (neural arch) elements sustain considerable force during extension has been demonstrated by Lin *et al.* (1978)[747] (p. 501).

Shah *et al.* (1978))[1108] subjected the 4th lumbar vertebra and L4–L5 discs, of six cadaveric spines, to controlled compressive loading.

With central compressive loads, the maximal strain was found to occur near the base of the pedicles, and the superficial and deep surfaces of the pars interarticularis. The importance of the posterior vertebral elements, in transmitting load, was thus emphasised. On applying loads with a posterior offset, both compressive and tensile strains on the pars interarticularis were increased, suggesting the probable genesis of stress fractures and group II spondylolisthesis.

Since the dominant feature is that of pain provocation by any posture which approximates the posterior joint structures, it will be plain that a flexion type of regime will suit them better, i.e.

a. When standing for long, one foot should be rested some 40–50 cm above the ground, and one or both elbows or hands rested on the raised knee, so that the low back is not hollow. If this is not feasible, the patient should tilt the pelvis backward from time to time, holding it so for some seconds at each use of the exercise.
b. Sitting with a somewhat curved posture in a semi-reclining position.
c. Lying supine with hips and knees flexed, and calves resting on a support.
d. Lying prone, so long as a pillow or two under the abdomen prevents lordosis.
e. Side-lying with the knees bent up (some may need a small pillow under the loin, to prevent overapproximation of the uppermost lumbosacral structures).
f. A comfortable *sleeping* posture, which diminishes joint strain during the night, is that of side-lying with the hips and knees bent, but the uppermost limb being less flexed, so that the uppermost thigh comes to lie across mid-thigh and mid-calf of the underneath limb (Fig. 18.5).

Patients with the clinical features of frank spinal stenosis, with bilateral limb pains and paraesthesiae aggravated by lordotic postures, belong to this group rather

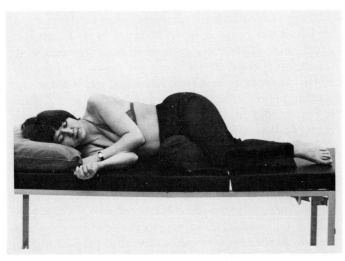

Fig. 18.5 A side-lying sleeping position, in which the usual disposition of lower limbs is reversed, puts less strain on the low lumbar region.

than the following one, as will those patients whose pain is assessed as being due to a mild or moderate degree of spondylolisthesis.

Conversely, a simplified 'B' group, whose painful recurrences are more likely to be provoked by prolonged sitting and bending, tend to present with:

a. A degree of loss of lordosis
b. Sometimes with slight listing to one or other side
c. The amount of pain on sitting and the preference for standing depends upon the severity of loss of lordosis
d. Severe but temporary incapacity after driving for more than 30–45 minutes
e. Less provocation of pain on bending backwards (which, if possible, they nevertheless do cautiously) than on flexion
f. Pain on side-flexion is variable, but is usually greater on bending towards the side of pain
g. Reduced straight-leg-raising, sometimes bilaterally and asymmetrically, but often on one side only
h. No neurological signs.

Akerblom (1949)[13] demonstrated that in sitting upright the lumbar spine is flexed.

Suitable resting postures for reducing painful episodes then are:

a. Standing normally with the weight on both feet; the patient should sit as soon as standing begins to bring on pain
b. Sitting with a support across the low back, if relaxed, and sitting upright in the neutral position if in a hard chair
c. Lying prone or supine on a hard surface
d. Sleeping on the side with the limbs disposed as described above, but with less flexion of both hips so that the neutral lumbar position is maintained.

The bed. The important factor is rest *in a position of comfort*, and not an arbitrarily imposed position unmodified by individual needs.

Lumbosacral joint problems are usually more comfortably rested on a firm mattress with boards beneath, but not invariably so. Mid-lumbar joint pain often responds to rest with the patient lying with knees flexed on a somewhat soft mattress. Patients should be encouraged to experiment and find for themselves what suits them, and perhaps should be advised not to expend large sums of money on specialised beds until they are satisfied that it is not possible to make arrangements using ordinary materials usually to hand.

(ii) Activities

Driving. An epidemiological study[646] has shown that commuters who drive some distance to and from work are twice as likely to experience severe back pain as those who do not drive daily; those who drive as a work occupation for most of the day are three times as likely to develop severe back pain.

With regard to driving posture and car seats, Anderson et al. (1975)[31] measured the e.m.g. activity of several back muscles, and the intravital lumbar disc pressures, of healthy subjects in automobile seats. The parameters were:

a. backrest inclination
b. degree of lumbar support
c. seat inclination
d. depression of the clutch
e. shifting gear.

The lowest level of both lumbar disc pressure and myoelectrical activity occurred when the backrest inclination was 120°, the lumbar support was 5 cm thick and the seat inclination 14°. A considerable increase was observed in lumbar disc pressure during depression of the clutch pedal; shifting of the gear lever also increased the disc pressure and influenced the myoelectrical activity. In general terms the lessons for the average driver are plain:

a. A seat which supports the low back so that it can *rest*, whether in neutral or in a degree of lordosis—whichever they find most comfortable.
b. A backrest inclined as above, and tall enough to support the upper thorax and shoulders, with a measure of 'wrap-around' support for the trunk and lateral buttocks. Car seats which allow a *lateral dipping* of one buttock can provoke otherwise latent lumbar pain.
c. A degree of hip and knee flexion which suits the driver (by fore and aft adjustment of the seat position).
d. A 'driving drill' of stopping and getting out for a stretch every hour or so during long journeys.
e. For commuter-drivers in heavy town traffic, automatic transmission, but also a more philosophical attitude to

traffic jams. Involuntary tensing of low back and pelvic girdle muscles, through the daily frustrations of driving in city streets, may be a more potent cause of 'driving backache' than is realised.

The above study on four adult volunteers[30] is a valuable pointer to car-seat design, but there is always a group of individuals who seem to prefer, because they are only comfortable then, a hunched-up attitude at the steering wheel, and it is unwise to try and impose, willy-nilly, arbitrary driving postures upon every patient. In the end, it is an amalgam of the car, the patient and what they know by experience is best for them.

The influence on lumbar spinal posture of the degree of backrest inclination when seated, and the presence of a localised lumbar support pad, has been radiographically studied in 38 healthy subjects by Anderson et al. (1979)[32]

Increases of the angle of the backrest, in four 10° steps from 80° to 110°, had only a minor effect upon the lumbar lordosis. The presence of a localised support pad had a significant influence on the lumbar curve, lordosis increasing with increased support, i.e. an increased distance between the plane of the backrest and the front of the lumbar pad.

The precise *position* of the lumbar support pad, with respect to the segmental level, did not significantly influence the angles measured.

Getting in and out of the car is a matter of choice—either lead with the fundament, sitting sideways with the legs together and then swinging them in together, or rely on a secure grip with one hand on the roof-edge and step in with the near leg so that the lumbar spine is unweighted during the manœuvre. If this method is preferred, the foot of the outer leg should be placed somewhat forward. Getting out is a reversal of these procedures; it is not wise to get in or out of a car while holding a heavy or awkward package.

Stooping and reaching. These two activities, when the back is used like a derrick, whether the individual is kneeling, sitting or standing, are probably responsible for far more back disability than the plain lifting of weights, e.g.

a. using a vacuum cleaner
b. reaching to lift a battery from a car
c. stooping over furniture to clean windows
d. making beds
e. kneeling while bathing a baby
f. reaching across desks, to lift weights
g. stooping and reaching, or kneeling and reaching, while gardening.

Remedies are:
a. remembering not to do it—get closer to the work
b. getting forward support from one hand when standing, or one foot forward as in half-kneeling
c. utensils with long handles
d. place the work at waist height if you can.

When changing from sitting to standing, and vice versa, an important principle is to keep the body's centre of gravity over the feet, e.g. lumbar strain is lessened when standing up if the pelvis is moved forward during the earliest phase of hip and knee extension; this is not always feasible for the elderly patient. On sitting down, there is less strain if hips and knees are flexed while still over the feet, so that the pelvis is moved backwards in the chair as the last phase of the manœuvre. When reaching forward in a stoop, flexion of the forward knee (where feasible) reduces lumbar strain.

The strain of reaching to the bottom drawer of a filing cabinet, or tucking in bedclothes, is reduced if a backward step is followed by dropping to the rear knee, so that flexion can then occur from the hips while the body is supported on forward foot and rear knee.

Lifting Shah (1976)[1107] mentions that in establishing a complete pattern of loading in the lumbar spine, the following forces must be considered:

a. gravitational force
b. muscular force
c. forces due to ligaments
d. forces due to abdominal pressure.

However, force vectors cannot be calculated from e.m.g. measurements by methods presently available; e.m.g. studies of the spinal musculature are incomplete, thus force diagrams for *in vivo* loading of the spine cannot be drawn. Also, no completely satisfactory attempt has been made to evaluate tensile loads due to the configuration of ligaments.

For these reasons accurate force diagrams, which depict the directions and magnitudes of the various loadings, cannot yet be drawn. Yet the research findings of Nachemson[889b] and his colleagues, by which intravital lumbar disc manometry recorded great differences according to the subject's posture when handling weights, in sitting as well as in standing, provide some factual evidence that most of our few timeless principles of lifting are probably correct, at least in so far as they reduce intradiscal pressure and myoelectrical activity of back muscles to the minimum, but whether this is actually going to reduce the incidence of low back pain remains to be seen.[1338, 253]

It is for this reason that the writer would stress very strongly the need to educate young people in physiologically efficient ways of using their bodies,[29] which is not the same as learning how to lift.

We should not leave out of consideration the need, not so much to teach people how to lift, but during school years to instil instinctive proprioceptive knowledge of the difference between a clumsy jerky movement and a sweet, flowing movement 'which fulfils its function efficiently with a minimum of effort and the minimum of cumulative strain'. (Anderson, 1971.)[29] The analogy between a furious swipe at the golf ball and a sweet, flowing and powerful swing, is too tempting to omit.

If the writer may be allowed a hobby-horse, perhaps the genesis of back injuries to adults at work (and, in passing, a proportion of arthrotic jip joints)[880] lies in the fiercely competitive atmosphere of the school playground, the school gymnasium, the athletic field, and the sports club gymnasium, e.g. touching the toes at all costs, lying supine and raising both legs slowly off the floor, while the feet hold a heavy medicine ball, lying prone and vigorously raising head, arms and legs.

Being qualified to make observations by reason of long experience in times past, as a regular RN Physical Educator at a Naval Engineering College, the writer believes the youthful emphasis on strength, virility and 'success' may perhaps present its account in later life. Might physical educators and athletic coaches also hold out to the young and eager the goals of mobility, extensibility and the harmonious development of co-ordination with sweet movement within the reasonable capabilities of each? It is not so glamorous as athletic success, but then neither is backache and disablement, especially when a wife and children have become interested parties.

With regard to lifting as such, after a simple exposition of the natural reaction of living tissues to physical insult, and the particular way in which this applies to the individual concerned, perhaps patients should receive no more written advice than can be contained on one side of a postcard.

For those with recurrent back pain, here indeed is the suggested postcard:

> *Analyse* your work—relate your pain to what you do and how you do it
> No lifting if too heavy—get help
> No lifting without secure foothold
> No lifting by stooping with legs almost straight
> Stand close and grip well
> *Always* keep seat lower than head
> Hold low back in neutral position
> Lift without jerking
> Change foot position to turn with weight
> Don't stoop or reach to put it down

Where the hazards of specific industrial lifting and handling duties are well understood, and safety measures can be incorporated into preventive training, instructions can be highly specific,[168] but for most individuals it is a matter of grasping and applying principles.

Sexual difficulties. The present-day rash of official and semi-official institutions, eager to give advice and guidance to the citizens on almost every aspect of their daily lives (however intimate), has tended to generate in its wake a fair proportion of people who, having grown up in this milieu, seem to be losing the ability, the will or the wit to shift for themselves, and to resourcefully tackle their own intimate domestic difficulties according to their means and the circumstances. 'Sexual activity may precipitate recurrent pain or aggravate existing pain in the same manner as lifting, pushing, pulling or any other physical activity, if performed too early or too vigorously in the course of recovery from neck, back, or radicular pain syndromes.'[1064] This much is plain to patients, and having perceived the dilemma, a proportion of them have acted on the principle, 'If it hurts, I'll find another way of doing it—or I'll stop for a bit, and put up with it.'

For those with back pain who require advice and guidance on sexual intercourse, Fahrni (1976)[336] (Fig. 18.6) has presented some charmingly sedate illustrations of positions from one to seven. He makes the sensible suggestion that, upon the stable footing of a firm, non-sprung mattress over a 2 cm plywood board:

... advances are made with the prior agreement that nothing painful is to be persisted in, and that the advent of pain should require the immediate notification of the other partner. This may result in several false starts but once the proper course has been tenderly explored and established, the memory of the initial disappointment will soon be clouded over by the impact of the pleasant results. All such preliminary skirmishings should work towards a position where the partner with the backache maintains an S-shaped attitude and the other assumes a position, one way or another, to conform to this necessity.

Stoddard (1979)[1183b] includes some sensible advice on sexual intercourse in his admirable booklet on advice for back sufferers.

Nursing mothers, the low back and the sacroiliac joint. After delivery it will be many weeks before the connective tissues of the lumbar spine and pelvic joints lose the softening and extensibility which occur during the last stages of pregnancy (p. 283).

At a time when these structures are at their most vulnerable, they are often subjected to the greatest stress—of sitting and bending to feed the baby and to change it, bending over the washtub, placing the baby in and picking it up from cot and pram, wheeling it and shopping (often up slopes and negotiating steps and pavements).

In conjunction with postnatal exercises, it is important to avoid prolonged sitting, and in the early postnatal phase to avoid those exercises or functional activities which stress the pelvis asymmetrically, e.g. stepping up high with one foot, leaping over a ditch or puddle and landing the body weight on one foot, getting awkwardly out of a bath. Carrying bulky or awkward objects, shifting furniture, taking muscular and boisterous dogs on a lead or sitting on the floor with both legs curled to one side are all likely to give rise to lumbar and pelvic joint stress.

A frequent cause of low back and sacroiliac joint problems is that of attending to the toenails, while sitting on

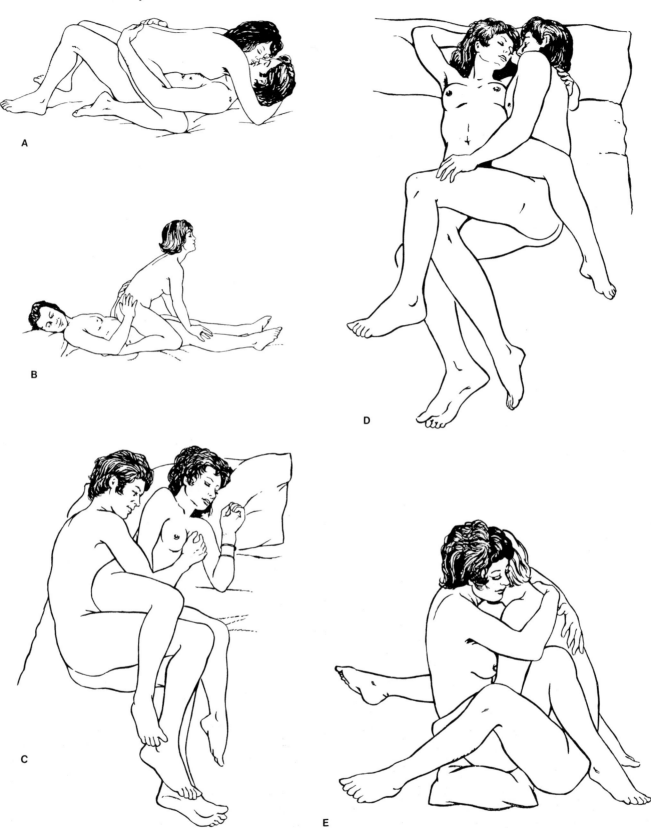

Fig. 18.6 (A–G) The difficulties of sexual intercouse with back pain may be diminished by partners arranging a position whereby the one with backache 'maintains an S-shaped attitude and the other assumes a position, one way or another, to conform to this necessity'.

(Figures reproduced from 'Backache: Assessment and Treatment', 1976, by kind permission of W. Harry Farhni MD FRCS MCh Orth and Musqueam Publishers Ltd.)

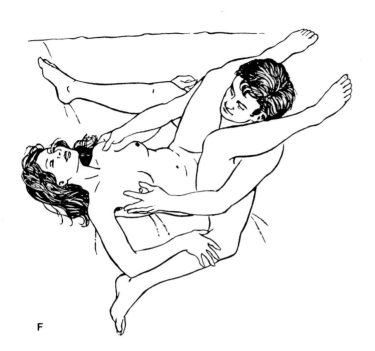

F

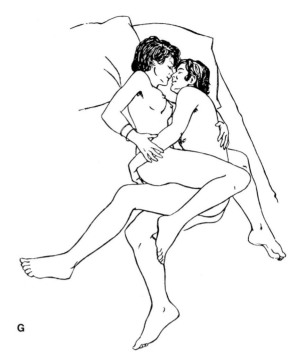

G

the floor after a bath, when normally strained positions feel easier to assume.

Stooping and reaching, while standing on one leg with the other extended at the hip to retain balance, is also unwise (see p. 499).

(iii) Preventive exercises

Aside from habitual occupational stresses and/or single episodes of exciting trauma to which everybody is liable, low back pain appears generally more common in those with weak trunk musculature, somewhat tight hamstrings, a tendency to lordosis because of lax abdominal muscles, shortening of the psoas muscle and also the lumbosacral soft tissues. For these reasons preventive exercises should, in general terms, include those for:

a. Joint mobility, with an emphasis on flexion and extension
b. Abdominal and dorsal muscle strengthening
c. Stretching of the psoas muscle
d. Elongation of shortened hamstrings (to a degree normal for each individual)
e. Ability to correct forward pelvic tilt
f. Physical endurance (again to varying degrees suitable for the individual).

a. *Joint mobility*. The exercise of pulling the knees onto the chest (Fig. 14.7) and its progressions (p. 457) will assist in maintaining flexion mobility, and in preventing tightness of the lumbodorsal fascia. Extension mobility can be maintained by standing with the feet a little apart, supinating the forearms to place the palms on the lumbar region or iliac spines, and then leaning backwards as the pelvis

is pushed forwards, so that the body's centre of gravity remains over the support area. Placing the palms higher or lower makes a slight but negligible difference to the effect (Fig. 14.8). Vigorous flexion exercises, and passive hyperextension regimes in prone-lying (when the trunk musculature is relaxed) should not be given until such time as a passive physiological-movement test (PP-MT) has determined that there is no hypermobile segment at the lower thoracic or lumbar spines, e.g. T10–T11, L1–L2 or L4–L5.

b. *Abdominal and dorsal muscle strengthening*. Those exercises described in the treatment of a hypermobile lumbar segment (pp. 452–454) are also suitable as preventive exercises.

c. *Stretching of the psoas muscle*. When sitting and standing, *in vivo* manometry of the middle lumbar discs reveals that they support heavier loads than can be attributed to gravitational compression, e.g. in a 70 kg man sitting upright, the L3 disc is carrying 140 kg, and when standing upright the load on L3 is 100 kg.[884]

Besides acting as a hip flexor, the vertebral portion of the psoas muscle also appears to take part in maintaining the upright posture, and by this activity adds a compressive effect upon the lumbar discs, in addition to that of gravitational force alone.

A simple 'maintenance' stretch of the left psoas muscle is achieved by lying supine on a firm surface and, grasping the right knee, pulling the knee onto the chest by full hip and knee flexion. The left lower limb is pressed onto the surface along its whole length. Repeat to opposite side (Fig. 18.7).

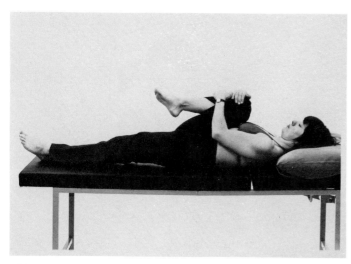

Fig. 18.7 A 'sustained hold' position for maintaining extensibility of the psoas major muscle. While one hip and knee are fully flexed, the patient endeavours to approximate the back of the other knee to the surface of the plinth.

d. *Elongation of shortened hamstrings.* The flexion exercises (*vide supra*) will assist this aim, but a more specific exercise is necessary. From standing with both feet parallel and a little apart, one heel is placed forward onto a support (stool, chair seat, desk) as high as stability allows—the height will vary according to the individual. The hamstring muscles of the raised leg will be stretched as the standing-leg knee is bent, while both hands reach down the shin to the foot of the raised leg. Repeat to opposite side (Fig. 18.8).

e. *Backward pelvic tilting.* These exercises need no description here.

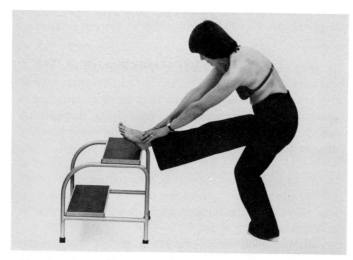

Fig. 18.8 A stretching exercise for the left hamstring muscles. The knee of the supported leg must be kept straight. The foot of the standing leg has been incorrectly illustrated, and it should be parallel with the supported foot. The exercise has a powerful effect and should not be repeated more than four times at a session, although it may be done two or three times a day.

f. *Physical endurance.* The physically active person appears less likely to get backache. Recreation or work which involves 'global' mobility of joints is preferable to that which repetitively stresses one aspect of joints.

A more comprehensive scheme of exercises is given by Buswell (1978).[145]

The nature of prophylactic advice

One important aspect, which seldom appears to enter into consideration, is the likelihood of changing a reasonably back-conscious patient into a decidedly back-happy patient. An overcautious state of mind about back problems, roughly proportional to (i) the size of the detailed instructions and (ii) the severity of the admonition to 'take care', often slowly becomes transposed into an underlying loss of confidence in the durability of the vertebral column and in its inherent ability to recover and to stand up to the stresses of life (p. 261).

One would hesitate to be responsible for inducing such a state of mind in an otherwise fit individual, yet for many patients the process has probably begun the moment they peruse and digest an interminable list of do's and don'ts upon which, they may be given to understand, the health and welfare of their lumbar spine depends. Over many years of clinical practice, the writer has seen this again and again.

Prophylaxis is important, but it cannot prevent steady progression, to varying degrees, of the changes of degeneration. Degeneration as such is not disease, and the patients should never be given the notion that they have got a 'disease'.

The evidence is all around us—individuals who have survived a back-pain episode, got over it and pressed on regardless, albeit by sensibly avoiding the more gross type of physical insult, but by no means thinking carefully before they do anything at all.

It is gratifying to feel that our advice and detailed guidance may have been responsible for this happy state of affairs—but when we encounter cheerful, durable people who have got over a back episode and got on with their lives and no such advice or guidance has been given, there is food for thought. This is not to say that we should neglect our professional duties by ignoring potential hazard, but that while giving the patient instruction, we should instil confidence and not unwittingly undermine it. Thus the 'Lifting advice' postcard referred to above (p. 509) might have on its reverse side a further injunction:

Do the preventive exercise given
Avoid prolonged periods in one position (sitting, standing, driving, bending, decorating ceilings)
If you cannot, do the reverse for a bit, every so often
Your back is not falling to bits and will last as long as you do; get on with your life and don't become overconcerned about your back.

Naturally excluded from these observations are those with significant mechanical defects, gross hypermobility, spinal stenosis and conditions other than degenerative change as such.

A change of job may be desirable or necessary, but is not always possible.

Ergonomic guidance—home or workplace visit

A comprehensive analysis, of occupational and domestic-duty stresses imposed upon one individual, is a formidable undertaking, and more usually the patient is questioned about occupational, sporting, domestic and other physical stresses and the applicable prophylactic guidance given. This should be recorded. Where group training is given, this must also be recorded.

Adaptation of the height of working surfaces and more suitable arrangement of work situations help to reduce stress on the low back.

Supports and appliances

The fact that a patient has been given an 'instant' lumbar support, which is to be worn for 5 to 10 days and no more, or is to be used only for gardening and long car trips, should be recorded, as should be a note of the effects, for future reference.

Comment

As 'Nature follows art', it may well be that the current enormous expansion of interest in common vertebral joint problems, nationally and internationally, will be accompanied by a great deal more of them—not necessarily for the obvious reasons, since truth is stranger than fiction, the human animal is indeed a strange device and that which is fashionable sways all of us much more than we care to admit, even to the extent of having a 'real' backache with physical signs!

Wood (1976)[1338] has posed a relevant question: 'Does back pain *have* a pathology?' [my italics] and also draws attention to the finding that persons with back pain appear to have an increased propensity to use health services.[894]

These observations are not meant to suggest that there is no relation between back pain and degenerative change or tissue-reaction to stress, but that its multifactorial nature and our limited knowledge should not lead us to suppose that there *is*, necessarily, a one-to-one relationship between back pain and something we call pathological changes, in all cases.

PROPHYLAXIS FOR SPORTS INJURIES

Vertebral strains, during family and competitive sport, can occur for many reasons, not least insecure footholds.

1. Do not stint on good shoes. Feet and ankles should be well supported with plenty of room for toes.
2. Bundle up warmly, since warm muscles are less prone to injury. Older people should wear enough to start perspiring *before* playing, and following the activity should bundle up immediately to avoid chill.
3. Start slowly—the more precompetitive tension, the greater the need for warming-up by gentle rhythmic exercises, gradually progressed before the competitive stress.
4. Re-educate and co-ordinate 'rusty' muscles—train first, play later. For example, the lower limbs can best be strengthened by walking groin-deep in water. For upper limbs, throw and catch an increasingly heavy medicine ball; then increase the speed of doing it.
5. For simple or moderately severe *acute* musculoskeletal injuries, apply ice immediately. For injuries which have been ignored for several days but become persistent, warm heat pads or warm soaks. Seek help if the injury is persistent.

19. Invasive procedures

These can be considered under the two divisions of (A) those minor invasive techniques which are usually conducted on an outpatient (or short instay) basis, such as injections and rhizotomy or rhizolysis procedures, and (B) major surgical procedures.

A. MINOR INVASIVE TECHNIQUES

A list of injection and other techniques cannot be definitive, since the variety of procedures is so great and the techniques are constantly changing; they might be summarised as follows:

1. Injection of soft-tissue 'trigger' points with local anaesthetic
2. Peripheral nerve block with anaesthetic and neurolytic agents
3. Hydrocortisone-derivative and local anaesthetic injection of attachment-tissues
4. Sclerosant injection of attachment-tissues
5. Injection into joint cavities or synovial spaces
6. Epidural or extradural injections
7. Rhizotomy and rhizolysis by tenotome and radiofrequency, respectively
8. Chemonucleolysis by chymopapain injection.

(Acupuncture is mentioned on p. 484.)

1. INJECTION OF SOFT-TISSUE 'TRIGGER' POINTS WITH LOCAL ANAESTHETIC

Non-articular rheumatism is an 'umbrella' name for a number of syndromes, some poorly defined and others well recognised. In some patients the clinical features can be attributed with confidence to defined systemic disease or some local pathological process, but there remains a large group of patients in whom the connection is difficult to demonstrate. Clinicians offer a variety of explanations and, despite vocal assertions that the problem is simple and has been solved, many remain unconvinced.

Smythe and Maldofsky (1978)[1151] propose a set of criteria for 'fibrositis' or 'non-articular rheumatism' as the invariable association of:

a. Symptoms of chronic aching
b. A non-restorative sleep pattern with marked morning stiffness and fatigue
c. The e.e.g. finding of alpha intrusion in non-REM sleep
d. Localised tenderness at 12 or more of 14 specific sites.

Among the sites mentioned are the lateral epicondyle attachments, the cervical intervertebral ligaments joining transverse processes C4 to C6 and the L4 to S1 interspinous ligaments—the possibility of an association, between vertebral changes and those in the soft tissues of more proximal peripheral joints, is not pursued.

The generic label 'non-articular rheumatism' may be convenient, but is perhaps unsuitable. Clinical impressions suggest that much localised pain arising from the attachment-tissues around larger peripheral joints is due to chronic secondary changes initiated there primarily by degenerative change in the associated vertebral segments.

Thus, while the 'trigger' point areas of referred pain and referred tenderness in *muscle bellies*, and localised painfully tender points in *attachment-tissues near joints*, may not be quite the same thing, the production of these changes may have much more to do with vertebral joint changes than the phrase 'non-articular rheumatism' may suggest.

Mooney and Cairns (1978)[869] have briefly summarised the rationale of these procedures as follows:

One of the most poorly understood phenomena related to chronic pain syndromes is the focal hyperirritability of tissues related to painful areas of the body. These areas are generally classed as trigger points and frequently represent areas of referred pain and autonomic nerve dysfunction. By a poorly understood mechanism, local injection with anaesthetic can provide pain relief at a distant location for far longer than can be explained by the pharmacological action of the drug. Probably the most simplistic explanation of this phenomenon is the break-up of a cycle of neurological action and response.

Travell (1942[1233] 1949,[1236] 1954,[1239] 1960,[1240] 1968[1241]) has written extensively on this subject (considered in some detail on pp. 118–119) and in 1952[1238] published detailed charts of predictable patterns of pain associated with tender trigger points.

Wilkinson (1971)[1316] observes that, in cervical spondylosis, injections into painful areas may give relief of pain and spasm, and improved cervical movement. The technique is usually that of injecting an 0.5 per cent procaine or 0.25 per cent xylocaine solution into the soft tissues at the site of maximum tenderness;[356] there is considerable variation in the solutions employed.

Mehta (1973)[839] employs local infiltration of painful tissues with dilute local anaesthetic (0.25 per cent lignocaine or bupivacaine) as a simple means of relieving symptoms. He observes that while relief is seldom permanent it frequently outlasts the duration of local analgesia, and that this effect may be consequent upon relief of muscle spasm (see p. 196) and vasomotor changes associated with an irritable focus in superficial soft tissues; he suggests local infiltration in detecting trigger areas for referred pain, for temporary relief of chronic pain, muscle injuries and strains, muscle spasm in muscle-tension headache, wry neck (torticollis) and lumbago.

Bourdillon (1973)[105] describes his use of 1 per cent lignocaine as the local anaesthetic when infiltrating muscles, preferring this to the mixture of 2 per cent lignocaine in equal parts with hydrocortisone (25 mg in 1 ml) because his results have been very satisfactory in the majority of patients, using the local anaesthetic alone.

He describes effects which sometimes occur and are difficult to explain:

a. Patients with back and leg pain, accompanied by acutely tender fibrositic areas which when injected with local anaesthetic are dramatically relieved together with the back and leg pain.
b. Somewhat similar effects produced by local injections into the muscles and ligaments around the spinal joint which is causing symptoms.

Stoddard (1969)[1180b] also describes the infiltration of painful soft-tissue sites by local anaesthetic, as a method of inducing relaxation of muscle hypertonus which is self-perpetuating because of chronic mechanical faults.

In low back pain, impressive improvement follows intramuscular injection, and Burnell (1974)[143] infiltrates the tender bands and nodules which are so often found in association with vertebral pain.

The injection technique for a tender piriformis muscle (Kirkaldy-Willis and Hill, 1979)[662] is that of inserting one finger in the rectum so that its tip overlies the sensitive belly of the muscle (p. 296). With the other hand a long needle is inserted posteriorly, halfway between the lateral margin of the sacrum and the greater trochanter. The needle tip is inserted further until its tip can be felt beneath the rectal mucosa. After withdrawal for 1 cm, 2–3 ml of 0.5 per cent lidocaine are injected, to ensure that the needle does not lie in the vicinity of the sciatic nerve. A further 2–3 ml of 0.75 per cent marcaine are then injected, and if the diagnosis is correct dramatic relief of pain occurs within 10 minutes.

2. PERIPHERAL NERVE BLOCK

The use of analgesic or neurolytic block of nerve conduction is almost a century old.[98] Sensory block relieves pain, motor neurone block relieves spasm and sympathetic neurone block can relieve vasomotor, sudomotor and visceral disturbances.

Nerve blocks may help to determine the pathways and mechanism of pain, the cause of the pain and the patient's reaction to elimination of pain. After full investigation of the nature of the pain, temporary interruption of conduction in nociceptor fibres often produces relief which persists appreciably longer than the duration of the anaesthetic block. The analgesia is not due to nerve destruction.

Mehta (1973)[839] observes that one or more peripheral nerve blocks may be needed. He mentions a series of patients (some of whom had compression of spinal roots from orthopaedic conditions) who remained comfortable for up to 21 days after peripheral nerve block. It is ill-understood how completely reversible local analgesia provides sustained relief, and suggestions are that the effect may not depend entirely upon simple and temporary interruption of the peripheral nociceptor pathway, but that modulation of the substantia gelatinosa 'pain-gate' mechanism (see p. 168) may allow freer use of the body part and, because of this, persistence of the modulation effect.

The advantages of the procedure are that pain relief is complete and, in comparison with analgesic drugs, the side effects are fewer. Depending upon the concentrations employed, some differential effect is possible, i.e. sympathetic neurone block with low concentrations, somatic sensory block with slightly higher concentration and a block of motor neurones as well with still higher concentrations.

Technique

Accurate needle placement requires care, and difficulties can be unrecognisable landmarks, anomalies of nerves, obese patients and those who may be unable to communicate or are unco-operative; also, individual susceptibility to local anaesthetic is variable.

Aids which can assist accurate needle placement include the initial production of paraesthesia in the nerve distribution, image-intensification fluoroscopy, nerve stimulator locators and a 'block-aid monitor', in which the close approximation of the needle to the nerve is demonstrated by an electrical stimulus producing a muscle twitch.

The technique is especially valuable when attempting to block nerves which are not related to bony landmarks.

Mehta's description of block techniques and their indications, from the cranial to the anococcygeal nerves, includes the following:

a. Spinal accessory nerve for spasm of trapezius and sternomastoid
b. C1 and C2 a.p.r., when these nerves are damaged in trauma
c. The greater occipital nerve in intractable headache
d. Brachial plexus block for compressive syndromes of the cervical region
e. Paravertebral space injections for peripheral thoracic nerves, and mid-axillary intercostal blocks
f. Injection of intercostal nerves at the point of traversing the rectus sheath (see pp. 100, 241)
g. Paravertebral block of lumbar nerves in vertebral anomalies and disc protrusion
h. Injection of the lateral cutaneous nerve of thigh in meralgia paraesthetica and more proximal degenerative trespass upon the nerve root (see p. 268)
i. Sciatic nerve block, providing analgesia and interruption of autonomic function in those rare cases where sciatic pain may have a vascular origin
j. Trans-sacral block of sacral and coccygeal nerves in intractable sciatica
k. Block of the anococcygeal nerves in coccydynia.

Among the treatments for internal derangement, Cyriax (1974)[217] mentions sinuvertebral nerve block for the lumbar and thoracic joints.

The value of lignocaine intercostal block, in abdominal pain of spinal origin, has been demonstrated by Ashby (1977),[46] yet there are alternative methods of successful treatment.[452] In his series, the most commonly involved intercostal nerve was T11 on the right.

Neurolysis

More prolonged effects are produced by neurolytic agents such as alcohol, phenol, chlorocresol and ammonium salt, and they produce a patchy destruction of all types of fibre in the nerve root injected. Placement of the needle must be very accurate, and the pain relief may last for a matter of weeks or may be permanent; the average period is a few months.

Alcohol blocks of somatic nerves may be followed by chemical neuropathy and severe neuralgia, which can be more distressing than the pain which they are intended to relieve.[98]

3. HYDROCORTISONE-DERIVATIVE AND LOCAL ANAESTHETIC INJECTION OF ATTACHMENT-TISSUES

Mention has been made (pp. 116, 188) of the great importance of attachment-tissues in vertebral pain syndromes. The attachments of ligaments, muscles and aponeuroses are peculiarly liable to undergo changes which are a fruitful source of musculoskeletal pain. While the true genesis and nature of these changes remains debatable, their accurate localisation by painstaking examination and their relief by localised procedures have improved beyond measure over the last three decades.

Much attachment-tissue pain arising from the vertebral column itself, the limb-girdle regions (i.e. bicipital tendinitis) and around the more peripheral joints (e.g. medial or lateral epicondylitis) can frequently be relieved by a single, accurately placed injection.

Hydrocortisone reduces inflammation at tissue-level and is potent in the connective tissues; because the natural hormone is too soluble and disperses too quickly, hydrocortisone acetate (HCA) was employed. Longer lasting preparations are methylprednisolone and triamcinolone. The addition of hyaluronidase, to the mixture of hydrocortisone and local anaesthetic, is sometimes employed when injecting the soft tissues, but since it is a foreign protein an allergy may develop following repeated injections.

The instant analgesic effect of the local anaesthetic wears off in two or more hours, and the corticosteroid component may take one to two days to become fully effective; thus the pain may soon return and also be provoked for a day. Patients should be warned of this.

Common sites for injection are the bicipital and supraspinatus tendons, the common flexor and extensor attachments on the humeral epicondyles, the second and third costochondral junctions in Tietze's disease and, in low back pain, the supraspinous and interspinous vertebral ligaments, the tips of the lumbar transverse processes and muscle attachments along the iliac crest. Burnell (1974)[143] observes that if painful apophyseal joints can be numbed, even temporarily, the patient has a chance to mobilise them by doing active exercises immediately afterwards.

If automobilisation is not possible by the patient, the relaxation obtained may allow more effective localised passive movement.

Cyriax (1974)[217] describes the technique of injection for ligamentous and tendon strains, and for those joints and ligaments which are unsupported by muscle, e.g. the sacroiliac joint.

In the ill-defined but large group of patients with what is variously called low back strain, iliolumbar strain, sacroiliac strain or lumbosacral strain, Ingpen and Burry (1970[591] had considerable success by combining one, and at the most, two injections with lumbar isometric exercises. They infiltrated the region of maximum tenderness, between the L5 spinous process and the posterior superior iliac spine, with a suspension of 1 ml of prednisolone acetate (25 mg/ml) and 2 ml of procaine HCl 2 per cent.

4. SCLEROSANT INJECTION OF ATTACHMENT-TISSUES

Segmental instability, where a degenerating vertebral segment is functionally incompetent because of insufficient soft tissue control (whether muscle, ligament or disc) can be an intractable problem.

In 1957, a monograph entitled *Joint Ligament Relaxation* (Hackett)[478] described a method of injecting sclerosant solutions into spinal and pelvic ligaments which had become attenuated or slack through degenerative processes, trauma and stress. He described weakening of the fibro-osseous junction as 'a condition in which the strength of the ligamentous fibres has become impaired so that a stretching of the fibrous strands occurs when the ligament is submitted to normal or less than normal tension'. Hackett used a phenol-glucose solution for what he termed 'prolotherapy', to encourage fibro-osseous proliferation at the site of insufficient soft-tissue control.

Stoddard (1969)[1180b] employs 1 ml of ethanolamine oleate with 1 ml of 2 per cent procaine. Three injections are given, at fortnightly intervals, and a lumbosacral support is worn for three months to ensure that the maximum fibrous tissue reaction occurs in the connective tissue. A fourth and fifth injection may need to be given in some; after the final injection, six weeks should elapse before final assessment of results.

There is considerable variation in the amount of pain caused by these injections, ranging from no pain at all to an intense reaction. Barbor (1974)[58] describes in detail the technique at each site and employs a solution of:

Phenol	2.0–2.5 per cent
Dextrose	20.0–25.0 per cent
Glycerine	20.0–25.0 per cent
Pyrogen-free water to 100 per cent	

mixed in 1:200 procaine in saline to a proportion of 4 ml sclerosant to 6 ml procaine, and gives *the indications* as:

a. Prevention of recurrent disc protrusion (after reduction)
b. Stabilisation of the sacroiliac joint (after reduction of subluxation)
c. Pure ligamentous strain
d. Stabilisation of spondylolisthesis.

Ligaments which he commonly injects, at the ligamento-periosteal junction rather than the whole length, are the L4 and L5 supraspinous ligaments, the iliolumbar ligaments, the posterior sacroiliac and interosseous ligaments and the sacral attachments of the sacrotuberous and sacrospinous ligaments.

A strong and disagreeable reaction after the local anaesthetic wears off is said to presage a good result. Barbor injects at weekly intervals, and three weeks after the final injection the patient must walk two miles a day for a fortnight.

Stoddard also employs the procedure for the lower cervical joints. Some physicians use the technique for superficial ligaments but are understandably reluctant to inject substances which initiate an inflammatory reaction into the deep spinal ligaments.

Whether the good results are due to actually improving ligamentous laxity is regarded as unproven by some,[143, 357] and even when the clinical results are satisfactory the radiographic evidence is often disappointing. Hackett has suggested that the sclerosant produces a firmer attachment to bone, rather than an actual reduction of excessive mobility.

5. INJECTION INTO JOINT CAVITIES AND SYNOVIAL SPACES

Intervertebral facet-joints are a significant source of pain.[870] The introduction of stable suspensions of hydrocortisone into a joint cavity, so that the microcrystalline deposit would remain for some weeks and exert an anti-inflammatory effect, is some 30 years old and now standard procedure in orthopaedic and rheumatology clinics. Injection into the cavity of a vertebral facet-joint is a more recent practice, at least on a wide scale.

Following injection, under fluoroscopy control, of hypertonic saline into the lumbar facet-joint cavities of 20 subjects (5 normal individuals and 15 patients with chronic low back pain), Mooney and Robertson (1976)[867] noted a painful reaction after about 5 seconds. An initial deep, dull, vague discomfort, which increased after 20 seconds, radiated over the buttock and down the posterior thigh. In two patients the pain transgressed the midline and in three patients the pain spread in a sciatic radiation to the whole leg and foot.

Following an injection of saline irritant into his own low lumbar facet-joint, Mooney (1977)[870] experienced pain of sciatic distribution, i.e. into buttock, posterior thigh and calf. Overall, there was a relationship between the distance of radiation and the amount, the duration and the volume of the irritant fluid.

A further test, of the responses to irritant material in synovial facet-joint cavities, showed marked myoelectrical activity in the hamstring muscles and a reduction of straight-leg-raising to some 70°. Three of the patients in the group had depressed deep tendon reflexes. Both the pain and the hamstring hypertonus were obliterated in all 20 subjects by a second injection of 2 to 5 cc of 1 per cent xylocaine; the previously depressed tendon reflexes also returned to normal as compared with the normal limb.

The authors then formulated a diagnostic-therapeutic procedure of facet block, and in 100 patients who potentially had a facet-joint problem as a part of the source of their pains, the synovial facet cavities were injected with steroid and local anaesthetic under fluoroscopy control. Therapeutic success was assessed on the basis of subjective description of pain relief, and results were tabulated as follows:

Patients with initial relief	62
Continued complete relief a six months review	20
Partial relief at six months review	32
No relief at six months review	10
Return to normal work activities	55
Seen by other physicians for back care	8
Currently requiring pain medicines for back	30

Their findings suggest that injections of synovial facet-joint cavities can produce long-term relief in some 20 per cent of patients with low back pain, and partial relief in a further third of the patients.

Mooney (1977)[870] describes a postsurgical patient with chronic low back pain who had been unable to work for six months. A consistent physical sign was a painful 'hitch', or arc of pain, on bending forward; this was associated with increased myoelectrical activity in both multifidus and the regional musculature of the erector spinae.

Immediately after injection into the facet-joint the e.m.g. was quiescent and the pain relieved—the patient went back to work. A week later the findings remained improved.

The technique of facet block was originally used as a diagnostic procedure prior to facet-joint rhyzolysis by the method of Shealey (1974)[1118] and it became apparent that many of the patients needed no further treatment, since the period of pain relief extended far beyond the anticipated 14-day action of the corticosteroid injected.

Periarticular injections, and those into facet-joint cavities, in the cervical spine are not without hazard.

As the facet syndrome becomes more commonly diagnosed, injection of the involved areas is becoming a widely used technique. In the treatment of headaches, especially those involving the suboccipital region or the upper cervical facet-joints, injection of these areas may have severe, permanent and even fatal complications . . . [we] report the association of injection of these structures with brain stem ischaemia and the sequelae of this phenomenon. (Gottesman, Harris and Olshan, 1975.)[428]

Relief of pain by injection of facet-joints has been criticised on the basis that the procedure is merely another form of 'trigger' point injection,[870] yet the comparison is a little unjust—the injection of a tender locality in soft tissues is not the same as depositing hydrocortisone and local anaesthetic into the synovial cavity of a joint. Injection of a painful point, in the tender muscle mass of the quadriceps of a painfully arthrotic knee, is not the same as suffusing the joint cavity.

6. EPIDURAL ANALGESIA

Infiltration of the epidural or extradural space is not a new technique; it was described by French physicians in 1901 and 1909.[201, 1374]

Evans (1930)[321] employed an epidural block for the treatment of low back pain with sciatic radiation. He injected 60 to 145 cc of 1 to 2 per cent novocaine or saline, with immediate or complete relief in over 60 per cent of 40 patients.

There are a number of variations of injection method and solutions employed. In severe low back or sciatic pain it is effective as an outpatient procedure in temporarily blocking transmission of impulses in a large proportion of thinly myelinated or unmyelinated neurones (without disturbance of larger diameter fibres) when dilute solutions of 10 ml or more are introduced by lumbar injection, or 20–50 ml by caudal injection via the sacral hiatus.

Mehta (1973)[839] observes that mechanical stretching of nerve roots, by the physical mass of fluid volumes greater than 40 ml, is unnecessary and potentially dangerous, although Cyriax (1975)[218] and others employ 50 ml as a routine.

As with injections of local anaesthetic into the attachment-tissues around joints, relief of pain may long outlast the duration of pharmacological effect. Two groups of 20 patients, in severe sciatic pain, were studied by Coomes (1961)[201] who treated one group by epidural injection and the other by bedrest, after full clinical and radiological assessment. Simple analgesics were not effective in controlling the pain and the patients were only comfortable in bed. The duration of symptoms prior to treatment was comparable; a mean duration of 37 days in the epidural group, and of 31 days in the bedrest group, who were rested either at home on fracture-boards or in hospital.

Epidural injections were given via the sacral hiatus with a solution of 50 ml 0.5 per cent procaine. The mean time for recovery in the bedrest group was 31 days, and in the epidural group 11 days; the epidural group had a greater improvement in neurological signs than the bedrest group.

a. Lumbar technique

The epidural space may be entered in the midline, between the lumbar spinous processes, or by a lateral or paramedian approach. For sciatica and low back pain, Mehta advocated up to 10 ml of 1 per cent lignocaine or 0.25 per cent bupivacaine (plain) injected at L2–L3 level, and prefers this method when the pain lies in the distribution of the upper roots of the sciatic nerve.

Burn and Langdon (1967)[142] employed the lumbar

method in 138 patients on an outpatient basis, by injecting 40 ml of 0.75 per cent lignocaine, to which was added 80 mg of methylprednisolone (in 20 ml) and 25 mg of hydrocortisone acetate (in 20 ml).

The solution was infiltrated at the 3rd–4th lumbar interspace with the patient lying on the side and conscious. Following this, a brief general anaesthesia of one to two minutes was induced by intravenous injection; the lumbar spine was then rotated and the sciatic nerve stretched. After resting under observation in the recovery ward for one to two hours, the patient waited a further hour, and left the hospital.

Patients with gross neurological deficit were not accepted, but those with minor deficits such as depressed reflexes or diminished sensibility were included. The overall success rate was 66 per cent, and it appeared that the best results were achieved in those over 40 years whose current episode was under 12 months duration, whose straight-leg-raising was over 45 degrees and in whom there was no paresis, paraesthesiae or anaesthesia.

For pseudoradicular (referred) pain, i.e. that distributed to low back and thigh but not below the knee, relieved by rest and often associated with unilateral paraesthesiae, Oudenhoven (1979)[960] suggests diagnostic local anaesthetic injections of the posterior primary rami, bilaterally at L3, L4 and L5. Relief of pain inculpates the posterior primary rami as the pain source, and specifically *excludes* the ramus meningeus, or sinuvertebral nerve (q.v.) as the source.

In passing, it should be mentioned that while eradication of a local pain (from attachment-tissues of muscle and/or ligament) around the limb girdle areas does not necessarily indicate its source (see Referred Pain, p. 189) this phenomenon of referred pain and referred tenderness is less likely to be so misleading when the diagnostic local anaesthetic is injected at the vertebral column itself.

Oudenhoven suggests that referred pain mechanisms which involve the posterior primary ramus are 'best relieved by a properly performed radiofrequency denervation', and for those cases where pain is presumed to arise from the recurrent sinuvertebral nerves, the specific treatment is epidural injection of 30 cc of 0.5 per cent procaine, with 80 mg Depo-Medrol. His series of over 4000 such injections were all done between L3 and L4. He regards epidural injections as specific for pain which is secondary to degenerative discs without herniation, and it is particularly effective in sciatic scoliosis without neurological deficit; it may also help in early degenerative (group III) spondylolisthesis. He describes the injections as having both a neural effect, upon the sinuvertebral nerve, and a ligamentous effect upon the posterior longitudinal ligament, and suggests that intradiscal steroids are only effective in a chemical discitis, while intrathecal steroids are only effective in residual radiculitis or root sleeve inflammation.

Repeat epidural injections at 18–24-month intervals may be necessary.

b. Sacral technique

With the patient prone, the fluid is introduced into the epidural space, at the rate of 5–10 ml per minute, by an ordinary lumbar puncture needle with stylet (Cyriax, 1975)[218] via the sacral hiatus, after anaesthetising the superficial tissues overlying it. The majority of patients experience a sacral ache, sometimes including the posterior thighs, as the fluid enters the epidural space.

Fluid ascends cranially for a distance which is proportional to the force and volume of the injection, the amount of leakage through the intervertebral foramina, the height of the individual, the capacity of the sacral canal and the amount of connective tissue within it.[839] Following the injection patients are as a rule quite composed after lying for 20–30 minutes, and can get up and go home.

Some patients are virtually pain-free for two days, after which the pain returns; in others, pain may increase for a day or two and following this it quickly diminishes. Generally, a week is allowed before assessment of results, but those with severe sciatic pain and root signs are seen in about five days for a further injection; those with longstanding root pain should be left for a fortnight.

An improvement in either signs or symptoms, or both, indicates a further injection,[218] but a proportion do not need the second procedure.

Epidural corticosteroid injection, of 50 successive patients with sciatica, was reported by Harley (1966)[502] Most patients received one or two injections, which were sufficient to produce significant benefit in those who were likely to respond. He observed that the greatest incidence of benefit occurred in those patients who had pain but no sensation abnormalities, no abnormal physical signs and normal X-ray findings. Twenty of the group were completely relieved, 13 considerably improved and 17 unchanged.

Burnell (1974)[143] finds that it is rarely necessary to use epidural injections for an acute low back pain episode, since manipulation combined with relaxation techniques usually proves effective. On the occasions when he does employ the injection technique, the solution is one-quarter per cent citanest combined with 20–50 ml of prednisone. Others use lesser amounts of local anaesthetic, i.e. 20 ml or less for small patients, to secure relaxation of the spinal muscles, so that the operator can then use manipulation with a better likelihood of success.[105] For low thoracic joint problems somewhat larger quantities are needed.

With the patient under brief general anaesthesia, orthopaedic surgeons may use an injection of local anaesthetic and hydrocortisone via the sacral hiatus, followed by passive straight-leg-raising and passive hip-extension-with-knee-flexion, to mobilise the roots of the sciatic and femoral nerves. The procedure may be indicated for possible root adhesions following surgery or as the sole therapeutic measure.

The effect of solutions employed

In support of the rationale for using steroids in epidural block, Cho (1970)[172] refers to the study by Lindhal and Rexed (1950)[749] who described the inflammatory changes in nerve roots, and hyperplasia of the perineurium, which were observed in biopsies of nerve roots in ten patients.

Cyriax[218] observed that adding hydrocortisone to the anaesthetic solution does not enhance the effect; Coomes[201] has suggested that the hydrostatic effect of the extradural fluid mass of the local anaesthetic, together with the anaesthetised nerve sheath and the painless lumbar movement, must bring about improvement. He pointed out that the improvement may occur either by relieving pressure on the nerve root, or increasing it, both of which are capable of relieving pain, though by different mechanisms. Since that time, research findings have supported 'a growing feeling that sciatic pain and limited straight-leg-raising may not be an indicator of root compression, but instead may be due to muscle spasm in paraspinal muscles or referred pain from the posterior joints or paraspinal ligaments. It is therefore not valid to equate relief of radicular pain with reduction in nerve compression.'[487]

Haldeman (1978),[487] Lewit (1978)[743] and Sunderland (1978)[1194] reiterate that mere nerve compression usually produces numbness rather than pain, and that damage to sensory nerve fibres is not necessarily painful. In some patients, the injection of a weak solution of local anaesthetic will abolish pain before there is any effect upon the nerve roots,[105] and it has been suggested that the effect is upon the ramus meningeus or sinuvertebral nerve.

A comparison of the solutions employed for epidural injections was made by Yates (1978).[1374]

Four different injection-solutions of 50 ml were randomly used in a series of patients with low back pain and sciatica, over a period of one year, the solutions being:

(i) 50 ml of normal saline
(ii) 50 ml of 0.5 per cent lignocaine
(iii) 47 ml normal saline and 3 ml lederspan
(iv) 47 ml 0.5 per cent lignocaine and 3 ml lederspan.

The patients graded their symptoms before and 30 minutes after the weekly injections, and the subjective assessments were compared with changes in signs. The changes in mobility were greatest after the injections containing lederspan.

The indications are given by Yates (1976)[1373] as: very severe lumbago, agonising sciatica, chronic sciatica and for differential diagnosis.

The long-term response to epidural local anaesthetic is extremely variable, and the degree and duration of relief differs from a virtually immediate and dramatic response to partial and only transitory relief.

Epidural analgesia will only be produced in: (a) structures innervated by the sinuvertebral nerve; (b) the nerve sheath; (c) the dura mater; (d) the posterior longitudinal ligament; (e) the apophyseal joint, and in diagnostic problems this can help in distinguishing pain from other structures.

The dangers (Cyriax, 1975)[218] include local sepsis, sensitivity to procaine and the use of an excessive volume of fluid. It is dangerous to give an epidural injection while the patient is under general anaesthesia, and difficulties arise when the neural canal is filled with dense fibrosis.

7. RHIZOTOMY AND RHIZOLYSIS

The procedures of rhizotomy (attempted cutting of nerve root or primary ramus) and rhizolysis (neurolysis of nerve by radiofrequency or thermister probe) have, by their success rate in relieving lumbar symptoms and signs, stimulated a great deal of interest in changes in the vertebral facet-joints and/or paraspinal soft tissues as likely to be a common cause of low back and sciatic pain.

The severe pain which is so characteristic of the 'intervertebral disc syndrome' may more often be related to the sensory distribution of the posterior rami of segmental nerves, which are distributed to fascia, ligaments and periosteum of the posterior intervertebral joints. It is unlikely that the intervertebral discs, which have a different sensory innervation through the sinuvertebral nerves, are commonly involved in this pain mechanism. (Rees, 1971.)[1019]

King (1977)[658] has observed, '... it is difficult to escape the conclusion that structures innervated by the posterior primary rami play an important role in generating the back *and* leg pain which accompanies acute disc rupture, as well as the chronic pain of many patients suffering from intervertebral disc degeneration'.

The essentials of this view were put forward by Putti (1927)[1003] and significant support for these observations lies in the subjective and objective relief regularly and consistently provided by minor invasive procedures involving the facet-joints and paravertebral soft tissues, but not directly involving the intervertebral disc.

From about 1966, Rees[1019] used the technique of multiple, bilateral, subcutaneous rhizotomy for the relief of vertebral joint pain; the technique may also be used for the relief of pain arising from degenerative changes in the neck.

Essentially, lumbar rhizotomy is performed with the patient lying prone under epidural anaesthesia. Through stab incisions at the points of maximum tenderness over the facet-joint regions, some 2–3 cm from the midline, a long narrow blade is inserted to the hilt, directing the point of the blade towards the facet-joint. The blade is then swept backwards and forwards through an arc of 80°, for the purpose of deep sagittal cutting of the posterior rami of segmental nerves. This is done bilaterally, and usually four to six segments are incised. There may be a brisk haemorrhage which is controlled by digital pressure; no sutures are required and a sterile dressing under adhesive plaster completes the procedure.

'Relief of pain is immediate; the patient walks back to the ward for two hours rest in bed and then gets up and begins prescribed exercises, all movement-limiting prostheses being discarded.' (Rees, 1971.)[1019]

Some patients go home the next day but most remain in hospital for 48 hours. There may be a mild sunburn sensation across the buttocks, probably due to cutaneous nerve irritation by extravasated blood, and occasionally there is reduced sensibility in those who have a large haematoma. Leg pain may be exacerbated for a few hours.

Rees reported no complications in 1000 patients whose ages ranged from 12 to 84 years; 95 per cent of these had previously received unavailing treatment. In 1972, more than 3000 patients in Australia had received treatment since 1966, with no major complications recorded. There was no clinical or radiological evidence of the formation of Charcot's joints, or any other pathological change, resultant on the operation.

With three years experience of the technique, Francis (1974)[372] mentions that rhizotomy is not considered until other pathology is ruled out by full clinical and radiological examination and blood tests, and manipulative treatment tried. He gives the indications as:

(i) *History:* chronic low back pain, often needing bed-rest, which is provoked by sitting, driving, standing, bending over a basin, lying in bed and intercourse. Some have buttock and thigh pain, and some report pain in the ankle.

(ii) *Signs:* limitation of flexion and lateral tenderness in the lumbar region; straight-leg-raising reduced, reflexes usually unaffected.

An assessment of 200 cases (116 males and 84 females) was reported by Toakley (1973).[1221] Preoperatively, the average duration of pain was 9 years, and varied from 9 months of constant pain to 30 years. Most were never free from pain, the distribution of which was:

Back	200 patients
Buttock(s)	111 patients
Thigh/groin	152 patients
Calf, and to ankle	60 patients

Neurological deficit was present in 90 patients, and X-ray examination revealed:

Disc narrowing	176 patients
Spondylolisthesis (grade 1–2)	14 patients
Lumbar facet-joint sclerosis	83 patients

Generalised osteoarthritis or ankylosing spondylitis	5 patients
Normal appearance	18 patients

The number with prior operations was 48.

Apart from modifying the mode of anaesthesia, the rhizotomy procedure was essentially that described by Rees (1971)[1019] and was followed by mobilisation exercises.

With a minimum follow-up period of two months, the results were as follows:

Good	—70 per cent or more improved	125 patients
Fair	—50 to 70 per cent improved	37 patients
No change	—less than 50 per cent improved	36 patients
Subjectively worse		2 patients
		200 patients

Reoperation, in 20 patients from the 'Fair' and 'No change' groups, achieved an 80 per cent improvement figure.

Toakley[1221] remarks that, '... true disc protrusion with sciatica of dermatome distribution, and changes in reflexes and sensation, do not appear to be helped by the procedure.'

Postoperative mobilisation exercises are necessary to gain maximum mobility, a physiotherapist visiting the patient 12 hours after the rhizotomy. Common to all cases were (i) heavy bleeding in spite of pressure dressings, and (ii) an aggravation of local pain on completion of exercises; an immediate return to maximum mobility required encouragement.

Of a group of 74 patients, 31 were contacted 6 to 12 months after their lumbar rhizotomies. It was notable (Shanahan, 1974)[1109] that those whose pain relief was accompanied by increased mobility, and who continued their exercise regimes, continued to improve. Those whose pain was not relieved but whose mobility increased showed no later improvement in their pain and often lost the earlier gains in movement.

Following e.m.g. investigation of patients who had undergone rhizotomy procedures, Burnell (1974)[143] reported that quite large segments of the sacrospinalis had been denervated, and suggested that denervation of muscle may be a factor responsible for the pain relief after rhizotomy.

In the lumbar region, the medial branch of the posterior primary ramus winds backward around the base of the superior articular facet of the subjacent vertebra; it passes beneath a strong ligament connecting the mamillary and accessory processes to supply the facet-joint, and also provides a branch to the joint below as well as innervating the segmental musculature, i.e. multifidus, rotatores and interspinales.

The mean depth, of the most dorsal aspects of the target

for the Rees procedure, is greater than the length of the tenotome blade,[658] and lateral X-rays taken at the time of the surgical procedure showed that the knife-blade had not reached the facets. Since the tenotome blade cannot, with the technique described, reach the nerve supplying the facet-joints,[101] denervation of those joints (in the patients reported upon) cannot be the mechanism of pain relief.

Francis[372] suggests, on the basis of cadaver experiments, that what is being cut are the branches of the posterior primary rami which *pass laterally* to innervate paravertebral muscle, i.e. sacrospinalis and intertransversarii. His hypothesis, of the possible cause of much back pain and its relief by rhizotomy, may be summarised sequentially as follows:

synovial meniscoid villus impacted between joint surfaces of hypermobile facet-joint
↓
stretching of joint capsule and stimulation of type IV nociceptors
↓
regional spasm, i.e. polysynaptic reflex contraction of the related portions of paravertebral muscle
↓
synovial effusion within the joint, with anterior bulging of the thinnest part of capsule, and thus trespass upon its anterior relation, i.e. the nerve root
↓
possible root pain by localised hyperaemia as well as physical trespass upon the root
↓
persisting muscle spasm irritating (i) those joint-nociceptor neurones which traverse the paravertebral musculature, and (ii) biochemical irritation of nociceptors in the walls of blood vessels in hypertonic muscle.

Following rhizotomy, e.m.g. studies demonstrated a reduction in myoelectrical activity in paravertebral muscle.

King (1977)[658] studied the effects of radiofrequency rhizolysis at (a) the level reached by a tenotome and (b) the dorsal aspect of the facets. In a third placebo group (c), the radiofrequency probe was introduced through the anaesthetised skin close to the point of maximum tenderness, and a stimulating instead of a coagulating current was passed through the probe for two minutes at each point.

In groups (a) and (b), a coagulation lesion (10 mm × 7 mm) was produced by a two-minute current producing a temperature of 80°C.

In group (a) (Rees procedure): Of 21 patients, 15 (71 per cent) experienced satisfactory pain relief, the figure dropping to 10 in 6 months.

In group (b) (Shealy procedure): Of 25 patients, 18 (72 per cent) experienced satisfactory relief, the number falling to 6 in 6 months.

In group (c) (placebo): Of 14 patients, 7 (50 per cent) had satisfactory pain relief, but all had regressed after 5 weeks.

A pre- and postoperative review of signs indicated that the only consistent change was in the straight-leg-raising test. In about 40 per cent of those in group (b), the straight-leg-raising test improved considerably. One patient, who was not included in the study because of sciatic pain of acute onset, showed myelographic evidence of a large right extradural defect at L4–L5; his right extensor hallucis longus was weak. Immediately after radiofrequency rhizolysis his pain was relieved and his toe strength was normal. Some months later, a large sequestrum of disc material was removed. Of a further seven patients with symptoms, signs and compatible, large myelographic defects indicating disc trespass, six experienced total pain relief after radiofrequency myotomy. In three patients, large sequestra were subsequently removed when pain recurred. After six months, the remaining four had not required surgical attention.

Together with the studies reported by Hitselburger and Whitten (1968)[552] these findings have important implications, and raise considerable doubts about the common notion that discogenic trespass and pain have a one-to-one relationship.

On the basis of these findings King (1977)[658] suggests that the backache and sciatica which may be *initiated* by discogenic change is largely *generated* by the pain–muscle–spasm cycle of structures innervated by the primary posterior rami. On interruption of this neurological circuit, either at the deep soft-tissue trigger points as in the rhizotomy procedure, or at the p.p.r. as in the rhizolysis procedure, pain relief and improved signs can be achieved in many.

It has been demonstrated that myelographic evidence of lumbar disc trespass exists in one-third of asymptomatic people.

Studies of the effects of radiofrequency rhizolysis, and Depo-Medrol-with-xylocaine injections with needle-placement exactly similar to the radiofrequency probe, were made by Oudenhoven (1977)[958] in 129 patients. All had mechanical low back and leg pain, positive articular signs and restricted straight-leg-raising.

All responded positively to diagnostic local anaesthesia of the facet articular nerves, with resolution of back and leg symptoms and disappearance of leg signs for the short duration of the anaesthesia. Following this, 20 patients (controls) had Depo-Medrol-with-xylocaine injections of articular nerves, with the result that 3 had marginally abnormal electromyograms and no relief of pain, while 17 had a normal e.m.g. yet relief of pain; in none of the 20 did the pain relief last longer than 33 days.

The remaining 109 patients underwent bilateral radiofrequency rhizolysis at the segments L3, L4 and L5. The e.m.g. was *bilaterally* abnormal in 89 (81 per cent); 9 (10 per cent) of these had had previous surgery. Of the remaining 80 without previous surgery:

21 (26 per cent) had excellent relief of pain
43 (54 per cent) had good pain relief
16 (20 percent) were considered treatment failures.

The author's conclusions are that facet rhizolysis *does* denervate the structures supplied by the posterior primary ramus, and there is a direct correlation between the degree of denervation and the quality of pain relief. Pain relief without denervation is only temporary, and *unilateral* denervation of the dorsal ramus is ineffective in controlling mechanical low back pain and leg pain.

Thus, the facet-joint mechanoreceptors must exert facilitatory and/or inhibitory influences in both ipsilateral and contralateral facet structures and musculature. Patients with normal electromyograms after rhizolysis will not have their pain relieved.

Oudenhoven (1979)[960] reported the effect of radiofrequency denervation on a group of 337 patients, all of whom met the criteria of pseudoradicular pain which could be relieved by an initial local anaesthetic injection of posterior primary rami. All had been occupationally disabled for over four weeks.

Following denervation, 279 (83 per cent) had continuing good-to-excellent pain relief and were occupationally re-abled.

Pain relief correlated directly wth abnormal post-denervation electromyography. Average follow-up was 26 months, and it was noted that unilateral denervation did not control pain.

The incidence of denervation of paravertebral musculature, following major spinal surgery, has been studied by Macnab *et al.* (1977)[780] and in this connection it is interesting to recall a paper by Scott-Charlton (1972),[1100] who drew attention to the significance of the posterior primary rami, and suggested that the pain relief achieved by sacro-iliac joint fusions may well be due to the simple cutting of dorsal nerves during the surgical approach to the joint.

8. CHEMONUCLEOLYSIS BY CHYMOPAPAIN INJECTION

The feasibility of injecting a discolytic enzyme into the intervertebral space was discussed in 1959[357] and on the basis of experiments on rabbits and dogs, the technique was used on human patients after 1963.

Chymopapain is a proteolytic substance extracted from the paw-paw tree (*Carica papaya latex*), a vegetable enzyme with a quite selective action on chondromuco-protein; it will rapidly cause disintegration of the nucleus pulposus of the disc without any effect upon the retaining annulus fibrosus, the ligaments, nerve fibres or dura mater.

Before the injection of chymopapain was employed,

some clinicians injected steroids; others used the enzyme *coagulase*.

In experimental discolysis with injection of the enzyme collagenase (clostridium histolyticum) into dogs, Sussman and Mann (1969)[1195] showed that while the enzyme had an overwhelming effect upon the nucleus pulposus, it had only slightly less activity against fibrocartilage. Massive intrathecal injection produced no effect.

Chymopapain has a much more selective action upon the nuclear material.[143] Its mode of action is to attack the keratosulfate, chrondroitin sulfate and protein of the nucleus, hydrolysing and dissolving the non-collagenous protein which connects long-chain mucopolysaccharides. It is very specific and is effective in a dose some 20 times less than that which would affect the fibrous tissue of the annulus.[709]

Smith and Brown (1967)[1147] gave the first comprehensive account of the procedure, and all 75 patients selected were considered as candidates for existing surgical operations, on the basis of a presumptive diagnosis of lumbosacral nerve root compression. Most patients had spinal listing, muscle spasm, articular signs, limitation of straight-leg-raising and neurological deficit. Attempts were made to choose only those patients who were emotionally stable, and all had undergone prolonged conservative treatment.

The first patient was injected under local analgesia, but after this a routine general anaesthetic was employed.

With the patient lying on the left side, a 6-inch (15-cm) 18-gauge spinal needle with stylet is introduced at an angle of 45° or more, with the help of a portable image-intensifier. The needle is directed just lateral to the articular facet and just above the transverse process, and its position is checked by rotating the portable intensifier. The needle in the 4th lumbar disc is used as a surface guide to the lateral approach for the 5th lumbar disc.

After needle placement is completed, X-rays in two projections are taken to confirm the position, and for record.

After injection of 1 ml of radio-opaque material (only 0.5 ml of which would be accepted, under considerable injection pressure, by a normal disc) the degenerate nucleus is outlined by a discogram. Following this, 2 mg of chymopapain in 0.5 ml of distilled water is slowly injected into the disc.

Assessments, at 4 to 30 months after injection, were as follows:

Result	No previous spinal surgery	Previous spinal surgery	Total
Good	46	11	57
Fair	5	6	11
Poor	2	5	7
	53	22	75

Postoperatively, almost all patients were relieved of sciatica; after injection back pain was severe in 28 patients and analgesic drugs were necessary. Most patients were free of symptoms after three to four weeks.

When the fine structures of chondromucoprotein has been disrupted, the degraded material is then of sufficiently small molecular size to diffuse out of the disc. Smith and Brown[1147] observed that: '... the rapid loss of sciatica in most of our patients can best be explained by this mechanism.'

The fate of the chymopapain has been studied by Kapsalis et al. (1974),[632] who observe that the direct result of chymopapain injection is rapid loss of the nucleus pulposus with the annulus remaining essentially intact. Disruption of the central protein cores of protein–polysaccharide complexes decreases the water-trapping properties of the nucleus pulposus, and reduces the accompanying intradiscal presure.

After radio-immuno-assay of plasma, and other studies, the authors suggest the following sequence of events on chymopapain injection in man:

(i) Immediately, relatively high concentrations of enzyme depolymerise the soluble, high molecular weight glycosamino–glycan–protein complexes, and bind to less soluble complexes.

(ii) Some solubilised components, combined with some of the then inactive chymopapain, diffuse rapidly out of the disc into the circulation. (The milky fluid, which can be aspirated from the nucleus immediately after injection, is a combination of soluble disc component and chymopapain.)

(iii) Over several hours, residues of the enzyme may remain in the disc, acting as a catalyst in the slow decomposition of the less soluble, non-collagenous residues.

(iv) Over a period of several days, degraded nucleus pulposus and chymopapain gradually diffuse out of the disc.

(v) This diffusion is made good by extracellular fluid containing inhibitory macroglobulin, and thus residual enzyme bound in the disc is inactivated.

(vi) Finally, as antibodies are developed, residual chymopapain protein is removed by the reticuloendothelial system.

There is the risk of severe allergic reaction[143] and this occurs in about 1 per cent of patients. The rapid diffusion of immunoreactive chymopapain out of the disc space is probably the reason for the swift anaphylaxis in those patients with hypersensitivity to the enzyme.[632] This is the main hazard of the procedure.[172]

With regard to toxicity, experiments show that the toxic dose far exceeds the therapeutic dose.[709]

Direct injections into lumbar discs after an extraperitoneal approach have been employed[1271] on two patients, but subsequently, injections were given under X-ray control.

Graham (1974)[432] reported on 90 patients treated by chymopapain ('Discase') injection and suggested, on the basis of his results, that the procedure gives the patient a one-in-three chance of complete cure. Improvement was noted in the majority of those not completely relieved, but this group were not entirely free from some lumbar stiffness. Those with two segments involved did less well than those with a solitary lesion.

An accurate diagnosis of the intervertebral level at fault, and of the *type* of disc problem, are important factors for good results, and the difficulty with a technique which relies on X-ray localisation is that there is no absolute certainty of the *extent* of the changes. Where there is complete extrusion of disc material, injection of the enzyme is unlikely to be effective.[709]

Burnell (1974)[143] suggests that the main indication for the procedure is when there is increased intradiscal pressure, with or without early prolapse of disc substance. Advanced degenerative change, sequestration of disc material and sciatica caused by osteophytic trespass are unlikely to be helped by chymopapain injection. Macnab (1977)[780] considers that the procedure should be employed as the last resort of conservative treatment, and if a patient has not improved significantly after two weeks of bedrest, the injection should be employed before surgical intervention is considered.

In 1974, the preliminary data of a double-blind study at four institutions were reviewed,[357] and the results of a placebo injection were not significantly different from the chymopapain injection.

On the basis of a review of laboratory and clinical reports, Sussman (1975)[1195] believes that chymopapain is toxic for muscular and neural tissue.

Rydevik et al. (1978)[1071] have suggested that a spinal nerve compressed by discogenic trespass is probably already injured, and thus has a lower threshold for tissue injury:

... consequently, even concentrations of chymopapain below 0.4 per cent might be expected to cause nerve injury, but such an effect may not necessarily become clinically manifest, due to overlapping innervation from different spinal segments. ... Obviously chemonucleolysis with possible leakage of intradiscally injected chymopapain is a pathophysiologically and anatomically highly complex situation. It is our opinion that (i) chymopapain at clinically used concentrations has a potential for affecting nerve tissue, and (ii) the rare clinical occurrence of neurologic sequelae as seen after chymopapain injection may be explained by various factors cooperating to counteract the side-effects of the enzyme, e.g. the dura barrier, inactivation of enzyme and possibly also the phenomenon 'hidden nerve injury'.

B. MAJOR INVASIVE PROCEDURES

Measured against the totality of patients with musculo-skeletal spinal joint problems, and the numbers and types of treatment procedures, the important step of major surgical intervention is most uncommon. Yet, with specialised investigation methods, it is the clinical assessment by surgeons and surgical procedures which have provided such a wealth of important information; for this reason, discussion of common spinal joint conditions is not complete without a section on surgery.

The indications for seeking a surgical opinion are more proper to this text than writing in detail of surgery itself, which is summarised below in general terms only, with such detail as may be of special interest.

THE INDICATIONS FOR SEEKING A SURGICAL OPINION

Factors which may influence the surgeon's decision are the severity of symptoms, the lack of response to conservative treatment, the passage of time and the degree of functional restriction imposed by the lesion.[926]

The indications for surgery and the type of surgical procedure are the prerogative of surgeons, but for those whose daily work is the conservative treatment of vertebral joint problems, it is important to know when a surgical opinion may be indicated. *In some clinical states, the need may be urgent.**

In addition to *the factors which may provide warning of the possibility of neoplastic disease* (p. 302), the salient indications for seeking opinion may be set out as follows:

Cervical region

a. Instability of the craniovertebral joint complex (C0–C1–C2) due to rheumatoid disease, trauma, stress or congenital anomaly (pp. 208, 209)
b. Persistent symptoms of vertebrobasilar insufficiency, e.g. vertigo, tinnitus, or nausea related to head movements, and particularly 'drop' attacks (p. 200)
c. Long-continued and intractable unilateral neck and arm pain which is resistant to adequate conservative treatment
d. Difficulties of walking and/or other lower limb involvement, in mature patients with cervical spondylosis (p. 228)
e. Bilateral neurological deficit and root pain in upper limbs (this does not include transient nocturnal 'glove' paraesthesiae)
f. A degree of dysphagia which is greater than mild discomfort or compulsive throat-clearing.

Cervicothoracic region

a. Persistent oedema or other vascular changes of one or both hands or upper limb (other than early morning puffiness of fingers) (p. 229)
b. 'Light-headedness', dizziness and visual disturbances on active use of an upper limb (p. 528)
c. Horner's syndrome associated with upper limb symptoms of C8–T1 distribution (p. 300).

Thoracic spine

*a. Girdle pain, bizarre and unpleasant paraesthesiae of lower limbs, walking difficulties, or *any* involvement of lower limbs in association with thoracic joint problems (p. 249)
b. Frank instability of a thoracic segment which is resistant to adequate conservative treatment.

Lumbar spine

*a. Sphincter disturbance associated with low back and bilateral leg pain, usually due to central disc prolapse (p. 257)
*b. Extrasegmental root signs in *one* lower limb (p. 107) associated with a back pain episode.
   NB: With regard to the *recovery of motor function*, operative treatment appears to give no better prognosis than conservative treatment,[1293] although patients with evidence of multisegmental but unilateral root deficit may stand a better chance of optimum recovery of power if operative intervention is speedy.[1369]
c. Failure of adequate conservative treatment, e.g. in relieving severe limitation of unilateral or bilateral straight-leg-raising, with or without neurological deficit in one or both lower limbs.
d. Increase in neurological involvement despite adequate conservative treatment
e. Recurrent and disabling sciatica
f. Intermittent claudication, associated with low back pain (p. 276)
g. Segmental instability, of whatever cause, e.g. intractable nagging low back pain provoked by *any* activity, associated with an arc of lumbar pain on sagittal movement (p. 259).

AMONG THE SURGICAL PROCEDURES FOR COMMON VERTEBRAL JOINT PROBLEMS ARE:

Vertebral region

C0–C1–C2. (a) Occipitocervical fusion[491, 925]
   (b) Transpharyngeal fusion of atlantoaxial joint, for traumatic rupture of transverse ligament of atlas, rheumatoid arthritis, un-united fracture of odontoid and rotatory subluxation at the atlantoaxial joint.[103, 354, 829, 1213, 1346]

Occipitocervical fusion is employed in stabilising an unstable atlantoaxial joint, the main cause of which is rheumatoid arthritis. Inclusion of the occipitoatlantoid joint in the fusion adds only a minor degree of movement limitation, and does not materially affect the amount of rotation restriction.[491, 925]

Fusion of the atlantoaxial joint alone may be done by the Gallie[396] method of wiring which holds in place a cortical graft from the iliac crest, the graft being notched to conform to the C2 spinous process and the posterior tubercle of C1.

McGraw and Rusch (1973)[829] and Fielding et al (1976)[354] discuss the indications for including the occiput or the C3 segment. When the remainder of the spine is diseased in its full length, as in some cases of rheumatoid disease and ankylosing spondylitis, transpharyngeal fusion may be the method of choice.[103, 1213]

Simmons and Bhalla (1969)[1132] emphasise that in handling patients with mechanical disorders of the cervical spine, operation is rarely required.

Middle and lower cervical.
(a) Vertebral body fusion by bone graft to immobilise an unstable segment, by anterior approach;[117] also discectomy and removal of osteophytes[1102, 1103, 1319, 1132, 1087]

(b) Decompression by facetectomy or foraminotomy, with or without incision of dural root sleeve and adhesions, to relieve pressure upon a nerve root, by posterior approach[117]

(c) Laminectomy, with foraminotomy if necessary, to relieve spinal cord compression in cervical myelopathy[117, 316]

(d) Decompression of the vertebral artery, in basilar artery insufficiency and spinal cord ischaemia[117, 221, 656]

(e) Removal of spondylotic osteophytes and soft-tissue calcium deposits causing dysphagia, by anterior approach[89, 102, 141, 1075]

(f) Vertebral artery ligation in the subclavian steal syndrome.[991, 1377]

In 1955, Robinson and Smith[1051] described a comparatively simple anterior approach to the cervical spine, this method being said[1132] to be easier than the posterior approach, with a higher fusion rate and simpler postoperative management. Yet the operation of anterior interbody decompression and fusion of the cervical spine by Cloward's technique[183] is now an established surgical method in treating chronic, incapacitating cervicobrachial pain, cervical myelopathy and other conditions.

Schaeffer (1976)[1087] mentions that the Cloward procedure is not indicated unless radicular brachialgia exists.

There may be difficulties in localising the segmental level of the lesion, since a single nerve root can be affected by pathological change at any of three different levels.[1103] Myelography, tomography and e.m.g. conduction studies are necessary, but even with thorough neurological examination, e.m.g. studies, discography and cervical phlebography, localisation of the correct segmental level for surgical intervention is not always certain.[751]

Selecki (1971)[1102] observes that the procedure is most suitable for the lower cervical spine and that a posterior approach is more suitable for the levels above C4.

After postoperative periods ranging from two to nine years, Williams et al. (1968)[1319] compared the signs, symptoms and X-ray appearances of 60 patients who had undergone cervical discectomy and interbody fusion, and concluded that:

a. Those with radicular symptoms had a higher rate of improvement than those without.

b. Men tended to have much better results than women.

c. Those with occipital headaches as a dominant symptom tended on the whole to do less well—although some were greatly improved (see Keuter, below).

d. Those with correlated signs and symptoms of root involvement did better than those in whom good fusion was manifest '... suggesting that the selection of patients for cervical discectomy may be more important than the obtaining of a bone fusion.'

e. Patients with apparently normal X-ray appearances did less well than those with frank osteophytosis and/or reduced disc space.

After follow-up of one to eight years on 84 patients, Simmons and Bhalla[1132] suggested that those who require the operation often give a history of significant injury; they have a mechanical type of pain which is consistently provoked by activity and coughing and sneezing, and somewhat improved by rest, support and traction.

Some surgeons perform the discectomy without the bone graft,[812] and in 51 patients with cervical disc disease, the standard Cloward procedure was used for 25 patients and radical discectomy with foraminotomy for the remaining 26 patients. Ninety-two per cent of the patients in each group were improved after surgery.

Epstein et al. (1969)[316] observe that:

The ideal operation should relieve the spinal cord and nerve roots from pressures in all quadrants, including those exerted ventrally by osteophytes and dorsally by infolded yellow ligaments, lamina, or osteophytes on the posterior facets ... Adequate circumferential decompression of the spinal canal, by means of laminectomy, foraminotomy, and excision of osteophytes over as many as four or more interspaces, is possible only through a posterior approach.

Yet Sim et al. (1970)[1129] mention that there is a risk of late instability with so-called swan-neck deformity which may require surgical stabilisation.

In cervical arthrosis with vascular symptoms, Jung and Kehr (1972)[623] reported the technique of opening the intervertebral foramen via an anterior approach, i.e. an anterior foraminectomy or an uncoforaminectomy, and in 57 patients with Barré-Lieou-like symptoms due to arthrosis, achieved the following results:

Headache ceased in 91 per cent
Vertigo attacks ceased in 90 per cent
Hearing abnormalities ceased in 83 per cent
Psychic disturbances ceased in 70 per cent.

In 5 of 6 patients with previous 'drop attacks', these no longer occurred.

In a further group of 21 patients with post-traumatic cervicoencephalic syndromes, they reported 17 successes (7 'very good', 5 'good' and 5 'fairly good').

Since the surgical procedure is limited to removal of the uncus at one or more segments, they emphasise the especially damaging effect of uncoarthrosis in the aetiology of cervical pain and cervicoencephalic syndromes (see p. 5).

Dan (1976)[221] has also drawn attention to the frequent involvement of the uncovertebral joint in cervical degenerative change, and to the bony spur thus developed which may displace the artery laterally and sometimes anteriorly. 'When vertigo, tinnitus, nausea or syncope occurs in relation to head movements, significant encroachment on the vertebral artery may be suspected.' He describes a more limited surgical decompression procedure without fusion: '... in the light of the long-term effects of fusion in spondylotic necks.'

Keuter (1970)[656] studied the pathogenesis of clinical features due to lesions of trespass upon the vertebrobasilar vascular system. He commented upon the difficulties of segmental localisation of the trespass, due to the enormous variability of the vascular arrangement.[704]

Degenerative changes in the lower neck, producing vascular disturbances of the spinal cord, may give rise to syndromes with an upper limit of effect at about the C4 level; these are considered due to flow impedence in the lower cervical portion of the anterior spinal artery, and sometimes by partial impedence of a major radicular artery.

In some cases, neurological involvement occurs at a higher level because of a diminished blood supply in the *upper* cervical cord. In six patients, Keuter demonstrated a combination of neurological abnormalities both above and below the level of lower cervical lesions, with the two regions separated by a pectoral area of normal function. Of the two involved areas, the higher level disturbance is not topographically consistent with the segmental level of the lesion, and suggests ischaemic changes affecting the spinal trigeminal nucleus (see p. 11).

Williams and Wilson (1962)[1318] have drawn attention to the vulnerability of this spinal nucleus to ischaemic changes.

With regard to the more distal changes, cervical myelopathy presents most often as unilateral or bilateral corticospinal and spinothalamic tract involvement, corresponding to the postmortem findings of widespread demyelination and neuronal loss, occurring mainly in the lateral and anterior columns. Less commonly, the posterior columns may suffer most.

The Brown–Sequard syndrome[175]

Ipsilaterally	Contralaterally
Cutaneous anaesthesia in the involved segment	Zone of hyperaesthesia in the segment involved
Hyperaesthesia below the anaesthetic zone	Loss of pain and temperature sense below the segment involved
Loss of proprioceptive, vibratory and two point discrimination below the involved segment	
Lower motor neurone paralysis in the involved segment	
Upper motor neurone paralysis below the involved segment	

While the Brown–Sequard syndrome has been linked, *inter alia,* to cervical trauma and extramedullary neoplasms, a rapidly progressive myelopathy of the Brown–Sequard type may be associated with cervical spondylosis (Jabbari *et al.,* 1977).[596] The authors have presented a series of six patients with a rapidly progressive myelopathy of this type. The surgical procedure employed was bilateral cervical laminectomy and foraminotomy.

Breig (1978)[121b] describes the cervicolordodesis procedure in which transplantation of fascia lata to the posterior aspect of the neck, in a patient with cervical myelopathy and Brown–Sequard's syndrome, prevents flexion and thus cord, and meningeal and nerve root traction. He observes:

To prevent flexion of the cervical spine when there is a risk of pathological tension and hence over-stretching of the nerve fibres and blood vessels, a brake may be inserted in the neck, an operation that has been designated *cervicolordodesis.* This procedure also prevents separation of intramedullary wound surfaces in the case of tissue rupture due to compression. It has now been employed in a score of patients for the relief of symptoms in various types of myelopathy and rhizopathy and to promote approximation of the intramedullary wound surfaces after compressive cervical spinal cord injury.

To eliminate compression of the nervous tissues in the cervical canal by means of bilateral laminectomy it is mandatory to use a protective technique which avoids introducing any part of an instrument into the lumen of the canal and thus exerting even the slightest momentary pressure on the dura and the cord. For this purpose the techniques of *protective bilateral laminectomy* and *protective arcocristectomy* have been designed. The latter consists in sawing out only the upper rims of the laminae and then raising them carefully from the canal. This type of partial superior bilateral laminectomy maintains spinal stability; it is therefore recommended wherever it is practicable.

Vertebral artery ligation. If either subclavian artery is occluded proximal to the vertebral artery branch, and the resultant decrease of distal subclavian arterial pressure is sufficient to create an arterial pressure gradient, a reversal of blood flow will occur in the vertebral artery of the same side, and blood is shunted from the vertebrobasilar (and thus cerebral) system to the ipsilateral upper limb.[1377]

The tendency to dysequilibrium, blurring of vision and headache will be intensified by use of the limb, and the condition could possibly be mistaken for a degenerative cervicoencephalic syndrome.

The most common cause is an atherosclerotic plaque in the subclavian vessel, and vertebral artery ligation is a surgical method of providing relief.

Dysphagia

Cervical osteophytosis may be causally related to difficulty in swallowing[141, 1075] and the bony mass trespassing upon the oesophagus may be excised via a transoral approach in the upper neck, or an anterolateral external approach.[102]

Cervicothoracic region.
(a) Excision of an anomalous cervical rib[702] or malformations of first thoracic rib[1060]
(b) Division of supernumary fascial bands[1210]
(c) Scalenotomy, to reduce soft-tissue trespass upon the neurovascular bundle[1128]
(d) Vascular surgery for aneurysmal dilatations, etc.[764]

Notes on surgical intervention are included on pages 136 and 230.

Thoracic spine.
(a) Posterolateral rhachiotomy with rib resection and discectomy, for thoracic disc prolapse[82, 1116, 1131]
(b) Thoracic discectomy by anterior extrapleural approach[957]
(c) Decompression for thoracic spinal stenosis[430]
(d) Surgical fusion of hypermobile segment[721](p. 239).

'There is no characteristic clinical syndrome that typifies all thoracic disc herniations.' (Simeone, 1971.)[1131] 'The type of surgical operation most suited to thoracic disc removal does not appear clear cut.' (Benson and Byrnes, 1975.)[82]

Shaw (1975)[1116] discussed the dangers of laminectomy in treating thoracic disc lesions, and mentioned the first choice of a posterolateral approach.

'The blood supply of the spinal cord is shown to be least rich, and the spinal canal narrowest, from the T4 to approximately the T9 vertebral level. This is named the "critical vascular zone of the spinal cord", the zone in which interference with the circulation is most likely to result in paraplegia.' (Dommisse, 1974.)[266]

Hume (1960)[581] advocated a posterolateral approach to the thoracic spine, and Ranshoff (1969)[1011] suggested the importance of preoperative intercostal angiography, if the lesion were above T9, to determine the location and the size of the *arteria radicularis magna*, or artery of Adamkiewicz (p. 14).

Otani *et al.* (1977)[957] reported six surgical cases in which an anterior extrapleural approach was used, these comprising 1.7 per cent of a total of 348 disc operations at all levels over a period of 11 years. The authors suggest that the past notoriously unfavourable results of surgery may be due to the fact that the compressive lesion lies in front of the spinal cord and is commonly in the midline. They suggest that removal of the posterior structures by laminectomy allows an abnormal increase in spinal motion.

In a report of the surgical decompression of developmental stenosis of T9 vertebra, Govoni (1971)[430] mentions that among 594 thoracic vertebrae, and 11 complete spines in a department of anatomy, there was a moderate dorsoventral narrowing of the spinal canal in only four vertebrae, and in one the narrowing was severe. Osteophytic projections from the neural arch protruded into the spinal canal in two vertebral bodies.

A series of six patients with herniated thoracic discs, all of whom did well after disc removal by the anterolateral transthoracic approach, is described by Allbrand and Corkill (1979).[15] In four patients the affected segment was T11–T12, the others being T10–T11 and T5–T6. All exhibited neurological abnormalities in lower limbs either clinically or on e.m.g. Three patients with T11–T12 lesions had bladder dysfunction, as did the patient with the T5–T6.

Lumbar spine. The results of surgical treatment for low back pain depend upon diagnostic accuracy and the nature of the pathology. There are few controlled prospective studies comparing surgical treatment with conservative management, since the decision for surgical intervention is usually initiated by a period of failed conservative treatment, or by the need to deal with a significant mechanical defect like spondylolisthesis.

When a proven herniated disc is associated with nerve root compression, its surgical removal gives an initial success rate of over 90 per cent in the relief of sciatic pain, yet long-term follow-up shows the need for reoperation in about 10 per cent of cases, and a recurrence of symptoms, especially back pain, in 20 to 30 per cent.

As an adjunct to disc removal, the role of primary fusion remains uncertain; there is conflicting evidence in the literature, although it is claimed by some authors that primary fusion improves the long-term results by 10 per cent. Certainly, a higher incidence of indifferent results is associated with poor patient selection, unsettled claims for compensation, and reoperation.

The three main objectives of lumbar surgery[926] are: (1) removal of space-occupying lesion, (2) stabilisation, (3) decompression. As in other spinal regions, techniques vary between surgeons and once operation is undertaken each surgeon, on the basis of his own experience and the nature of the findings, usually includes some individual modification or extension of textbook procedures.[1195]

For detailed descriptions of technique, with indications, the literature should be consulted.

'There is some confusion in the nomenclature used for the different operative procedures on the low back.' (Newman, 1973.)[926]

Laminectomy describes the excision of a lamina, or two or more laminae; also the excision of a neural arch on one side, between spinous process and pedicle, or the whole neural arch between pedicles, or multiple neural arches. The term has no other meaning.

Fenestration indicates exploration of the spinal canal and lateral recess through an inspection aperture, avoiding severance of the neural arch and with minimum disturbance of the facet-joint.

Spondylotomy (or rhachiotomy) indicates cutting into soft tissue and/or bone of the vertebral column; it includes all surgical opening of the intervertebral canal.

Procedures for lumbar spine[926]

Fenestration operation via interlaminar exposure for lateral disc prolapse.

Adequate exposure by laminectomy of one or more vertebrae, for excision of massive central disc prolapse.

Disc removal with or without stabilisation by fusion, in chronic and severe disc degeneration, instability and arthrosis of facet-joints.

Stabilisation for instability, by transarticular screws and posterior laminar arthrodesis, when neural arch and articular facets are intact.

Stabilisation for instability, with decompression of lateral recess by lateral laminectomy or facetectomy, when the neural arch is defective. The transverse processes are fused by bone slivers from the ilium.

Stabilisation for group I (congenital) spondylolisthesis, by fusion with autogenous bone slivers bilaterally in the paravertebral gutters, from L4 to the sacral alae. Decompression is added if there is significant cauda equina involvement.

Fusion for group II (isthmic) spondylolisthesis, with decompression added if true sciatica due to nerve entrapment is present. Transarticular screw fusion is not used, and the stabilisation is achieved by intertransverse or anterior intercorporeal fusion.[378]

Decompression of theca and both L5 roots, for group

III (degenerative) spondylolisthesis, most often at the L4–L5 segment. Partial bilateral laminectomy, with partial bilateral vertical facetectomy, occasionally with removal of the whole neural arch of L4. Stabilisation is necessary and may be included during the procedure, with intertransverse autogenous bone graft, or fusion of vertebral bodies may be done at a second operation by extraperitoneal exposure.

During a review of surgery for 21 patients with degenerative (group III) spondylolisthesis, Reynolds and Wiltse (1979)[1033] found that those who had had a midline decompression only, in which the articular processes and the pars interarticularis were preserved but the lateral recesses enlarged, did better than those in whom the articular processes were completely sacrificed to accomplish decompression.

Patients with a midline decompression had 78 per cent good or excellent results while those with articular processes removed had only a 33 per cent good or excellent result.

The difference was attributed to the instability consequent upon removal of articular processes.

Decompression by multiple laminectomy and facetectomy for spinal stenosis; stabilisation may be added if there is instability.

Decompression of the first sacral root, in chronic lumbosacral disc degeneration, by partial laminectomy and partial vertical facetectomy, and fusion of the segment by transarticular screws and posterior laminar graft.

Decompression of the lateral recess by laminectomy and facetectomy, for root pain in elderly patients with lumbar scoliosis and progressive stenosis on the concave side.[318]

The lateral or posterolateral prolapsed lumbar disc

Naylor (1977)[910] observes that disc disorders, in many cases, are 'contained within the annulus', i.e. a biochemical disturbance of the nucleus causes increased intradiscal pressure or minor incomplete rupture, resulting in defective function of the disc and the vertebral mobility segment. He suggests that, in these cases, surgical enucleation of the disc has no place in the treatment of the associated back and buttock pain.

There is no common agreement on the choice of surgical exposure,[199] and the nature of surgical problems is clearly stated in the following paragraph:

The close anatomical relationship of the axial skeleton and the central and immediately peripheral nerve system brings its particular problems and this provides the surgeon's dilemma. Minimal exposure of the affected nerve root via the interlaminar approach does not seriously affect the stability of the spine, but certainly carries the risk of failure to find the effective cause, whereas wide exposure will usually, with patience, satisfactorily demonstrate the source of mechanical interference; but we are then confronted with significant joint instability. [Bell, 1974.][81]

Preoperative assessment

A lumbar-disc-surgery predictive score card has been developed to assist accurate appraisal (Finneson, 1978)[358] in selecting the patients most likely to do well, and those likely to fare indifferently. The predictive method refers only to those patients with prolapsed lumbar discs, who have had no previous surgery. The score card is summarised as follows:

Positive points		Negative points	
5	Incapacitating back pain and sciatica	Back pain principally	15
15	Sciatica more severe than back pain	Gross obesity	10
5	Sitting and bending provoke the pain—bedrest relieves it	Entire leg numb. Simultaneous weakness of toe extensors and flexors. Extension of pain into areas not explained by an organic lesion	10
25	Neurological examination reveals single root involvement	Poor psychological background—unrealistically high expectations, hostility to environment—spouse—employer. Much time off work for medical reasons	15
25	Myelogram corroborates neurological findings	Secondary gain—work-connected accident—medicolegal adversary factors—eligibility for pension if symptoms persist	20
10	Positive straight-leg-raising test		
20	Crossed straight-leg-raising test		
10	Realistic self-appraisal of future capabilities	History of previous medicolegal problems	10
Positive total		Negative total	

The negative total is subtracted from the positive total to give the predictive number.

Predictive scoring:

Points	Prospects
75 and over	good
65–75	fair
55–65	marginal
below 55	poor

Finneson and Cooper (1979)[359] determined the validity of the predictive score card by reviewing the charts of 596 patients who had undergone lumbar disc surgery between 1962 and 1974. Two hundred and eighty patients responded to the mailed request form, and it was evident that the outcome of lumbar disc surgery seems directly related to patient selection, at least during the first five postoperative years. Because of the everchanging state of the lumbar spine, the outcome is less critical after five years.

Notwithstanding the personality of the patient, intractable sciatic pain with spinal rigidity, reduced straight-leg-raising and a positive myelogram often responds dramatically to surgical removal of the disc prolapse.[912]

The operation over, it is psychologically important to regard the procedure as a relatively minor one. Walking in a few days and flexion and extension movement of the spine after ten days are important for two reasons; to mobilise the nerve tissues and to build up the intrinsic intersegmental muscles. Flexion accounts for the former, recovery by extension for the latter. [Newman, 1973.][926]

When frank disc trespass is myelographically evident, and is currently underlying sciatic pain with neurological deficit, the results of conservative treatment may not be quite as gratifying as those of surgical treatment, although an important variable may be the nature of conservative treatment. Over a period varying from 4 to 8 years, with a mean observation period of 5.5 years, Weber (1970)[1293] compared the conservative and surgical treatment of lumbar disc protrusions, the presence of which had been verified by positive myelographic appearances in all patients. Patients in both groups were between 20 and 50 years of age, had radiating pains in the leg and all had neurological signs of nerve root involvement. The segments involved were equally distributed as to sides; 10 were at L3–L4, 93 were at L4–L5 and 87 were at L5–S1.

Conservative group. 108 patients, of whom 101 were assessed at follow-up. A good or fairly good result was obtained in 70 per cent of this group.

Surgical group. 95 patients, of whom 89 were assessed at follow-up. A good or fairly good result was obtained in 95 per cent of this group.

After consideration of the factors involved, it was concluded that the difference in results could mainly be ascribed to the treatment itself. In the *surgical* group, there were no variables which significantly affected the results. In the *conservative* group, however, there were three variables which appeared to influence the outcome: mental disturbance, a long period of incapacity prior to hospitalisation and a leptosome body type.

Experienced manual workers will be familiar with the introspective, light, thin patient whose responses are less gratifying than in those who are somewhat better covered.

In 400 consecutive patients with low back pain, Froning and Frohman (1968)[388] made 565 X-ray films of the lumbar flexion/extension ranges: 92 of these patients underwent surgical procedures. Among 72 patients in this group, 52 had a laminectomy for partial disc removal and 20 had fusion of the lumbosacral spine. The group of 72 was followed up postoperatively at 3, 6 and 12 months, and were re-examined by X-ray. Diminished segmental movement after disc herniation and partial discectomy appeared to be related to a good operative outcome.

The findings demonstrated restricted flexion and extension in most of the patients in whom disc-substance removal was a success; where virtually normal mobility persisted the operative result was poor. Mobility X-rays often demonstrated increase flexion/extension ranges in segments adjacent to the stiff one, especially in arthrodesed segments.

Regarding the local sequelae of removal of the prolapsed material and enucleation of the disc, Brown (1971)[137] mentions the growth of granulation tissue into the avascular disc as a beneficial process, with rapid clearing of polysaccharide molecules and subsequent fibrosis being a factor in relieving back pain; he suggests that perforation of the cartilaginous end-plates allows granulation tissue to enter and rapidly produce fibrosis.

It is interesting that laboratory discectomy, i.e. thorough removal of nuclear material from fresh postmortem discs by a technique resembling that of the clinical procedure, still left almost half of the nucleus remaining (Markolf and Morris, 1974).[807]

These authors' research findings suggest that the annulus is much more important for the compressive behaviour of the disc than was believed. By repetitive loading of fresh autopsy specimen discs, and recording changes by a bulge transducer, they observed:

1. An apparent self-healing phenomenon in discs with experimental lesions through the annular wall. They suggest that the first loading cycle reflected a flow of the remaining nuclear material into the channel; the return to normal compressive behaviour after only a few loading cycles showed how rapidly a temporary repair could take place, long before *in vivo* repair could occur by scarring and the formation of fibrous tissue.

2. Following a laboratory discectomy, the new response to repetitive loading was very nearly that of the intact specimen—this observation perhaps explains the postoperative improvement of patients following lumbar disc surgery.

3. A similarity of behaviour between that of the isolated annulus and the intact disc. Without the nucleus, the disc responded normally to compression in load-deflection, load-relaxation and creep tests, demonstrating that the viscoelastic behaviour of the disc as well as its static stiffness are *determined by the annulus*. 'In these tests, the annulus was the major structure determining the compressive characteristics of the disc ... concluded that the nucleus plays a less important mechanical role in determining compressive deformations.'

The discs showed a wide variety of degenerative states, yet the degree of degeneration did not appear to influence the compressive characteristics observed.

Since Naylor (1977)[910] remarks that in only 12 to 14 per cent of patients is injury a prime factor in the onset of disc prolapse, that injury is usually only a precipitating factor and that an underlying biochemical defect is the basic cause on which mechanical stresses are superimposed, it may possibly be that the surgical correction of simple lateral discogenic trespass has more than purely mechanical effects. Expressed otherwise, have the procedures of chemonucleolysis (p. 523) and surgical disc enucleation more in common than is expected?

Spencer and De Wald (1979)[1161] have described a technique of simultaneous anterior and posterior surgical approach to the thoracic and lumbar spine; the procedure entails two teams of surgeon and assistant surgeon, and is applicable where combined anterior and posterior instability needs reduction, internal stabilisation and circumferential fusion. In some fixed deformities, circumferential osteotomy, correction and fusion may be required, as in ankylosing spondylitis, for example.

Sciatica and back pain

It is well known that removal of prolapsed disc material is more effective in relieving severe limb pain than it is in relieving the backache, and following surgery some 60 to 70 per cent of patients will still have some back pain at times.[889b]

Another estimate is that while seven or eight out of ten patients will have their sciatica completely relieved, backache will also be relieved in about two out of three.[912]

Mooney (1977)[870] observes that where chronic degenerative changes are responsible for both sciatica and backache, both backache and sciatica are relieved by including the decompression procedure of hemifacetectomy.

Naylor (1974)[909] reviewed 204 cases of surgery for prolapsed intervertebral disc by (in the majority) unilateral exposure with excision of one lamina and ligamentum flavum, with or without removal of the spinous process to expose two roots. He observed that backache was the most frequent disability after operation (17 per cent), and is related to the degree of degenerative change before and after the operation. The surgical procedure of itself does not produce backache.

Types of root trespass

In a minority of patients with clinical evidence of root involvement, further exploration for the cause may be necessary during the surgical procedure.[775]

Among 842 patients, there were 68 in whom surgical exposure did not reveal any disc herniation, until the operative field was further explored and five causes of root tension were revealed:

(i) Migration of a fragment of disc into the intervertebral foramen.
(ii) Kinking of the nerve root by the pedicle above.
(iii) Compression of a nerve root between a superior articular process and the pedicle above.
(iv) Diffuse annular bulge by loss of disc height, with subluxation of posterior joints, marked osteophytosis

and ligamentum flavum bulging. In all of this group the lesion was at L4–L5.

(v) Extraforaminal lateral disc herniation.

In 18 of the 68 patients, no abnormality could be found.

Postoperative management

The rate at which the patient is mobilised, the time before walking is permitted and the relative vigour of rehabilitation exercises, varies with the surgeon and the degree of surgical exposure.[723]

Microsurgical technique

For the 'virgin' herniated lumbar disc, a *conservative discectomy* by microsurgical technique has recently been described (Williams, 1978).[1322] There is no laminectomy or disturbance of facet-joint structure, no disturbance of the epidural fat and no sacrifice of healthy disc material. The technique of blunt perforation of the annulus, rather than scalpel incision, appears to minimise reherniation and the formation of adhesions.

The small operative field is approached through a one-inch midline incision. Perforation of the 'virgin' annulus is made gently by blunt dissector, producing a small dilated opening which can be seen to close in a sphincter-like fashion after the decompression procedure. A portion of the herniated disc, which is compressing the nerve root, is removed by repeated small evacuations with micro-lumbar forceps. The perineural extradural fat is preserved, thus minimising the risk of postoperative adhesions. Operating time averages 37 minutes.

Straight-leg-raising begins on the second postoperative day, and on average the patient goes home on the third day. No car-riding or sitting is allowed for three weeks postoperatively.

A series of 530 patients is reported, and on the basis of recovery to being physically comfortable and economically productive, satisfactory results were achieved in 91 per cent. The average time for return to work in non-compensation cases was 5.2 weeks.

It is interesting that slow onset, recurrent sciatica occurred in the same root distribution in three patients who ceased the twice-daily straight-leg-raising exercise several years after the initial operation.

Re-exploration after negative myelography showed an annulus well sealed by fibrous reaction, plentiful epidural fat but a nerve root immobile to straight-leg-raising testing in the theatre. Dense adhesions on the ventral root surface were tethering the root, which became freely mobile after their release; these patients were asymptomatic two years later and were continuing their twice-daily straight-leg-raising exercise.

After a follow-up study of 147 patients over a two-and-a-half year period, Goald (1978)[415] mentions that a transfusion was never necessary, and that the procedure is safe,

effective and economic. The surgical cure rate was 96 per cent, and one year after surgery all non-compensation cases were working, as were 80 per cent of the compensation cases. Unless the patient's work was heavy labour, they returned to their usual activities within four to six weeks.

Fusion

There are several procedures:

a. Posterior laminae fusion
b. Screw-fusion[104]
c. Intertransverse fusion
d. Interbody fusion
e. Posterior H-graft fusion
f. Facet block fusion or posterolateral fusion.[326]

A common technique is transfacet screw fusion and posterior laminae fusion by bone graft.[923]

'Surgical procedures tend to produce certain irreversible effects on the intervertebral joints. Spinal fusion, when successful, tends to produce permanent stability in the treated joint ... but limitation of movement may precipitate problems with neighbouring joints.' (Farfan, 1973.)[326]

Aside from the techniques of spinal fusion and indications for particular modifications of technique, which are not the concern of this text, there appears much less disagreement about surgical fusion for frank lumbar instability than about fusion procedures as an accompaniment to excision of prolapsed disc material, when this is the sole reason for surgical intervention.

'Over 80 per cent of neurosurgeons and 60 per cent of orthopaedic surgeons consider fusion rarely or never indicated ... spinal fusion in lumbar-disc surgery is one of the most disputed fields in orthopaedics; some urge routine fusion to improve functional results, others agree that trials in alternate cases show that it is never required.' (Le Vay, 1967.)[723]

After 10 years, Frymoyer *et al.* (1978)[393] evaluated 79 per cent of 312 patients who had undergone lumbar disc surgery, some with fusion and some without.

Functional restrictions, back symptoms and nerve root problems were just as common among the 143 patients on whom fusion was carried out, as they were among the 64 patients who did not have the fusion procedure with disc excision. Of those whose spines were fused, 30 per cent were considered long-term failures; of those without fusion the figure was 37.7 per cent. Symptoms at the bone-graft donor site persisted in 37 per cent of the fusion patients.

After reviewing other studies, the authors conclude that there is slight but statistically insignificant benefit in combining fusion with disc excision.

Freebody (1964)[378] described the procedure of trans-peritoneal anterior interbody fusion, and later (1971)[379] reviewed the results of 252 operations over a 12-year period; 243 patients were followed-up and are tabulated as follows:

Degenerative disc lesions	66	patients excellent or good results in 60
Retrospondylolisthesis	10	patients excellent or good results in 10
Spondylolisthesis (mostly group II)	167	patients excellent or good results in 152

Analysis revealed no close relationship between the clinically less good patients and radiological evidence of partial union or non-union.

The presence of postoperative symptoms may be related to something less than good bony fusion, but analysis of the 'satisfactory' and 'failure' patients revealed that other factors are also important and may contribute to failure.

A consecutive series of 83 patients treated by anterior disc excision and interbody fusion was reported by Stauffer and Coventry (1972)[1163] with a good clinical result in only 36 per cent, and X-ray evidence of fusion at all levels grafted in only 56 per cent. They concluded that the reported differences in success rates with this technique were attributable chiefly to interpretation of clinical and X-ray factors by different authors, and to the type of patient selected for the procedure.

In this respect it is noteworthy that Rolander (p. 41)[1055] has suggested that while a 'solid' fusion corrects instability it does not completely immobilise a vertebral segment.

Further, bony union is not necessary for subjective relief of symptoms; fibrous union may be enough (Shaw and Taylor, 1956).[1115]

Weber (1970)[1293] has shown, over a mean follow-up period of 5.5 years after discectomy and spinal fusion from L4 to S1, that with mobility at the fusion levels or visible fractures in the bone graft a 'good' or 'fair' result may be achieved. X-ray films were taken at full flexion and extension.

Adkins (1955)[7] suggested that estimations of fusion by mobility X-rays may be unreliable in that no distinction can be made between bony union and fibrous ankylosis.

A stereophotogrammetric X-ray method[1104] can be used to detect and measure all movement between segments which have not fused with complete bony union, and among a small series of three patients with a total of seven mobility segments operated on, only one segment had healed with a solid bony union. Three of the segments operated on had retained their mobility, and the three remaining segments were comparatively rigid though still mobile.

The patient with the one solidly fused segment still had a painful stiff back after 275 days; the other two patients without solid fusion were largely relieved of their pain, one at 285 days and the other after a year.

It is suggested by Goldner et al. (1971)[418] that assessment of bone union by X-ray may not be accurate until a postoperative year has elapsed.

Kokan et al. (1974)[670] mention that solid lumbar fusion is not the only requirement for relief of disabling low back pain, and that successful pain relief is more likely when degenerative changes are limited to one or two levels only; there is freedom from neuroticism; the history of back pain is short.

Continuous chronic or episodic pain following spinal fusion may be due to several factors, e.g.

a. Disc prolapse and root involvement at a segment below the fusion
b. Iatrogenic stenosis, by overgrowth of new tissue into the neural canal or trespass upon the foraminal contents
c. Extensive fibrosis around nerve roots
d. Dural cysts forming adjacent to or below the fusion site.

Goldner et al. (1971)[418] refer to these factors when advocating, for certain cases, the technique of anterior disc excision and interbody fusion. They suggest that the fusion rate is at least as good as that with other methods of operation, give the indications for the anterior approach and recommend discography under local anaesthesia as a useful diagnostic procedure.

Farfan (1973)[326] considers it primarily important to regard *facet fusion* as an antitorsion device, and by the technique of denuding the facet-planes of articular cartilage, and wedging the joints open with blocks of cancellous bone, the length of the neural arch is maintained, the articular processes are preserved and the neural arch is strengthened.

Occasional cases of acquired spondylosis, following lumbar and lumbosacral fusion procedures, are reviewed by Harris and Wiley (1963),[510] who suggest that the lesion may be more common than brief references in the literature may indicate.

Spinal stenosis

... the elderly individual crippled by spondylotic caudal radiculopathy can be given a new lease of life by adequate surgical decompression, just as can younger individuals with lumbar stenosis. As our knowledge expands and experience increases in these areas, it is hoped that diagnosis will become even more sophisticated and treatment even safer and more effective. Recent developments leading to application of techniques of axial spinal tomography and microsurgery with high-speed drills suggest that this may indeed be the case.[1300]

It has been suggested[714] that the recent emphasis upon *acquired* abnormality, such as space-occupying trespass by herniated disc and tumours, as a cause of spinal stenosis has overshadowed the importance of *developmental stenosis* (see p. 275).

Three types of developmental stenosis are described:

(i) Concentric
(ii) Sagittal flattening
(iii) Unilateral or bilateral abnormal articular processes.

Occasionally, type (iii) coexists with either of types (i) or (ii).

The authors observe that adequate relief requires decompression of the neural contents in all three dimensions, sagittal, coronal and vertical length of spinal canal; they have not yet encountered any significant spinal instability after total resection of posterior structures for developmental stenosis.

The multiply-operated back

Mooney and Cairns (1978)[869] suggest that multiple operations do not increase the success rate in controlling chronic low back pain, and that the chances are only 1 in 10 that improvement will occur after two operations in the industrial case of back pain (see p. 491).

> ... the assumption that we are treating a progressive degenerative disease ... episodic complaints of pain reflect a process of injury which exceeds the rate of repair ... loss of soft tissue control has occurred in the degenerating segment ... our goal is to return soft tissue control to the highest level feasible and to train the patient to avoid reinjury, but we must add to this various psychogenic factors which tend to potentiate the pain initiated by structural disorders. These significant factors are often poorly measured by the clinician.

Perhaps the outlook need not be so gloomy.

Saunders and Jacobs (1976)[1084] report the outcome in 50 patients who had undergone previous back surgery. In all, the vertebral structures were explored and the procedure completed by posterolateral fusion; those with nerve root involvement had thorough decompression including wide laminectomy where indicated. Back pain was relieved in 44 out of 50 patients and sciatic pain was relieved in 38 of 43 patients. Of 30 patients in whom assessment of fundamental ability was possible, 24 returned to work.

In a review of 60 patients who required repeat surgery after lumbar disc excision,[160] 49 were found to be suffering recurrent root pain, 20 suffered back pain and 8 had other problems such as infection and extradural cysts. In the group with recurrent sciatica, perineural fibrosis and recurrent herniation were the most common factors. Most patients presented within the first year following the initial procedure, but some were delayed for as long as five years.

Recurrent sciatica was usually early, on the same side and at the same level; involvement of other levels usually indicated extensive degenerative disc disease.

Lumbosacral arachnoiditis. This is not as rare as previously thought, but common in patients with severe back and/or leg pain—the 'failed-back-surgery syndrome'. The condition is a definable pathological entity, although its relationship to pain is at present poorly defined (Burton, 1978).[144a] It represents a reaction to a number of causal factors, and the presence of Pantopaque in the subarachnoid space is probably the most significant of these.

The long-term failure rate of back surgery is variously reported as being between 10 and 40 per cent, so the number of patients with chronic pain and functional disablement is significant.

In a series of 100 failed-back-surgery patients who had been referred for intractable pain, 280 myelograms with Pantopaque had been performed prior to referral. The group studied averaged 3.6 back operations and 2.8 myelograms per patient.

Arachnoiditis may be suspected in some, but since diagnosis requires direct observation at open operation or an unequivocal myelographic appearance, its incidence is difficult to document.

Burton proposes the following stages in development of the condition:

(i) *Radiculitis*—inflammation of the pia-arachnoid with hyperaemia and swelling of the nerve roots of the cauda equina. Strands of collagen begin to appear between roots and the pia-arachnoid.

(ii) *Arachnoiditis*—the decreased nerve root swelling is accompanied by fibroblast proliferation and increased collagen deposits.

(iii) *Adhesive arachnoiditis*—the end of the inflammatory stage is marked by dense fibrosis, completely encapsulating the nerve roots, which are now ischaemic and progressively atrophied.

In the majority of patients studied, the observed changes included loculated cysts containing spinal fluid and/or Pantopaque.

When the dural cavity is opened, there may be exposed apparently empty space; atrophied nerve roots are enmeshed in solid collagenous scar tissue and are 'plastered' to the dura and to each other.

It is suggested by the author that this pathological entity will fade from the clinical scene when reliable, non-invasive diagnostic techniques are developed, and in this respect, the technique of computerised transverse axial tomography scanning (p. 371) shows promise.

References

1. Adams C B T, Logue V 1971 Studies in cervical spondylotic myelopathy I. Brain 94: 557
2. Adams C B T, Logue V 1971 Studies in cervical spondylotic myelopathy II. Brain 94: 569
3. Adams C B T, Logue V 1971 Studies in cervical spondylotic myelopathy III. Brain 94: 587
3a. Adams M A, Hutton W C 1980 Correspondence. Spine 5: 483
4. Adams P, Muir H 1976 Qualitative changes with age of proteoglycans of human lumbar disc. Ann Rheum Dis 35: 289
5. Adams R 1857 A treatise on chronic rheumatic arthritis. Publisher unnamed, London
6. Adams-Ray J, Pernow B 1949 Some new observations concerning the symptom 'pallor' in the inflammation syndrome. Acta Chir Scand 98: 221
7. Adkins E W 1955 Lumbosacral arthrodesis after laminectomy. J Bone & Jt Surg 37B: 208
8. Adler I 1900 Muscular rheumatism. Med. Rec 57: 529
9. Agarival A, Lloyd K N, Dovey P 1970 Thermography of the spine and sacro-iliac joints in spondylitis. Rheum & Phys Med 10: 349
10. Agnoli A L 1975 Myelotomography in the diagnosis of lumbo-sacral disc prolapse. Acta Neurochirurg 32: 113
11. Agnoli A L 1976 Anomalies in the pattern of lumbo-sacral nerve roots and its clinical significance. J Neurol 211: 217
12. Aho A J et al 1969 Analysis of cauda equina symptoms in patients with lumbar disc prolapse. Acta Chir Scand 135: 413
13. Åkerblom B 1949 Standing and sitting posture. AB Nordiska Bokhandeln, Stockholm
14. Alarcón-Segovia D, Cetina J A, Díaz-Jouanen E 1973 Sacro-iliac joints in primary gout. Amer J Roentgen 188: 438
15. Albrand O W, Corkill G 1979 Thoracic disc herniation: treatment and prognosis. Spine 4: 41
16. Albuquerque J E et al 1974 The effects of vinblastine and colchicine on neural regulation of muscle. Ann NY Acad Sci 228: 224
17. Alexander F M 1932 The use of self. Methuen, London
18. Allbrook F M 1957 Movements of the lumbar spinal column. J Bone & Jt Surg 39B: 339
19. Allen F M 1938 Effects of ligations on nerves of the extremities. Ann Surg 108: 1088
20. Allison D R 1950 Pain in the chest wall simulating heart disease. British Medical Journal 1: 332
21. American Academy of Orthopaedic Surgeons 1969 Symposium on the spine. C V Mosby, St Louis
22. Amsler F R, Wilber M C 1967 Interosseous vertebral venography as a diagnostic aid in evaluating intervertebral-disc disease of the lumbar spine. J Bone & Jt Surg 49A: 703
23. Anderson I F, Corrigan A B, Champion G D 1972 Rib erosions in rheumatoid arthritis. Ann Rheum Dis 31: 16
24. Anderson J A D 1976 Back pain in industry. In Jayson M (ed) The lumbar spine and back pain. Sector Publishing, London, ch 2
25. Anderson J A D 1977 Problems of classification of low back pain. Rheum & Rehab 16: 34
26. Anderson P, Eccles J C, Sears J C 1964 Cortically evoked depolarization of primary afferent fibres in the spinal cord. J Neurophysiol 27: 63
27. Anderson S A et al 1976 Evaluation of the pain suppressive effect of different frequencies of peripheral electrical stimulation in chronic pain conditions. Acta Orthop Scand 47: 149
28. Anderson T M 1955 Manual lifting and handling. Industrial Welfare Society, London
29. Anderson T M 1971 Human kinetics and good movement. Physio 57: 169
30. Andersson B J G, Ötengren R et al 1974 On myoelectric back muscle activity and lumbar disc pressure in sitting postures. Scand J Rehab Med Suppl
31. Andersson B J G, Ötengren R et al 1975 The sitting posture: an electromyographic and discometric study. Orth Clin N Amer 6: 1
32. Andersson B J G, Murphy R W et al 1979 The influence of back rest inclination and lumbar support on lumbar lordosis. Spine 4: 52
33. Annartone G, Pavetto G C 1975 Eleven cases of scalenous syndrome. Excerpta Med 18: 217
34. Appenzeller O 1978 Somato-autonomic reflexology–normal and abnormal. In Korr I (ed) Neurobiologic mechanisms in manipulative therapy. Plenum Press, London, p 179
35. Arbuthnot Lane, W 1886 Some points in the phsyiology and pathology of the changes produced by pressure in the bony skeleton of the trunk and shoulder girdle. Guy's Hospital Reports 43: 321
36. Arieff A J, Tigay E L et al 1961 The Hoover sign. Arch Neurol 5: 109
37. Arlen A 1977 Die 'paradox kippbewegung der atlas' in der funktiondiagnostik der halswirbelsäule. Man Med 1: 16
38. Arlen, A 1979 Röntgenologische Funktiondiagnostik der Halswirbelsäule. Man Med 2: 24
39. Armour Pharmaceutical Co undated Radiological atlas of Paget's disease of bone. Eastbourne
40. Armstrong J R 1965 Lumbar disc lesions, 3rd edn. Livingstone, Edinburgh, p. 170
41. Arnold N, Harriman D G F 1970 The incidence of abnormality in control human peripheral nerves studied by single axon dissection. J Neurol Neurosurg Psychiat 33: 55
42. Arnoldi C C 1972 Intravertebral pressures in patients with lumbar pain: a preliminary communication. Acta Orthop Scand 43: 109
43. Arnoldi C C, Lindblom H, Mussbichler H 1972 Venous engorgement and intraosseous hypertension in patients with degenerative arthrosis of the hip. J Bone & Jt Surg 54B: 409
44. Arnoldi C C 1976 Intraosseous hypertension: a possible cause of back pain? Clin Orth & Rel Res 115: 30
45. Arseni C, Nash F 1963 Protrusion of thoracic intervertebral disc. Acta Neurochirurg 11: 1

46. Ashby E C 1977 Abdominal pain of spinal origin. Ann Roy Coll Surg Eng 59: 242
47. Åström J 1975 Pre-operative effect of fenestration upon intraosseous pressures in patients with osteoarthrosis of the hip. Acta Orthop Scand 46: 963
48. Atkinson B W 1978 A new concept in traction tables: Kaltenborn three-dimensional treatment table. Aust J Physio 24: 4
49. Baarstrup C 1933 On the spinous processes of the lumbar vertebrae and the soft tissues between them, and on pathological changes in that region. Acta Radiol 14: 52
50. Bache F 1826 Cases illustrative of the remedial effects of acupuncture. N Amer Med & Surg J 1: 311
51. Bacsich P, Wyburn G M 1945 The effect of interference with the blood supply on the regeneration of peripheral nerves. J Anat 79: 74
52. Baddeley H 1976 Radiology of spinal stenosis. In Jayson M (ed) The lumbar spine and back pain. Sector, London, ch 8
53. Badgley C E 1941 The articular facets in relation to low back pain and sciatic radiation. J Bone & Jt Surg 23: 481
54. Bailey H W, Beckwith C G 1937 Short leg and spinal anomalies. J Amer Osteop Assoc 36: 7
55. Ball J, Sharp J 1971 Rheumatoid arthritis of the cervical spine. In Modern trends in rheumatology II. Butterworth, London, p 117
56. Ballard C F 1956 Affections of the temperomandibular joint. Proc Roy Soc Med 49: 994
57. Bankart A S B 1932 Manipulative surgery. Constable, London
58. Barbor R 1974 Sclerosant therapy. In Cyriax J (ed) Textbook of orthopaedic medicine, 8th edn. Baillière Tindall, London, vol 2, p 292
59. Barbor R 1975 Symptomatology and treatment of disturbance of ligaments in the low back. Rehabilitacia Suppl VIII: 182
60. Barbor R 1978 Personal communication
61. Barker M E 1977 Pain in the back and leg: a general practice survey. Rheum & Rehab 16: 37
62. Barlow E D, Pochin E E 1948 Slow recovery from ischaemia in human nerves. Clin Sci 6: 303
63. Barlow W (1952) Postural homeostasis. Ann Phys Med 1: 77
64. Barnett C H, Cobbold A F 1962 Lubrication within living joints. J Bone & Jt Surg 44B: 662
65. Barnett C H, Cobbold A F 1969 Muscle tension and joint mobility. Ann Rheum Dis 28: 652
66. Barnett C H 1971 The mobility of synovial joints Rheum Phys Med 11: 20
67. Barr J S 1951 Protruded discs and painful backs. J Bone & Jt Surg 33B: 3
68. Barré J-A 1924 Troubles pyramideaux et arthrite vertebral chronique. Médecine, Paris 5: 358
69. Barron D H, Mathews B H C 1935 Intermittent conduction in the spinal cord. J Physiol (London) 85: 73
70. Barron D H, Mathews B H C 1938 The interpretation of potential changes in the spinal cord. J Physiol (London) 92: 276
71. Barson A J 1970 The vertebral level of termination of the spinal cord during normal and abnormal development. J Anat 106: 489
72. Bartelink D L 1957 The role of abdominal pressure in relieving the pressure on the lumbar intervertebral disc. J Bone & Jt Surg 39B: 718
73. Basmajian J V 1976 A fresh look at the intrinsic muscles of the back. The American Surgeon 42: 9
73a. Basmajian J V (ed) 1979 Biofeedback: principles and practice for clinicians. Williams & Wilkins, Baltimore
74. Bathe Rawling L 1940 Landmarks and surface markings of the human body. Lewis, London
75. Baum J, Ziff M 1971 The rarity of ankylosing spondylitis in the black race. Arth & Rheum 14: 12
76. Beadle O A 1931 The intervertebral disc. London: MRC Special Report Series no 161
77. Becks J W F, ter Weeme C A 1975 Herniated lumbar discs in teenagers. Acta Neurochirurg 31: 195
78. Beecher H K 1960 Increased stress and effectiveness of placebo and 'activity' drugs. Science 132: 91

79. Begg A G, Falconer M A 1949 Plain radiographs in intraspinal protrusion of lumbar intervertebral discs: a correlation with operative findings. Brit J Surg 36: 225
80. Bell C 1830 The nervous system of the human body, Appendix P. CXXVII, no LXIV. Longman, London
81. Bell F G 1974 The place of surgery in acute low back pain. In Twomey L T (ed) Symposium: Low back pain. Western Aust Inst Tech, Perth, p 132
82. Benson M K D, Byrnes D P 1975 The clinical syndromes and surgical treatment of thoracic intervertebral disc prolapse. J Bone & Jt Surg. 57B: 471
83. Bentley F H, Schlapp W 1943 Experiments on the blood supply of nerves. J Physiol 102: 62
84. Bentley F H, Schlapp W 1943 The effects of pressure on conduction in peripheral nerves. J Physiol 102: 72
85. Bergquist-Ullman M, Larsson U 1977 Acute low back pain in industry. Acta Orthop Scand Suppl 170
86. Berkovitz B K B, Holland G R, Moxham B J 1978 A colour atlas and text-book of oral anatomy. Wolfe Medical Publications, London
87. Berlin L 1971 A peroneal muscle stretch reflex. Neurol 21: 11
88. Berman L, Isaacs H, Pickering A 1976 Structural abnormalities of muscle tissue in ankylosing spondylitis. SA Med J 50: 1238
89. Bernstein S A 1975 Acute cervical pain associated with soft-tissue calcium deposit anterior to the interspace of the first and second cervical vertebrae. J Bone & Jt Surg 57A: 426
90. Bhalla S K 1968 Cervical spine: recent observations on anatomy and clinical applications. J Can Physio Assoc 20: 2
91. Bianco A J 1968 Low back pain and sciatica: diagnosis and indications for treatment. J Bone & Jt Surg 50A: 170
92. Bick E M, Copel J W 1951 The ring apophysis of the human vertebra: a contribution to human osteogeny II. J Bone & Jt Surg 33A: 803
93. Bickel W H, Romness J O 1957 True diastasis of the sacro-iliac joints with hypermobility. J Bone & Jt Surg 39A: 1381
94. Biemond A, de Jong J M B 1969 On cervical nystagmus and related disorders. Brain 92: 437
95. Bihaug, Oddbjørn 1975 Erfaring med autotraksjon. Fysioterapeuten 42: 434
96. Bishop B 1974 Abdominal muscle activity during respiration. In Wyke B D (ed) Ventilatory and phonatory control systems. Oxford University Press, London
96a. Bishop B 1980 Pain: its physiology and rationale for management. Part 1. Phys Ther 60: 13
97. Bistrom O 1954 Congenital anomalies of the lumbar spine of persons with painless backs. Ann Chir Gyn Fenn 43: 102
98. Black R G, Bonica J J 1973 Analgesic blocks. Postgrad Med 53: 105
99. Boasson M, Forrestier J, Certonciny A et al 1969 Durée des manifestations douloureuses dans les arthroses vertébrales. Rev Rheum Mal Osteoporic 36: 151
100. Bohl W R, Steffee A D 1979 Lumbar spinal stenosis: a cause of continued pain and disability in patients after total hip arthroplasty. Spine 4: 168
101. Bokduk N, Calman R R, Winer C E 1977 An anatomical assessment of the percutaneous rhizolysis procedure. Med J Aust 1: 379
102. Bone R C, Nahum A M, Harris A S 1974 Evaluation and correction of dysphagia-producing cervical osteophytosis. Laryngoscope 84: 2045
103. Bonney G 1970 Stabilisation of the upper cervical spine by the transpharyngeal route. Proc Roy Soc Med 63: 896
104. Boucher H H 1959 A method of spinal fusion. J Bone & Jt Surg 41B: 248
105. Bourdillon J F 1973 Spinal manipulation, 2nd edn. Heinemann, London
106. Braakman R, Vinken P J 1967 Unilateral facet locking in the lower cervical spine. J Bone & Jt Surg 49B: 249
107. Braddock G T F 1979 Personal communication
108. Bradford D S, Garcia A 1971 Lumbar intervertebral disc herniations in children and adolescents. Orth Clin N Amer 2: 583

109. Bradley K C 1967 The importance of anatomical knowledge: Symposium on manipulative treatment. Med J Aust 1: 1274

110. Bradley K C 1974 The anatomy of backache. Aust & NZ J Surg 44: 227

111. Bradshaw P, Parsons M 1965 Hemiplegic migraine: a clinical study. Quart J Med 34: 65

112. Bradshaw P 1957 Some aspects of cervical spondylosis. Quart J Med 26: 177

113. Brailsford J F 1929 Deformities of the lumbo-sacral region of the spine. Brit J Surg 16: 562

114. Brain W R, Northfield D W C, Wilkinson M 1952 The neurological manifestations of cervical spondylosis. Brain 75: 187

115. Brain, Lord 1956 Some aspects of the neurology of the cervical spine. J Fac Radiol 8: 74

116. Brain, Lord 1957 The treatment of pain. SA Med J 31: 973

117. Brain, Lord, Wilkinson M (eds) 1967 Cervical spondylosis. Heinemann, London

118. Breathnach A S 1965 Frazer's anatomy of the human skeleton, 6th ed. Churchill, London

119. Breig A 1960 Biomechanics of the central nervous system: Some basic normal and pathological phenomena. Almqvist & Wiksell, Stockholm

120. Breig A, Turnbull I, Hassler O 1966 Effects of mechanical stress on the spinal cord in cervical spondylosis. J Neurosurg 15: 45

121a. Breig A 1970 Overstretching of, and circumscribed pathological tension in, the spinal cord—a basic cause of symptoms in cord disorders. J Biomech 3: 7

121b. Breig A 1978 Adverse mechanical tension in the central nervous system. Almqvist & Wiksell, Stockholm

121c. Breig A, Troup J D G 1979 Biomechanical considerations in the straight-leg-raising test. Spine 4: 242

122. Bremner R A 1958 Manipulation in the management of chronic low backache due to lumbo-sacral strain. Lancet 1: 20

123. Brendler S J 1968 The human cervical myotomes: functional anatomy studied at operation. J Neurosurg 28: 105

124. Brendstrupp P, Jaspersen K, Asboe-Hansen G 1957 Morphological and chemical connective tissue changes in fibrositic muscles. Ann Rheum Dis 2: 114

125. Brewerton D A et al 1973 Ankylosing spondylitis and HL-A27. Lancet 1: 904

126. Brewerton D A 1977 The doctor's role in diagnosis and prescribing vertebral manipulation. In Maitland G D Vertebral manipulation, 4th edn. Butterworth, London

127. British Association of Physical Medicine 1966 Pain in the neck and arm: a multicentre trial of the effects of physiotherapy. British Medical Journal 1: 253

128. Brocher J E W 1955 Die Occipito-cervical Gegend. Thieme, Stuttgart

129. Brodal A 1965 The cranial nerves—anatomy and anatomicoclinical correlations. Blackwell Scientific, Oxford

130. Brodal A 1969 Neurological anatomy in relation to clinical medicine, 2nd edn. Oxford University Press, London

131. Broderick T W et al 1978 Enostosis of the spine. Spine 3: 167

132. Brodsky A E, Binder W F 1979 Lumbar discography: its value in diagnosis and treatment of lumbar disc lesions. Spine 4: 110

133. Brody I A, Wilkins R H 1969 The signs of Kernig and Brudzinski. Arch Neurol 21: 215

134. Bronowski J 1973 The ascent of man. BBC, London

135. Brooke R 1924 The sacro-iliac joint. Journal of Anatomy 58: 299

136. Brown F R 1949 Testicular pain: its significance and localisation. Lancet 1: 994

137. Brown M D 1971 The pathophysiology of disc disease. Orth Clin N Amer 2: 359

138a. Brown T, Hansen R T, Yorra A J 1957 Some mechanical tests on the lumbo-sacral spine with particular reference to the intervertebral discs. J Bone & Jt Surg 39A: 1135

138b. Bruhn J G 1978 The doctor's touch: tactile communication in the doctor–patient relationship. Southern Med J 71: 1469

139. Buckwalter J A, Cooper R R, Maynard J A 1976 Elastic fibres in human intervertebral discs. J Bone & Jt Surg 58A: 73

140. Bulgen D Y, Hazleman B L, Voak D 1976 HLA-B27 and frozen shoulder. Lancet May 15: 1042

141. Bulos S 1974 Dysphagia caused by cervical osteophyte. J Bone & Jt Surg 56B: 148

142. Burn J M B, Langdon L 1967 Lumbar epidural injection for the treatment of chronic sciatica. Rheum & Phys Med 10: 368

143. Burnell A 1974 Injection techniques in low back pain. In Twomey L T (ed) Symposium: Low back pain. Western Aust Inst Tech, Perth, p 111

144a. Burton C V 1978 Lumbosacral arachnoiditis. Spine 3: 24

144b. Burton C V 1979 Computed tomography scanning and the lumbar spine. Spine 4: 353

145. Buswell J 1978 A manual of home exercises for the spinal column. NZ Manip Ther Assoc, Auckland

146. Butler R W 1955 The nature and significance of vertebral osteochondritis. Proc Roy Soc Med 48: 895

147. Byers P D 1974 What is osteoarthrotic cartilage? In Ali S Y, Elves M W, Leaback D H (eds) Symposium: Normal and osteoarthrotic articular cartilage. Inst of Orthop, London

148. Caccese L F, Aliperta G 1969 I disturbi del sistema nervosa vegetitivo in portatori di ernia dicale. La Clin Orthop 21: 119

149. Cailliet R 1964 Neck and arm pain. Davis, Philadelphia

150. Cailliet R 1966 Low back pain syndrome. Davis, Philadelphia

151. Cailliet R 1977 Rehabilitation management of the patient with low back pain. In Buerger A A, Tobis J S (eds) Approaches to the validation of manipulation therapy. Thomas, Springfield, Illinois, p 94

152. Cairns D, Thomas L et al 1976 A comprehensive treatment approach to chronic low back pain. Pain 2: 301

153. Calin A, Fries J F 1975 Striking prevalence of ankylosing spondylitis in 'healthy' W27 positive males and females: a controlled study. New England J Med 293: 835

154. Callahan M, Sternbach R A et al 1978 Changes in somatic sensitivity during transcutaneous electrical analgesia. Pain 5: 115

155. Calne D B, Pallis C A 1966 Vibratory sense: a critical review. Brain 89: 723

156. Campbell D G, Parsons C M 1944 Referred head pain and its concomitants. J Nerv Ment Dis 99: 544

157. Caplan P S et al 1962 Degenerative joint disease of the lumbar spine in coal miners: a clinical and X-ray study. Arthritis & Rheumatism 5: 288

158. Carson J, Gumpert J, Jefferson A 1971 Diagnosis and treatment of thoracic intervertebral disc protusions. J Neurol Neurosurg Psychiat 34: 68

159. Carstairs L S 1959 Radiology. In: Nassim R, Burrows H J (eds) Modern trends in diseases of the vertebral column. Butterworth, London, p 210

160. Cauchoix J, Girard B 1978 Recurrent surgery after disc excision. Spine 3: 256

161. Causey G, Palmer E 1949 The effect of pressure on nerve conduction and nerve-fibre size. J Physiol 109: 220

162. Cautilli R A et al 1972 Congenital elongation of the pedicles of the sixth cervical vertebra in identical twins. J Bone & Jt Surg 54A: 653

163. Cavaziel H 1973 Beitrag zur kenntnis des iliosakralsyndrome. Man Med 5: 74

164. Cavaziel H 1974 Beitrag zur kenntnis der rippengelenksläsionen. Man Med 5: 110

165. Cavaziel H 1977 Acute torticollis: clinical features and treatment. Man Med 4: 58

166. Cave A J E, Griffiths J D, Whiteley M M 1955 Osteoarthritis deformans of the Luschka joints. Lancet 1: 176

167. Chakravorty B G 1967 Arterial supply of the cervical spinal cord and its relation to cervical myelopathy in spondylosis. Ann Roy Coll Surg Eng 45: 232

168. Charlesworth D, Hayne C R, Troup J D G 1978 Lifting instructor's manual Back Pain Association, Teddington

169. Charnley J 1951 Orthopaedic signs in the diagnosis of disc protrusion. Lancet 1: 186

170. Charnley J 1959 Lubrication of animal joints. Proceedings: Symposium—Biomechanics. Inst Mech Engineers, London

171. Cheatum D E 1976 Ankylosing spondylitis without sacro-ilitis in a woman without the HLA B27 antigen. J Rheum 3: 420

172. Cho K O 1970 Therapeutic epidural block with a combination of a weak local anaesthetic and steroids in management of complicated low back pain. The Amer Surg 36: 303

173. Chrissman D O, Gervais R F 1962 Otologic manifestations of the cervical syndrome. In: De Palma A (ed) Clinical orthopaedics, vol 24. Pitman, London, p 34

174. Chrissman D O et al 1964 Results following rotatory manipulation in the lumbar intervertebral disc syndrome. J Bone & Jt Surg 46A: 517

175. Chusid J G 1973 Correlative neuroanatomy and functional neurology, 15th edn. Lange Medical, Los Altos, California

176. Clark G R, Willis L A et al 1975 Preliminary studies in measuring range of motion in normal and painful stiff shoulder. Rheum & Rehab 14: 39

177. Clark K 1969 Significance of the small lumbar spinal canal: cauda equina compression syndromes due to spondylosis. J Neurosurg 31: 495

178. Clarke A K et al 1977 Ascending lumbar venography in the diagnosis of lumbar disc lesions. Rheum & Rehab 16: 83

179. Clarke G R, Stenner L 1976 Use of therapeutic ultrasound. Physio 62: 185

180. Clarke N G, Kardachi B J 1977 The treatment of myo-fascial pain-dysfunction syndrome using the biofeedback principle. J Periodontal 48: 643

181. Clayson C J et al 1962 Evaluation of mobility of hip and lumbar vertebrae of normal young women. Arch Phys Med 43: 1

182. Clifton H C, Oakley E M 1978 Correspondence: Therapeutic ultrasound. Physio 64: 374

183. Cloward R B 1958 The anterior approach for ruptured cervical discs. J Neurosurg 15: 602

184. Cloward R B 1959 Cervical diskography. Ann Surg 150: 1052

185. Cöers C, Woolf A L 1959 The innervation of muscle. Blackwell, Oxford

186. Cohen A S, McNeil J M et al 1967 The 'normal' sacro-iliac joint. Amer J Roentgenol Rad Ther & Nuc Med 100: 559

187. Cohen H 1947 Visceral pain. Lancet 2: 933

188. Cohen L A 1961 Role of eye and neck proprioception mechanism in body orientation and motor co-ordination. J Neurophysiol 24: 1

189. Cohen L M et al 1976 Increased risk for spondylitis stigmata in apparently healthy HL-AW27 men. Ann Int Med 84: 1

190. Colachis S C, Warden R E et al 1963 Movement of the sacro-iliac joint in the adult male. Arch Phys Med Rehab 44: 490

191. Colachis S C, Strohm B R 1965 Cervical traction: relationship of traction time to varied tractive force with constant angle of pull. Arch Phys Med Rehab 46: 815

192. Colachis S C, Strohm B R 1965 A study of tractive forces and angle of pull on vertebral interspaces in the cervical spine. Arch Phys Med Rehab 46: 820

193. Colachis S C, Strohm B R 1966 Effect of duration of intermittent cervical traction on vertebral separation. Arch Phys Med Rehab 47: 353

194. Collins D H 1949 The pathology of articular and spinal disease. Edward Arnold, London

195. Collins D H 1959 Degenerative diseases. In: Nassim R, Burrows H J (eds) Modern trends in diseases of the vertebral column. Butterworth, London, p 101

196. Collins W F, Nulsen F E, Randt C T 1960 Relation of peripheral nerve size and sensation in man. Arch of Neurol (Chicago) 3: 381

197. Colson J H C 1947 The rehabilitation of the injured, vol 2: Remedial gymnastics. Cassell, London

198. Conlon P W, Isdale I C, Rose B S 1966 Rheumatoid arthritis of the cervical spine. Ann. Rheum Dis 25: 120

199. Connolly R Campbell, Newman P H 1971 Lumbar spondylotomy. J Bone & Jt Surg 53B: 575

200. Cooke A M 1955 Osteoporosis. Lancet 1: 877 and 929

201. Coomes E N 1961 A comparison between epidural anaesthesia and bed rest in sciatica. British Medical Journal 1: 20

202. Cope S, Ryan G M S 1959 Cervical and otolith vertigo. J Laryng & Otolog 73: 113

203. Copeman W S C, Ackerman W L 1947 Oedema or herniations of fat lobules as a cause of lumbar and gluteal 'fibrositis'. Arch Int Med 79: 22

204. Copland J 1954 Abnormal muscle tension and mandibular joint. Dent Rec 74: 331

205. Coppola A R 1968 Neck injury: a reappraisal. Internat Surg 50: 510

206. Cossette J W et al 1971 The instantaneous centre of rotation of the third lumbar intervertebral joint. J Biomech 4: 149

207. Coventry M B, Taper E M 1972 Pelvic instability. J Bone & Jt Surg 54A: 83

208. Coutts M B 1934 Atlanto-epistropheal subluxation. Arch Surg 29: 297

209. Cramer von A 1965 Iliosakralmechanik. Asklepios 9: 1

210. Cregan J C F 1966 Internal fixation of the unstable rheumatoid cervical spine. Ann Rheum Dis 25: 242

211. Crock H V 1970 A re-appraisal of intervertebral disc lesions. Med J Aust 1: 983

212. Crock H V et al 1973 Observations on the venous drainage of the human vertebral body. J Bone & Jt Surg 55B: 528

213. Crock H V 1974 The planning of treatment in spondylolisthesis. In: Twomey L T (ed) Symposium: Low back pain. Western Australia Institute of Technology, Perth, p 117

214. Crock H V 1976 Isolated lumbar disc resorption. Clin Orthop & Rel Res 115: 109

215. Cuello A C, Polak J M, Pearse A G 1976 Substance P: a naturally-occurring transmitter in the human spinal cord. Lancet 2: 1054

216. Curwen I H M 1952 The therapeutic use of ultrasound. Physio 38: 202

217. Cyriax J 1974 Textbook of orthopaedic medicine, vol II, 8th edn. Baillière Tindall, London

218. Cyriax J 1975 Textbook of orthopaedic medicine, vol I, 6th edn. Baillière Tindall, London

219. Dale B B 1973 The clinical findings in 200 low back cases. Brit Osteop J 6: 10

220. Dalseth I 1974 Anatomical studies of the osseous cranio-vertebral joints. Man Med 6: 130

221. Dan N G 1976 The management of vertebral artery insufficiency in cervical spondylosis: a modified technique. Aust NZ J Surg 46: 164

222. Dan N G 1976 Entrapment syndrome. Med J Aust 1: 528

223. Danbury R 1971 Functional anatomy of the intervertebral disc. Man Med 6: 128

224. Dandy D J, Shannon M J 1971 Lumbo-sacral subluxation: Group I spondylolisthesis. J Bone & Jt Surg 53B: 578

225. Dandy W E 1929 Loose cartilage from intervertebral disc simulating tumour of the spinal cord. Arch Surg 19: 660

226. Davis J B, Blair H C 1950 Spurs of the calcaneus in Strümpell–Marie disease: report of fifteen cases. J Bone & Jt Surg 32A: 838

227. Davis P, Lentle B C 1978 Evidence for sacro-iliac disease as a common cause of low backache in women. Lancet 2: 496

228. Davis P R 1955 The thoraco-lumbar mortice joint. J Anat 89: 370

229. Davis P R 1959 Posture of the trunk during the lifting of weights. British Medical Journal 1: 87

230. Davis P R 1963 Some effects of lifting, pulling and pushing on the human trunk. Ergonomics 6: 303

231. Davis P R, Troup J D G 1964 Pressures in the trunk cavities when pulling, pushing and lifting. Ergonomics 7: 466

232. Davis P R, Troup J D G 1966 Human thoracic diameters at rest and during activity. J Anat 100: 397

233. Davis P R, Troup J D G 1966 Effects on the trunk of erecting pit props at different working heights. Ergonomics 9: 475

234. Davis P R 1972 The physical causation of disease. Roy Soc Health J 92: 63

235. Davis P R 1979 Personal communication

236. de Domenico G 1979 Tonic vibratory reflex. Physio 65: 44

237. de Jarnette B 1967 The philosophy, art and science of sacro-occipital technique, de Jarnette, Nebraska

238. de Jong P and J M, Cohen B, Jonkees L B 1977 Ataxia and nystagmus induced by injection of local anaesthetics in the neck. Ann Neurol 1: 240

239. de Palma A F, Rothman R H 1970 The intervertebral disc. W B Saunders, London

240. de Puky P 1935 The physiological oscillation of the length of the body. Acta Orthop Scand 6: 338

241a. De Sèze S, Levernieux J 1951 Les tractions vertébrales; premières études expérimentales et resultats thérapeutiques d'après une experience de quatre années. Semaine des Hôpitaux (de Paris) 27: 2085

241b. De Sèze S 1955 Les attitudes antalgiques dans le sciatique disco-radiculaire commune. Sem Hop Paris 31: 2291

242. Decher H 1969 The cervical syndrome in ENT practice (Die Zervikalen Syndrome in der Hals-Nasen-Ohren Heilkunde). Thieme, Stuttgart

243. Decroix G et al 1965 Electronystagmography and cupulometry as an objective means of symptomatological evaluation and control of vertebral manipulations in the 'Vertebral artery syndrome'. Ann de Méd Physique 8: 12

244. Dee R 1969 Structure and function of hip-joint innervation. Ann Roy Coll Surg Eng 45: 357

245. Dee R 1978 The innervation of joints. In: Sokoloff L (ed) The joints and synovial fluid I. Academic Press, London

246. Dehner J R 1971 Seatbelt injuries of the spine and abdomen. Amer J Roentgen Rad Ther & Nuc Med 111: 833

247. Delmas J, Laux G, Guerrier Y 1947 Comment atteindre les fibres vaso-motrices préganglionaires du membre supérieur. Gaz Méd de France 54: 703

248. Delvin D 1977 You and your back. Pan Books, London

249. Denny-Brown D, Brenner C 1944 Lesions in peripheral nerves resulting from compression by spring-clip. Arch Neurol Psychiat 51: 1

250. Denny-Brown D, Kirk E J, Yanagisawa N 1973 The tract of Lissauer in relation to sensory transmission in the dorsal horn of the spinal cord in the macaque. J Comp Neurol 151: 175

251. Denslow J S, Hassett C C 1942 Central excitatory state associated with postural abnormalities. J Neurophysiol 5: 393

252. Denslow J S 1944 An analysis of the variability of spinal reflex threshold. J Neurophysiol 7: 207

253. Dept. of Health and Social Security 1979 Report of working group on back pain. HMSO, London

254. Deshayes P et al 1977 Rheumatic signs in 80 cases of Crohn's disease. Rev du Rheum 43: 345

255. Devlin B H, Goldman M 1966 Backache due to osteoporosis in an industrial population. Irish J Med Sci 484: 141

256. Dexler H 1893 Weiner Med Presse 34: 1997

257. Dible J H, Davie T B 1950 Pathology, 3rd edn. Churchill, London

258. Dietzel G 1978 Befunderhebung von funktionellen störungen der sakro-iliakal-gelenke nach sell. Man Med 3: 54

259. Dintenfasse L 1963 Lubrication in synovial joints. J Bone & Jt Surg 50B: 1241

260. Dionne J 1974 Neck torsion nystagmus. Can J Otolaryng 3: 37

261. Dixon A S J, Campbell-Smith S 1969 Long-leg arthropathy. Ann Rheum Dis 28: 359

262. Dixon A S J 1976 Diagnosis of low back pain: sorting the complainers. In: Jayson M (ed) The lumbar spine and back pain. Sector, London, p 77

263. Dixon A S J 1978 The diagnosis of polymyalgia rheumatica. EULAR Bulletin (English edn) 7: 93

264. Dixon B (ed) 1979 Technology. New Scientist 82: 122

265. Dombrowski E T 1970 Personal communication

266. Dommisse G F 1974 The blood supply of the spinal cord. J Bone & Jt Surg 56B: 225

267. Donald H R 1965 The carpal tunnel syndrome. Lancet 2: 740

268. Donisch E W, Basmajian J V 1972 Electromyography of deep muscles of the back in man. Amer J Anat 133: 25

269. Doran D M L 1969 Mechanical and postural causes of chest pain. Proc Roy Soc Med 62: 876

270. Doran D M L, Newell D J 1975 Manipulation in treatment of low back pain: a multi-centre study. British Medical Journal 2: 161

271. Doran F S A, Ratcliffe A H 1954 Physiological mechanisms of referred shoulder-tip pain. Brain 77: 427

272. Doran F S A 1967 The sites to which pain is referred from the common bile-duct in man and its implication for the theory of referred pain. Brit J Surg 54: 599

273. Dott N M 1951 Facial pain. Proc Roy Soc Med 44: 1034

274. Downie W W, Leatham P A et al 1978 Studies with pain rating scales. Ann Rheum Dis 37: 378

275. Dowson D 1973 Lubrication and wear in joints. Physio 59: 104

276. Doyle J R 1960 Narrowing of the intervertebral disc space in children. J Bone & Jt Surg 42A: 1191

277. Draheim J H, Johnson L C, Helwig E B 1959 A clinico-pathologic analysis of 'rheumatoid' nodules occurring in 54 children. Amer J Path 35: 678

278. Driver A F M 1964 Sensitivity to heat and cold of summer and winter preferers. Ergonomics 7: 475

279. Drum D C 1975 The vertebral motor unit and intervertebral foramen. In: The research status of spinal manipulative therapy. US Dept of Health NINCDS Monograph no 15, Bethesda

280. Duffin D 1978 Acupuncture past and present. Physio 64: 203

281. Duncan C P, Shim S S 1977 The autonomic nerve supply to bone. J Bone & Jt Surg 59B: 323

282. Duncan D 1948 Alterations in the structure of nerves caused by restricting their growth with ligatures. J Neuropath & Exp Neurol 7: 261

283. Dunham W F 1949 Ankylosing spondylitis: measurement of hip and spine movement. Brit J Phys Med 12: 126

284a. Durey A, Rodineau J 1976 Les lésions pubiennes des sportifs. Ann de Méd Physique 3: 282

284b. du Toit G T 1973 Knee joint-ligament injuries. South Afr J Surg 11: 261

285. Dutton C B, Riley L H 1969 Cervical migraine: not merely a pain in the neck. Amer J Med 47: 141

286. Dyson M, Pond J B 1970 The effect of pulsed ultrasound on tissue regeneration. Physio 56: 136

287. Dyson M, Pond J B 1976 Biological effects of therapeutic ultrasound. Rheum & Rehab 12: 209

288. Dyson M, Suckling J 1978 Stimulation of tissue repair by ultrasound: a survey of the mechanisms involved. Physio 64: 105

289. Ebbetts J 1971 Autonomic pain in the upper limb. Physio 57: 270

290. Ebner M 1978 Connective tissue massage. Physio 64: 208

291. Eckerson L B, Roberts G H, Howard T 1928 Thoracic pain persisting after coronary thrombosis. J Amer Med Assoc 90: 1780

292. Edds M V, Small W T 1951 The behaviour of residual axons in partially denervated muscles of the monkey. J Exp Med 93: 207

293. Edeiken J, Pitt M J 1971 The radiologic diagnosis of disc disease. Orth Clin N Amer 2: 405

294. Eder M 1975 Die krankengymnastiche rehabilitation in rhamen der manuelle medizin. Man Med 2: 41

295. Ederling J 1974 Migraine and other chronic headaches. Physio S Africa 30: 2

296. Ederling J 1975 The abandoned headache syndrome. Proceedings: Golden Jubilee Congress. SA Physio Assoc, Johannesburg

297. Edgar M A, Nundy S 1966 Innervation of the spinal dura mater. J Neurol Neurosurg Psychiat 25: 530

298. Edgar M A, Park W M 1974 Induced pain patterns on passive straight-leg-raising in lower lumbar disc protrusion. J Bone & Jt Surg 56B: 658

299. Edgar M A, Ghadially J A 1976 Innervation of the lumbar spine. Clin Orth & Rel Res 115: 35

300. Editorial 1972 Rheumatological remedies. The Practitioner 208: 1

301. Editorial 1978 Concern for care. Physio 64: 33

302. Editorial 1978 Apophyseal joints and back pain. Lancet July 29: 247

303. Editorial 1979 Back pain: what can we offer? British Medical Journal 1: 706

304. Editorial 1979 Technology. New Scientist 82: 122

305. Editorial 1979 Stay young by good posture. New Scientist 82: 544

306. Editorial 1979 Scanning for X-ray hazards. New Scientist 82: 932

307. Edwards B C 1969 Low back pain and pain resulting from lumbar spine conditions: a comparison of treatment results. Aust J Physio 15: 3

308a. Edwards W L J 1955 Musculo-skeletal chest pain following myocardial infarction. Amer Heart J 49: 713

308b. Egund N et al 1978 Movements in the sacro-iliac joints demonstrated with roentgen stereo-photogrammetry. Acta Radiol (Diagn) 19: 833

309. Eis, N 1964 Combined extirpation and spinal fusion in lumbar intervertebral disc herniation. J Oslo City Hosp 14: 149

310. Elbe J N 1960 Pattern of responses of the paravertebral musculature to visceral stimulation. Amer J Physiol 198: 429

311. Emmett J L, Love J G 1971 Vesical dysfunction caused by protruded lumbar disc. J Urol 105: 86

312. Emminger E 1968 Die wirbelgelenk luxation. Machr Unfallheilk 71: 181

313. Emminger E 1972 Les articulations inter-apophysaires et leurs structures ménisciodes vues sous l'angle de la pathologie. Ann de Méd Physique 15: 219

314. Epstein B S 1966 An anatomic, myelographic and cinemyelographic study of the dentate ligaments. Amer J Roentgen 98: 704

315. Epstein B S 1969 The spine: a radiological text and atlas, 3rd edn. Lea & Febiger, Philadelphia

316. Epstein J A et al 1969 The importance of removing osteophytes as part of the surgical treatment of myeloradiculopathy in cervical spondylosis. J Neurosurg 30: 219

317. Epstein J A 1973 Lumbar root compression at the intervertebral foramina caused by arthritis of the posterior facets. J Neurosurg 39: 362

318. Epstein J A et al 1974 Surgical treatment of nerve root compression caused by scoliosis of the lumbar spine. J Neurosurg 41: 449

319. Epstein J A et al 1979 Total myelography in the evaluation of lumbar discs: with the presentation of three cases of thoracic neoplasms simulating nerve root lesions. Spine 4: 121

320. Evans J A 1947 Reflex sympathetic dystrophy: report on 57 cases. Ann Int Med 26: 417

321. Evans W 1930 Intra-sacral epidural injections in the treatment of sciatica. Lancet 2: 1225

322. Eyring E J et al 1964 Intervertebral disc calcification in children: a distinct clinical syndrome. J Bone & Jt Surg 46A: 1432

322a. Fairbanks J C T, O'Brien J P 1980 The abdominal cavity and thoraco-lumbar fascia as stabilisers of the lumbar spine. In: Conference proceedings: Engineering aspects of the spine. Mechanical Engineering Publications Ltd, London, p 83

323. Fallet G H, Mason M et al 1976 Rheumatoid arthritis and ankylosing spondylitis occurring together. British Medical Journal 1: 804

324. Farfan H F 1969 Effects of torsion on the intervertebral joints. Can J Surg 12: 336

325. Farfan H F et al 1972 Lumbar intervertebral disc degeneration: the influence of geometrical features on the pattern of disc degeneration. J Bone & Jt Surg 54A: 492

326. Farfan H F 1973 Mechanical disorders of the low back. Lea & Febiger, Philadelphia

327. Farfan H F 1975 Paper read at the meeting of the international society for the study of the lumbar spine. London

328. Farfan H F 1975 Muscular mechanisms of the lumbar spine and the position of power and efficiency. Orth Clin N Amer 6: 135

329. Farfan H F et al 1976 The mechanical aetiology of spondylolysis and spondylolisthesis. Clin Orth & Rel Res 117: 40

330. Farfan H F 1977 Pathological basis for manipulative therapy. In: Kent B (ed) Proceedings: Third Seminar: Internat Fed Orthop Manip Therapists, IFOMT. Hayward, California, p 135

331. Farfan H F, Lamy C 1977 A mathematical model of the soft tissue mechanisms of the lumbar spine. In: Buerger A A, Tobis J S (eds) Approaches to the validation of manipulative therapy. Thomas, Springfield, Illinois, p 5

332. Farhion S L 1977 Autogenic biofeedback training for migraine. Mayo Clin Proc 52: 776

333. Farhni W H, Trueman G E 1965 Comparative radiological study of the spines of a primitive population with North Americans and Southern Europeans. J Bone & Jt Surg 47B: 552

334. Farhni W H 1966 Observations on straight-leg-raising with special reference to nerve-root adhesions. Can J Surg 9: 44

335. Farhni W H 1976 Backache and primal posture. Musqueam Publishers, Vancouver

336. Farhni W H 1976 Backache: assessment and treatment. Musqueam Publishers, Vancouver

337. Farhni W H 1977 Postural concepts in back pain. In: Kent B (ed) Proceedings: Third Seminar: Internat Fed Orthop Manip Therapists. IFOMT, Hayward, California, p. 35

338. Farkas A 1950 On the pathomechanism and therapy of the low back syndrome with special reference to osteoporosis of the spine. Rheumatism 6: 157

339. Farkas J 1932 Über einen fall von luxation des 5 halswirbels. Zentr-Org ges Chir 60: 36

340. Farrow R C 1961 Shoulder pain and stiffening. Physio 47: 326

341. Fein R S 1967 Are synovial joints squeeze-film lubricated? Proc Inst Mech Eng 181: Part 3J: 125

342. Feinstein B et al 1954 Experiments on referred pain from deep somatic tissues. J Bone & Jt Surg 36A: 981

343. Feinstein B 1977 Referred pain from paravertebral structures. In: Buerger A A, Tobis J F (eds) Approaches to the validation of manipulation therapy. Thomas, Springfield, Illinois, p 139

344. Fenlin J M 1971 Pathology of degenerative disease of the cervical spine. Orth Clin N Amer 2: 371

345. Fentem P H, Shakir I 1977 Vibration, blood pressure and heart rate. Physio 63: 364

346. Fetz E E 1968 Pyramidal tract effects on interneurons in the cat lumbar dorsal horn. J Neurophysiol 31: 69

347. Fick R 1911 Handbuch der Anatomie und Mechanik der Gelenke. unter: Berucksichtigung der Beweegenden Muskein. Bardeleben, Jena

348. Fielding J W 1954 Cineroentgenography of the normal cervical spine. J Bone & Jt Surg 39A: 1280

349. Fielding J W 1964 Normal and selected abnormal motion of the cervical spine from the second cervical vertebra to the seventh cervical vertebra: based on cineroentgenography. J Bone & Jt Surg 46A: 1779

350. Fielding J W, Zickel R E 1964 Accessory lamina: a cause of lumbar nerve root pressure. J Bone & Jt Surg 46A: 837

351. Fielding J W, Reddy K 1969 Atlanto-axial rotatory deformity. J Bone & Jt Surg 51A: 1672

352. Fielding J W, Reddy K, Pappalardo P 1971 Fixed atlanto-axial rotatory subluxation. J Bone & Jt Surg 53A: 1031

353. Fielding J W, Hohl M (1974) Tears of the transverse ligament of atlas: a clinical and biomechanical study. J Bone & Jt Surg 56A: 1683

354a. Fielding J W, Hawkins R J, Ratzan S A 1976 Spine fusion for atlanto-axial instability. J Bone & Jt Surg 58A: 400

354b. Fielding J W, Hawkins R J 1977 Atlanto-axial rotatory fixation. J Bone & Jt Surg 59A: 37

354c. Fielding J W, Hawkins R J et al 1978 Atlanto-axial rotatory deformities. Orth Clin N Amer 9: 995

355. Fielding J W et al 1978 Use of computed tomography for the diagnosis of atlanto-axial rotatory fixation. J Bone & Jt Surg 60A: 1102

356. Finneson B E 1969 Diagnosis and management of pain syndromes, 2nd edn. W B Saunders, London

357. Finneson B E 1977 A summary of the clinical approaches to back pain. In: Buerger A A, Tobis J S (eds) Approaches to the validation of manipulation therapy, ch 3. Thomas, Springfield, Illinois

358. Finneson B E 1978 A lumbar disc surgery predictive score card. Spine 3: 186

359. Finneson B E, Cooper V R 1979 A lumbar disc surgery predictive score card: a retrospective evaluation. Spine 4: 141

360. Fischer-Wasels J 1959 Über die atlasfehestellung mit einer kritischen bemerkung zu der arbeit von H Felton. Z Orthop 91: 3

361. Fisher T 1922 A contribution to the pathology and aetiology of osteo-arthritis. Brit J Surg 10: 73

362. Fisk J W 1971 Manipulation in general practice. NZ Med J 74: 172
363. Floyd W F, Silver P H S 1950 Electromyographic study of patterns of activity of the anterior abdominal wall muscles in man. J Anat 84: 132
364. Floyd W F, Silver P H S 1955 Functions of erector spinae muscles in certain movements and postures in man. J Physiol 129: 184
365. Flowers R S 1968 Meralgia paraesthetica—a clue to retroperitoneal malignant tumour. Amer J Surg 116: 89
366. Fordyce W E et al 1973 Operant conditioning in the treatment of chronic pain. Arch Phys Med Rehab 54: 399
367. Fordyce W E 1973 An operant conditioning method for managing chronic pain. Post-grad Med 53: 123
368. Forrest A J, Wolkind S N 1974 Masked depression in men with low back pain. Rheum & Rehab 13: 148
369. Fossgreen J, Foldspang A 1974 Das iliosakralgelenk nach bekenfraktur. Man Med 2: 32
370. Fox E J, Melzack R 1976 Transcutaneous electrical stimulation and acupuncture: comparison of treatment for low back pain. Pain 2: 141
371. Fox M, Saunders N R 1978 The significance of loin pain in women. Lancet 1: 115
372. Francis J 1974 Posterior rhizotomy in low back pain. In: Twomey L T (ed) Symposium: Low back pain. Western Aust Inst Tech, Perth, p 156
373. Frankel V H, Burstein A H 1965 Biomechanics and related engineering topics. In: Kenedi R M (ed) Load capacity of tubular bones. Pergamon Press, London
374. Frankel V H, Yi-Shiong H 1975 Recent advances in the biomechanics of sports injuries. Acta Orthop Scand 46: 484
375. Franks A S T 1968 Cervical spondylosis presenting as the facial pain of tempero-mandibular joint disorder. Ann Phys Med 9: 193
376. Fraser D M 1976 Post-partum backache: a preventable condition? Can Fam Phys 22: 1434
377. Fraser F W 1978 Persistent post-sympathetic pain treated by connective tissue massage. Physio 64: 211
378. Freebody D 1964 Treatment of spondylolisthesis by anterior fusion via the transperitoneal route. J Bone & Jt Surg 46B: 788
379. Freebody D, Bendall R, Taylor R D 1971 Anterior transperitoneal lumbar fusion. J Bone & Jt Surg 53B: 617
380. Freeman W, Watts J W 1946 Pain of organic disease relieved by pre-frontal lobotomy. Proc Roy Soc Med 39: 445
381. Friburg S 1939 Studies on spondylolisthesis. Acta Chirurg Scand 82: Suppl 55
382. Friburg S 1948 Anatomical studies on lumbar disc degeneration. Acta Orthop Scand 17: 224
383. Friburg S, Hirsch C 1949 Anatomical and clinical studies on lumbar disc degeneration. Acta Orthop Scand 19: 222
384. Fried L C, Doppman J L, Chiro G 1970 Direction of blood flow in the primate cervical spinal cord. J Neurosurg 33: 325
385. Friedenberg Z B et al 1959 Degenerative changes in the cervical spine. J Bone & Jt Surg 41A: 61
386. Friedman A P 1975 Migraine. Psychiat Ann 5: 29
387. Frigerio N A, Stowe R R, Howe J W 1974 Movement of the sacro-iliac joint. Clin Orthop & Rel Res 100: 370
388. Froning E C, Frohman B 1968 Motion of the lumbo-sacral spine after laminectomy and spinal fusion. J Bone & Jt Surg 50A: 897
389. Froriep A 1843 Ein Beitrag zur pathologie und therapie des rheumatismus. Weimar
390. Fryette H H 1954 Principles of osteopathic technique. Academy of Applied Osteopathy, Carmel, California
391. Frykholm R 1951 Cervical nerve root compression resulting from disc degeneration and root sleeve fibrosis. Acta Chir Scand Suppl 160
392. Frykholm R 1971 The clinical picture. In: Hirsch C, Zotterman Y (eds) Cervical pain. Pergamon Press, Oxford, p 5
393. Frymoyer J W et al 1978 Disc excision and spine fusion in the management of lumbar disc disease. Spine 3: 1
394. Fung Y B 1968 Biomechanics: its scope, history and some problems of centenuum mechanics in physiology. Appl Mech Rev 21: 1
395. Galenus: Opera Bd IV Venetia 1625 quoted by Schiotz E H (1968) Manipulation treatment of the spinal column from the medico-historical viewpoint (NIH Library translation). Tidsskr Nor Laegeform 78: 359
396. Gallie W E 1939 Fractures and dislocations of the cervical spine. Amer J Surg 46: 495
397. Ganne J-M 1972 Why do physical treatments relieve pain? Aust J Physio 18: 117
398. Gardner D L, Woodward D 1969 Scanning electron microscopy and replica studies of articular surfaces of guineapig synovial joints. Ann Rheum Dis 28: 379
399. Gardner E 1950 Physiology of movable joints. Physiol Rev 30: 127
400. Gardner E 1963 Physiology of joints. J Bone & Jt Surg 45A: 1061
440a. Greenman P E 1979 Lift therapy: use and abuse. J Amer Osteop Assoc 79: 238
401. Gasser H S 1935 Conduction in nerves in relation to fibre types. Res Publ Ass Nerv Ment Dis 15: 35
402. Gaymans F 1973 New mobilisation principles and techniques for the vertebral column. Man Med 2: 28
403. Gelfan S, Tarlov I M 1956 Physiology of spinal cord, nerve root and peripheral nerve compression. Amer J Physiol 185: 217
404. Gershen-Cohen J 1946 Phantom nucleus pulposus. Amer J Roentgen 56: 43
405. Ghadially F N 1978 The fine structure of joints. In: Sokoloff L (ed) The joints and synovial fluid 1. Academic Press, London
406. Ghormley R K 1933 Low back pain: with special reference to the articular facets. J Amer Med Assoc 101: 1773
407. Gilchrist I C 1976 Psychiatric and social factors related to low back pain in general practice. Rheum & Rehab 15: 101
408. Gillet H, Liekens M 1968 Belgian chiropractic research notes, 7th edn. Gillet & Liekens, Brussels
409. Gilliatt R W 1975 Peripheral nerve compression and entrapment, 11th symposium: Advanced medicine. Pitman Medical, Tunbridge Wells
410. Glick E N, Lucas M 1970 Ice therapy. Ann Phys Med 10: 70
411. Glogowski G, Wallraff J 1951 Ein beitrag zur klinik und histologie der muskelhärten (myogelosen). Z Orthop 80: 237
412a. Glover J 1960 Back pain and hyperaesthesia. Lancet 1: 1165
412b. Glover J R 1971 Occupational health research and the problem of back pain. Trans Soc Occup Med 21: 2
413. Glover J R, Morris J G, Khosola T 1974 Back pain: a randomized clinical trial of rotational manipulation of the trunk. Brit J Indust Med 31: 59
414. Glyn J H 1971 Rheumatic pains: some concepts and hypotheses. Proc Roy Soc Med 64: 354
415. Goald H J 1978 Microlumbar discectomy: follow-up of 147 patients. Spine 3: 183
416. Goddard M D, Reid J D 1965 Movements induced by straight leg raising in the lumbo-sacral roots, nerves and plexus, and in the intra-pelvic portion of the sciatic nerve. J Neurol Neurosurg Psychiat 28: 12
417. Golding D N 1969 Cervical and occipital pain as presenting symptoms of intracranial tumour. Ann Phys Med 10: 1
418. Goldner J L et al 1971 Anterior disc excision and interbody spinal fusion for chronic low back pain. Orth Clin N Amer 2: 543
419. Goldstein M J, Korr I 1948 Dematomal autonomic activity in relation to segmental motor reflex threshold. Fed Proc 7: 67
420. Goldthwait J E 1911 The lumbo-sacral articulation: an explanation of many cases of lumbago, sciatica and paraplegia. Boston Med & Surg J 164: 365
421. Goldthwait J E et al 1952 Essentials of body mechanics. Lippincott, London
422. Golub B S, Silverman B 1969 Transforaminal ligaments of the lumbar spine. J Bone & Jt Surg 51A: 947
423. Gomez J M, Cunill M A B, Querol J R 1977 Correlation between pseudospondylolisthesis and arthrosis of the hands. Rheum & Rehab 16: 30
424. Good A E 1967 Non-traumatic fracture of the thoracic spine in ankylosing spondylitis. Arth & Rheum 10: 467

425. Gooding M R 1964 MSc thesis, University of London
426. Gooding M R 1974 Pathogenesis of myelopathy in cervical spondylosis. Lancet Nov 16: 1180
427. Goor C, Ongerboor de Visser B W 1976 Jaw and blink reflexes in trigeminal nerve lesions. Neurol 26: 95
428. Gottesman J R, Harris D H, Olshan N H 1975 Suboccipital and cervical facet-joint injection complications. Arch Phys Med & Rehab 56: 539
429. Goulden E A 1921 The treatment of sciatica by galvanic acupuncture. British Medical Journal April 9: 523
430. Govoni A F 1971 Developmental stenosis of a thoracic vertebra resulting in narrowing of the spinal canal. Amer J Roentgen Rad Ther & Nuc Med 112: 401
431. Gowers W R 1904 Lumbago: its lessons and analogues. British Medical Journal 1: 117
432. Graham C E 1974 Back ache and sciatica: a report of 90 patients treated by intradiscal injection of chymopapain (discase). Med J Aust 1: 5
433. Grant A P, Keegan D A J 1968 Rib pain—a neglected diagnosis. Ulster Med J 37: 162
434. Grant J C B 1958 Method of anatomy. Williams & Wilkins, Baltimore
435. Grantham V A 1977 Backache in boys—a new problem? The Pract 218: 226
436. Gratz C M 1931 Tensile strength and elasticity tests on human fascia lata. J Bone & Jt Surg 13: 334
437. Warwick R, Williams P (eds) 1973 Gray's anatomy, 35th edn. Longman, London
438. Green D, Joynt R J 1959 Vascular accidents to the brain stem associated with neck manipulation. J Amer Med Assoc 170: 522
439. Greenfield J G 1963 Neuropathology, 2nd edn. Williams & Wilkins, Baltimore
440. Greenman P E 1978 Manipulative therapy in relation to total health care. In: Korr I (ed) The neurobiologic mechanisms in manipulative therapy. Plenum Press, London, p 83
440a. Greenman P E 1979 Lift therapy: use and abuse. J Amer Osteop Assoc 79: 238
441. Gregersen G, Lucas D B 1967 An in vivo study of axial rotation of the human thoraco-lumbar spine. J Bone & Jt Surg 49A: 247
442. Grieve G P 1958 Manual lifting and handling. Physio 44: 1
443. Grieve G P 1967 The rationale of manipulation. Physio 53: 338
444. Grieve G P 1970 The post-graduate teaching of manipulation. Physio 56: 21
445. Grieve G P 1970 Sciatica and the straight-leg-raising test in manipulative treatment. Physio 56: 337
446. Grieve G P 1970 The application of manual mobilising technique. Prog in Phys Ther 1: 321
447. Grieve G P 1971 The hip. Physio 57: 212
448. Grieve G P 1973 Post-graduate manipulation courses. Physio Canada 25: 1
449. Grieve G P 1974 Manual mobilising techniques in degenerative arthrosis of the hip. In: Proceedings: WCPT Congress. WCPT, London, p 262
450. Grieve G P 1975 Manipulation. Physio 61: 11
451. Grieve G P 1976 The sacro-iliac joint. Physio 62: 384
452. Grieve G P 1977 Abdominal pain of spinal origin (letter). Lancet 2: 455
453. Grieve G P 1978 Sacroiliacaleddet. Danske Fysio-terapeuter 4: 7 and 5: 5
454. Grieve G P 1978 Manipulation: a part of physiotherapy. Physio 64: 358
455. Grieve G P 1979 Manipulation therapy for neck pain. Physio 65: 5
456. Grieve G P 1979 Mobilisation of the spine, 3rd edn. Churchill Livingstone, Edinburgh
457. Griffin G A 1973 Osteopathy in general practice. Proc Roy Soc Med 66: 423
458. Grisel P 1930 Énucleation de l'atlas et torticollis nasopharyngien. Press Méd 38: 50
459a. Gross D 1974 Pain and the autonomic nervous system. In: Bonica J J (ed) Advances in neurology. Raven Press, New York, IV, 92
459b. Gross D 1977 Multifactorial diagnosis and treatment of low back pain. Munch Med Wochenschr 119: 1263
460. Grundfest H 1936 Effects of hydrostatic pressures upon the excitability, the recovery and potential sequence in frog nerve. Cold Harbour Symposia on Quantitative Biology 4: 179
461. Guerrier Y 1944 Le sympathique cervical. Imprimière de la Charité, Montpelier
462. Gunn C C, Milbrandt, W E 1975 Review of 100 patients with 'low back sprain' treated by surface electrode stimulation of acupuncture points. Amer J Acupunct 3: 224
463. Gunn C C, Milbrandt W E 1976 Transcutaneous neural stimulation, needle acupuncture and 'tech-i' phenomenon. Amer J Acupunct 4: 317
464. Gunn C C et al 1976 Acupuncture loci; a proposal for their classification according to their relationship to known neural structures. Amer J Chin Med 4: 183
465. Gunn C C, Milbrandt W E 1976 Tenderness at motor points: a diagnostic and prognostic aid for low back injury. J Bone & Jt Surg 58A: 815
466. Gunn C C, Milbrandt W E 1976 Tennis elbow and the cervical spine. Can Med Ass J 114: 803
467. Gunn C C, Milbrandt W E 1977 The neurological mechanism of needle-grasp in acupuncture. Amer J Acupunct 5: 115
468. Gunn C C, Milbrandt W E 1977 Shoulder pain, cervical spondylosis and acupuncture. Amer J Acupunct 5: 121
469. Gunn C C, Milbrandt W E 1977 Tennis elbow and acupuncture. Amer J Acupunct 5: 61
470. Gunn C C, Milbrandt W E 1977 Tenderness at motor points: an aid in diagnosis of pain in the shoulder referred from the cervical spine. J Amer Osteop Assoc 77: 196
471. Gunn C C, Milbrandt W E 1977 Utilizing trigger points. The Osteop Phys March 29
472. Gunn C C, Milbrandt, W E 1978 Early and subtle signs in low back sprain. Spine 3: 267
473. Guthrie-Smith O F 1949 Rehabilitation, re-education and remedial exercises, 2nd edn. Baillière, Tindall, & Cox, London
474. Gutmann von G 1967–68 Zur stellung der chirotherapie in der medezin. Man Med 4: 1
475. Gutmann von G 1970 X-ray diagnosis of spinal dysfunction. Man Med 4: 73
476. Gutmann von G 1970 Statische aspekte bei der coxarthrose. Man Med 5: 111
477. Gutmann von G 1973 Haltungsfehler und kopfschmerz. Man Med 4: 76
478. Hackett J S 1957 Joint ligament relaxation. Thomas, Springfield, Illinois
479. Hadley L A 1936 Apophyseal subluxation: disturbances in and around the intervertebral foramen causing back pain. J Bone & Jt Surg 18: 428
480. Hadley L A 1961 Anatomico-roentgenographic studies of the posterior spinal articulations. Amer J Roentgen 86: 270
481. Hagen R 1974 Pelvic girdle relaxation from an orthopaedic point of view. Acta Orthop Scand 45: 550
482. Haines R W 1946 Movements of the first rib. J Anat 80: 94
483a. Hakelius A et al 1969 The cold sciatic leg. Acta Orthop Scand 40: 614
483b. Hakelius A 1970 Prognosis in sciatica. Acta Orthop Scand Suppl 129
484. Hakim N, King A 1976 Programmed replication of in situ (whole body) loading conditions during in vitro (substructure) testing of a vertebral column segment. J Biomech 9: 629
485. Haldeman S, Meyer B J 1970 The effect of constriction on the conduction of the action potential in the sciatic nerve. SA Med J 44: 903
486. Haldeman S 1977 Why one cause of back pain? In: Buerger A A, Tobis J S (eds) Approaches to the validation of manipulation therapy. Thomas, Springfield, Illinois, ch 10
487. Haldeman S 1978 The clinical basis for discussion of mechanics of manipulative therapy. In: Korr I (ed) The neurobiologic mechanisms in manipulative therapy. Plenum Press, London, p 53
488. Hall M C 1965 The locomotor system: functional anatomy. Thomas, Springfield, Illinois

489. Halliday H V 1957 Applied anatomy of the spine. Year Book: Academy of Applied Osteopathy, Carmel, California
490. Halsted W S 1916 An experimental study of circumscribed dilation of an artery immediately distal to a partially occluding band, and its bearing on the dilatation of the subclavian artery observed in certain cases of cervical rib. J Exp Med 24: 271
491. Hamblen D L 1967 Occipito-cervical fusion. Indications, technique and results. J Bone & Jt Surg 49B: 33
492. Hammond M J 1969 Clinical examination and the physiotherapist. Aust J Physio 15: 47
493. Hampson W G J, Shah J S 1973 Perspectives in biomaterials science. Physio 59: 120
494. Hankey G T 1954 Temperomandibular arthrosis: an analysis of 150 cases. Brit Dent J 97: 249
495. Hankey G T 1956 Affections of the temperomandibular joint. Proc Roy Soc Med 49: 983
496. Hannington-Kiff J G 1977 The c.n.s. mechanisms of pain perception. In: Lonbay E L (ed) The anatomy of pain, Book I. Dista Ltd, Basingstoke
497. Hansen H-J 1959 Comparative views on the pathology of disc degeneration in animals. Lab Invest 8: 1242
498. Hansen K, Schliak D 1962 Segmental Innervation: ihre Bedeuting für Klinic und Praxis. Thieme, Stuttgart
499. Happey F 1976 A biophysical study of the human intervertebral disc. In: Jayson M (ed) The lumbar spine and back pain. Sector, London, ch 13
500. Harding M E 1977 The 'I' and the 'Not-I': a study in the development of consciousness. Coventure, London
501. Hardingham T E, Muir H 1974 The function of hyaluronic acid in proteoglycan aggregation. In: Ali S Y, Elves M W, Leaback D H (eds) Symposium: Normal and arthrotic articular cartilage. Institute of Orthopaedics, London, p 51
502. Harley C 1966 Extradural corticosteroid infiltration. Ann Phys Med 9: 22
503. Harman J B 1948 The localisation of deep pain. British Medical Journal 1: 188
504. Harman J B 1951 Angina in the analgesic limb. British Medical Journal 2: 521
505. Harris N H 1974 Lesions of the symphysis pubis in women. British Medical Journal 4: 209
506. Harris N H, Murray R O 1974 Lesions of the symphysis in athletes. British Medical Journal 4: 211
507. Harris R I 1951 Spondylolisthesis. Ann Roy Coll Surg Eng 8: 259
508. Harris R I, Macnab I 1954 Structural changes in the lumbar intervertebral discs. J Bone & Jt Surg 36B: 304
509. Harris R I 1959 Congenital anomalies. In: Nassim R, Burrows H J (eds) Modern trends in diseases of the vertebral column. Butterworth, London, p 52
510. Harris R I, Wiley J J 1963 Acquired spondylolysis as a sequel to spine fusion. J Bone & Jt Surg 45A: 1159
511. Hart F D, Taylor R T, Huskisson E C 1970 Pain at night. Lancet April 25: 881
512. Hart F D, Huskisson E C 1972 Pain patterns in the rheumatic disorders. British Medical Journal 4: 213
513. Hart F D (1972) Analgesics and non-steroid anti-inflammatory agents in rheumatic disease. The Practitioner 208: 10
514. Hart F D 1977 Nice, simple, revealed truth. World Med Aug. 10: 24
515. Hartman J T, Dohn D F 1966 Paget's disease of the spine with cord or nerve root compression. J Bone & Jt Surg 48A: 1079
516. Harvey B R, Elphick A M 1969 Electrotherapy. Physio 55: 198
517. Harvey P G 1978 Biofeedback—trick or treatment? Physio 64: 333
518. Haugen F P 1968 The autonomic nervous system and pain. Anaesthesiol 29: 785
519. Hawkins R J et al 1976 Os odontoideum: congenital or acquired. J Bone & Jt Surg 58A: 413
520. Haxton H A 1954 Sympathetic nerve supply of the upper limb in relation to sympathectomy. Ann Roy Coll Surg Eng 14: 247
521. Hay M C 1974 The incidence of low back pain in Busselton. In: Twomey L T (ed) Symposium: Low back pain. Western Aust Inst Tech, Perth, p 7
522. Hazelman B, Bulgen D 1979 Low back pain. Medicine Series 3: 13: 649
523. Hazlett J W 1975 Low back pain with femoral neuritis. Clin Orthop & Rel Res 108: 19
524. Head H, Rivers W H R, Sherren J 1905 The afferent nervous system from a new aspect. Brain 28: 99
525. Head H, Sherren J 1905 The consequences of injury to peripheral nerves in man. Brain 28: 116
526. Head H 1920 Studies in neurology. Oxford Medical Publications, London, p 653
527. Hearn E 1975 You are as young as your spine. Heinemann, London
528. Heinz E R, Goldman R L 1972 The role of gas myelography in neuroradiologic diagnosis. Radiol 102: 629
529. Heinz G J, Zavala D C 1977 Slipping rib syndrome diagnosis using the hooking manœuvre. J Amer Med Assoc 237: 794
530. Hekelius A 1970 Prognosis in sciatica. Acta Orthop Scan Suppl 129
531. Helbing R (1978) The sacro-iliac joint after hip arthrodesis. Z Orthop 116: 113
532. Henriques C Q 1962 Veins of the vertebral column. Ann Roy Coll Surg Eng 31: 1
533. Hensen R A, Parsons M (1967) Ischaemic lesions of the spinal cord. Quart J Med 36: 205
534. Herbert C M et al 1975 Changes in the collagen of human intervertebral discs during ageing and degenerative disc disease. J Mol Med 1: 79
535. Herlihy W F 1947 Revision of the venous system: the role of the vertebral veins. Med J Aust 1: 661
536. Herman R 1979 A chemical clue to disease: nuclear magnetic resonance. New Scientist 81: 874
537. Hewitt W 1970 The intervertebral foramen. Physio 56: 332
538. Heylings D J A 1978 Supraspinous and interspinous ligaments of the human lumbar spine. J Anat 125: 127
539. Hicklin J A 1968 Erosive vertebral disease in ankylosing spondylitis. Ann Phys Med 9: 206
540. Hidayet M A et al 1973 Investigations on the innervation of the human diaphragm. Anat Record 179: 507
541. Hilton R C, Ball J, Benn R T 1976 Vertebral end-plate lesions (Schmorl's nodes) in the dorso-lumbar spine. Ann Rheum Dis 35: 127
542. Hiltz D L 1976 The sacro-iliac joint as a source of sciatica. Phys Ther 56: 1373
543. Hinoki M, Teremaya K 1966 Physiological role of neck muscles in the occurrence of optic eye nystagmus. Acta Otolaryng 62: 157
544. Hinsey J C, Phillips R A 1940 Observations on diaphragmatic sensation. J Neurophysiol 3: 175
545. Hinz P, Erdmann H 1968 Zur manuellen unterschung der halswirbelsäule in der gutachterpraxis. Z Orthop 104: 28
546. Hirsch C, Schajowicz F 1953 Studies on the structural changes in the lumbar annulus fibrosus. Acta Orthop Scand 22: 184
547. Hirsch C, Bobechko W P 1965 Auto-immune response to nucleus pulposus in the rabbit. J Bone & Jt Surg 47B: 574
548. Hirsch C, Schajowicz F, Galante J 1967 Structural changes in the cervical spine. Acta Orthop Scand Suppl 109
549. Hirsch C 1971 Reflections on the use of surgery in lumbar disc disease. Orth Clin N Amer 2: 493
550. Hirsch C, Zotterman Y 1971 Cervical pain. Pergamon Press, Oxford
551. Hirsch D, Ingelmark B, Miller M 1963 The anatomical basis for low back pain. Acta Orthop Scand 33: 1
552. Hitselburger W E, Witten R M 1968 Abnormal myelograms in asymptomatic patients. J Neurosurg 28: 204
553. Hockaday J M, Whitty C W M 1967 Patterns of referred pain in the normal subject. Brain 90: 481
554. Hodge C J, Binet E F, Kieffer S A 1978 Intradural herniation of lumbar intervertebral discs. Spine 3: 346
555. Hodgson A R 1969 Cervical spondylosis. J West Pac Orthop Assoc 6: 1
556. Hoff J et al 1977 The role of ischaemia in the pathogenesis of cervical spondylotic myelopathy. Spine 2: 100

557. Hoffman P 1915 Ueber eine methode, den erfalgeiner nervenn aht zu beurteilen. Med Klin 11: 359

558. Hohl M, Baker H R 1964 The atlanto-axial joint: roentgenographic and anatomical study of normal and abnormal motion. J Bone & Jt Surg 46A: 1739

559. Hohl M 1974 Soft tissue injuries of the neck in automobile accidents: factors influencing prognosis. J Bone & Jt Surg 56A: 1675

560. Hollander J L 1978 Painful joints: clues to early diagnosis. Postgrad Med 64: 50

561. Hollin S A, Gross S W, Levin P 1965 Fracture of cervical spine in patients with rheumatoid arthritis. Amer Surg 31: 532

562. Hollinshead W H 1969 Anatomy for surgeons, 2nd edn. Harper & Row, New York, vol 3, p 176

563. Holman J F 1941 A study of the slipping-rib-cartilage syndrome. New Eng J Med 224: 928

564. Holt E P 1964 Fallacy of cervical discography: report of 50 cases in normal subjects. J Amer Med Assoc 188: 799

565. Holt S, Yates P O 1966 Cervical spondylosis and nerve root lesions. J Bone & Jt Surg 48B: 407

566. Homewood A E 1963 The neurodynamics of the vertebral subluxation. Chiropractic Publishers, Willowdale

567. Homma S H 1973 A survey of Japanese research on muscle vibration. In: Desmedt J (ed) New developments in e.m.g. and clinical neurophysiology. Karger, Basel, vol 3

568. Hood L B, Chrissman D 1968 Intermittent pelvic traction in the treatment of ruptured intervertebral disc. J Amer Phys Ther Assoc 48: 21

569. Hoover B B 1970 Value of polyphasic potentials in diagnosis of lumbar root lesions. Arch Phys Med Rehab 51: 546

570. Hoppenfeld S 1979 Physical examination of the knee joint by complaint. Orthop Clin N Amer 10: 3

571. Horack H M 1967 Cervical root syndrome. Med Clin N Amer 51: 1027

572. Horal J 1969 The clinical appearance of low back disorders in the city of Gothenburg, Sweden. Acta Orthop Scand Suppl 118

573. Horner D B 1964 Lumbar back pain arising from stress fractures of the lower ribs. J Bone & Jt Surg 46A: 1553

574. Hovind H, Nielsen S L 1974 Local blood flow after short-wave diathermy. Arch Phys Med Rehab 55: 217

575. Howe J F et al 1977 Mechanosensitivity of dorsal root ganglia and chronically injured axons: a physiological basis for the radicular pain of nerve root compression. Pain 3: 25

576. Howes R G, Isdale I C 1971 The loose back: an unrecognised syndrome. Rheum Phys Med 11: 72

577. Hudgins C V 1933 Conditioning and voluntary control of the pupillary light reflex. J Gen Psychol 8: 3

578. Hudgins W R 1977 The crossed straight-leg-raising test. New Eng J Med 297: 1127

579. Huft R 1975 EMG and X-ray evaluation of pelvic traction. Orthopaedic seminars, vol 7. Rancho Los Amigos Hosp, Downey, California

580a. Hult L 1954 The Munkfors investigation. Acta Orthop Scand 16: 30

580b. Hult L 1971 Frequency of symptoms for different age groups and professions. In: Hirsch C, Zotterman Y (eds) Cervical pain. Pergamon Press, Oxford, p 17

581. Hume A 1960 The surgical approach to thoracic intervertebral disc protrusion. J Neurol Neurosurg Psychiat 23: 133

581a. Hurrell M 1980 Electromyographic feedback in rehabilitation. Physiotherapy 66: 293

582. Hursch J B 1939 Conduction velocity and diameter of nerve fibres. Amer J Physiol 127: 131

583. Huskisson E C, Hart F D 1973 Joint diseases: all the arthropathies. Wright, Bristol

584. Huskisson E C 1974 Recent drugs and the rheumatic diseases. Report on Rheum Dis no 54. Arthritis & Rheumatism Council, London

584a. Hutton W C, Adams M A 1980 The forces acting on the neural arch and their relevance to low back pain. In: Conference proceedings: Engineering aspects of the spine. Mechanical Engineering Publications Ltd, London, p 49

585. Huwyler J 1952 Hernias discales. Rev Chir Orthop 38: 219

586. Igarashi M et al 1969 Role of the neck proprioceptors for the maintenance of dynamic bodily equilibrium in the squirrel monkey. Laryngoscope 79: 1713

587. Igarashi M et al 1972 Nystagmus after experimental cervical lesions. Laryngoscope 82: 1609

588. Iggo A 1955 Tension receptors in the stomach and urinary bladder. J Physiol (London) 128: 593

589. Iggo A 1966 Cutaneous receptors with a high sensitivity to mechanical displacement. In: de Reuck A V S, Knight K (eds) Touch, heat and pain: Ciba Foundation Symposium. Churchill, London

590. Illouz von G, Coste F 1965 Das 'dreiben-zeichen' bei der untersuchung der iliosakral gelenke. Asklepios 9: 255

591. Ingpen M L, Burry H C 1970 A lumbo-sacral strain syndrome. Ann Phys Med 10: 270

592a. Inman V T, Saunders J B 1942 The clinico-anatomical aspects of the lumbo-sacral region. Radiol 38: 669

592b. Inman V T, Saunders J B 1944 Referred pain from skeletal structures. J Nerv & Ment Dis 90: 660

593. Inman V T, Saunders J B 1947 Anatomico-physiological aspects of injuries to the intervertebral disc. J Bone & Jt Surg 29: 461

594. Irstam L, Rosencrantz M 1972 Water soluble contrast media and adhesive arachnoiditis. Acta Radiol Diag Reprint 1

595. Irstam L, Sundström R, Sigstedt B 1974 Lumbar myelography and adhesive arachnoiditis. Acta Radiol 15: 356

596. Jabbari B et al 1977 Brown-Sequard syndrome and cervical spondylosis. J Neurosurg 47: 556

597. Jackson A M et al 1978 Lytic spondylolisthesis above the lumbo-sacral level. Spine 3: 260

598. Jackson R 1966 The cervical syndrome, 3rd edn. Thomas, Springfield, Illinois

599. Jackson R 1967 Headaches associated with disorders of the cervical spine. Headache 6: 175

600. Jacobson M 1970 The neural control of differentiation of skeletal muscle. In: Developmental neurobiology. Holt, Rinehart & Wilkinson, New York, p 281

601. Jacobson R E, Gargano F P, Rasomoff H L 1975 Transverse axial tomography of the spine: Part I. Axial anatomy of the normal lumbar spine. J Neurosurg 42: 406

602. Jacobson R E, Gargano F P, Rasomoff H L 1975 Transverse axial tomography of the spine: Part II. The stenotic spinal canal. J Neurosurg 42: 412

603. Jacoby R K et al 1976 Radiographic stereo-plotting. Ann Rheum Dis 35: 168

604a. Jaffe H L 1956 Benign osteoblastoma. Bull Hosp Jt Dis 17: 141

604b. Jaffe L F, Poo M 1979 Neurites grow faster towards the cathode than the anode in a steady field. J Exp Zool 209: 115

605. James C C, Lassman L P 1972 Spinal dysraphism. Butterworth, London

606. Janda V 1976 The muscular factor in the pathogenesis of back pain syndrome. Physiotherapy Symposium, Oslo

607. Janda V 1978 Muscles, central nervous motor regulation and back problems. In: Korr I (ed) The neurobiologic mechanisms in manipulative therapy. Plenum Press, London, p 27

608. Jayson M et al 1973 Intervertebral discs: nuclear morphology and bursting pressures. Ann Rheum Dis 32: 308

608a. Jayson M I V 1980 Structure and function of the human spine. In: Conference proceedings: Engineering aspects of the spine. Mechanical Engineering Publications Ltd, London, p 9

609. Jenness M E 1975 The role of thermography and postural measurement in structural diagnosis. In: The research status of spinal manipulative therapy. US Dept of Health NINCDS, Bethesda, Monograph No 15, p 255

610. Jennett W B 1956 A study of 25 cases of compression of the cauda equina by prolapsed intervertebral discs. J Neurol Neurosurg Psychiat 19: 109

611. Jirout J 1971 Pattern of changes in the cervical spine in lateroflexion. Neuroradiol 2: 164

612. Johnson C, Kersley C D, Airth G R 1970 Rib lesions in rheumatoid disease. Brit J Radiol 43: 269

613. Johnson E W, Melvin J L 1971 Value of electromyography in lumbar radiculopathy. Arch Phys Med Rehab 52: 239

614. Johnson E W, Wolfe C V 1972 Bifocal spectacles in the etiology of cervical radiculopathy. Arch Phys Med Rehab 53: 201

615. Jones E S 1934 Joint lubrication. Lancet 1: 1426

616. Jones L H 1964 Spontaneous release by positioning. Doct Osteop 4: 109

617. Jones M D, Wise B L 1967 Contribution of venous obstruction to experimentally-induced Scheuermann's disease. Radiol Clin (Basel) 36: 91

618. Jones R A C, Thompson J L G 1968 The narrow lumbar canal. J Bone & Jt Surg 50B: 595

618a. Jones A I, Wolf S L 1980 Treating chronic low back pain: emg biofeedback training during movement. Phys Ther 60: 58

619. Jowett R L, Fidler M W 1975 Histochemical changes in the multifidus in mechanical derangements of the spine. Orth Clin N Amer 6: 145

620. Judovich B D 1954 Lumbar traction therapy and dissipated force factors. Lancet 74: 411

621. Judovich B D 1955 Lumbar traction therapy: elimination of physical factors that prevent lumbar stretch. J Amer Med Assoc 159: 549

622. Judovich B D, Nobel G R 1957 Traction therapy: a study of resistance forces. Amer J Surg 93: 108

623. Jung A, Kehr P 1972 Das zerviko-enzephale syndrom bei arthrosen und nach traumen der halswirbelsäule. Man Med 6: 86

624. Junghanns H 1930 Spondylolisthesen ohne spalt im zwischengelenkstück (pseudospondylolisthesen). Arch Orthop und Unfall-Chirurg 29: 118

625. Junghanns H 1974 Die bedentung der insufficienta intervertebralis für die wirbelsäulenforschung. Man Med 5: 93

626. Kahn E A 1947 The role of the dentate ligaments in spinal cord compression and the syndrome of lateral sclerosis. J Neurosurg 4: 191

627. Kaltenborn F, Lindahl O 1969 Reproducerbarheten vid rörelseundersökning av enskilda kotor. Läkartidningen 66: 962

628. Kamieth H, Reinhardt K 1955 Der ungleiche symphysenstand ein wichtiges symptom der beckenringlockerung. Fortsch Roentgen 83: 530

629. Kane R L et al 1974 Manipulating the patient. Lancet 1: 1333

630. Kanshepolsky J, Danielson H, Flynn R E 1972 Vertebral artery insufficiency and cerebeller infarct due to manipulation of the neck. Bull LA Neurol Soc 37: 62

631. Kapandji I A 1974 The physiology of joints III: The trunk and vertebral column. Churchill Livingstone, London

632. Kapsalis A A, Stern I J, Bornstein I 1974 The fate of chymopapain injected for therapy of intervertebral disc disease. J Lab & Clin Med 83: 532

633. Kazarian L 1974 NASA (unpublished data). USA

634. Keele C A, Armstrong D 1964 Substances producing pain and itch. Edward Arnold, London

635. Keele C A, Neil E (eds) 1971 Samson Wright's applied physiology, 12th edn. Oxford University Press, London

636. Keene G C R, Hone M R, Sage M R 1978 Atlas fracture: demonstration using computerized tomography. J Bone & Jt Surg 60A: 1106

637. Keidel W D 1972 The problem of subjective and objective quantification of pain. In: Janzen R, Keidel W D, Herz A, Steichele C (eds) Pain, basic principles, pharmacology, therapy. Thieme, Stuttgart, p 16

638. Keith A 1948 Human embryology and morphology. Edward Arnold, London

639. Keller G 1959 Die arthrose der wirbelgelenke in ihrer beziehung zum rückenschmerz. Z Orthop 91: 538

640. Kellgren J H 1938 Observations on referred pain arising from muscle. Clin Sci 3: 175

641. Kellgren J H 1939 On the distribution of pain arising from deep somatic structures with charts of segmental pain areas. Clin Sci 4: 35

642. Kellgren J H 1940 Somatic simulating visceral pain. Clin Sci 4: 303

643. Kellgren J H, Lawrence J S 1958 Osteo-arthritis and disc degeneration in an urban population. Ann Rheum Dis 17: 388

644. Kellgren J H (ed) 1963 Atlas of standard radiographs of arthritis. Blackwell Scientific, London, vol 2

645. Kellgren J H 1977 The anatomical source of back pain. Rheum & Rehab 16: 3

646. Kelsey J L, Hardy R J 1975 Driving of motor vehicles as a risk factor for acute herniated lumbar intervertebral disc. Amer J Epidemiol 102: 63

647. Kemp H, Worland J 1974 Infections of the spine. Physio 60: 2

648. Kendall P H 1955 A history of lumbar traction. Physio 41: 177

649. Kendall P H, Jenkins J M 1968 Exercises for backache: a double-blind controlled trial. Physio 54: 154

650. Kennard M A, Haugen F P 1955 The relation of subcutaneous focal sensitivity to referred pain of cardiac origin. Anaesthesiol 16: 297

651. Keon-Cohen B 1968 Abnormal arrangement of the lower lumbar and first sacral nerves within the spinal canal. J Bone & Jt Surg 50B: 261

652. Kern E B 1972 Referred pain to the ear. Minn Med Oct: 896

653. Kerr F W L 1975 Pain: a central inhibitory balance theory. Mayo Clin Proc 50: 685

654. Kéry L, Vizkeletey T, Woutters H W 1971 Recherches expérimentales à propos de l'effect de la stase veineuse sur los, le cartilage et le disque intervertebral. Rev de Chir Orthop 57: 8

655. Kettunen K, Kabjalainen J 1969 External counting of radio-strontium in differential diagnosis of osteochondrosis of the spine. Ann Chir Gynae Fenn 58: 9

656. Keuter E J W 1970 Vascular origin of cranial sensory disturbances caused by pathology of the lower cervical spine. Acta Neurochirurg 23: 249

657. Kimmel D L 1961 Innervation of the spinal dura mater and dura mater of the posterior cranial fossa. Neurology (Minneapolis) 11: 800

658. King J S 1977 Randomised trial of the Rees and Shealy methods for the treatment of low back pain. In: Buerger A A, Tobis J S (eds) Approaches to the validation of manipulation therapy. Thomas, Springfield, Illinois, p 70

659. Kirk E J, Denny-Brown D 1970 Functional variations in dermatomes in the macaque monkey following dorsal root lesions. J Comp Neurol 139: 307

660. Kirkaldy-Willis, W H et al 1974 Lumbar spinal stenosis. Clin Orth 99: 30

661a. Kirkaldy-Willis W H, Wedge J H et al 1978 Pathology and pathogenesis of lumbar spondylosis and stenosis. Spine 3: 319

661b. Kirkaldy-Willis W H 1978 Five common back disorders: how to diagnose and treat them. Geriatrics 33: 32

662. Kirkaldy-Willis W H, Hill R J 1979 A more precise diagnosis for low-back pain. Spine 4: 102

663. Kirveskari P 1978 Credibility of morphologic and psychologic theories of T-M joint pain-dysfunction aetiology. J Oral Rehab 5: 201

664. Klafta L A, Callis J S 1969 The diagnostic inaccuracy of the pain response in cervical discography. Clev Clin Quart 36: 35

665. Kleiner S B 1924 Fracture of ribs by muscular action, with report of a case. Boston Med & Surg J 190: 1034

666. Knottson E, Mattson E 1969 Effects of local cooling on monosynaptic reflexes in man. Scand J Rehab Med 1: 126

667. Knuttson F 1942 Vacuum phenomenon in intervertebral discs. Acta Radiol 23: 173

668. Knuttson F 1944 Instability associated with disc degeneration of the lumbar spine Acta Radiol 25: 593

669. Kogstad O et al 1977 Cervico-brachialgia: a controlled trial of conventional therapy and manipulation. Proceedings: 5th congress: Internat Fed Manipulative Med. FIMM, Copenhagen

670. Kokan P J et al 1974 Factors associated with failure of lumbar spine fusion. Can J Surg 17: 294

671. Kopell H P 1972 Help for your aching back. Wolfe, London

672. Korr I et al 1947 Quantitative studies of chronic facilitation in human motor neurone pools. Amer J Physiol 105: 229

673. Korr I, Thomas P E, Wright H M 1955 The functional implication of segmental facilitation. J Amer Osteop Assoc 54: 1

674. Korr I et al 1967 Axonal delivery of neuroplasmic components to muscle cells. Science 155: 342

675. Korr I 1976 The spinal cord as organiser of disease processes: some preliminary perspectives. J Amer Osteop Assoc 76: 89

676. Korr I (ed) 1978 What is manipulative therapy? Preface to: The neurobiologic mechanisms in manipulative therapy. Plenum Press, London, p xvi

677. Kos J, Wolf J 1972 Les ménisques intervertébraux et leur rôle possible dans les blocages vertébraux. Ann de Méd Physique 15: 203

678. Kosary I Z et al 1973 Lumbosacral myelography with Dimer-X. J Neurosurg 39: 359

679. Kosoy J, Glassman A L 1974 Audiovestibular findings with cervical spine trauma. Tex Med 70: 66

680. Kostyuk P G 1968 Presynaptic and post-synaptic changes produced in spinal neurones by an afferent volley from visceral afferents. In: von Euler C, Skoglund S, Söderberg U (eds) Structure and function of inhibitory neuronal mechanisms. Pergamon Press, Oxford

681. Kraft G H, Johnson E W, Laban M M 1968 The fibrositis syndrome. Arch Phys Med 49: 155

682. Kraft G L, Levinthal D H 1951 Facet synovial impingement: a new concept in the etiology of lumbar vertebral derangement. Surg Gyn & Obst 93: 439

683. Krausova L, Lewit K 1965 The mechanism and the measuring of mobility in the cranio-cervical joints during lateral inclinations. Acta Univers Carol Med Suppl 21: 119

684. Kräuzl B, Kranzl C 1976 The role of the autonomic nervous system in trigeminal neuralgia. J Neurol Trans 38: 77

685. Kreel L 1975 The EMI body scanner—CT5000. Therapy Nov 21: 3

686. Kunert W 1965 Functional disorders of internal organs due to vertebral lesions. Ciba Symposium 13: 85

687. Kunert W 1975 Brust-und herzschmerz bei wirbelsäulenerkrankungen. Diagnostik 8: 16

688. Kuntz A 1945 Anatomic and physiologic properties of cutaneous-visceral vasomotor reflex arcs. J Neurophysiol 8: 421

689. Laban M M, Meerschaert J R 1975 Lumbosacral anterior pelvic pain associated with pubic symphysis instability. Arch Phys Med Rehab 56: 548

690. Laban M M et al 1978 Symphyseal and sacro-iliac joint pain associated with pubic symphysis instability. Arch Phys Med Rehab 59: 470

691. Lance J W 1969 Mechanisms and management of headache. Butterworth, London

692. Lange F 1925 Die muskelhärten der beinmuskeln. Münch Med Wochenschr 72: 1626

693. Lange F 1931 Die muskelhärten (myogelosen). J F Lehmann, München

694. Langley H V 1945 The migraine lesion. Research Books, London

695. Lansche W E, Ford L T 1960 Correlation of the myelogram with clinical and operative findings in lumbar disc lesions. J Bone & Jt Surg 42A: 193

696. Lanyon L E 1971 Strain in sheep lumbar vertebrae recorded during life. Acta Orthop Scand 42: 102

697. La Rocca H, Macnab I 1969 Value of pre-employment radiographic assessment of the lumbar spine. Can Med Assoc J 101: 383

698. La Rocca H 1971 New horizons in research on disc disease. Orth Clin N Amer 2: 521

699. Laruelle N L 1940 Les bases anatomique du système autonome cortical et bulbo-spinal. Rev Neurol 72: 349

700. Law W A 1976 Ankylosing spondylitis and spinal osteotomy. Proc Roy Soc Med 69: 715

701. Lawrence J S 1976 Radiological cervical arthritis in populations. Ann Rheum Dis 35: 365

702. Lawrence M S, Rossi N P, Tidrick R T 1967 Thoracic-outlet compression syndrome. J Iowa Med Soc June: 561

703. Lazorthes G 1972 Les branches postérieures des neufs rachidiens et le plan articulaire vertebral postérieur. Ann de Méd Physique 15: 192

704. Leading article 1967 Infarction of the spinal cord. Lancet 11: 143

705. Leading article 1968 Hypermobile joints. British Medical Journal Mar 9: 596

706. Leading article 1970 Entrapment neuropathies. British Medical Journal Mar 14: 645

707. Leading article 1972 Signs and symptoms in cervical spondylosis. Lancet 2: 7767

708. Leading article 1973 Physiotherapy or psychotherapy. Lancet Dec 29: 1483

709. Leading article 1975 Chemonucleolysis. Lancet May 3: 1022

710. Leading article 1976 Trial by traction. British Medical Journal Jan 3: 1

711. Leading article 1977 Rel.ability of tests for rheumatism. Brit J Clin Pract 31: 173

712. Leading article 1977 Abdominal pain of spinal origin. Lancet 1: 1190

713. Leading article 1977 Ankylosing spondylitis and its early diagnosis. Lancet Sept 17: 591

714. Lee C K, Hansen H T, Weiss A B 1978 Developmental lumbar spinal stenosis: pathology and surgical treatment. Spine 3: 246

715. Lee D, Lishman R 1975 Vision in movement and balance. New Scientist 65: 59

716. Lee Peng C H et al 1978 Endorphin release: a possible mechanism of acupuncture analgesia. Comp Med East West 6: 57

717. Lehmann J F, Warren C G, Scham S M 1974 Therapeutic heat and cold. Clin Orthop & Rel Res 99: 207

718. Leitch O W 1955 The first lumbar root syndrome. Med J Aust Nov 19: 842

719. Lendrum F C 1951 The patho-physiology of the upright posture. In: Studies of medicine. Thomas, Springfield, Illinois, ch 20

720. Lettin A W F 1967 Diagnosis and treatment of lumbar instability. J Bone & Jt Surg 49B: 520

721. Lettin A W F 1978 Personal communication

722. Lettvin M 1976 Maggie's back book. Houghton Mifflin Co, Boston

723. Le Vay D 1967 A survey of surgical management of lumbar disc prolapse in the United Kingdom and Eire. Lancet June 3: 1211

724. Levine J D, Gormley J, Fields H L 1976 Observations on the analgesic effects of needle puncture (acupuncture). Pain 2: 149

725. Lewin R 1979 Ancient footprints mark time. New Scientist 82: 931

726. Lewin T, Moffet B, Vüdik A 1962 The morphology of the lumbar synovial intervertebral joints. Acta Morph Neerland-Scand 4: 299

727. Lewin T 1964 Osteoarthrosis in lumbar synovial joints. Orstadius Bokryckeri Aktiebolag, Göteborg

728. Lewis M M, Arnold W D 1976 Complete anterior dislocation of the sacro-iliac joint. J Bone & Jt Surg 58A: 136

729. Lewis T, Kellgren J H 1939 Observations relating to referred pain, viscero-motor reflexes and other associated problems. Clin Sci 4: 47

730. Lewis T 1942 Pain. Macmillan, London

731. Lewit K, Krausova L 1962 Beitrag zur flexion der halswirbelsäule. Fortschr Röentgenstr 97: 38

732. Lewit K 1965 Sacro-iliac dislocation and disturbance of muscle function. Asklepios 9: 274

733. Lewit K 1967 The coccyx and lumbago (sacral pain). Man Med 4: 2

734. Lewit K 1969 The course of impaired function in the spinal column and its possible prevention. In: Proceedings: Faculty of Medicine & Hygiene, Charles University, Prague

735. Lewit K, Knobloch V, Faktorova X 1970 Vertebral disorders and obstetric pain. Man Med 4: 79

736. Lewit K, Wolff H D 1970 Conference on the pelvis. Man Med 6: 150

737. Lewit K 1971 Ligament pain and anteflexion headache. Europ Neurol 5: 365

738. Lewit K 1971 The reposition effect: an unfavourable prognostic sign. Man Med 1: 8

739. Lewit K 1972 Functional diagnosis as the basis of manual treatment. Man Med 3: 41

740. Lewit K 1974 The functional pathology of the motor system. Proceedings: IVth Congress: Internat Fed Man Med, Prague

741. Lewit K 1976 Manuelle Medizin im Rahmen der Medizinischen Rehabilitation. Barth, Leipzig

742. Lewit K 1977 Pain arising in the posterior arch of atlas. Europ Neurol 16: 263

743. Lewit K 1978 The contribution of clinical observation to neurological mechanisms in manipulative therapy. In: Korr I (ed) The neurobiologic mechanisms in manipulative therapy. Plenum Press, London, p 3

744. Lewit K 1979 The needle effect in the relief of myofascial pain. Pain 6: 83

745. Lichtblau S 1962 Dislocation at the sacro-iliac joint. J Bone & Jt Surg 44A: 193

746. Lidstrom A, Zachrisson M 1970 Physical therapy on low back pain and sciatica. Scand J Rehab Med 2: 37

747. Lin H S et al 1978 Mechanical response of the lumbar intervertebral joint under physiological (complex) loading. J Bone & Jt Surg 60A: 41

748. Lind G A M 1974 Auto-traction treatment of low back pain and sciatica (Thesis). University Med Diss, Linkopings

749. Lindahl O, Rexed B 1950 Histologic changes in spinal nerve roots of operated cases of sciatica. Acta Orthop Scand 20: 215

750. Lindahl O 1966 Hyperalgesia of the lumbar nerve roots in sciatica. Acta Orthop Scand 37: 367

751. Lindberg L 1970 Anterior cervical fusion for cervical rhizopathies. Acta Orthop Scand 41: 312

752. Lindblom K 1948 Diagnostic puncture of intervertebral discs in sciatica. Acta Orthop Scand 17: 231

753. Lindblom K, Rexed B 1948 Spinal nerve injury in dorso-lateral protrusions of lumbar discs. J Neurosurg 5: 413

754. Lincoln N B 1978 Behaviour modification in physiotherapy. Physio 64: 265

755. Lipson S J, Mazur J 1978 Antero-posterior spondyloschisis of the atlas revealed by computerized tomography scanning. J Bone & Jt Surg 60A: 1104

756. Lissiman M 1974 Clinical application of lumbar traction. In: Twomey L T (ed) Symposium: Low back pain. Western Aust Inst Tech, Perth

757. Little T, Freeman M, Swanson A 1969 Experiments on friction in the human hip joint. In: Wright V (ed) Lubrication and wear in joints. Sector, London, p 110

758. Livingston M C P 1968 Spinal manipulation in medical practice: a century of ignorance. Med J Aust 2: 552

759. Livingston M C P 1971 Spinal manipulation causing injury Clin Orth 81: 82

760. Loebl W Y 1967 Measurement of spine and range of spinal movement. Ann Phys Med 9: 103

761. Long C H 1955 and 1956 Myofascial pain syndromes. Henry Ford Hosp Med Bull Part I 3: 189 (1955) Part II 4: 22 (1956) Part III 4: 102 (1956)

762. Long D M 1977 Electrical stimulation for the control of pain. Arch Surg 112: 884

763. Longmire W T (Moderator) 1976 Keys to treating acute neck or back pain. J Pract Fam Med 10: 18

764. Lord J W, Rosati L M 1971 Thoracic outlet syndrome. Ciba Clin Symposia 23: 3

765. Love J G 1955 Clinical neurology. Baker A B (ed). Hoeber-Harper, New York, vol 2, p 1398

766. Love J G, Emmett J L 1967 'Asymptomatic' protruded lumbar disc as a cause of urinary retention: preliminary report. Mayo Clin Proc 42: 249

767. Low S A 1974 Acupuncture in low back pain. In: Twomey L T (ed) Symposium: Low back pain. Western Aust Inst Tech, Perth

768. Lövgren O, Dowèn S-A 1969 Strontium (85_{SR}) scintigrams of the sacro-iliac joints. Acta Rheum Scand 15: 327

769. Lumsden R M, Morris J M 1968 An in vivo study of axial rotation and immobilisation of the lumbo-sacral joint. J Bone & Jt Surg 50A: 1591

770. Luschnitz F et al 1967 Tableau clinique et radiologique de l'ostéo-nécrose post-traumatique du pubis ches joueurs de football. Fortsch Gebiet Roentgenspr 107: 113

771. Macallister A 1889 A textbook of human anatomy. Griffin, London

772. Mace B E W 1976 Vertebral venography in disc disorders. Proc Roy Soc Med 69: 433

773. Macnab I 1969 Pathogenesis of symptoms in discogenic low back pain. Symposium: The spine. Amer Acad Orthop Surgeons. C V Mosby, St Louis, ch 6

774. Macnab I 1971 The traction spur. J Bone & Jt Surg 53A: 663

775. Macnab I 1971 Negative disc exploration. J Bone & Jt Surg 53A: 891

776. Macnab I 1971 The painful shoulder due to rotator cuff tendinitis. Rhode Isl Med J 54: 367

777. Macnab I 1971 The mechanism of spondylogenic pain. In: Hirsch C, Zotterman Y (eds) Cervical pain. Pergamon Press, Oxford

778. Macnab I et al 1976 Selective ascending lumbo-sacral venography in the assessment of lumbar disc herniation. J Bone & Jt Surg 58A: 1093

779. Macnab I, Cuthbert H, Godfrey C M 1977 The incidence of denervation of the sacrospinalis muscles following spinal surgery. Spine 2: 294

780. Macnab I 1977 Backache. Williams & Wilkins, Baltimore

781. MacConaill M A 1932 The function of intra-articular fibrocartilages. J Anat 66: 210

782. MacConaill M A 1964 Joint movement. Physio 50: 359

783. MacConaill M A, Basmajian J V 1969 Muscles and movements. Williams & Wilkins, Baltimore

784. Madders J 1974 Relax: the relief of tension through muscle control, 2nd edn. BBC, London

785. Magora F et al 1974 An electromyographic investigation of the neck muscles in headache. Electromyog Clin Neurophysiol 14: 453

786. Magoun H W 1975 Summary of neuroscience studies. In: The research status of spinal manipulative therapy, US Dept of Health NINCDS Monograph No 15, Bethesda, p 209

787. Maigne R 1965 The concept of painlessness and opposite motion in spinal manipulations. Amer J Phys Med 44: 55

788. Maigne R, Le Corre F 1969 New ideas on the mechanism of common adult dorsalgia. Man Med 4: 73

789. Maigne R 1972 La sémeiologie clinique des dérangements intervértébraux mineurs. Ann de Méd Physique 15: 275

790. Maigne R 1972 Sacro-iliac joints: the problem of their 'blockings' and strains. In: Douleurs d'origine vertébrale et traitements par manipulations, 2nd edn. Expansion Scientifique, Paris, p 294

791. Maigne R 1972 Douleurs d'origine vertébrale et traitements par manipulations, 2nd edn. Expansion Scientifique, Paris

792. Maigne R 1976 Un signe évocateur et inattendu de céphalée cervicale: 'la douleur au pincé-roulé du sourcil'. Ann de Méd Physique 19: 416

793. Maisel E 1974 The Alexander techniques: the essential writings of F. Mathias Alexander. Thames & Hudson, London

794. Maitland G D 1961 Some observations on sciatic scoliosis. Aust J Physio 7: 84

795. Maitland G D 1969 A friction-free couch. Physio 55: 22

796. Maitland G D 1972 Manipulation: individual responsibility. Physio South Africa 28: 2

797. Maitland G D 1977 Vertebral manipulation, 4th edn. Butterworth, London

798. Maitland G D 1977 Peripheral manipulation, 2nd edn. Butterworth, London

799. Maitland G D 1978 Musculo-skeletal examination and recording guide. Lauderdale Press, Adelaide

799a. Maitland G D 1978 Movement of pain sensitive structures in the vertebral canal. In: Proceedings: Manipulative Therapists of Australia Congress, Sydney

800. Mankin H J 1974 Biochemical abnormalities in articular cartilage in osteoarthrosis. In: Ali S Y, Elves M W, Leaback D H (eds) Symposium: Normal and arthrotic articular cartilage. Inst of Orthop, London

801. Malawista S E et al 1965 Sacro-iliac gout. J Amer Med Assoc 194: 954

802. Mann F 1966 Atlas of acupuncture. Heinemann, London

803. Mann F 1967 The treatment of disease by acupuncture. Heinemann, London
804. Mann F et al 1973 The treatment of intractable pain by acupuncture. Lancet 1: 57
805. Mannheim H 1930 Freier körper in einen zwischenwirbelgelenk nach trauma. Mechr Unfallheilk 37: 67
806. Marinacci A A, Courville C B 1962 Radicular syndromes simulating intra-abdominal surgical conditions. Amer Surg 28: 59
807. Markolf K L, Morris J H 1974 The structural components of the intervertebral disc. J Bone & Jt Surg 56A: 675
808. Maroudas A 1967 Lubrication and wear in living and artificial joints. Symposium Proceedings 181: part 3J: 122. Inst Mech Engineers, London
809. Maroudas A 1974 Transport through articular cartilage and some physiological implications. In: Ali S Y, Elves M W, Leaback D H (eds) Symposium: Normal and arthrotic articular cartilage. Inst of Orthop, London
810. Marr J T 1953 Gas in the intervertebral discs. Amer J Roentgenol 70: 804
811. Marshall L L, Trethewie E R 1973 Chemical irritation of nerve root in disc prolapse. Lancet 2: 320
812. Martins A N 1976 Anterior cervical discography with and without interbody bone graft. J Neurosurg 44: 290
813. Maruta T, Swanson D W 1977 Psychiatric consultation in the chronic pain patient. Mayo Clin Proc 52: 793
814. Mastný V 1974 Einflub der vibration auf die funktion der gelenke. Man Med 2: 36
815. Masturzo A 1955 Vertebral traction for treatment of sciatica. Rheum 11: 62
816. Mathews B H C 1934 Impulses leaving the cord by dorsal roots. J Physiol (London) 81: 29
817. Mathews J A 1968 Dynamic discography: a study of lumbar traction. Ann Phys Med 9: 275
818. Mathews J A 1969 Atlanto-axial subluxation in rheumatoid arthritis. Ann Rheum Dis 28: 260
819. Mathews J A, Hickling J 1975 Lumbar traction: a double-blind controlled study for sciatica. Rheum & Rehab 14: 222
820. Mathews J A 1976 Epidurography—a technique for diagnosis and research. In: Jayson M (ed) The lumbar spine and back pain. Sector, London, p 173
821. Maxwell T D 1978 The piriformis muscle and its relation to the long-legged syndrome. J Can Chir Assoc July: 51
822. McAllister V L, Sage M A 1976 The radiology of thoracic disc protrusion. Clin Radiol 27: 291
823. McBeath A A, Keene J S 1975 The rib-tip syndrome. J Bone & Jt Surg 57A: 795
824. McCloughlin D P, Wortzman G 1972 Congenital absence of a cervical vertebral pedicle. J Can Assoc Radiol 23: 195
825. McCutchen C W 1959 Mechanism of animal joints: sponge hydrostatic and weeping bearings. Nature 182: 1284
826. McCutchen C W 1966 Boundary lubrication by synovial fluid: demonstration and possible osmotic explanation. Fed Proc 25: 1061
827. McCutchen C W 1978 Lubrication of joints. In: Sokoloff L (ed) Joints and synovial fluid I. Academic Press, London, p 438
828. McEwin C, Ditata D et al 1972 Ankylosing spondylitis and spondylitis accompanying ulcerative colitis, regional enteritis, psoriasis and Reiter's disease. Arth & Rheum 14: 291
829. McGraw R W, Rusch R M 1973 Atlanto-axial arthrodesis. J Bone & Jt Surg 55B: 482
830. McGregor M 1948 The significance of certain measurements of the skull in the diagnosis of basilar impression. Brit J Radiol 21: 171
831. McKee G K 1956 Traction-manipulation and plastic corsets in the treatment of disc lesions of the lumbar spine. Lancet 1: 473
832. McKenzie J 1909 Symptoms and their interpretation. Shaw, London
833. McKenzie R A 1972 Manual correction of sciatic scoliosis. NZ Med J 76: 194
834. McKenzie R A 1977 Prophylaxis in recurrent low back pain. Proceedings: Int Fed Man Med Congress, Copenhagen
835. McKenzie R A 1979 Prophylaxis in recurrent low back pain. NZ Med J 89: 22
836. McKibbin B 1974 The nutrition of articular cartilage and its relationship to development. In: Ali S Y, Elves M W, Leaback D H (eds) Symposium: Normal and arthrotic articular cartilage. Inst of Orthop, London
837. McQueen P M 1977 The piriformis syndrome. Physio Soc Manip Newsletter 8: 1, Melbourne
838. Meckel J F 1816 Handbuch der Menschlichen Anatomie. Halle, Berlin, vol 2
839. Mehta M 1973 Intractable pain. W B Saunders, London, p 147
840. Melnick J C, Silverman F N 1963 Intervertebral disc calcification in childhood. Radiol 80: 399
841. Melzack R, Wall P D 1962 On the nature of cutaneous sensory mechanisms. Brain 85: 331
842. Melzack R, Wall P D 1965 Pain mechanisms: a new theory. Science 150: 971
843. Melzack R, Casey K L 1968 Sensory, motivational and central control determinants of pain: a new conceptual model. In: Kenshalo D R (ed) The skin sense. Thomas, Springfield, Illinois, p 423
844. Melzack R, Torgenson W S 1971 On the language of pain. Anaesthesiol 34: 50
845. Melzack R 1972 Mechanisms of pathological pain. In: Critchley M, O'Leary J L, Jennett B (eds) Scientific foundations of neurology. Heinemann, London, p 153
846. Melzack R 1973 The puzzle of pain. Penguin, London
847. Melzack R 1973 Pain control. Physio Can 25: 47
848. Melzack R, Stillwell D M, Fox E J 1977 Trigger points and acupuncture points for pain: correlations and implications. Pain 3: 23
849. Meyerding H W 1941 Low backache and sciatic pain associated with spondylolisthesis and protruded intervertebral disc: incidence, significance and treatment. J Bone & Jt Surg 23: 461
850. Mennell J B 1945 Physical treatment by movement, manipulation and massage, 5th edn. Churchill, London
851. Mennell J B 1952 The science and art of joint manipulation. Churchill, London, vol 2
852. Mennell J McM 1960 Back pain. Little Brown, Boston
853. Mennell J McM 1972 Treatment of myofascial pain, secondary to facet-joint dysfunction, by cold. Man Med 4: 76
854. Merskey H, Boyd D 1978 Emotional adjustment and chronic pain. Pain 5: 173
855. Meyer G H 1878 Der mechanismus der symphysis sacroiliaca. Archiv für Anatomie und Physiologie: Leipzig 1: 1
856. Middleton G S, Teacher H J 1911 Injury to spinal cord due to rupture of an intervertebral disc during muscular effort. Glasgow Med J 76: 1
857. Miehkle K, Schulze G, Eger W 1960 Klinische und experimentelle untersuchungen zum fibrositissyndrom. Z Rheumaforsch 19: 310
858. Miller A 1958 Testicular pain. The Med Press 240: 877
859. Miller J 1978 How do you feel? The Listener 100: 665
860. Miller M R, Kasahara M 1963 Observations on the innervation of human long bones. Anat Rec 145: 13
861. Minagi H, Gronner A T 1969 Calcification of the posterior longitudinal ligament: a cause of cervical myelopathy. Amer J Roent Rad Ther Nuc Med 105: 365
862. Mitchell F 1965 Structural pelvic function. Year Book: Academy of Applied Osteopathy. Carmel, California
863. Mixter W J, Barr J S 1934 Rupture of intervertebral disc with involvement of the spinal cord. New England J Med 211: 210
864. Moles A, Cook J, Stoker D J 1977 Diagnosis. In: Rowe J, Dyer L (eds) Care of the orthopaedic patient. Blackwell, London
865. Moll J M H, Wright V 1971 Normal range of spinal mobility. Ann Rheum Dis 30: 381
866. Moll J M H, Haslock I et al 1975 Associations between ankylosing spondylitis, psoriatic arthritis, Reiter's disease, the interstinal arthropathies and Bechet's syndrome. Excerpt Med (Sect 19) 18: 216
867. Mooney V, Robertson J 1976 The facet syndrome. Clin Orth & Rel Res 115: 149

868. Mooney V, Cairns D, Robertson J 1976 A system for evaluating and treating chronic back disability. West J Med 124: 370

869. Mooney V, Cairns D 1978 Management in the patient with chronic low back pain. Orth Clin N Amer 9: 543

870. Mooney V T 1977 Facet pathology. In: Kent B (ed) Proceedings: Third Seminar: Internat Fed Orthop Manip Therapists. IFOMT, Hayward, California

871. Morgan E H, Hill L B 1954 Objective identification of chest pain of oesophageal origin. J Amer Med Assoc 187: 921

872. Morgan F P, King T 1957 Primary instability of the lumbar vertebrae as a common cause of low back pain. J Bone & Jt Surg 39B: 6

873. Morris J M 1973 Biomechanics of the spine. Arch Surg 107: 418

874. Moseley I 1976 Neural arch dysplasia of the sixth cervical vertebra: 'congenital cervical spondylolisthesis'. Brit J Radiol 49: 81

875. Morvin A 1966 Myelographic appearances of disc protrusions in different positions. Acta Radiol 6: 524

876. Mulholland R 1974 Lateral hydraulic permeability and morphology of articular cartilage. In: Ali S Y, Elves M W, Leaback D H (eds) Symposium: Normal and arthrotic articular cartilage. Inst of Orthop, London

877. Müller A 1912 Der untersuchungsbefund am rheumatisch erkrankten muskel Z Klin Med 74: 34

878. Munro A 1972 The psychosomatic approach. The Practitioner 208: 162

879. Murray J G, Thompson J W 1957 The occurrence and function of collateral sprouting in the sympathetic nervous system of the cat. J Physiol 135: 133

880. Murray R O, Duncan C 1971 Athletic activity in adolescence as an aetiological factor in degenerative hip disease. J Bone & Jt Surg 53B: 406

881. Murray R O, Jacobson H G 1977 The radiology of skeletal disorders, 2nd edn. Churchill Livingstone, London

882. Murrey-Leslie C F, Wright V 1976 Carpal tunnel syndrome, humeral epicondylitis and the cervical spine. British Medical Journal 1: 1439

883. Nachemson A 1964 *In vivo* measurement of intra-discal pressure. J Bone & Jt Surg 46A: 1077

884. Nachemson A 1966 Electromyographic studies on the vertebral portion of the psoas muscle. Acta Orthop Scand 37: 177

885. Nachemson A 1968 Some mechanical properties of the third human interlaminar ligament (ligamentum flavum). J Biomech 1: 211

886. Nachemson A 1969 Intradiscal measurement of pH in patients with lumbar rhizopathies. Acta Orthop Scand 40: 23

887. Nachemson A, Lindh M 1969 Measurement of abdominal and back muscle strength with and without low back pain. Scand J Rehab Med 1: 60

888. Nachemson A, Elfström G 1970 Intravital dynamic pressure measurements in lumbar discs. Scand J Rehab Med Suppl no 1

889a. Nachemson A 1975 Towards a better understanding of low back pain: a review of the mechanics of the lumbar disc. Rheum & Rehab 14: 129

889b. Nachemson A 1976 The lumbar spine: an orthopaedic challenge. Spine 1: 59

890. Nachemson A 1976 Lumbar intradiscal pressures. In: Jayson M (ed) The lumbar spine and back pain. Sector, London, ch 11

891. Nachemson A 1976 A critical look at conservative treatment for low back pain. In: The lumbar spine and back pain. Sector, London, ch 17

892. Nachemson A, Schultz A B, Berkson M H 1979 Mechanical properties of human lumbar spine motion segments: influence of age, sex, disc level and degeneration. Spine 4: 1

893. Nagant de Deuxchaisnes C, Haux J P et al 1974 Ankylosing spondylitis, sacro-iliitis, regional enteritis and HL-A27. Lancet June 15: 1238

894. Nagi S Z, Riley L R, Newby L G 1973 A social epidemiology of back pain in a general population. J Chron Dis 26: 769

895. Nash C L, Moe J M 1969 A study of vertebral rotation. J Bone & Jt Surg 51A: 223

896. Nassim R, Burrows H J (eds) 1959 Modern trends in diseases of the vertebral column. Butterworth, London

897. Nassim R 1959 Osteoporosis. In: Nassim R, Burrows H J (eds) Modern trends in diseases of the spinal column. Butterworth, London, p 125

898. Nathan H 1959 The para-articular processes of the thoracic vertebrae. Anat Record 4: 605

899. Nathan H, Alkalaj I, Aviad I 1960 Spondylolysis in the aged. Geriatrics 15: 187

900. Nathan H 1962 Osteophytes of the vertebral column. J Bone & Jt Surg 44A: 243

901. Nathan H, Schwartz A 1962 Inverted pattern of development of thoracic vertebral osteophytosis in situs inversus and in other instances of right descending aorta. Radiol Clin 31: 150

902. Nathan H et al 1964 The costovertebral joints: anatomico-clinical observations in arthritis. Arth & Rheum 7: 228

903. Nathan H 1968 Compression of the sympathetic trunk by osteophytes of the vertebral column in the abdomen: an anatomical study with pathological and clinical consideration. Surgery 63: 609

904. Nathan H, Feuerstein M 1970 Angulated course of spinal nerve roots. J Neurosurg 32: 349

905. Nathan P W, Sears T A 1963 Susceptibility of nerve fibres to analgesics. Anaesthesia 18: 467

906. Nathan P W 1973 The nervous system. Penguin, London, p 73

907. Nathan P W 1976 The gate-control theory of pain. Brain 99: 123

908. Naylor A 1971 Biochemical changes in the human intervertebral disc in degeneration and nuclear collapse. Orthop Clin N Amer 2: 343

909. Naylor A 1974 The late results of laminectomy for lumbar disc prolapse. J Bone & Jt Surg 56B: 17

910. Naylor A 1977 Surgical treatment in lumbar disc protrusion. British Medical Journal 1: 567

911. Nelson M A 1973 Lumbar spinal stenosis. J Bone & Jt Surg 55B: 506

912. Nelson M A 1976 Surgery of the spine. In: Jayson M (ed) The lumbar spine and back pain. Sector, London, ch 18

913. Nelson M A et al 1979 Reliability and reproducibility of clinical findings in low-back pain. Spine 4: 97

914. Nemiah J C, Freyberger H, Sifneos P E 1976 Alexithymia: a view of the pyschosomatic process. In: Hill O W (ed) Modern trends in psychosomatic medicine 3. Butterworth, London, p 154

915. Neugebauer F L 1888 A new contribution to the history and aetiology of spondylolisthesis (translated by F. Barnes). Selected Monographs vol 121. The New Sydenham Society, London

916. Neuwirth E 1952 Headaches and facial pain in cervical discopathy. Ann Int Med 37: 75

917. Neuwirth E 1960 Current concepts of the cervical portion of the sympathetic nervous system. Lancet 80: 337

918. Newill R G 1963 Epidemic cervical myalgia: an outbreak in Hertfordshire. J Coll Gen Pract 6: 344

919. Neuwirth E 1952 Headaches and facial pain in cervical J Roy Coll Gen Pract 15: 51

920. Newman P H 1952 Sprung back. J Bone Jt Surg 34B: 30

921. Newman P H 1955 Spondylolisthesis: its cause and effect. Ann Roy Coll Surg Eng 16: 305

922. Newman P H 1959 Low back pain. In: Nassim R, Burrows H J (eds) Modern trends in diseases of the vertebral column. Butterworth, London, ch 13

923. Newman P H 1963 The aetiology of spondylolisthesis. J Bone & Jt Surg 45B: 39

924. Newman P H 1968 The spine, the wood and the trees. Proc Roy Soc Med 61: 35

925. Newman P H, Sweetnam R 1969 Occipito-cervical fusion. An operative technique and its indications. J Bone & Jt Surg 51B: 423

926. Newman P H 1973 Surgical treatment for derangement of the lumbar spine. J Bone & Jt Surg 55B: 7

927. Newman P H 1974 Spondylolisthesis. Physio 60: 14

928. Newton D R L 1957 Clinical aspects of sacro-iliac disease. Proc Roy Soc Med 50: 850

929. Newton T H 1958 Cervical intervertebral disc calcification in children. J Bone & Jt Surg 40A: 107
930. Nicholas J A et al 1978 Factors influencing manual muscle tests in physical therapy. J Bone & Jt Surg 60A: 186
931. Nicholls P J R 1960 Short-leg syndrome. British Medical Journal June 18: 1863
932. Nicholson J T, Sherk H H 1968 Anomalies of the occipito-cervical articulation. J Bone & Jt Surg 50A: 295
933. Nordenbos W 1959 Pain: problems pertaining to the transmission of nerve impulses which give rise to pain. Elsevier, London
934. Norman G F, May A 1956 Sacro-iliac conditions simulating intervertebral disc syndrome. Western J Surg 64: 461
935. Norman G F 1968 Sacro-iliac disease and its relationship to lower abdominal pain. Amer J Surg 116: 54
936. Norman W J, Johnson C 1973 Congenital absence of pedicle of a lumbar vertebra. Brit J Radiol 46: 631
937. Norris C W, Eakins K 1974 Head and neck pain: the T-M joint syndrome. The Laryngoscope 84: 1466
938. Northupp G W 1978 Discussion. In: Korr I (ed) The neurobiologic mechanisms in manipulative therapy. Plenum Press, London, p 286
939. Norton P L, Brown T 1957 The immobilising effect of back braces: their effect on the posture and motion of the lumbo-sacral spine. J Bone & Jt Surg 39A: 111
940. Novotny A, Dvorak V 1971 Functional disturbances of the vertebral column after gynaecological operations. Man Med 3: 65
941. Nümi K, Inoshita H 1971 Cortical projections of the lateral thalamic nuclei in the cat. Proc Jap Acad 47: 664
942. Nurick S 1975 Cervical spondylosis and the spinal cord. Brit J Hosp Med Dec: 668
943. Nykamp P W et al 1978 Computed tomography for a bursting fracture of the lumbar spine. J Bone & Jt Surg 60A: 1108
944. Oakley E M 1978 Application of continuous beam ultrasound at therapeutic levels. Physio 64: 169
945. O'Brien J P 1979 Anterior spinal tenderness in low back pain syndromes. Spine 4: 85
946. Ochs S 1975 A brief review of material transport in nerve fibres. In: The research status of spinal manipulative therapy. US Dept of Health NINCDS, Bethesda, Monograph no 15, p 189
947. O'Connor J F, Cohen J 1978 Computerized tomography (CAT Scan—CT Scan) in orthopaedic surgery. J Bone & Jt Surg 60A: 1096
948. O'Dell C W et al 1977 Ascending lumbar venography in lumbar disc disease. J Bone & Jt Surg 59A: 159
949. Ogston A G, Stanier J E 1953 The physiological function of hyaluronic acid in synovial fluid: viscous, elastic and lubricant properties. J Physiol 119: 244
950. Olsson O 1942 Arthrosis deformans des vorderen zahngelenkes. Fortschr Röentgen 66: 233
951. Olsson Y 1966 Studies on vascular permeability in peripheral nerves. Acta Neuropath Berl 17: 114
952. Olsson Y, Sourander P, Kristensson K 1971 Neuropathological aspect of root affections in the cervical region. In: Hirsch C, Zotterman Y (eds) Cervical pain. Pergamon Press, Oxford, p 81
953. Ongerboor de Visser B W, Goor C 1976 Jaw reflexes and masseter electromyograms in mesencephalic and pontine lesions: an electrodiagnostic study. J Neurol Neurosurg Psychiat 39: 90
954. Onji Y et al 1967 Posterior paravertebral ossification causing cervical myelopathy. J Bone & Jt Surg 49A: 1314
955. Orsini A 1972 Récherches anatomiques sur l'innervation de le jonction sacroiliaque. Ann de Méd Physique 15: 257
956. Osborne G 1974 Spinal stenosis. Physio 60: 7
957. Otani K, Manzoku S et al 1977 The surgical treatment of thoracic and thoracolumbar disc lesions using the anterior approach. Spine 2: 266
958. Oudenhoven R C 1977 Paraspinal electromyography following facet rhizotomy. Spine 2: 299
959. Oudenhoven R C 1978 Gravitational lumbar traction. Arch Phys Med Rehab 59: 11: 510

960. Oudenhoven R C 1979 The role of laminectomy, facet rhizotomy, and epidural steroids. Spine 4: 145
961. Pace J B, Nagle D 1976 The piriformis syndrome. West J Med 124: 435
962. Paige M J 1959 Manipulation in the management of the first lumbar root syndrome. Aust J Physio 5: 47
963. Paine K W E 1976 Clinical features of lumbar spinal stenosis. Clin Orthop & Rel Res 115: 77
963a. Paine K W E 1972 Lumbar disc syndrome. J Neurosurg 37: 75
964. Palazzi A S 1957 On the operative treatment of arthritis deformans of the hip joint. Acta Orthop Scand 27: 291
965. Pallie W, Manuel J K 1968 Intersegmental anastomoses between dorsal spinal rootlets in some vertebrates. Acta Anat 70: 341
966. Palmer D D 1910 The science, art and philosophy of chiropractic. Printing House Co, Portland
967. Pang L Q 1971 The otological aspects of whiplash injuries. Laryngoscope 81: 1381
968. Panjabi M M 1973 Three-dimensional mathematical model of the human spine structure. J Biomechanics 6: 671
969. Pare A 1582 Opera Liber XV, 440–441 Paris (1582). Quoted by Schiötz E H 1958 Manipulation treatment of the spinal column from the medico-historical viewpoint (NIH Library translation). Tidsskr Nor Laegeform 78: 359
970. Park W M 1976 Radiological investigation of the intervertebral disc. In: Jayson M (ed) The lumbar spine and back pain. Sector, London, p 116
971. Parke W W, Schiff D C M 1971 The applied anatomy of the intervertebral disc. Orth Clin N Amer 2: 309
972. Parker N 1977 Accident litigants with neurotic symptoms. Med J Aust 2: 318
973. Parsons W B, Cumming J D A 1957 Mechanical traction in lumbar disc syndrome. J Can Med Assoc 77: 7
974. Patrick M K 1978 Applications of therapeutic pulsed ultrasound. Physio 64: 103
975. Pauwels F 1965 Gessamelte Abhandlugen zur Funktionellen Anatomie des Bewengungsapparatis. Springer, Berlin
975a. Paxton S L 1980 Clinical use of TENS: a survey of physical therapists. Phys Ther 60: 38
976. Payne E E, Spillane J D 1957 The cervical spine: an anatomical study of 70 specimens with particular reference to the problem of cervical spondylosis. Brain 80: 571
977. Pearson H 1960 The life of Oscar Wilde. Penguin, Harmondsworth
978. Peck D F 1976 Operant conditioning and physical rehabilitation. Eur J of Behav Anal & Mod 3: 158
979. Pedersen H E, Blunck C F J, Gardner E 1956 The anatomy of lumbosacral posterior rami and meningeal branches of spinal nerves (sinu-vertebral nerves). J Bone & Jt Surg 38A: 377
980. Pennal G F et al 1972 Motion studies of the lumbar spine. J Bone & Jt Surg 54B: 442
981. Penning L 1968 Functional pathology of the cervical spine. Excerpta Med Foundation, Amsterdam
982. Perkins G 1958 Fractures and dislocations. Athlone Press, London, p 93
983. Perkins G 1961 Orthopaedics. Athlone Press, London
984. Perl E R 1971 Mode of action of nociceptors. In: Hirsch C, Zotterman Y (eds) Cervical pain. Pergamon Press, Oxford, p 157
985. Perl E R 1971 Is pain a specific sensation? J Psychiat Res 8: 273
986. Perl E R 1975 Pain: spinal and peripheral factors. In: Research status of spinal manipulative therapy. US Dept of Health, Bethesda, Monograph No 15, p 173
987. Perry J 1970 The use of external support in the treatment of low back pain. J Bone & Jt Surg 52A: 1440
988. Phillips D G 1975 Upper limb involvement in cervical spondylosis. J Neurol Neurosurg Psychiat 38: 386
989. Phillips E L 1964 Some psychological characteristics associated with orthopaedic complaints. In: Current practice in orthopaedic surgery. C V Mosby, St Louis, vol 2, p 165
990. Piedallu P 1952 Problémes sacro-iliaque. Bière (ed) Homme Sain No 2, Bordeaux

991. Pineda A, Smith J J 1966 True and false subclavian steal syndrome. Arch Surg 92: 258

992. Pitkin H C, Pheasant H C 1936 Sacrarthrogenetic telalgia. J Bone & Jt Surg 18: 365

993. Pizzarelo L D, Golden S T, Shaw A 1974 Acute abdominal pain caused by osteitis pubis. Amer Surgery 40: 660

994. Platts R G S 1977 Spinal mechanics. Physio 63: 224

995. Pleasure D 1975 Nerve root compression: effects on neural chemistry and metabolism. In: The research status of spinal manipulative therapy. US Dept of Health, Bethesda, NINCDS Monograph No 15, p 197

996. Plomer W 1938 Cecil Rhodes. Nelson, London

997. Plotz C M, Spiera H 1978 Polymyalgia rheumatica. EULAR Bulletin (English edn) 7: 95

998. Polacek P 1966 Receptors of the joints. University Press, Brno, Czechoslovakia

999. Pomeranz B, Wall P D, Weber W V 1968 Cord cells responding to fine myelinated afferents from viscera, muscle and skin. J of Physiol 199: 511

1000. Porter R W, Wicks M, Ottewell D 1978 Measurement of the spinal canal by diagnostic ultrasound. J Bone & Jt Surg 60B: 481

1001. Porter R W, Hibbert C S, Wicks M 1978 The spinal canal in symptomatic lumbar disc lesions. J Bone & Jt Surg 60B: 485

1001a. Porter R W, Hibbert C et al 1980 The shape and size of the lumbar canal. In: Conference proceedings: Engineering aspects of the spine. Mechanical Engineering Publications Ltd, London, p 19

1002. Prinzmetal M, Massumi R A 1955 The anterior chest wall syndrome: chest pain resembling pain of cardiac origin. J Amer Med Assoc 159: 177

1003. Putti V 1927 New conceptions in the pathogenesis of sciatic pain. Lancet 2: 53

1004. Rådberg C, Wennberg E 1973 Late sequelae following lumbar myelography with water-soluble contrast media. Acta Radiol 14: 507

1005. Radin E L, Paul I L, Lowry M 1970 A comparison of the dynamic force transmitting properties of subchondral bone and articular cartilage. J Bone & Jt Surg 52A: 444

1006. Radin E L et al 1971 Joint lubrication with artificial lubricants. Arth & Rheum 14: 126

1007. Radin E L, Paul I L 1972 A consolidated concept of joint lubrication. J Bone & Jt Surg 54A: 607

1008. Radin E L et al 1972 Role of mechanical factors in pathogenesis of primary osteoarthrosis. Lancet Mar 4: 519

1009. Radin E L 1973 Response of joints to impact loading—III. J Biomech 6: 51

1010. Radin E L 1976 Mechanical aspects of osteo-arthrosis. Bull Rheum Dis 26: 862

1011. Ranshoff J, Spencer F et al 1969 Transthoracic removal of thoracic disc. J Neurosurg 31: 459

1012. Rana N A et al 1973 Atlanto-axial subluxation in rheumatoid arthritis. J Bone & Jt Surg 55B: 458

1013. Rana N A et al 1973 Upward translocation of the dens in rheumatoid arthritis. J Bone & Jt Surg 55B: 471

1014. Rasmussen G G 1979 Manipulation in the treatment of low back pain: a randomized clinical trial. Man Med 1: 8

1015. Rawlings M S 1962 The rib syndrome. Dis of the Chest 41: 432

1016. Ray B Wolff H 1940 Experimental studies on headache: pain sensitive structures of the head and their significance in headache. Arch Surg 41: 813

1017. Reading A E 1977 Biofeedback training—an evaluation. Hosp Update 3: 669

1018. Rees L 1970 Attitudes and emotional reactions to illness St Bart Hosp J 74: 259

1019. Rees W S 1971 Multiple bilateral subcutaneous rhizolysis of segmental nerves in the treatment of the intervertebral disc syndrome. Ann Gen Pract 16: 126

1020. Reeves D L, Brown H A 1968 Thoracic intervertebral disc protrusion with spinal cord compression. J Neurosurg 28: 24

1021. Reid D 1969 The shoulder girdle: its function as a unit in abduction. Physio 55: 57

1022. Reid D C, Cummings G E 1973 Factors in selecting the dose of ultrasound. Physio Can 25: 5

1023. Reid D C, Cummings G E 1977 Efficiency of ultrasound coupling agents Physio 63: 255

1024. Reid J D 1960 Effects of flexion-extension movements of the head and spine upon the spinal cord and nerve roots. J Neurol Neurosurg Psychiat 23: 214

1025. Reimann I, Christensen S B 1977 A histological demonstration of nerves in subchondral bone. Acta Orthop Scand 48: 345

1026. Resnick D 1974 Temperomandibular joint involvement in ankylosing spondylitis. Radiol 112: 587

1027. Resnick D, Dwosh I L, Niwayama G 1975 Sacro-iliac joint in renal osteodystrophy. J Rheumatol 2: 287

1028. Resnick D et al 1976 Clinical and radiographic abnormalities in ankylosing spondylitis: a comparison of men and women. Radiol 119: 213

1028a. Resnick D 1980 Disorders of the axial skeleton which are lesser known, poorly recognised or misunderstood. Eular Bulletin (English edn) 9: 70

1029. Rewald J 1973 The history of impressionism, 4th edn. Secker & Warburg, London

1030. Rexed B 1954 A cytoarchitectonic atlas of the spinal cord in the cat. J Comp Neurol 100: 297

1031. Rexed B A, Wennström K G 1959 Arachnoid proliferation and cystic formation in the spinal nerve root pouches in man. J Neurosurg 16: 73

1032. Reynolds P M G 1975 Measurement of spinal mobility: a comparison of three methods. Rheum & Rehab 14: 180

1033. Reynolds J B, Wiltse L L 1979 Surgical treatment of degenerative spondylolisthesis. Spine 4: 148

1034. Ricard A, Masson R 1951 Complications médullaires des discopathies cervicales (à propos 24 cas opérés). Rev Neurol 85: 420

1035. Ricciadi J E et al 1976 Acquired os odontoideum following acute ligament injury. J Bone & Jt Surg 58A: 410

1036. Richards H J 1954 Causes of coccydynia. J Bone & Jt Surg 36B: 142

1037. Richards R L 1951 Ischaemic lesions of peripheral nerves: review. J Neurol Neurosurg Psychiat 14: 76

1038. Richardson A T 1952 A standard technique for clinical electrodiagnosis. Ann Phys Med 1: 88

1039. Richardson A T 1975 The painful shoulder. Proc Roy Soc Med 68: 731

1040. Richardson J (ed) 1960 The practice of medicine. Churchill, London

1041. Rissanen P M 1960 The surgical anatomy and pathology of the supraspinous and interspinous ligaments of the lumbar spine, with special reference to ligament ruptures. Acta Orthop Scand Suppl 46

1042. Rissanen P M 1962 'Kissing spine' syndrome in the light of autopsy findings. Acta Orthop Scand 32: 132

1043. Rissanen P M 1964 Comparisons of pathological changes in intervertebral discs and interspinous ligaments of lower part of the lumbar spine. Acta Orthop Scand 34: 54

1044. Ritchie J H, Farhni W H 1970 Age changes in lumbar intervertebral discs. Can J Surg 13: 65

1045. Roaf R 1978 Posture. Academic Press, London

1046. Roberts A D 1971 Role of electrical repulsive forces in synovial fluid. Nature 231: 434

1047. Roberts G M et al 1978 Lumbar spine manipulation on trial 11: radiological assessment. Rheum & Rehab 17: 54

1048. Roberts H J 1977 Abdominal pain of spinal origin. Lancet July 23: 195

1049. Robertson J A, Edgar M, Mooney V 1975 Facet arthropathy. Lecture to British Orthopaedic Assoc, Cambridge

1050. Robinson P R G 1965 Massive protrusions of lumbar discs. Brit J Surg 52: 858

1051. Robinson R A, Smith G W 1955 Anterolateral cervical disc removal and interbody fusion for cervical disc syndrome. Bull Johns Hopkins Hosp 96: 233

1052. Roca P D 1972 Ocular manifestations of whiplash injuries. Ann of Ophth 4: 63

1053. Rocabado M 1977 Relationship of the tempero-mandibular joint to cervical dysfunction. In: Kent B (ed) Proceedings: Third Seminar: Internat Fed Orthop Manip Therapists. IFOMT, Hayward, California, p 103

1054. Rogers L F 1971 The roentgenographic appearance of transverse or chance fractures of the spine: the seat-belt fracture. Amer J Roentgen Rad Ther & Nuc Med 111: 844

1055. Rolander S D 1966 Motion of the lumbar spine with special reference to the stabilising effect of posterior fusion. Acta Orthop Scand Suppl 90

1056. Rose M B 1974 Effects of weather on rheumatism. Physio 60: 306

1057. Rosemeyer B 1971 Electromyographische untersuchungen de rücken-und schultermuskulatur im stehen und sitzen unter berücksichtigung der haltung des autofahrers. Arch Orthop Unfallchir 71: 59

1058. Rosenberg N J 1975 Degenerative spondylolisthesis. J Bone & Jt Surg 57A: 467

1059. Rosomoff H L et al 1970 Cystometry as an adjunct in the evaluation of lumbar disc syndromes. J Neurosurg 33: 67

1060. Ross C A, Vyas U S 1972 Thoracic outlet syndrome due to congenital anomalous joint of the first thoracic rib. Can J Surg 15: 1

1061. Ross J 1888 On the segmental distribution of senory disorders. Brain 10: 333

1062. Ross J C, Jameson R M 1971 Vesical dysfunction due to prolapsed disc. British Medical Journal Sept 25: 752

1063. Roy-Camille R, Le Lievre J F 1975 Non-union after fracture of the vertebral bodies at the thoraco-lumbar level. Rev. Chirurg Orthop 61: 249

1064. Rubin D 1970 The no!—or the yes and the how—of sex for patients with neck, back and radicular pain syndromes. Calif Med 113: 12

1065. Ruch T C 1960 Pathophysiology of pain. In: Ruch T C, Fulton J F (eds) Medical physiology and biophysics. W B Saunders, Philadelphia, ch 15

1066. Rugtviet A 1966 Juvenile lumbar disc herniations. Acta Orthop Scand 37: 348

1067. Ruhmann W 1932 Über das wesen der rheumatischen muskelhärte. Dtsch Arch Klin Med 173: 645

1068. Rule L G 1977 Understanding back pain. Heinemann, London

1069. Rutowski B, Niedzialkowska T, Otto J 1977 Electrical stimulation in chronic low back pain. Brit J Anaesth 49: 629

1070. Ryan G M S, Cope S 1955 Cervical vertigo. Lancet 2: 1355

1071. Rydevik B et al 1978 Correspondence on chymopapain. Spine 3: 282 and 283

1072. Sachs B, Fraenkel J 1900 Progressive ankylotic rigidity of the spine. J Nerv & Ment Dis 27: 1

1073. Sadjera S W 1974 The structure of proteoglycans in cartilage. In: Ali S Y, Elves M W, Leaback D H (eds) Symposium: Normal and arthrotic articular cartilage. Inst of Orthop, London, p 41

1074. Sadowska-wrobleska M et al 1976 Analysis of results of thermographic investigations of lumbo-sacral region in healthy subjects and patients with ankylosing spondylitis. Rhumatol 6: 565

1075. Saffouri M H, Ward P H 1974 Surgical correction of dysphagia due to cervical osteophytes. Ann Otol Rhin Laryngol 83: 65

1076. Sager P 1969 Spondylosis cervicalis: a pathological and osteo-archaeological study. Munksgaard, Copenhagen

1077. Saltin B, Nazar K et al 1976 The nature of the training response: peripheral and central adaptations to one-legged exercise. Acta Physiol Scand 96: 289

1078. Samson F 1978 Axonal transport: the mechanisms and their susceptibility to derangement; anterograde transport. In: Korr I (ed) Neurobiologic mechanisms of manipulative therapy. Plenum Presss, London, p 291

1079. Sandifer P 1967 Neurology in orthopaedics. Butterworth, London

1080. Sandström C 1951 Calcifications of the intervertebral discs and the relationship between various types of calcification in the soft tissues of the body. Acta Radiol 36: 217

1081. Saporta L, Simon F et al 1970 Les ostéites pubiennes en milieu rheumatologie. Rev de Rhum 37: 451

1082. Sashin D 1930 A critical analysis of the anatomy and pathological changes of the sacro-iliac joints. J Bone & Jt Surg 12: 891

1083. Sato A 1975 The somato-sympathetic reflexes: their physiological and clinical significance. In: The research status of spinal manipulative therapy. US Dept of Health, Bethesda, NINCDS Monograph No 15, p 163

1084. Saunders E A, Jacobs R R 1976 The multiply-operated back: fusion of the postero-lateral spine with and without nerve root compression. South Med J 69: 868

1085. Savastano A A, Stutz S J 1978 Traumatic sterno-clavicular dislocation. Int Surg 63: 10

1086. Schade H 1919 Beiträge zur umgrenzung und klärung einer lehre von der erkältung. Z Ges Exp Med 7: 275

1087. Schaeffer H 1976 A neurosurgeon looks at spinal conditions. Med J Aust 1: 267

1088. Schatzker J, Pennal G F 1968 Spinal stenosis: a cause of cauda equina compression. J Bone & Jt Surg 50B: 606

1089. Scheuermann H 1921 Zur röntgensymptomatologie der juvelinen osteochondritis dorsi. Z Orthop Chir 41: 305

1090. Schey W L 1976 Vertebral malformations and associated somatovisceral abnormalities. Clin Rad 27: 341

1091. Schiötz E H, Cyriax J 1975 Manipulation past and present. Heinemann, London

1092. Schmorl G, Junghanns H 1956 Clinique radiologie de la colonne vertébrale normale et pathologique: confrontation anatomico-pathologique. Doin et Cie, Paris, p 137

1093. Schmorl G, Junghanns H 1971 The human spine in health and disease, 2nd American edn. Grune & Stratton, New York

1094. Schorstein J, Scott R 1968 Fixed skull traction in cervical spondylosis. Brit J Surg 55: 257

1095. Schunke G B 1938 The anatomy and development of the sacro-iliac joint in man. Anat Rec 72: 313

1096. Schwartz G A, Geiger J K, Spano A V 1956 Posterior inferior cerebellar artery syndrome of Wallenberg after chiropractic manipulation. Arch Int Med 97: 352

1097. Schwartz G E, Beatty J (eds) 1977 Biofeedback theory and research. Academic Press, London

1098. Scott B O 1968 The principles of micro-wave diathermy. Physio 54: 150

1099. Scott M E 1974 Spinal osteoporosis in the aged. Aust Fam Phys 3: 281

1100. Scott-Charlton W, Roebuck D J 1972 The significance of posterior primary divisions of spinal nerves in pain syndromes. Med J Aust 2: 945

1101. Seddon H J 1954 Peripheral nerve injuries. MRC Report, HMSO, London

1102. Selecki B R 1971 Diagnostic assessment and indications for anterior interbody decompression and fusion of the cervical spine. Med J Aust 2: 1233

1103. Selecki B R 1971 Complications and limitations of anterior decompression and fusion of the cervical spine (Cloward's technique). Med J Aust 2: 1235

1104. Selvick G 1974 A röentgen stereophotogrammetric method for the study of the kinematics of the skeletal system. Thesis, Lund

1105. Shafar J 1966 The syndromes of the third neurone of the cervical sympathetic system. Amer J Med 40: 97

1106. Shafiroff B G P, Sava A F 1935 Low back pain in women. New York State J Med 35: 722

1107. Shah J S 1976 Experimental stress analysis of the lumbar spine. In: Jayson M (ed) The lumbar spine and back pain. Sector, London, p 271

1108. Shah J S, Hampson W G J, Jayson M I V 1978 The distribution of surface strain in the cadaveric lumbar spine. J Bone & Jt Surg 60B: 246

1109. Shanahan B 1974 Rhizolysis—a physiotherapist's report. Aust J Physio 20: 96

1110. Sharp J 1957 Differential diagnosis of ankylosing spondylitis. British Medical Journal 1: 975

1111. Sharp J, Purser D W 1961 Spontaneous atlanto-axial dislocation in ankylosing spondylitis and rheumatoid arthritis. Ann Rheum Dis 20: 47

1112. Sharpless S K 1975 Susceptibility of spinal roots to compression block. In: The research status of spinal manipulative therapy. US Dept of Health, Bethesda, NINCDS Monograph No 15, p 155

1113. Sharr M M et al 1976 Lumbar spondylosis and neuropathic bladder: investigation of 73 patients with chronic urinary symptoms. British Medical Journal Mar 20: 695

1114. Shaumburg H H, Spencer P S 1975 Pathology of spinal root compression. In: The research status of spinal manipulative therapy. US Dept of Health, Bethesda, NINCDS Monograph No 15, p 141

1115. Shaw E G, Taylor J G 1956 The results of lumbo-sacral fusion for low back pain. J Bone & Jt Surg 39B: 485

1116. Shaw N E 1975 The syndrome of the prolapsed thoracic intervertebral disc. J Bone & Jt Surg 57B: 412

1117. Shealy C N, Mortimer J T, Hagfors N R 1970 Dorsal column electroanalgesia. J Neurosurg 32: 560

1118. Shealy C N 1974 Facets in back and sciatic pain. Minn Med 57: 199

1119. Shealy C N 1977 The development of neuromodulation. Kent B (ed) Proceedings: Third Seminar: Internat Fed Orthop Manip Therapists. IFOMT, Hayward, California, p 165

1120. Sheldon K W 1967 Headache patterns and cervical nerve root compression—a 15-year study of hospitalization for headache. Headache Jan: 180

1121. Sherk H H, Nicholson J T, Nixon J E 1978 Vertebra plana and eosinophilic granuloma of the cervical spine in children. Spine 3: 116

1122. Sherrington C S 1893 Experiments in the examination of the peripheral distribution of the fibres of the posterior roots of some spinal nerves. Phil Trans B 184: 641

1123. Sherrington C S 1906 The integrative action of the nervous system. Scribner, New York. Reprinted by Yale University Press 1947

1124. Shober P 1937 The lumbar vertebral column and backache. Münch Med Wschr 84: 336

1125. Shore L R 1935 On osteo-arthritis in the dorsal intervertebral joints. Brit J Surg 22: 833

1126. Silver C M, Simon S D, Litchman H M 1971 Tempero-mandibular joint disorders. Amer Fam Phys 3: 90

1127. Silver R A et al 1969 Intermittent claudication of neurospinal origin. Arch Surg 98: 523

1128. Silversten B, Christensen J H 1977 Pain relieving effect of scalenotomy. Acta Orthop Scand 48: 158

1129. Sim F H et al 1970 Swan-neck deformity following extensive cervical laminectomy. J Bone & Jt Surg 56A: 564

1130. Sim F H, Dahlin D C 1977 Primary bone tumours simulating lumbar disc syndrome. Spine 2: 65

1131. Simeone F A 1971 The modern treatment of thoracic disc disease. Orth Clin N Amer 2: 453

1132. Simmons E H, Bhalla S K 1969 Anterior cervical discectomy and fusion. J Bone & Jt Surg 51B: 225

1133. Simons D G 1975 Muscle pain syndromes: Part I. Amer J Phys Med 54: 289

1134. Simons D G 1976 Muscle pain syndromes: Part II. Amer J Phys Med 55: 15

1135. Sims-Williams H, Jayson M, Baddeley H 1977 Rheumatoid involvement of the lumbar spine. Ann Rheum Dis 36: 524

1136. Sims-Williams H, Jayson M, Baddeley H 1978 Small spinal fractures in back pain patients. Ann Rheum Dis 37: 262

1137. Sims-Williams H et al 1978 Controlled trial of mobilisation and manipulation for patients with low back pain in general practice. British Medical Journal 2: 1338

1138. Sinclair D 1973 The anatomy and physiology of pain. Brit J Hosp Med 9: 568

1139. Sinclair D C, Weddell G, Feindel W H 1948 Referred pain and associated phenomena. Brain 71: 184

1140. Sissons H A 1959 Tumours of the vertebral column. In: Nassim R, Burrows H J (eds) Modern trends in diseases of the vertebral column. Butterworth, London, p 192

1141. Sjöstrand J et al 1978 Impairment of intraneural microcirculation, blood-nerve barrier and axonal transport in experimental nerve ischaemia and compression. In Korr I (ed)

The neurobiologic mechanisms of manipulative therapy. Plenum Press, London, p 337

1142. Skalpe I O et al 1973 Lumbar myelography with Metrizamide. Acta Radiol Suppl 335: 367

1143. Skalpe I O, Talle K 1973 Lumbar radiculography with meglumine iocarmate (Dimer-X). J Oslo City Hosp 23: 121

1144. Smith A J 1974 Medicine in China: best of the old and the new. British Medical Journal 2: 343

1145. Smith B H 1969 Anatomy of facial pain. Headache 9: 7

1146. Smith G R, Beckly D E, Abel M S 1976 Articular mass fracture: a neglected cause of post-traumatic neck pain? Clin Radiol 27: 335

1147. Smith L, Brown J E 1967 Treatment of lumbar intervertebral disc lesions by direct injection of chymopapain. J Bone & Jt Surg 49B: 502

1148. Smith R A, Estridge M N 1962 Neurologic complications of head and neck manipulations. J Amer Med Assoc 182: 528

1148a. Smith O G, Langworthy, S M, Paxson M C 1906 Modernized chiropractic. Laurence Press, Cedar Rapids, Iowa

1149. Smyth M J, Wright V 1958 Sciatica and the intervertebral disc. J Bone & Jt Surg 40A: 1401

1150. Smythe H A 1972 Non-articular rheumatism and the fibrositis syndrome. In: Hollander J L, McCarty D J (eds) Arthritis and allied conditions, 8th edn. Lea & Febiger, Philadelphia, p 874

1151. Smythe H A, Moldofsky H 1978 Two contributions to understanding of the 'fibrositis' syndrome. EULAR Bulletin (English edn) 4: 73

1152. Snyder S H 1977 Opiate receptors and internal opiates. Sci Amer 236: 44

1153. Soholt S T 1951 Tuberculosis of the sacro-iliac joint. J Bone & Jt Surg 33A: 119

1154. Sokoloff L 1974 The general pathology of osteoarthrosis. In: Ali S Y, Elves M W, Leaback D H (eds) Symposium: Normal and arthrotic articular cartilage. Inst of Orthop, London, p 111

1155. Sokoloff L (ed) 1978 The joints and synovial fluid I. Academic Press, London

1156. Sola A E, Williams R L 1956 Myofascial pain syndromes. Neurol 6: 91

1157. Solonen K A 1957 The sacro-iliac joint in the light of anatomical röentgenological and clinical studies. Acta Orthop Scand Suppl 26

1158. Somerville B 1976 Migraine: the serotonin theory re-examined. Hemicrania 7: 2

1159. Soo Y S, Ang A H 1973 The value of the lateral cervical myelogram in the evaluation of cervical spondylosis. Australas Radiol 17: 371

1160. Soren A 1965 Evaluation of ultrasound treatment in musculo-skeletal disorders. Physio 51: 214

1161. Spencer D L, De Wald R L 1979 Simultaneous anterior and posterior surgical approach to the thoracic and lumbar spine. Spine 4: 29

1162. Spisak J 1972 Bedentung des segments C2–C3 im Klinischen bild des akuten tortikollis. Man Med 6: 87

1162a. Squires J W, Pinch L W 1979 Heparin-induced spinal fractures. J Amer Med Assoc 241: 2417

1163. Stauffer R N, Coventry M B 1972 Anterior interbody lumbar spine fusion. J Bone & Jt Surg 54A: 756

1164. St Clair Strange F G 1966 Debunking the disc. Proc Roy Soc Med 59: 925

1165. Steel H H 1968 Anatomical and mechanical considerations of the atlanto-axial articulations. J Bone & Jt Surg 50A: 1481

1166. Steinbrocker O 1947 The shoulder–hand syndrome: associated painful humo-lateral disability of shoulder and hand with swelling and atrophy of the hand. Amer J Med 3: 402

1167. Steinbrocker O, Argyros T G 1958 The shoulder–hand syndrome: present status as a diagnostic and therapeutic entity. Med Clin N Amer Nov: 1533

1168. Steinbrocker O 1968 The shoulder–hand syndrome: present perspective. Arch Phys Med Rehab 49: 388

1169. Steindler A, Luck J V 1938 Differential diagnosis of pain low in the back. J Amer Med Assoc 110: 106

1170. Steindler A 1954 The reversibility of low back and sciatic symptoms and their relation to the antalgic attitude. Schweiz Med Wchnschr 84: 1016

1171. Steindler A 1962 Ilio-psoas. Thomas, Springfield, Illinois

1172. Stevenson H G 1970 Back injury and depression—a medico-legal problem. Med J Aust 1: 1300

1173. Stewart D Y 1962 Current concepts of the Barré syndrome or the posterior cervical sympathetic syndrome. In: De Palma A F (ed) Clinical Orthopaedics No 24, Pitman Medical, London, p 40

1174. Stewart J D, Eisen A 1978 Tinel's sign and the carpal tunnel syndrome. British Medical Journal 2: 1225

1175. Stewart T D 1953 Age incidence of neural arch defects in Alaskan natives. J Bone & Jt Surg 35A: 937

1176. Still A T 1899 Philosophy of osteopathy. Still, Kirksville

1177. Stillwell D 1956 Nerve supply of the vertebral column and its associated structures in the monkey. Anat Record 125: 129

1178. Stockman R 1904 The causes, pathology and treatment of chronic rheumatism. Edin Med J 15: 107

1179. Stoddard A 1958 Conditions of the sacro-iliac joint and their treatment. Physio 44: 97

1180a. Stoddard A 1962 Manual of osteopathic technique, 2nd edn. Hutchinson, London

1180b. Stoddard A 1969 Manual of osteopathic practice. Hutchinson, London

1181. Stoddard A 1970 Cervical spondylosis and cervical osteo-arthritis. Man Med 2: 31

1182. Stoddard A 1977 Acute spinal pain. Brit Osteop J 10: 3

1183a. Stoddard A, Osborn J F 1979 Scheuermann's disease or spinal osteochondrosis. J Bone & Jt Surg 61B: 56

1183b. Stoddard A 1979 The back—relief from pain, Dunitz, London

1184. Strauss H 1898 Über die sogenannte 'rheumatische muskelschweile'. Klin Wochenschr 35: 89

1184a. Stripp W J 1980 Special techniques in orthopaedic radiography. Churchill Livingstone, Edinburgh

1185. Sturge W A 1883 The phenomena of angina pectoris and their bearing upon the theory of counter irritation. Brain 5: 492

1186. Sturrock R D et al 1973 Spondylometry in a normal population and in ankylosing spondylitis. Rheum & Rehab 12: 135

1187. Südek P 1900 Über die akute enzündliche knochenatrophie. Arch Klin Chir 62: 147

1188. Sullivan M 1976 Low back pain. Brit J Hosp Med 15: 25

1189. Sunderland S, Bradley K C 1952 Perineurium of peripheral nerves. Anat Rec 113: 125

1190. Sunderland S, Bradley K C 1961 Stress-strain phenomena in human spinal roots. Brain 84: 121

1191. Sunderland S 1968 Nerves and nerve injuries. Churchill Livingstone, London

1192. Sunderland S 1974 Meningeal-neural relations in the intervertebral foramen. J Neurosurg 40: 756

1193. Sunderland S 1975 Anatomical perivertebral influences on the intervertebral foramen. In: The research status of spinal manipulative therapy. US Dept of Health, Bethesda, NINCDS Monograph No 15, p 129

1194. Sunderland S 1978 Traumatised nerves, roots and ganglia: musculo-skeletal factors and neuropathological consequences. In: Korr (ed) The neurobiologic mechanisms in manipulative therapy. Plenum Press, London, p. 137

1195. Sussman B J, Mann M 1969 Experimental intervertebral discolysis with collagenase. J Neurosurg 31: 628

1196. Sussman B J 1975 Inadequacies and hazards of chymopapain injections as treatment for intervertebral disc disease. J Neurosurg 42: 389

1197. Swann D A et al 1974 Role of hyaluronic acid in lubrication. Ann Rheum Dis 33: 318

1198. Swann D A 1978 Macromolecules of synovial fluid. In: Sokoloff L (ed) The joints and synovial fluid I. Academic Press, London, p 407

1199. Swanson S A V, Freeman M A R 1969 The mechanism of human joints. Science Journal 5: 73

1200. Swezey R L, Silverman T R 1971 Radiographic demonstration of induced vertebral facet displacement. Arch Phys Med Rehab 52: 244

1201. Swinson D R et al 1972 Vertical subluxation of the axis in rheumatoid arthritis. Ann Rheum Dis 31: 359

1202. Sylvén B 1950 On the biology of the nucleus pulposus. Acta Orthop Scand 20: 275

1203. Sylvest J et al 1977 Ultrastructure of prolapsed disc. Acta Orthop Scand 48: 32

1204. Symon L 1971 Surgical treatment. In: Wilkinson M (ed) Cervical spondylosis, 2nd edn. Heinemann Medical, London

1205. Tanz S S 1953 Motion of the lumbar spine. Amer J Roentgen 69: 399

1206. Taylor A R 1953 Mechanism and treatment of spinal cord disorders associated with cervical spondylosis. Lancet 1: 717

1207. Taylor T K F, Weiner M 1969 Great-toe extensor reflexes in the diagnosis of lumbar disc disorder. British Medical Journal 2: 487

1208. Tegner W 1959 'Functional' backache. In: Nassim R, Burrows H J (eds) Modern trends in diseases of the vertebral column. Butterworth, London, p 281

1209. Telford E D, Stopford J S 1931 Vascular complications of cervical rib. Brit J Surg 18: 557

1210. Telford E D, Mottershead S 1947 The costo-clavicular syndrome. British Medical Journal Mar 15: 4497

1211. Thoenon H et al 1978 Transfer of information from effector organs to innervating neurons by retrograde axonal transport of macromolecules. In: Korr I (ed) The neurobiologic mechanisms in manipulative therapy. Plenum Press, London, p 311

1212. Thomas P K 1974 Neurological aspects of pain. Physio 60: 101

1213. Thompson H 1970 Transpharyngeal fusion of the upper cervical spine. Proc Roy Soc Med 63: 893

1213a. Thompson M 1980 Low back pain and sciatica. Eular Bulletin (English edn) 9: 67

1214. Thompson S 1969 A temporary lumbo-sacral support. Physio 55: 67

1215. Tichauer E R 1977 The objective corroboration of back pain. Journal of Occupational Medicine 19 (Part II): 727

1216. Tidy N M 1968 Massage and remedial exercises, 11th edn. Revised by Wale J O. Wright & Sons, Bristol

1217. Tietze A 1921 Ueber eine eigenartige haufung von fallen mit dystrophie der rippenknorpel. Berlin Klin Wchnischr 58: 829

1218. Till D 1969 Cold therapy. Physio 55: 461

1219. Tinel J 1915 Le signe du 'fourmillement' dans les lésions des nerfs périphériques. Presse Méd 23: 388

1220. Tinel J 1937 Le système nerveux végétatif. Masson, Paris

1220a. Tkach S 1970 Gouty arthritis of the spine. Clin Orthop Rel Res 71: 81

1221. Toakley J G 1973 Subcutaneous lumbar rhizolysis—an assessment of 200 cases. Med J Aust 2: 490

1222. Todd R C, Freeman M A R, Pirie C J 1972 Isolated trabecular fatigue fractures in the femoral head. J Bone & Jt Surg 54B: 723

1223. Todd T W 1912 Hinder end of the brachial plexus in man and animals. Anat Anz 42: 129

1224. Toglia J U, Rosenberg P E, Ronis M L 1969 Vestibular and audiological aspects of whiplash injury and head trauma. J Forens Sci 14: 219

1225. Toglia J U, Rosenberg P E, Ronis M L 1970 Post-traumatic dizziness. Arch Otolaryng 92: 485

1226. Toglia J U 1972 Vestibular and medico-legal aspects of closed cranio-cervical trauma. Scand J Rehab Med 4: 126

1227. Toller P A 1973 Osteo-arthrosis of the mandibular condyle. Brit Dent J 134: 223

1228. Toller P A 1977 The use and mis-use of intra-articular cortico-steroids in the treatment of tempero-mandibular joint pain. Proc Roy Soc Med 70: 461

1229. Tondury G 1971 The behaviour of cervical discs during life. In: Hirsch C, Zotterman Y (eds) Cervical pain. Pergamon Press, Oxford

1230. Tondury G 1972 Anatomie fonctionelle des petite articulations du rachis. Ann de Méd Physique 15: 173

1231. Torres F, Shapiro S K 1961 Electroencephalograms in whiplash injury. Arch Neurol 5: 40

1232. Trauner D A, Conner J D 1975 Radio-active scanning in diagnosis of acute sacro-iliac osteomyelitis. J Paediat 87: 751

1233. Travell J, Rinzler S H, Hermann M 1942 Pain and disability of the shoulder and arm. J Amer Med Assoc 120: 417

1234. Travell J, Berry C, Bigelow N 1944 Effects of referred somatic pain on structures in the reference zone. Fed Proc 3: 49

1235. Travell J, Rinzler S H 1946 Relief of cardiac pain by local block of somatic trigger areas. Proc Soc Exp Biol Med 63: 480

1236. Travell J 1949 Rapid relief of acute 'stiff neck' by ethylchloride spray. Amer Med Wom Assoc 4: 89

1237. Travell J 1952 Ethyl chloride spray for painful muscle spasm. Arch Phys Med 33: 291

1238. Travell J, Rinzler S H 1952 The myofascial genesis of pain. Post-Grad Med 11: 425

1239. Travell J 1954 Introduction. In: Ragan C (ed) Transactions: Vth Conference on Connective Tissues. Josiah Macy Foundation, New York

1240. Travell J 1960 Temperomandibular joint pain referred from muscles of head and neck. J Prosth Dent 10: 745

1241. Travell J 1968 Office hours: day and night. World Publishing Co, New York

1242. Trevor-Jones R 1964 Osteo-arthritis of the paravertebral joints of the second and third cervical vertebrae as a cause of occipital headaches. SA Med J 38: 392

1243. Trott P H, Goss A N 1978 Physiotherapy in diagnosis and treatment of the myofascial pain dysfunction syndrome. Int J Oral Surg 7: 360

1244. Trotter M 1937 Accessory sacro-iliac articulations. Amer J Phys Anthropol 22: 247

1245. Troup J D G 1970 Some problems of measurement in clinical trials of physiotherapy with particular reference to the assessment of pain. Physio 56: 491

1246. Troup J D G 1970 Spinal biomechanics. World Med 5: 48

1247. Troup J D G 1975 A method for assessing the ankle jerk response electromyographically: preliminary results from patients with lumbar spinal disorders. Electromyog Clin Neurophysiol 15: 403

1248. Troup J D G 1975 The biology of back pain. New Scientist 65: 17

1249. Troup J D G 1975 Personal communication

1250a. Troup J D G 1977 The etiology of spondylolysis. Orth Clin N Amer 8: 57

1250b. Troup J D G 1979 Biomechanics of the vertebral column. Physio 65: 238

1251. Tucker W E, Armstrong J R 1964 Injury in sport. Staples Press, London, p 575

1252. Tucker W E 1973 Home treatment and posture. Churchill Livingstone, London

1253. Tulsi R S 1974 Sacral arch defect and low backache. Australas Radiol 18: 43

1254. Turnbull I M, Breig A 1966 Blood supply of the cervical spinal cord in man. J Neurosurg 24: 951

1255. Turner R H, Bianco A J 1971 Spondylolysis and spondylolisthesis in children and teenagers. J Bone & Jt Surg 53A: 1298

1256. Twomey L T, Furniss B I 1978 The life-cycle of the intervertebral discs and vertebral bodies: a review. Aust J Physio 24: 209

1257. Ueke T, Ueda F 1969 Dysfunction of the autonomic nervous system in whiplash injury. J West Pac Orthop Assoc 6: 1

1258. Unsworth A, Dowson D, Wright V 1971 Cracking joints: a bioengineering study of cavitation in the metacarpophalangeal joint. Ann Rheum Dis 30: 348

1259. Urban B J, Nashold B S 1978 Percutaneous epidural stimulation of the spinal cord for relief of pain: long term results. J Neurosurg 48: 323

1260. Valtonen E J et al 1968 Comparative radiographic study of the effect of intermittent and continuous traction on elongation of the cervical spine. Ann Med Int Fenn 57: 143

1261. Valtonen E J, Kiuru E 1970 Cervical traction as a therapeutic tool: a clinical analysis based on 212 patients. Scand J Rehab Med 2: 29

1262. Van Adrichem J A M, Van der Korst G 1973 Assessment of the flexibility of the lumbar spine. Scand J Rheum 2: 87

1263. Van Harreveld A 1952 Re-innervation of paretic muscle by collateral branching of residual motor innervation. J Comp Neurol 97: 385

1264. Van Laere M, Vays E M, Mielants H 1972 Strontium 87m scanning of the sacro-iliac joints in ankylosing spondylitis. Ann Rheum Dis 31: 201

1265. Van Leuven R M, Troup J D G 1969 The 'Instant' lumbar corset. Physio 55: 499

1266. Venables C S, Stuck A 1946 Muscle flap transplant for the relief of painful monarticular arthritis (aseptic necrosis) of the hip. Ann Surg 123: 641

1267. Verbeist H 1954 A radicular syndrome from developmental narrowing of the lumbar vertebral canal. J Bone & Jt Surg 36B: 230

1268. Vermillon C D et al 1971 Urinary retention due to asymptomatic protruded lumbar disc. Aust & NZ J Surg 41: 182

1269. Vernon-Roberts B, Pirie C J 1973 Healing trabecular microfractures in the bodies of lumbar vertebrae. Ann Rheum Dis 32: 406

1270. Vernon-Roberts B 1976 Pathology of degenerative spondylosis. In: Jayson M (ed) The lumbar spine and back pain. Sector, London, p 55

1271. Vincent Y N 1969 Experience with chymopapain injection into lumbar discs. J West Pac Orthop Assoc 6: 1

1272. Vogelsang H 1970 Interosseous spinal venography. Excerpta Medica, Amsterdam

1273. Vogler P, Krauss H 1975 Periostbehandlung, 2nd edn. Thieme, Leipzig

1274. Von Torklus D, Gehle W 1972 The upper cervical spine. Butterworth, London

1275. Von Zicha K 1970 Manuelle therapie bei spondylarthritis ankylopoetica. Man Med 5: 97

1276. Vrettos X C, Wyke B D 1974 Articular reflexogenic systems in the costo-vertebral joints. J Bone & Jt Surg 56B: 382

1277. Waghemacker R 1968 Functional troubles of minor cervical injuries. Ann de Méd Physique 3: 45

1278. Walker P S et al 1968 Boosted lubrication in synovial joints by fluid entrapment and enrichment. Ann Rheum Dis 27: 512

1279. Wall P D 1967 The laminar organisation of dorsal horn and effects of descending impulses. J Physiol (London) 188: 403

1280. Wall P D, Sweet W H 1967 Temporary abolition of pain in man. Science (New York) 155: 108

1281. Wall P D 1971 The mechanisms of pain associated with cervical vertebral disease. In: Hirsch C, Zotterman Y (eds) Cervical pain. Pergamon Press, Oxford, p 201

1282. Wall P D et al 1974 Ongoing activity in peripheral nerve injury discharge. Exp Neurol 45: 576

1283. Wall P D 1974 Acupuncture revisited. New Scientist Oct 31: 31

1284. Wall P D, Noordenbos W 1977 Sensory functions which remain in man after complete transection of dorsal columns. Brain 100: 641

1285. Wall P D 1978 The gate control theory of pain mechanisms: a re-examination and restatement. Brain 101: 1

1286. Waller A 1862 On the sensory, motory and vaso-motory symptoms resulting from refrigeration and compression of the ulnar and other nerves in man. Proc Roy Soc Lond. 12: 89

1287. Walmsley R 1959 Anatomy and development. In: Nassim R, Burrows H J (eds) Modern trends in diseases of the vertebral column. Butterworth, London, p 1

1288. Walshe F M R 1951 Diseases of the nervous system, 6th edn. Livingstone, Edinburgh

1289. Walshe F M R 1951 The hypothesis of cybernetics (Discussion). Brit J Philos Sci

1290. Walters R L, Norris J M 1970 The effects of spinal supports on the electrical activities of the trunk. J Bone & Jt Surg 52A: 51

1291. Webb J H, Craig W M, Kernohan J W 1953 Intraspinal neoplasms in the cervical region. J Neurosurg 10: 360

1292. Weber F A, De Klerk D J 1973 Spinal stenosis. SA Med J 47: 207

1293. Weber H 1970 An evaluation of conservative and surgical treatment of lumbar disc protrusion. J Oslo City Hosp 20: 81

1294. Weber H 1973 Traction therapy in sciatica due to disc prolapse. J Oslo City Hosp 23: 167

1295. Weber H 1975 The effect of delayed disc surgery on muscular paresis. Acta Orthop Scand 46: 631

1296. Wees S R, Raskind R 1968 The teen-age lumbar disc syndrome. Int Surg 49: 528

1297. Weightman B O et al 1973 Fatigue of articular cartilage. Nature 244: 303

1298. Weinstein C J 1974 Acupuncture and its application to physical therapy. Phys Ther 54: 12

1299. Weinstein M A et al 1975 Computed tomography in diastematomyelia. Radiol 117: 609

1300. Weinstein P R, Ehni G, Wilson C B 1977 Lumbar spondylosis: diagnosis, management and surgical treatment. Year Book Medical Publications, London

1301. Weisl H 1955 The movements of the sacro-iliac joint. Acta Anatomica 23: 80

1302. Weiss P, Davis H 1953 Pressure block in nerves supplied with arterial sleeves. J Neurophysiol 6: 269

1303. Werne S 1957 Studies in spontaneous atlas dislocation. Acta Orthop Scand Suppl 23

1304. Whaley K, Dick W C 1968 Fatal sub-axial dislocation of cervical spine in rheumatoid arthritis. British Medical Journal 2: 31

1305. White A A 1969 Analysis of the mechanics of the thoracic spine in man. Acta Orthop Scand Suppl 127

1306. White A A et al 1974 Practical biomechanics of the spine for the orthopaedic surgeon. Instructional Course Lectures. Amer Acad of Orthop Surg 23: 62

1307. White A A, Punjabi M M 1978 The basic kinematics of the human spine. Spine 3: 12

1308. White A G 1972 Prolonged elevation of serum protein-bound iodine following myelography with Myodil. Brit J Radiol 45: 21

1309. White A W M 1966 The compensation back. Appl Ther 8: 971

1310. White J C, Poppel M H, Adams R 1945 Congenital malformations of the first thoracic rib: cause of brachial neuralgia which simulates cervical rib syndrome. Surg Gynaecol Obst 81: 643

1311. White J C, Sweet W H 1969 Control of pain by activation of inhibitory mechanisms. In: Pain and the neurosurgeon. Thomas, Springfield, Illinois

1312. Wiberg G 1949 Back pain in relation to the nerve supply of the intervertebral disc. Acta Orthop Scand 19: 211

1313. Wiles P 1965 Essentials of orthopaedics, 4th edn. Churchill, London

1314. Wilkins R H, Brody I A 1969 Lasègue's sign. Arch Neurol 21: 219

1315. Wilkinson M 1960 The morbid anatomy of cervical spondylosis and myelopathy. Brain 83: 589

1316. Wilkinson M 1971 Cervical spondylosis, 2nd edn. Heinemann, London

1317. Wilkinson M 1975 A neurological perspective. Rheum & Rehab 14: 162

1318. Williams D, Wilson T G 1962 The diagnosis of the major and minor syndrome of basilar insufficiency. Brain 85: 741

1319. Williams J L, Allen M B, Harkness J W 1968 Late results of cervical discectomy and interbody fusion: some factors influencing the results. J Bone & Jt Surg 50A: 277

1320. Williams P C 1932 Lumbar spine: reduced lumbo-sacral joint space: its relation to sciatic nerve irritation. J Amer Med Assoc 99: 1677

1321. Williams P C 1974 Low back and neck pain. Thomas, Springfield, Illinois

1322. Williams R W 1978 Micro-lumbar discectomy: a conservative surgical approach to the virgin herniated lumbar disc. Spine 3: 175

1323. Williams S J 1977 The 'back school'. Physio 63: 90

1324. Willie C D 1969 Interferential therapy. Physio 55: 503

1325. Wilson M E 1974 The neurological mechanisms of pain. Anaesthesia 29: 407

1326. Wiltse L L 1969 Spondylolisthesis: classification and aetiology. In: Proceedings: Symposium on the spine. Amer Acad Orthop Surg. C V Mosby, St Louis, p 143

1327. Wiltse L L 1971 The effect of common anomalies at the lumbar spine upon disc degeneration and low back pain. Orthop Clin of N Amer 2: 569

1328. Wiltse L L, Rocchio P D 1975 Pre-operative psychological tests as predictors of success of chemonucleolysis in the treatment of the low-back syndrome. J Bone & Jt Surg 57A: 4

1329. Wiltse L L, Newman P H, Macnab I 1976 Classification of spondylolysis and spondylolisthesis. Clin Orthop & Rel Res 117: 23

1330. Wing L W, Hargrave-Wilson W 1974 Cervical vertigo. Aust NZ J Surg 44: 275

1330a. Wingerson L 1980 Gut feelings about neuropeptides. New Scientist 86: 16

1331. Woesner M E, Mitts M G 1972 The evaluation of cervical spine motion below C2: a comparison of cineroentgenographic and conventional roentgenographic methods. Amer J Roentgen Rad Ther & Nuc Med 115: 148

1332. Wolbrink A J et al 1974 Occult roentgenographic changes in the cervical spine. Mayo Clin Proc 49: 879

1333. Wolf S 1970 Emotions and the autonomic nervous system. Arch Int Med 126: 1024

1334. Wolkind S N 1974 Psychiatric aspects of low back pain. Physio 60: 75

1335. Wolkind S N 1976 Psychogenic low back pain. Brit J Hosp Med 15: 17

1336. Wood E J 1972 Anatomical aspects of some vertebral anomalies. SA J Physio 28: 10

1337. Wood P H N, McLeish C L 1974 Statistical appendix—digest of data on the rheumatic diseases: 5. Morbidity in industry, and rheumatism in general practice. Ann Rheum Dig 33: 93

1338. Wood P H N 1976 The epidemiology of back pain. In: Jayson M (ed) The lumbar spine and back pain. Sector, London, p 13

1339. Wood P H N (ed) 1977 The challenge of arthritis and rheumatism: report of problems and progress in health care for rheumatic disorders. British League Against Rheumatism, London

1340. Wood P H N 1977 Editorial. Rheum & Rehab 16: 1

1340a. Wood P H N 1980 Undergraduate education in rheumatology in Great Britain. Eular Bulletin (English edn) 9: 61

1341. Woods W W, Compere W E 1969 Electronystagmography in cervical injuries. Internat Surg 51: 251

1342. Woolf D 1974 Shoulder-hand syndrome. The Practitioner 213: 176

1343. Woollam D H M, Millen J W 1958 Discussion on vascular disease of the spinal cord. Proc Roy Soc Med 51: 540

1344. Worcester J N, Green D P 1968 Osteoarthritis of the acromio-clavicular joint. Clin Orth Rel Res 58: 69

1345. World Health Organisation 1967 International statistical classfication of diseases, Geneva, vols I and II

1345a. Worth D, Selvik G, Glover J 1978 Kinematics of the cranio-vertebral joints. In: Proceedings: Manipulative Therapists of Australia Congress, Sydney

1346. Wortzman G, Dewar F P 1966 Rotatory fixation of the atlanto-axial joint: rotational atlantal subluxation. Radiol 90: 479

1347. Wright F G, Rennels D C 1964 A study of the elastic properties of plantar fascia. J Bone & Jt Surg 46A: 482

1348. Wright F W et al 1971 Some observations on the value and techniques of myelography in lumbar disc lesions. Clin Radiol 22: 33

1349. Wright J 1944 Mechanics in relation to derangement of the facet joints of the spine. Arch Phys Ther 25: 201

1350. Wright V (ed) 1969 Lubrication and wear in joints. Sector, London

1351. Wright V 1972 Joint mechanics. Physio 58: 367

1352. Wright V, Dowson D 1976 Lubrication and cartilage. J Anat 121: 107

1353. Wright V, Hopkins R 1978 What the patient means. Physio 64: 146

1354. Wyke B D 1967 The neurology of joints. Ann Roy Coll Surg Eng 41: 25

1355. Wyke B D 1968 The neurology of face pain. Brit J Hosp Med Oct: 46

1356. Wyke B D 1970 The neurological basis of thoracic spinal pain. Rheum & Phys Med 10: 356

1357. Wyke B D 1972 Articular neurology—a review. Physio 58: 94

1358. Wyke B D, Molina F 1972 Articular reflexology of the cervical spine. Abstracts: Proc Int Fed Phys Med, Barcelona

1359. Wyke B D 1974 Neurological aspects of the diagnosis and treatment of facial pain. In: Cohen B, Kramer I (eds) Scientific foundations of dentistry. Heinemann, London

1360. Wyke B D 1974 Clinical physiology of peripheral nerve fibres. In: Wells C et al (eds) Scientific foundations of surgery. Heinemann, London, p 242

1361a. Wyke B D 1975 Morphological and functional features of the innervation of the costovertebral joints. Folia Morphologica 23: 296

1361b. Wyke B D, Polácek P 1975 Articular neurology: the present position. J Bone & Jt Surg 57B: 401

1362. Wyke B D 1976 Neurological aspects of low back pain. In: Jayson M (ed) The lumbar spine and back pain. Sector, London, p 189

1363. Wyke B D 1979 Neurology of the cervical spinal joints. Physio 65: 72

1364. Wyke M 1965 Comparative analysis of proprioception in left and right arms. Quart J Exp Psych 17: 149

1365. Wynne-Davies R 1971 Familial joint laxity. Proc Roy Soc Med 64: 29

1366. Wynn-Parry C B 1966 Management of ankylosing spondylitis. Proc Roy Soc Med 59: 619

1367a. Wyper D J, McNiven D R 1976 Effects of some physiotherapeutic agents on skeletal muscle blood flow. Physio 62: 83

1367b. Yarom R, Rabin G C 1979 Studies on spinal and peripheral muscle from patients with sciatica. Spine 4: 12

1368. Yates D A H 1962 Unilateral sciatica with neurological involvement: a correlated clinical and electrodiagnostic study. MD thesis, London

1369. Yates D A H 1964 Unilateral lumbo-sacral root compression. Ann Phys Med 7: 169

1370. Yates D A H 1969 Cervical spine. British Medical Journal 2: 807

1371. Yates D A H, Mathews J A 1969 Reduction of lumbar disc prolapse by manipulation. British Medical Journal 3: 696

1372. Yates D A H 1972 The treatment of osteoarthrosis. In: Rheumatological remedies. The Practitioner 208: 43

1373. Yates D A H 1976 Treatment of back pain. In: Jayson M (ed) The lumbar spine and back pain. Sector, London, ch 16

1374. Yates D A H 1978 A comparison of the types of epidural injection commonly used in the treatment of low back pain and sciatica. Rheum & Rehab 17: 181

1375. Youel M A (1967) Effectiveness of pelvic traction. J Bone & Jt Surg 49A: 204

1376. Young H H 1952 Non-neurological lesions simulating protruded intervertebral disc. J Amer Med Assoc 148: 1101

1377. Yum K Y, Myers R N 1969 Vertebral artery ligation. Arch Surg 98: 199

1378. Zachs S I, Langfitt T W, Elliott F A 1964 Herpetic neuritis. Neurol 14: 744

1379. Zanca P 1971 Shoulder pain: involvement of the acromio-clavicular joint. Amer J Roentgen Rad Ther Nuc Med 112: 493

1380. Zeidses des Plantes B G 1933 Planigraphie. Röfo 47: 407

1381. Zuckner J, Baldassere A 1976 The non-specific rheumatoid subcutaneous nodule: its presence in fibrositis and scleroderma. Amer J Med Science 271: 69

1382. Zukschwerdt L 1956 Die akute blocklerung von halswirbelgelenken. Med Klin 51: 508

Index